# Neurocritical Care Management of the Neurosurgical Patient

# Neurocritical Care Management of the Neurosurgical Patient

**Monisha Kumar, MD**

Assistant Professor
Departments of Neurology, Neurosurgery, and Anesthesiology & Critical Care
Associate Director of Neurocritical Care Fellowship Program
Perelman School of Medicine at the University of Pennsylvania
Philadelphia, PA, USA

**W. Andrew Kofke, MD, MBA, FCCM, FNCS**

Professor, Director Neuroscience in Anesthesiology and Critical Care Program
Co-Director Neurocritical Care
Co-Director Perioperative Medicine and Pain Clinical Research Unit
Department of Anesthesiology and Critical Care
Department of Neurosurgery
University of Pennsylvania
Philadelphia, PA, USA

**Joshua M. Levine, MD, FANA, FNCS**

Chief, Division of Neurocritical Care, Department of Neurology
Co-Director, Neurocritical Care Program
Associate Professor, Departments of Neurology, Neurosurgery, and Anesthesiology and Critical Care
Perelman School of Medicine at the University of Pennsylvania
Philadelphia, PA, USA

**James Schuster, MD, PhD**

Associate Professor, Department of Neurosurgery
Director of Neurotrauma
Perelman School of Medicine at the University of Pennsylvania
Philadelphia, PA, USA

ELSEVIER

Edinburgh   London   New York   Oxford   Philadelphia   St Louis   Sydney   Toronto

ELSEVIER

**ISBN: 978-0-323-32106-8**

Printed in China
Last digit is the print number: 9  8  7  6  5  4  3  2  1

**Content Strategist:** Charlotta Kryhl
**Content Development Specialist:** Sharon Nash, Trinity Hutton
**Project Manager:** Julie Taylor
**Design:** Christian Bilbow
**Illustration Manager:** Brett MacNaughton, Amy Faith Heyden
**Illustrator:** Victoria Heim, TNQ Books & Journals Private Limited
**Marketing Manager:** Michele Milano

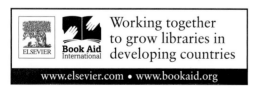

# Contents

# *Foreword*

In medicine there are a few nodes of care where over a short period of time a person's life lies in the balance. The neurocritical care unit (NICU) is one such node. Though postoperative care units for neurosurgical patients have existed for many decades the multidisciplinary neurocritical care field is still very young, dating back only to the 1980s. As a result, the evidence-base that underlies much of the decision-making in the NICU is still being assembled. The lessons-learned from experienced neurointensivists remains the bedrock of the art of neurocritical care.

This textbook incorporates the wisdom of an impressive cadre of dedicated physicians who clearly communicated their art, as well as describing the evidence-base for their craft. The focus on the neurosurgical patient places the book in a special position in medical literature. Close working relationships between the patient's neurosurgeon, neuroanesthesiologist, and the neurointensivist is crucial for good patient care in the NICU, but is not by itself a replacement for a working knowledge of each others concerns, abilities, and processes. Understanding the neurosurgery is as essential for the neurointensivist, as neurointensive care is to the neurosurgeon. It would be impossible to provide quality care for the person transferred to the NICU from the emergency department without knowledge of what occurred in the emergency department. A similar knowledge of the events that occur in the operating room is equally essential. However, the emergency department is a much more familiar environment for the neurointensivist than the operating room. This textbook, written by neurosurgeons, neuroanesthesiologists, and neurointensivists, defines the key issues needed to meld these two approaches.

Dr. Kumar and her co-authors bring a unique viewpoint that mimics the reality of the NICU where the patient care is a complicated dance with multiple caregivers, the patient and family. From my position at NIH it's also important to note that many of the chapters identify the evidence gaps that need to be addressed to inform decision-making in the NICU. Outlining these should enable neurointensivists to engage in research to understand those interventions associated with clinically important outcomes in specific patients. Though professional agendas differ among caregivers, a good final clinical outcome is shared by all, and the body of knowledge displayed in the text is a wonderful guide to the care of the neurosurgical patient in the NICU.

*Walter Koroshetz, MD*
*Director, National Institute of*
*Neurological Disorders and Stroke*

# Preface

Neurocritical Care is a burgeoning field dedicated to the management of patients with life-threatening neurological and neurosurgical illness as well as those at risk for neurological complications of systemic disease. Much of neurointensive care unit (Neuro ICU) management focuses on the postoperative neurosurgical patient. Treating neurosurgical patients without a comprehensive understanding of what occurs in the operating room (OR) may severely hinder the intensivist in the provision of optimal care. It is imperative that neuro-intensivists be aware of the relevant neuroanatomical structures, surgical approach, and anesthetic considerations as well as the range of known complications of elective and non-elective neurosurgery. This is fundamental to the practice of neurocritical care. However, the preoperative evaluation, perioperative assessment and intraoperative management are not comprehensively taught in the neurocritical care curriculum. This book is intended to grant deeper insight into perioperative neurosurgical evaluations and anesthetic considerations that may affect the intensive care management of these patients.

It is critical that this knowledge gap be sealed as the field of neurocritical care matures. The knowledge gap is further compounded by the fact that practitioners of neurocritical care hail from a wide variety of primary specialties including Internal Medicine, Emergency Medicine, General Surgery, Anesthesiology and Neurology. The diversity of specialties allows practitioners a varied skill set; however, a standard and comprehensive set of skills may be elusive. Although a fundamental understanding of neurosurgery, including proper patient positioning, operative techniques and relevant neuroanatomy, remain a prerequisite for those caring for postoperative neurosurgical patients, it is an oft-overlooked segment of clinical training.

Transitions in care and patient handoffs have evolved dramatically over the last decade. Hand-offs in surgical specialties often focus on the operative intervention, whereas hand-offs in medical specialties focus on the history of present illness. These distinct approaches intersect in the Neuro ICU, which is frequently a mixed medical-surgical ICU. Surgical ICU sign-out rounds involves a review of the anatomy, anesthesia and complications of the surgery performed for each postoperative patient, in contradistinction to the individual patient's initial presentation and symptom chronology as is often done in the Neuro ICU. Although reviewing the patient's initial symptomatology may be important, it is likely that the early ICU course might be as much related to the operative procedure, as to the presenting signs and symptoms. We are unaware of a reference for the intensivist that provides this type of perioperative information regarding neurosurgical patients in a clear and concise manner. This was the impetus for this textbook.

Furthermore, the options and methods for intraoperative monitoring have grown over the past decade and will continue to do so. Physiological data gleaned from novel monitors provide critical information about the individual patient's response to surgery and anesthesia. Understanding the advantages and disadvantages of these monitoring techniques is imperative to the provision of exemplary care of the neurocritically-ill patient. Similarly, mounting evidence suggests that critical information is progressively omitted during points of transitions of care. Anticipatory inquiry may enhance communication between OR and ICU staff *if* providers receiving the patients are knowledgeable enough to ask probing questions and to elicit details that may be lost in translation.

The aim of this text, *Neurocritical Care Management of the Neurosurgical Patient*, is to serve as the premier reference for the intensive care management of neurosurgical patients. Many available neurocritical care textbooks have focused on particular disease states, pathophysiological conditions, or medical complications. However, none has described the specific neurosurgical procedures or anesthetic considerations that impact the critical care management of these patients.

This textbook is divided into 6 sections. **Section 1** offers a review of core neuroanesthesiology principles applied to the operative care of neurosurgical patients. Chapters in this section focus on neurophysiological effects of anesthetic agents, procedural patient positioning, specific anesthetic considerations for brain, spinal cord and endovascular neurosurgery, intraoperative neuromonitoring, and intraoperative catastrophes.

The lion's share of the volume is contained within **Sections 2-5**. For the most part, a neurosurgeon or neuro-interventionalist collaborated with a neurointensivist to write each chapter. **Section 2** focuses on types of craniotomy procedures, including vascular neurosurgery, neuro-oncologic surgery, epilepsy surgery, functional neurosurgery and trauma neurosurgery. **Section 3** is devoted to spinal surgery and **Section 4** focuses on endovascular neurosurgery. **Section 5** is dedicated to specialty procedures including ventricular shunts and neuro-monitor placement, combined neurosurgical procedures (e.g. with Otorhinolaryngology or Plastic Surgery) and peripheral neurosurgery.

Chapters in **Sections 2-5** adhere to a prescribed structure and format. Each chapter is divided into 3 parts: Neuroanatomy and Procedure, Perioperative Considerations, and ICU Complications. The first part, *Neuroanatomy and Procedure*, reviews the relevant neuroanatomy and operative steps of the procedure. The second part, Perioperative Considerations, describes the related neuro-monitoring, operative position and anesthetic choices for the procedure. The remainder of the chapter, *ICU Complications*, comprises an evidence-based review of the potential procedural complications and the relevant critical care management strategies. **Section 6** is exclusively devoted to potential ICU complications of neurosurgery including delayed emergence, intracranial hypertension, hemodynamic complications, intracranial hypertension, or status epilepticus.

The editors are grateful that the Neuro ICUs at the University of Pennsylvania foster collaborative endeavors between Neurology, Neurosurgery and Anesthesiology. It is likely due to the fact that from its inception, the Penn Neuro ICU represented a shared vision of the chairpersons of the Departments of Neurology, Neurosurgery and Anesthesiology & Critical Care. The inherent nature of this Neuro-ICU program has borne fruitful clinical, academic and research programs that are nationally and internationally recognized. These academic and clinical endeavors have resulted in partnerships with experts in neuroanesthesia, neurocritical care and neurosurgery, many of whom have graciously contributed to this volume. We believe that this textbook will have broad applicability and will serve neurosurgeons, anesthesiologists, medical intensivists, surgical intensivists as well as neurointensivists. We hope that it will also serve as a reference for trainees of varied backgrounds.

*M. A. Kumar, MD*
*W. A. Kofke, MD, MBA*
*J. M. Levine, MD*
*J. M. Schuster, MD, PhD*

# List of Contributors

**Manish K. Aghi, MD, PhD**
Department of Neurological Surgery, Center for Minimally Invasive Skull Base Surgery, University of California, San Francisco, CA, USA

**Zarina S. Ali, MD**
Assistant Professor, Department of Neurosurgery, University of Pennsylvania, Philadelphia, PA, USA

**Dorothea Altschul, MD**
Clinical Assistant Professor of Neurology, Neurological Surgery, Columbia University College of Physicians and Surgeons, New York, NY, USA

**Zirka H. Anastasian, MD**
Assistant Professor of Anesthesiology, Department of Anesthesiology, Columbia University Medical Center, New York, NY, USA

**Safdar Ansari, MD**
Assistant Professor, Chief, Division of Neurocritical Care, Department of Neurology, University of Utah School of Medicine, Salt Lake City, UT, USA

**William J. Ares, MD**
Department of Neurological Surgery, University of Pittsburgh Medical Center, Pittsburgh, PA, USA

**Mark Attiah, BA**
Medical Student, Perelman School of Medicine, University of Pennsylvania, Philadelphia, PA, USA

**Anthony M. Avellino, MD, MBA**
Chief Executive Officer, OSF HealthCare Neuroscience Service Line and Illinois Neurological Institute; Professor of Neurosurgery and Pediatrics, University of Illinois College of Medicine at Peoria, Peoria, IL, USA

**Rafi Avitsian, MD**
Section Head, Neurosurgical Anesthesiology, Associate Professor of Anesthesiology, Neuroanesthesia Fellowship Program Director, Anesthesiology and Neurological Institutes, Cleveland Clinic, Cleveland, OH, USA

**Neeraj Badjatia, MD, MSc**
Chief of Neurocritical Care, Program in Trauma, Associate Professor of Neurology, Neurosurgery, Anesthesiology, University of Maryland School of Medicine, Baltimore, MD, USA

**Robert L. Bailey, BS, MD**
Physician, Department of Neurosurgery, Paoli Hospital, Paoli, IN, USA

**Nicholas Bastidas, MD, FAAP**
Attending, Plastic Surgery, Assistant Professor, Surgery, Hofstra Northwell School of Medicine, Manhasset, NY, USA

**Paulomi Bhalla, MD**
Neurocritical Care Fellow, Department of Neurology, Hospital of the University of Pennsylvania, Philadelphia, PA, USA

**Adarsh Bhimraj, MD**
Head, Section of Neurologic Infectious Diseases, Cleveland Clinic, Cleveland, OH, USA

**Joshua T. Billingsley, MD, MS**
Cerebrovascular Surgery, Department of Neurosurgery, University of Florida at Orlando Health, Orlando, FL, USA

**Thomas P. Bleck, MD**
Professor and Associate Chief Medical Officer, Departments of Neurological Sciences, Neurosurgery, Anesthesiology, and Medicine, Rush University Medical Center, Chicago, IL, USA

**Christine Boone, BS**
MD, PhD Candidate, Department of Neurosurgery, The Johns Hopkins University School of Medicine, Baltimore, MD, USA

**Steven Brem, MD**
Chief, Neurosurgical Oncology, Co-Director, Penn Brain Tumor Center, Department of Neurosurgery, Abramson Cancer Center, Perelman School of Medicine, University of Pennsylvania, Philadelphia, PA, USA

**Vivek Buch, MD**
Neurosurgery Resident, Department of Neurosurgery, Hospital of the University of Pennsylvania, Philadelphia, PA, USA

**Richard W. Byrne, MD**
Professor and Chairman, Department of Neurosurgery, Rush University Medical Center, Chicago, IL, USA

**Daniel P. Cahill, MD, PhD**
Associate Professor, Department of Neurosurgery, Massachusetts General Hospital, Boston, MA, USA

**Justin M. Caplan, MD**
Resident Department of Neurosurgery, Johns Hopkins
  University School of Medicine, Baltimore, MD, USA

**Nohra Chalouhi, MD**
Department of Neurological Surgery, Thomas Jefferson
  University Hospital, Philadelphia, PA, USA

**Catherine S. Chang, MD**
Resident Division of Plastic Surgery, University of
  Pennsylvania, Philadelphia, PA, USA

**Jason J. Chang, MD**
Assistant Professor of Neurological Surgery, Oregon Health
  & Science University, Center for Health & Healing,
  Portland, OR, USA

**Steven D. Chang, MD**
Robert C. and Jeannette Powell Professor, Director,
  Stanford Neuromolecular Innovations Program,
  Director, Stanford Neurogenetics Oncology Program,
  Co-Director, Stanford CyberKnife Program, Department
  of Neurosurgery, Stanford University School of
  Medicine, Stanford, CA, USA

**Navjot Chaudhary, MD**
Clinical Assistant Professor, Department of Neurosurgery,
  Stanford University, Stanford, CA, USA

**H. Isaac Chen, MD**
Assistant Professor, Department of Neurosurgery, Hospital
  of the University of Pennsylvania, Philadelphia, PA,
  USA

**Randall M. Chesnut, MD, FCCM, FACS**
Department of Neurological Surgery and Orthopaedics
  and Sports Medicine, University of Washington School
  of Medicine, Harborview Medical Center, University of
  Washington School of Global Health, Seattle, WA,
  USA

**E. Antonio Chiocca, MD, PhD, FAANS**
Harvey W. Cushing Professor of Neurosurgery, Established
  by the Daniel E. Ponton Fund, Harvard Medical School,
  Neurosurgeon-in-Chief and Chairman, Department of
  Neurosurgery, Co-Director, Institute for the
  Neurosciences at the Brigham, Brigham and Women's/
  Faulkner Hospital, Surgical Director, Center for
  Neurooncology, Dana-Farber Cancer Institute, Boston,
  MA, USA

**Rohan Chitale, MD**
Assistant Professor, Department of Neurosurgery,
  Vanderbilt University Medical Center, Nashville, TN,
  USA

**Claudia F. Clavijo, MD**
Assistant Professor, Department of Anesthesiology,
  University of Colorado School of Medicine, Aurora, CO,
  USA

**William T. Curry, Jr., MD**
Associate Professor and Attending Neurosurgeon, Director
  of Neurosurgical Oncology, Department of
  Neurosurgery, Massachusetts General Hospital,
  Harvard Medical School, Boston, MA, USA

**Andrew Dailey, MD**
Associate Professor, Department of Neurosurgery,
  University of Utah School of Medicine, Salt Lake City,
  UT, USA

**Rahul Damani, MD, MPH**
Assistant Professor, Division of Vascular Neurology and
  Neurocritical Care, Department of Neurology, Baylor
  College of Medicine, Houston, TX, USA

**Daniel J. DiLorenzo, MD, PhD, MBA**
Functional and Epilepsy Neurosurgery Fellow, Department
  of Neurosurgery, Rush University Medical Center,
  Chicago, IL, USA

**Christopher F. Dowd, MD**
Professor, Department of Radiology and Biomedical
  Imaging, University of California, San Francisco, San
  Francisco, CA USA

**Emad N. Eskanadar, MD**
Professor in Surgery, Charles Anthony Pappas Chair of
  Neurosciences, Harvard Medical School, Department of
  Neurosurgery, Massachusetts General Hospital, Boston,
  MA, USA

**James J. Evans, MD**
Professor, Department of Neurological Surgery, Thomas
  Jefferson University, Philadelphia, PA, USA

**Brenda G. Fahy, MD, MCCM**
Associate Chair and Chief, Division of Critical Care,
  Department of Anesthesiology, University of Florida,
  Gainesville, FL, USA

**Christopher J. Farrell, MD**
Assistant Professor, Department of Neurological Surgery,
  Thomas Jefferson University, Philadelphia, PA, USA

**Anna K. Finley Caulfield, MD**
Clinical Associate Professor, Department of Neurology and
  Neurological Sciences, Stanford University, Stanford,
  CA, USA

**Alana M. Flexman, MD**
Assistant Professor, Department of Anesthesiology,
  Pharmacology and Therapeutics, University of British
  Columbia, Vancouver, BC, Canada

**Sunil V. Furtado, MS, MCh, DNB**
Clinical Instructor, Department of Neurosurgery,
  Stanford University School of Medicine, Stanford,
  CA, USA

**Alexander J. Gamble, DO**
Resident in Neurosurgery, Hofstra Northwell School of
Medicine, Manhasset, NY, USA

**Paul A. Gardner, MD**
Associate Professor, Department of Neurological
Surgery, University of Pittsburgh School of Medicine,
Co-Director, Center for Cranial Base Surgery,
University of Pittsburgh Medical Center, Pittsburgh,
PA, USA

**John G. Gaudet, MD**
Assistant Professor of Anesthesiology, Department of
Anesthesiology, Columbia University Medical Center,
New York, NY, USA

**Emily J. Gilmore**
Assistant Professor of Neurology, Department of
Neurology, Yale University School of Medicine, New
Haven, CT, USA

**C. Rory Goodwin, MD, PhD**
Neurosurgery Resident, Department of Neurosurgery, The
Johns Hopkins University School of Medicine, Baltimore,
MD, USA

**William B. Gormley, MD, MPH**
Director, Neurosurgical Critical Care, Brigham and
Women's Hospital, Department of Neurosurgery,
Harvard Medical School, Boston, MA, USA

**M. Sean Grady, MD**
Charles Harrison Frazier Professor and Chairman,
Department of Neurosurgery, The University of
Pennsylvania, Philadelphia, PA, USA

**Ramesh Grandhi, MD**
Department of Neurological Surgery, University of
Pittsburgh Medical Center, Pittsburgh, PA, USA

**Benjamin F. Gruenbaum, MD**
Resident Physician, Department of Anesthesiology, Yale
University School of Medicine, New Haven, CT, USA

**Shaun E. Gruenbaum, MD**
Clinical Fellow, Neurosurgical Anesthesiology,
Department of Anesthesiology, Yale University School of
Medicine, New Haven, CT, USA

**James S. Harrop, MD**
Professor of Neurological and Orthopedic Surgery, Thomas
Jefferson University, Philadelphia, PA, USA

**J. Claude Hemphill, III, MD**
Professor, Department of Neurology and Neurological
Surgery, Kenneth Rainin Chair in Neurocritical Care,
University of California, San Francisco, Co-Director,
Brain and Spinal Cord Injury Center, Director,
Neurocritical Care, San Francisco General Hospital, San
Francisco, CA, USA

**Todd M. Herrington, MD, PhD**
Instructor in Neurology, Fellow in Movement Disorders,
Department of Neurology, Massachusetts General
Hospital, Boston, MA, USA

**Lawrence J. Hirsch**
Professor of Neurology, Department of Neurology,
Yale University School of Medicine, New Haven,
CT, USA

**Kyle S. Hobbs, MD**
Neurocritical care fellow, Division of Neurocritical Care
and Stroke, Department of Neurology, Stanford
University School of Medicine, Stanford, CA, USA

**Brian L. Hoh, MD**
James and Newton Eblen Professor, Department of
Neurosurgery, Chief, Division of Cerebrovascular
Surgery, University of Florida, Gainesville, FL, USA

**Yin C. Hu, MD**
Assistant Professor, Westchester Neurovascular
Institute, Westchester Medical Center, Department
of Neurosurgery, New York Medical College,
Valhalla, NY, USA

**Christina Huang, MD**
Department of Neurological Surgery, Keck School of
Medicine, University of Southern California, Los
Angeles, CA, USA

**Judy Huang, MD**
Professor of Neurosurgery, Program Director,
Neurosurgery Residency Program, Fellowship Director,
Cerebrovascular Neurosurgery, Johns Hopkins
University School of Medicine, Department of
Neurosurgery, Baltimore, MD, USA

**Robert W. Hurst, MD**
Professor of Radiology, Department of Radiology, Hospital
of the University of Pennsylvania, Children's Hospital of
Philadelphia, Philadelphia, PA, USA

**Michael E. Ivan, MD**
Department of Neurological Surgery, University of Miami,
Chief of Service, Cranial and Neuro-oncology, JSCH,
Director of Research, University of Miami Brain Tumor
Initiative, Miami, FL, USA

**Pascal Jabbour, MD**
Division Director of Neurovascular Surgery and
Endovascular Neurosurgery, Department of
Neurological Surgery, Thomas Jefferson University
Hospital, Philadelphia, PA, USA

**Ian Kaminsky, MD**
Assistant Professor, Department of Radiology, Tufts
University, School of Medicine, Interventional
Neuroradiologist, Lahey Hospital & Medical Center,
Burlington, MA, USA

**Suhail Kanchwala, MD**
Assistant Professor of Surgery, Division of Plastic Surgery, University of Pennsylvania, Philadelphia, PA, USA

**Gregory Kapinos, MD, MS, FASN**
Attending, Neurocritical Care, Assistant Professor, Neurosurgery and Neurology, Hofstra Northwell School of Medicine, Manhasset, NY, USA

**Craig Kilburg, MD**
Resident, Department of Neurosurgery, University of Utah School of Medicine, Salt Lake City, UT, USA

**Koffi M. Kla, MD**
Assistant Professor, Department of Anesthesiology, Vanderbilt University School of Medicine, Nashville, TN, USA

**W. Andrew Kofke, MD, MBA, FCCM, FNCS**
Professor, Director Neuroscience in Anesthesiology and Critical Care Program, Co-Director Neurocritical Care, Co-Director Perioperative Medicine and Pain Clinical Research Unit, Department of Anesthesiology and Critical Care, Department of Neurosurgery, University of Pennsylvania, Philadelphia, PA, USA

**David Kung, MD**
Fellow, Neurovascular Surgery and Endovascular Neurosurgery, Thomas Jefferson University, Philadelphia, PA, USA

**Shih-Shan Lang, MD**
Instructor, Division of Neurosurgery, Children's Hospital of Philadelphia, Philadelphia, PA, USA

**Sean D. Lavine, MD**
Clinical Associate Professor in Neurological Surgery, Columbia College of Physicians and Surgeons, New York, NY, USA

**Peter Le Roux, MD, FACS**
Brain and Spine Center, Lankenau Medical Center, Wynnewood, PA, USA

**Lorri A. Lee, MD**
Professor, Departments of Anesthesiology and Neurological Surgery, Vanderbilt University School of Medicine, Nashville, TN, USA

**Vincent Lew, MD**
Department of Anesthesia and Perioperative Care, University of California, San Francisco, CA, USA

**Caitlin Loomis, MD**
Assistant Professor, Department of Neurology, Yale University, New Haven, CT, USA

**Timothy Lucas, MD, PhD**
Assistant Professor of Neurosurgery, Department of Neurosurgery, Hospital of the University of Pennsylvania, Philadelphia, PA, USA

**K.H. Kevin Luk, MD, MS**
Assistant Professor, Department of Anesthesiology and Pain Medicine, University of Washington, Seattle, WA, USA

**Tracy S. Ma, MD**
Neurosurgery Resident, Department of Neurosurgery, Perelman School of Medicine, University of Pennsylvania, Philadelphia, PA, USA

**Brian Mac Grory**
Resident Physician Department of Neurology, Yale University School of Medicine, New Haven, CT, USA

**Luke Macyszyn, MD, MA**
Assistant Professor of Neurosurgery and Orthopedics, David Geffen School of Medicine at UCLA, Los Angeles, CA, USA

**Stephen T. Magill, MD, PhD**
Resident Physician, Department of Neurological Surgery, University of California, San Francisco, San Francisco, CA, USA

**Geoffrey T. Manley, MD, PhD**
Professor, Vice-Chairman, Department of Neurological Surgery, University of California, San Francisco, Chief, Neurological Surgery, Co-Director, Brain and Spinal Cord Injury Center, San Francisco General Hospital, San Francisco, CA, USA

**Edward M. Manno, MD FCCM, FANA, FAAN, FAHA**
Head, Neurological Intensive Care Unit, Cleveland Clinic, Cleveland, OH, USA

**Neena I. Marupudi, MD, MS**
Neurosurgery Resident, Wayne State University School of Medicine, Detroit, MI, USA

**Hesham Masoud, MD**
Assistant Professor of Neurology, Neurosurgery and Radiology, SUNY Upstate Medical University, Syracuse, NY, USA

**Christopher M. Maulucci, MD**
Assistant Professor, Department of Neurosurgery, Tulane University, New Orleans, LA, USA

**Christopher Melinosky, MD**
Neurocritical Care Fellow, Department of Neurology, University of Maryland School of Medicine, Baltimore, MD, USA

**Jennifer Gutwald Miller, MD**
Attending, Neurocritical Care, Christiana Care Health System, Newark, DE, USA

**Bradley J. Molyneaux, MD, PhD**
Assistant Professor, Departments of Neurology and Critical Care Medicine, University of Pittsburgh Medical Center, Pittsburgh, PA, USA

**Bryan Moore, MD**
Hospital of the University of Pennsylvania, Division of
Neurocritical Care, Department of Neurology,
Philadelphia, PA, USA

**Patricia L. Musolino, MD, PhD**
Instructor, Department of Neurology, Massachusetts
General Hospital, Boston, MA, USA

**Raj K. Narayan, MD, FACS**
Professor and Chairman, Department of Neurosurgery,
Hofstra Northwell School of Medicine and Executive
Director, Northwell Neuroscience Institute,
Manhasset, NY, USA

**Sandra Narayanan, MD, FAHA**
Assistant Professor, Depts. of Neurosurgery and
Neurology, Wayne State University School of
Medicine, Detroit, MI, USA

**Neeraj Naval, MD**
Assistant Professor of Neurology, Neurosurgery and
Anesthesiology and Critical Care Medicine, Johns
Hopkins University School of Medicine, Department
of Neurology, Director, Neurosciences Critical Care,
Johns Hopkins Bayview Medical Center, Baltimore,
MD, USA

**Cuong Nguyen, MD**
Hospital of the University of Pennsylvania, Division of
Interventional Neuroradiology, Department of
Radiology, Philadelphia, PA, USA

**Peggy Nguyen**
Department of Neurology, Keck School of Medicine,
University of Southern California, Los Angeles,
CA, USA

**Thanh Nguyen, MD, FRCP**
Associate Professor, Departments of Neurology, Radiology
and Neurosurgery, Boston University School of
Medicine, Boston, MA, USA

**Raul G. Nogueira, MD**
Professor of Neurology, Neurosurgery and Radiology,
Emory University School of Medicine, Marcus Stroke &
Neuroscience Center, Grady Memorial Hospital,
Atlanta, GA, USA

**Alexander Norbash, MD, MHCM**
Professor and Chairman, Department of Radiology,
University of California, San Diego CA, USA

**David Okonkwo, MD, PhD**
Associate Professor, Department of Neurological
Surgery, University of Pittsburgh Medical Center,
Pittsburgh, PA, USA

**Mark E. Oppenlander, MD**
Clinical Assistant Professor, Department of Neurosurgery,
University of Michigan, Ann Arbor, MI, USA

**Santiago Ortega Gutierrez, MD, MSc**
Clinical Assistant Professor, Departments of
Neurology, Anesthesia, Neurosurgery &
Radiology, University of Iowa Hospitals & Clinics,
Iowa City, IA, USA

**Bryan A. Pukenas, MD**
Assistant Professor of Radiology, Department of
Radiology, Hospital of the University of Pennsylvania,
Children's Hospital of Philadelphia, Philadelphia,
PA, USA

**Alfredo Quiñones-Hinojosa, MD, FAANS, FACS**
William J. and Charles H. Mayo Professor, Neurologic
Surgery Chair, Mayo Clinic College of Medicine,
Jacksonviille, FL, USA

**Preethi Ramchand, MD**
Neurology Resident, Department of Neurology, Perelman
School of Medicine, University of Pennsylvania,
Philadelphia, PA, USA

**Jordina Rincon-Torroella, MD**
Post-doctoral Fellow, Department of Neurosurgery, The
John Hopkins University, Baltimore, MD, USA

**Jonathan Rosand, MD, MSc**
Professor and Medical Director of the Neurosciences
Intensive Care Unit, Chief, Division of Neurocritical Care
and Emergency Neurology, Department of Neurology,
Massachusetts General Hospital, Harvard Medical
School, Boston, MA, USA

**Robert H. Rosenwasser, MD**
Chairman, Department of Neurological Surgery,
Thomas Jefferson University Hospital, Philadelphia,
PA, USA

**W. Caleb Rutledge, MD**
Department of Neurological Surgery, Center for Minimally
Invasive Skull Base Surgery, University of California,
San Francisco, CA, USA

**R. Alexander Schlichter, MD**
Chief of Neuroanesthesia, Department of Anesthesiology
and Critical Care, Perelman School of Medicine,
University of Pennsylvania, Philadelphia, PA, USA

**James M. Schuster, MD, PhD**
Associate Professor of Neurological Surgery, Director of
Neurotrauma, University of Pennsylvania,
Philadelphia, PA, USA

**Daniel M. Sciubba, MD**
Director, Spine Tumor and Spine Deformity Research,
Co-Director, Spinal Column Biomechanics and Surgical
Outcomes, Associate Professor of Neurological Surgery,
Oncology, Orthopaedic Surgery, Radiation Oncology
and Molecular Radiation Sciences, Department of
Neurosurgery, The Johns Hopkins University School
of Medicine, Baltimore, MD, USA

**Benjamin K. Scott, MD**
Assistant Professor, Department of Anesthesiology,
University of Colorado School of Medicine, Aurora,
CO, USA

**Alfred Pokmeng See, MD**
Neurosurgery Resident, Brigham and Women's Hospital,
Department of Neurosurgery, Harvard Medical School,
Boston, MA, USA

**Ganesh M. Shankar, MD, PhD**
Instructor, Department of Neurosurgery, Massachusetts
General Hospital, Boston, MA, USA

**Yoram Shapira, MD, PhD**
Professor and Chairman, Department of Anesthesiology
and Critical Care, Ben-Gurion University of the Negev,
Beer-Sheva, Israel

**Deepak Sharma, MBBS, DM, MD**
Professor and Division Chief, Neuroanesthesiology &
Perioperative Neurosciences, Department of
Anesthesiology and Pain Medicine, University of
Washington, Seattle, WA, USA

**Kevin N. Sheth, MD**
Chief, Division of Neurocritical Care and Emergency
Neurology; Chief, Clinical Research, Department of
Neurology; Director, Neurosciences Intensive Care Unit,
Yale School of Medicine and Yale New Haven Hospital,
New Haven, CT, USA

**Lori A. Shutter, MD, FCCM, FNCS**
Professor, Departments of Critical Care Medicine,
Neurology and Neurosurgery, University of Pittsburgh
School of Medicine, Medical Director, Neurovascular
Intensive Care Unit, University of Pittsburgh Medical
Center, Pittsburgh, PA, USA

**James E. Siegler, MD**
Resident Physician, Department of Neurology, Hospital
of the University of Pennsylvania, Philadelphia,
PA, USA

**Michelle J. Smith, MD**
Hospital of the University of Pennsylvania, Department of
Neurosurgery, Philadelphia, PA, USA

**Carl H. Snyderman, MD, MBA**
Professor, Departments of Otolaryngology and
Neurological Surgery, University of Pittsburgh School of
Medicine, Co-Director, Center for Cranial Base Surgery,
University of Pittsburgh Medical Center, Pittsburgh,
PA, USA

**Gary K. Steinberg, MD, PhD**
Bernard and Ronni Lacroute–William Randolph
Hearst Professor of Neurosurgery and the
Neurosciences, Chairman, Department of
Neurosurgery, Stanford University School of
Medicine, Stanford, CA, USA

**Michael F. Stiefel, MD, PhD, FAANS**
Director, Capital Institute for Neurosciences, Director,
Stroke and Cerebrovascular Center, Capital Health
System, Pennington, NJ, USA

**Geoffrey P. Stricsek, MD**
Resident Physician, Department of Neurological
Surgery, Thomas Jefferson University, Philadelphia,
PA, USA

**Jose I. Suarez, MD**
Professor and Head, Division of Vascular Neurology and
Neurocritical Care, Department of Neurology, Baylor
College of Medicine, Houston, TX, USA

**Gene Sung, MD, MPH**
Department of Neurology, Keck School of Medicine,
University of Southern California, Los Angeles, CA, USA

**Peter Syre, MD**
Chief Resident, Department of Neurosurgery, University of
Pennsylvania, Philadelphia, PA, USA

**Pekka O. Talke, MD**
Professor, Department of Anesthesia and Perioperative
Care, University of California, San Francisco, San
Francisco, CA, USA

**Rafael J. Tamargo, MD**
Walter E. Dandy Professor of Neurosurgery, Professor of
Neurosurgery and Otolaryngology-Head and Neck
Surgery, Director of Cerebrovascular Neurosurgery,
Neurosurgical Co-Director, The Johns Hopkins
Neurocritical Care Unit, Johns Hopkins University
School of Medicine, Department of Neurosurgery,
Baltimore, MD, USA

**Robert Taylor, MD**
Stroke and Neurovascular Center of Central California,
Santa Barbara, CA, USA

**Anurag Tewari, MD**
Neuroanesthesia Fellow, Anesthesia Institute, Cleveland
Clinic, Cleveland, OH, USA

**Stavropoula Tjoumakaris, MD**
Department of Neurological Surgery, Thomas Jefferson
University Hospital, Philadelphia, PA, USA

**Chitra Venkatasubramanian, MBBS, MD, MSc**
Clinical Associate Professor, Division of Neurocritical
care and Stroke, Department of Neurology,
Stanford University School of Medicine, Stanford,
CA, USA

**Andrew S. Venteicher, MD, PhD**
Resident physician, Department of Neurosurgery,
Massachusetts General Hospital, Harvard Medical
School, Boston, MA, USA

**Michael S. Weinstein, MD**
Associate Professor of Surgery and Critical Care
Medicine, Thomas Jefferson University, Philadelphia,
PA, USA

**Peggy White, MD**
Assistant Professor of Anesthesiology, Department of
Anesthesiology, University of Florida, Gainesville,
FL, USA

**Anthony J. Wilson, MD**
Resident, Division of Plastic Surgery, University of
Pennsylvania, Philadelphia, PA, USA

**James M. Wright, MD**
Department of Neurological Surgery, Case Western
Reserve School of Medicine, Cleveland, OH, USA

**Debbie Yi, MD**
Assistant Professor, Department of Emergency Medicine,
UC San Francisco, San Francisco, CA, USA

**Patricia Zadnik, MD**
Resident Physician, Department of Neurosurgery, Hospital
of the University of Pennsylvania, Philadelphia, PA, USA

**Eric L. Zager, MD**
Professor of Neurosurgery, Department of
Neurosurgery, University of Pennsylvania,
Philadelphia, PA, USA

**Mario Zanaty, MD**
Senior Clinical Research Fellow, Department of
Neurological Surgery, Thomas Jefferson
University Hospital, Philadelphia, PA, USA

**Alexander Zlotnik, MD, PhD**
Associate Professor, Department of Anesthesiology
and Critical Care, Ben-Gurion University of the
Negev, Beer-Sheva, Israel

# Acknowledgements

We would like to express our sincere gratitude and appreciation to all the contributors to this volume. We also thank the editorial, design and production staff at Elsevier, in particular: Charlotta Kryhl, Sharon Nash, Trinity Hutton, and Julie Taylor who have been particularly helpful in producing this volume. We would like to thank Dr. Rae Allain, formerly of the Massachusetts General Hospital, for planting the seed that would grow into this textbook. Also we would like to thank the nurses in the clinic, operating room and intensive care unit who care for our patients as we could not do our job without them. Finally, we would like to thank our patients and their families; we are grateful for the opportunity to be a part of their treatment, cure and recovery.

Acknowledgments

# *Dedications*

*To the nurses in the clinic, operating room and intensive*
*care unit who care for our patients.*
*Monisha Kumar*
*W. Andrew Kofke*
*Joshua M. Levine*
*James M. Schuster*


*To my parents who motivated me, my girls who*
*inspire me, my husband who encourages me and CC*
*who supports me.*


*To RJS: for teaching me, training me, and giving me*
*the confidence to accomplish, one ML at a time.*
*Monisha Kumar*

# Neuroanesthesia and Perioperative Care

# 1 Effects of Anesthetics, Operative Pharmacotherapy, and Recovery from Anesthesia

ZIRKA H. ANASTASIAN and JOHN G. GAUDET

## Introduction

Even after completion of a neurosurgical intervention, intraoperative factors, including anesthetic agents, pharmacotherapy, and surgery, may have lasting effects that persist through recovery. The goal of this chapter is to discuss the effects of intraoperative factors, such as anesthetic effect and surgical manipulation, on postoperative recovery, including respiratory function, nausea and vomiting, glucose control, temperature variations, pain management, and delirium and cognitive dysfunction.

### Key Concepts

- Anesthetics, sedatives, and opioids impair respiratory arousal by reducing chemoresponsiveness to hypoxemia and hypercarbia.
- The effect of anesthetics on respiratory muscles depends on the agent, the dose, the patient's state of consciousness, and the specific muscle group.
- Risk factors for postoperative respiratory depression in patients with obstructive sleep apnea include the severity of sleep apnea, the dose of systemic opioids, the use of sedatives, the site and invasiveness of surgical procedure, and the potential for apnea during rapid eye movement (REM) rebound.
- When neuromuscular blockade is employed, it is necessary to monitor the degree of neuromuscular blockade and consider adequacy and potential side effects of reversal of neuromuscular blockade.

## Respiratory Muscle Effects

The muscles involved in respiration are skeletal muscles and can be classified by their anatomical function into two groups: (1) upper airway dilators and (2) respiratory pump muscles. Upper airway dilator muscles counterbalance the negative inspiratory pressure generated by the respiratory pump muscle to permit airflow during inspiration.[1]

Surgery itself can have direct effects on respiratory pump muscles by functional disruption (injury of muscle), postoperative pain leading to restrictions on ventilation, and phrenic nerve injury resulting in diaphragm dysfunction. Other factors that affect diaphragmatic dysfunction postoperatively include inflammation[2] and reflex vagal inhibition.[3] Indirect effects of abdominal surgery may increase intraabdominal pressure. Increased intraabdominal pressure decreases chest wall compliance and increases the work of breathing, further taxing the muscles of the respiratory pump.[1]

Upper airway muscles are generally more sensitive to anesthetics and sedatives than respiratory pump muscles. Animal trials have shown that although volatile anesthetics, barbiturates, and benzodiazepine anesthetics all decrease neural input to both upper airway (hypoglossal nerve) and respiratory pump muscles (phrenic nerve), the decrease of upper airway neural input is much more than respiratory pump muscles.[4] In human clinical studies, even subhypnotic concentrations of propofol, isoflurane, and sevoflurane increase the incidence of pharyngeal dysfunction. This places patients at increased risk for aspiration of pharyngeal contents during recovery of anesthesia. The effect on the pharyngeal contraction pattern may be most pronounced in patients treated with propofol because propofol use results in markedly reduced pharyngeal contraction.[5] In contrast, ketamine reduces neural input to both the upper airway and respiratory muscles equally. Reduction in neural input to the upper airway muscles is much less with ketamine relative to the other classes of anesthetics.[4] Ketamine has no inhibitory effect on genioglossus activity. Unlike other anesthetics, ketamine preserves a high level of upper airway dilator muscle activity, similar to that of conscious patients.[6] Ketamine, however, is a sialagogue, a property that can occasionally be problematic.

Opioid analgesics cause respiratory depression via both upper airway dilator and respiratory pump muscle dysfunction. Opioids reduce genioglossus activity in animals, decrease vagal motor neuron activity in the laryngeal abductors, and increase vagal motor neuronal activity in adductors.[7-9] These changes result in increased upper airway resistance and possibly vocal cord closure, as well as pharyngeal airflow obstruction.[9] Opioid analgesia also increases abdominal muscle activity, which produces a rapid decrease in end-expiratory lung volume and functional residual capacity, contributing to a higher degree of atelectasis.[10] Chest wall rigidity also occurs with the use of opioids, even when dosed conservatively.[11]

### Clinical Pearl

Upper airway muscles are generally more affected by anesthetics and sedatives than respiratory pump muscles.

Controlled ventilation immobilizes the diaphragm and disrupts diaphragmatic function. Controlled ventilation is associated with proteolysis in the diaphragm, which over a long period leads to diaphragmatic atrophy and dysfunction.[12] As little as 18 hours of controlled ventilation results in diaphragmatic atrophy and decreases contractile function.[13] Duration of controlled ventilation correlates with thinning, injury, and atrophy of the diaphragm.[14,15]

Neuromuscular blocking agents (NMBAs) are often used during surgery to provide immobility and optimal operating conditions. Train-of-four (TOF) ratios are customary measures to assess neuromuscular blockade at muscle groups. The TOF ratio value is determined by the ratio of the last twitch height to the first twitch height after a TOF twitches. Recovery at the adductor pollicis is often used for this assessment because the hand is generally convenient and available for monitoring purposes. A TOF ratio of 0.6 or more predicts acceptable recovery of forced vital capacity,[16,17] and for many years recovery to a TOF ratio of 0.7 was considered indicative of adequate recovery of neuromuscular function.[18] Recovery from NMBA generally occurs sooner at the diaphragm than peripheral muscles, such as the hand muscles. Therefore tidal volumes are usually preserved, whereas residual paralysis may still be noted by peripheral monitoring.[19,20] However, a TOF ratio of 0.6 and even 0.8 may be insufficient to ensure recovery of respiratory function. TOF ratios of <1.0 are associated with decreased forced inspiratory volume in one second (FIV1), upper airway obstruction, and impaired pharyngeal function and impaired ability to swallow.[16,21]

Even when nerve stimulators are used, subjective tactile or visual evaluation of the evoked response to indirect nerve stimulation is notoriously inaccurate. Once the TOF ratio exceeds 0.4, most clinicians cannot detect the presence of any fade in the twitches upon four stimuli.[22] A very strong case can be made for the routine administration of a nondepolarizing reversal agent (cholinesterase inhibitor), unless it can be objectively demonstrated that complete recovery (TOF ratio >0.9) has occurred spontaneously.[23,24] As little as 0.015 to 0.025 mg/kg of neostigmine is required at a TOF count of four with minimal fade, whereas 0.04 to 0.05 mg/kg is needed at a TOF count of two or three.[23]

Neuromuscular blockade reversal is not without consequence, however. Neostigmine, in clinically recommended doses, can actually cause neuromuscular transmission failure when given to patients who have already recovered from neuromuscular block.[25] Cholinesterase inhibitors may cause neuromuscular transmission failure by various mechanisms, including the desensitization of acetylcholine receptors,[26] block of neuromuscular transmission, or open channel block.[27,28] Neostigmine, when given in the absence of postsynaptic neuromuscular block, also impairs upper airway dilator volume, genioglossus muscle function, and diaphragmatic function.[28] Thus patients fully recovered from the effects of NMBAs given unwarranted reversal may develop secondary neuromuscular impairment. Neostigmine can also have other systemic effects, including bradycardia, bronchorrhea, bronchospasm, and alimentary peristalsis, muscarinic cholinergic effects that require concomitant administration of an anticholinergic drug such as atropine or glycopyrrolate.

**Clinical Pearl**

Monitoring of neuromuscular blockade is necessary to evaluate for residual blockade when muscle relaxants have been used. Clinical examination for fade in TOF ratio is not dependable.

## Anesthetic Effect on Respiratory Control

At 1 minimum alveolar concentration (MAC), the concentration at which 50% of patients do not move in response to a painful stimulus, all volatile anesthetics (in absence of other depressants) increase respiratory rate, decrease tidal volume, decrease minute ventilation, and increase the arterial $P_{CO_2}$. The order of the respiratory depressant effect, as measured by the increase in arterial $P_{CO_2}$n is enflurane > desflurane ≥ isoflurane > sevoflurane ≥ halothane.[29] Volatile anesthetics abolish the ventilatory response to hypoxia in animals and humans in a dose-dependent manner.[30,31] The peripheral chemoreceptors are the site responsible for this action.[32] Volatile anesthetics also decrease the ventilatory response to hypercapnia, but the response to hypercapnia is more resistant than the response to hypoxia.[33] At subanesthetic concentrations, similar to those that would be found in patients recovering from anesthesia (0.1 MAC), volatile anesthetics reduce the acute hypoxic response by 30% to 50%. The order of potency is halothane > enflurane > sevoflurane > isoflurane > desflurane. This is reflective of the extent to which these agents are metabolized. This effect is probably mediated through a preferential action on the peripheral chemoreflex loop.[34] Low-dose volatile anesthetics also uncouple the association between peripheral chemoreceptor activity and hypoxic ventilatory depression.[34] The effect of subanesthetic volatile anesthetics on the hypercapnic ventilatory response is minimal or absent.[35]

**Clinical Pearl**

At subanesthetic concentrations, volatile anesthetics reduce the acute hypoxic response.

## Anesthetic Effects on Bronchial Tree, Mucociliary Function, and Surfactant Production

Volatile anesthetics are potent bronchodilators that relax airway smooth muscle by directly depressing smooth muscle contractility. This effect is thought to result from direct effects on bronchial epithelium and indirect inhibition of reflex neural pathways. Animal models suggest that halothane (1 MAC), enflurane (1 MAC), and isoflurane (1.5 MAC) produce a similar reduction in bronchial airway resistance.[36] In vitro models demonstrate that isoflurane preferentially relaxes the bronchiole versus the bronchus.[37] Halothane, enflurane, sevoflurane, and isoflurane do not affect baseline pulmonary resistance and dynamic pulmonary compliance, but do attenuate increases in resistance and decreases in compliance due to histamine.[38] In addition to volatile anesthetics, intravenous anesthetics affect bronchial tone. Ketamine has a bronchodilator effect that may be due to inhibition of catecholamine reuptake and action as a sympathomimetic agent.[39] Propofol also has bronchoprotective properties by reducing basal airway tone and histamine-induced bronchoconstrictions in animal studies. Propofol also has a vagolytic effect on the airway.[40,41]

Foreign matter is removed from the tracheobronchial tree by the upward clearance of the ciliated respiratory epithelium. Impaired ciliary motility in anesthetized or intensive care patients may predispose them to respiratory complications, including infections and atelectasis. Poorly humidified inspiratory gases, cuffed endotracheal tubes, high fractional inspired $O_2$, and positive pressure ventilation are known to reduce ciliary movement and decrease mucus production. Halothane, enflurane, nitrous oxide with halothane, and nitrous oxide with opioid all produce dose-dependent decreases of mucociliary movement in dogs.[42,43] Human studies with isoflurane show no inhibition in mucus production; however, data are conflicting regarding the impact on ciliary motion.[44,45] Intravenous anesthetics, including propofol, dexmedetomidine, and thiopental, have no effect on ciliary function. Administration of ketamine and fentanyl at high doses increases ciliary beat frequency.

Lastly, volatile anesthetics cause a progressive, reversible reduction in phosphatidylcholine, the main lipid component of surfactant. The reversibility was within 2 hours in culture.[46]

## Anesthesia Effects on Respiratory Arousal from Sleep, Rapid Eye Movement Rebound, and Obstructive Sleep Apnea

Anesthetics, sedatives, and opioids impair respiratory arousal, defined as arousal from sleep due to respiratory stimuli. These agents reduce chemoresponsiveness to hypoxia[47] and hypercarbia,[48] suppress the reflexive responsiveness to negative upper airway pressure,[49] and depress the magnitude of wakefulness.

During REM sleep, there is hypotonia of voluntary muscles. Electromyogram activity is at the lowest level of any stage of sleep.[50] Neural drive to the upper airway dilators is decreased, and this predisposes the patient to airway instability and episodes of hypoxemia.[51] REM sleep also reduces the hypoxic ventilatory drive and the hypercarbic ventilatory response. Therefore REM rebound (i.e., increased REM sleep due to sleep deprivation or anesthetic inhibition of REM sleep) results in more episodes of hypoxemia due to impaired respiratory arousal[52] (see Fig. 1.1). The effect of anesthetics on REM rebound varies according to the specific agent. Six hours of treatment with volatile anesthesia in mice caused REM rebound,[53] but 3 hours of isoflurane in human volunteers had no effect on REM

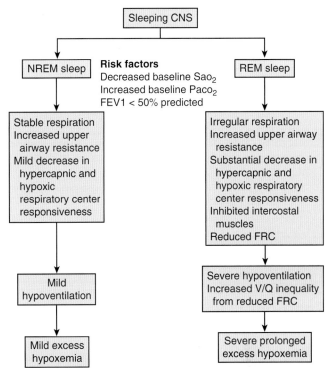

Fig. 1.1 Effect of nonrapid eye movement (NREM) and rapid eye movement (REM) sleep on nocturnal arterial hemoglobin saturation in patients with severe to very severe COPD, with FEV₁ generally less than 50% predicted. Boldface type indicates differences between NREM and REM sleep contributing to hypoxemia. *CNS,* central nervous system; *COPD,* chronic obstructive pulmonary disease; *FRC,* functional residual capacity (end-expiratory lung volume); *Paco₂,* partial arterial pressure of carbon dioxide; *Sao₂,* arterial oxygen saturation (%) of hemoglobin, usually expressed in as a percentage; *V̇/Q̇,* pulmonary alveolar/pulmonary capillary ventilation/perfusion inequality. (Adapted from Barkoukis, TJ & Littner, MR. *Therapy in Sleep Medicine.* Copyright © 2012 Elsevier, Inc. All rights reserved.)

sleep.[54] Benzodiazepines and opioids cause REM rebound upon discontinuation.[55] Propofol has no effect on REM rebound.[56]

Obstructive sleep apnea (OSA) is a syndrome characterized by periodic, partial, or complete obstruction in the upper airway during sleep. This, in turn, causes repetitive arousal from sleep to restore airway patency. The airway obstruction may also cause episodic sleep-associated oxygen desaturation, episodic hypercarbia, and cardiovascular dysfunction. In the postoperative period, patients with OSA, even if asymptomatic, present special challenges that must be addressed to minimize the risk of perioperative morbidity and mortality. Risk factors for postoperative respiratory depression may include the severity of the underlying sleep apnea, administration of opioids or sedatives, site and extent of the surgical procedure, and the potential for apnea during REM rebound. Postoperative interventions to manage OSA patients who may be susceptible to the aforementioned risks should take into consideration (1) postoperative analgesia, (2) oxygenation, (3) patient positioning, and (4) monitoring. Recently published guidelines[57] relevant to the postoperative management of patients with OSA include the following:

A. Provide evidence supporting the use of postoperative continuous positive airway pressure (*Category A3-B evidence*).[58]
B. Suggest consideration of a regional anesthesia technique. This is in the setting of insufficient literature to evaluate outcomes associated with different types of postoperative analgesia (regional versus systemic analgesia and effects of basal rates of analgesia) on patients with OSA.
C. Suggest consideration of providing supplemental oxygenation, but this is in the setting of insufficient literature.
D. Support positioning patients in a nonsupine fashion (*Category B1-B evidence*).[59]
E. Support using postoperative pulse oximetry monitoring (*Category B3-B evidence*).[60]

# Effects of Anesthetics and Surgery on Postoperative Nausea and Vomiting

## Key Concepts

- Postoperative nausea and vomiting (PONV) is multifactorial involving anesthetic risk factors, surgical risk factors, and individual risk factors.
- Prevention and treatment of PONV should focus on identification of risk factors, reduction of baseline risk factors, and intervention based on a multimodal prophylaxis and treatment regimen.
- Some neurosurgical procedures, particularly those involving the posterior fossa, are at higher risk of PONV.

General anesthesia using volatile anesthetics is associated with an average incidence of PONV ranging between 20% and 30% for general surgery patients, 50% for craniotomy patients, and even higher for infratentorial craniotomy.[61,62] Development of PONV is multifactorial, involving anesthetic, surgical, and individual risk factors (see Fig. 1.2). Anesthetic risk factors include the use of volatile anesthetics, nitrous oxide, and intraoperative and postoperative opioids. The emetogenic effect of the inhaled anesthetics and opioids appears to be dose related.[61,63] The duration of surgery also affects the likelihood of PONV. For each 30-minute increase in duration, the risk of PONV increases by 60% from baseline. However, patient-specific factors, including female sex, nonsmoking status, and history of PONV, may be the most important determinants. A validated scoring system based on risk factors includes female gender, nonsmoker, history of PONV, and administration of postoperative opioids, with a corresponding risk of 10% for no risk factors, 20% for one risk factor, 40% for two, 60% for three, and 80% for four risk factors[64] (see Table 1.1).

Nausea and vomiting after neurosurgery may increase the risk of systemic hypertension, vagal maneuvers, and increased venous postoperative bleeding. Anesthesiology guidelines to prevent PONV focus on identification of risk factors, reduction of exacerbating factors, and

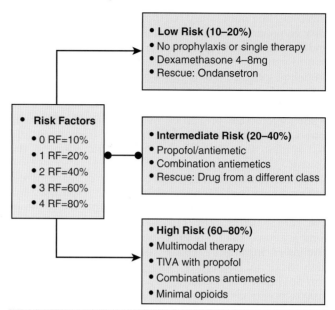

**Fig. 1.2** Risk factors and PONV management strategy. (Adapted from Keyes, M. Management of postoperative nausea and vomiting in ambulatory surgery: the big little problem. *Clinics in Plastic Surgery.* Copyright © 2013 Elsevier, Inc.)

**Table 1.1** Risk of PONV

| Risk Factors | Female sex<br>Nonsmoker<br>History of PONV<br>Use of post op opioids |
| --- | --- |
| Risk of PONV | 10%: No risk factor<br>20%: One risk factor<br>40%: Two risk factors<br>60%: Three risk factors<br>80%: Four risk factors |

administration of appropriate prophylaxis.[65] Antiemetics that are commonly used, the classes, mechanisms, and common side effects are as follows:

5-hydroxytryptamine (5-HT$_3$) receptor antagonists (ondansetron, dolasetron, granisetron, and tropisetron).[66] There are no effects on cerebral hemodynamics or intracranial pressure with minimal added sedation.[67] Side effects include the potential to produce a headache, dizziness,[68] and a possibility to produce a dystonic/encephalopathic reaction.[69]

Metoclopramide is a D2 and 5-HT$_3$ antagonist.[70] It increases gastric motility.[71] It can produce dystonic reactions, which can include respiratory insufficiency and extrapyramidal symptoms. It is therefore contraindicated in patients with Parkinson's disease.

Corticosteroids (dexamethasone) have an unclear mechanism on decreasing nausea and vomiting, but it is thought to be related to antiinflammatory effects, a direct effect on the solitary tract nucleus, interaction with serotonin and receptor proteins NK1 and NK2, regulation of the hypothalamic–pituitary–adrenal axis, and reduction of pain and thus the use of opioids.[72] Side effects include blood glucose abnormalities and genital pain/burning upon administration.

Propofol in low doses is an antiemetic of an unclear mechanism. The residual antiemetic properties postoperatively make propofol a popular choice or adjunct for an anesthetic in a patient who is at high risk for nausea and vomiting postoperatively.[68]

Phenothiazines (promethazine and prochlorperazine) are D2 antagonists with moderate antihistamine and anticholinergic properties.[70] They can produce extrapyramidal reactions.[68]

Phenylethylamine (ephedrine) is a sympathomimetic agent that has been used as an antiemetic in the obstetrical and abdominal surgery populations.[73] It does increase heart rate and blood pressure.

Butyrophenones (droperidol, haloperidol) are D2 receptor antagonists.[70] They have minimal effect on cerebral hemodynamics or intracranial pressure and tend to decrease blood pressure. Side effects include mild sedation, dysphoria, and extrapyramidal side effects. It is therefore contraindicated in patients with Parkinson's disease and prolonged QT interval.

Antihistamines (dimenhydrinate, hydroxyzine) block histamine receptors in the nucleus of the solitary tract. They can produce some sedation.[68]

Anticholinergic (transdermal scopolamine) medications act centrally and block impulses from vestibular nuclei to higher areas in the central nervous system and reticular activating system.[68,74] The central cholinergic antagonism can lead to delirium, which can be reversed with physostigmine, a centrally acting cholinesterase inhibitor. It also can result in mild sedation and dizziness.

Neurokinin antagonists (aprepitant) act by blocking the binding of substance P (a regulatory neuropeptide) to NK1 receptors in vagal afferents in the gastrointestinal tract and in regions of the central nervous system. Common side effects include fatigue, headache, and constipation.[75]

In general, combination therapy has superior efficacy compared with monotherapy for PONV prophylaxis, and drugs with different mechanisms of action should be used in combination to optimize efficacy.[76]

Postoperatively, when a prophylactic dose of an antiemetic has failed, a rescue dose should be chosen from another mechanistic class. To repeat a prophylactic dose in the first 6 hours after administration has not been shown to be effective.[77]

# Effects of Anesthetics and Surgery on Postoperative Glycemic Control

## Key Concept

Optimal glucose management, particularly in patients with acute brain insult, remains a controversial issue because both hypoglycemia and hyperglycemia appear to result in critical adverse effects.

Many preclinical studies conclusively demonstrate the deleterious effects of hyperglycemia in the ischemic brain.[78,79] Also numerous retrospective studies have reported an association between hyperglycemia and adverse outcomes in humans with various types of neurological problems.[80] Sieber et al. reported that routine elective neurosurgery was associated with levels of hyperglycemia thought to be high enough to exacerbate ischemic brain damage.[81] Thus the stage was set for needed prospective randomized studies. In 2001 Van den Berghe et al. reported on the use of intensive insulin therapy targeted to tight blood glucose control (target range 80–110 mg/dL) in critically ill surgical patients. This and subsequent studies from her group resulted in recommendations calling for the widespread use of intensive insulin therapy (IIT) in critically ill patients.[82] To address the safety of IIT administered to postoperative neurosurgical patients, tight blood glucose control with IIT resulted in a three-fold increase in the risk of iatrogenic hypoglycemia.[83] The Normoglycemia in Intensive Care Evaluation-Survival Using Glucose Algorithm Regulation trial, a large (6104 patients), multicenter, international, randomized trial, reported that in adult intensive care unit (ICU) patients, IIT targeted to tight blood glucose control (target range 81–108 mg/dL), compared with conventional glucose control (target <144–180 mg/dL), resulted in higher mortality.[84]

Optimal glucose management, particularly in patients with acute brain injury and those undergoing neurosurgery, remains a controversial issue. Both hypoglycemia and hyperglycemia appear to result in critical adverse effects. Although there may be benefit in controlling hyperglycemia in neurocritical care and neurosurgical ICU patients,[85–87] the actual incidence and impact of hypoglycemia remain unknown. This may be due to the fact that the temporal relationship to ictus, optimal level of control, and the impact of confounding factors such as stress or steroid administration remains unknown. More information is needed about the correlation of peripheral glucose levels with intracellular levels in the brain, particularly in the ischemic or potentially ischemic brain. Current guidelines suggest that hyperglycemic levels above 180 to 200 mg% warrant insulin therapy.[88]

The widespread use of glucocorticoids in the neurosurgical ICU affects optimal glucose management. Glucocorticoids stabilize the blood–brain barrier and increase absorption of cerebrospinal fluid. They are beneficial when administered in low doses (e.g., 10 mg of dexamethasone) in preventing PONV and are commonly used in neurosurgery to reduce vasogenic edema in primary and metastatic tumors. The administration of a single dose of dexamethasone will, however, increase blood glucose concentration significantly in both diabetic and nondiabetic patients.[89,90]

## Clinical Pearl

Although hyperglycemia has negative consequences, hypoglycemia can be regional in the injured brain and should be avoided.

# Effects of Anesthetics and Surgery on Temperature Regulation

## Key Concepts

- Hypothermia has both deleterious and potentially neuroprotective effects when performed intraoperatively and postoperatively.
- Rewarming should be done gradually and with caution to avoid complications.

Abnormal body temperature results from an imbalance between heat loss and heat production. Radiation, conduction, convection, and evaporation mechanisms contribute to heat loss.[91] The hypothalamus is responsible, in large part, for maintaining core temperature within a normal range (35.0–37.5°C, 95.0–99.5°F).[92] It receives afferent peripheral input from C (warm) and Aδ (cold) fibers and regulates both heat production (basal metabolic rate, shivering) and heat distribution (peripheral vasomotor tone, sweat) via efferent autonomic and endocrine signals.[93] Disruption of afferent or efferent signaling, as well as hypothalamic dysfunction, may lead to hypothermia (any core temperature below 35°C) or hyperthermia (any core temperature above 37.5°C) as measured centrally (pulmonary artery, bladder, nasopharynx, lower esophagus, tympanic membrane) or peripherally (axilla, mouth, rectum). Core temperature is usually higher than peripheral temperature. Core hypothermia is graded as mild (32–35.0°C, 90–95.0°F), moderate (28–32°C, 82–90°F), severe (20–28°C, 68–82°F), or profound (less than 20°C, 68°F). Severe hyperthermia (any core temperature above 40.0°C, 104.0°F) is sometimes referred to as *hyperpyrexia*.[94]

Whereas hypothermia is frequently observed following administration of general anesthesia, the onset of hyperthermia is rare but should prompt immediate investigation because it may be the expression of anaphylaxis or abnormal drug reaction.[95] Malignant hyperthermia is most concerning and potentially lethal, but quite rare. Most general anesthetic drugs affect both peripheral vasomotor tone and hypothalamic function but preserve sweat mechanisms and afferent hypothalamic input.[96] Initially after induction of general anesthesia, heat loss is accelerated due to redistribution of blood flow to peripheral tissues. Skin warming before induction attenuates this phenomenon by reducing the thermic gradient between the central and peripheral compartments.[97] Drugs such as ketamine[98] and midazolam,[99] as well as nitrous oxide[100] may help preserve vasomotor tone and decrease heat loss. During maintenance of general anesthesia, the hypothalamic temperature set point gets readjusted to a lower temperature due to drug-related effects. Inhibition of shivering by muscle relaxants further decreases heat production.[101] During neuraxial anesthesia, the combination of sympatholytic vasoplegia and altered afferent signaling leads to hypothermia from accelerated heat loss and abnormal elevation in apparent temperature, respectively.[102] Under such circumstances, skin warming may fail to prevent hypothermia.[103] Heat loss is also exacerbated by the frequent administration of hypnotic drugs to produce sedation in combination with neuraxial anesthesia.

The effects of general and/or neuraxial anesthesia may either balance or exacerbate temperature changes commonly observed in brain or spinal cord injury. After brain injury, hypothalamic dysfunction or stress-induced immune modulation may result in hypothermia or hyperthermia.[104] In patients with altered mental status, fever is also commonly due to environmental exposure and bronchoaspiration. After spinal cord injury, although prolonged immobility may present with hyperthermia due to infectious or thrombotic complications, neurogenic vasoplegia can be responsible for significant heat loss.[105]

Fever is clearly associated with worse clinical outcomes in patients with neurological injury.[106] Although hypothermia has multiple systemic deleterious side effects, it may also have neuroprotective effects in patients with traumatic brain injury (TBI) or massive stroke.[107,108] Mild hypothermia attenuates secondary cerebral insults due to intracranial hypertension after TBI.[109] In stroke patients, therapeutic effects of hypothermia are equivocal despite robust benefits in animal models. In absence of strong evidence from clinical trials, therapeutic hypothermia should be considered for treatment of massive stroke with intracranial hypertension.[110] Unclear benefits of therapeutic hypothermia in a clinical setting are due in part to the deleterious effects of rewarming.[111] Patients with brain or spinal cord injury should be rewarmed carefully before initiation of emergence. As a general rule, the more severe the injury and/or degree of hypothermia, the more progressive and closely monitored rewarming should be. In all cases of brain or spinal cord injury, hyperthermia should be avoided, as it is clearly deleterious.[112]

## Clinical Pearl

Hypothermia is common during and after surgery and may be neuroprotective in some cases, but hyperthermia is clearly deleterious and should be avoided.

# Effects of Anesthetics and Surgery on Pain and Pain Control

## Key Concepts

- Multimodal analgesia, including acetaminophen, nonsteroidal antiinflammatory drugs (NSAIDs), local anesthetics, gabapentinoids, ketamine, and opioids, should be considered in chronic pain patients or patients at risk of developing chronic pain.
- Whenever necessary, collaboration with a pain specialist should be considered.

Up to two-thirds of patients suffer from postoperative pain after craniotomy.[113] Compared with supratentorial procedures, patients undergoing infratentorial craniotomy report more severe pain scores. Such poor outcomes are at least in part due to avoidance or underutilization of opioids to reduce the sedation associated with their use. They also result from a presumed lack of need for analgesics, as well as difficulties in assessing pain during recovery from brain surgery.

Pain after spine surgery represents a particularly difficult challenge. These patients often have chronic pain, significant disability, and psychological distress, and many have had prior neurosurgery.[114] The challenge in managing pain after spine surgery resides in treating patients with multiple predictors of severe postoperative pain and analgesic consumption.[115] Factors clearly associated with difficult postoperative pain management include chronic pain independent of opioid tolerance, significant disability with psychological distress, major surgery, or reoperation after failed surgery.[114] In the presence of such risk factors, the perioperative analgesic plan should be made and adjusted in collaboration with a pain specialist.

Opioids remain the mainstay of analgesia after neurosurgical procedures. Although most share common pharmacodynamical properties (μ receptor agonism), their pharmacokinetic profiles tend to differ significantly.[116] Whenever rapid neurological recovery from anesthetic effect is required, drugs with shorter half-lives are usually favored. Unless complemented with other nonopioid analgesics, use of such short-acting drugs may result in suboptimal postoperative analgesia. Alternatively, drugs with longer half-lives may be preferred to optimize analgesia during emergence and recovery whenever pain management is anticipated to be problematic. Opioid-induced side effects include respiratory depression, sedation, and prolonged immobilization. Perioperative analgesia should be managed in collaboration with a pain specialist in presence of respiratory risk factors such as obesity, sleep apnea, or obstructive or restrictive lung disease. Nausea, vomiting, constipation, and slow gastric emptying with delayed enteral nutrition may also complicate their use.[117] Prolonged duration of high opioid plasma levels has been associated with increasing sensitivity to noxious stimuli (opioid-induced hyperalgesia)[118] and immunosuppression.[119] In order to reduce the incidence and severity of opioid-induced side effects, modern analgesic management relies on a multimodal approach that combines opioids with coanalgesics.[120]

Acetaminophen may be used as an adjunctive to treat mild to moderate postoperative pain. In patients with fever, it may also induce a significant decrease in temperature within 15 minutes. Compared with the oral or rectal routes, IV acetaminophen may be beneficial. However, due to the relatively high cost of the IV formulation, physicians remain hesitant to use it.[121]

The use of NSAIDs such as ketorolac after neurosurgical procedures remains controversial. On one hand, ketorolac is a nonsedating drug with potent analgesic activity that has been demonstrated to reduce postoperative opioid requirements.[122] On the other hand, ketorolac has an inhibitory effect on both platelet function[123] and bone formation,[124] a key determinant for the success of spinal fusion procedures. In the absence of strong clinical evidence, ketorolac should be used cautiously, if at all, after intracranial surgery[125] or spinal fusion procedures.[126] In addition, NSAIDs should be avoided in patients with, or at risk for, renal dysfunction and gastrointestinal bleeding.[127]

Ketamine has potent antinociceptive effects in the spinal cord at subanesthetic concentrations.[128] It may also have beneficial antiinflammatory effects.[129] The combination of a low-dose bolus (0.1–0.5 mg/kg preferably administered before incision) and a continuous infusion (2–5 mcg/kg/min) may improve postoperative pain management while decreasing opioid consumption without increasing the risk of aberrant excitatory cortical, hippocampal, and limbic hallucinogenic activity observed at higher dosages. Although the use of ketamine during craniotomy remains very controversial, there is preliminary clinical evidence indicating ketamine may be beneficial in sedated, ventilated patients with severe traumatic brain injury.[130] It should be considered for patients with chronic pain and opioid dependence undergoing spine surgery.[131]

Gabapentinoids, such as gabapentin and pregabalin, are oral anticonvulsant drugs. They block calcium channels, which are upregulated in dorsal root ganglia and contribute to neuropathic pain symptoms (hyperalgesia, allodynia) after nerve injury. A heterogeneous body of clinical studies shows they may also have antinociceptive, opioid-sparing, and anxiolytic properties.[128] Their use as analgesic premedication before craniotomy is very controversial due to a high incidence of dizziness and sedation, most commonly in the elderly and/or in patients with renal dysfunction.[132] Gabapentinoids appear to be most beneficial in patients undergoing major spine surgery; however, timing and optimal dosage remain unclear.[133]

Finally, postoperative pain may also be attenuated using local anesthetics to reduce transmission of the nociceptive signal from the peripheral to the central nervous system. During craniotomy, regional scalp block using lidocaine, bupivacaine, or ropivacaine before incision has been shown to reduce postoperative pain and opioid consumption. Addition of low-dose epinephrine to the local anesthetic solution may help prolong duration of the block without systemic hemodynamic effects.[134] Local anesthetics may also be administered in the epidural space or intravenously in patients undergoing major spine surgery. Combined epidural/general anesthesia with postoperative epidural analgesia may produce better pain control and a lower surgical stress response than general anesthesia with postoperative systemic opioid analgesia. However, patients with epidural catheters should be carefully monitored and referred to a pain specialist postoperatively due to the potential significant side effects of sympathetic blockade.[135] Alternatively, perioperative IV administration of lidocaine may improve postoperative pain management after complex spine procedures. The evidence supporting this strategy remains limited; further research is needed to confirm preliminary results, demonstrate safety, and clarify dosage.[136]

## Effects of Anesthetics and Surgery on Consciousness and Cognition

### Key Concepts

- Postoperative delirium (POD) and postoperative cognitive decline (POCD) are frequently encountered in the elderly after surgery.
- Management should rely on early identification of patients at risk and avoidance of any disruption of cerebral physiology until the mechanisms leading to POD and POCD are elucidated.
- Treatment can include reduction of psychological and physiological perioperative stress and use of dexmedetomidine and antipsychotics.

POD and POCD are two distinct forms of brain dysfunction that are frequently encountered mostly in the elderly after major surgery.[137] Although it is unclear whether both disorders share common pathophysiological mechanisms, they have clearly been associated with an increased risk of complications leading to longer hospital stays, significantly higher costs, and higher mortality rates.[138]

Rapid, often fluctuant alterations of consciousness are the hallmark of POD. Psychomotor changes (agitation or, more commonly, hypoactivity) and acute cognitive disturbances are other important signs frequently observed alongside an abnormal sleep/wake cycle or disturbed visual/auditory perception. POD typically presents 1 to 3 days after surgery; it may persist for several days to weeks. Several diagnostic scales using *Diagnostic and Statistical Manual of Mental Disorders* criteria are available for use in multiple settings, including the ICU.[139] In some situations of an apparent hypoactive cognitive state, consideration should be given to nonconvulsive seizures, which have been reported in up to 19% of ICU patients.[140]

POCD has a subtler, subacute presentation dominated by memory loss and executive dysfunction leading to inability to perform simple activities of daily living. POCD usually presents weeks to months after surgery; it may be only partially reversible over a period of several months. The diagnosis of POCD must be confirmed by the results of a time-consuming battery of neurocognitive tests, administered by trained personnel, showing significant decline from baseline evaluation.[141] Education and awareness of POCD are of considerable importance because many patients and their families may not be aware of the potential scope of this disease.

Because the stress response to surgery appears to play a central role in development of postoperative brain dysfunction, strategies aimed at reducing tissue injury and/or limiting its impact on the brain may be beneficial. Minimally invasive surgical techniques are associated with lower rates of POD.[142] Their role in decreasing the risk of POCD remains unclear. Similarly, effective attenuation of the pain-induced stress response using a multimodal, opioid-sparing analgesic strategy may be beneficial during and after surgery.[143] Other neuroprotective strategies targeting the perioperative inflammatory activation or the neuroendocrine response are being investigated.[144] Finally, reduction of psychological perioperative stress using reassurance, orientation, and maintenance of sensory input from visual or auditory aids has been shown to be as efficient as, if not more than, other strategies.[145]

Clearly, management should rely on early identification of patients at risk (Table 1.2) and avoidance of any disruption of cerebral physiology until the mechanisms leading to POD and POCD are elucidated. Patient management relying on a multimodal, multidisciplinary strategy is most successful when initiated before surgery and continued postoperatively.[146] Overall, conditions associated with insufficient cerebral oxygen or energy delivery (hypoxemia, anemia, hypotension, hypoglycemia, stroke), excessive cerebral metabolism (hyperthermia, seizure activity, substance withdrawal), and any acute homeostatic imbalance (renal or hepatic dysfunction, drug toxicity, systemic inflammation) should be identified as early as possible and treated promptly. Whereas most hypnotic drugs have

**Table 1.2** Predisposing and Precipitating Factors for Postoperative Delirium

| Predisposing factors | Precipitating factors |
| --- | --- |
| Reduced cognitive reserve (advanced age, cognitive impairment) | Polymedication<br>Drugs affecting the central nervous system |
| Sensory impairment (visual, auditory) | Pain<br>Urinary obstruction/catheterization |
| Frailty (malnutrition, dehydration) | Hypoxemia<br>Hypotension |
| Substance dependence (alcohol, drugs) | Infection<br>Electrolyte abnormalities |
| Severe illness with organ dysfunction | Environmental changes |
| Apolipoprotein E4 genotype | Sleep/wake disturbances |

been shown to increase the risk of POD irrespective of dose or duration of administration, dexmedetomidine may be advantageous and should be considered for sedation or as a complement for general anesthesia in patients at risk.[147] Interestingly, recent evidence indicates excessive depth of anesthesia, as measured with electroencephalography, may correlate with a higher risk of both POD and POCD.[148]

Anticholinergic drugs used for reversal of muscle paralysis have been suspected to contribute to the development of POD and POCD; however, recent reports have failed to confirm this hypothesis.[149] Antipsychotic medications have been successfully used for prevention and treatment of hyperactive POD. The precise underlying mechanism remains unclear; some authors suggest it may convert hyperactive episodes of POD into hypoactive ones without resolving the issue.[150] In absence of a reversible cause for brain dysfunction, they may be administered cautiously. Atypical antipsychotics such as risperidone or olanzapine have a better side effect profile but are available for oral administration only. Alternatively, haloperidol may be administered intravenously or intramuscularly.[151]

**Clinical Pearl**

Management of POD and POCD should focus on early identification of patients at risk and minimizing disruption of cerebral physiology.

## Summary

The effects of anesthetics, agents given during surgery, and surgery itself can have an effect on the recovering patient. Patients who are at an increased risk for postoperative respiratory dysfunction, PONV, hyperglycemia, hypothermia, pain, and cognitive dysfunction should be identified by preoperative risk factors, and the postoperative management should take into consideration the intraoperative course and management.

## References

1. Sasaki N, Meyer MJ, Eikermann M. Postoperative respiratory muscle dysfunction: pathophysiology and preventive strategies. *Anesthesiology*. 2013;118(4):961–978.
2. Krause KM, Moody MR, Andrade FH, et al. Peritonitis causes diaphragm weakness in rats. *Am J Respir Crit Care Med*. 1998;157(4 Pt 1):1277–1282.
3. Ford GT, Grant DA, Rideout KS, Davison JS, Whitelaw WA. Inhibition of breathing associated with gallbladder stimulation in dogs. *J Appl Physiol (1985)*. 1988;65(1):72–79.
4. Nishino T, Shirahata M, Yonezawa T, Honda Y. Comparison of changes in the hypoglossal and the phrenic nerve activity in response to increasing depth of anesthesia in cats. *Anesthesiology*. 1984;60(1):19–24.
5. Sundman E, Witt H, Sandin R, et al. Pharyngeal function and airway protection during subhypnotic concentrations of propofol, isoflurane, and sevoflurane: volunteers examined by pharyngeal videoradiography and simultaneous manometry. *Anesthesiology*. 2001;95(5):1125–1132.
6. Eikermann M, Grosse-Sundrup M, Zaremba S, et al. Ketamine activates breathing and abolishes the coupling between loss of consciousness and upper airway dilator muscle dysfunction. *Anesthesiology*. 2012;116(1):35–46.
7. Hajiha M, DuBord MA, Liu H, Horner RL. Opioid receptor mechanisms at the hypoglossal motor pool and effects on tongue muscle activity in vivo. *J Physiol*. 2009;587(Pt 11):2677–2692.
8. Campbell C, Weinger MB, Quinn M. Alterations in diaphragm EMG activity during opiate-induced respiratory depression. *Respir Physiol*. 1995;100(2):107–117.
9. Lalley PM. Mu-opioid receptor agonist effects on medullary respiratory neurons in the cat: evidence for involvement in certain types of ventilatory disturbances. *Am J Physiol Regul Integr Comp Physiol*. 2003;285(6):R1287–R1304.
10. Chawla G, Drummond GB. Fentanyl decreases end-expiratory lung volume in patients anaesthetized with sevoflurane. *Br J Anaesth*. 2008;100(3):411–414.
11. Vaughn RL, Bennett CR. Fentanyl chest wall rigidity syndrome: a case report. *Anesth Prog*. 1981;28(2):50–51.
12. Shanely RA, Zergeroglu MA, Lennon SL, et al. Mechanical ventilation-induced diaphragmatic atrophy is associated with oxidative injury and increased proteolytic activity. *Am J Respir Crit Care Med*. 2002;166(10):1369–1374.
13. Levine S, Nguyen T, Taylor N, et al. Rapid disuse atrophy of diaphragm fibers in mechanically ventilated humans. *N Engl J Med*. 2008;358(13):1327–1335.
14. Grosu HB, Lee YI, Lee J, Eden E, Eikermann M, Rose KM. Diaphragm muscle thinning in patients who are mechanically ventilated. *Chest*. 2012;142(6):1455–1460.
15. Jaber S, Petrof BJ, Jung B, et al. Rapidly progressive diaphragmatic weakness and injury during mechanical ventilation in humans. *Am J Respir Crit Care Med*. 2011;183(3):364–371.
16. Eikermann M, Groeben H, Husing J, Peters J. Accelerometry of adductor pollicis muscle predicts recovery of respiratory function from neuromuscular blockade. *Anesthesiology*. 2003;98(6):1333–1337.
17. Ali HH, Wilson RS, Savarese JJ, Kitz RJ. The effect of tubocurarine on indirectly elicited train-of-four muscle response and respiratory measurements in humans. *Br J Anaesth*. 1975;47(5):570–574.
18. Ali HH, Savarese JJ, Lebowitz PW, Ramsey FM. Twitch, tetanus and train-of-four as indices of recovery from nondepolarizing neuromuscular blockade. *Anesthesiology*. 1981;54(4):294–297.
19. Donati F, Meistelman C, Plaud B. Vecuronium neuromuscular blockade at the diaphragm, the orbicularis oculi, and adductor pollicis muscles. *Anesthesiology*. 1990;73(5):870–875.
20. Eikermann M, Vogt FM, Herbstreit F, et al. The predisposition to inspiratory upper airway collapse during partial neuromuscular blockade. *Am J Respir Crit Care Med*. 2007;175(1):9–15.
21. Cedborg AI, Sundman E, Boden K, et al. Pharyngeal function and breathing Pattern during Partial Neuromuscular Block in the Elderly: Effects on Airway Protection. *Anesthesiology*. 2014;120(2):312–325.
22. Viby-Mogensen J, Jensen NH, Engbaek J, Ording H, Skovgaard LT, Chraemmer-Jorgensen B. Tactile and visual evaluation of the response to train-of-four nerve stimulation. *Anesthesiology*. 1985;63(4):440–443.
23. Kopman AF, Eikermann M. Antagonism of non-depolarising neuromuscular block: current practice. *Anaesthesia*. 2009;64(Suppl 1):22–30.
24. Viby-Mogensen J. Postoperative residual curarization and evidence-based anaesthesia. *Br J Anaesth*. 2000;84(3):301–303.
25. Caldwell JE. Reversal of residual neuromuscular block with neostigmine at one to four hours after a single intubating dose of vecuronium. *Anesth Analg*. 1995;80(6):1168–1174.
26. Yost CS, Maestrone E. Clinical concentrations of edrophonium enhance desensitization of the nicotinic acetylcholine receptor. *Anesth Analg*. 1994;78(3):520–526.
27. Legendre P, Ali DW, Drapeau P. Recovery from open channel block by acetylcholine during neuromuscular transmission in zebrafish. *J Neurosci*. 2000;20(1):140–148.
28. Eikermann M, Fassbender P, Malhotra A, et al. Unwarranted administration of acetylcholinesterase inhibitors can impair genioglossus and diaphragm muscle function. *Anesthesiology*. 2007;107(4):621–629.
29. Teppema LJ, Baby S. Anesthetics and control of breathing. *Respir Physiol Neurobiol*. 2011;177(2):80–92.
30. Hirshman CA, McCullough RE, Cohen PJ, Weil JV. Depression of hypoxic ventilatory response by halothane, enflurane and isoflurane in dogs. *Br J Anaesth*. 1977;49(10):957–963.
31. Knill RL, Gelb AW. Ventilatory responses to hypoxia and hypercapnia during halothane sedation and anesthesia in man. *Anesthesiology*. 1978;49(4):244–251.
32. Morray JP, Nobel R, Bennet L, Hanson MA. The effect of halothane on phrenic and chemoreceptor responses to hypoxia in anesthetized kittens. *Anesth Analg*. 1996;83(2):329–335.
33. Pandit JJ. The variable effect of low-dose volatile anaesthetics on the acute ventilatory response to hypoxia in humans: a quantitative review. *Anaesthesia*. 2002;57(7):632–643.
34. Teppema LJ, Dahan A. The ventilatory response to hypoxia in mammals: mechanisms, measurement, and analysis. *Physiol Rev*. 2010;90(2):675–754.
35. Pandit JJ. Effect of low dose inhaled anaesthetic agents on the ventilatory response to carbon dioxide in humans: a quantitative review. *Anaesthesia*. 2005;60(5):461–469.
36. Hirshman CA, Edelstein G, Peetz S, Wayne R, Downes H. Mechanism of action of inhalational anesthesia on airways. *Anesthesiology*. 1982;56(2):107–111.
37. Mazzeo AJ, Cheng EY, Stadnicka A, Bosnjak ZJ, Coon RL, Kampine JP. Topographical differences in the direct effects of isoflurane on airway smooth muscle. *Anesth Analg*. 1994;78(5):948–954.
38. Katoh T, Ikeda K. A comparison of sevoflurane with halothane, enflurane, and isoflurane on bronchoconstriction caused by histamine. *Can J Anaesth*. 1994;41(12):1214–1219.
39. Cook DJ, Carton EG, Housmans PR. Mechanism of the positive inotropic effect of ketamine in isolated ferret ventricular papillary muscle. *Anesthesiology*. 1991;74(5):880–888.
40. Hashiba E, Hirota K, Suzuki K, Matsuki A. Effects of propofol on bronchoconstriction and bradycardia induced by vagal nerve stimulation. *Acta Anaesthesiol Scand*. 2003;47(9):1059–1063.
41. Hirota K, Sato T, Hashimoto Y, et al. Relaxant effect of propofol on the airway in dogs. *Br J Anaesth*. 1999;83(2):292–295.
42. Forbes AR. Halothane depresses mucociliary flow in the trachea. *Anesthesiology*. 1976;45(1):59–63.
43. Forbes AR, Horrigan RW. Mucociliary flow in the trachea during anesthesia with enflurane, ether, nitrous oxide, and morphine. *Anesthesiology*. 1977;46(5):319–321.
44. Raphael JH, Butt MW. Comparison of isoflurane with propofol on respiratory cilia. *Br J Anaesth*. 1997;79(4):473–475.
45. Lichtiger M, Landa JF, Hirsch JA. Velocity of tracheal mucus in anesthetized women undergoing gynecologic surgery. *Anesthesiology*. 1975;42(6):753–756.
46. Molliex S, Crestani B, Dureuil B, et al. Effects of halothane on surfactant biosynthesis by rat alveolar type II cells in primary culture. *Anesthesiology*. 1994;81(3):668–676.
47. Zhang Z, Zhuang J, Zhang C, Xu F. Activation of opioid mu-receptors in the commissural subdivision of the nucleus tractus solitarius abolishes the ventilatory response to hypoxia in anesthetized rats. *Anesthesiology*. 2011;115(2):353–363.
48. Zhang Z, Xu F, Zhang C, Liang X. Activation of opioid mu receptors in caudal medullary raphe region inhibits the ventilatory response to

hypercapnia in anesthetized rats. *Anesthesiology.* 2007;107 (2):288–297.

49. Eastwood PR, Szollosi I, Platt PR, Hillman DR. Collapsibility of the upper airway during anesthesia with isoflurane. *Anesthesiology.* 2002;97(4):786–793.

50. Roth T, Roehrs T. Sleep organization and regulation. *Neurology.* 2000;54(5 Suppl 1):S2–S7.

51. Cherniack NS. Respiratory dysrhythmias during sleep. *N Engl J Med.* 1981;305(6):325–330.

52. Rosenberg J, Wildschiodtz G, Pedersen MH, von Jessen F, Kehlet H. Late postoperative nocturnal episodic hypoxaemia and associated sleep pattern. *Br J Anaesth.* 1994;72(2):145–150.

53. Pick J, Chen Y, Moore JT, et al. Rapid eye movement sleep debt accrues in mice exposed to volatile anesthetics. *Anesthesiology.* 2011;115(4):702–712.

54. Moote CA, Knill RL. Isoflurane anesthesia causes a transient alteration in nocturnal sleep. *Anesthesiology.* 1988;69(3):327–331.

55. Kay DC, Eisenstein RB, Jasinski DR. Morphine effects on human REM state, waking state and NREM sleep. *Psychopharmacologia.* 1969;14 (5):404–416.

56. Tung A, Lynch JP, Mendelson WB. Prolonged sedation with propofol in the rat does not result in sleep deprivation. *Anesth Analg.* 2001;92 (5):1232–1236.

57. Practice guidelines for the perioperative management of patients with obstructive sleep apnea: an updated report by the American Society of Anesthesiologists task force on perioperative management of patients with obstructive sleep apnea. *Anesthesiology.* 2014;120 (2):268–86.

58. Neligan PJ, Malhotra G, Fraser M, et al. Continuous positive airway pressure via the Boussignac system immediately after extubation improves lung function in morbidly obese patients with obstructive sleep apnea undergoing laparoscopic bariatric surgery. *Anesthesiology.* 2009;110(4):878–884.

59. Pevernagie DA, Shepard Jr JW. Relations between sleep stage, posture and effective nasal CPAP levels in OSA. *Sleep.* 1992;15 (2):162–167.

60. Bolden N, Smith CE, Auckley D, Makarski J, Avula R. Perioperative complications during use of an obstructive sleep apnea protocol following surgery and anesthesia. *Anesth Analg.* 2007;105(6): 1869–1870.

61. Gan TJ, Meyer TA, Apfel CC, et al. Society for Ambulatory Anesthesia guidelines for the management of postoperative nausea and vomiting. *Anesth Analg.* 2007;105(6):1615–1628. table of contents.

62. Fabling JM, Gan TJ, El-Moalem HE, Warner DS, Borel CO. A randomized, double-blinded comparison of ondansetron, droperidol, and placebo for prevention of postoperative nausea and vomiting after supratentorial craniotomy. *Anesth Analg.* 2000;91(2): 358–361.

63. Roberts GW, Bekker TB, Carlsen HH, Moffatt CH, Slattery PJ, McClure AF. Postoperative nausea and vomiting are strongly influenced by postoperative opioid use in a dose-related manner. *Anesth Analg.* 2005;101(5):1343–1348.

64. Apfel CC, Laara E, Koivuranta M, Greim CA, Roewer N. A simplified risk score for predicting postoperative nausea and vomiting: conclusions from cross-validations between two centers. *Anesthesiology.* 1999;91(3):693–700.

65. Gan TJ, Meyer TA, Apfel CC, et al. Society for Ambulatory Anesthesia guidelines for the management of postoperative nausea and vomiting. *Anesth Analg.* 2007;105(6):1615–1628. table of contents.

66. Seynaeve C, Verweij J, de Mulder PH. 5-HT3 receptor antagonists, a new approach in emesis: a review of ondansetron, granisetron and tropisetron. *Anticancer Drugs.* 1991;2(4):343–355.

67. Jacot A, Bissonnette B, Favre JB, Ravussin P. The effect of ondansetron on intracranial pressure and cerebral perfusion pressure in neurosurgical patients. *Ann Fr Anesth.* 1998;17(3):220–226.

68. Kovac AL. Prevention and treatment of postoperative nausea and vomiting. *Drugs.* 2000;59(2):213–243.

69. Ritter MJ, Goodman BP, Sprung J, Wijdicks EF. Ondansetron-induced multifocal encephalopathy. *Mayo Clin Proc.* 2003;78 (9):1150–1152.

70. Hamik A, Peroutka SJ. Differential interactions of traditional and novel antiemetics with dopamine D2 and 5-hydroxytryptamine3 receptors. *Cancer Chemother Pharmacol.* 1989;24(5):307–310.

71. MacLaren R, Kiser TH, Fish DN, Wischmeyer PE. Erythromycin vs metoclopramide for facilitating gastric emptying and tolerance to intragastric nutrition in critically ill patients. *JPEN.* 2008;32 (4):412–419.

72. Chu CC, Hsing CH, Shieh JP, Chien CC, Ho CM, Wang JJ. The cellular mechanisms of the antiemetic action of dexamethasone and related glucocorticoids against vomiting. *Eur J Pharmacol.* 2014;722:48–54.

73. Rothenberg DM, Parnass SM, Litwack K, McCarthy RJ, Newman LM. Efficacy of ephedrine in the prevention of postoperative nausea and vomiting. *Anesth Analg.* 1991;72(1):58–61.

74. Crowell Jr EB, Ketchum JS. The treatment of scopolamine-induced delirium with physostigmine. *Clin Pharmacol Ther.* 1967;8(3): 409–414.

75. Curran MP, Robinson DM. Aprepitant: a review of its use in the prevention of nausea and vomiting. *Drugs.* 2009;69(13):1853–1878.

76. Eberhart LH, Morin AM, Bothner U, Georgieff M. Droperidol and 5-HT3-receptor antagonists, alone or in combination, for prophylaxis of postoperative nausea and vomiting. A meta-analysis of randomised controlled trials. *Acta Anaesthesiol Scand.* 2000;44 (10):1252–1257.

77. Kovac AL, O'Connor TA, Pearman MH, et al. Efficacy of repeat intravenous dosing of ondansetron in controlling postoperative nausea and vomiting: a randomized, double-blind, placebo-controlled multicenter trial. *J Clin Anesth.* 1999;11(6):453–459.

78. Siemkowicz E. Hyperglycemia in the reperfusion period hampers recovery from cerebral ischemia. *Acta Neurol Scand.* 1981;64 (3):207–216.

79. Prado R, Ginsberg MD, Dietrich WD, Watson BD, Busto R. Hyperglycemia increases infarct size in collaterally perfused but not end-arterial vascular territories. *J Cereb Blood Flow Metab.* 1988;8 (2):186–192.

80. Pulsinelli WA, Levy DE, Sigsbee B, Scherer P, Plum F. Increased damage after ischemic stroke in patients with hyperglycemia with or without established diabetes mellitus. *Am J Med.* 1983;74(4): 540–544.

81. Sieber F, Smith DS, Kupferberg J, et al. Effects of intraoperative glucose on protein catabolism and plasma glucose levels in patients with supratentorial tumors. *Anesthesiology.* 1986;64(4):453–459.

82. van den Berghe G, Wouters P, Weekers F, et al. Intensive insulin therapy in critically ill patients. *N Engl J Med.* 2001;345 (19):1359–1367.

83. Bilotta F, Caramia R, Paoloni FP, Delfini R, Rosa G. Safety and efficacy of intensive insulin therapy in critical neurosurgical patients. *Anesthesiology.* 2009;110(3):611–619.

84. Finfer S, Chittock DR, Su SY, et al. Intensive versus conventional glucose control in critically ill patients. *N Engl J Med.* 2009;360 (13):1283–1297.

85. Rostami E. Glucose and the injured brain-monitored in the neurointensive care unit. *Front Neurol.* 2014;5:91.

86. Kruyt ND, Biessels GJ, DeVries JH, et al. Hyperglycemia in aneurysmal subarachnoid hemorrhage: a potentially modifiable risk factor for poor outcome. *J Cereb Blood Flow Metab.* 2010;30(9): 1577–1587.

87. Latorre JG, Chou SH, Nogueira RG, et al. Effective glycemic control with aggressive hyperglycemia management is associated with improved outcome in aneurysmal subarachnoid hemorrhage. *Stroke.* 2009;40(5):1644–1652.

88. Van den Berghe G. What's new in glucose control in the ICU? *Intensive Care Med.* 2013;39(5):823–825.

89. Pasternak JJ, McGregor DG, Lanier WL. Effect of single-dose dexamethasone on blood glucose concentration in patients undergoing craniotomy. *J Neurosurg Anesthesiol.* 2004;16(2):122–125.

90. Hans P, Vanthuyne A, Dewandre PY, Brichant JF, Bonhomme V. Blood glucose concentration profile after 10 mg dexamethasone in non-diabetic and type 2 diabetic patients undergoing abdominal surgery. *Br J Anaesth.* 2006;97(2):164–170.

91. Sessler DI. Temperature monitoring and perioperative thermoregulation. *Anesthesiology.* 2008;109(2):318–338.

92. Clapham JC. Central control of thermogenesis. *Neuropharmacology.* 2012;63(1):111–123.

93. Nomoto S, Shibata M, Iriki M, Riedel W. Role of afferent pathways of heat and cold in body temperature regulation. *Int J Biometeorol.* 2004;49(2):67–85.

94. Hernandez M, Cutter TW, Apfelbaum JL. Hypothermia and hyperthermia in the ambulatory surgical patient. *Clin Plast Surg.* 2013;40(3):429–438.

95. Herlich A. Perioperative temperature elevation: not all hyperthermia is malignant hyperthermia. *Paediatr Anaesth*. 2013;23(9): 842–850.

96. Lenhardt R. The effect of anesthesia on body temperature control. *Front Biosci (Schol Ed)*. 2010;2:1145–1154.

97. Roberson MC, Dieckmann LS, Rodriguez RE, Austin PN. A review of the evidence for active preoperative warming of adults undergoing general anesthesia. *AANA J*. 2013;81(5):351–356.

98. Ikeda T, Kazama T, Sessler DI, et al. Induction of anesthesia with ketamine reduces the magnitude of redistribution hypothermia. *Anesth Analg*. 2001;93(4):934–938.

99. Bjelland TW, Dale O, Kaisen K, et al. Propofol and remifentanil versus midazolam and fentanyl for sedation during therapeutic hypothermia after cardiac arrest: a randomised trial. *Intensive Care Med*. 2012;38(6):959–967.

100. Lenhardt R, Negishi C, Sessler DI, Ozaki M, Tayefeh F, Kurz A. Paralysis only slightly reduces the febrile response to interleukin-2 during isoflurane anesthesia. *Anesthesiology*. 1998;89(3):648–656.

101. Imamura M, Matsukawa T, Ozaki M, et al. Nitrous oxide decreases shivering threshold in rabbits less than isoflurane. *Br J Anaesth*. 2003;90(1):88–90.

102. Arkilic CF, Akca O, Taguchi A, Sessler DI, Kurz A. Temperature monitoring and management during neuraxial anesthesia: an observational study. *Anesth Analg*. 2000;91(3):662–666.

103. Butwick AJ, Lipman SS, Carvalho B. Intraoperative forced airwarming during cesarean delivery under spinal anesthesia does not prevent maternal hypothermia. *Anesth Analg*. 2007;105. (5):1413–1419. table of contents.

104. Childs C. Human brain temperature: regulation, measurement and relationship with cerebral trauma: part 1. *Br J Neurosurg*. 2008;22(4): 486–496.

105. Price MJ. Thermoregulation during exercise in individuals with spinal cord injuries. *Sports Med*. 2006;36(10):863–879.

106. Greer DM, Funk SE, Reaven NL, Ouzounelli M, Uman GC. Impact of fever on outcome in patients with stroke and neurologic injury: a comprehensive meta-analysis. *Stroke*. 2008;39(11):3029–3035.

107. Choi HA, Badjatia N, Mayer SA. Hypothermia for acute brain injury–mechanisms and practical aspects. *Nat Rev Neurol*. 2012;8(4): 214–222.

108. Rivera-Lara L, Zhang J, Muehlschlegel S. Therapeutic hypothermia for acute neurological injuries. *Neurotherapeutics*. 2012;9(1):73–86.

109. Urbano LA, Oddo M. Therapeutic hypothermia for traumatic brain injury. *Curr Neurol Neurosci Rep*. 2012;12(5):580–591.

110. Jeon SB, Koh Y, Choi HA, Lee K. Critical care for patients with massive ischemic stroke. *J Stroke*. 2014;16(3):146–160.

111. Povlishock JT, Wei EP. Posthypothermic rewarming considerations following traumatic brain injury. *J Neurotrauma*. 2009;26(3): 333–340.

112. Badjatia N. Hyperthermia and fever control in brain injury. *Crit Care Med*. 2009;37(7 Suppl):S250–S257.

113. Flexman AM, Ng JL, Gelb AW. Acute and chronic pain following craniotomy. *Curr Opin Anaesthesiol*. 2010;23(5):551–557.

114. Ip HY, Abrishami A, Peng PW, Wong J, Chung F. Predictors of postoperative pain and analgesic consumption: a qualitative systematic review. *Anesthesiology*. 2009;111(3):657–677.

115. Cahana A, Dansie EJ, Theodore BR, Wilson HD, Turk DC. Redesigning delivery of opioids to optimize pain management, improve outcomes, and contain costs. *Pain Med*. 2013;14(1):36–42.

116. Drewes AM, Jensen RD, Nielsen LM, Droney J, Christrup LL, Arendt-Nielsen L, et al. Differences between opioids: pharmacological, experimental, clinical and economical perspectives. *Br J Clin Pharmacol*. 2013;75(1):60–78.

117. Benyamin R, Trescot AM, Datta S, Buenaventura R, Adlaka R, Sehgal N, et al. Opioid complications and side effects. *Pain Physician*. 2008;11(2 Suppl):S105–S120.

118. Brush DE. Complications of long-term opioid therapy for management of chronic pain: the paradox of opioid-induced hyperalgesia. *J Med Toxicol*. 2012;8(4):387–392.

119. Rittner HL, Roewer N, Brack A. The clinical (ir)relevance of opioid-induced immune suppression. *Curr Opin Anaesthesiol*. 2010;23 (5):588–592.

120. Young A, Buvanendran A. Recent advances in multimodal analgesia. *Anesthesiol Clin*. 2012;30(1):91–100.

121. O'Neal JB. The utility of intravenous acetaminophen in the perioperative period. *Front Public Health*. 2013;1:25.

122. De Oliveira Jr GS, Agarwal D, Benzon HT. Perioperative single dose ketorolac to prevent postoperative pain: a meta-analysis of randomized trials. *Anesth Analg*. 2012;114(2):424–433.

123. Bauer KA, Gerson W, Wright CT, et al. Platelet function following administration of a novel formulation of intravenous diclofenac sodium versus active comparators: a randomized, single dose, crossover study in healthy male volunteers. *J Clin Anesth*. 2010;22 (7):510–518.

124. Pountos I, Giannoudis PV, Jones E, English A, Churchman S, Field S, et al. NSAIDS inhibit in vitro MSC chondrogenesis but not osteogenesis: implications for mechanism of bone formation inhibition in man. *J Cell Mol Med*. 2011;15(3):525–534.

125. Magni G, La Rosa I, Melillo G, Abeni D, Hernandez H, Rosa G. Intracranial hemorrhage requiring surgery in neurosurgical patients given ketorolac: a case-control study within a cohort (2001-2010). *Anesth Analg*. 2013;116(2):443–447.

126. Li Q, Zhang Z, Cai Z. High-dose ketorolac affects adult spinal fusion: a meta-analysis of the effect of perioperative nonsteroidal anti-inflammatory drugs on spinal fusion. *Spine (Phila Pa 1976)*. 2011;36(7):E461–E468.

127. Davies NM, Reynolds JK, Undeberg MR, Gates BJ, Ohgami Y, Vega-Villa KR. Minimizing risks of NSAIDs: cardiovascular, gastrointestinal and renal. *Expert Rev Neurother*. 2006;6(11):1643–1655.

128. Weinbroum AA. Non-opioid IV, adjuvants in the perioperative period: pharmacological and clinical aspects of ketamine and gabapentinoids. *Pharmacol Res*. 2012;65(4):411–429.

129. Dale O, Somogyi AA, Li Y, Sullivan T, Shavit Y. Does intraoperative ketamine attenuate inflammatory reactivity following surgery? A systematic review and meta-analysis. *Anesth Analg*. 2012;115 (4):934–943.

130. Chang LC, Raty SR, Ortiz J, Bailard NS, Mathew SJ. The emerging use of ketamine for anesthesia and sedation in traumatic brain injuries. *CNS Neurosci Ther*. 2013;19(6):390–395.

131. Grathwohl KW. Does ketamine improve postoperative analgesia? More questions than answers. *Pain Med*. 2011;12(8):1135–1136.

132. Ture H, Sayin M, Karlikaya G, Bingol CA, Aykac B, Ture U. The analgesic effect of gabapentin as a prophylactic anticonvulsant drug on postcraniotomy pain: a prospective randomized study. *Anesth Analg*. 2009;109(5):1625–1631.

133. Khurana G, Jindal P, Sharma JP, Bansal KK. Postoperative pain and long-term functional outcome after administration of gabapentin and pregabalin in patients undergoing spinal surgery. *Spine (Phila Pa 1976)*. 2014;39(6):E363–E368.

134. Guilfoyle MR, Helmy A, Duane D, Hutchinson PJ. Regional scalp block for postcraniotomy analgesia: a systematic review and meta-analysis. *Anesth Analg*. 2013;116(5):1093–1102.

135. Ezhevskaya AA, Mlyavykh SG, Anderson DG. Effects of continuous epidural anesthesia and postoperative epidural analgesia on pain management and stress response in patients undergoing major spinal surgery. *Spine (Phila Pa 1976)*. 2013;38(15):1324–1330.

136. Farag E, Ghobrial M, Sessler DI, et al. Effect of perioperative intravenous lidocaine administration on pain, opioid consumption, and quality of life after complex spine surgery. *Anesthesiology*. 2013;119(4):932–940.

137. Krenk L, Rasmussen LS. Postoperative delirium and postoperative cognitive dysfunction in the elderly - what are the differences? *Minerva Anestesiol*. 2011;77(7):742–749.

138. Rudolph JL, Marcantonio ER. Review articles: postoperative delirium: acute change with long-term implications. *Anesth Analg*. 2011;112(5):1202–1211.

139. Luetz A, Heymann A, Radtke FM, et al. Different assessment tools for intensive care unit delirium: which score to use? *Crit Care Med*. 2010;38(2):409–418.

140. Claassen J, Mayer SA, Kowalski RG, Emerson RG, Hirsch LJ. Detection of electrographic seizures with continuous EEG monitoring in critically ill patients. *Neurology*. 2004;62(10):1743–1748.

141. Rudolph JL, Schreiber KA, Culley DJ, et al. Measurement of postoperative cognitive dysfunction after cardiac surgery: a systematic review. *Acta Anaesthesiol Scand*. 2010;54(6):663–677.

142. Salata K, Katznelson R, Beattie WS, Carroll J, Lindsay TF, Djaiani G. Endovascular versus open approach to aortic aneurysm repair surgery: rates of postoperative delirium. *Can J Anaesth*. 2012;59 (6):556–561.

143. Sieber FE, Mears S, Lee H, Gottschalk A. Postoperative opioid consumption and its relationship to cognitive function in

older adults with hip fracture. *J Am Geriatr Soc.* 2011;59 (12):2256–2262.

144. Bilotta F, Gelb AW, Stazi E, Titi L, Paoloni FP, Rosa G. Pharmacological perioperative brain neuroprotection: a qualitative review of randomized clinical trials. *Br J Anaesth.* 2013;110(Suppl 1):i113–i120.

145. Colombo R, Corona A, Praga F, et al. A reorientation strategy for reducing delirium in the critically ill. Results of an interventional study. *Minerva Anestesiol.* 2012;78(9):1026–1033.

146. Deschodt M, Braes T, Flamaing J, et al. Preventing delirium in older adults with recent hip fracture through multidisciplinary geriatric consultation. *J Am Geriatr Soc.* 2012;60(4):733–739.

147. Zhang H, Lu Y, Liu M, et al. Strategies for prevention of postoperative delirium: a systematic review and meta-analysis of randomized trials. *Crit Care.* 2013;17(2):R47.

148. Radtke FM, Franck M, Lendner J, Kruger S, Wernecke KD, Spies CD. Monitoring depth of anaesthesia in a randomized trial decreases the rate of postoperative delirium but not postoperative cognitive dysfunction. *Br J Anaesth.* 2013;110(Suppl 1):i98–i105.

149. Watne LO, Hall RJ, Molden E, et al. Anticholinergic activity in cerebrospinal fluid and serum in individuals with hip fracture with and without delirium. *J Am Geriatr Soc.* 2014;62(1):94–102. http://dx.doi.org/10.1111/jgs.12612. Epub 2014 Jan 2.

150. Butterfield S. Clearing or clouding the mind? Debate over antipsychotics as delirium treatment. *ACPHospitalist [Internet];* 2011. Available from: http://www.acphospitalist.org/archives/2011/11/delirium.htm.

151. Popp J, Arlt S. Prevention and treatment options for postoperative delirium in the elderly. *Curr Opin Psychiatry.* 2012;25(6):515–521.

# 2  Patient Positioning for Neurosurgical Procedures

SHAUN E. GRUENBAUM, BENJAMIN F. GRUENBAUM, YORAM SHAPIRA, and ALEXANDER ZLOTNIK

## Introduction

Perhaps more so than in any other surgical specialty, patient positioning is a critical component of neurosurgical procedures. Whereas most other surgeries are performed in the supine position with little input or assistance from the anesthesiologist, positioning for neurosurgical procedures requires cooperation between the surgeon, anesthesiologist, and nursing staff.

Correct patient positioning is essential to ensure adequate surgical access, surgeon comfort, and minimal risk for patient injury. There are several positions commonly employed for neurosurgical procedures. It is essential that all operating room personnel have a comprehensive understanding of the various positions employed for neurosurgical procedures, as well as the unique risks and possible postoperative implications associated with that position.

The four major positions utilized for neurosurgical procedures include the supine, lateral, prone, and sitting positions. Patients should be carefully evaluated prior to surgery, and the benefits of a particular position as they pertain to surgical access and comfort for the surgeon should be weighed against the specific risks.

Each step of positioning the patient should be a cooperative effort and should be accomplished in an efficient and safe manner. Communication is vital to minimize patient risk. Care and diligence should be taken when fixing the patient's head in a stereotaxic frame, positioning the head and neck, and positioning the patient's body. The general principles of patient positioning are discussed at length in the literature. In this chapter, we will focus our discussion on the specific considerations that pertain to positioning patients for neurosurgical procedures.

## General Principles

### Key Concepts

- Positioning the patient is an important part of the neurosurgical procedure and should be planned during the preoperative evaluation.
- Positioning the extremities should be done under the guidelines of the American Society of Anesthesiologists Practice Advisory for the Prevention of Perioperative Peripheral Neuropathies.

- Temporary disconnection of the patient's monitors, lines, and ventilator may be necessary during positioning and when turning the head of the bed; this should be done efficiently and with the coordination of the operating room staff.

The general goals of patient positioning for neurosurgical procedures are to provide optimal surgical exposure while maintaining patient safety. Positioning the patient is an important component of the neurosurgical procedure, and this step is perhaps more critical than in any other specialty. Whereas positioning for most other surgical specialties usually involves little input by anesthesiologists, positioning the patient for neurosurgical procedures should be a collaborative effort between the surgical, anesthesia, and nursing staff.[1] Especially in long surgeries, poor positioning may result in significant comorbidity secondary to direct effects of positioning or indirect effects related to suboptimal anatomical orientation.

Many patient positions have unique associated risks, which must be appreciated by the surgical, nursing, and anesthesia staff.[2] The risks of a particular position must be weighed against the benefits of surgical access and comfort. The patient should be thoroughly evaluated in the preoperative clinic, and the optimal position should be considered and planned at that time. The operating room nurses and anesthesiologist should be notified as early as possible about the planned patient position so they can prepare all necessary equipment. The anesthesiologist should be able to anticipate potential complications associated with the planned position and be prepared to treat accordingly.

The basic principles of patient positioning with regard to appropriate padding and positioning the extremities should be based on the American Society of Anesthesiologists Practice Advisory for the Prevention of Perioperative Peripheral Neuropathies[3] (Table 2.1). The patient's eyes should be taped after induction of general anesthesia, and eye lubrication should be considered for long procedures. The arms should be maintained in a neutral position, with arm abduction limited to 90 degrees. The bony prominences of the extremities should be padded well to prevent compression and breakdown of the skin, as well as peripheral neuropathies.

After induction of general anesthesia and placement of arterial and venous lines, the operating room table is typically rotated 90 degrees or 180 degrees away from the anesthesiologist. For a brief period, the patients may be disconnected from the monitoring devices, vascular lines, and ventilation circuit. This requires careful coordination

**Table 2.1** Positioning Strategies of the Upper and Lower Extremities to Reduce the Risk of Perioperative Peripheral Neuropathies

| A. UPPER EXTREMITY | |
|---|---|
| | **Positioning Strategy** |
| BRACHIAL PLEXUS NEUROPATHY | Arm abduction should not exceed 90 degrees |
| ULNAR NEUROPATHY (ELBOW) | Avoid pronation of the hands or forearms |
| RADIAL NEUROPATHY (ARM) | Avoid pressure in the spiral groove of the humerus from prolonged contact with a hard surface |
| MEDIAN NEUROPATHY (ELBOW) | Avoid extending the elbow beyond what is comfortable for the patient during the preoperative examination |
| **B. LOWER EXTREMITY** | |
| | **Positioning Strategy** |
| SCIATIC NEUROPATHY | Avoid stretching the hamstring muscle beyond what is comfortable for the patient during the preoperative examination |
| | Avoid extreme hip flexion |
| PERONEAL NEUROPATHY | Avoid pressure near the fibular head from contact with a hard surface or rigid support |

Adapted from the American Society of Anesthesiologists Practice Advisory for the Prevention of Perioperative Peripheral Neuropathies. *Anesthesiology.* 2011 Apr;114(4):741–54.

between the surgery and anesthesia team to ensure patient safety, and the patient should be reconnected to the ventilator and monitors in a timely manner.

### Clinical Pearl

Rotating the bed 90 to 180 degrees often necessitates that monitors, vascular lines, and ventilation circuit be disconnected from the patient; this is a moment of risk and should be accomplished efficiently and with the cooperation of the surgical and anesthesia teams.

## Head Fixation and Positioning

### Key Concepts

- Fixing the head with pins in a Mayfield frame is profoundly stimulating, and severe hypertension and tachycardia can ensue if not anticipated and pharmacologically prevented.
- Positioning the head and neck is one of the most important considerations when positioning patients for neurosurgical procedures, and proper positioning ensures optimal surgical approach and exposure.
- To facilitate venous and lymphatic drainage and minimize the chance of endotracheal tube kink when the neck is flexed, a distance of at least 2–3 fingerbreadths must be maintained between the mandibular protuberance and the manubrium of the sternum at all times.

## HEAD FIXATION

Fixing the head in a stereotaxic Mayfield frame is commonly done prior to neurosurgical procedures. Placing the stereotaxic frame requires the placement of 3–4 external pins on the patient's scalp at a pressure of 60–80 pounds per square inch (psi). Head pinning has a profoundly stimulating effect, similar to that of a surgical incision. If not properly anticipated and treated, pinning can result in a large catecholamine release and associated hypertension and tachycardia. Furthermore, if the patient's head moves after being fixed in the stereotaxic frame, this can result in significant lacerations to the patient's scalp or cervical spine injury.

The severe hypertension that results from head pinning may result in exacerbation of cerebral edema or hemorrhage at the surgical site or, rarely, at another intracranial site remote from the surgical area.[4,5] If the hemorrhage is large enough, it may require surgical evacuation. Worsening edema due to fixation-related hypertension may compromise exposure during an intracranial procedure. It is therefore very important to anticipate the sequelae of head pinning, ensure adequate pain control, and maintain the blood pressure within the normal range. This is especially important for patients with vascular lesions in the brain (such as arteriovenous malformations or cerebral aneurysm), known coagulation disorders or on anticoagulants, and disrupted blood–brain barrier function. Blood pressure should be frequently monitored, preferably with an arterial line, during head pinning.

Patients with chronically uncontrolled hypertension are at particularly high risk of severe hypertension during pinning. Head fixation requires constant communication between the surgical and anesthesia teams, and the hemodynamic responses associated with head pinning should be anticipated and preemptively treated. Prior to head pinning in both the awake and anesthetized patient, the patient's scalp should be infiltrated with local anesthetic.[6] The anesthesia should be deepened, and when appropriate, muscle relaxation should be administered to anesthetized patients. When one plans to administer an opioid infusion during the neurosurgical procedure, it should ideally be started prior to head pinning to further blunt the response to pinning.

It is important to note that the hemodynamic response from pinning is typically short lived, and after the patient's head is fixed, the stereotaxic frame is no longer stimulating. For this reason, a bolus of a short-acting opioid (such as remifentanil 1 mcg/kg), with or without propofol, may be advantageous over large doses of propofol or volatile anesthetics that may result in profound hypotension after the head is fixed.

Fixing the head in the Mayfield frame is associated with several additional complications.[7] In children or adults with thin skulls, the use of excessive force may cause a depressed skull fracture. Occasionally, the fracture may be so severe that it results in a poor outcome. Similarly, in trauma patients with a known or suspected skull fracture, fixing the head should be done with extreme caution.

In the immediate postoperative period, the clinician should be cognizant of potential complications related to head pinning (Table 2.2). When the pins are removed at the end of the procedure, bleeding is common at the pin sites. Typically, a pressure dressing with gauze is sufficient

**Table 2.2** Postoperative Complications That May Result from Neurosurgery in the Various Positions

| Risk Factor | Postoperative Complications |
| --- | --- |
| Head Pinning | ■ Bleeding at the pin sites<br>■ VAE |
| Head and Neck Positioning | ■ Neck discomfort or pain<br>■ Brachial plexus injury<br>■ Postoperative airway obstruction from inadequate cerebral venous or lymphatic drainage<br>■ Cervical spine ischemia and quadriplegia from vertebral or carotid artery obstruction |
| Supine Position | ■ Lower back pain and peripheral neuropathies (especially ulnar) from inadequate padding of pressure points<br>■ Complications related to neck rotation or flexion (see earlier) |
| Lateral Position | ■ Brachial plexus injury from axillary artery compression<br>■ Pressure and stretch palsies (especially peroneal nerve and lateral femoral cutaneous nerve injury due to improper positioning of the lower extremities) |
| Prone position | ■ Postoperative blindness (most commonly due to OIN)<br>■ Pressure sores<br>■ Brachial plexus injuries<br>■ Vascular compression with subsequent quadriplegia |
| Sitting position | ■ Pneumocephalus<br>■ Quadriplegia (due to cervical spine ischemia from extreme head and neck flexion)<br>■ Pressor support and mechanical ventilation for severe VAE |

OIN, optic ischemic neuropathy; VAE, venous air embolism.

to stop the bleeding. Occasionally, the holes may require closure with sutures or staples. Furthermore, the removal of the pins may increase the risk of venous air embolism (VAE). For procedures in the sitting position, where the risk of VAE is highest, the placement of antibiotic ointment on the pins is advocated to prevent VAE.[6]

## HEAD AND NECK POSITIONING

The positioning of the head and neck is one of the most important aspects of patient positioning for neurosurgical procedures[8] because the orientation of the head provides the neurosurgeon with the appropriate surgical approach and exposure. There are a few basic principles of positioning the head and neck that are important to consider, and vigilance on the part of the surgeon and anesthesiologist are vital in preventing complications. First, the patient's neck mobility and stability should be assessed prior to surgery and should dictate the extent of intraoperative head and neck positioning. If a patient reports neurological symptoms associated with neck mobility, one should avoid or minimize hyperflexion, hyperextension, lateral flexion, or rotation.[6]

Extreme hyperflexion of the neck may result in obstruction of venous and lymphatic drainage from the head, resulting in tongue and face swelling, and increased intracranial pressure. Extreme hyperflexion can also cause

compression of the vertebral arteries, resulting in cerebral ischemia, and difficulties in oxygenation and ventilation. It is therefore recommended that a distance of at least 2–3 fingerbreadths be maintained between the mandibular protuberance and the manubrium of the sternum at all times. Furthermore, the surgical and anesthesia team should be cognizant to avoid a position that maintains pressure on the patient's chin, which can result in skin breakdown or pressure necrosis.

Complications related to head and neck positioning might present in the immediate postoperative period[6] (Table 2.2). Excess strain of the neck may cause brachial plexus injury or postoperative discomfort or pain. Skin breakdown or pressure necrosis may result from prolonged pressure on the patient's chin. Swelling of the neck and airway from inadequate cerebral venous or lymphatic drainage may result in postoperative airway obstruction. Furthermore, if the vertebral or carotid arteries were obstructed during surgery for a prolonged period, cervical spine ischemia and quadriplegia may ensue.

## Body Positioning

### Key Concepts

- The supine position is the easiest, most common position used for neurosurgical procedures and does not require any special equipment.
- Risks of neurosurgical procedures in the lateral position include kinking of the jugular vein and brachial plexus injury, peripheral nerve injury, and ventilation-perfusion mismatch.
- Turning a patient prone may necessitate being disconnected from monitors, vascular lines, and the ventilator and should be done carefully but efficiently.
- VAE is a potentially catastrophic complication that can occur in the sitting position, and the risk-to-benefit ratio of performing procedures in this position has been heavily debated.

Neurosurgical procedures are generally performed with the patient in the supine, lateral, prone, or sitting position or in a variation of one of these positions. Each of these positions has unique associated benefits and risks that should be considered in the preoperative assessment (Table 2.3). A comprehensive understanding of the risks associated with each of these positions is essential for ensuring patient safety during the neurosurgical procedure. Especially after long procedures, an incorrectly positioned patient may be at increased risk of postoperative complications.

### SUPINE POSITION

The supine position is the most common position employed for neurosurgical procedures.[8] The supine position is easily achieved and is arguably associated with the lowest risk of complications. Moreover, the supine position does not require any special equipment.

For patients in the supine position, special attention should be paid to the extremities. The arms are typically

**Table 2.3**    Advantages and Risks Associated with the Four Primary Patient Positions Employed in Neurosurgical Procedures

| | Advantages | Risks |
|---|---|---|
| **SUPINE** | ▪ Simplest position<br>▪ Does not require any special equipment<br>▪ Lowest risk of complications<br>▪ Access to patient's airway | ▪ Peripheral neuropathies<br>▪ Lower back injury<br>▪ May require moderate neck rotation and shoulder traction, which can result in kinking of the internal jugular vein or brachial plexus injury |
| **LATERAL** | ▪ Best surgical access for temporal lobe<br>▪ Three-quarter prone position allows for access to the posterior cranial fossa with less risk of venous air embolism and increased surgeon comfort (compared with the sitting position) | ▪ Kinking of the jugular vein and brachial plexus injury<br>▪ Peripheral nerve injury<br>▪ Ventilation/perfusion mismatch<br>▪ Fluid accumulation in the dependent lung |
| **PRONE** | ▪ Best surgical access to the suboccipital region or posterior spine<br>▪ Low risk of venous air embolism compared with the sitting position | ▪ Typically necessitates disconnection from monitors, vascular lines, and ventilator<br>▪ Potential injury when turning prone<br>▪ Decreased pulmonary compliance with increased peak airway pressure<br>▪ Increased intracranial pressure<br>▪ Poor airway access<br>▪ If arms are tucked at the patient's sides, vascular access may be lost<br>▪ Postoperative blindness |
| **SITTING** | ▪ Best surgical access for posterior cranial fossa<br>▪ Reduced tissue retraction results in improved exposure and reduced risk of cranial nerve damage<br>▪ Improved cerebrospinal fluid drainage, resulting in reduced intracranial pressure<br>▪ Improved cerebral venous drainage, resulting in potentially reduced surgical blood loss<br>▪ Good airway access | ▪ Significant hypotension and reduced cerebral perfusion pressure<br>▪ Highest risk of venous air embolism (compared with other positions)<br>▪ Many clinicians advocate for screening for a patent foramen ovale |

placed neutrally at the patient's sides and are often tucked, making them poorly accessible during the procedure. Prior to sterile draping, the anesthesiologist should confirm that the arterial and venous lines are functioning well. Pressure points should be padded well, according to the recommendations of the American Society of Anesthesiologists Task Force on Prevention of Perioperative Peripheral Neuropathies.[3] In the supine position, the ulnar nerve and lower back are particularly vulnerable to injury. The arms should be supinated and padded, and knees should be elevated with pillows to relieve pressure from the lower back.

Due to the low pressure in the venous system, venous return to the heart is highly dependent on the patient's position. The effects of gravity on venous drainage are minimal in the supine position. For intracranial procedures, head elevation or reverse Trendelenburg position up to 30 degrees is often recommended to facilitate venous return, decrease intracranial pressure, and improve cerebral perfusion pressure.[9,10] However, some studies suggest that the reverse Trendelenburg position may actually reduce cerebral perfusion pressure by decreasing the hydrostatic pressure at both the cranial and cardiac level.[11] Furthermore, the head-up position decreases intrathoracic pressure and improves respiratory mechanics during mechanical ventilation. It should be noted that the degree of head elevation determines the height of the surgical site relative to the level of the heart. As such, the degree of head elevation determines the relative risk of VAE. The sitting position, which results in the maximum difference in height between the surgical site and the heart, confers the highest risk of VAE.

## Clinical Pearl

For intracranial procedures in the supine position, head elevation or reverse Trendelenburg up to 30 degrees may facilitate venous return and decrease intracranial pressure, but may reduce cerebral perfusion pressure by decreasing hydrostatic pressure at the cranial and cardiac levels.

The biggest risk associated with the supine position is that it often requires moderate neck rotation to achieve optimal surgical conditions.[6] Neck rotation is typically achieved by elevating the ipsilateral shoulder with a rolled blanket or pillow.[12] Neck rotation can be especially problematic in elderly patients, in whom kinking of the internal jugular vein or arteries in the neck may occur. Additionally, if there is excessive traction on the shoulder, the brachial plexus can be stretched and injured.

Postoperative complications that result from the supine position are rare (Table 2.2). Lower back pain and peripheral neuropathies (especially the ulnar nerve) may result from inadequate padding of pressure points. Most complications that result from the supine position are related to head rotation or flexion.

## LATERAL POSITION

The lateral position (Fig. 2.1) provides the best access for surgery on the temporal lobe and can be useful for surgery on the lateral skull base, posterior fossa, or lateral suboccipital area.[6,8] In the supine position, the patient's head and

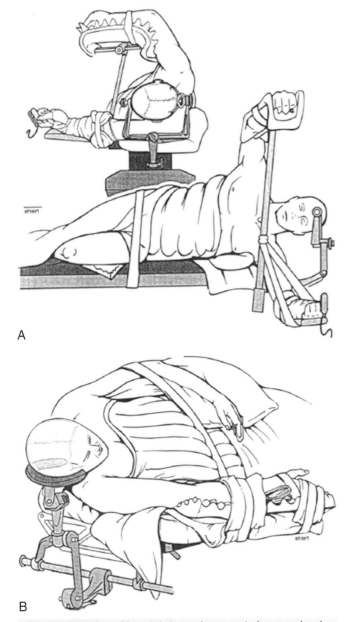

A

B

**Fig. 2.1 Lateral position. (A)** Dependent arm is hung under the operating table; an upper arm is placed on the arm board. **(B)** Dependent arm is positioned on the operating table and an arm board; an upper arm is placed over the trunk on the pillow. (Adapted from Goodkin R, Mesiwala A. General principles of operative positioning. In: Winn RH, ed. *Youmans Neurological Surgery*, 5th ed. Philadelphia: Saunders; 2004; with permission.)

dependent arm is placed on a padded armrest. The nondependent arm is placed on a padded, raised armrest that is secured to the operating room table in front of the patient. The nondependent shoulder is slightly abducted, and the elbow is minimally flexed. A beanbag or some other support mechanism is used to secure the patient's torso in the lateral position.

When placed in the lateral position, special attention should be given to positioning the patient's dependent arm.[6] Perhaps the most important feature of the lateral position is the proper placement of the axillary roll to prevent brachial plexus compression or pressure on the dependent shoulder. The axillary roll should be placed under the upper part of the chest rather than the axilla. Incorrect placement of the axillary roll can actually cause, instead of prevent, injury to the brachial plexus.[12] The patient's head should be fixed and adequately supported to prevent any injury to the cervical spine. A pillow should be placed between legs, and the dependent knee should be flexed to avoid compression over the fibular head and peroneal nerve. Care should also be taken to avoid extreme flexion of the neck, which is sometimes necessary in the lateral position. Extreme flexion can result in kinking of the jugular vein, delayed face swelling, and brachial plexopathy.[13]

### Clinical Pearl

When placing patients in the lateral position, one should be especially careful to place an axillary roll under the upper part of the chest to prevent brachial plexus injury.

Due to gravitational forces, perfusion is best in the dependent part the lungs (West zone 3), where vascular pressure exceeds alveolar pressure. In the anesthetized, mechanically ventilated patient, the lung areas 18 cm above the bed are poorly perfused but receive the largest inspired volumes. In the lateral position, there is a worsening mismatch between ventilation and perfusion.[14] Furthermore, if a large volume of fluid is administered to the patient, the fluid may accumulate in the dependent lung over time. If this occurs, peak airway pressures may increase, and adequately ventilating and oxygenating the patient may prove difficult. Indeed, the increased airway pressures can become so pronounced that adding positive end-expiratory pressure in response to hypoxemia may encourage increased blood flow to the dependent lung, resulting in worsened hypoxemia.

The park bench position is a modification of the lateral position (Fig. 2.2) and is used to allow access to the posterior fossa without need for the sitting position.[8,12] In this position, the patient is placed superiorly enough on the operating table that the dependent arm, which is slightly flexed, can hang over the edge of the bed. The dependent arm is then secured with a sling. The patient's neck is flexed toward the floor, and the head is rotated toward the floor. Patients in the park bench position are particularly susceptible to venous stasis and deep vein thrombosis.[7] Compression boots should be used when feasible and should be applied when the patient enters the operating room.

body can approach the lateral position when a shoulder bolster is used and the head is turned. A true lateral position, however, requires that the patient's hips be perpendicular to the floor. The risks associated with the lateral approach include kinking of the jugular vein and brachial plexus injury, peripheral nerve injury, and mismatch in ventilation and perfusion.

The lateral position is achieved by first inducing general anesthesia with the patient lying supine on the operating room table. The patient is rolled laterally, an axillary roll is placed under the patient's upper chest to minimize compression of important structures in the upper arm, and the

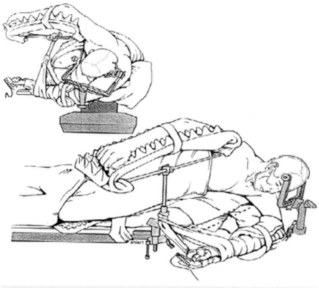

**Fig. 2.2 Three-quarters (lateral oblique) positioning.** The principles of three-quarter positioning resemble those for the lateral position, but the head may be placed on the table or in pins, and the dependent (lower) arm may be placed behind the body or in a sling below the face for a so-called *park bench modification*. If a suboccipital approach is required, the nondependent (upper) shoulder may need to be taped down toward the foot. However, this can cause additional stretching of the brachial plexus with associated risk of postoperative neuropathy. (Adapted from Goodkin R, Mesiwala A. General principles of operative positioning. In: Winn RH, ed. *Youmans Neurological Surgery*, 5th ed. Philadelphia: Saunders; 2004; with permission.)

The three-quarter prone position (Fig. 2.2) is similar to the prone position in many ways and may be utilized to access the parietooccipital cranial region and posterior cranial fossa. The three-quarter prone position offers several advantages over the sitting position. Even though the head is above the level of the heart, there is a lower risk of VAE compared with the sitting position. Furthermore, the three-quarter prone position offers more comfort for the surgeon, with decreased fatigue of the surgeon's arms and shoulders.[8]

Postoperative complications that result from surgery in the lateral position include brachial plexus injury due to axillary artery compression, pressure palsies, and stretch injuries[6] (Table 2.2). In particular, symptoms related to peroneal nerve injury and lateral femoral cutaneous nerve injury might result from improper positioning of the lower extremities.

## PRONE POSITION

The prone position is often preferred for surgical access to the suboccipital region or posterior spine.[12] A variety of prone configurations and support frames are used (Fig. 2.3). Prior to turning the patient prone, the patient is typically induced under general anesthesia on the hospital bed in the supine position. Venous and arterial access is established, and the bladder is catheterized. The head is then fixed in the Mayfield frame (for intracranial and cervical spine procedures), and the patient is subsequently

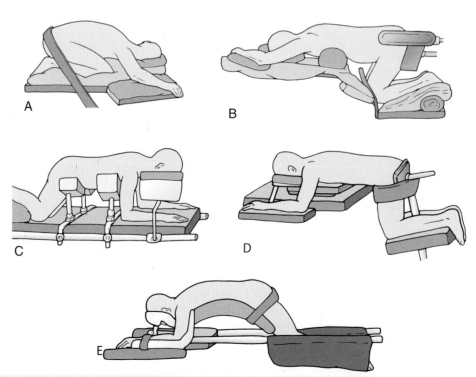

**Fig. 2.3** Examples of positioning frames for spinal surgery designed to minimize vertebral venous distension: **(A)** Tuck position; **(B)** Canadian frame; **(C)** Relton Hall type frame; **(D)** Andrews frame; **(E)** Wilson frame. (Adapted from Schonauer C, Bocchetti A, Barbagallo G, Albanese V, Moraci A. Positioning on surgical table. *European Spine Journal.* 2004;13(Suppl. 1):S50–S5.)

turned onto the operating room table. Alternatively, special operating tables (such as the RotoProne) have the ability to rotate the patient prone without having to transfer the patient to a different bed.

Turning the patient prone should be done with extreme caution and with the coordination of several staff members. The surgeon, not the anesthesiologist, should be responsible for controlling the head and spine during the turn as the anesthesiologist ensures security of the endotracheal tube. The surgeon must be especially careful to maintain the head in a stable and neutral position during the turn to prevent any spinal injury. Turning the patient prone may require that the patient be disconnected from the ventilator circuit and monitors, causing a brief temporary period of no monitoring or ventilation. During the turn, special care must be made to monitor all lines, urinary catheter, and endotracheal tube. There must be cooperation between the surgical and anesthesia team to ensure that the patient is efficiently turned and reconnected to the ventilator and monitors in a timely fashion.

Once the patient is turned and reconnected to the ventilator circuit and monitors, the patient's body, extremities, and eyes should be examined. When positioning the body, special care should be taken to avoid excessive intraabdominal pressure. Pressure on the abdomen may occlude the inferior vena cava, thereby decreasing venous return and increasing bleeding for lumbar surgery (Chapter 7), and may prevent or impair optimal diaphragmatic excursion during ventilation. Providing adequate chest support may reduce pressure on the abdomen. The arms and knees should be padded over the bony prominences to prevent skin breakdown due to mechanical pressure. The shoulders should not be abducted more than 90 degrees, and the arms should be flexed. The knees should be flexed, and one should avoid excessive plantar flexion of the feet. Male genitalia should hang freely, the eyes should be taped shut and free from orbital compression, and the breasts should be adequately padded. The head should be fixed in the neutral or flexed position as indicated by the surgery.

If the patient's head is not fixed in a Mayfield frame, a prone foam pillow with cutouts for the eyes, nose, and airway should be used. It should be noted that a prone pillow is only available in one height, and neck hyperextension may occur in smaller patients.[7] During the procedure, the eyes should be checked at least every 15 minutes to ensure that there is no orbital compression.[15] During long procedures in the prone position, there may be significant facial edema that occurs. After letting the endotracheal tube cuff down, the absence of a leak around the cuff may necessitate postoperative ventilation.

Compared with the supine position, the prone position may lower the patient's pulmonary compliance, resulting in higher peak airway pressure. Furthermore, the prone position results in decreased venous return to the heart, with increased systemic and pulmonary vascular resistance.[6] The prone position also increases intracranial pressure and should be used with caution in patients with reduced intracranial compliance.[16] The prone position is advantageous in that it improves matching of ventilation and perfusion, resulting in improved arterial oxygenation and cerebral tissue oxygenation, as well as increased cerebral perfusion pressure. Compared with the sitting position, surgery in the prone position may provide excellent posterior access with a significantly lower risk of VAE.

## Clinical Pearl

The most common risk factors associated with postoperative visual loss include the prone position, length of surgery over 6 hours, intraoperative hypotension, and significant blood loss.

Postoperative visual loss is a rare but devastating complication after surgery in the prone position (Table 2.2). The incidence and mechanism of visual loss are poorly understood.[17] The four causes of postoperative visual loss include ischemic optic neuropathy (most common cause, accounting for approximately 89% of cases of postoperative visual loss), central retinal artery occlusion, cortical infarction, and external ocular injury. The most common risk factors associated with postoperative visual loss include the prone position, length of surgery over 6 hours, intraoperative hypotension, and significant blood loss. It should be noted, however, that the risk factors are speculative based on associations made in retrospective reports.[18] There is no effective treatment for ischemic optic neuropathy (see also Chapter 4). Other potential postoperative complications include pressure sores, brachial plexus injuries, and vascular compression with subsequent quadriplegia.[6]

## SITTING POSITION

The sitting position (Fig. 2.4) has traditionally been the preferred position to surgically access the posterior cranial fossa or posterior cervical spine.[12] Although the prone and lateral positions may also be used when operating on the posterior cranial fossa, the sitting position offers several physiological advantages. The effects of gravity facilitate an improvement in cerebrospinal fluid drainage, consequently lowering intracranial pressure more than any other position.[19] Compared with other positions, there is improved exposure of the posterior cranial fossa due to less tissue retraction, and there is a reduced risk of cranial nerve damage. Cerebral venous drainage is also improved, thereby draining blood away from the surgical field. This results in optimal surgical conditions and potentially less surgical blood loss than other positions.

Compared with the prone position, the patient's airway is easily accessible to the anesthesiologist when in the sitting position. Furthermore, intrathoracic pressure is lower in the sitting position, allowing for easier ventilation. In the event of cardiac arrest, cardiopulmonary resuscitation (CPR) in the sitting position is easier than in the prone position, and the bed can be positioned to facilitate CPR.

Neurosurgery in the sitting position is associated with significant and potentially life-threatening risks. The effects of gravity on venous drainage make patients prone to potentially significant hypotension, thereby reducing cerebral perfusion pressure. The drop in blood pressure may be partially ameliorated by a fluid bolus prior to positioning,

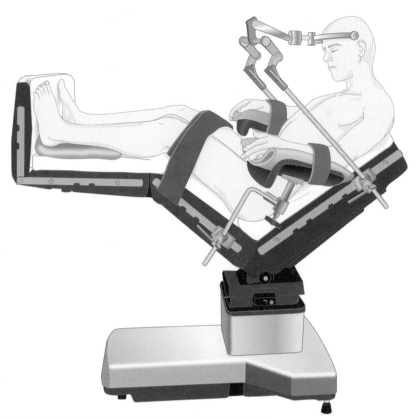

**Fig. 2.4** "Sitting" position with Mayfield head pins. This is actually a modified recumbent position because the legs are kept as high as possible to promote venous return. Arms must be supported to prevent shoulder traction. Note that the head holder support is preferably attached to the back section of the table so that the patient's back may be adjusted or lowered emergently without first detaching the head holder. If the head holder is connected to the thigh section of the table, this cannot be done. (Reprinted from Cassorla L, Lee J-W. Patient positioning and anesthesia. In: Miller RD, ed. *Miller's Anesthesia*. Maryland Heights: Churchill-Livingstone; 2009: pp. 1151–70.).

administration of vasopressors, application of elastic bands to the lower extremities, and positioning the patient to the sitting position in increments. Furthermore, the sitting position is associated with an increase in pulmonary and systemic vascular resistance.[20]

VAE is a potentially catastrophic complication that can occur when neurosurgery is performed in the sitting position. VAE can occur when there is an open vein and a pressure gradient between the surgical site and the heart. The risk of VAE in the sitting position greatly varies depending on the type of procedure. The noncollapsible venous sinuses are exposed during posterior cranial fossa surgery, making these procedures particularly high risk. The presence of a patent foramen ovale (PFO) further increases the risk of introducing a paradoxical embolism into the systemic circulation. Stendel and colleagues[21] demonstrated a prevalence of PFO in 27% of patients with a posterior cranial fossa lesion. They further demonstrated the presence of VAE in 75% of patients during posterior cranial fossa surgery in the sitting position. It should be noted that the risk of VAE is not unique to the sitting position and can occur during surgery in the prone or lateral position as well, providing the venous pressure in the surgical bed is subatmospheric, which typically can arise when the level of the surgery is above the heart.

VAE is typically detected with end-tidal $CO_2$, precordial Doppler, or transesophageal echocardiogram, although no single monitoring modality will accurately predict all cases of VAE.[22] In the event of a VAE, hypoxemia can quickly ensue due to an increase in dead space in the lungs. Right heart strain can further result in cardiac ischemia and significant hypotension and cardiac arrest. A paradoxical air embolism can lead to significant neurological sequelae, including stroke and quadriplegia. Patients with VAE can also develop thrombocytopenia, increasing the patient's risk of bleeding.[23]

Due to the increased risk of VAE in patients with a PFO, many clinicians advocate for routine preoperative screening with contrast-enhanced transesophageal, transthoracic echocardiography. In recent years, transcranial Doppler has emerged as an inexpensive, noninvasive, and easy method of assessing for PFO.[21] In short, a contrast agent with a small amount of air is injected into the antecubital vein. If a right to left shunt is present, the contrast will bypass the pulmonary circulation and result in microembolic signals in the basal cerebral arteries. The quantity of microbubbles indicates the severity of PFO. When a neurosurgical procedure is preferred in the sitting position and a PFO is found on screening, some authors recommend that the PFO be surgically closed prior to surgery.[24]

Postoperative tension pneumocephalus can occur in up to 3% of posterior cranial fossa surgeries in the sitting position.[25] Tension pneumocephalus may result when air enters the epidural space in large enough volumes to cause a mass effect, which can result in life-threatening brain herniation. Some authors recommend that minute ventilation be decreased to allow for brain expansion as the dura is closed,[26] and nitrous oxide should be avoided in the first 14 days after posterior cranial fossa surgery. The risk is further decreased by the placement of a ventriculostomy drain, which is commonly placed after major posterior fossa surgeries in the sitting position.

Extreme neck flexion, in which the chin rests on the chest, combined with the use of an oropharyngeal airway or transesophageal probe that obstructs venous and lymphatic drainage, can result in significant postoperative tongue edema.[26] This can result in postoperative airway obstruction and hypoxemia. Careful positioning of the neck and proper placement of a bite block rather than an oropharyngeal airway may reduce this risk.

Rarely, peripheral neuropathies can result from neurosurgical procedures in the sitting position. The most commonly injured nerve in the sitting position is the common peroneal nerve, resulting in foot drop. Injury to the common peroneal nerve may be due to ischemic compression or from stretching the sciatic nerve.

The risk-to-benefit ratio of neurosurgical procedures in the sitting position has been considerably debated.[24,27] In recent years, the sitting position has largely fallen out of favor in the United States due to fear of its associated complications. Today, the most common procedure done in the sitting position in the United States is an insertion of a deep-brain stimulator[8] or occasionally for difficult-to-access lesions such as pineal tumors. In Europe, the sitting position is still very popular and is the preferred position for surgery of the posterior cranial fossa.[28]

It has never been firmly established that neurosurgical procedures in the lateral or prone position are safer than the sitting position. Many authors have argued that the fear of catastrophic complications related to the sitting position seems unwarranted.[29] With an experienced surgical and anesthesia team, neurosurgery in the sitting position may be done safely and may be advantageous to the prone position.[22,30,31] Orliaguet and colleagues[32] retrospectively analyzed 85 pediatric patients undergoing craniotomy for posterior fossa tumor in either the sitting or prone position and found that patients in the sitting position actually experienced fewer intraoperative and postoperative complications, with a shorter intensive care and hospital stay. When the sitting position is preferred for a neurosurgical procedure, the surgical and anesthesia team must cooperate in the early detection of VAE. The presence of a right to left intracardiac shunt has generally been considered an absolute contraindication to surgery in the sitting position, although this premise has been challenged in recent years. Limited data suggest that even patients with a PFO may be safely operated on in the sitting position, with minimal risk of VAE.[33–35] Relative contraindications include severe atherosclerotic coronary artery disease and severe hypotension or hypertension.

In the immediate postoperative period, pneumocephalus is common and may persist for weeks after surgery[6] (Table 2.2). Pneumocephalus after surgery in the sitting position may occur with or without the use of nitrous oxide. With extreme head and neck flexion, quadriplegia may result from cervical spine ischemia. In the event of a significant VAE, continued pressor support and mechanical ventilation may be needed in the postoperative period.

## Summary

The long duration of neurosurgical procedures and the fact that patients are completely covered by drapes makes proper patient positioning especially critical. When deciding the patient's position during surgery, the benefits of optimal surgical access and surgeon comfort should be weighed against the risks of a particular position. A comprehensive preoperative assessment is vital, and the position decided on should be communicated to the anesthesiologist and nursing staff as early as possible. Proper patient positioning requires the cooperation and communication between all operating room personnel.

Fixing the patient's head in a Mayfield stereotaxic frame, positioning the head and neck, and positioning the body all deserve special attention and consideration. Pinning the head may result in significant hypertension and tachycardia and should be anticipated by the anesthesiologist. Prior to pinning, patients should be preemptively treated with an opioid or anesthetic agent, and blood pressure should be carefully monitored during this time. During positioning of the head and neck, a patient's preoperative mobility should be considered. Extreme hyperflexion is discouraged, and at least 2–3 fingerbreadths should be maintained between the mandibular protuberance and manubrium at all times.

Each patient position is associated with unique benefits and risks and should be considered for all neurosurgical patients. Peripheral nerve injury is possible in all positions, and care should be taken when positioning the extremities. Similarly, there is a risk of VAE in all procedures in which the operative site is above the heart, with the highest risk in the sitting position.

## References

1. Kroll DA, Caplan RA, Posner K, Ward RJ, Cheney FW. Nerve injury associated with anesthesia. *Anesthesiology.* 1990;73(2):202–207.
2. McCaig C. Review: positioning for neurosurgery. *AORN J.* 1978;28(6):1053–1060.
3. American Society of Anesthesiologists Task Force on Prevention of Perioperative Peripheral N. Practice advisory for the prevention of perioperative peripheral neuropathies: an updated report by the American Society of Anesthesiologists Task Force on prevention of perioperative peripheral neuropathies. *Anesthesiology.* 2011;114(4):741–754.
4. Brisman MH, Bederson JB, Sen CN, Germano IM, Moore F, Post KD. Intracerebral hemorrhage occurring remote from the craniotomy site. *Neurosurgery.* 1996;39(6):1114–1121. discussion 21–2.
5. Koller M, Ortler M, Langmayr J, Twerdy K. Posterior-fossa haemorrhage after supratentorial surgery—report of three cases and review of the literature. *Acta Neurochir.* 1999;141(6):587–592.
6. Rozet I, Vavilala MS. Risks and benefits of patient positioning during neurosurgical care. *Anesthesiol Clin.* 2007;25(3):631–653.
7. Silverman RB. Ruskin KJ, Rosenbaum SH, Rampil IJ, eds. *Positioning for Neurosurgery.* New York: Oxford University Press; 2014.
8. Lapointe G, Kemp J, Rajan G, Walter GE, Abdulrauf SI. Ellenbogen RG, Abdulrauf SI, Sekhar LN, eds. *Principles of Surgical Positioning.* Philadelphia: Saunders; 2012.

9. Fan JY. Effect of backrest position on intracranial pressure and cerebral perfusion pressure in individuals with brain injury: a systematic review. *J Nurosci Nurs: Journal of the American Association of Neuroscience Nurses.* 2004;36(5):278–288.

10. Winkelman C. Effect of backrest position on intracranial and cerebral perfusion pressures in traumatically brain-injured adults. *Am J Crit Care: An Official Publication, American Association of Critical-Care Nurses.* 2000;9(6):373–380. quiz 81–2.

11. Rosner MJ, Coley IB. Cerebral perfusion pressure, intracranial pressure, and head elevation. *J Neurosurg.* 1986;65(5):636–641.

12. Du R, Lee CZ. Gupta AK, Gelb AW, eds. *Surgical Positioning.* Philadelphia: Elsevier; 2008.

13. Shimizu S, Sato K, Mabuchi I, Utsuki S, Oka H, Kan S, et al. Brachial plexopathy due to massive swelling of the neck associated with craniotomy in the park bench position. *Surg Neurol.* 2009;71(4):504–508. discussion 8–9.

14. Nyren S, Mure M, Jacobsson H, Larsson SA, Lindahl SG. Pulmonary perfusion is more uniform in the prone than in the supine position: scintigraphy in healthy humans. *J Appl Physiol.* 1999;86(4):1135–1141.

15. American Society of Anesthesiologists Task Force on Perioperative B. Practice advisory for perioperative visual loss associated with spine surgery: a report by the American Society of Anesthesiologists Task Force on Perioperative Blindness. *Anesthesiology.* 2006;104(6):1319–1328.

16. Nekludov M, Bellander BM, Mure M. Oxygenation and cerebral perfusion pressure improved in the prone position. *Acta Anaesthesiol Scand.* 2006;50(8):932–936.

17. Uribe AA, Baig MN, Puente EG, Viloria A, Mendel E, Bergese SD. Current intraoperative devices to reduce visual loss after spine surgery. *Neurosurg Focus.* 2012;33(2).

18. Goepfert CE, Ifune C, Tempelhoff R. Ischemic optic neuropathy: are we any further? *Curr Opin Anaesthesiol.* 2010;23(5):582–587.

19. Gale T, Leslie K. Anaesthesia for neurosurgery in the sitting position. *J Clin Neurosci: Official Journal of the Neurosurgical Society of Australasia.* 2004;11(7):693–696.

20. Ueki J, Hughes JM, Peters AM, et al. Oxygen and 99mTc-MAA shunt estimations in patients with pulmonary arteriovenous malformations: effects of changes in posture and lung volume. *Thorax.* 1994;49(4):327–331.

21. Stendel R, Gramm HJ, Schroder K, Lober C, Brock M. Transcranial Doppler ultrasonography as a screening technique for detection of a patent foramen ovale before surgery in the sitting position. *Anesthesiology.* 2000;93(4):971–975.

22. Lindroos AC, Niiya T, Randell T, Romani R, Hernesniemi J, Niemi T. Sitting position for removal of pineal region lesions: the Helsinki experience. *World Neurosurg.* 2010;74(4–5):505–513.

23. Schafer ST, Sandalcioglu IE, Stegen B, Neumann A, Asgari S, Peters J. Venous air embolism during semi-sitting craniotomy evokes thrombocytopenia. *Anaesthesia.* 2011;66(1):25–30.

24. Fathi AR, Eshtehardi P, Meier B. Patent foramen ovale and neurosurgery in sitting position: a systematic review. *Br J Anaesth.* 2009;102(5):588–596.

25. Standefer M, Bay JW, Trusso R. The sitting position in neurosurgery: a retrospective analysis of 488 cases. *Neurosurgery.* 1984;14(6):649–658.

26. Porter JM, Pidgeon C, Cunningham AJ. The sitting position in neurosurgery: a critical appraisal. *Br J Anaesth.* 1999;82(1):117–128.

27. Engelhardt M, Folkers W, Brenke C, et al. Neurosurgical operations with the patient in sitting position: analysis of risk factors using transcranial Doppler sonography. *Br J Anaesth.* 2006;96(4):467–472.

28. Schaffranietz L, Gunther L. The sitting position in neurosurgical operations. Results of a survey. *Anaesthesist.* 1997;46(2):91–95.

29. Ammirati M, Lamki TT, Shaw AB, Forde B, Nakano I, Mani M. A streamlined protocol for the use of the semi-sitting position in neurosurgery: a report on 48 consecutive procedures. *J Clin Neurosci: Official Journal of the Neurosurgical Society of Australasia.* 2013;20(1):32–34.

30. Kaye AH, Leslie K. The sitting position for neurosurgery: yet another case series confirming safety. *World Neurosurg.* 2012;77(1):42–43.

31. Rath GP, Bithal PK, Chaturvedi A, Dash HH. Complications related to positioning in posterior fossa craniectomy. *J Clin Neurosci: Official Journal of the Neurosurgical Society of Australasia.* 2007;14(6):520–525.

32. Orliaguet GA, Hanafi M, Meyer PG, et al. Is the sitting or the prone position best for surgery for posterior fossa tumours in children? *Paediatr Anaesth.* 2001;11(5):541–547.

33. Misra BK. Neurosurgery in the semisitting position in patients with a patent foramen ovale. *World Neurosurg.* 2014 Jul-Aug;82(1–2):e41–e42. http://dx.doi.org/10.1016/j.wneu.2013.07.098. Epub 2013 Aug 3.

34. Feigl GC, Decker K, Wurms M, et al. Neurosurgical procedures in the semisitting position: evaluation of the risk of paradoxical venous air embolism in patients with a patent foramen ovale. *World Neurosurg.* 2014;81(1):159–164.

35. Nozaki K. Selection of semisitting position in neurosurgery: essential or preference? *World Neurosurg.* 2014;81(1):62–63.

# 3 Anesthetic Considerations for Craniotomy

DEEPAK SHARMA and K.H. KEVIN LUK

## Introduction

Anesthetic management of craniotomy incorporates preoperative, intraoperative, and postoperative considerations based on the neurological pathophysiology, planned surgical procedure, and systemic comorbidities. Although specific anesthetic considerations depend on the nature and clinical presentation of the neurological condition, this chapter addresses general considerations for craniotomy. The neuroanesthesiologist's goal preoperatively is to evaluate and optimize the patient's condition and synthesize a suitable anesthetic plan consistent with the neurosurgical plan. The primary intraoperative considerations are to render the patient unconscious and insensitive to surgical and psychological trauma, minimize the stress response to the surgical procedure, optimize physiological function, and provide optimal surgical conditions. The postoperative considerations involve adequate pain control, hemodynamic stability, adequacy of ventilation/oxygenation, correction of electrolyte imbalance, and facilitation of neurological assessment.

## Preanesthesia Evaluation and Optimization

### Key Concepts

- Proper preanesthesia evaluation is critical for anesthetic management.
- The American Society of Anesthesiologists (ASA) classification is used for stratification of a patient's preoperative health status.
- Consultation with an internist and routine screening tests do not replace preanesthesia evaluation by a neuroanesthesiologist. "Medical clearance" for surgery without the underlying data and rationale is not an appropriate or useful consultation.

Anesthesia care starts with a preanesthesia evaluation designed to assess and to optimize the patient's medical condition and to formulate a suitable anesthesia plan. Other potential benefits of preanesthesia evaluation include improved safety and coordination of perioperative care, optimal resource utilization, improved outcomes, and patient satisfaction. An important aspect is to arrange for essential investigations and consultations to eliminate unnecessary preoperative standing "screening tests." The patient's preexisting medical condition may require more intense scrutiny than the specific neuropathological process being treated. For example, implanted cardiac devices such as pacemakers may need to be interrogated preoperatively to ensure optimal perioperative functioning. Yet a consultation with an internist does not replace preanesthesia evaluation by a neuroanesthesiologist.

The use of preanesthesia clinics has been shown to improve operating room efficiency and minimize unexpected delays and cancellations because of poorly prepared patients.[1] For emergency surgeries, a brief, focused evaluation is performed just before surgery. The ASA classification of physical status is a universally accepted system used for stratification of a patient's preexisting health status (Table 3.1) and correlates with perioperative morbidity and mortality.[2] The ASA physical status 3–5 independently predicts increased risk of perioperative cardiovascular complications in intracranial surgical patients and is also a risk factor for perioperative mortality.[3] Coexisting cardiopulmonary, hepatic, renal, and other diseases have specific anesthetic implications. The cardiac evaluation follows the American College of Cardiology/American Heart Association guidelines.[4] The overall risk of cardiac patients undergoing a noncardiac surgery is assessed using the Revised Cardiac Risk Index,[5] according to which, the presence of three or more of the following factors is associated with a cardiac morbidity rate of 9%, which affects postoperative management in the neurology intensive care unit (ICU): (i) high-risk surgery, (ii) history of ischemic heart disease, (iii) history of congestive heart failure, (iv) history of cerebrovascular disease, (v) preoperative treatment with insulin, and (vi) preoperative serum creatinine level greater than 2.0 mg/dL. The risk factors for postoperative pulmonary complications include advanced age, ASA class 2 or greater, functional dependence, chronic obstructive pulmonary disease, and congestive heart failure.[6]

A review of current medications is critical because of significant anesthetic implications. For example, anticonvulsant therapy is associated with increased resistance to nondepolarizing muscle relaxants and hence an increased requirement under anesthesia.[7] Steroid administration might be associated with intraoperative hyperglycemia and adrenal suppression.[8] Beta-blocker therapy is typically continued through the perioperative period,[9] whereas angiotensin-converting enzyme inhibitors and angiotensin receptor blockers are often avoided on the morning of major craniotomy to avoid intraoperative hypotension. Interruption of antiepileptic therapy may affect susceptibility to

**Table 3.1** ASA Classification of Physical Status

| ASA Physical Status | Disease State |
| --- | --- |
| 1 | A normal healthy patient |
| 2 | A patient with mild systemic disease |
| 3 | A patient with severe systemic disease |
| 4 | A patient with severe systemic disease that is a constant threat to life |
| 5 | A moribund patient who is not expected to survive without the operation |
| 6 | A patient declared brain-dead whose organs are being removed for donor purposes |

*ASA,* American Society of Anesthesiologists.
Excerpted from the Relative Value Guide 2008 of the American Society of Anesthesiologists. A copy of the full text can be obtained from ASA, 520 N. Northwest Highway, Park Ridge, IL 60068-2573.

perioperative seizure. Discussion of relevant social/religious background (e.g., Jehovah's Witnesses, who may not want to receive blood transfusion), as well as personal preferences (such as "do not resuscitate" orders), is imperative to anesthetic planning. Establishing a rapport with the patient preoperatively is invaluable if an awake craniotomy is being planned.

A comprehensive physical examination is critical for anesthetic planning. Preoperative correction of dehydration in patients with reduced intake of fluids, vomiting, or the use of diuretics and contrast agents can prevent hypotension after induction of anesthesia. Recording of preoperative vital parameters provides baseline values to direct hemodynamic management. Assessment of the airway is mandatory to ensure the ability to adequately oxygenate and ventilate under anesthesia. Modified Mallampati scoring, thyromental distance, presence of overbite or underbite, and the range of neck flexion-extension collectively provide an estimate of the risk for difficult intubation. Difficult airway should be anticipated in patients who have recently undergone a frontotemporal craniotomy and may have developed a pseudoankylosis of the temporomandibular joint,[10] acromegalic patients undergoing pituitary surgery,[11] and patients with cervical spine lesions or with cervical immobilization devices (internal or external). Recognition of potential airway difficulty allows proper planning with the availability of equipment and resources and formulation of a backup plan. Patients with depressed level of consciousness are likely to have a reduced need for anesthetic agents and are more likely to emerge from anesthesia slowly postoperatively. The presence of brainstem lesions or lower cranial nerve dysfunction predisposes patients to an increased risk of aspiration, and extubation of the trachea may electively be delayed. Patients with ruptured intracranial aneurysms with higher Hunt and Hess grades are more likely to have impaired cerebral autoregulation (and, hence, susceptibility to hemodynamic fluctuations) in addition to the higher chance of associated diminished airway reflexes and cardiopulmonary, metabolic, and electrolyte imbalances compared with patients with lower Hunt and Hess grades.[12]

Cushing's reflex (hypertension, bradycardia, and irregular breathing) in a patient with intracranial mass lesions triggers rapid intervention to acutely decrease the intracranial pressure (ICP). Finally, preexisting motor deficits are identified to avoid life-threatening hyperkalemia secondary to succinylcholine.[13]

Review of neuroimaging is pertinent to anesthetic management. Computed tomography (CT) and magnetic resonance imaging scans are reviewed to predict intraoperative brain swelling and risk of bleeding. The degree of midline shift, peritumoral edema, and a diagnosis of glioblastoma multiforme or metastasis are independent predictors of brain swelling.[14] The presence of subdural hematoma on imaging is associated with intraoperative hyperglycemia, as well as intraoperative hypotension, during emergent craniotomy.[15,16] Cerebral angiograms provide information regarding collateral vessels, which is helpful in anticipating the risk of cerebral ischemia (and hence the need for neuroprotective interventions) during temporary clipping for aneurysm surgery. Tumors adjacent to the superior sagittal sinus or other dural sinuses suggest a risk of hemorrhage and venous air embolism.

## Clinical Pearl

Proper preanesthesia evaluation is critical—a consultation with an internist and routine screening tests do not replace preanesthesia evaluation.

## Goals of Anesthetic Management

The general goal of intraoperative anesthetic management is to render the patient unconscious and immobile to facilitate surgery, to provide adequate analgesia, and to maintain homeostasis and vital functions. The anesthetic goals specific to craniotomy are listed in Box 3.1. These goals are accomplished by selection of appropriate pharmacological agents, careful titration of hemodynamic and ventilation parameters, and vigilant neuromonitoring and will be described in detail later.

## Box 3.1   Anesthetic Goals for Craniotomy

1. Provide adequate amnesia, analgesia, and immobility
2. Optimize cerebral blood flow and oxygenation
3. Control intracranial pressure
4. Avoid secondary physiological insults (hypotension, hypoxia, hyper-/hypoglycemia, hyper-/hypocarbia, hyperthermia, seizures)
5. Provide optimal operating conditions (brain relaxation)
6. Facilitate intraoperative neurophysiological monitoring
7. Provide intraoperative neuroprotection
8. Avoid positioning-related complications
9. Accomplish early emergence after surgery to facilitate neurological assessment

# Airway Management for Craniotomy

## Key Concepts

- Airway should be carefully secured in patients with intracranial disease, while avoiding hypoxemia, hypercapnia, and hemodynamic perturbations.
- Difficult intubation should be anticipated in patients with acromegaly, cervical spine disease or fixation, and when access to airway is limited (awake craniotomy and stereotactic surgery).

Airway management in patients with intracranial pathology is a delicate balance between safe and expeditious placement of the endotracheal tube and offsetting the sympathetic surge due to laryngoscopy and its effect on ICP and blood pressure. Difficulty in airway management may be anticipated in patients with acromegaly presenting for resection of pituitary tumors and situations where access to the airway may be limited during craniotomy—for example, awake craniotomy and stereotactic neurosurgery. Awake fiberoptic intubation is often considered the safest approach in patients with advanced acromegaly. In patients presenting for emergent craniotomy who may have a full stomach, and in patients with acutely increased ICP where gastric emptying may be altered, increasing the risk of aspiration during intubation, a rapid sequence intubation is performed. Although there are few data suggesting potential increased ICP with succinylcholine, the clinical significance of the transient increase in ICP is unknown.[17] Hypertension during laryngoscopy and intubation can cause rupture/rebleeding of unsecured aneurysms and is attenuated by using one or more of the following: opioids, lidocaine, beta-blockers, calcium channel blockers, or additional bolus of propofol. Neuroanesthesiologists often place an arterial line to monitor arterial blood pressure prior to induction of anesthesia.

For patients undergoing awake craniotomy, typically an asleep-awake-asleep anesthetic technique is used where a scalp block is placed and general anesthesia is induced during the initial phase of surgical exposure, then the patient is woken up for neurocognitive testing and then reanesthetized to complete the surgical resection and closure. During the initial exposure, a laryngeal mask airway (LMA) is frequently inserted to maintain the patency of the airway. Some neuroanesthesiologists prefer not to orally instrument the airway in this phase, and the patient breathes spontaneously using a nasopharyngeal airway as needed. For neurocognitive testing, the patient is smoothly emerged from anesthesia and the LMA is removed. For the final resection and surgical closure, the LMA may be reinserted to facilitate adequate gas exchange in order to avoid hypercapnia and brain swelling.

## Clinical Pearl

Hypoxemia and hypercarbia must be avoided during airway management in patients with neurological disease.
Familiarity with the ASA "difficult airway" algorithm and availability of backup airway devices are critical.

# Choice of Anesthetic Agents

## Key Concepts

- The choice of anesthetic agent is based on the patient's neurological condition, planned procedure, and neurophysiological monitoring.
- In general, propofol decreases cerebral blood flow (CBF) and maintains the coupling between cerebral metabolic rate (CMR) and CBF, whereas inhaled anesthetics have a dose-dependent potential to increase CBF.
- Brainstem-evoked potentials are the most resistant to the effect of anesthetic agents, whereas cortical motor–evoked potentials are the most sensitive.

The most commonly used intravenous anesthetic agent is propofol. The commonly used inhalational anesthetic agents are isoflurane, sevoflurane, and desflurane. The anesthetic agents that provide for both loss of consciousness and amnesia (so-called *balanced anesthesia*) are typically combined with potent opioids to provide analgesia (remifentanil, fentanyl, morphine, or hydromorphone) and neuromuscular blocking agents (typically vecuronium, rocuronium, or cis-atracurium) to provide immobility. Dexmedetomidine, an $\alpha_2$-adrenoceptor agonist with sedative properties, is increasingly being used for craniotomies, particularly awake craniotomies. The properties that make it suitable as an adjunct for craniotomy include sedation and analgesia without respiratory depression, attenuation of neuroendocrine and hemodynamic responses, and reduction of anesthetic and opioid requirements, in addition to favorable pharmacokinetics facilitating rapid wash-out after termination of infusion.[18] The intravenous and inhaled anesthetic agents differ substantially in their pharmacodynamics and pharmacokinetic properties, and the choice of anesthetic agents is based on the patient's neurological condition, proposed procedure, coexisting diseases, and planned neurophysiological monitoring.

Most anesthetic agents decrease the CMR. However, in general terms, propofol decreases CBF and maintains the coupling between CMR and CBF, whereas inhaled anesthetics have a dose-dependent effect on the CBF.[19,20] Inhaled anesthetics decrease CBF when used in <1.0 minimum alveolar concentration (MAC) doses, but tend to cause cerebral vasodilation at higher concentrations, leading to increase in CBF and uncoupling between flow and metabolism in the brain,[20] but with preservation of some reactivity to changes in $Paco_2$. This "luxury perfusion" may increase ICP and brain swelling in patients with already reduced intracranial compliance.[21]

There is also significant difference among various inhaled anesthetics. Isoflurane causes more cerebral vasodilation than an equipotent concentration of sevoflurane.[22] The diseased/injured brain with preexisting intracranial hypertension may be more sensitive to the cerebral vasodilatory effects of inhaled agents even at lower concentrations. However, the cerebral vasodilatory effect of inhalational agents can be avoided by hyperventilation to decrease the partial pressure of carbon dioxide ($Paco_2$). On the other hand, institution of hypocapnia in patients under propofol anesthesia may lead to excessive cerebral vasoconstriction and can cause cerebral ischemia.[23]

Positron emission tomography studies demonstrate that although both sevoflurane and propofol similarly reduce CMR in all brain areas, sevoflurane decreases CBF in some and propofol in all brain structures, and only propofol reduces cerebral blood volume in the cortex and cerebellum.[19] In an open-label study of patients with supratentorial cerebral tumors randomized to propofol-fentanyl, isoflurane-fentanyl, or sevoflurane-fentanyl anesthesia, the ICP was significantly lower and cerebral perfusion pressure (CPP) higher in patients who received propofol anesthesia.[21] The cerebral swelling after opening of the dura was also lower in patients who received propofol, but the arteriovenous oxygen difference was higher and jugular venous saturation and carbon dioxide reactivity lower in patients anesthetized with propofol.[21] Moreover, cerebral autoregulation is impaired at 1.5 MAC by isoflurane and desflurane, whereas propofol preserves it.[24] These and similar other findings indicate the potential benefit of propofol anesthesia in patients with intracranial tumors. Importantly, propofol-induced burst suppression after traumatic brain injury (TBI) may not reduce the level of regional ischemic burden measured by arterial-jugular venous oxygen differences.[25] However, low-dose inhaled agents as part of balanced anesthesia are often effectively used by neuroanesthesiologists to provide optimal operative conditions during craniotomy.[26]

Numerous other factors, such as the effect on evoked potential signal quality, are considered in selecting an anesthetic agent. Although the inhalational agents cause dose-dependent increases in latency and decreases in amplitude of somatosensory-evoked potentials (SSEPs), less than 1.0 MAC concentration is generally compatible with monitoring of cortical SSEPs, although propofol anesthesia does not affect SSEPs.[27] However, if motor-evoked potential monitoring is contemplated, many neuroanesthesiologists prefer propofol anesthesia, especially in patients who may have preexisting neurological deficits. It should be noted that despite the apparent preference for propofol, <0.5 MAC of desflurane is also compatible with motor-evoked potentials.[28,29] Ketamine is also often added to support motor-evoked potentials, but its use requires consideration of potential for increased CMR and CBF. Motor-evoked potentials also preclude the use of neuromuscular blocking agents, whereas brainstem-evoked potentials are, in general, most resistant to the effect of anesthetic agents. The choice of anesthetic agents is also determined by the need for intraoperative electrocorticography or motor mapping. There is growing evidence regarding potential epileptogenicity of sevoflurane.[30]

## Clinical Pearl

Volatile anesthetic agents cause cerebral vasodilatation only in concentrations above 1.0 MAC.
Low-concentration volatile anesthetics may be safely used in combination with mild hyperventilation without causing brain swelling.

# Hemodynamic Management under Anesthesia

## Key Concepts

- According to the Brain Trauma Foundation guidelines, the recommended CPP for TBI is 50 to 70 mm Hg.
- Hypertension should be avoided in patients with unsecured aneurysms.
- Blood pressure is actively decreased after resection of large arteriovenous malformations to prevent normal perfusion pressure breakthrough and hyperemia.
- Emerging data suggest that the lower and upper limits of cerebral autoregulation may be more variable and the range of autoregulation narrower than previously believed.
- Warm, nonglucose-containing isotonic fluids are preferred during craniotomy.

Optimization of hemodynamic parameters is important to ensure adequate cerebral perfusion during craniotomy. Patients with neurosurgical disorders are likely to have impaired cerebral autoregulation[31] and, hence, increased susceptibility to hemodynamic fluctuations. The hemodynamic goals differ depending on the intracranial pathology as well as comorbid conditions. The current guidelines recommend maintaining CPP between 50 and 70 mm Hg and mean arterial pressure above 90 mm Hg in patients with severe TBI. Intraoperative hypotension is anticipated in patients with multiple lesions on the CT, subdural hematoma, and thickness of lesion[15] and is frequently encountered after decompression of the brain. Hypotension is also undesirable in patients with occlusive cerebrovascular disease such as Moyamoya and intracranial arterial stenosis. Conversely, in patients undergoing craniotomy for aneurysm clipping, the goal is to avoid acute increases in blood pressure that may risk rebleeding due to increase in the transmural pressure. Calcium channel blockers such as nicardipine and short-acting beta-blockers like esmolol are sometimes used to actively decrease the blood pressure. However, during the periods of temporary clipping, the blood pressure may be actively raised to ensure blood flow through the collateral channels to avoid cerebral ischemia. Once the aneurysm is secured, the blood pressure goals are normalized. Occasionally, in order to facilitate clipping of giant basilar tip aneurysms, intraoperative temporary cardiac standstill is provided using high-dose adenosine (0.2–0.3 mg/kg).[32] Blood pressure is actively reduced after the resection of arteriovenous malformation to prevent hyperemia and normal perfusion pressure breakthrough.

Invasive arterial blood pressure monitoring is used to titrate hemodynamic goals during craniotomy. Myocardial stunning is not uncommon after aneurysmal subarachnoid hemorrhage, which can result in a Takotsubo-like cardiomyopathy. Myocardial dysfunction has also been described in the setting of TBI. Although the effects of vasopressor agents on cerebral vasculature have not been fully deciphered, the inotropic and vasopressor medication choices can contribute to such comorbidities. The arterial pressure transducer is zeroed and positioned at the level of the external auditory meatus to ensure adequate CPP and CBF, and is especially prudent in patients undergoing craniotomy in the sitting position.

Patients undergoing craniotomy typically receive nonglucose-containing warm, isotonic intravenous fluids. Hypotonic fluids like lactated Ringer's solution are avoided because they can worsen cerebral edema and brain swelling. Despite the use of diuretics to facilitate brain relaxation, the goal is to maintain normovolemia during the procedure. Albumin may be associated with poor outcomes in patients with TBI and hence is often avoided.[33] Because cerebral salt wasting, diabetes insipidus, hypokalemia, and hypocalcemia are often associated with intracranial disease, electrolytes are periodically monitored under anesthesia and corrected accordingly. Surgical blood loss can sometimes be substantial, requiring blood transfusion. Some typical examples include resection of a large arteriovenous malformation or meningioma, intraoperative rupture of an aneurysm, and inadvertent vascular injury. The transfusion triggers for neurosurgical patients are somewhat elusive, although historically, a hemoglobin level of 10 g/dL was often considered to be a balance between optimal oxygen-carrying capacity and rheology of blood to facilitate perfusion of cerebral microvasculature. However, more recently, lower hemoglobin values have been advocated in neurosurgical patients. Anemia in neurosurgical patients is associated with poor outcomes, but so is the use of transfusion of blood. Intraoperative decision to transfuse blood is often made based on overall fluid and hemodynamic status, hemoglobin value, and rapidity of blood loss, taking into account the patient's cardiac comorbidity and neurological dysfunction, including estimates of cerebrovascular reserve (i.e., capability to vasodilate in compensation for anemia). Although the safety of acute normovolemic hemodilution during craniotomy has been demonstrated,[34] the practice has not gained substantial popularity.

---

> **Clinical Pearl**
>
> Nonglucose-containing warm, isotonic intravenous fluids are preferable during craniotomy. Strict hemodynamic control is critical.

---

## Intraoperative Monitoring

The details of intraoperative neuromonitoring are discussed in Chapter 6. Briefly, the ASA recommends monitoring electrocardiography, blood pressure, pulse oximetry, capnography, temperature, and anesthetic concentration monitoring for inhaled anesthetics. Arterial lines are also useful for hemodynamic monitoring and to sample $PaO_2$, $PaCO_2$, glucose levels, and electrolytes. Evoked potential monitoring and electroencephalography are increasingly being used. In addition, monitoring for venous air embolism may include transesophageal echocardiography or precordial Doppler. Monitoring cerebral blood flow velocity using transcranial Doppler ultrasonography may provide useful information in surgeries where probe placement is

feasible.[35] Jugular venous oximetry can be used intraoperatively to optimize oxygen delivery to the brain.[36] Jugular venous saturation maintained between 50% and 70% serves as a surrogate for the balance between the global cerebral oxygen delivery and metabolic requirement and is useful in individualizing blood pressure and ventilation parameters intraoperatively.[36]

## Intracranial Pressure Management and Brain Relaxation

---

### Key Concepts

- Hyperventilation should be used selectively—prolonged and excessive hyperventilation must be avoided.
- Steroids should not be administered to patients with TBI.

---

Patients presenting for craniotomy often have elevated ICP. In addition, brain relaxation is desirable to facilitate surgical exposure and brain retraction. The various interventions used intraoperatively for brain relaxation and ICP reduction are listed in Box 3.2. Briefly, maintenance of adequate anesthesia and analgesia is essential to avoid cerebral metabolic demand associated with increase in CBF, which may cause swelling of a poorly compliant brain. Volatile anesthetic agents are used in low concentrations to avoid direct cerebral vasodilation, and in patients where brain swelling is anticipated, intravenous anesthesia with propofol (but avoiding hypotension) is often preferred.[21] Optimal patient positioning is critical because excessive flexion or rotation of the neck can lead to obstruction of cerebral venous drainage, resulting in brain swelling. Slight head elevation is desirable to facilitate cerebral venous drainage. Avoidance of hypercarbia with controlled ventilation is critical, and moderate hypocarbia ($PaCO_2$

---

> **Box 3.2  Strategies for Intraoperative Brain Relaxation and Control of Intracranial Pressure**
>
> 1. Maintenance of adequate depth of anesthesia and analgesia
> 2. Selection of appropriate anesthetic agents (intravenous anesthetics for patients with anticipated brain swelling)
> 3. Optimal positioning with slight head elevation and avoiding excessive neck flexion or rotation
> 4. Optimization of hemodynamic parameters
> 5. Controlled ventilation with normocarbia to moderate hypocarbia ($PaCO_2$ 30–35 mm Hg)*
> 6. Mannitol (osmotic diuretic)
> 7. Furosemide
> 8. Hypertonic saline
> 9. Cerebrospinal fluid drainage (external ventricular drainage)
> 10. Steroids in patients with tumors/vasogenic edema#
> 11. Treatment of fever/seizures
> 12. Burst suppression with propofol/thiopental bolus
>
> *Brief periods of hypocarbia with $PaCO_2 < 30$ mm Hg should be used only in emergent conditions or when other ICP reduction maneuvers have failed.
> #Steroids should not be administered in patients with traumatic brain injury.

30–35 mm Hg) is used judiciously to facilitate surgical exposure. In patients with supratentorial brain tumors, intraoperative hyperventilation improves surgeon-assessed brain bulk and is associated with a decrease in ICP.[37] However, excessive/prolonged hyperventilation can lead to cerebral ischemia and must be avoided.[38]

Hemodynamic stability and avoidance of hypertension in patients with impaired cerebral autoregulation is critical to the intracranial milieu. Mannitol (0.25–1.0 g/kg) causes osmotic diuresis and provides brain relaxation. Three percent hypertonic saline is associated with similar brain relaxation and arteriovenous oxygen and lactate difference.[39] Occasionally, furosemide is administered to potentiate the brain-relaxing effect of mannitol. The volume of urine output from mannitol- and/or furosemide-induced diuresis is generally replaced with isotonic crystalloid or normal saline. In patients with ventricular drainage devices, drainage of cerebrospinal fluid may be an effective and convenient method for rapid ICP reduction and brain relaxation, but should be used cautiously, considering the potential risk of aneurysm rebleeding or intracranial hypotension/brain sag. Steroids help reduce vasogenic edema and may be helpful in patients with tumors, but should not be administered to patients with TBI, in whom they have been shown to worsen outcomes. Finally, fever and seizures should be promptly treated, and in refractory cases, burst suppression with thiopental or propofol may be attempted.

### Clinical Pearl

Steroids should not be administered to patients with TBI. Prolonged and excessive hyperventilation must be avoided. Brain relaxation using mannitol/furosemide can result in continued electrolyte imbalance postoperatively and should be monitored and corrected aggressively.

## Glycemic Management

### Key Concepts

- Glucose levels may fluctuate intraoperatively and must be monitored.
- Both hyperglycemia and hypoglycemia are detrimental for the brain—normoglycemia is targeted.

Given the association of both hypoglycemia and hyperglycemia with poor outcomes in neurosurgical patients, the goal of anesthetic management is to maintain normoglycemia. The surgical stress response and perioperative steroid use often contribute to intraoperative hyperglycemia. In fact, new-onset intraoperative hyperglycemia may be observed during craniotomy in patients who had normal blood glucose levels preoperatively.[40,41] Because the benefits of tight glucose control in neurosurgical patients have not been demonstrated conclusively and glucose levels may fluctuate substantially under anesthesia,[40,41] neuroanesthesiologists monitor glucose regularly and maintain the blood glucose level in the range of 150 to 200 mg/dL.

## Temperature Management

### Key Concept

Intraoperative hypothermia should be avoided by using forced-air warming blankets, warming intravenous fluids, and adjusting room temperature.

General anesthesia is associated with a decrease in the body temperature due to peripheral vasodilatation and redistribution of the body heat from the core. Forced-air warming blankets, warmed intravenous fluids, and adjustment of the operating room temperature are some strategies used to maintain normothermia under anesthesia. However, the detrimental effects of hyperthermia on the brain are well known. Although laboratory studies and animal data suggest that mild hypothermia (33–35°C) is protective against cerebral dysfunction in ischemic and TBI models, clinical data on effectiveness of hypothermia are not equally encouraging. The International Hypothermia in Aneurysm Surgery Trial failed to demonstrate a difference in Glasgow Outcome Score, Rankin Score, Barthel's Index, or National Institute of Health Stroke Scale Score between the normothermic (33°C) and hypothermic (36.5°C) groups.[42] In addition, there was a higher incidence of postoperative bacteremia in the hypothermic group. Clinical benefits of intraoperative hypothermia in other neurosurgical conditions have also not been demonstrated. Hence, although the temperature may spontaneously decrease under anesthesia, the neuroanesthesiologist's aim is intraoperative normothermia and certainly to avoid hyperthermia.

## Emergence from General Anesthesia

### Key Concepts

- Emergence from craniotomy should be rapid and smooth, with minimal hemodynamic changes and straining on the tracheal tube.
- Emergence response may be decreased using esmolol, lidocaine, or dexmedetomidine.

The goal for emergence from anesthesia for craniotomy is to have an awake patient so that a neurological examination may be performed reliably. Patients who were intubated preoperatively, those with poor neurological status, and patients undergoing prolonged surgery around the brainstem are likely to remain intubated. Emergence from anesthesia requires diligent planning to accomplish a timely, smooth emergence with minimal hemodynamic perturbation and straining on the tracheal tube. Anesthetic agents are gradually weaned, and the patients are trialed on spontaneous ventilation to determine if their respiratory drive and minute ventilation are appropriate. With the modern short-acting anesthetic agents, rapid emergence can be accomplished in most cases.[43,44] Despite the popular belief, systematic studies show no benefit of using total intravenous anesthesia with an ultrashort-acting opioid over the conventional balanced volatile technique in terms of recovery and cognitive functions after craniotomy.[43,44] However, patients who receive desflurane are likely to have a shorter extubation and recovery time compared with those who receive sevoflurane.[44] Desflurane also provides earlier postoperative cognitive recovery and reversal to normocapnia and normal pH in overweight and obese patients after craniotomy. Incorporation of dexmedetomidine in the anesthetic regimen is another strategy to facilitate shorter emergence and recovery time in neurosurgical patients[45] with attenuation of delirium, and scalp blocks have been shown to improve recovery profiles.

The adrenergic surge associated with emergence may be treated with a short-acting opioid or an antihypertensive such as esmolol or nicardipine. Coughing and straining on the tracheal tube during emergence can be prevented with lidocaine or judicious use of remifentanil. Dexmedetomidine has both sedative and analgesic properties, but does not cause respiratory depression and is also useful in facilitating timely and smooth emergence. Perioperative hypertension has been associated with increased incidence in postoperative intracranial hemorrhage in patients undergoing craniotomy and should be avoided.[46] Unexpected delay in emergence mandates ruling out potential confounding factors such as nonconvulsive status epilepticus, drug overdose, hypothermia, and hypoglycemia before an imaging study will be performed to rule out an intracranial cause.

## Clinical Pearl

Patients should almost never be extubated under deep anesthesia after craniotomy. Extubation should be smooth and without hemodynamic response with a patient who can yield a valid neurological examination.

# Immediate Postoperative Management

## Key Concepts

- Opioids are the mainstay of postcraniotomy pain control but should be used judiciously to avoid respiratory and neurological depression.
- Regional scalp block prevents and attenuates the postcraniotomy pain and stress responses.
- Selective serotonin (5-HT3) receptor antagonists are first-choice drugs for prophylaxis of postoperative nausea and vomiting (PONV).
- Patients with neurological deterioration, respiratory distress, copious oropharyngeal secretions, or seizures may need reintubation.
- Effective hand-off with adequate communication is critical for patient safety.

Immediate postoperative recovery arises in the postanesthesia care unit or neurology ICU, where the patients are closely monitored for adequacy of oxygenation and ventilation, hemodynamic stability, pain control, neurological recovery, and any complications. Data on the effect of craniotomy site on the severity of pain are somewhat conflicting. Despite the associated risk of overdosing-related adverse effects such as respiratory depression with hypoxemia and/or carbon dioxide retention and increased CBF and ICP, judicious use of potent opioids such as fentanyl, morphine, and hydromorphone, including patient-controlled analgesia (PCA), remains the cornerstone of postoperative pain management.[47] The use of scheduled tramadol in addition to narcotics may provide better pain control in some patients, decrease the side effects associated with narcotic pain medications, encourage earlier postoperative ambulation, and reduce total hospitalization costs.[48] Importantly, tramadol does present a small increased risk of seizure in addition to the high incidence of vomiting. The cyclooxygenase-2 inhibitor parecoxib has been found to offer no benefit in addition to local anesthetic scalp infiltration, intravenous paracetamol, and morphine PCA after supratentorial craniotomy.[49] Preoperative oral gabapentin used for antiepileptic prophylaxis in patients undergoing craniotomy for supratentorial tumor resection can decrease the postoperative pain scores and the total morphine consumption, albeit with increased sedation postoperatively. Regional scalp blocks attenuate the postcraniotomy pain and stress responses but appear to remain underutilized. Although the published randomized controlled trials of regional scalp block are small and of limited methodological quality, metaanalysis shows reduced postoperative pain.[50]

PONV after elective craniotomy may affect up to two thirds of patients. Selective serotonin (5-HT3) receptor antagonists are considered first-choice drugs for prophylaxis of PONV due to their favorable safety profile. Ondansetron 4 mg given at the time of dural closure is safe and effective in preventing emetic episodes after elective craniotomy. However, the effectiveness may be substantially variable. Granisetron 1 mg provides comparable prevention of emesis after supratentorial craniotomy. Metaanalysis of published data indicates that the cumulative incidence of emesis but not nausea is significantly reduced with 5-HT3 receptor antagonists at 24 and 48 hours.[51] A single 600-mg dose of gabapentin also reduces the 24-hour incidence of PONV. Other options, based on disparate antiemetic mechanisms, for rescue of PONV include metoclopramide, droperidol, and scopolamine.

Maintenance of adequate ventilation and oxygenation postoperatively is critical. Some common indications for reintubation are neurological deterioration, respiratory distress, copious oropharyngeal secretions, and seizures. The neurological deterioration may be related to residual tumor with surrounding edema, intracerebral hemorrhage, or cerebral infarction. Patients who are not extubated at the end of surgery or require reintubation usually undergo imaging followed by transfer to the ICU. A systematic and detailed hand-off communication is critical to facilitate a smooth transition of care from the anesthesia providers to the ICU. Table 3.2 summarizes some possible perioperative complications related to craniotomy that may require special attention while transitioning to intensive care.

**Table 3.2** Possible Perioperative Complications Related to Craniotomy That may Require Special Attention While Transitioning to Intensive Care

| Complications | Possible Mechanisms |
|---|---|
| Delayed emergence | ■ Residual anesthetic<br>■ Hypothermia<br>■ Hypoglycemia<br>■ Cerebral ischemia<br>■ Pneumocephalus<br>■ Intracranial hematoma |
| Respiratory depression/inadequate ventilation | ■ Overdose of opioid analgesics<br>■ Residual neuromuscular blockade<br>■ Surgical causes (particularly after surgery near brainstem) |
| Hypoxemia | ■ Postoperative atelectasis<br>■ Fluid overload |
| Hypotension | ■ Inadequate fluid replacement<br>■ Adrenal suppression due to the use of etomidate |
| Anemia/coagulopathy | ■ Inadequate replacement of surgical blood loss with packed red blood cells/blood products |
| Electrolyte abnormalities | ■ Use of osmotic or loop diuretics for intraoperative brain relaxation<br>■ Diabetes insipidus<br>■ Syndrome of inappropriate antidiuretic hormone secretion<br>■ Cerebral salt wasting |
| Hypothermia | ■ Anesthesia-induced redistribution of body heat<br>■ Induced hypothermia for cerebral protection |
| Postcraniotomy pain | ■ Inadequate analgesia |
| Postoperative nausea and vomiting | ■ Exposure to anesthesia/surgery |
| Peripheral neuropathy/skin damage | ■ Patient positioning during surgery |
| Tongue swelling/tongue damage | ■ Combination of pressure due to bite block and tracheal tube and neck flexion for surgical positioning |

**Clinical Pearl**

Narcotics must be used judiciously after craniotomy to avoid the risk of respiratory or neurological depression.

## Summary

Successful anesthetic management of craniotomy requires careful integration of physiological and pharmacological principles with judicious use of monitoring modalities to implement a comprehensive perioperative management plan. The critical elements of anesthesia care include comprehensive preanesthetic evaluation and optimization; delivery of anesthesia care in the operating room integrating amnesia, analgesia, hemodynamic, and ventilatory control; facilitation of surgical exposure and intraoperative neuromonitoring; and immediate postoperative care incorporating neurological recovery with control of pain, PONV, and hemodynamic stability before the patient is transferred to the ICU.

## References

1. Fischer SP. Development and effectiveness of an anesthesia preoperative evaluation clinic in a teaching hospital. *Anesthesiology.* 1996;85(1):196–206.
2. Wolters U, Wolf T, Stützer H, et al. ASA classification and perioperative variables as predictors of postoperative outcome. *Br J Anaesth.* 1996;77(2):217–222.
3. Akavipat P, Ittichaikulthol W, Tuchinda L, et al. The Thai Anesthesia Incidents (THAI Study) of anesthetic risk factors related to perioperative death and perioperative cardiovascular complications in intracranial surgery. *J Med Assoc Thai.* 2007;90(8):1565–1572.
4. American College of Cardiology/American Heart Association Task Force on Practice Guidelines (Writing Committee to Revise the 2002 Guidelines on Perioperative Cardiovascular Evaluation for Noncardiac Surgery); American Society of Echocardiography; American Society of Nuclear Cardiology; Heart Rhythm Society; Society of Cardiovascular Anesthesiologists; Society for Cardiovascular Angiography and Interventions; Society for Vascular Medicine and Biology; Society for Vascular Surgery. Fleisher LA, Beckman JA, Brown KA, et al. ACC/AHA 2007 guidelines on perioperative cardiovascular evaluation and care for noncardiac surgery: executive summary: a report of the American College of Cardiology/American Heart Association Task Force on Practice Guidelines (Writing Committee to Revise the 2002 Guidelines on Perioperative Cardiovascular Evaluation for Noncardiac Surgery. *Anesth Analg.* 2008;106(3):685–712.
5. Lee TH, Marcantonio ER, Mangione CM, et al. Derivation and prospective validation of a simple index for prediction of cardiac risk of major noncardiac surgery. *Circulation.* 1999;100(10):1043–1049.
6. Smetana GW, Lawrence VA, Cornell JE. American College of Physicians. Preoperative pulmonary risk stratification for noncardiothoracic surgery: systematic review for the American College of Physicians. *Ann Intern Med.* 2006;144(8):581–595.
7. Wright PM, McCarthy G, Szenohradszky J, et al. Influence of chronic phenytoin administration on the pharmacokinetics and pharmacodynamics of vecuronium. *Anesthesiology.* 2004;100(3):626–633.
8. Pasternak JJ, McGregor DG, Lanier WL. Effect of single-dose dexamethasone on blood glucose concentration in patients undergoing craniotomy. *J Neurosurg Anesthesiol.* 2004;16(2):122–125.
9. Fleisher LA, Beckman JA, Brown KA, et al. 2009 ACCF/AHA focused update on perioperative beta blockade incorporated into the ACC/AHA 2007 guidelines on perioperative cardiovascular evaluation and care for noncardiac surgery: a report of the American College of Cardiology Foundation/American Heart Association Task Force on Practice Guidelines. *Circulation.* 2009;120(21):e169–e276.
10. Kawaguchi M, Sakamoto T, Furuya H, et al. Pseudoankylosis of the mandible after supratentorial craniotomy. *Anesth Analg.* 1996;83(4):731–734.
11. Sharma D, Prabhakar H, Bithal PK, et al. Predicting difficult laryngoscopy in acromegaly: a comparison of upper lip bite test with modified Mallampati classification. *J Neurosurg Anesthesiol.* 2010;22(2):138–143.
12. Tenjin H, Hirakawa K, Mizukawa N, et al. Dysautoregulation in patients with ruptured aneurysms: cerebral blood flow measurements obtained during surgery by a temperature-controlled thermoelectrical method. *Neurosurgery.* 1988;23(6):705–709.
13. Yentis SM. Suxamethonium and hyperkalaemia. *Anaesth Intensive Care.* 1990;18(1):92–101.
14. Rasmussen M, Bundgaard H, Cold GE. Craniotomy for supratentorial brain tumors: risk factors for brain swelling after opening the dura mater. *J Neurosurg.* 2004;101(4):621–626.
15. Sharma D, Brown MJ, Curry P, et al. Prevalence and risk factors for intraoperative hypotension during craniotomy for traumatic brain injury. *J Neurosurg Anesthesiol.* 2012;24(3):178–184.
16. Pecha T, Sharma D, Hoffman NG, et al. Hyperglycemia during craniotomy for adult traumatic brain injury. *Anesth Analg.* 2011;113(2):336–342.
17. Brown MM, Parr MJ, Manara AR. The effect of suxamethonium on intracranial pressure and cerebral perfusion pressure in patients with severe head injuries following blunt trauma. *Eur J Anaesthesiol.* 1996;13(5):474–477.

18. Tanskanen PE, Kyttä JV, Randell TT, et al. Dexmedetomidine as an anaesthetic adjuvant in patients undergoing intracranial tumour surgery: a double-blind, randomized and placebo-controlled study. *Br J Anaesth.* 2006;97(5):658–665.

19. Kaisti KK, Långsjö JW, Aalto S, et al. Effects of sevoflurane, propofol, and adjunct nitrous oxide on regional cerebral blood flow, oxygen consumption, and blood volume in humans. *Anesthesiology.* 2003;99(3):603–613.

20. Kaisti KK, Metsähonkala L, Teräs M, et al. Effects of surgical levels of propofol and sevoflurane anesthesia on cerebral blood flow in healthy subjects studied with positron emission tomography. *Anesthesiology.* 2002;96(6):1358–1370.

21. Petersen KD, Landsfeldt U, Cold GE, et al. Intracranial pressure and cerebral hemodynamic in patients with cerebral tumors: a randomized prospective study of patients subjected to craniotomy in propofol-fentanyl, isoflurane-fentanyl, or sevoflurane-fentanyl anesthesia. *Anesthesiology.* 2003;98(2):329–336.

22. Matta BF, Heath KJ, Tipping K, et al. Direct cerebral vasodilatory effects of sevoflurane and isoflurane. *Anesthesiology.* 1999;91(3):677–680.

23. Kawano Y, Kawaguchi M, Inoue S, et al. Jugular bulb oxygen saturation under propofol or sevoflurane/nitrous oxide anesthesia during deliberate mild hypothermia in neurosurgical patients. *J Neurosurg Anesthesiol.* 2004;16(1):6–10.

24. Strebel S, Lam AM, Matta B, et al. Dynamic and static cerebral autoregulation during isoflurane, desflurane, and propofol anesthesia. *Anesthesiology.* 1995;83(1):66–76.

25. Johnston AJ, Steiner LA, Chatfield DA, et al. Effects of propofol on cerebral oxygenation and metabolism after head injury. *Br J Anaesth.* 2003;91(6):781–786.

26. Talke P, Caldwell JE, Brown R, et al. A comparison of three anesthetic techniques in patients undergoing craniotomy for supratentorial intracranial surgery. *Anesth Analg.* 2002;95(2):430–435.

27. Boisseau N1, Madany M, Staccini P, et al. Comparison of the effects of sevoflurane and propofol on cortical somatosensory evoked potentials. *Br J Anaesth.* 2002;88(6):785–789.

28. Sloan TB, Toleikis JR, Toleikis SC, et al. Intraoperative neurophysiological monitoring during spine surgery with total intravenous anesthesia or balanced anesthesia with 3% desflurane. *J Clin Monit Comput.* 2014;19 [Epub ahead of print].

29. Chong CT, Manninen P, Sivanaser V, et al. Direct comparison of the effect of desflurane and sevoflurane on intraoperative motor-evoked potentials monitoring. *J Neurosurg Anesthesiol.* 2014;30 [Epub ahead of print].

30. Pilge S, Jordan D, Kochs EF, et al. Sevoflurane-induced epileptiform electroencephalographic activity and generalized tonic-clonic seizures in a volunteer study. *Anesthesiology.* 2013;119(2):447.

31. Sharma D, Bithal PK, Dash HH, et al. Cerebral autoregulation and CO2 reactivity before and after elective supratentorial tumor resection. *J Neurosurg Anesthesiol.* 2010;22(2):132–137.

32. Bendok BR, Gupta DK, Rahme RJ, et al. Adenosine for temporary flow arrest during intracranial aneurysm surgery: a single-center retrospective review. *Neurosurgery.* 2011;69(4):815–820.

33. SAFE Study Investigators; Australian and New Zealand Intensive Care Society Clinical Trials Group; Australian Red Cross Blood Service; George Institute for International Health. Myburgh J, Cooper DJ, Finfer S, et al. Saline or albumin for fluid resuscitation in patients with traumatic brain injury. *N Engl J Med.* 2007;357(9):874–884.

34. Oppitz PP, Stefani MA. Acute normovolemic hemodilution is safe in neurosurgery. *World Neurosurg.* 2013;79(5-6):719–724.

35. Sharma D, Ellenbogen RG, Vavilala MS. Use of transcranial Doppler ultrasonography and jugular oximetry to optimize hemodynamics during pediatric posterior fossa craniotomy. *J Clin Neurosci.* 2010;17(12):1583–1584.

36. Sharma D, Siriussawakul A, Dooney N, et al. Clinical experience with intraoperative jugular venous oximetry during pediatric intracranial neurosurgery. *Paediatr Anaesth.* 2013;23(1):84–90.

37. Gelb AW, Craen RA, Rao GS, et al. Does hyperventilation improve operating condition during supratentorial craniotomy? A multicenter randomized crossover trial. *Anesth Analg.* 2008;106(2):585–594.

38. Curley G, Kavanagh BP, Laffey JG. Hypocapnia and the injured brain: more harm than benefit. *Crit Care Med.* 2010;38(5):1348–1359.

39. Rozet I, Tontisirin N, Muangman S, et al. Effect of equiosmolar solutions of mannitol versus hypertonic saline on intraoperative brain relaxation and electrolyte balance. *Anesthesiology.* 2007;107(5):697–704.

40. Pecha T, Sharma D, Hoffman NG, et al. Hyperglycemia during craniotomy for adult traumatic brain injury. *Anesth Analg.* 2011;113(2):336–342.

41. Sharma D, Jelacic J, Chennuri R, et al. Incidence and risk factors for perioperative hyperglycemia in children with traumatic brain injury. *Anesth Analg.* 2009;108(1):81–89.

42. Todd MM, Hindman BJ, Clarke WR, et al. Intraoperative Hypothermia for Aneurysm Surgery Trial (IHAST) Investigators. Mild intraoperative hypothermia during surgery for intracranial aneurysm. *N Engl J Med.* 2005;352(2):135–145.

43. Lauta E, Abbinante C, Del Gaudio A, et al. Emergence times are similar with sevoflurane and total intravenous anesthesia: results of a multicenter RCT of patients scheduled for elective supratentorial craniotomy. *J Neurosurg Anesthesiol.* 2010;22(2):110–118.

44. Magni G1, Rosa IL, Melillo G, et al. A comparison between sevoflurane and desflurane anesthesia in patients undergoing craniotomy for supratentorial intracranial surgery. *Anesth Analg.* 2009;109(2):567–571.

45. Soliman RN, Hassan AR, Rashwan AM, et al. Prospective, randomized study to assess the role of dexmedetomidine in patients with supratentorial tumors undergoing craniotomy under general anaesthesia. *Middle East J Anesthesiol.* 2011;21(3):325–334.

46. Basali M, Mascha EJ, Kalfas I, et al. Relation between perioperative hypertension and intracranial hemorrhage after craniotomy. *Anesthesiology.* 2000;93(1):48–54.

47. Sudheer PS, Logan SW, Terblanche C, et al. Comparison of the analgesic efficacy and respiratory effects of morphine, tramadol and codeine after craniotomy. *Anaesthesia.* 2007;62(6):555–560.

48. Rahimi SY, Alleyne CH, Vernier E, et al. Postoperative pain management with tramadol after craniotomy: evaluation and cost analysis. *J Neurosurg.* 2010;112(2):268–272.

49. Williams DL, Pemberton E, Leslie K. Effect of intravenous parecoxib on post-craniotomy pain. *Br J Anaesth.* 2011;107(3):398–403.

50. Guilfoyle MR, Helmy A, Duane D, et al. Regional scalp block for post-craniotomy analgesia: a systematic review and meta-analysis. *Anesth Analg.* 2013;116(5):1093–1102.

51. Neufeld SM, Newburn-Cook CV. The efficacy of 5-HT3 receptor antagonists for the prevention of postoperative nausea and vomiting after craniotomy: a meta-analysis. *J Neurosurg Anesthesiol.* 2007;19(1):10–17.

# 4 Perioperative Anesthetic and ICU Considerations for Spinal Surgery

KOFFI M. KLA and LORRI A. LEE

## Introduction

More spinal surgeries are performed in the United States than any other country in the world. Over the last 3 decades, lumbar spinal fusion rates have risen dramatically, with rates increasing 2-fold in the 1980s, 3-fold in the 1990s, and 2.4 fold from 1998 to 2008.[1,2] The steep rise in spinal surgery is attributed to many changes, including a rapidly aging population with degenerative spinal disease, advanced surgical techniques and equipment, and a change in practice toward more instrumented spinal fusion procedures for diagnoses that were previously treated with a simple decompression.[3] Multilevel spinal reconstruction may take up to 8 to 12 hours or more and lose more than the patient's entire estimated blood volume. These cases are frequently performed on and near vital structures and in the prone or lateral position, making airway edema and positioning injuries more likely. The highest rate of increase in spinal fusion surgery has been in patients over the age of 60 years who have more comorbidities and experience higher complication rates.[1,4] The combination of prolonged surgery with high blood loss in locations that can result in severe neurological injury or airway compromise and older patients with more coexisting disease frequently results in the need for intensive care with ongoing resuscitation postoperatively. This chapter is geared toward the neurointensivist and divided into subheadings discussing complications or issues related to all spine procedures as well as a focus on site-specific complications.

### PREOPERATIVE PLANNING: SURGICAL SPINE PATHWAY

> **Key Concept**
>
> Prehabilitation, spine clinical pathways, and rehabilitation should be considered as early as possible for all spine patients to improve outcomes and decrease length of stay and increase patient satisfaction.

Preoperative planning before spine surgery can be helpful in optimizing patients for surgery and managing postoperative expectations. Many hospitals have developed clinical pathways for spine surgery, which can involve a multidisciplinary team of physical therapists, nutritionists, and pain management physicians who help with planning for preoperative and postoperative therapies. Studies have shown that preoperative analgesic optimization, protein supplementation, and exercise programs (prehabilitation) along with early postoperative rehabilitation led to less postoperative pain, earlier hospital discharge, and cost savings of several thousand dollars.[5–7]

> **Clinical Pearls**
>
> Develop spine clinical care pathways with a multidisciplinary team
>
> - Consultation with anesthesiologist for patients with severe coexisting diseases
>   - Consider conservative management
>   - Consider staging prolonged procedures
> - Consider prehabilitation with physical therapy
>   - Enlist family support for exercises at home
> - Improved nutrition preoperatively
>   - For morbidly obese, may need significant weight loss prior to elective procedure
> - Pain specialist consultation if on chronic opioids
>   - Consider weaning from high-dose opioids
>   - Consider starting nonopioid analgesics
>   - Patients on buprenorphine require special analgesic regimens—may require weaning preoperatively
> - Develop multimodal analgesia regimen
> - Assess likelihood of inpatient physical therapy/occupational therapy
> - Assess nutrition postoperatively
>   - May need swallow evaluation
>   - Protein supplementation
> - Assess likelihood of need for discharge to rehabilitation center or skilled nursing facility
> - Constantly reevaluate status of patient to anticipate postacute care needs

### PAIN CONTROL

> **Key Concepts**
>
> - Chronic opioid use is common in patients presenting for elective spinal procedures and can complicate the postoperative course with respiratory depression, increased length of stay, and patient dissatisfaction.
> - Consultation with the pain management service and development of multimodal analgesic algorithms that minimize the use of opioids may improve short- and long-term outcomes.

Pain control can be a major issue delaying recovery for spine patients. Patients taking opioid medications prior to surgery may have increased opioid requirements postoperatively. A study of spine surgery patients found that 20% were opioid dependent, with the highest rates in lumbar decompression and fusion cases (23.8%) and among women (22.8%).[8] A study of 2378 lumbar fusion patients found that analgesic-related deaths were responsible for 21% of all deaths long term and 31.4% of all potential life lost.[9] Enlisting the pain service prior to admission to provide recommendations or to manage patients perioperatively with chronic pain issues and high-dose opioid requirements is recommended. This can be particularly problematic with the high rates of obesity in spine patients and associated obstructive sleep apnea.[10] Use of multimodal analgesia in the perioperative period with adjuncts such as gabapentin, acetaminophen, ketamine, nonsteroidal antiinflammatory drugs (if not contraindicated), and other drugs should be utilized to minimize the dosages of opioids required.[11]

## ACUTE SPINE INJURY: PREOPERATIVE ASSESSMENT AND OPTIMIZATION BY THE NEUROINTENSIVIST AND ANESTHESIOLOGIST

### Key Concepts

- Stabilization of traumatic spine injuries is critical for early mobilization.
- Neurogenic shock with acute spinal cord injury may require volume resuscitation and atropine/vasopressor/inotropic support to maintain adequate spinal cord perfusion.
- In patients with poor intracranial compliance (e.g., traumatic brain injury) from coexisting intracranial pathology, the prone position for acute spinal cord injury will increase intracranial pressure (ICP) because the prone position increases intraabdominal and intrathoracic pressure and reduces venous return, cardiac output, and renal perfusion.
- Preoperative communication with the anesthesiologist and surgeon for optimization of the patient's hemodynamics, oxygenation, and coagulation and transfusion parameters is recommended to improve outcomes.

The neurocritical care unit may manage spine patients both preoperatively and postoperatively. Knowledge of the procedure and potential complications will enable the intensivist to better prepare the patient for surgery. Patients who are cared for in the neurocritical care unit preoperatively prior to major spine surgery may have associated major traumatic injuries, acute lung injury, acute spinal cord injury, and/or a traumatic brain injury. Stabilizing the spine in trauma patients is critical for optimal mobilization, and surgery should be done as soon as is safely possible. Careful neurological examination of patients immediately prior to their operative interventions is important to provide a baseline neurological assessment so that any new neurological injuries postoperatively may be

addressed quickly. Goals for the management of acute spinal cord injuries include limiting secondary injury and maximizing spinal cord perfusion. Neurogenic shock can cause hemodynamic instability, resulting in bradycardia, cardiac dysfunction, hypotension, and decreased systemic vascular resistance and often requires atropine, volume resuscitation, and vasopressor/inotropic support to maintain spinal cord perfusion.[12]

## TRANSFUSION THRESHOLD AND CORRECTION OF COAGULOPATHY

### Key Concepts

- The transfusion threshold in the intensive care unit (ICU) may need to be adjusted by anticipated events in the operating room and concerns for vascular reserve during surgery.
- Coagulopathy, thrombocytopenia, and thrombocytopathia must be avoided during spinal surgery.

Numerous studies have demonstrated reduced morbidity and mortality with lower transfusion thresholds in the ICU in a nonoperative setting. For minor operative procedures in areas at low risk for hemorrhage, transfusion is rarely required in the operating room. However, for major spine operations, hemorrhage may be relatively rapid. Preoperative hematocrit levels of greater than 21% may provide a margin of safety. The risk of transfusion should be weighed against the risk of rapid hemorrhage. Knowledge of the procedure, the patient's disease, local surgical practice, and ready availability of blood products are critical elements in assessing the transfusion threshold. Coagulopathy in major spine surgery can be very detrimental because there are large surfaces of decorticated bone that can be difficult to completely cauterize. In this regard, many anesthesiologists administer antifibrinolytics during the procedure in addition to optimizing the international normalized ratio and platelet count. Antifibrinolytics have been shown to decrease total blood loss and transfusions during spine surgery. Although they do not appear to increase the risk of thrombotic events, caution is warranted in patients at high risk for clotting.[13] The decision to use antifibrinolytics should be made in conjunction with the surgical team and on an individual patient basis.

# Perioperative Concerns in Management of Patients Undergoing Spinal Surgery

### Key Concepts

- Fluid management should be goal directed to maintain euvolemia.
- Target mean arterial pressure (MAP) for acute spinal cord injuries should be close to baseline MAP or higher.

- Intraoperative emboli from air, fat, bone marrow, and cement are common, particularly during pedicle screw insertion and injection of cement.
- Increased surgical duration of 5 or more hours correlates with significant increases in multiple medical and surgical complications.
- Positioning injuries are common with major spine operations and may include pressure sores, facial and airway edema requiring postoperative mechanical ventilation, nerve injuries, and postoperative visual loss (POVL).

Major spine procedures involve numerous considerations by the anesthesiologist. For patients admitted to the ICU preoperatively, neurointensivists can facilitate perioperative care by ensuring euvolemia prior to the operation, optimizing any end organ dysfunction, correcting coagulopathy, and having cross-matched blood available for transfusion. A detailed conversation preoperatively with the anesthesiologist regarding the patient will ensure good transition of care.

## Clinical Pearls

- Neurological status/stability of spine
  - Avoid succinylcholine for spinal cord injury patients with motor deficits present greater than 48 hours
  - Neurogenic shock
- Urgency of procedure
- Coexisting illnesses or conditions of heightened concern
  - Severe cardiac conditions with prone position or large resuscitation
  - Severe COPD with $CO_2$ retention or restrictive lung disease and anterior thoracic procedures
  - Elevated intracranial pressure and prone position
  - Acute kidney injury and prone position
- Prone vs. supine position
- Airway issues and spine disease
  - Cervical spine instability, severe cervical stenosis, or acute cervical spinal cord injury
- Pain management
- Expected EBL
  - A function of procedure, surgical technique, patient conditions, and anesthetic/coagulation management
- Coagulopathy
  - Tighter control than for intraabdominal or extremity surgery because there is diffuse bleeding with possibly high EBL, and postoperative hematoma may cause severe permanent neurological disability
- Availability of blood and blood products and patient acceptance of transfusion
- Adequate intravenous access
- Arterial line monitoring
  - Pulse pressure variation (PPV) and stroke volume variation (SVV) indicate fluid responsiveness in the prone position with positive pressure ventilation
- Fluid management
  - Crystalloid vs. colloid
    - Consider potential for edema formation in prone position
    - Risk of ischemic optic neuropathy increased in prone position with lower % colloid administration
  - Goal-directed fluid therapy
- Transfusion threshold

- Consider potential for rapid blood loss and cardiac conditions that may not tolerate rapid infusion of products
- Cases with large EBL will frequently lose 1–2 units of PRBCs in their drains overnight.
- Target MAP range
  - Close to baseline MAP if acute spinal cord injury
  - Increase MAP to baseline for any significant change in motor-evoked potentials (MEP) or somatosensory-evoked potentials (SSEP)
- Expected operative duration
  - Both surgical and operative complications increase with increasing operative time.
- Intraoperative neuromonitoring and impact on anesthetic
- Positioning injuries
  - SSEPs are nearly 100% specific and can detect early nerve injury
  - Prone superman and lateral positions at increased risk of nerve injury
  - Skin pressure sores common—consider padding high-risk sites for prone position
  - Use biteblock between molars (not oral airway) to prevent tongue getting caught between teeth—critical with MEP neuromonitoring and to prevent endotracheal tube obstruction
  - Perform and document frequent and regular eye and nose checks
- Likelihood of postoperative ventilation
- Availability of ICU bed
- Site-specific complications

*COPD*, chronic obstructive pulmonary disease; *EBL*, estimated blood loss; *PRBC*, packed red blood cell; *MAP*, mean arterial pressure; *ICU*, intensive care unit.

## FLUID AND HEMODYNAMIC MANAGEMENT

Several retrospective studies have demonstrated poorer outcomes in spine surgery with increased total volume of fluids administered, but these high volumes are frequently related to high estimated blood loss (EBL).[14] There is a paucity of data using goal-directed fluid therapy for major spine surgery in the prone position with respect to outcomes. Pulse pressure variation (PPV) and stroke volume variation (SVV) obtained from the arterial line pressure tracing are useful indicators of fluid responsiveness but the prone position has slightly higher thresholds (e.g., 14%–15% PPV prone versus 9%–11% PPV supine), indicating volume responsiveness compared with the supine position.[15]

The optimal MAP needed during major spine operations remains controversial. Blood pressure goals for patients with acute spinal cord injuries aim to maintain the MAP near baseline levels to optimize spinal cord perfusion and minimize secondary injury. Several case reports and series have shown that deterioration of evoked potentials, signifying an impending nerve injury, can be reversed with elevation of the MAP in some situations.[16] In addition, the lowest MAP is one of the three determinants of the surgical Apgar score (along with the lowest heart rate and EBL) that has correlated with poorer outcomes in spine surgery patients.[17] However, adequate cardiac output and oxygen delivery are equally, if not more, important than MAP, as demonstrated in a hemorrhagic swine model utilizing motor-evoked potentials.[18]

## INTRAOPERATIVE EMBOLI

Although intraoperative emboli can occur in other types of spine operations, they are particularly common during major thoracolumbar scoliosis revisions. The large venous channels in the thoracolumbar spine, the numerous vertebral levels involved in these procedures, and the high number of pedicle screws inserted may explain their frequency in these procedures. One study utilizing transesophageal echocardiography in the prone position found an 80% incidence of moderate- to high-grade emboli in instrumented spines, particularly during pedicle screw insertion.[19] Injection of cement that is sometimes used for vertebral augmentation, vertebroplasty, or kyphoplasty can leak out into a vessel and cause a pulmonary embolus with acute cardiovascular collapse or embolize paradoxically through a patent foramen ovale to the brain or other vital organs. Most patients do not have obvious hemodynamic effects from these thousands of microemboli, but it is possible that they contribute to surgical inflammation and other complications.

## OPERATIVE DURATION AND COMPLICATIONS

Longer surgical duration has been associated with an increase in the incidence of complications.[20] Kim et al. analyzed 4588 lumbar fusion cases and found that as operative duration increased, the overall complication risk increased (Table 4.1). Operations lasting 5 or more hours were associated with increased reoperation rates, surgical site infections, sepsis, wound dehiscence, deep vein thrombosis (DVT), and postoperative transfusion compared with those less than 2 hours in duration.

## POSITIONING-RELATED COMPLICATIONS

### Physiological Changes

Intensivists and anesthesiologists should be aware of the physiological changes incurred with prone positioning in the operating room, including increased intraabdominal and intrathoracic pressures, reduced venous return and cardiac output, reduced renal perfusion, and elevation of the ICP in a noncompliant cranium. Hypovolemia will exaggerate these changes. Conservative management or postponement of surgery should be considered for patients with poorly controlled intracranial hypertension or extremely tenuous cardiopulmonary conditions.

An important consideration in evaluating effects of prone positioning is the integrity of the airway. Use of some prone pillows can predispose to endotracheal tube kinks with associated airway obstruction. Prone patients in pins or prone head rests may be susceptible to inadvertent extubation. Most anesthesiologists pay extra attention to securing the airway with tape and securing the breathing circuit to the bed or head frame to avoid tension on the airway.

---

### Clinical Pearls

**Physiological Changes with Prone Position**

- Increased intraabdominal pressure
  - Decreased renal perfusion
- Increased intrathoracic pressure
  - Increased peak airway pressures
  - Increased central venous pressure
    - Increased venous pressure in the head
    - Increased intracranial pressure with poor intracranial compliance
    - Increased interstitial edema
- Decreased venous return
  - Decreased cardiac output
    - Decreased end organ perfusion
  - Increased systemic vascular resistance

**Possible Complications from Physiological Changes of Prone Position**

- Hypotension
- Relative hypovolemia from reduced venous return
  - May affect patients who are preload dependent such as severe pulmonary hypertension, critical aortic stenosis, etc.
- Acute kidney injury if relative hypovolemia and hypotension persist
- Inadequate oxygenation and ventilation from high intrathoracic pressure
  - Oxygenation typically improves in the prone position if adequate tidal volumes can be achieved
- Elevated intracranial pressure with poor intracranial compliance (e.g., traumatic brain injury)
- Facial edema
  - Chemosis and inadequate closure of eyelids
- Airway edema
  - Postoperative ventilation
- Ischemic optic neuropathy (vision loss)

---

**Table 4.1** Risk of Complications with Increased Operative Duration*

|  | Odds ratio | 95% CI | p value |
|---|---|---|---|
| All complications | 5.73 | 3.69–8.89 | <0.001 |
| Postoperative transfusions | 12.19 | 5.33–27.87 | <0.001 |
| Sepsis | 4.41 | 1.72–11.31 | 0.002 |
| Reoperation rates | 2.17 | 1.25–3.79 | 0.006 |
| Deep venous thrombosis | 17.22 | 2.20–134.65 | 0.007 |
| Wound dehiscence | 10.98 | 1.32–91.37 | 0.027 |
| Deep surgical site infections | 9.72 | 1.18–80.22 | 0.035 |

*Comparison of single-level lumbar fusion procedures lasting 5 or more hours to those lasting less than 2 hours.
Adapted with permission from Kim BD, Hsu WK, De Oliveira GS, Saha S, Kim JYS. Operative duration as an independent risk factor for postoperative complications in single-level lumbar fusions. *Spine.* 2014;39(6):510–20.

### Facial and Oropharyngeal Edema Requiring Postoperative Mechanical Ventilation

Edema of the face and oropharynx can occur after procedures done in the prone position. This is especially true for longer cases in which greater amounts of intravenous fluids are administered. Facial and oropharyngeal edema may lead to airway issues postoperatively. Some patients

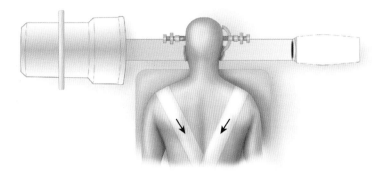

**Fig. 4.1** The shoulders are gently pulled caudad by adhesive tape. (Reprinted from Vaccaro AR, Baron EM. *Operative techniques: spine surgery*, 2nd ed. Philadelphia, PA: Elsevier/Saunders; 2012.)

need to remain intubated in the postoperative period until swelling subsides. Airway edema can be evaluated by direct laryngoscopy or fiberoptic examination. Checking for leaks around the endotracheal tube with the cuff deflated can also be done, with lesser leaks being more predictive of post-extubation stridor and increased risk of reintubation.[21] In extubated patients, edema can make mask ventilation and reintubation difficult even if the preoperative intubation was uncomplicated.

### Peripheral Nerve and Skin Positioning Injuries

Brachial plexus stretch injuries may occur from taping the shoulders (Fig. 4.1) to increase exposure of the cervical and high thoracic spine while the arms are tucked. Injuries to the brachial plexus can also occur from direct compression from chest supports. The ulnar nerve is at risk for injury from direct pressure or stretch injury. A study by Kamel et al. showed that changes in somatosensory-evoked potentials, which are nearly 100% specific for impending nerve injury, occurred in 7.5% of procedures in the lateral decubitus position and in 7% of operations in the prone superman position, and are easily reversed with repositioning or loosening of tape.[22] Skin necrosis from pressure points in the prone position is a common problem; however, it is frequently underreported because of its quick resolution. Areas at risk in the prone position include the forehead, chin, cheeks, nose, tongue, chest, and iliac crests. Padding some of these skin areas at risk may reduce the risk of pressure sores, but definitive data are lacking.

### Postoperative Visual Loss

POVL is a rare, but potentially catastrophic, complication associated with major spine surgery in the prone position. Its diagnosis, risk factors, and workup are discussed in more detail at the end of this chapter.

## Specific Operative Procedures and Complications

### Key Concepts

- The overall complication rate in all spinal fusion procedures is approximately 10%, but certain procedures, such as major spinal reconstruction for scoliosis, may have complication rates as high as 61%.

### Key Concepts

- Knowledge of the specific procedure in terms of anatomy and potential complications, as well as the patient population, is critical for prevention or early detection of complications.
- Elderly patients with cervical fractures from falls from standing may have early mortality as high as 13% to 50% depending on the presence of a neurological deficit.
- Patients in the ICU preoperatively may have higher complication rates than published data suggest, given the high presurgical acuity.

Knowledge of the most common types of complications in spine surgery patients informs the entire perioperative management with preventative measures and heightened scrutiny preoperatively, intraoperatively, and postoperatively. The overall complication rate for spinal fusion procedures in 5887 patients in the National Surgical Quality Improvement Project (NSQIP) from 2005 to 2010 was 10%,[23] although rates for major thoracolumbar surgery for scoliosis are as high as 61%.[24] Certain patient populations, such as elderly patients with odontoid fractures and neurological deficit, may have an early mortality rate up to 50%.[25]

Significant complications for major spine surgery that may be diagnosed in the ICU or lead to an ICU admission are shown in Table 4.2. Knowledge of the surrounding anatomy for these spine procedures, as well as the muscles and dermatomes innervated by the spinal cord and peripheral nerves at risk during a procedure, are critical for anticipating, diagnosing, and treating complications (Figs. 4.2a and 4.2b).

Many of these complications will be discussed in further detail in subsequent chapters covering different approaches to the spine (Chapters 31–33).

## ANTERIOR CERVICAL SPINE PROCEDURES

### Key Concepts

- Dysphagia is common after anterior cervical procedures and may be related to edema or nerve injury. Swallowing studies are recommended for symptomatic patients.
- Hoarseness from vocal cord paralysis from recurrent laryngeal nerve (RLN) injury is symptomatic in approximately 2% to 3% of patients, but occurs without symptoms more commonly.
- Reintubation occurs in up to 5% to 6% of patients, with symptom onset approximately 24 hours postoperatively. Risk factors from one study included surgical duration more than 5 hours, blood loss more than 300 mL, surgery on C4 or higher, and more than three levels of exposure.

**Table 4.2**  Complications Associated with Spinal Fusion Surgery

| Complication | Anterior Cervical Discectomy and Fusion[26-37,39-42] | Posterior Cervical Spine Surgery[37-40,43,54] | Thoracolumbar Fusion for Scoliosis[24,45-50] | Odontoid Fracture Surgery in the Elderly[25,51-53] (higher ranges with neurological deficits) |
|---|---|---|---|---|
| | range (%) | range (%) | range (%) | range (%) |
| In-hospital mortality or 90-day mortality | 0.1–0.3 | 0.7 | 0.5–3.5 | 10–50 |
| 1-yr mortality | 0.2–2 | | | 5–36 |
| Pneumonia | 1 | 6.2 | 10.5* | 5–90 |
| Respiratory failure | 1 | | | 3–40 |
| Tracheotomy | | | | 3–25 |
| Prolonged intubation or reintubation | 1–6 | | | 1–13 |
| Recurrent laryngeal nerve palsy | 2–24 | NA | NA | 3 |
| Wound hematoma | 0.6–0.7 | 1.3 | 2.7 | 1–5 |
| Cardiac (failure, infarction, arrhythmia) | 0.3–3 | 0.8 | 2.8 | 2–38 |
| Deep venous thrombosis/embolism | 0.6–2 | 0.8 | 1–4 | 2–6 |
| Stroke | | | 1.4 | 0–3 |
| Vertebral artery injury | 0.3 | 4.1 | NA | |
| Dysphagia | 10–79 | 0–21 | 0 | 7–13 |
| New or worsened neurological deficit | 0.2 | 0.03–12 | 4–7.4 | 4 |
| C5 palsy | 7–8.5 | 4.8–9.5 | NA | |
| Epidural hematoma | 0.2 | 1.5 | 4.5 | |
| Lateral femoral cutaneous nerve injury | NA | | 20 | |
| Esophageal/pharyngeal perforation | 0.3–1.5 | NA | NA | |

*Described as "pulmonary complications," not including pulmonary embolus.
*NA*, not applicable.

Anterior cervical spine surgery is a commonly performed procedure used to treat a wide variety of cervical pathologies. Structures at risk during this approach include the superior laryngeal nerve, RLN, sympathetic trunk, spinal accessory nerve, esophagus, trachea, carotid artery, and jugular vein (Fig. 4.3). Anterior cervical spine procedures carry a relatively low complication rate of approximately 3%, with the exception of dysphagia, which is very common in these procedures.[26] Injuries reported include cerebrospinal fluid leak, RLN injury, nerve root injury, quadriplegia, and death.

## Nerve Injuries

The rate of worsened myelopathy (0.2%) or new-onset neurological injury postoperatively after anterior cervical spine surgery is relatively low,[27] although procedures for myelopathy around the C4–5 level have up to 8.5% incidence of delayed onset of C5 palsy.[28] Intraoperative somatosensory-evoked potential (SSEP) monitoring, which is approximately 50% sensitive and nearly 100% specific, can detect surgical- and positioning-related impending nerve injuries. Intraoperative positioning-related injuries may frequently be corrected with loosening of the shoulder tape, removal of the weight attached to the cranial tongs, or

repositioning of the head or arms. If a nerve injury in the operative site is suspected postoperatively, surgeons will frequently obtain computed tomography (CT) scans to ensure that the pedicle screws are not near the nerve roots. For nonoperative site injuries, evaluation by a neurologist should occur as early as possible. Electrophysiological testing may be done; however, it may have to be delayed several weeks to ensure accuracy.

## Recurrent Laryngeal Nerve Injury

RLN injury usually presents postoperatively with voice changes and/or hoarseness. Symptomatic incidence varies between 2.3% and 24.2%, and most patients recover within 1 year.[29] Either unilateral or bilateral (seen with revision surgery approached from the contralateral side) vocal cord paralysis can cause airway compromise and should be considered early in the differential if patients exhibit respiratory distress after extubation. Consultation with an otolaryngologist can be helpful in diagnosing vocal cord dysfunction. If present, evaluation of speech and swallowing should be done to minimize the risk of aspiration. Patients with significant respiratory compromise should be reintubated and may require tracheostomy if bilateral nerve injuries are present.

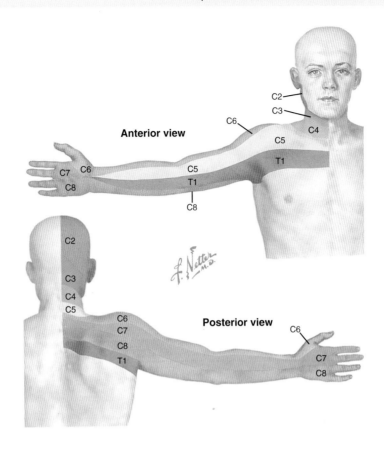

| LEVEL | MOTOR | SENSORY | REFLEX | COMMENT |
|---|---|---|---|---|
| **CERVICAL ROOTS** | | | | |
| C1 | Geniohyoid Thyrohyoid Rectus capitus | None | None | Part of cervical plexus, contributes to ansa cervicalis |
| C2 | Longus colli/capitis | Parietal scalp | None | Muscle innervation via the dorsal rami |
| C3 | Diaphragm | Occipital scalp | None | Contributes to phrenic & dorsal scapular nerves |
| C4 | Diaphragm | Base of neck | None | Branches to phrenic and dorsal scapular nerves & levator scapula muscle |
| C5 | Deltoid | Lateral shoulder and arm | Biceps | Dorsal scapular n. branches from C5 root |
| C6 | Biceps brachii ECRL, ECRB | Lateral forearm and thumb | Brachioradialis | Most commonly compressed cervical nerve root |
| C7 | Triceps brachii FCR, FCU | Posterior forearm, central hand, and middle finger | Triceps | Exits above C7 vertebra |
| C8 | FDS, FDP | Medial forearm, ulnar fingers | None | Exits below C7 vertebra |
| T1 | Interosseous | Medial arm | None | Only thoracic root in brachial plexus |

A

**Fig. 4.2AB** Knowledge of the dermatomes and muscles innervated by the area of the spinal cord at risk, as well as the anatomical structures located near the site of operation such as major blood vessels, esophagus, recurrent laryngeal nerve, and others will inform the neurointensivist of potential complications postoperatively. **(A)** Upper extremity dermatomes. (Reprinted from Thompson JC, ed. *Netter's concise orthopaedic anatomy*, 2nd ed. Philadelphia, PA: Saunders, Elsevier; 2010: pp. 62–3.)

*(continued)*

## Reintubation and Airway Obstruction from Edema or Hematoma

One of the most potentially life-threatening complications is postoperative airway obstruction due to hematoma or pharyngeal edema. Hematomas can expand quickly and cause distortion of the anatomical structures, which can make airway management more difficult. The incidence of hematomas after anterior cervical discectomy and fusion surgery ranges from 0.6% to 0.7%, and risk factors include presence of diffuse idiopathic skeletal hyperostosis, presence of ossification of the posterior longitudinal ligament, therapeutic heparin use, longer operative time, and greater number of surgical levels.[30]

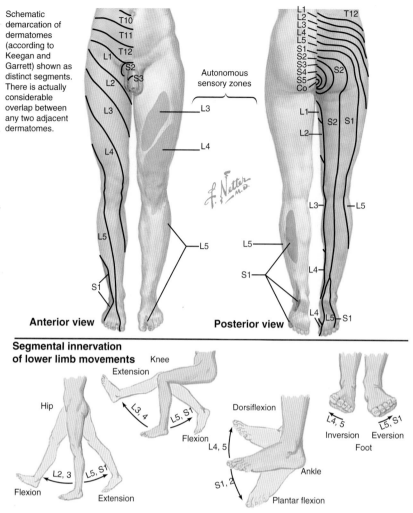

Schematic demarcation of dermatomes (according to Keegan and Garrett) shown as distinct segments. There is actually considerable overlap between any two adjacent dermatomes.

| LEVEL | MOTOR | SENSORY | REFLEX | COMMENT |
|---|---|---|---|---|
| | | **LUMBOSACRAL ROOTS** | | |
| L1 | Transversus abdominis Internal oblique | Inguinal region | None | Rarely injured nerve root |
| L2 | Psoas | Upper thigh | None | Test with hip flexion |
| L3 | Quadriceps | Anterior and medial thigh | None | L3 & L4 tested with quadriceps |
| L4 | Tibialis anterior | Medial leg, ankle, foot | Patellar | Test with ankle dorsiflexion |
| L5 | Extensor hallux longus | Dorsal/plantar foot, 1st web space, lateral leg | Hamstring | Most commonly compressed lumbar root; test with hallux dorsiflexion |
| S1 | Gastrocnemius | Lateral foot, posterior leg | Achilles | Test with ankle plantar flexion/toe walking |
| S2-4 | Sphincter | Perianal sensation | Anal wink | Test tone to evaluate for cauda equina syndrome |

**Fig. 4.2AB, cont'd** **(B)** Lower extremity dermatomes.

One of two small studies on anterior cervical procedures found that 6.1% of 311 patients had an airway complication, with six patients requiring reintubation.[31] The second study found 7 of 133 patients (5.2%) required reintubation. Mean time to symptom onset was 24 hours for patients requiring reintubation in the first study, and an average of 3 hours to reintubation in the second. Risk factors for airway complications were operative duration more than 5 hours; blood loss greater than 300 mL; exposure of more than three vertebral levels; or surgery on C2, C3, or C4 in the first study and preoperative myelopathy and multilevel corpectomy in the second.[31] Both studies attributed the airway compromise to edema and not hematoma.[31,32] Careful assessment of the patient's ventilation and airway prior to transfer out of the ICU, particularly on the first postoperative day, is recommended in light of these findings. A recent

**Anterior Approach to Cervical Spine**

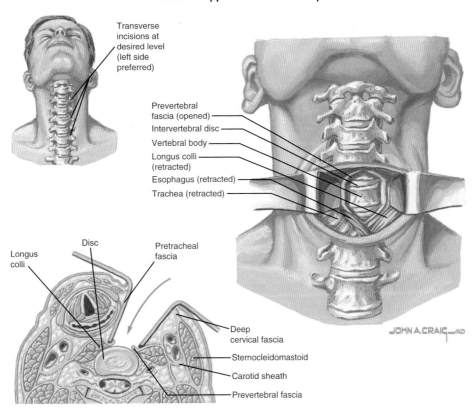

| USES | INTERNERVOUS PLANE | DANGERS | COMMENT |
|---|---|---|---|
| **ANTERIOR APPROACH** | | | |
| • Anterior cervical dis-kectomy & fusion (ACDF) for cervical spondylosis and/or HNP<br>• Tumor or biopsy | **Superficial**<br>Deep cervical fascia: SCM goes lateral<br>Pretracheal fascia: carotid sheath goes lateral<br>**Deep**<br>Prevertebral fascia be-tween longus collis muscles (right & left) | • Recurrent laryngeal n.<br>• Sympathetic n.<br>• Carotid artery<br>• Internal jugular<br>• Vagus nerve<br>• Inferior thyroid artery | • Access C3 to T1<br>• Right recurrent laryngeal nerve more susceptible to injury; many surgeons approach on left side<br>• Thyroid arteries limit extension of the approach |

**Fig. 4.3** Operative approach for anterior cervical discectomy and fusion. Note the numerous structures at risk for injury, including the carotid artery, internal and external jugular veins, pharynx, esophagus, recurrent laryngeal nerve, pleura, and others. (Reprinted from Thompson JC, ed. *Netter's concise orthopaedic anatomy*, 2nd ed. Philadelphia, PA: Saunders, Elsevier; 2010: p. 73.)

analysis of the Nationwide Inpatient Sample database from 2002 to 2011 examining airway compromise in 262,425 anterior cervical spine surgery patients found a 0.56% incidence (n = 1464) of reintubation during admission.[33] Corpectomies may further increase the risk of postoperative upper airway obstruction.[32]

Emergency intubation for airway obstruction from hematoma or edema can be challenging. Opening the neck at the bedside will relieve pressure from a rapidly expanding hematoma but may be less helpful for edema or a hematoma tracking cephalad. Awake or asleep intubation with a variety of airway devices, including direct laryngoscopy, may be utilized depending on the situation and degree of airway compromise. Emergency airway equipment (e.g., fiberoptic scopes, video-laryngoscopes, tracheostomy tray), anesthesiologists, and airway surgeons should be available when possible for intubating

these very high-risk patients. A similar level of support may be considered when extubating such patients in the context of lack of certainty regarding success of extubation.

## Pharyngeal and Esophageal Perforations

Pharyngeal and esophageal perforations are rare but potentially fatal complications of anterior cervical spine surgery that can result in pneumothorax, mediastinitis, sepsis, and respiratory failure. Reported incidence is between 0.25% and 1.49%, and mortality is as high as 19%.[34] Perforations may be immediate with symptoms developing within the first few days, or delayed by years with erosion of hardware into the esophagus. The three most common signs and symptoms are dysphagia, neck abscess, and aspiration pneumonia.[34]

## Dysphagia

Dysphagia is the most common complication after anterior cervical spine surgery. A recent literature review found that 1% to 79% of patients have dysphagia in the first week after surgery, 50% to 56% at 1 month, and 8% to 21% at 6 months.[35] The incidence progressively decreases over time, but as many as 11% to 13% of patients may have dysphagia at 2 years after surgery. Swallowing evaluations should be obtained for more clinically symptomatic cases to reduce the risk of aspiration. In some cases tube feeding is indicated postoperatively, and if intractable and severe, a gastrostomy may be needed.

## POSTERIOR CERVICAL SPINE PROCEDURES

### Key Concepts

- C5 palsies occur in 4.8% to 9.5% of posterior cervical procedures with average symptom onset at 7 days postoperatively.
- Vertebral artery injuries may occur in more than 4% of C1–2 fusions with transarticular screws.

The posterior approach to the cervical spine can be used to decompress neural elements and treat instability with fusion. The overall incidence for neurological injury after posterior cervical spine fusion is 0.03%.[36] C5 palsy is relatively common and varies from 4.8% after laminoplasty to 9.5% after laminectomy and fusion, with average symptom onset at 7 days postoperatively.[37] Compared with anterior cervical spine surgery, dysphagia is less common[38]; thromboembolic events are approximately the same frequency,[39] and there is a trend for a higher incidence of pneumonia in posterior cervical procedures[40] (Table 4.2).

### Vertebral Artery Injuries

Injury to the vertebral artery during cervical spine surgery can be devastating and lead to severe problems such as fistulas, pseudoaneurysm, dissection, bleeding and thrombosis, embolism, cerebral ischemia, and even death. Stroke from this complication generally involves the posterior circulation and thus can lead to issues related to brainstem or occipital cortex function. Vertebral artery injuries occur in approximately 0.3%[41] of anterior cervical procedures and up to 4.1% with the posterior approach and placement of C1–2 transarticular screws.[42] Intraoperative or postoperative angiography can be useful in assessing repair and need for further intervention. Postoperative management includes close neurological monitoring and may include obtaining a magnetic resonance image (MRI) or CT angiogram to rule out a pseudoaneurysm or other anatomical abnormality or occlusion. Anticoagulation and antiplatelet therapy may also be needed to help prevent thromboembolic events.

## THORACIC AND LUMBAR SPINE

### Key Concepts

- Blood loss can be significant, increasing with revision surgeries, costotransversectomies, osteotomies, and with more levels fused.

- Ongoing resuscitation, correction of coagulopathy, and prolonged mechanical ventilation in the ICU may be necessary.

Surgery on the thoracic and lumbar spine can be approached posteriorly, anteriorly, or laterally. Detailed descriptions of these approaches can be found in subsequent chapters. Injury to large vessels such as the iliac arteries and veins, bowel, pleura, and other structures can result in life-threatening complications. Prolonged posterior fusions in the thoracolumbar region are associated with many postoperative complications from positioning, high EBL, large fluid shifts, prolonged operative duration, and proximity to vital structures. Complication rates vary among studies, ranging from 17.8% to 80%, with risk factors including age of the patients, number of levels fused, EBL, and operative duration.[43,44]

### Blood Loss

Blood loss can be significant regardless of approach and can continue into the postoperative period. Although major vascular injuries are rare with anterior lumbar procedures, blood loss will be rapid and difficult to control if the iliac vessels are injured. Posteriorly, epidural venous bleeding is one of the more common causes of rapid blood loss. Certain aspects of these operations, such as costotransversectomies and osteotomies, have the potential for greater blood loss because of segmental intercostal vessels and the complex system of venous drainage of the vertebrae. Anterior or anterolateral approaches to low cervical or high thoracic vertebrae are at risk for injury to the major vascular structures in the neck and chest. Achieving surgical hemostasis can be challenging. EBL may vary from 1.5 to 6 liters or more depending on surgical technique, number of levels fused, and patient condition.[45,46] Resuscitation with fluids and blood products may be needed into the postoperative period to achieve normovolemia, as reviewed later, while also correcting any temperature or coagulation issues.

### Postoperative Neurological Complications and Causes for Reoperation

Worsened myelopathy may be present in up to 4% of these procedures.[5] Lateral femoral cutaneous nerve injuries (meralgia paresthetica) from prone positioning or iliac crest graft harvesting may occur in up to 20% of patients, but the vast majority of patients recover within 3 months.[47] Postoperative neurological deficits can also be caused by malpositioned hardware or inadvertent nerve injury during surgery. These deficits may resolve without reoperation; however, some patients may need to return to the operating room for repositioning of the hardware. Pedicle screws may also need to be repositioned because of their proximity to major blood vessels such as the aorta. Rod or pedicle screw breakage or loosening is common in the first 2 years postoperatively and can require reoperation. Surgeons will typically obtain CT scans postoperatively for unexpected new or worsened neurological deficits within the operative site to evaluate for malpositioned hardware. Rapidly evolving neurological deficits within or near the operative site should raise alarm for a potential epidural hematoma (see section on epidural hematoma later in this chapter for workup).

## ANTERIOR-POSTERIOR AND STAGED SPINE OPERATIONS

### Key Concepts

- Controversy exists in the literature regarding complication rates for planned staging of anterior-posterior spine surgery compared with unstaged surgery.
- Intraoperative deterioration may force staging a procedure in order to correct life-threatening derangements from blood loss, coagulopathy, hemodynamic instability, or acidosis.

Some patients will require a staged spine procedure performed on separate days, typically because of an expected prolonged procedure with high blood loss or a combined anterior and posterior approach to the spine. If the procedure is done in a staged fashion, the patient may require postoperative controlled ventilation between stages if the interval between operations is very short. Varied results have been obtained for complication rates related to staging major spinal procedures. An analysis of 11,265 patients who underwent circumferential spine surgery[48] showed that the overall complication rate was significantly higher in patients undergoing staged versus same-day procedures with overall complication rates of 28.4% vs. 21.7%, respectively (p < 0.0001). These data were taken from a national database, and it is unclear if the staged procedures were planned or performed because of life-threatening complications. In contrast, other studies either reported no difference in complications between staged and unstaged procedures[46] or found that staging anterior-posterior procedures more than 21 days apart decreased transfusion requirements and improved patient functionality.[49] Given these conflicting data, more research is needed to clarify this issue. However, if intraoperative patient condition is rapidly deteriorating and cannot be corrected with respect to blood loss, coagulopathy, acidosis, hypotension, and other physiological parameters, staging the procedure may be a lifesaving maneuver.

## CERVICAL SPINE FRACTURE IN THE ELDERLY

### Key Concepts

- Elderly patients with cervical spine fractures after a fall from standing have very high in-hospital morbidity and mortality. Presence of neurological injury increases the early mortality rate up to 50%.
- Controversy exists regarding surgical versus conservative management, and patients should be considered on a case-by-case basis.
- Aspiration and fall precautions should be instituted for all patients.

Elderly patients with cervical spine fractures sustained after a fall from standing have a very high complication rate (62%) and early mortality rate (13%).[50-52] The mortality rate may be as high as 50% when there is an associated acute spinal cord injury.[25] Complications ensue from cardiac failure, respiratory failure, pneumonia, liver failure, stroke, DVT, and infection. Conservative management should be strongly considered, but halo vests are not tolerated well in these elderly patients who may already suffer from bulbar dysfunction and dysphagia. Aspiration risk and impaired mobility may be increased with these vests. Aspiration precautions should be in place for all patients. Decisions regarding power of attorney, advanced directives, and do not resuscitate orders should be solicited regardless of treatment choice.

# Other Complications and Postoperative Management Issues

### Key Concepts

- Major spine surgery can lead to significant blood loss both intraoperatively and postoperatively and require ongoing resuscitation in the ICU.
- Symptomatic postoperative epidural hematoma is most common after thoracic procedures and can cause spinal cord compression that requires emergent decompression. MRI or CT myelography should be performed immediately because symptom onset–to–decompression times of less than 6 to 8 hours correlate with better neurological outcomes.
- Any complaint of POVL should prompt an urgent ophthalmological consultation to rule out very rare causes of POVL that are reversible and require immediate treatment.

## RESUSCITATION MANAGEMENT IN THE NEUROLOGY INTENSIVE CARE UNIT

Many patients undergoing spine surgery will have significant blood loss intraoperatively. These patients may require large amounts of fluids and blood products intraoperatively, and resuscitation may continue well into the postoperative period. One of the goals of postoperative care in the ICU is to restore volume status, ensure adequate oxygen-carrying capacity, and correct acid–base derangements. Special attention to the intraoperative blood loss and postoperative losses through drain output will be needed. Frequent laboratory assessment of hematocrit, coagulation parameters, and acid–base status with attention to the hemodynamic condition can help guide resuscitation efforts. A more detailed review of the approach to postoperative management of exsanguination is reviewed in Chapter 7.

## POSTOPERATIVE EPIDURAL HEMATOMAS

Postoperative epidural hematoma is a potentially devastating complication of spine surgery, which can lead to spinal cord compression and permanent neurological disability. Immediate diagnosis and decompression are needed to minimize spinal cord injury related to expanding hematoma. It is considered a surgical emergency and thus warrants frequent neurological assessment postoperatively. Signs and symptoms can include a spectrum from inordinate surgical site pain to paresis to paralysis. Reported incidence varies from 0% for lumbar laminectomy to 4.5% for thoracic laminectomy.[53] Symptoms of epidural hematoma after lumbar surgery manifest shortly after surgical wound drain removal in almost half of patients. Time to decompression correlates with neurological recovery, with better outcomes for symptom-to-decompression times of 6 to 8 hours.

MRI or CT myelography is the preferred diagnostic study because plain CT imaging will not demonstrate the hematoma.

## POSTOPERATIVE VISUAL LOSS

POVL is a dreaded perioperative complication associated with spine surgery in the prone position. Its incidence is relatively rare, with the highest reported rate of 1 in 500 spine operations (0.2%).[54] National rates are lower at 0.03% for spinal fusion procedures, but the incidence varies depending on the procedure and center examined. The most common cause of POVL after spine surgery in adults is ischemic optic neuropathy (ION). A multicenter retrospective case-control study identified six risk factors for ION: male sex, obesity, use of the Wilson frame, prolonged operative duration, high EBL, and lower use of colloid for fluid replacement.[54] The leading theory regarding the pathophysiology of ION is that the prone position increases the venous pressure in the head and promotes edema formation that eventually compromises optic nerve perfusion. The American Society of Anesthesiologists developed a practice advisory for prevention of this complication primarily based on case series, case reports, case-control studies, and expert opinion.[55] Cortical blindness and central retinal artery occlusion (CRAO) are less common causes of POVL associated with spine surgery in adults. Cortical blindness is caused by embolic phenomenon or profound and prolonged hypotension. CRAO is most commonly associated with spine procedures in the prone position with pressure on the globe, but may be a result of embolic phenomena. CRAO caused by globe compression can easily be prevented by frequent and regular eye checks throughout the procedure. These different POVL etiologies can be distinguished from each other by an ophthalmological examination including fundoscopy (Table 4.3). ION, cortical

**Table 4.3** Features of the Three Major Causes of POVL Associated with Spine Surgery in the Prone Position*

|  | Ischemic Optic Neuropathy | Central Retinal Artery Occlusion | Cortical Blindness |
|---|---|---|---|
| Associated factors | Posterior and anterior ION with prone spine surgery: elevated venous pressure/prone position/Wilson frame/obesity/male sex/high EBL/prolonged duration/lower % of colloid in volume administration<br>Anterior ION: may have small cup:disc ratio | Emboli; globe compression | Emboli; profound hypotension/hypoperfusion |
| Onset of symptoms | PION: immediate on awakening<br>AION: may be delayed by 1–3 days postoperatively | Immediate on awakening | Immediate on awakening |
| Visual deficit | Altitudinal field cuts, scotomas, complete loss of vision with no light perception | Nearly complete or complete loss of vision in the affected eye | Unilateral infarction: contralateral homonymous hemianopsia; bilateral infarction: complete loss of vision or small central island of spared vision |
| Pupillary light reflex | Abnormal: RAPD if unilateral; may be absent | Sluggish to absent; RAPD | Normal |
| Other signs/symptoms |  | If caused by globe compression, may have ipsilateral periocular trauma (corneal abrasion, bruising, ophthalmoplegia, etc.) |  |
| Funduscopic examination | PION: normal<br>AION: optic disc swelling, attenuated vessels, splinter hemorrhages | Pale ischemic retina; usually cherry-red spot at macula; attenuated vessels | Normal |
| Special tests | Visual-evoked potentials | Electroretinogram |  |
| Imaging | Head CT or MRI to rule out intracranial mass/hemorrhage | Head CT or MRI to rule out intracranial mass/hemorrhage | Head CT or MRI to evaluate watershed infarction vs. embolic pattern |
| Treatment | No proven benefit: Consultants usually recommend optimizing blood pressure/oxygen delivery. | No proven benefit: Consultants may recommend optimizing perfusion; use of inhaled $CO_2$, acetazolamide. Intraarterial thrombolysis is controversial in postop patients. | Consultants may recommend optimizing perfusion and oxygen delivery. |
| Recovery | Little recovery | Little recovery | Better than ION, but rarely to baseline vision |

*Any complaint of POVL should prompt an urgent ophthalmology consultation to rule out extremely rare causes of POVL that are reversible if provided prompt treatment (acute angle closure glaucoma, retrobulbar hematoma, posterior reversible encephalopathy syndrome, and pituitary apoplexy).
*EBL,* estimated blood loss; *ION,* ischemic optic neuropathy; *PION,* posterior ION; *AION,* anterior ION; *RAPD,* relative afferent pupillary defect; *CT,* computed tomography; *MRI,* magnetic resonance imaging.

blindness, and CRAO have no proven effective therapy, although consultants typically recommend optimization of the hemodynamics and oxygen delivery, which may involve transfusion. Recovery is typically poor, with return to baseline vision uncommon. Any complaint of POVL should result in an urgent ophthalmological consultation and CT or MRI of the head to rule out exceedingly rare cases of intracranial masses or hemorrhage. Much rarer causes of POVL that are reversible and require immediate treatment include acute angle closure glaucoma, retrobulbar hematoma, posterior reversible encephalopathy, and pituitary apoplexy.

## Summary

Spinal surgeries have increased in number dramatically over the last three decades. As patient comorbidities and complexity of surgical interventions increase, so does the need for critical care management of these patients in both the preoperative and postoperative periods. Optimization of patients preoperatively will improve outcomes. Rehabilitation and pain management can be a major impediment to a smooth postoperative recovery, and consultations with these specialists should be initiated as early as possible. Postsurgical spine patients will have a multitude of critical care issues that will require attention, including frequent ongoing resuscitation in the ICU setting. Knowledge of site-specific complications is crucial to the management of spine surgery patients. Complex spine surgery is associated with a relatively high incidence of prolonged mechanical ventilation or reintubation, particularly after anterior cervical spine surgery. Ongoing communication between the ICU, anesthesiologists, and surgical teams regarding patient needs is paramount for successful outcomes in high-acuity patients undergoing complex spine surgery and should be maximized whenever possible.

### References

1. Deyo RA, Mirza SK. Trends and variations in the use of spine surgery. *Clin Orthop Relat Res.* 2006;443:139–146.
2. Rajaee SS, Bae HW, Kanim LE, et al. Spinal fusion in the United States: analysis of trends from 1998 to 2008. *Spine.* 2012;37 (1):67–76.
3. Deyo RA, Mirza SK, Martin BI, et al. Trends, major medical complications, and charges associated with surgery for lumbar spinal stenosis in older adults. *JAMA.* 2010;303(13):1259–1265.
4. Li G, Patil CG, Lad SP, et al. Effects of age and comorbidities on complication rates and adverse outcomes after lumbar laminectomy in elderly patients. *Spine.* 2008;33(11):1250–1255.
5. Nielsen PR, Jorgensen LD, Dahl B, et al. Prehabilitation and early rehabilitation after spinal surgery: randomized clinical trial. *Clin Rehabil.* 2010;24(2):137–148.
6. Nielsen PR, Andreasen J, Asmussen M, et al. Costs and quality of life for prehabilitation and early rehabilitation after surgery of the lumbar spine. *BMC Health Serv Res.* 2008;8:209–215.
7. McGregor AH, Probyn K, Cro S, et al. Rehabilitation following surgery for lumbar spinal stenosis. *Cochrane Database Syst Rev.* 2013 Dec 9;12. http://dx.doi.org/10.1002/14651858.CD009644.pub2.
8. Walid MS, Hyer L, Ajjan M, et al. Prevalence of opioid dependence in spine surgery patients and correlation with length of stay. *J Opioid Manag.* 2007;3(3):127–128 30–2.
9. Juratli SM, Mirza SK, Fulton-Kehoe D, et al. Mortality after lumbar fusion surgery. *Spine.* 2009;34(7):740–747.
10. Patel N, Bagan B, Vadera S, et al. Obesity and spine surgery: relation to perioperative complications. *J Neurosurg Spine.* 2007;6(4):291–297.
11. Porhomayon J, Leissner KB, El-Solh AA, Nader ND. Strategies in postoperative analgesia in the obese obstructive sleep apnea patient. *Clin J Pain.* 2013;29(11):998–1005.
12. Stevens RD, Bhardwaj A, Kirsch JR, et al. Critical care and perioperative management in traumatic spinal cord injury. *J Neurosurg Anesthesiol.* 2003;15(3):215–229.
13. Gill JB, Chin Y, Levin A, Feng D. The Use of antifibrinolytic agents in spine surgery: a meta-analysis. *J Bone Joint Surg Am.* 2008;90 (11):2399–2407.
14. Siemionow K, Cywinski J, Kusza K, Lieberman I. Intraoperative fluid therapy and pulmonary complications. *Orthopedics.* 2012;35 (2):e184–e191.
15. Biais M, Bernard O, Ha JC, et al. Abilities of pulse pressure variations and stroke volume variations to predict fluid responsiveness in prone position during scoliosis surgery. *Br J Anaesth.* 2010;104(4):407–413.
16. Jarvis JG, Strantzas S, Lipkus M, et al. Responding to neuromonitoring changes in 3-column posterior spinal osteotomies for rigid pediatric spinal deformities. *Spine.* 2013;38(8):E493–E503.
17. Ziewacz JE, Davis MC, Lau D, et al. Validation of the surgical Apgar score in a neurosurgical patient population. *J Neurosurg.* 2013 Feb;118(2):270–279.
18. Lieberman JA, Feiner J, Lyon R, Rollins MD. Effect of hemorrhage and hypotension on transcranial motor-evoked potentials in swine. *Anesthesiology.* 2013;119(5):1109–1119.
19. Takahashi S, Kitagawa H, Ishii T. Intraoperative pulmonary embolism during spinal instrumentation surgery. A prospective study using transoesophageal echocardiography. *J Bone Joint Surg Br.* 2003;85(1):90–94.
20. Kim BD, Hsu WK, De Oliveira Jr GS, et al. Operative duration as an independent risk factor for postoperative complications in single-level lumbar fusion: an analysis of 4588 surgical cases. *Spine.* 2014;39 (6):510–520.
21. Wittekamp BH, van Mook WN, Tjan DH, et al. Clinical review: postextubation laryngeal edema and extubation failure in critically ill adult patients. *Crit Care.* 2009;13(6):233.
22. Kamel IR, Drum ET, Koch SA, et al. The use of somatosensory evoked potentials to determine the relationship between patient positioning and impending upper extremity nerve injury during spine surgery: a retrospective analysis. *Anesth Analg.* 2006;102(5):1538–1542.
23. Schoenfeld AJ, Carey PA, Cleveland 3rd AW, et al. Patient factors, comorbidities, and surgical characteristics that increase mortality and complication risk after spinal arthrodesis: a prognostic study based on 5,887 patients. *Spine J.* 2013;13(10):1171–1179.
24. Smith JS, Sansur CA, Donaldson 3rd WF, et al. Short-term morbidity and mortality associated with correction of thoracolumbar fixed sagittal plane deformity: a report from the Scoliosis Research Society Morbidity and Mortality Committee. *Spine.* 2011;36(12):958–964.
25. Patel A, Smith HE, Radcliff K, et al. Odontoid fractures with neurologic deficit have higher mortality and morbidity. *Clin Orthop Relat Res.* 2012;470(6):1614–1620.
26. Gruskay JA, Fu M, Basques B, et al. Factors affecting length of stay and complications following elective anterior cervical discectomy and fusion: a study of 2164 patients from the American College of Surgeons National Surgical Quality Improvement Project Database (ACS NSQIP). *Clin Spine Surg.* 2016;29(1):E34–E42.
27. Fountas KN, Kapsalaki EZ, Nikolakakos LG, et al. Anterior cervical discectomy and fusion associated complications. *Spine.* 2007;32 (21):2310–2317.
28. Hashimoto M, Mochizuki M, Aiba A, et al. C5 palsy following anterior decompression and spinal fusion for cervical degenerative diseases. *Eur Spine J.* 2010;19(10):1702–1710.
29. Tan TP, Govindarajulu AP, Massicotte EM, et al. Vocal cord palsy following anterior cervical spine surgery: a qualitative systematic review. *Spine J.* 2014;14(7):1332–1342.
30. O'Neill KR, Neuman B, Peters C, et al. Risk factors for postoperative retropharyngeal hematoma after anterior cervical spine surgery. *Spine.* 2014;39(4):E246–E252.
31. Sagi HC, Beutler W, Carroll E, et al. Airway complications associated with surgery on the anterior cervical spine. *Spine.* 2002;27(9):949–953.
32. Emery SE, Smith MD, Bohlman HH. Upper-airway obstruction after multilevel cervical corpectomy for myelopathy. *J Bone Joint Surg Am.* 1991;73(4):544–551.
33. Marquez-Lara A, Nandyala SV, Fineberg SJ, et al. Incidence, outcomes, and mortality of reintubation after anterior cervical fusion. *Spine.* 2014;39(2):134–139.

34. Phommachanh V, Patil YJ, McCaffrey TV, et al. Otolaryngologic management of delayed pharyngoesophageal perforation following anterior cervical spine surgery. *Laryngoscope.* 2010;120(5):930–936.
35. Riley 3rd LH, Vaccaro AR, Dettori JR, et al. Postoperative dysphagia in anterior cervical spine surgery. *Spine.* 2010;35(9 Suppl):S76–S85.
36. Marquez-Lara A, Nandyala SV, Hassanzadeh H, et al. Sentinel events in cervical spine surgery. *Spine.* 2014;39(9):715–720.
37. Nassr A, Eck JC, Ponnappan RK, et al. The incidence of C5 palsy after multilevel cervical decompression procedures: a review of 750 consecutive cases. *Spine.* 2012;37(3):174–178.
38. Smith-Hammond CA, New KC, Pietrobon R, et al. Prospective analysis of incidence and risk factors of dysphagia in spine surgery patients: comparison of anterior cervical, posterior cervical, and lumbar procedures. *Spine.* 2004;29(13):1441–1446.
39. Oglesby M, Fineberg SJ, Patel AA, et al. The incidence and mortality of thromboembolic events in cervical spine surgery. *Spine.* 2013;38(9):E521–E527.
40. Anastasian ZH, Gaudet JG, Levitt LC, et al. Factors that correlate with the decision to delay extubation after multilevel prone spine surgery. *J Neurosurg Anesthesiol.* 2014;26(2):167–171.
41. Burke JP, Gerszten PC, Welch WC. Iatrogenic vertebral artery injury during anterior cervical spine surgery. *Spine J.* 2005;5(5):508–514 discussion 14.
42. Wright NM, Lauryssen C. Vertebral artery injury in C1-2 transarticular screw fixation: results of a survey of the AANS/CNS section on disorders of the spine and peripheral nerves. *J Neurosurg.* 1998;88(4):634–640.
43. Nasser R, Yadla S, Maltenfort MG, et al. Complications in spine surgery. *J Neurosurg Spine.* 2010;13(2):144–157.
44. Carreon LY, Puno RM, Dimar 2nd JR, et al. Perioperative complications of posterior lumbar decompression and arthrodesis in older adults. *J Bone Joint Surg Am.* 2003;85-A(11):2089–2092.
45. Smorgick Y, Baker KC, Bachison CC, et al. Hidden blood loss during posterior spine fusion surgery. *Spine J.* 2013;13(8):877–881.
46. Maddox JJ, Pruitt DR, Agel J, et al. Unstaged versus staged posterior-only thoracolumbar fusions in deformity: a retrospective comparison of perioperative complications. *Spine J.* 2014;14(7):1159–1165.
47. Mirovsky Y, Neuwirth M. Injuries to the lateral femoral cutaneous nerve during spine surgery. *Spine.* 2000;25(10):1266–1269.
48. Passias PG, Ma Y, Chiu YL, et al. Comparative safety of simultaneous and staged anterior and posterior spinal surgery. *Spine.* 2012;37(3):247–255.
49. Hassanzadeh H, Gjolaj JP, El Dafrawy MH, et al. The timing of surgical staging has a significant impact on the complications and functional outcomes of adult spinal deformity surgery. *Spine J.* 2013;13(12):1717–1722.
50. Schoenfeld AJ, Bono CM, Reichmann WM, et al. Type II odontoid fractures of the cervical spine: do treatment type and medical comorbidities affect mortality in elderly patients? *Spine.* 2011;36(11):879–885.
51. White AP, Hashimoto R, Norvell DC, Vaccaro AR. Morbidity and mortality related to odontoid fracture surgery in the elderly population. *Spine.* 2010 Apr 20;35(9 Suppl):S146–S157.
52. Vaccaro AR, Kepler CK, Kopjar B, et al. Functional and quality-of-life outcomes in geriatric patients with type-II dens fracture. *J Bone Joint Surg Am.* 2013 Apr 17;95(8):729–735.
53. Aono H, Ohwada T, Hosono N, et al. Incidence of postoperative symptomatic epidural hematoma in spinal decompression surgery. *J Neurosurg Spine.* 2011;15(2):202–205.
54. Postoperative Visual Loss Study Group. Risk factors associated with ischemic optic neuropathy after spinal fusion surgery. *Anesthesiology.* 2012;116:15–24.
55. American Society of Anesthesiologists Task Force on Perioperative Visual Loss. Practice advisory for perioperative visual loss associated with spine surgery: an updated report by the American Society of Anesthesiologists Task Force on Perioperative Visual Loss. *Anesthesiology.* 2012;116(2):274–285.

# 5 Anesthetic Considerations for Endovascular Neurosurgery

PEKKA O. TALKE, ALANA M. FLEXMAN, and CHRISTOPHER F. DOWD

## Introduction

Interventional neuroradiology (INR) procedures continue to increase in volume and complexity and are used to treat numerous different intracranial pathologies.[1] The patients who require these procedures range from the neurologically intact outpatient population to the neurologically devastated critically ill population. Endovascular neuroradiology procedures may be elective, such as an embolization of an unruptured intracranial aneurysm. In contrast, these procedures may be emergent, such as for endovascular treatment of acute ischemic stroke. Factors related to the patient and procedure will guide the decision as to whether the patient receives general anesthesia or sedation. Despite this variability, there are several common themes regarding the anesthetic considerations for endovascular procedures performed in the INR suite. The aim of this chapter is to discuss specific concerns related to the provision of anesthesia in the INR suite, as well as to review anesthetic management of commonly performed INR procedures.

## The Interventional Neuroradiology Suite

### Key Concepts

- Anesthesiologists should be part of modern INR suite design.
- Anesthesiologists often have limited access to the patient during the procedure.
- Anesthesiologists are at high risk of radiation exposure during interventional neuroradiology procedures.

State-of-the-art INR suites are designed specifically for INR procedures. These sophisticated spaces utilize biplane digital angiography equipment and software to produce high-resolution and three-dimensional images. Inside the INR suite there is a large panel of flat-screen displays that allow the proceduralists (radiologists or surgeons) to view both real-time and previously acquired images throughout the procedure. Adjacent to the INR suite is a control room that is separated from the INR suite by a leaded window to protect against radiation exposure. Radiologists in the control room are able to control the fluoroscopy equipment. The control room contains displays that are used to view real-time images and to review previous images. Ideally, the anesthesia team should have a workstation or physiological monitor in the control room to minimize exposure to radiation during the procedure.

The typical arrangement of the INR suite has unique implications for the anesthesiologist. For example, the anesthesiologist has extremely limited access to the patient during the procedure (Fig. 5.1). Typically, the anesthesiologist is positioned on the opposite side of the patient as the proceduralist, with the anesthesia equipment far off to one side to minimize interference with movement of equipment during the procedure. A large panel of flat screens occupies the space opposite the proceduralist, and large biplane fluoroscopy equipment surrounds the patient's head. Anesthesiologists need to anticipate the logistics relating to this arrangement, including adding extensions to monitoring equipment and intravenous/arterial tubing.

Ideally, the INR suite should be thoughtfully designed with input from the procedural, anesthesia, and support staff. The anesthesiologist should be able to observe the patient and have easy access to the anesthesia machine and equipment such as infusion pumps. The anesthesia team should have access to the monitors that display real-time fluoroscopy images in order to follow the procedure and anticipate periods of increased risk to the patient. Recently increased attention has been placed on optimizing the design of these suites to minimize radiation exposure to anesthesia team as well as the proceduralists, which is often not the case.[2]

### Clinical Pearl

Anesthesiologists should be able to follow the procedure in order to anticipate high-risk time periods.

### RADIATION EXPOSURE

Although advances in modern fluoroscopy equipment have resulted in a reduced potential for radiation exposure among medical personnel, care should be taken to minimize radiation exposure. INR procedures are associated with an increased potential for radiation exposure compared with other radiology procedures due to increased complexity and duration, as well as the need for frequent continuous radiation exposure. A recent study demonstrated that anesthesia personnel were exposed to a threefold greater amount of radiation to the face than radiology

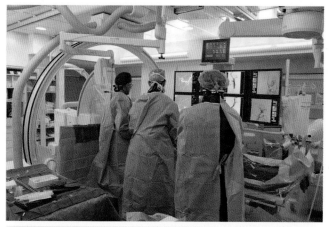

**Fig. 5.1** One of the University of California San Francisco interventional neuroradiology suites with state-of-the-art biplane angiography equipment. Patient is supine under the drapes between the flat-screen monitors and interventional radiologists. The fluoroscopy tubes surround the patient's head. The photo illustrates the limited access anesthesiologists have to the patient in the INR suite.

personnel during neurointerventional angiographic procedures due to the typical configuration of INR suites.[2] The increased exposure in this study was associated with the higher number of pharmacological interventions (e.g., administration of medication or changes in infusion rates) that were required during these complex neurological procedures. All personnel working in INR suites need to be educated on radiation safety and use protective clothing and devices such as lead aprons, thyroid shields, protective eyewear, and leaded screens.

## Interventional Neuroradiology Procedures

### Key Concepts

- During INR procedures, endovascular access is typically via femoral arteries.
- Closure devices can be used to close arteriotomy sites.
- Intravascular contrast dye is nephrotoxic and may cause allergic reactions.

Although INR procedures are varied, there are several common components. All are performed using endovascular techniques with access through a major vessel, typically through the femoral artery and occasionally the femoral vein (e.g., to treat some dural arteriovenous fistulas). After vascular access is achieved with a larger sheath, catheters of various sizes and designs are inserted through the sheath in order to delineate the vascular anatomy and perform interventions. Normally the endovascular catheters are removed at the end of the procedure, and hemostasis is achieved either by applying pressure to the femoral artery or use of a specially designed closure device. Hemostasis is achieved much more quickly with a closure device, even in patients heparinized after the procedure. Regardless of the

method to achieve hemostasis, patients should remain supine for several hours after the procedure and monitored for hemorrhage from the vascular puncture site.

### CONTRAST DYE

Virtually all INR procedures require that the patient receive intravascular contrast dye. The use of intravascular contrast dye has several implications for the anesthesiologist. First, these contrast dyes are nephrotoxic and have the potential to cause deterioration of renal function. Hydration with intravenous fluids may reduce this risk, and patients with poor renal function may not be able to tolerate use of contrast dyes. Second, patients are at risk for having an allergic reaction to contrast dye, although this is rare with newer formulations. Allergic reactions can range from a rash to life-threatening anaphylactic reaction. Patients with known allergies to contrast dye may be pretreated with steroids (e.g., prednisone) and antihistamines (e.g., diphenhydramine and ranitidine).[3] Pretreatment may reduce but does not eliminate the risk of allergic reactions, nor does a previous uneventful exposure; thus the anesthesiologist must always be vigilant for these reactions.

### Clinical Pearls

- Patients with known contrast allergy should be pretreated.
- Patients with poor renal function may not be candidates for INR procedures.

## Anesthesia in the Neurointerventional Suite

### Key Concepts

- Patients who require tight hemodynamic control should have continuous intraarterial blood pressure monitoring.
- Many procedures may be done using sedation or general anesthesia. The choice depends on patient condition and institutional preferences.
- Patients may be anticoagulated with heparin during INR procedures. Heparin effect may or may not be reversed with protamine.

### PREOPERATIVE ASSESSMENT

Patients presenting for INR procedures should be assessed with a thorough history, physical examination, and review of laboratory investigations. Baseline neurological symptoms and signs should be documented. Hemoglobin and coagulation status should be reviewed, as well as the patient's renal function given the use of contrast dye. When appropriate, patients should be assessed for suitability for local anesthesia and sedation. Patients with significant anxiety, those with significant neurological compromise, and those who cannot reliably cooperate during a potentially lengthy procedure may be poor candidates for local anesthesia/sedation. Patients must also be able to tolerate supine positioning for a potentially long procedure.

## MONITORING

Ideally the anesthesiologist should be able to simultaneously observe the patient, have easy access to the anesthesia machine and monitors, and be able to follow the procedural images in order to anticipate high-risk time periods. All patients under general anesthesia should be monitored using standard anesthetic monitors such as noninvasive blood pressure, pulse oximeter, electrocardiography, temperature, neuromuscular monitoring, and end-tidal carbon dioxide and anesthetic gas analysis. Similar monitors are required if the patient is sedated, including respiratory rate monitoring via end-tidal carbon dioxide sampling. Intracranial pressure is often monitored in critically ill patients, typically through an external ventricular drain (EVD). A bladder catheter is often inserted, given the length of the procedure as well as the contrast load and intravenous fluid loading. Blood loss is typically minimal, and one intravenous catheter is sufficient.

Many patients having INR procedures benefit from continuous, invasive arterial blood pressure measurement. For example, close hemodynamic monitoring is essential for patients with subarachnoid hemorrhage (SAH), acute ischemic stroke, or Moyamoya disease. Finally, some procedures are associated with significant hemodynamic changes, such as during endovascular intraarterial treatment of cerebral vasospasm after SAH.[4] Invasive blood pressure monitoring is typically achieved through insertion of a catheter into the radial artery, but may occasionally be done through the side port of a femoral artery sheath inserted for the procedure.

The patient with an EVD for increased intracranial pressure (ICP) warrants particular care both during transport and the procedure itself. The management plan for the EVD must be clearly communicated to the anesthesia team because the patient will likely spend several hours away from the intensive care unit (ICU) in a supine position. Similarly the anesthesia team needs to communicate how the EVD was managed in the INR suite when the patient is transferred back to the ICU. Often the EVD is clamped for safety during transport because the drain may not be reliably positioned intraprocedure; nonetheless care must be taken to ensure that the EVD is not left clamped and unobserved for prolonged periods given the risk of increased ICP. In the INR suite ICP should be monitored continuously and cerebrospinal fluid (CSF) drained periodically as necessary.

## ANESTHETIC TECHNIQUE

Goals of sedation and general anesthesia during INR procedures are to provide patient comfort, minimize patient movement, and provide optimal circumstances for good quality image acquisition. Many procedures can be performed using local anesthesia and sedation, but the decision to choose general anesthesia or local anesthesia is patient specific and depends on many factors, including patient preference, institutional preference, patient comorbidities, and procedural requirements (Table 5.1). After the procedure, the patient should emerge rapidly from anesthesia when possible to facilitate early neurological assessment.

Local anesthesia requires that the patient be cooperative lying flat for a prolonged period and is commonly used for

**Table 5.1** General Anesthesia vs. Sedation for INR Procedures

| General Anesthesia | Sedation |
|---|---|
| PRO | PRO |
| Improved comfort | Ability to assess neurological status |
| Immobile patient | Takes less time |
| Better image quality | May not need an anesthesia team |
| Secure airway | |
| Less aspiration risk | |
| Better ability to control blood pressure | |
| Better ability to control ventilation | |
| | |
| CON | CON |
| Unable to assess neurological status | More discomfort |
| Risks of general anesthesia | More anxiety |
| Increases hemodynamic lability | More patient movement |
| Takes more time | Reduced image quality |
| | Respiratory depression |
| | Risk for airway complications |
| | Risk for aspiration |

simpler procedures such as a diagnostic cerebral angiogram. Obtaining vascular access through the femoral artery can be accomplished with relatively little discomfort with aid of local anesthetic infiltration. Various anxiolytics can be used to improve patient comfort, and drug selection is based on personal and institutional preferences. Sedated patients should remain awake and cooperative so that they can breath-hold and remain still during image acquisition. A combination of midazolam and fentanyl is commonly used. Excessive sedation should be avoided because this can lead to respiratory depression and airway obstruction, as well as an uncooperative patient. In addition, neurologically compromised patients may deteriorate with sedation, resulting in somnolence, inadequate airway protection, and aspiration. During stroke treatment about 3% of the procedures done under sedation are converted to general anesthesia.[5]

General anesthesia is often used for complex endovascular neuroradiology procedures and has several advantages, including improved patient comfort, a reliably immobile patient, and superior image quality.[6] The disadvantages of general anesthesia are the risks related to general anesthesia itself, time delays, and the inability to assess the patient's neurological status during the procedure.[6] In addition, general anesthesia is associated with greater hemodynamic variability compared with sedation.[7] At our institution, we prefer general anesthesia for uncooperative patients or those unable to protect their airway. In addition, general anesthesia is used for procedures that require prolonged immobility (e.g., spinal angiograms) or for which immobility is critical to avoid catheter-induced perforations (e.g., aneurysm coiling). General anesthesia can be achieved using intravenous or inhalation anesthetics or a combination of both. Anesthetic management should aim for a rapid emergence from anesthesia after the procedure to allow for timely neurological evaluation. Neuromuscular relaxants are frequently used to ensure immobility during critical time periods to reduce the risk of catheter-induced blood vessel perforation. Ventilation is suspended during image acquisition to reduce artifact from respiratory movement.

## ANTICOAGULATION

The anesthesiologist will manage anticoagulation if required and be prepared to treat possible complications. Many patients are anticoagulated during their INR procedures, although basic diagnostic cerebral angiography may be done without anticoagulation. When endovascular catheters are advanced into smaller cerebral arteries, patients are usually anticoagulated to reduce the incidence of catheter-induced thrombus formation. This is achieved by administering a bolus of intravenous heparin (70 U/kg), followed by hourly supplemental heparin doses or by a heparin infusion. Heparin effect is monitored by the activated clotting time with a target of 250 to 300 seconds (two to three times normal).[8] Heparin may or may not be reversed at the end of the procedure using protamine. Use of heparin, protamine, or other anticoagulants should be clearly communicated to the ICU team when transferring care of the patient.

## Postprocedure Care of INR Patients

### Key Concepts

- Postoperative care varies significantly. Some patients go home the same day; some are critically ill and go to ICU for management and/or observation.
- Anesthesia and ICU teams need to communicate clearly what was done during INR procedures, which drugs were administered, and any complications.

Clear communication about the patient's status is essential and should involve neuroradiologists, neurosurgeons, neurovascular neurologists, neurointensivists, and intensive care nurses as necessary. Interdisciplinary communication should include the patient's baseline neurological status and diagnosis, hemodynamic management, management of ICP/EVD, and need for postoperative ventilation. Transfer between the INR suite and other locations should be done with appropriate hemodynamic monitors, medications, and personnel.

Postoperative care of INR patients varies tremendously depending on the patient and the procedure. Patients undergoing elective diagnostic angiograms are often expected to go home the same day. Most patients who come for elective INR procedures, such as coiling of intracranial aneurysms, spend one night in the ICU for neurological monitoring but need minimal postoperative care. Conversely, emergency patients who come to the INR suite typically go to the ICU after the procedure and require intense postprocedure care.

Although morbidity and mortality associated with endovascular neurointerventional procedures may be lower than with intracranial surgery, complications can occur (Box 5.1). Procedure-related intracranial hemorrhage is a major complication and may present with sudden bradycardia and hypertension. This complication may be diagnosed by angiographic extravasation of contrast dye during the procedure and may require immediate reduction of ICP such as with an EVD. In the event of intracranial hemorrhage, any remaining heparin effect should be reversed immediately with protamine. Other catheter-induced complications

### Box 5.1   Endovascular Neurosurgery–Related Complications

Cerebral artery perforation
Dissection of an artery
Arterial occlusion
Cerebral edema
Thromboembolism
Allergic reaction to contrast dye
Contrast dye–related nephrotoxicity
Vasospasm
Embolization of normal tissue (brain, lung)
Hematoma (arteriotomy site)
Hemorrhage (arteriotomy site and retroperitoneal)
Limb ischemia
Pseudoaneurysm formation (arteriotomy)
Arteriotomy site infection
Aspiration
Upper airway obstruction

include blood vessel spasm, dissection and rupture, and thromboembolism. Many patients receive transdermal nitroglycerin ointment in the beginning of the procedure to prevent catheter-induced spasm. The patient should be monitored postoperatively for complications of vascular access through the femoral arteries, including hematoma formation (including retroperitoneal) and limb ischemia. Use of embolic materials is associated with risk of embolization of these materials into both the cerebral and systemic vasculature.

## Common INR Procedures

### DIAGNOSTIC CEREBRAL ANGIOGRAM

Diagnostic cerebral angiography is performed to define the cerebrovascular anatomy and to investigate potential cerebrovascular pathology. During this procedure, contrast dye is injected into internal carotid and vertebral arteries to study the anterior and posterior circulations, respectively (Fig. 5.2). Contrast dye may also be injected into external carotid arteries to study the extracranial circulation. As mentioned earlier, choice of sedation or general anesthesia is driven largely by institutional preference because little evidence exists to support one type of anesthesia over another. Any planned endovascular interventions in addition to diagnostic angiography should be clearly communicated in advance of the procedure because general anesthesia may be required. Generally, neurologically intact, cooperative patients tolerate the procedure with local anesthesia with sedation to alleviate anxiety. In contrast, uncooperative patients, those with inadequate airway protection, or those with significant neurological deficits may require general anesthesia. Patients for diagnostic angiography of spinal cord lesions will also typically receive general anesthesia in order to minimize movement-related deterioration of image quality. If a decision is made to pursue further intervention after the diagnostic angiogram, general anesthesia may be induced at this point if not already done. During image acquisition, ventilation is suspended to reduce movement.

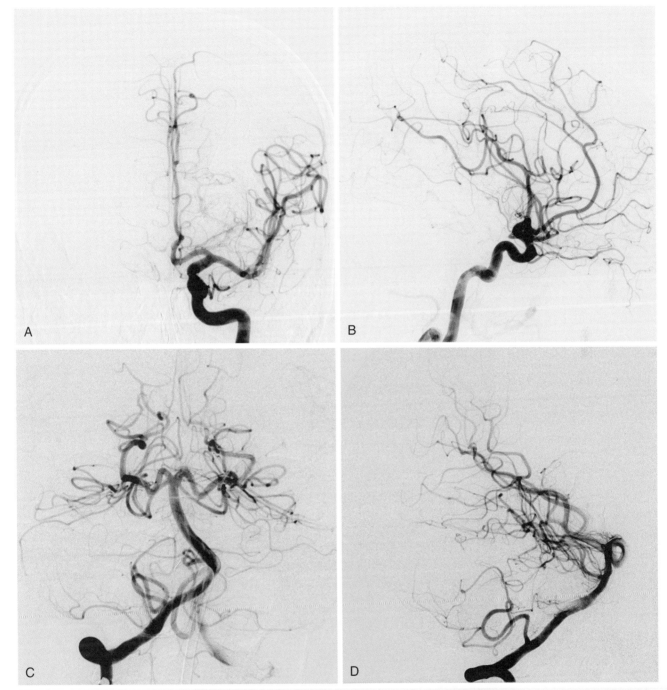

**Fig. 5.2** Examples of normal diagnostic angiogram images. Angiographic images of the anterior and posterior cerebral circulation. **(A–B)** Anteroposterior (AP) and lateral images after left internal carotid artery injection of contrast dye. **(C–D)** AP and lateral images after right vertebral artery injection of contrast dye.

**Clinical Pearl**

Patients do not need to be anticoagulated for diagnostic INR procedures.

## COILING OF INTRACRANIAL ANEURYSMS

Endovascular treatment of intracranial aneurysms is done with increasing frequency and involves filling the aneurysmal sac with detachable platinum coils.[9] A guide catheter is advanced through a femoral sheath (a coaxial system) selectively into a cerebral artery so that the tip of the guide catheter is within the aneurysm sack. Detachable platinum coils are inserted into the aneurysm through the guide catheter (Fig. 5.3). During this procedure, patient immobility is critical because both the guide catheter and the coils can perforate the aneurysm. For this reason, general anesthesia is typically used during aneurysm coiling. Catheter-induced intracranial hemorrhage may present with an abrupt increase in blood pressure or bradycardia, and extravasation of intravascular contrast

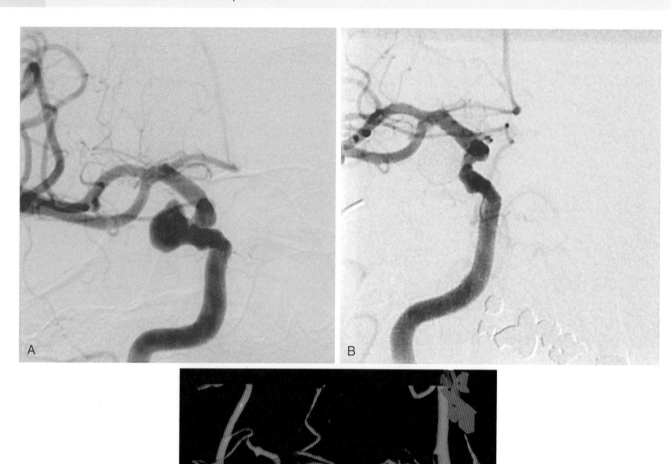

**Fig. 5.3** Right carotid artery aneurysm before **(A)** and after **(B)** coiling of the aneurysm. **(C)** A three-dimensional reconstructed rotational angiographic image of the aneurysm before coiling.

dye may be seen on imaging. Anesthesiologists should be vigilant for this complication, particularly when the guide catheter is advanced into the aneurysm sac and coils are inserted, and communicate immediately any abrupt hemodynamic changes.

Occasionally endovascular coiling of the aneurysm may be challenging due to anatomical features, such as a wide aneurysm neck. Coiling can still be achieved by first inserting a perforated endovascular stent into the cerebral vessel across the

aneurysm neck. The aneurysm is coiled through the spaces between the stent struts, a procedure called *stent-assisted coiling*, or by inserting the tip or the guide catheter into the aneurysm sac before deploying the stent. Alternatively, an intraarterial balloon may be temporarily inflated across the aneurysm neck to retain the coils within the aneurysm sac.

Patients treated with coil embolization may have an unruptured aneurysm, a ruptured aneurysm, or multiple aneurysms. Because patients may be sedated or intubated when they arrive to the INR suite, their last known neurological status should be communicated to the anesthesia team. Good hemodynamic control is essential for all patients with intracranial aneurysms, as even brief periods of hypertension may cause rupture or rebleeding of the aneurysm. In contrast, hypotension should also be avoided because cerebral autoregulation is often disrupted in these patients and some patients may have post-SAH vasospasm. Induction of anesthesia, intubation, and emergence from anesthesia are the most hemodynamically labile periods. Blood pressure management goals and radiological findings should be communicated clearly. During the procedure, blood pressure goals are maintained by altering anesthetic depth and vasopressor infusions (e.g., phenylephrine). Once the aneurysm is secured, or coiled, permissive hypertension is allowed; however, hypertension should be avoided if not all aneurysms have been treated.

> ### Clinical Pearls
>
> - SAH patients may have vasospasm.
> - Hemodynamic management depends on multiple factors.
> - Anesthesiologists should be prepared to treat iatrogenic ICH.

## ENDOVASCULAR TREATMENT OF CEREBRAL VASOSPASM

Cerebral vasospasm and delayed cerebral ischemia are common after SAH and are associated with increased morbidity and mortality.[10] The treatment of cerebral vasospasm often includes a combination of induced hypertension, avoidance of hypovolemia, and treatment of anemia, as well as prophylactic use of nimodipine, a calcium channel blocker.[10] In addition to these medical therapies, endovascular treatment of cerebral vasospasm in the INR suite has been increasingly applied, particularly in patients who have persistent clinical vasospasm despite medical therapy. The endovascular treatment may include balloon angioplasty of more proximal vessels as well as intraarterial injection of cerebral vasodilators such as calcium channel blockers (verapamil, nicardipine) or milrinone. The anesthesiologist caring for these patients should continue the preoperative strategies, including induced hypertension, during the procedure. The anesthetic considerations for patients undergoing these procedures include not only those related to a patient with significant neurological compromise, but also the hemodynamic effects of these interventions. Previous research has demonstrated that intraarterial injection of calcium channel blockers has been associated with consistent and occasionally dramatic reductions in blood pressure.[4,11–13]

> ### Clinical Pearl
>
> Treatment of vasospasm using intraarterial vasodilators will have short- and long-term hemodynamic effects.

## ARTERIOVENOUS MALFORMATIONS

Arteriovenous malformations (AVMs) are an abnormal group of blood vessels that contain one or more arteries that directly drain into veins. As a result, the veins are "arterialized" and exposed to unusually high blood pressures. AVM hemorrhage typically occurs from the draining veins, nidus, or nidal aneurysms. During general anesthesia hypertensive episodes should be avoided to reduce the risk of rupture of AVM-associated aneurysms. Hypotension should be avoided in patients with ruptured AVMs who may have increased ICP and limited cerebral perfusion pressure.

AVMs can be treated surgically by radiosurgery (gamma knife) or by endovascular embolization. Embolization of an AVM is performed mainly to reduce intraoperative blood loss, but can occasionally be a sole therapy. Patients will initially have a diagnostic cerebral angiogram to identify the anatomy and the feeding and draining vessels of the AVM (Fig. 5.4). The diagnostic angiogram will also identify any aneurysms associated with the AVM. The information from the diagnostic angiogram is pivotal to evaluate the relative risks of the various treatment options, as well as to plan surgical resection. Endovascular embolization of the AVM can be done by using coils, particles, or glues (polyvinyl alcohol particles [PVA], N-butyl cyanoacrylate glue [NBCA], ethylene vinyl alcohol in dimethyl sulfoxide with tantalum [Onyx]). Embolization is performed by selectively inserting microcatheters into arteries feeding the AVM.

The diagnostic angiogram can be done under sedation. However, general anesthesia is preferred if embolization is likely. Because microcatheters are inserted selectively into small cerebral arteries, patients will receive heparin to reduce catheter-induced thromboembolism. Patients with a ruptured AVM may be intubated prior to the procedure depending on their neurological status. The anesthetic considerations include not only the management of patients with intracranial hemorrhage, but also the potential for inadvertent systemic embolism of the injected material. Some of the material used to embolize the AVM may pass through the high-flow shunt into the pulmonary circulation. During long embolization procedures, enough embolization material may deposit in the lungs and produce an acute pulmonary embolism and hypoxemia. Embolization material may also go to normal areas of the brain, resulting in neurological deficits after the procedure. Finally, if a significant portion of the AVM is embolized, the patient may be at risk for normal perfusion pressure breakthrough–related cerebral edema and possibly hemorrhage. This is thought to be due to inadequate autoregulation in adjacent brain tissue that had previously been exposed to relatively low perfusion pressure.

> ### Clinical Pearl
>
> Material used for embolization may pass through the AVM and embolize pulmonary tissue, resulting in poor oxygenation.

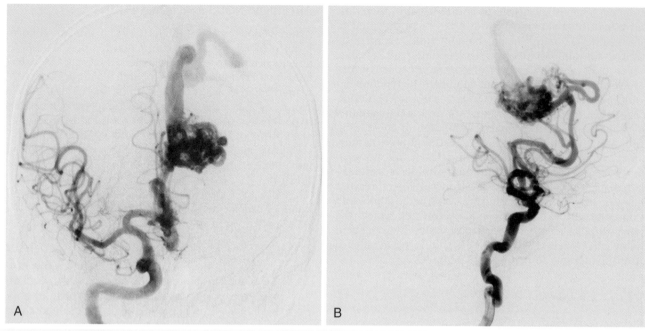

**Fig. 5.4** Angiographic images of an AVM. The AP **(A)** and lateral **(B)** images show the feeding arteries, AVM nidus, and draining vein.

## THERAPY FOR ACUTE ISCHEMIC STROKE

### Key Concepts

- Time is of essence. Time is brain.
- It is currently controversial whether sedation or general anesthesia is better.
- ICH rates are high. ICH may happen postprocedure.

Endovascular treatment of acute ischemic stroke is a true emergency, and endovascular recanalization of the occluded artery should be attempted within 6 hours from the onset of the stroke symptoms.[14] Patients typically arrive directly from the emergency room to the INR suite, and some may have received intravenous tissue plasminogen activator in the emergency room without clinical improvement. Time is of essence during these procedures to minimize neuronal cell death, and any delay to reperfusion should be minimized.[15] This patient population is commonly elderly, with comorbidities such as hypertension and vascular disease. Endovascular treatment to recanalize the cerebral vessels involves pharmacological intraarterial thrombolysis or mechanical thrombectomy (Fig. 5.5). Several thrombectomy devices are available such as stent and

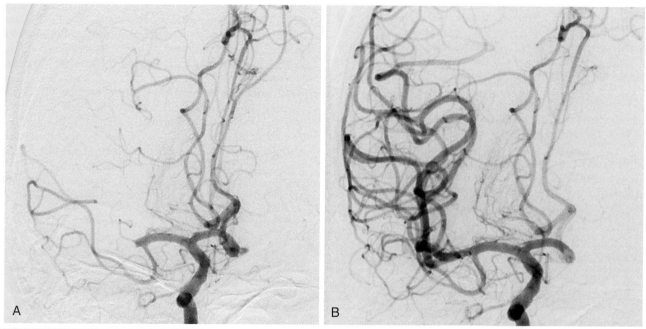

**Fig. 5.5** Middle cerebral artery ischemic stroke before **(A)** and after **(B)** successful mechanical thrombectomy of the middle cerebral artery.

coil retrievers. Removal of the thrombus may cause patient discomfort in sedated patients due to traction on the cerebral vessels.

The literature has scant information regarding anesthetic management of these cases. Recently the Society for Neuroscience in Anesthesiology and Critical Care created an expert consensus statement on anesthetic management of acute ischemic stroke.[16] The choice between sedation and general anesthesia during these procedures is controversial. Several retrospective studies have suggested an association between general anesthesia or deep sedation and poor neurological outcome. However, these studies must be interpreted cautiously due to the inherent limitations of retrospective design and inclusion bias, because patients with more severe strokes are more likely to receive general anesthesia.[17] Currently, the choice of anesthesia is based on patient and procedural factors as well as institutional preferences.

Blood pressure management in patients with acute ischemic stroke is critical and a primary concern for the anesthesiologist. Use of invasive blood pressure monitoring is recommended, provided it does not cause significant delays to reperfusion. A U-shaped relationship is seen between baseline blood pressure and death and dependency, suggesting that both excessive hypertension and hypotension should be avoided.[18,19] If general anesthesia is used, even brief episodes of hypotension should not be tolerated. A recent study found that a systolic blood pressure of less than 140 mm Hg was an independent predictor of poor neurological outcome in patients undergoing endovascular therapy for acute ischemic stroke.[7] Once the occluded cerebral artery is successfully recanalized, lowering blood pressure targets should be discussed with the neurointerventionalist and neurocritical care teams.

There is an inherent risk of hemorrhagic transformation during and after the procedure. Endovascular treatment of acute ischemic stroke is associated with a moderate incidence (3%–10%) of periprocedural intracranial hemorrhage.[14] If this complication occurs, any heparin effect should be reversed immediately with protamine and systolic blood pressure should be maintained between 140 and 180 mm Hg. If necessary, an EVD may be placed in the INR suite for management of increased ICP.

Postoperatively, these patients require intensive care and may or may not remain intubated depending on their neurological status prior to the procedure as well as the success of the intervention. Interdisciplinary communication is again pivotal to ensure optimal patient care, as often the intensive care team is not involved until after the procedure.

## ENDOVASCULAR CAROTID AND CEREBRAL ARTERY STENTING

Patients with symptomatic or severe carotid stenosis may present to the INR suite for endovascular balloon angioplasty and stenting of the carotid and proximal intracranial arteries. These procedures can be done using local anesthesia and sedation or general anesthesia depending on the characteristics of the lesion, patient comorbidities, and institutional preferences. If general anesthesia is selected, hypotension should be avoided to preserve adequate collateral cerebral circulation and cerebral blood flow.

The anesthesiologist must be prepared to treat the complications of carotid and cerebral artery stenting. Because these procedures are associated with high incidence of thromboembolism, protective devices are used to capture embolic material distal to the dilated blood vessel during the procedure. Other procedural risks include dissection or occlusion of the artery, which may require further operative intervention. Finally, dilation in close proximity to the carotid sinus may result in severe bradycardia or even asystole. If the risk of bradycardia is high, such as with dilation of carotid bulb, transcutaneous pacing pads or anticholinergic agents (glycopyrrolate, atropine) may be used either prophylactically or therapeutically. When insertion of an intraarterial stent is planned, patients are typically premedicated with antiplatelet agents (e.g., aspirin and clopidogrel) to reduce stent-associated thrombus formation. Antiplatelet drugs may also be administered during the procedure, and protamine, a reversal agent for heparin, should be readily available in case of vascular injury. Postoperatively, patients undergoing carotid or cerebral artery dilation should be evaluated frequently due to the risk of arterial occlusion or thromboembolism. In addition, dilation of a stenotic artery may increase cerebral perfusion beyond autoregulatory control, leading to hyperperfusion and neurological deterioration.

### Clinical Pearl

Patients undergoing stent procedures typically are premedicated with antiplatelet agents.

## INTRACRANIAL TUMORS

Embolization of vascular tumors before surgery is often undertaken to reduce intraoperative blood loss, induce tumor softening, and reduce operating time.[20] Once the blood supply to the tumor is determined through cerebral angiography, these vessels may be embolized using coils, particles, or glues (PVA, NBCA, or ethylene vinyl alcohol in dimethyl sulfoxide with tantalum [Onyx]). Meningiomas are commonly embolized preoperatively due to their dual intracranial and extracranial vascular supply. Again, embolization can be done using coils, particles, or glues (PVA, NBCA, or ethylene vinyl alcohol in dimethyl sulfoxide with tantalum [Onyx]). The entire vascular supply of the tumor is rarely embolized because the risk of inadvertent embolization and vascular compromise of normal brain structures is too high. These procedures are typically done under general anesthesia due to the need for patient immobility and the potentially long duration of the procedure. Anesthetic considerations are related to the tumor itself, and risks of the procedure are similar to the general risks of all endovascular procedures.

## ARTERIOVENOUS FISTULAS

Arteriovenous fistulas are abnormal connections between arteries and veins. The most common intracranial fistulas are dural arteriovenous fistulas and carotid cavernous fistulas. Patients may present with a variety of symptoms depending on the anatomical location. Fistulas can be treated using endovascular or surgical techniques. Endovascular access to treat fistulas may be from the arterial or venous side, or both. Anesthetic concerns during these procedures are mainly related to the procedure itself. The procedures are often lengthy, and general anesthesia is preferred for patient comfort. These procedures are associated with risk of intracranial hemorrhage if the blood pressure on the venous side of the fistula increases unintentionally.

## Summary

Patients undergoing procedures in the interventional neuroradiology suite present with a wide range of diagnoses for a wide spectrum of procedures. The choice of general or local anesthesia is influenced by factors related to the patient's neurological status and tolerance for lying still for a long period, the level of discomfort expected, and institutional preferences. Evidence to support one anesthetic technique over another is lacking. Potential complications from endovascular neuroradiology procedures include nephrotoxicity and allergic reactions related to contrast dye exposure, intracranial hemorrhage, stroke or emboli to healthy brain, and complications from the femoral vascular puncture site. Postoperatively, most patients require intensive care monitoring, although the level of intervention varies. Excellent communication between the neurocritical care, anesthesia, and interventional radiology teams is essential.

## References

1. Hughey AB, Lesniak MS, Ansari SA, et al. What will anesthesiologists be anesthetizing? Trends in neurosurgical procedure usage. *Anesth Analg.* 2010;110:1686–1697.
2. Anastasian ZH, Strozyk D, Meyers PM, et al. Radiation exposure of the anesthesiologist in the neurointerventional suite. *Anesthesiology.* 2011;114:512–520.
3. Tramer MR, von Elm E, Loubeyre P, et al. Pharmacological prevention of serious anaphylactic reactions due to iodinated contrast media: systematic review. *BMJ.* 2006;333:675.
4. Flexman AM, Ryerson CJ, Talke PO. Hemodynamic stability after intraarterial injection of verapamil for cerebral vasospasm. *Anesth Analg.* 2012;114:1292–1296.
5. Jumaa MA, Zhang F, Ruiz-Ares G, et al. Comparison of safety and clinical and radiographic outcomes in endovascular acute stroke therapy for proximal middle cerebral artery occlusion with intubation and general anesthesia versus the nonintubated state. *Stroke.* 2010;41:1180–1184.
6. McDonagh DL, Olson DM, Kalia JS, et al. Anesthesia and sedation practices among neurointerventionalists during acute ischemic stroke endovascular therapy. *Front Neurol.* 2010;1:118.
7. Davis MJ, Menon BK, Baghirzada LB, et al. Anesthetic management and outcome in patients during endovascular therapy for acute stroke. *Anesthesiology.* 2012;116:396–405.
8. Lee CZ, Young WL. Anesthesia for endovascular neurosurgery and interventional neuroradiology. *Anesthesiol Clin.* 2012;30:127–147.
9. Brown Jr RD, Broderick JP. Unruptured intracranial aneurysms: epidemiology, natural history, management options, and familial screening. *Lancet Neurol.* 2014;13:393–404.
10. Connolly Jr ES, Rabinstein AA, Carhuapoma JR, et al. Guidelines for the management of aneurysmal subarachnoid hemorrhage: a guideline for healthcare professionals from the American Heart Association/American Stroke Association. *Stroke.* 2012;43:1711–1737.
11. Linfante I, Delgado-Mederos R, Andreone V, et al. Angiographic and hemodynamic effect of high concentration of intra-arterial nicardipine in cerebral vasospasm. *Neurosurgery.* 2008;63:1080–1086.
12. Schmidt U, Bittner E, Pivi S, et al. Hemodynamic management and outcome of patients treated for cerebral vasospasm with intraarterial nicardipine and/or milrinone. *Anesth Analg.* 2010;110:895–902.
13. Avitsian R, Fiorella D, Soliman MM, et al. Anesthetic considerations of selective intra-arterial nicardipine injection for intracranial vasospasm: a case series. *J Neurosurg Anesthesiol.* 2007;19:125–129.
14. Jauch EC, Saver JL, Adams HP, et al. Guidelines for the early management of patients with acute ischemic stroke: a guideline for healthcare professionals from the American Heart Association/American Stroke Association. *Stroke.* 2013;44:870–947.
15. Saver JL. Time is brain—quantified. *Stroke.* 2006;37:263–266.
16. Talke PO, Sharma D, Heyer EJ, et al. Society for neuroscience in anesthesiology and critical care expert consensus statement: anesthetic management of endovascular treatment for acute ischemic stroke: endorsed by the society of neuroInterventional surgery and the neurocritical care society. *J Neurosurg Anesthesiol.* 2014;26:95–108.
17. Flexman AM, Donovan AL, Gelb AW. Anesthetic management of patients with acute stroke. *Anesthesiol Clin.* 2012;30:175–190.
18. Castillo J, Leira R, Garcia MM, et al. Blood pressure decrease during the acute phase of ischemic stroke is associated with brain injury and poor stroke outcome. *Stroke.* 2004;35:520–526.
19. Leonardi-Bee J, Bath PM, Phillips SJ, et al. Blood pressure and clinical outcomes in the International Stroke Trial. *Stroke.* 2002;33:1315–1320.
20. Shah AH, Patel N, Raper DM, et al. The role of preoperative embolization for intracranial meningiomas. *J Neurosurg.* 2013;119:364–372.

# 6 Intraoperative Neuromonitoring for Specific Neurosurgical Procedures

CLAUDIA F. CLAVIJO and BENJAMIN K. SCOTT

## Introduction

Intraoperative neurophysiological monitoring involves continuous evaluation of the electrical activity of one or more neural pathways in an anesthetized patient. The goal of these monitoring modalities is to detect surgical or physiological insults to the nervous system while they are still reversible, or in cases where prevention is not an option, to minimize the damage done to these structures during surgical resection. In recent decades, monitoring of the central nervous system has become a fundamental part of neurocritical care, a discipline primarily oriented around prevention of secondary brain and spinal cord injury. Monitoring of cerebral metabolism, brain oxygen tension, cerebral perfusion, and intracranial pressure are discussed elsewhere (see Chapter 47). In this chapter, we will focus on functional intraoperative monitoring of the primary sensory and motor pathways and the ways these monitoring techniques are commonly applied and interpreted during specific neurosurgical procedures. Intraoperative neuromonitoring findings, especially changes from baseline, should be communicated as part of the postoperative transfer of care and may help the intensivist make early decisions about imaging or focused clinical evaluations after a procedure.

## Evoked Potentials

### Key Concepts

- Evoked potential refers to an electrophysiological response obtained after stimulation of a targeted neural pathway.
- Somatosensory evoked potentials (SSEPs) are the most commonly used modality and allow continuous direct monitoring of the dorsal column–medial lemniscus pathway.
- Motor evoked potentials (MEPs) monitor the efferent pathways from the motor cortex via corticospinal and corticobulbar tracts.
- MEPs cannot be run continuously. Instead, they are performed at specified intervals or when there is concern for a potential injury. Changes will not be detected between tests.
- SSEP monitoring relies on temporal summation. Changes in SSEP waveforms may lag behind changes in MEPs.
- Auditory brainstem responses (ABRs) are relatively unaffected by anesthetic drugs.

- The use of visual evoked potentials is controversial when they are performed in patients under general anesthesia due to large variability between individuals and instability of the signals during exposure to anesthetic drugs.
- A multimodal approach, tailored to the anatomical pathways at risk, improves sensitivity and can overcome the weaknesses of individual modalities.

### SOMATOSENSORY EVOKED POTENTIALS

SSEPs are measured cortical or subcortical electrophysiological responses to stimulation of a peripheral sensory or mixed nerve. They provide direct monitoring of the dorsal column–medial lemniscus pathway. SSEPs were first described in the late 1970s,[1] and they remain the most widely used modality for intraoperative neuromonitoring (IONM). SSEPs can be measured from almost any nerve containing sensory fibers, but in practice, arms are generally monitored using the median or ulnar nerves, and legs using the common peroneal or posterior tibial nerves. Peripheral electrical stimulation, using a needle or contact electrode and current in the range of 200 to 400 mA, activates fast-conducting Ia muscle afferent fibers and group II cutaneous nerve fibers, producing two types of transmission: orthodromic (impulse propagation in the normal direction) and antidromic (propagation in the reverse direction). Orthodromic motor stimulation can be seen as twitching of the foot or hand, whereas orthodromic sensory stimulation produces the SSEP. The cortical response is detected on the scalp over the corresponding contralateral primary somatosensory cortex (Fig. 6.1). In some cases, a subcortical intracranial response may be measured over the posterior neck. These responses are recorded as deflections or peaks—positive and negative—and serial measurements are then plotted in a graph of voltage versus time, which can be quantified for comparison throughout the procedure in terms of strength of response, or amplitude (microvolts), and time from stimulus to response, referred to as *latency* (milliseconds) (Figs 6.2 and 6.3).[2]

Latencies are a function of patient height and limb length; are generally prolonged with age; and are influenced by neuropathy, temperature, and drug effects. Amplitude is also affected by patient factors. Because there are no true population-based normal values, the patient serves as his or her own baseline during monitoring. It is important to recognize that these measured electrical signals are very low amplitude relative to muscle artifact,

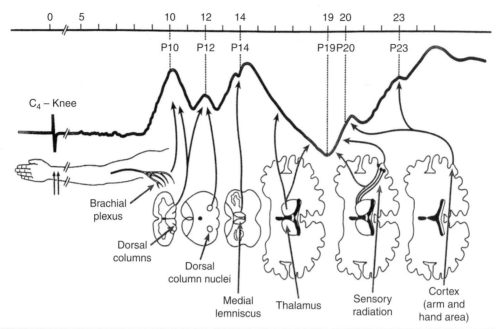

**Fig. 6.1** Somatosensory evoked potentials. Image shows the anatomy of the sensory cortex (C4) and the correspondent somatosensory evoked potential peaks using the international 10 to 20 system. Positive peaks are labeled "P" followed by the time in milliseconds. (Reprinted from Wiederholt WC, et al., Stimulating and recording methods used in obtaining short-latency somatosensory evoked potentials (SEPs) in patients with central and peripheral disorders. *Ann N Y Acad Sci.* 1982;388:349–58.)

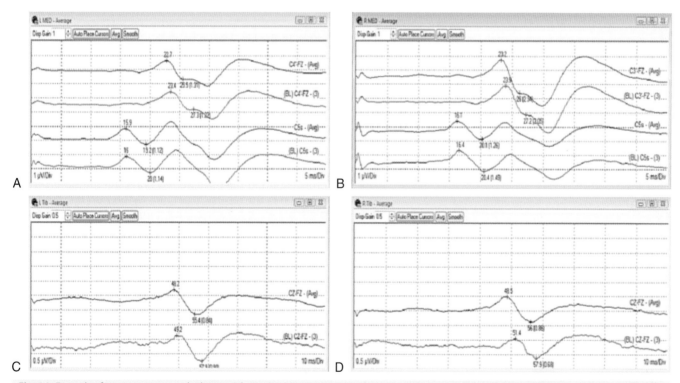

**Fig. 6.2** Example of somatosensory evoked potentials monitoring in a patient undergoing spine surgery. Recording from **(A)** left median nerve, **(B)** right median nerve, **(C)** left posterior tibial nerve, and **(D)** right posterior tibial nerve.

electroencephalogram (EEG) and electrocardiogram (ECG) activity, and environmental electrical interference. As a result, temporal summation is used to calculate averages of from 500 to 2000 repetitive stimulations, thereby allowing subtraction of electrical noise and reproduction of a meaningful signal.

SSEPs are used during surgeries in which the somatosensory pathways are at significant risk, and particularly when timely recognition of a new deficit may allow corrective action. Appropriate cases for SSEP monitoring include cervical and thoracic spine fusions, spinal cord tumor removal, arteriovenous malformations, surgeries that place peripheral

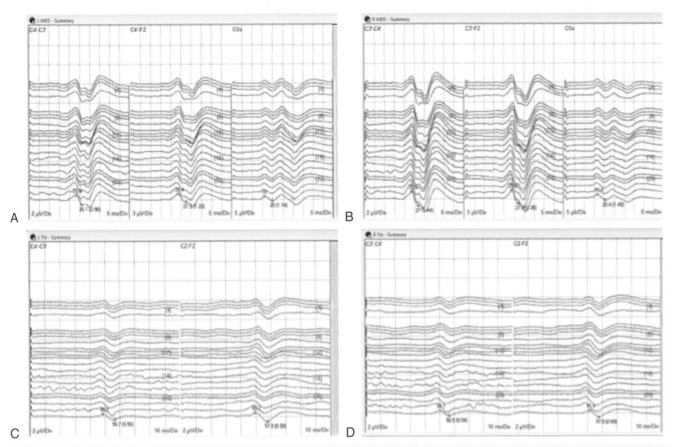

**Fig. 6.3** Summary or stack of somatosensory evoked potentials at the end of a spine surgery. Signals were recorded from (**A**) left median nerve, (**B**) right median nerve, (**C**) left posterior tibial nerve, and (**D**) right posterior tibial nerve. *Red line* at the bottom indicates baseline. *Black lines* represent signals at different time points throughout the case.

nerves and brachial plexus at risk (either because of the nature of the procedure or to avoid positioning-related neuropraxia), and thoracic and abdominal aneurysm repair. They can also be of paramount importance in the monitoring of the brainstem, subcortical, and cortical structures during tumor resection; carotid endarterectomy; cerebral aneurysm clipping; and hemispheric, deep brain, and posterior fossa surgeries. Spinal cord surveillance, however, is the most common application.

SSEP monitoring has several practical advantages. Although population-based normal values are lacking, for an individual patient under steady-state conditions, waveforms tend to be consistent and reproducible. Their amplitude and latency can be thus quantified, recorded, and assessed serially for comparison to the patient's preincision baseline. Because signals tend to be stable, changes in amplitude or latency correlate well with injury. Localization of the site of injury, that is, peripheral nerve, spinal cord, or brain, is also possible, because multiple recording sites can be ascertained concomitantly. Based on the available evidence, a significant change in SSEP is reported when the amplitude drops below 50% of baseline and/or the latency increases more than 10% (Fig. 6.4).[3]

Intraoperative degradation of the SSEP beyond the alert threshold is often due to relative hypothermia, anesthetic effects, or changes in carbon dioxide tension but should always prompt a search for reversible causes of neurotrauma, including positioning-related nerve stretch or

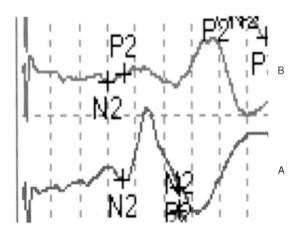

**Fig. 6.4** Example of changes in somatosensory evoked potentials in a patient undergoing aortic arch surgery. An increase in latency of somatosensory evoked potentials is noted at 26°C (**B**) in comparison with baseline signals at 37°C (**A**).

compression, ischemia or anoxic injury, acute surgical injury to the nerves or spinal cord itself, or hypoperfusion. Most anesthetic drugs cause a dose-dependent reduction in amplitude and can also prolong latency in higher doses. Close coordination between the surgical team, anesthesiologist, and neuromonitoring team is essential in order to minimize unnecessary anesthetic-mediated SSEP changes. Optimally a stable and minimally changing anesthetic paradigm is chosen that yields signals amenable to interpretation while ensuring suitable anesthetic goals.

The primary weakness of SSEP monitoring is related to the time it takes for changes to appear in a signal that relies on temporal summation. Evidence suggests that changes in SSEP waveforms may lag as far as 16 minutes behind changes in MEPs, well after an acute injury occurs, and possibly too late for corrective action.[4] SSEPs also have a lower likelihood of detecting nerve root injury from traction or hardware placement. As a result, many centers favor using SSEP monitoring in conjunction with other modalities.

Although definitive evidence demonstrating improved surgical outcomes due to SSEP monitoring has been elusive, benefits of SSEP monitoring have been reported in multiple studies. In 1995 the Scoliosis Research Society reported a 50% decrease in major neurological deficits associated with scoliosis surgeries after the introduction of IONM. SSEPs were found to be 92% sensitive and 98% specific to detect significant spinal cord insults. Not unexpectedly, a reduction of 50% in neurological deficits was described when experienced monitoring teams participated in the cases compared with inexperienced teams.[5] Based on the available evidence, SSEP monitoring has become standard of care in many centers, but specific indications are still a matter of some debate. Recent decisions by Medicaid and private insurers have challenged existing reimbursement paradigms and renewed concerns about the costs versus benefits of monitoring, particularly in lower-risk spine surgeries.

### Clinical Pearl

Single monitoring modalities are rarely used alone—a multimodal approach, tailored to the anatomical pathways at risk, improves sensitivity and can overcome the weaknesses of individual monitoring modalities.

## MOTOR EVOKED POTENTIALS

Motor dysfunction is probably the most feared form of spinal cord injury. Traditionally, SSEPs have been used to monitor spinal cord function, including motor dysfunction, even though SSEPs monitor the signals traveling through the dorsal columns of the spinal cord. However, because motor pathways lie in the anterior column, SSEPs can only indirectly evaluate motor function through coexisting dysfunction in sensory pathways. Anatomically, there is a separation between anterior (motor) and posterior (sensory) pathways. The vascular supply is also different, and the anterior columns are more susceptible to ischemia due to a weaker anastomotic network that provides less reserve for ischemia. In addition, gray-matter neurons are more sensitive to ischemia than those axons located in the white-matter dorsal columns. As a result of this anatomical context and the weaknesses of SSEP monitoring discussed earlier, MEPs have become common practice in surgical cases with a high probability of motor injury, such as correction of axial skeletal deformities, resection of intramedullary spinal cord and certain

intracranial tumors, and vascular procedures that threaten spinal cord perfusion. The most common scenario for MEP is in patients undergoing axial skeletal surgery above the terminal spinal cord. MEPs are combined with SSEPs and electromyography (EMG) monitoring to enhance the sensitivity and improve the confidence of these techniques and because they have better correlation with postoperative motor outcome. Several studies have demonstrated a correlation between a transient or permanent loss of MEP signals and long-term motor dysfunction.[6–8]

Monitoring of the motor pathways can be accomplished by stimulation of the motor cortex, using electrodes placed on the scalp, immediately above the motor cortex (transcranial MEP) or directly on the motor cortex (direct MEP), with the former being most common in clinical practice. Direct cortical stimulation is used for intraoperative motor mapping during surgical resection of tumors in the vicinity of the motor cortex. Two techniques have been described: the 60-Hz and the train of five technique. The 60-Hz technique applies 60-Hz-frequency stimuli over 1 to 3 seconds. On the other hand, in the train of five technique, five to seven high-frequency stimuli (256–512 Hz) are applied directly to the motor cortex to allow recording of muscle MEPs. Seizures have been reported with both techniques, being more common in the 60-Hz technique.[9] Although theoretically available since the 1980s,[10] early efforts to record MEPs were limited by the frailty of these signals. With the introduction of high-frequency, low-voltage multipulse stimulation in the mid-1990s, better reproducibility and increased anesthetic resistance made intraoperative MEP monitoring feasible.[11]

Transcranial stimulation of the motor cortex using electrical or magnetic techniques provokes a descending response that travels through the corticospinal tract (Fig. 6.5). This response generates either muscle activity that can be recorded near the muscle, as a compound muscle action potential (CMAP), or a spinal cord synaptic response in the anterior horn cells, which can be recorded with electrodes placed in the epidural or subdural space as a "direct wave" (D-wave).[12,13] The amplitudes of D-wave signals tend to be more stable and resistant to anesthetic effects. Unfortunately, they do not differentiate laterality of injury. On the other hand, muscle recordings can appropriately differentiate unilateral changes and evaluate specific nerves, but they are more affected by anesthetic techniques; therefore special anesthetic considerations are required when MEPs are going to be monitored.

Appropriate muscles must be selected to effectively localize motor deficits. It is recommended that at least two muscles from each side below the surgical level be monitored and at least one above it be utilized as a control. Some of the muscles commonly used are the abductor pollicis brevis, the tibialis anterior, and the abductor hallucis, but other muscles may be chosen according to the surgical needs (Figs. 6.6 and 6.7).

MEPs have been successful in multiple surgical scenarios. Recent studies have suggested that MEPs are a useful tool for intraoperative monitoring in intramedullary spinal cord tumor resection. They have been successfully used to determine the edge of the tumor, hence, maximizing the resection and minimizing the risk of motor injury. Both D-wave and CMAP are correlated with increased

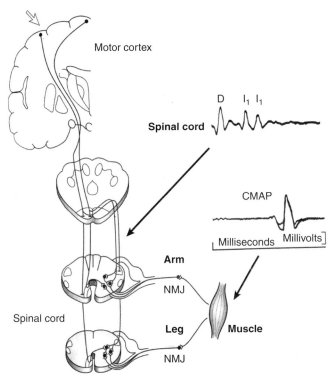

**Fig. 6.5** Motor evoked potentials. Image shows the motor pathway anatomy and the different modalities that can be used to record the response. The response can be recorded over the spinal cord (D wave). Responses can also be recorded near the muscle, as a compound muscle action potential (CMAP) after they have traveled via the anterior horn of the spinal cord and the neuromuscular junction. (Reprinted from Jameson LC, Sloan TB. Monitoring the brain and the spinal cord. *Anesthesiol Clin.* 2006 Dec;24(4):777–91.)

of ischemia and implementation of corrective actions. Examples of these cases include surgical or interventional radiological procedures for thoracoabdominal aneurysm repair and corrective anterior thoracic spinal surgery. During these procedures, inadequate perfusion due to insufficient collateral circulation, particularly through the artery of Adamkiewicz and pelvic supply to the caudal spinal cord, could occur and place the spinal cord at risk for ischemia.

In intracranial vascular surgery, and especially during clipping of aneurysms of the middle and anterior cerebral, basilar, and carotid territories, different components of the motor pathways, including the motor cortex, pyramidal cells, corticospinal tracts, and internal capsule, are at risk. In these cases MEPs have been used to detect intraoperative hypoperfusion (vasospasm or inadequate clip placement).[16,17]

Direct motor cortex stimulation is helpful to detect tumor boundaries during brain tumor resection, reducing the possibility of motor injury. In this particular case, transient motor changes have been shown to correlate with reversible postoperative motor weakness and permanent intraoperative changes of the MEP, with irreversible motor dysfunction.[18] In the same way, the magnitude of the change observed in motor signals is associated with the severity of the postoperative motor deficit.[18,19]

Common side effects of MEPs include muscle soreness, bruising, and bleeding at the place of needle insertion. More severe complications, including tongue lacerations, cardiac arrhythmias, scalp burns, awareness, and jaw fracture, have also been reported in the literature. The most feared complications are probably direct cortical thermal injury and brain injury due to the electrical overstimulation producing a seizure focus or triggering seizures in patients with epilepsy.[20] Fortunately in the last 17 years, only two cases of thermal injury have been reported. These complications are extremely rare, and MEPs are considered safe for the majority of patients. Relative contraindications for MEP include epilepsy, cortical lesions, skull defects, high intracranial pressure, and the presence of intracranial

likelihood of favorable motor outcome compared with SSEP alone.[14,15]

In cases where vascular supply of the spinal cord could be compromised, MEP monitoring allows rapid detection

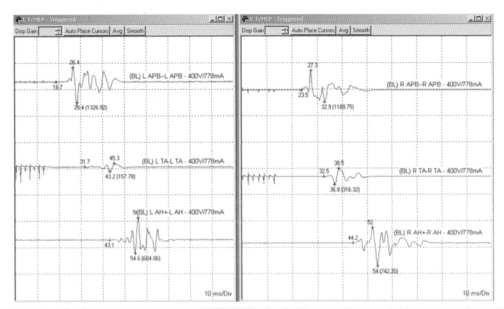

**Fig. 6.6** Example of transcranial evoked potentials (TcMEP) monitoring in a patient undergoing cervical spine surgery. Signals were obtained from right and left abductor pollicis brevis (APB), tibialis anterior (TA), and abductor hallucis (AH).

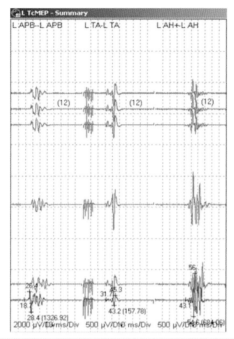

Fig. 6.7 Summary of transcranial motor evoked potentials. Abductor pollicis brevis (APB), tibialis anterior (TA), and abductor hallucis (AH) were monitored throughout the surgery. Signal in *red* at the bottom indicates baseline. Signals in *pink* indicate responses at different time points during the surgery.

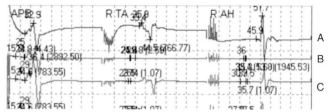

Fig. 6.8 Example of changes in motor evoked potentials. Baseline signals detected responses from abductor pollicis brevis (APB), tibialis anterior (TA), and abductor hallucis (AH) (A) in a patient undergoing endovascular repair of descending aortic aneurysm. The left iliac was occluded at some point during the procedure. Responses from the left leg were not detected (B). Signals returned after occlusion was removed (C).

devices. Implanted extracranial biomedical devices, such as pacemakers and defibrillators, vagal nerve stimulators, and drug-delivery pumps, are also considered a relative contraindication.[20,21]

As with SSEP monitoring, special anesthetic considerations are mandatory to obtain MEP. Coordination between anesthesia, surgical, and neuromonitoring teams is of paramount importance. The use of inhalational agents should be avoided in favor of total intravenous techniques when possible. Because MEPs rely on movement, neuromuscular blockade is incompatible with MEP monitoring. Aside from the fragility of the signals themselves, the primary disadvantage of MEPs is that they cannot be run continuously. Instead, they are performed at specified intervals or when there is concern for a potential injury. In either case, there is potential that a change may not be detected until well after an injury has occurred.

It has been difficult to establish standard criteria to determine when a change in motor responses is significant, because these vary substantially even in awake control subjects,[22] and that variability is intensified by general anesthesia.[23] As a result, various alert criteria have been suggested. The absence of a CMAP that was present at baseline is considered a definite change according to most authors (Fig. 6.8.). A rise in the stimulation strength >50 V, an increase in the number of stimuli required to obtain the same signal, and a reduction in the amplitude >80% from baseline have also been used to define a change in motor response. The degree of change has not been correlated with postoperative changes in motor function, but the absence of a signal should be promptly communicated to the surgeon and anesthesia provider so corrective actions can be implemented.

Specific anesthetic techniques may be required for patients undergoing intraoperative MEPs. Anesthetic goals generally include minimizing the use of inhaled agents and neuromuscular-blocking drugs and instead utilizing what is often referred to as *total intravenous anesthesia* (TIVA), which combines sedative hypnotics such as propofol, ketamine, dexmedetomidine, or etomidate to achieve amnesia and opioids such as sufentanil and remifentanil for analgesia. In combination, these infusions also act synergistically to minimize patient movement without the need for neuromuscular blockade.[24,25] As with any drug regimen, total intravenous techniques may have adverse intraoperative and postoperative effects. Patients who have received ketamine may develop postoperative hallucinations. Patients receiving etomidate may have issues with adrenal suppression or lactic acidosis from the drug vehicle, and cessation of remifentanil can result in significant and abrupt pain. Moreover, not using neuromuscular blockade may increase the risk of intraoperative coughing or movement that could result in surgical injury during critical portions of the operation and lead to residual postoperative deficits. Finally, the use of an intraoperative propofol infusion may precipitate hypotension, and patients undergoing total intravenous anesthesia for spine surgery are much more likely to be placed on an intraoperative phenylephrine infusion to mitigate this effect, which generally resolves by the time of extubation but may persist into the recovery room or intensive care unit.

## Clinical Pearl

Motor evoked potentials are extremely sensitive to anesthetic drugs. As a result, their proper application in the intraoperative setting requires careful selection of pharmacological agents and close coordination between the surgical, anesthesia, and monitoring teams.

## AUDITORY BRAINSTEM RESPONSES

ABRs are the evoked potential responses obtained from the brainstem after stimulation. They have also been called *brainstem auditory evoked responses* (BAER) and *brainstem auditory evoked potentials* (BAEP). These evoked potentials are relatively unaffected by anesthetic drugs and are

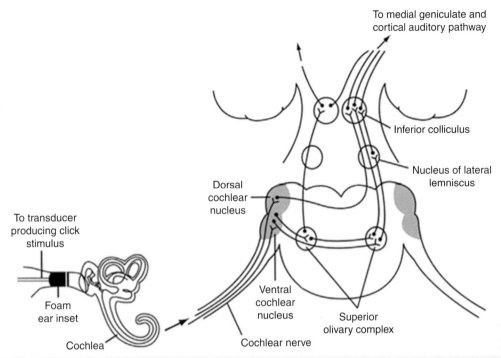

**Fig. 6.9** Auditory brainstem response. Image shows a representation of the normal brainstem response after stimulation and the correspondent peaks labeled by Roman numerals by convention: I. organ of Corti and extracranial nerve VII; II. cochlear nucleus; III. superior olivary complex; IV. lateral lemniscus; V. inferior colliculus; VI. medial geniculate body; VII. auditory radiation. (Reprinted with permission from Mahla ME. Neurological monitoring. In: Cucchiara RF, Black S, Michenfelder JD, eds. *Clinical neuroanesthesia*, 2nd ed. New York: Churchill Livingstone; 1998.)

usually obtained 10 msec after stimulation. Stimulation is undertaken with clicks or tone pips with frequencies in the 1000 to 4000 Hz range. This sound activates the auditory pathway. The middle ear is stimulated first. The vibration activates the hair cells in the cochlea, and the impulse travels, via the eighth cranial nerve, to the brainstem and then to the auditory cortex, producing a stereotyped series of evoked potential signals.

Peaks obtained are labeled I through VII, with peaks I, III, and V being the most useful for monitoring purposes (Figs 6.9 and 6.10). Wave I is produced by the extracranial portion of the cranial nerve VIII, whereas wave II is created by the intracranial portion of the same cranial nerve. Wave III is produced by the cochlear nuclei. Waves IV and V originate in the lateral lemniscus, the superior olivary complex, and the inferior colliculus and the contralateral lateral lemniscus, respectively. Wave VI arises in the medial geniculate nuclei, and wave VII in the thalamocortical radiations. The designations of the waveforms help identify the approximate location in case of injury.[26] Direct recording from the auditory neural pathways in the brainstem (cochlear microphonics from the promontorium) and recording from the exposed portion of cranial nerve VIII (cochlear action potentials) have also been utilized to monitor auditory function.

ABRs are mainly used in surgery involving the posterior fossa, because cochlear nerve involvement is not uncommon in tumors affecting this area. They are also helpful to monitor viability of the brainstem, mainly in cases where there is risk of injury by direct manipulation, positioning, or changes in vascular supply. Examples of these cases are tumors or vascular malformations of the cerebellum and microvascular decompression for trigeminal neuralgia.

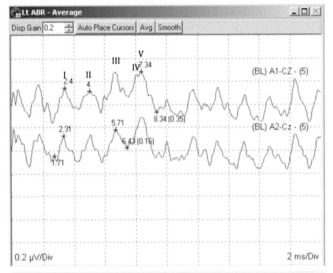

**Fig. 6.10** Example of auditory brainstem responses in a patient undergoing excision of acoustic neuroma. Classical waveforms were detected. The most common waveforms followed in surgical procedures are I, III, and V. The designations of the waveforms help to identify the approximate location in case of injury.

As in other evoked potential monitoring, the amplitude and the latency of the waveforms are followed and recorded, and changes are reported in real time to the surgical team. The most common changes seen are an increase in the latency in wave V and a rise in the interpeak latency from I through V. These changes are usually due to retractor placement in the posterior fossa and are reversible in nature. A complete loss of wave I can occur because of compromise of cochlear blood supply or transection of the nerve. Loss of hearing is the observed consequence. Wave V can be lost due to desynchronization in the hearing pathway and does not necessarily correlate with hearing loss. In most patients, if waves I and V are preserved, hearing is not compromised. When both are lost, hearing is usually affected.

## VISUAL EVOKED POTENTIALS

Visual evoked potentials (VEPs) are obtained as a response to ocular light stimulation. In patients under general anesthesia, flash stimulation through closed eyelids or stimulators placed in scleral caps has been described. Responses are generated by the visual cortex bilaterally. In practice, VEPs are difficult to employ clinically. Interindividual and intraindividual variability in the responses are commonly seen, as well as instability of MEP. Some authors have reported favorable outcomes when VEP are used,[27–30] but others have not been able to find a correlation between responses and postoperative functional outcomes.[31–37] Universal criteria have been difficult to determine due to the previously mentioned characteristics. Even though conflicting results are reported, VEPs are used to monitor the anterior visual pathways during craniofacial, pituitary, and occipital cortex surgeries, as well as during procedures of the retrochiasmatic visual tracts. Several anesthetic techniques have been studied to facilitate intraoperative monitoring of visual pathways. Most authors agree that VEPs are sensitive to inhalational agents in a dose-related manner. Both amplitude and latency are affected with different inhalational agents at high concentration—this is particularly true when nitrous oxide is added to the anesthetic regimen. Concentrations of nitrous oxide between 10% and 50% have no effect on latency but have a high impact on amplitude. The use of propofol-based anesthetics in conjunction with ketamine; opioids such as fentanyl, sufentanil, and remifentanil; and techniques targeting less than 0.5 mean alveolar concentration (MAC) of inhalational agent without nitrous oxide facilitate intraoperative VEPs.[38]

# Electromyography

## Key Concepts

- EMG is useful in the detection of peripheral nerve injury or irritation and can be done continuously (spontaneous) and/or with periodic stimulation.
- EMG signals are resistant to anesthetic effects and blood pressure changes, but they can be affected by the use of neuromuscular blockade.
- EMG is particularly useful in evaluating spinal nerve roots and is commonly performed for monitoring of the cranial nerves that have a motor component to avoid disability, deformities, and pain associated with injuries due to surgery.

EMG uses muscle responses to monitor neural tracts. EMG monitoring can be done by recording spontaneous activity or by recording the activity of motor pathways after proximal stimulation. Spontaneous activity can be continuously monitored using what is termed *free-running* EMG. To detect muscle activity, needles are placed near the targeted muscles and electrical activity from these muscles is recorded. Nerve irritation and injury produce spontaneous high-frequency bursts of motor unit potentials. Irritation may also originate from nerve retraction, thermal irritation, and mechanical or chemical stimulation.

During stimulated EMG (direct stimulation to locate/ identify a nerve or to test its distal motor function), a bipolar or monopolar electrode is used intentionally to activate a nerve. For identification of cranial nerves, low-intensity current and short-duration stimuli suffice. Short bursts of activity are concerning when they persist and have high amplitude. Impending nerve injury is suspected when continuous and synchronous long trains of activity are detected. Ischemia, compression, or traction of the nerve must be ruled out. Unfortunately, when a sharp transection has occurred, a response is not likely to be seen.

As with other modalities of IONM, coordination with the anesthesia team is indispensable. EMG signals are relatively resistant to inhalation agents, changes in blood pressure, and temperature fluctuations, but they can be affected by the use of neuromuscular blockade. Some experts argue that EMG can still be followed if at least 25% of the CMAPS are not suppressed,[39] but others claim that following nerve signals from weak or previously compromised nerves can be unacceptably difficult while the patient is under incomplete neuromuscular blockade; thus the use of neuromuscular blockade in EMG monitoring is controversial.

EMG is commonly used to monitor the motor function of cranial nerves (Table 6.1 summarizes the most commonly monitored cranial nerves). The facial nerve (VII) is the most common cranial nerve monitored. Its monitoring is particularly useful in vestibular schwannomas, also called *acoustic neuromas*. The facial nerve can be very closely adjacent to or involved with the tumor, and monitoring can help maintain its integrity. The National Institutes of Health (NIH) has recommended routine monitoring of cranial nerve VII in acoustic neuroma surgeries based on data demonstrating improved outcomes when monitoring was

**Table 6.1** EMG Cranial Nerves and Nerve Roots with Corresponding Muscles Most Commonly Monitored

| Cranial Nerves | Innervated Muscles |
| --- | --- |
| III | Extraocular |
| IV | Extraocular |
| V | Masseter, temporalis |
| VI | Extraocular |
| VII | Orbicularis oculus, orbicularis oris, mentalis, frontalis |
| IX | Stylopharyngeus |
| X | Pharyngeal and laryngeal |
| XI | Sternocleidomastoid, trapezius |
| XII | Tongue |

utilized.[40] Monitoring of the facial nerve is also used in other cerebellopontine angle procedures and in head and neck surgeries, such as removal of parotid tumors.

Stimulation of cranial nerves IX and X is also used to evaluate the integrity of these nerves during head and neck surgery. Stimulation of the recurrent laryngeal nerve and of the superior laryngeal branches of the vagus nerve is recommended in thyroidectomies, parathyroidectomies, anterior cervical spine fusions, and neck dissections—especially in reexplorations, second operations, malignancies, and when the anatomy is expected to be distorted. Electrodes may be placed directly in the cricothyroid or vocalis muscles, or more commonly, a specialized EMG endotracheal tube containing contact electrodes is used. Such endotracheal tubes are not magnetic resonance imaging (MRI) compatible. If an endotracheal tube is needed after surgery, it must be changed to a standard endotracheal tube prior to a postoperative MRI.

In spinal cord procedures, EMG is generally considered more sensitive than SSEP for the monitoring of nerve roots. The main reason is that cortical responses obtained in SSEP are the result of stimulation of multiple nerve roots, whereas EMG can monitor individual nerve roots by tracking the activity of specific muscles (Table 6.2 shows the nerve roots and muscles most commonly monitored). EMG has been particularly useful in guiding hardware placement during minimally invasive techniques. For pedicle screw placement, for example, EMG is recommended to evaluate the integrity of the pedicle wall and to detect pedicle breaches that might threaten nerve roots. Stimulation can be done through the screw hole or the screw itself. Because cortical bone has higher electrical resistance than soft tissue, the lower the stimulation threshold, the higher the possibility that the bone wall has been breached.

In interventions of the cauda equina, such as tumor resection or tethered-cord release, protecting the nerve roots that innervate the anal and urethral sphincters and the legs is of major concern. EMG may be helpful in differentiating nerves from nonfunctional tissue. Reflex arcs in the cauda equina, the spinal cord, and the nerve roots can also be monitored using nerve conduction studies. A peripheral nerve is stimulated (M wave is produced), and this stimulation activates the alpha motor neuron in the spinal gray matter (H reflex). The H reflex is therefore used to evaluate the sensory and motor-efferent pathway in the nerve and in the spinal gray matter, as well as the components of the reflex arc. The H reflex can be monitored from different nerve–muscle combinations. In the lower extremities, the combination of posterior tibial and gastrocnemius is commonly used. Some authors have reported that H reflexes are more sensitive for detection of spinal cord injury than SSEP. This signal can be lost within minutes before SSEP changes are detected. It has been reported that the extent of suppression correlates with the degree of injury.[41,42] H-reflex testing is most frequently used in combination with SSEP and MEP for monitoring in spine procedures.

As with SSEP and MEP monitoring, EMG offers advantages and disadvantages. Unlike MEP monitoring, free-running (spontaneous) EMG is continuous. However, EMG has high false-positive rates due to electrical

**Table 6.2** Nerve Roots with Corresponding Muscle Most Commonly Monitored

| Spinal Root | Innervated Muscle |
| --- | --- |
| C1 | None |
| C2 | Sternocleidomastoid |
| C3 | Sternocleidomastoid, trapezius |
| C4 | Trapezius, levator scapulae |
| C5 | Deltoid, biceps |
| C6 | Biceps, triceps, brachioradialis, pronator teres, flexor carpi radialis |
| C7 | Triceps, pronator teres, flexor carpis radialis, extensors of the forearm |
| C8 | Tricep, ulnar forearm muscles, hand intrinsic muscles |
| T1 | Hand intrinsic muscles, flexor carpi ulnaris |
| T2, T3, T4, T5, T6 | Intercostal, paraspinal |
| T6, T7, T8 | Upper rectus abdominis, intercostal, paraspinal |
| T8, T9, T10 | Middle rectus abdominis, intercostal, paraspinal |
| T10, T11, T12 | Lower rectus abdominis, intercostal, paraspinal |
| L1 | Quadratus lumborum, paraspinal, internal oblique, iliopsoas, cremaster |
| L2 | Iliopsoas, quadriceps, adductor longus, adductor magnus |
| L3 | Quadriceps, iliopsoas, adductor longus, adductor magnus |
| L4 | Quadriceps, tibialis anterior, adductor longus, adductor magnus, iliopsoas |
| L5 | Tibialis anterior, peroneus longus, adductor magnus |
| S1 | Gastrocnemius, abductor hallucis |
| S2 | Gastrocnemius, abductor hallucis |
| S2–S5 | Urethral sphincter, anal sphincter |

interference (as from cautery) and is affected by temperature changes. Stimulated EMG is not a direct test of nerve function, but rather a test of pedicle insulation and by proxy integrity, and thus may be falsely positive in cases where several screw passes must be made or conduction is altered by the presence of a bloody operative field. As a result of these strengths and weaknesses, a multimodal approach is generally used to monitor the spinal cord. SSEP, MEP, and EMG are usually combined to improve sensitivity and early detection of possible injuries, reducing the possibility of permanent damage.

## Clinical Pearl

EMG monitoring should be utilized when there is high risk of radicular or peripheral nerve injury during surgery.

# Electroencephalography

## Key Concepts

- Intraoperative EEG is often used to detect regional ischemia in addition to seizure foci and eloquent cortex during resection.
- Montages are often basic due to surgical priorities.
- Special attention is paid to asymmetrical changes or inappropriate slowing that may herald regional injury.
- EEG can be used to guide burst suppression during high-dose anesthetic administration, cooling, or after an intraoperative cardiac arrest.

The role of EEG in IONM is to measure cortical function and to detect widespread gross changes in real time. Even though cortical action potentials are larger in amplitude than postsynaptic potentials, EEG waveforms are the result of postsynaptic activity of cerebrocortical neurons. Montages are chosen according to surgical needs and sometimes have to be modified due to space limitation or interference with the sterile conditions of the surgical field. For intracranial procedures, scalp, subdural, or cortical electrode strips can be added to focus on a specific area. EEG is frequently used in combination with other monitoring techniques, such as SSEP. In these cases, standard electrode montages for SSEP can be used as part of the EEG montage. When the detection of gross changes is the goal, more complex high spatial resolution montages are generally not necessary.

EEG waveforms are classified according to their frequency: beta 13 to 30 Hz, alpha 8 to 12 Hz, theta 4 to 7 Hz, and delta <4 Hz. When a patient is awake and no anesthesia is administered, the frequency of the waves correlates with wakefulness. In patients under general anesthesia, however, the anesthesia depth influences the EEG frequency. During induction, beta activity is seen and then the frequency of the waves slows down. With increasing anesthetic depth, burst suppression and electric inactivity can be seen.

After a baseline EEG is obtained, subsequent waveforms need to be compared with the patient's own baseline signals. Special attention should be paid to symmetry throughout the case, as well as changes in amplitude and frequency, because they can lead to detection of surgically induced insults in the cerebral cortex. As in other modalities of neuromonitoring, coordination with the anesthesia provider is of major importance, particularly around the time of critical events. Anesthetic regimens should be stable to allow clinical interpretation of EEG, because boluses of anesthetics agents, for example, can produce a burst suppression pattern that is likely to interfere with the detection of changes.

EEG monitoring may be useful in procedures where the cerebral cortex is directly at risk. Examples include resection of arteriovenous malformations, carotid endarterectomy, and aneurysm repair, in which the vascular supply of the cortex can be compromised. EEG is also useful as a tool to evaluate anesthetic effects when cerebral protection is needed. Burst suppression and isoelectric cerebral silence are targeted when cerebral protection is intended as in procedures of the aortic arch. Monitoring of cerebral waves is also important for the detection of epileptogenic tissue in epilepsy surgery or to detect eloquent areas in cortex mapping techniques when resection of dysfunctional brain is needed.[13]

## SPECIFIC PROCEDURES REQUIRING NEUROMONITORING

Surgical procedures that commonly involve intraoperative neuromonitoring can be classified in four groups. Table 6.3 shows specific procedures and recommended neuromonitoring.

Spine skeletal procedures can be subdivided anatomically into cervical, thoracic, and lumbar procedures. For cervical spine interventions, the most common monitoring techniques are SSEP, MEP, and free-running EMG. In thoracic procedures, stimulated EMG is added to the previously mentioned neuromonitoring techniques. For lumbar instrumentation, SSEP and both free-running and stimulating EMG are indicated. In isolated lumbar discectomy, EMG alone may be considered sufficient.

The most common head and neck procedures requiring intraoperative monitoring are mastoid surgery, cochlear implant, parotidectomy, thyroidectomy, and radical neck dissection. For all of these procedures, free-running and stimulated EMG (primarily of cranial nerves VII and X) are recommended.

Neurosurgical procedures can be subclassified into procedures of the spine (tumors, vascular), the posterior fossa (acoustic neuroma, cerebellopontine angle, vascular), and supratentorial (middle cerebral artery aneurysms, tumors in the motor cortex). In cases of tumor- or vascular-related procedures of the spine, the combination of SSEP and MEP is recommended.

ABRs in combination with EMG are helpful in acoustic neuroma, cerebellopontine angle procedures, and other vascular interventions in the posterior fossa.

In supratentorial interventions such as aneurysms of the middle cerebral artery, the use of MEP is indicated. When a tumor in the cortex needs to be intervened, the addition of SSEP to MEP provides better sensitivity.

In neuroendovascular procedures, intraoperative neuromonitoring can detect evolving neural compromise and facilitate rapid intervention and correction of precipitating factors, including ischemia of the extremities and nerve impingement or stretch due to positioning, thereby minimizing the possibility of permanent neurological damage. Different modalities of neuromonitoring are recommended according to the area at risk. EEG monitoring is very sensitive to cortical ischemia but is less sensitive to changes in the subcortical area. SSEP and MEP are frequently used in combination with EEG to increase anatomical coverage.

Although beyond the scope of this chapter, intraoperative neuromonitoring has become routine in open cardiovascular procedures (aortic arch surgery, thoracoabdominal aortic aneurysm repair), as well as interventional radiology-based stenting of abdominal and thoracic aortic aneurysms.[43–46]

**Table 6.3**  Specific Procedures and Recommended Neuromonitoring

| Type of Surgery | RECOMMENDED MONITORING | | | | | |
| | SSEP | MEP | EMG free running | EMG stimulated | ABR | EEG |
|---|---|---|---|---|---|---|
| **SPINE SKELETAL** | | | | | | |
| Cervical | x | x | x | | | |
| Thoracic | x | x | x | x | | |
| Lumbar | x | | x | x | | |
| | | | | | | |
| **HEAD AND NECK** | | | | | | |
| Thyroid | | | x | x | | |
| Parathyroid | | | x | x | | |
| Neck dissection | | | x | x | | |
| Mastoid | | | x | x | | |
| Cochlear implant | | | x | x | | |
| | | | | | | |
| **NEUROSURGERY** | | | | | | |
| Spine | | | | | | |
| *Tumor* | x | x | | | | |
| *Vascular* | x | x | | | | |
| Posterior fossa | | | | | | |
| *Acoustic neuroma* | x | | x | x | x | |
| *Cerebellopontine* | x | x | x | x | x | |
| *Vascular* | x | x | x | | x | |
| Supratentorial | | | | | | |
| *Motor cortex tumor* | x | x | | | | |
| *Middle cerebral artery aneurysm* | | x | | | | |
| | | | | | | |
| **VASCULAR** | | | | | | |
| Aortic arch | x | | | | | x |
| Descending Aorta | x | x | | | | |
| Thoracic Endovascular Aortic Repair (TEVAR) | x | x | | | | |

# Conclusion

Although consensus regarding specific indications and alarm thresholds remains a challenge, intraoperative neurophysiological monitoring has become a de facto standard of care across a broad range of surgical procedures. Despite a lack of robust outcome data for every modality, the monitoring techniques reviewed have an important role to play in efforts to improve the safety and efficacy of neurological and vascular surgery. A multimodal approach, tailored to anatomical pathways at risk, is generally used to extend anatomical coverage and increase sensitivity in detecting impending operative injury to the central and peripheral nervous system. The goal of intraoperative neuromonitoring is to provide the surgeon and anesthesiologist with necessary and timely information to decrease the risk of permanent neurological damage. For some surgical interventions, neuromonitoring has been proven to be cost effective in decreasing morbidity and has become the standard of care. Refinement of these techniques and research on new modalities make it likely that other evidence-based indications are on the horizon.

## References

1. Nash Jr CL, Lorig RA, Schatzinger LA, et al. Spinal cord monitoring during operative treatment of the spine. *Clin Orthop Relat Res.* 1977;126:100–105.
2. Sloan TB, Jameson L, Janik D. Evoked potentials. In: Cottrell JE, Young WL, eds. *Neuroanesthesia.* Philadelphia: Mosby Elsevier; 2010:115–130.
3. Toleikis JR. Intraoperative monitoring using somatosensory evoked potentials. A position statement by the American Society of Neurophysiological Monitoring. *J Clin Monit Comput.* 2005;19(3):241–258.
4. Hilibrand AS, Schwartz DM, Sethuraman V, et al. Comparison of transcranial electric motor and somatosensory evoked potential monitoring during cervical spine surgery. *J Bone Joint Surg Am.* 2004;86-A (6):1248–1253.
5. Nuwer MR, Dawson EG, Carlson LG, et al. Somatosensory evoked potential spinal cord monitoring reduces neurologic deficits after scoliosis surgery: results of a large multicenter survey. *Electroencephalogr Clin Neurophysiol.* 1995;96(1):6–11.
6. MacDonald DB, Al Zayed Z, Khoudeir I, et al. Monitoring scoliosis surgery with combined multiple pulse transcranial electric motor and cortical somatosensory-evoked potentials from the lower and upper extremities. *Spine.* 2003;28(2):194–203.
7. Devlin VJ, Schwartz DM. Intraoperative neurophysiologic monitoring during spinal surgery. *J Am Acad Orthop Surg.* 2007;15(9):549–560.
8. Weinzierl MR, Reinacher P, Gilsbach JM, et al. Combined motor and somatosensory evoked potentials for intraoperative monitoring: intra- and postoperative data in a series of 69 operations. *Neurosurg Rev.* 2007;30(2):109–116, discussion 116.
9. Selenyi A, Joksimovic B, Seifert V. Intraoperative risk of seizures associated with transient direct cortical stimulation. *J Clin Neurophysiol.* 2007;24(1):39–43.
10. Merton PA, Morton HB. Stimulation of the cerebral cortex in the intact human subject. *Nature.* 1980;285(5762):227.
11. Taniguchi M, Nadstawek J, Langenbach U, et al. Effects of four intravenous anesthetic agents on motor evoked potentials elicited by magnetic transcranial stimulation. *Neurosurgery.* 1993;33(3):407–415.
12. Jameson LC. Transcranial motor evoked potentials. In: Koht A, Sloan TB, Toleikis JR, eds. *Monitoring the Nervous System for Anesthesiologist and Other Health Care Professionals.* New York: Springer; 2012:27–45.
13. Minahan RE, Mandir AS. Basic neurophysiologic intraoperative monitoring techniques. In: Husain AM, ed. *A Practical Approach to Neurophysiologic Intraoperative Monitoring.* New York: Demos Medical Publishing; 2008:21–44.
14. Lang EW, Chesnut RM, Beutler AS, et al. The utility of motor-evoked potential monitoring during intramedullary surgery. *Anesth Analg.* 1996;83(6):1337–1341.
15. Sala F, Palandri G, Basso E, et al. Motor evoked potential monitoring improves outcome after surgery for intramedullary spinal cord tumors: a historical control study. *Neurosurgery.* 2006;58 (6):1129–1143, discussion 1129–1143.
16. Neuloh G, Schramm J. Monitoring of motor evoked potentials compared with somatosensory evoked potentials and microvascular Doppler ultrasonography in cerebral aneurysm surgery. *J Neurosurg.* 2004;100(3):389–399.
17. Szelényi A, Langer D, Kothbauer K, et al. Monitoring of muscle motor evoked potentials during cerebral aneurysm surgery: intraoperative changes and postoperative outcome. *J Neurosurg.* 2006;105 (5):675–681.
18. Mikuni N, Okada T, Nishida N, et al. Comparison between motor evoked potential recording and fiber tracking for estimating pyramidal tracts near brain tumors. *J Neurosurg.* 2007;106(1):128–133.
19. Zhou HH, Kelly PJ. Transcranial electrical motor evoked potential monitoring for brain tumor resection. *Neurosurgery.* 2001;48 (5):1075–1080.
20. Sloan TB, Janik D, Jameson L. Multimodality monitoring of the central nervous system using motor-evoked potentials. *Curr Opin Anaesthesiol.* 2008;21(5):560–564.
21. Macdonald DB. Intraoperative motor evoked potential monitoring: overview and update. *J Clin Monit Comput.* 2006;20(5):347–377.
22. Wassermann EM. Variation in the response to transcranial magnetic brain stimulation in the general population. *Clin Neurophysiol.* 2002;113(7):1165–1171.
23. Koht A, Sloan TB. Intraoperative monitoring: recent advances in motor evoked potentials. *Anesthesiol Clin.* 2016;34(3):525–537.
24. Sloan TB, Toleikis JR, Toleikis SC, et al. Intraoperative neurophysiological monitoring during spine surgery with total intravenous anesthesia or balance anesthesia with 3% desflurane. *J Clin Monit Comput.* 2015;29(1):77–85.
25. Sloan TB. Muscle relaxant use during intraoperative neurophysiologic monitoring. *J Clin Monit Comput.* 2013;27(1):35–46.
26. Seubert CN, Herman M. Auditory evoked potentials. In: Koht A, Sloan TB, Toleikis JR, eds. *Monitoring the Nervous System for Anesthesiologist and Other Health Care Professionals.* New York: Springer; 2012:47–68.
27. Goto T, Tanaka Y, Kodama K, et al. Loss of visual evoked potential following temporary occlusion of the superior hypophyseal artery during aneurysm clip placement surgery. Case report. *J Neurosurg.* 2007;107(4):865–867.
28. Kodama K, Goto T, Sato A, et al. Standard and limitation of intraoperative monitoring of the visual evoked potential. 2010;152 (4):643–648.
29. Sasaki T, Itakura T, Suzuki K, et al. Intraoperative monitoring of visual evoked potential: introduction of a clinically useful method. *J Neurosurg.* 2010;112(2):273–284.
30. Herzon GD, Zealear DL. Intraoperative monitoring of the visual evoked potential during endoscopic sinus surgery. *Otolaryngol Head Neck Surg.* 1994;111(5):575–579.
31. Cedzich C, Schramm J, Mengedoht CF, et al. Factors that limit the use of flash visual evoked potentials for surgical monitoring. *Electroencephalogr Clin Neurophysiol.* 1988;71(2):142–145.
32. Cedzich C, Schramm J. Monitoring of flash visual evoked potentials during neurosurgical operations. *Int Anesthesiol Clin.* 1990;28 (3):165–169.
33. Lorenz M, Renella RR. Intraoperative monitoring: visual evoked potentials in surgery of the sellar region. *Zentralbl Neurochir.* 1989;50(1):12–15.
34. Chacko AG, Babu KS, Chandy MJ. Value of visual evoked potential monitoring during trans-sphenoidal pituitary surgery. *Br J Neurosurg.* 1996;10(3):275–278.
35. Wiedemayer H, Fauser B, Armbruster W. Visual evoked potentials for intraoperative neurophysiologic monitoring using total intravenous anesthesia. *J Neurosurg Anesthesiol.* 2003;15(1):19–24.
36. Wiedemayer H, Fauser B, Sandalcioglu IE, et al. Observations on intraoperative monitoring of visual pathways using steady-state visual evoked potentials. *Eur J Anaesthesiol.* 2004;21(6):429–433.
37. Neuloh G. Time to revisit VEP monitoring? *Acta Neurochir (Wien).* 2010;152(4):649–650.
38. Toleikis SC, Toleikis JR. VEP. In: *Monitoring the Nervous System for Anesthesiologist and Other Health Care Professionals.* Ney York: Springer; 2012:69–93.
39. Toleikis JR. Electromyography. In: Koht A, Sloan TB, Toleikis JR, eds. *Monitoring the Nervous System for Anesthesiologist and Other Health Care Professionals.* New York: Springer; 2012:137–164.
40. Acoustic Neuroma. *NIH Consens Statement.* 1991;9:1.
41. Leis AA, Zhou HH, Mehta M, et al. Behavior of the H-reflex in humans following mechanical perturbation or injury to rostral spinal cord. *Muscle Nerve.* 1996;19(11):1373–1382.
42. Leppanen RE. Intraoperative applications of the H-reflex and F-response: a tutorial. *J Clin Monit Comput.* 2006;20(4):267–304.
43. Barone FC, Feuerstein GZ, White RF. Brain cooling during transient focal ischemia provides complete neuroprotection. *Neurosci Biobehav Rev.* 1997;21(1):31–44.
44. Bachet J, Guilmet D, Goudot B, et al. Cold cerebroplegia. A new technique of cerebral protection during operations on the transverse aortic arch. *J Thorac Cardiovasc Surg.* 1991;102(1):85–93.
45. Bernard SA, Gray TW, Buist MD, et al. Treatment of comatose survivors of out-of-hospital cardiac arrest with induced hypothermia. *N Engl J Med.* 2002;346(8):557–563.
46. Bernard SA, Buist M. Induced hypothermia in critical care medicine: a review. *Crit Care Med.* 2003;7:2041–2051.

# 7  *Intraoperative Catastrophes*

W. ANDREW KOFKE

A variety of problems can arise during neurosurgery that can be characterized as medical catastrophes (Box 7.1). It is important to determine the culprit factors that resulted in a catastrophe and to limit the extent of injury once identified. A complete and thorough handoff between the anesthesia, neurosurgery, and intensive care unit (ICU) teams is of paramount importance to ensure optimal care. This chapter will review several types of intraoperative catastrophes that may precede neurology ICU admission.

## Exsanguination

Life-threatening exsanguination, defined as loss of >1 blood volume (about 75 mL/kg) or need for >10 units of blood cells,[1] is relatively uncommon in neurosurgery.[2] Factors predisposing to this problem are proximity of noncollapsible dural sinuses, arteries, aneurismal manipulation, vascularity of the surgical bed, and preexisting or acquired clotting abnormalities.

### NEUROANATOMY AND PROCEDURE

---

**Key Concepts**

Factors predisposing to exsanguination during neurosurgery:

- Sagittal or dural sinus laceration
- Aneurysmal rupture
- Carotid artery or other major artery laceration
- Vascular tumor surgery
- Distended vertebral veins
- Coagulopathy
- Inadequate venous access relative to volume of blood loss

---

Several neuroanatomical and hematological factors can predispose to problematic exsanguination during neurosurgery.

*Sagittal sinus.* The sagittal and other dural sinuses, when entered during surgery, can lead to rapid and high-volume blood loss. The dural sinuses are not easily compressed, and operative control can be very difficult. Occasionally, sinus ligation is required, but this is a highly morbid procedure and may lead to venous edema and infarction,[3] discussed later in this chapter (see Fig. 7.1).

*Aneurysms.* Aneurysmal clipping can be associated with an intraoperative rupture, which can lead to significant blood loss.[4,5] For this reason a common neurosurgical approach is to ensure proximal control of afferent blood flow. With this approach, a temporary clip may be placed on a feeding vessel or the feeding vessel is made available

for emergency access through prior dissection.[6] Occasionally this entails exposing the internal carotid artery through an additional neck incision[7] or preoperative radiological placement of a balloon-tipped catheter into a feeding artery.

*Pituitary.* The pituitary gland is nestled between the cavernous portion of the intracranial carotid arteries. This means that they are at risk of laceration during the transsphenoidal approach to hypophysectomy[8] (Fig. 7.2). In addition some tumors may be associated with the intercavernous sinuses.[9] These factors can produce exsanguination, which is relatively easily controlled with pressure; it may also result in intracranial hypertension or stroke.

*Vascular tumors.* Some tumors are hypervascular and do not shell out easily en masse. They may require tumoral incision, extensive dissection, and serial resection. Therefore highly vascular lesions, such as hemangiomas and some meningiomas, may result in extensive blood loss.[10,11] Preoperative embolization may be considered prior to surgical resection to minimize intraoperative blood loss.[12]

*Vertebral veins and spinal tumors.* Spine surgery may be associated with extensive blood loss. Significant bleeding may arise in the context of tumor resection[13] or with extensive bony dissection as may arise during multilevel corpectomies or fixation.[14,15] Typically these patients are in the prone position. Pressure from a prominent abdomen against the operative table may lead to increased venous congestion and contribute to bleeding (Fig. 7.3).[16] Placing a patient on a frame that allows the abdomen to hang unsupported may attenuate bleeding risk (see Chapter 2, Fig. 2.3).[17]

*Coagulopathy, thrombocytopenia, thrombocytopathia.* When there is dysfunction of the coagulation system, there may be life-threatening and unrelenting exsanguination arising from open vessels and oozing tissue beds. Problems may arise from endogenous or acquired deficiencies, dysfunction of coagulation proteins, dysfunctional or inadequate numbers of platelets, or multiple concomitant issues.[18]

*Venous access and fluid administration.* Venous access, although a basic consideration of anesthesia practice, can also be an extraordinary challenge. Generally for a procedure with high blood loss anticipated, at least two 16- or 14-gauge intravenous catheters are needed. Occasionally, even larger catheters may be placed in central veins. Data on comparative maximal pressurized flow rates with different cannulas and infusion systems are presented in Fig. 7.4.[19]

In cases of massive and rapid blood loss, simply hanging the blood is not sufficient. The infusion needs rapid and high-flow delivery, often requiring mechanical support. This is accomplished in several ways, varying from a high-pressure inflatable bag around the blood bag to any of several pump systems (Fig. 7.5).[19]

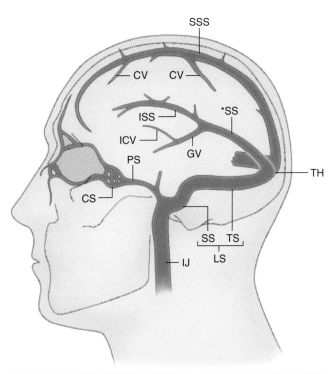

**Fig. 7.1** Venous drainage of intracranial structures. *CS* = cavernous sinus; *CV* = cortical veins; *GV* = great vein of Galen; *ICV* = internal cerebral vein; *IJ* = internal jugular vein; *ISS* = inferior sagittal sinus; *LS* = lateral sinus; *PS* = petrosal sinus; *SS* = sigmoid sinus; *\*SS* = straight sinus; *SSS* = superior sagittal sinus; *TH* = torcular Herophili; *TS* = transverse sinus. (Reprinted from Gates P, Barnett HJ, Mohr JP, et al., eds. *Stroke: Pathophysiology, Diagnosis and Management.* New York: Churchill Livingstone; 1986.)

## PERIOPERATIVE CONSIDERATIONS

Methods for estimating blood loss are approximations based on examination of soaked sponges; irrigation-mixed blood suctioned from the field; and blood on the surgical field, on the surgeons, and on the floor. The volume in suction canisters likely overestimates blood loss given irrigation contained. Estimated blood loss may also be gauged through serial hemoglobin assessment accounting for the amount of blood and fluids given and lost.[20]

Other perioperative considerations require making cost-conscious decisions regarding the amount of blood to have available before and during surgery. Other considerations include the need for preoperative platelets, fresh frozen plasma (FFP), cryoprecipitate, prothrombin complex concentrate (PCC), recombinant factor VIIa, or other factor-specific infusions.[18] Moreover, patients who are therapeutically anticoagulated require assessment as to the safety and duration of preoperative cessation of anticoagulation and the need for reversal. Dabigatran and analogs continue to be enigmatic, but some suggest preoperative infusion of activated PCC (factor VIII inhibitor bypassing agent). PCC was found to effectively reverse rivaroxaban but not dabigatran in human volunteers.[21] Another perioperative consideration on the part of the neurosurgeon is whether to employ preoperative embolization to decrease intraoperative hemorrhage.[9,12,22] Ultimately, the anesthesia team determines the need for activation of exsanguination protocols, availability and use of infusion pumps, and extent of venous access.

Surgical management of exsanguination, or damage control surgery, is the prevailing approach in trauma surgery and may be extrapolated to the neurosurgical patient with massive exsanguination. Damage control surgery is comprised of three elements. The first is aimed at urgently attenuating bleeding through maneuvers such as surgical packing and closure, planning for later definitive repair (Fig. 7.6).[1] When this occurs in neurosurgery, it is likely that significant neurological deficit will follow. The second element involves use of hemostatic aids, such as kaolin-impregnated gauze pads, surgiseal, bone wax, and other agents, which promote clot formation in the wound. The use of these aids is well described in trauma surgery and has been reported in neurosurgery.[23,24] The third element of damage control is the use of hypotensive resuscitation.[1] This aspect of damage-control surgery is controversial because, although low blood pressure may limit bleeding, it may promote irreversible ischemic brain damage in areas of edema or retraction.

## POSTOPERATIVE COMPLICATIONS

For a patient arriving in the neurology ICU after a massive neurosurgical exsanguination, many issues require attention. The first is determination of neurological deficits from local mass effect related to hematoma and interruption of arterial and venous flow. Mass effect can arise during surgery, and if feasible, the hematoma is removed. However, this may not be technically feasible, particularly in difficult-to-access locations.

*Source control.* Control of the source of bleeding is mandatory. Typically this arises during surgery under direct visualization by the neurosurgeon. However, occasionally rapid neuroradiological intervention is required to achieve control through endovascular means.

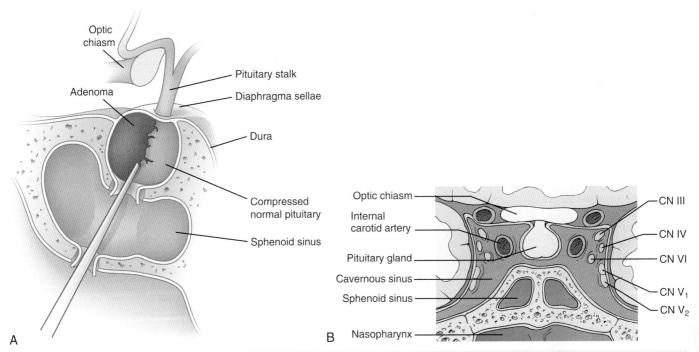

**Fig. 7.2** (**A**) Surgical approach to transsphenoidal resection of the pituitary gland. (**B**) Coronal depiction of pituitary gland and surrounding structures. Lateral aspects of pituitary gland are in close proximity to internal carotid artery and several cranial nerves. (**A**, Reprinted from Kronenberg, HM, et al., eds. *Williams Textbook of Endocrinology*, 11th ed. New York: Saunders, Elsevier; 2008: p. 177. **B**, Adapted from Foulad A, Bhandarkar N. Pituitary Gland Anatomy. Medscape Reference. 2001. Available from: emedicine.medscape.com/article/1899167-overview.)

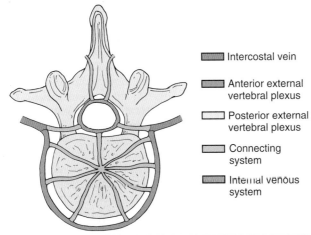

**Fig. 7.3** Batson's plexus. This figure depicts the venous interconnections by which obstructed blood flow from the lower body (e.g., with abdominal compression) can be diverted into the vertebral venous system to thus potentiate blood loss during lumbar surgery. (Adapted from Schonauer C, Bocchetti A, Barbagallo G, Albanese V, Moraci A. Positioning on surgical table. *Eur Spine J*. 2004;13(Suppl. 1):S50–S5.)

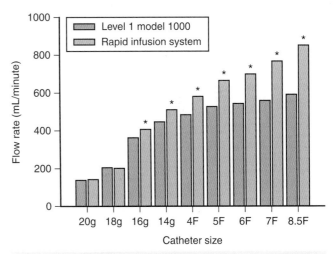

**Fig. 7.4** Flow rate and catheter size for the rapid infusion system versus Level 1 (L-1). Note that there is a minimal change in flow capacity with the L-1 device for all catheters 14 gauge (G). *$P <0.05$; F __French and also the significant apparently nonlinear increase in flow with 16 or larger catheters compared with 18 G or smaller. (From Barcelona SL, et al. A comparison of flow rates and warming capabilities of the level 1 and rapid infusion system with various-size intravenous catheters. *Anesth Analg*. 2003 Aug;97(2):358–63.)

*Surgical vs. nonsurgical bleeding.* It is important to bear in mind the distinction between surgical and nonsurgical bleeding.[1] Surgical bleeding connotes anatomical vascular bleeding generally responsive to surgical or endovascular therapy. Nonsurgical bleeding refers to bleeding from previously traumatized tissue beds, mucosa, and vascular access sites, suggesting superimposed coagulopathy or thrombocytopathia.

*Arterial infarct.* Arterial occlusion is sometimes necessary to achieve control of intraoperative hemorrhage.

Depending on collateral blood flow, this can lead to stroke and problematic edema.[5]

*Venous infarct.* Venous occlusion occasionally arises, particularly in the context of sagittal sinus manipulation from ligation or thrombosis, from inadvertent ligation of a draining vein in the context of an arteriovenous malformation

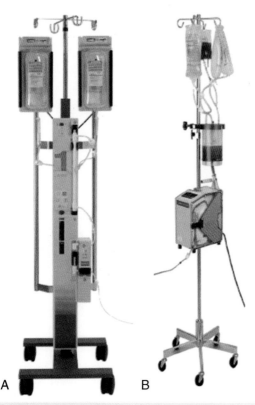

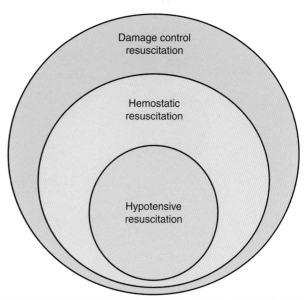

**Fig. 7.6** The relationship between hypotensive resuscitation, hemostatic resuscitation, and damage-control resuscitation. (Reprinted from Riha GA, Schreiber MA. Update and new developments in the management of the exsanguinating patient. *J Intensive Care Med.* 2013;28(1):46–57.)

**Fig. 7.5 (A)** Level 1 H-1200 Fast Flow Fluid Warmer. This device with figure provided by the vendor shows rigid pressure chambers accommodate standard blood and crystalloid bags, providing a constant 300 mm Hg pressure for rapid infusion; an on/off toggle switch used to quickly and easily pressurize chambers; an aluminum heat exchanger that transfers heat 1000 times faster than plastic; the countercurrent 42 °C circulating water bath, which ensures patients receive normothermic blood and IV fluids; and an integrated air detector/clamp that detects the presence of air in blood and crystalloid, alerts clinicians, and automatically stops the flow and allows quick removal of air without disconnecting from the patient or changing disposables. **(B)** The Belmont Rapid Infuser uses electromagnetic induction heating to heat to target temperature in a single pass, and intelligent software monitors and controls infusion. The touch screen allows for designating flow rate infusion from 2.5 to 1000 mL/min. The screen continuously displays total volume infused, infusion rate, fluid temperature, and system pressure. The disposable set is designed for easy setup and active air evacuation. (**A**, Reproduced from Level 1, © Smiths Medical, All rights reserved. Available from: http://www.smiths-medical.com/. **B**, Reproduced with permission of Belmont, Inc. Available from: www.belmontinstrument.com.)

(AVM) resection or mass effect from bleeding. This can lead to significant venous infarct[3] and brain edema.[25]

*Systemic consequences* of exsanguination and its treatment must be diagnosed and managed. Most important is the so-called lethal triad of hypothermia, acidosis, and coagulopathy.[1] Each of these factors potentiates the others,[1] presenting an important management challenge. *Hypothermia* is a well-known complication of massive transfusion.[26] Many blood products arrive in a chilled state, and blood warmers are employed as part of their administration. Nonetheless it can be difficult to maintain normothermia. This is extremely important because hypothermia induces a coagulopathy,[27] which can become part of a positive feedback cycle.

*Dilutional coagulopathy* and thrombocytopenia typically arise after massive transfusion.[28,29] Notably the decrease in

platelet count follows a standard washout equation supporting the notion of dilution as the primary cause.[28] Bleeding tends to be exacerbated when the platelet count drops to <65,000[29] and international normalized ratio >1.5,[30] although the threshold for bleeding in neurosurgery is thought to be <100,000.[31] Thus current protocols call for concurrent protocolized administration of FFP and platelets as part of massive transfusion therapy[32] complemented by point-of-care coagulation assessment.[33] Nonetheless this can be an ongoing issue postoperatively and requires vigilance. Moreover, disseminated intravascular coagulation (DIC) may arise in a delayed fashion, both from shock states[34] and release of tissue thromboplastin from brain tissue.[35] *Lactic acidosis* can be an ongoing problem postoperatively. It interferes with platelet function and potentiates degradation of fibrinogen.[1] Typically the most appropriate approach is to diminish production of lactate and improve hepatic clearance. This entails optimization of fluid status and cardiac output.

*Postoperative hematoma.* Because of the previously mentioned issues with coagulopathy, there is a need for ongoing concern for development of postoperative hematoma, which can compromise neural function. Particular concern exists for enlarging hematoma in the surgical bed, subdural hematoma,[36] and epidural spinal hematoma.[37]

*Transfusion-associated lung injury (TRALI).* TRALI can arise after infusion of blood products. The risk of TRALI varies from 1 case per 5000 units packed red blood cells (PRBCs) to 1 per 2000 units FFP to 1 per 400 units platelets.[26] The pathogenesis is ill defined but seems to be related to an antibody-associated inflammation of the lung, with an association with female donors.[26] The only therapy is supportive care.

*Electrolyte imbalances.* Several types of electrolyte abnormalities can arise with massive transfusion. *Potassium.* Packed cells typically are high in potassium but once infused with normalization of pH, the potassium moves intracellularly. Nonetheless extensive blood replacement can produce problematic hyperkalemia, especially if there is acute kidney injury related to the acute blood loss or in small or pediatric patients. *Calcium.* PRBC and FFP both contain citrate, which can bind calcium.[26] FFP particularly has high citrate levels. This is generally most problematic during the infusion or if there is hypoperfusion of the parathyroid glands. Thus careful monitoring of ionized calcium is important with replacement as needed. Inexplicable lack of blood pressure response to blood product infusion justifies empiric calcium administration. *Alkalosis.* The citrate that accompanies a massive transfusion is metabolized to bicarbonate such that metabolic alkalosis is very common in the days after massive transfusion.[26]

*Other systemic problems* can arise postoperatively from hypotension or shock states that may be associated with massive intraoperative blood loss. These include postischemic anoxic encephalopathy (especially if there was a cardiac arrest), lactic acidosis,[38] acute kidney or hepatic injury, DIC, acute respiratory distress syndrome (ARDS),[39] overresuscitation or underresuscitation, and multiple organ failure.[38]

### Clinical Pearl

Hypocalcemia may result from citrate binding incurred by massive transfusion.[26] The hypocalcemia may exacerbate hypotension already severe from hemorrhagic hypovolemia. Empiric calcium is indicated when low blood pressure is not responding to transfusion therapy.

## Venous Air Embolism

Venous air embolism (VAE) is a well-known complication of neurosurgery.[40,41]

### NEUROANATOMY AND PROCEDURE

### Key Concepts

- Factors predisposing to VAE
  - Sitting craniotomy
  - Very large head
  - Low venous pressure
  - Dural sinus laceration
  - Inadequate bone wax on exposed cranium diploic veins
  - Iatrogenic

The basic neuroanatomy and resultant pathophysiology of VAE are related to a vein or sinus being open in the surgical field, with the pressure in the vein or sinus being subatmospheric such that room air is entrained into the vein with dose (of air)–related systemic consequences. Venous pressure generally becomes low enough to produce entrainment of air when the surgical site is above the heart to an extent that is higher than the venous pressure (i.e., the surgical site in cm is above the venous pressure in cm). Thus very low tissue venous pressure, as may occur with hypovolemia, or very elevated surgical site, as may occur in the sitting position, can create the appropriate

conditions for VAE. The following are the most common situations where VAE may arise.

***Sitting craniotomy.***[42] Occasionally neurosurgery is most optimally accomplished with the patient in the sitting position. This can improve exposure of the surgical field and decrease bleeding. The decrease in bleeding is due to decreased venous blood pressure and volume, the very factors that lead to VAE.

***Large head.*** The neonatal and young pediatric patient's head is larger relative to the rest of the body than in adults. Thus neurosurgery, even done in the supine position, can create the conditions for VAE with the surgical site well above the level of the heart.[43] Moreover in such smaller patients less air is necessary to produce lethal results.

***Low central venous pressure (CVP).*** Even if the head is not well above the heart, the presence of hypovolemia with a low CVP can lead to VAE. This can include cases done in a typical 15- to 30-degree head elevation or even supine.[43] In addition to blood loss and preoperative fluid restriction, administration of diuretics such as mannitol, if not associated with maintenance of euvolemia, can produce such conditions.

***Sinus invasion.***[44] Most veins collapse on their own when lacerated, which may limit the extent of air entrainment. However, dural sinuses do not collapse or contract, further enhancing the subatmospheric pressure if the head is elevated.

***Bony air entrainment.*** Diploic veins in the skull are similar to sinuses because both are unable to collapse such that air can be entrained during entry into the skull.[45] For this reason the standard neurosurgical practice is to apply bone wax to open edges of a craniotomy in order to limit this problem.

***Fluid administration system errors.*** Iatrogenic factors can also lead to air embolism. These include mistakenly setting up IV sets without purging the air from them; using rapid infusion systems, which squeeze residual air from blood bags into veins; and leaving central cannula ports open, thus allowing air entrainment.

### PERIOPERATIVE CONSIDERATIONS

### Key Concepts

Venous air embolism monitors

- Esophageal stethoscope
- End-tidal $CO_2$ monitoring
- End-tidal $N_2$ monitoring
- Precordial Doppler
- Esophageal echocardiography

*Diagnosis and intraoperative approach.* The intraoperative approach entails placement of a multiorifice (e.g., Bunegin-Albin) central venous catheter into the right atrium.[46] This is most readily accomplished by placing the catheter with electrocardiogram guidance, typically from an antecubital vein.[41] Subsequently avoidance of hypovolemia is mandatory. Some anesthesiologists will transduce the CVP at the level of the surgery and infuse fluids or apply positive end-expiratory pressure (PEEP) to ensure that venous pressure at the surgical site remains above zero.[41]

The occurrence of VAE is generally monitored by the use of a precordial Doppler and end-tidal $CO_2$.[41,47] The presence of a VAE is heralded by harsh sounds on the Doppler with a sudden drop in end-tidal $CO_2$. Aspiration of the central catheter may yield air, confirming the diagnosis and contributing to the therapy. Some also use end-tidal nitrogen or echocardiography to aid in the diagnosis of VAE.

Hemodynamic compromise varies in relation to the dose of air that has been entrained. It can vary from no effect, to a modest decrease in cardiac output, to a full cardiac arrest. The development of an air lock in the heart and pulmonary artery can make standard resuscitation efforts futile.

*Intraoperative management.* One hundred percent oxygen is administered, and concomitantly the neurosurgeons are advised of the likely diagnosis. Their first move should be to flood the field with saline. If feasible, the site of surgery should be brought close to the level of the heart. Then efforts to increase the venous pressure should be implemented, including rapid fluid infusion, digital pressure to the jugular veins, and application of PEEP. The venous catheter should be aspirated in an effort to decrease the mechanical effects of the air and hemodynamic support as indicated is then used, including cardiopulmonary resuscitation (CPR). This is the sort of case where, if CPR is ineffective, cardiac surgical intervention with physical removal of an air lock or mechanical circulatory support may be appropriate.

## POSTOPERATIVE COMPLICATIONS

### Key Concepts

Postoperative issues after VAE

- Focal arterial occlusion of major organs
- Inflammatory response
- Coagulopathy
- Wound infection
- Hemodynamic instability
- Extracorporeal support

Postoperative issues are related to the severity of the VAE. For all severities of VAE there remains the possibility of a right-to-left shunt of the air, either via a cardiac septal defect or transpulmonary pathway.[48] Thus evaluation for evidence of organ ischemia of the brain, heart, viscera, and kidneys is needed. Cranial computed tomography (CT) scan may reveal arterial air.[49]

**For mild VAE** with minimal hemodynamic compromise, only observation for evidence of tissue injury is required. **For moderate to severe VAE with** evidence of organ ischemia, cardiopulmonary support is required and all available measures employed to provide support until the air is reabsorbed or removed. This may include hyperbaric therapy or extracorporeal membrane support. If neurological symptoms referable to likely air are present, consideration can be given also to artificially increased blood pressure and hyperbaric oxygen therapy,[50] although no evidence-based guidelines can be offered.

If surgery had to be abruptly stopped, then the wound may have been contaminated or not properly closed. Prophylactic antibiotics should be considered, and when stable,

a return visit to the operating room may be needed to complete the surgery or effect a proper closure. The interface between air and blood can induce an inflammatory response and DIC,[51] and monitoring for this should be done.

### Clinical Pearl

Severe VAE requires maximal life support and high levels of oxygen, with consideration given to hyperbaric oxygen and extracorporeal support.

## Massive Brain Swelling

Massive brain swelling can arise unexpectedly during neurosurgery,[52] affecting neurology ICU care. The main causes are venous occlusion, intraparenchymal hemorrhage, edema of brain tissue related to underlying disease or intraoperative brain trauma, arterial hypertension,[53,54] and extreme hypoxemia and hypercapnia.

## NEUROANATOMY AND PROCEDURE

### Key Concepts

- Factors predisposing to massive brain swelling
- Occlusion of draining veins
- Intraparenchymal hemorrhage
- Progressive brain edema from underlying disease process
- Extracranial increased venous pressure
- Hypoxemia
- Hypercapnia
- Osmolar gradients favoring ingress of water

The causes of acute intraoperative brain swelling are summarized next.

*Venous occlusion.* Several situations may arise during a craniotomy where venous outflow may be compromised. The first is sagittal sinus interruption, generally done to attenuate blood loss.[55] The second may arise in the process of AVM dissection. If there is still arterial inflow when a vein is permanently occluded, then massive venous edema and hemorrhage may arise. Occasionally a similar process may occur with resection of vascular tumors.[56] The third situation of venous occlusion arises when, once brain tissue herniates out a craniotomy from any cause, then venous drainage may be compromised from the herniated area, thus compounding the severity of the edematous herniated brain.

*Intraparenchymal hemorrhage* (IPH). This may arise during dissection for aneurysm or AVM surgery or arise spontaneously in deep nonsurgical tissue, typically associated with a hypertensive surge,[53,54] but not necessarily.

*Brain tissue edema.* During a craniotomy, cytotoxic or vasogenic edema leading to overt tissue swelling may arise from several causes.[57] It can arise as an expected progression of an underlying disease process, for example, traumatic brain injury contusion,[53,54] IPH,[58] or brain tumor.[56] Furthermore, additional brain edema can arise related to neurosurgical maneuvers during the procedure, typically related to retraction needed to gain access to a specific brain target of surgery.[59] Occasionally massive edema can follow drainage of a subdural hemorrhage or aneurismal rupture. Finally, after resection of a large AVM, if blood pressure is not well controlled, a postresection hyperemia can arise, which may cause brain swelling.[60,61]

*Extracranial increased venous pressure.* In order to produce or exacerbate brain edema, extracranial increased venous pressure needs to be significant. This may occur if there is some obstruction to cephalic venous outflow, either from disease or procedure.[62] Probably the most common cause, however, is unexpected severe coughing due to loss of neuromuscular blockade or inadequate opioid dose. When this arises and the skull is open, the combination of increased venous pressure from coughing with arterial hypertension can cause the brain to swell temporarily. However, if it produces herniation of brain through the craniotomy, venous occlusion can arise, leading to intractable edema that may require amputation of herniated brain tissue.

*Metabolic causes* or contributors to cerebral edema and swelling include hypoxemia, hypercapnia, hyponatremia, and osmolar gradients.

## PERIOPERATIVE CONSIDERATIONS

*Surgical.* The neurosurgeon prevents or attenuates procedure-related brain swelling through attention to venous drainage of surgical beds and minimizing brain retraction as much as feasible. Surgical resection of edematous brain or performance of a decompressive craniectomy may be needed.[63] Occasionally a ventriculostomy[64] or lumbar drain[65] is placed to produce brain relaxation sufficient to decrease the need for significant retraction.

*Occult IPH, hydrocephalus, or aneurysmal hemorrhage* is always a consideration when sudden unexplained brain swelling occurs. These are generally diagnosed intraoperatively with ultrasound.[66] The procedure may need to be aborted, followed by urgent CT with IPH removal or decompressive procedure done. Any arterial hypertension[53,54] needs to be appropriately managed.

*Anesthesia response.* Metabolic problems are generally under the control of the anesthesiologist and require their correction as a primary goal. This may mean correction of airway problems, diagnosis and management of gas exchange issues, avoidance of systemic hypertension, and evaluation and correction of osmolar factors. In any event, for all situations of intraoperative brain swelling, the anesthesia team may perform maneuvers to diminish the edema through induction of burst suppression with barbiturates or propofol,[67] hyperventilation, treatment of hypoxemia, and administration of hypertonic saline[68] or mannitol. As with management of intracranial hypertension, avoidance of hypotension and hypertension is also a component of intraoperative management of problematic brain edema.[53]

### Clinical Pearl

Immediate therapy of brain edema or swelling in the operating room includes hyperventilation, high-dose propofol or barbiturate, hyperosmolar therapy, and maintenance of nutritive cerebral perfusion pressure.

## POSTOPERATIVE COMPLICATIONS

### Key Concepts

Postoperative consequences of massive intraoperative brain swelling

- Progression of edema
- Brain ischemia
- Intracranial hypertension
- Delayed emergence from anesthetics
- Progression of intraparenchymal hemorrhage

The consequences of problems with intraoperative edema are related primarily to whether the team was able to rapidly resolve the problem. If not, the postoperative team will have to address several issues. These include the following:

*Progressive edema and intracranial hypertension.* Edema arising from ischemia, venous occlusion, or tissue trauma edema may progress.[69] This can produce or worsen focal deficits in the area of the edema or ischemia or, more globally, produce delayed emergence[70–72] or elevated intracranial pressure, requiring specific therapy directed to ICP control. If related to postoperative venous thrombosis,[73] consideration may be needed for anticoagulation or endovascular clot disruption.[74]

*Hemorrhage.* Intraoperative or possible new postoperative IPH will require serial CT to assess stability of the clot with appropriate blood pressure management, suggested <160 mm Hg, to prevent postoperative IPH. If of significant size, a return to the operating room may be necessary for decompression and/or clot removal.

# Cardiac Arrest

## NEUROANATOMY AND PROCEDURE

### Key Concepts

Factors predisposing to cardiac arrest during neurosurgery

- Medical errors
- Anesthesia
- Surgical position
- Exsanguination
- Venous air or thromboembolism
- Coronary artery or major valvular disease
- Excessive vagal tone
- Asphyxia
- Anaphylaxis
- Malignant hyperthermia

Intraoperative cardiac arrest arises primarily from iatrogenic, hemorrhagic, embolic, metabolic, medical, or airway-related causes.

*Iatrogenic.* Iatrogenic causes include cardiac arrests related to anesthetic problems/errors[75] or surgical errors or misadventures.[76] Examples of errors include drug errors,[77,78] such as excessive potassium administration; inappropriate succinylcholine use; rapid phenytoin administration; anesthetic overdose; central line placement–associated arterial puncture, pneumothorax, pericardial effusion, or hemothorax; inadvertent airway problems; human factors such as poor vigilance or teamwork[79]; or accidental intravenous air administration.[80]

*Hemorrhagic.* Excessive blood loss and/or hypovolemia with insufficient replacement will cause progressive hypotension, which can lead to cardiac arrest.[76,81,82]

*Embolic.* Intraoperative thromboembolism[76] or VAE[83] can both lead to cardiac arrest.

*Metabolic.* Problems related to organ dysfunction, drug effects, or toxic ingestions may cause lethal arrhythmias leading to cardiac arrest.[84] Moreover severe bradycardia can arise from brain irrigation or manipulation,[42,85] spinal cord injury,[86] or administration of adenosine.[87]

*Medical.* Preexisting cardiac problems may predispose to intraoperative cardiac arrest. Myocardial supply–demand imbalance in the context of coronary artery disease can predispose to acute myocardial dysfunction and lethal arrhythmia both during and after surgery. Severe cardiomyopathy can lead to cardiac arrest likely associated with variations in preload or afterload related to anesthetics, fluid administration, or hemorrhage. Some severe preexisting cardiac valvular abnormalities may lead to cardiac arrest. Most notable is severe aortic stenosis, which, with decreased intraoperative blood pressure, may lead to hypoperfusion of myocardium and consequent refractory cardiac arrest.[88]

*Postextubation or difficult intubation asphyxia.* Hypoxemia or asphyxia (hypoxemia plus hypercapnia) can arise related to endotracheal tube (ETT) placement or removal. Airway mishaps are reported to be a major cause of anesthesia morbidity and mortality.[89]

*Intubation* problems can be related to difficulty with mask ventilation or ETT placement. In addition, efforts to secure a difficult airway can produce airway trauma.[90,91] When difficulty with ventilation, inappropriate tube placement into the esophagus, or airway trauma produce severe hypoxemia, cardiac arrest can ensue.[92,93]

*Extubation.* Difficulties with extubation are typically associated with unexpected new airway abnormalities that may interfere with spontaneous or assisted ventilation.[94] Postextubation obstructive pharyngeal and laryngeal edema can arise related to dependent surgical positioning,[95,96] head position,[96] prolonged oropharyngeal airway or other devices,[97-99] and intubation trauma.[90] Also, unexpected angioedema can produce postextubation airway obstruction.[92]

Accidental extubation during surgery can lead to asphyxial cardiac arrest due to the patient being in a position that can make reintubation or mask/laryngeal mask airway (LMA) ventilation difficult. Examples include intraoperative extubation while prone or with the head in pins flexed forward or other position associated with difficult access to the airway. Rescue techniques with LMA[100] and fiberoptic bronchoscopy have been described.[101]

## PERIOPERATIVE CONSIDERATIONS

### Key Concepts

Non–Advanced Cardiac Life Support (ACLS) Considerations in Managing Perioperative Cardiac Arrest

- Manage bleeding and transfusion complications
- Consider VAE
- Airway problems in unusual position
- Anaphylaxis
- Local anesthetic toxicity
- Decision making for therapeutic hypothermia
- Role for extracorporeal support

Management of cardiac arrest during neurosurgery entails use of standard ACLS procedures. However, given that the circumstances of such a cardiac arrest are not within the usual context with which ACLS guidelines are typically associated, often variations or unproven approaches are required. This may include use of extracorporeal support[84] or unconventional chest compression techniques, for example, two-person front-back compressions used in the lateral position or back compression in the prone position.

*Position-related challenges.* Positioning of the patient to allow neurosurgery procedures (see Chapter 2) can create significant challenges in the management of cardiac arrest, challenges not typically taught in classic ACLS guidelines.

*Prone.* Cardiac arrest in the prone position generally mandates immediately placing the patient supine to enable proper chest compressions. The surgeon must effect a rapid covering of the wound, removal from head fixation pins if in place, and then turning onto a gurney or bed brought quickly into the operating room. The prone position typically entails loss of visual contact with many IVs such that placing in the supine position will facilitate identifying and fixing any IV access issues that might have contributed to the cardiac arrest. Nonetheless, there have been some discussion and case reports of efficacious CPR done in the prone position.[102]

If the cause of the cardiac arrest is inadvertent extubation, then the anesthesiologist may be able to rescue the situation through reestablishment of ventilation and oxygenation. Typically this would involve placement of an LMA.[100]

*Sitting or head elevated.* To ensure better perfusion to the brain during CPR, the head needs to be brought closer to heart level. If the procedure is being done in a full sitting position with anteriorly located pins and head fixation, then the bed needs to be adjusted to facilitate brain perfusion, cessation of VAE possibility, and chest compressions. Some have suggested an a priori specific bed configuration that can rapidly facilitate these goals without removing the pins.[103] The surgical wound needs to be rapidly covered.

*Lateral position or park bench position.* Cardiac arrest arising in these positions requires turning the patient on the operating room bed to the supine position while the surgeon rapidly covers the wound and controls the head position during the turn. This may be an awkward maneuver from the park bench position. Two-person front-back compressions in the lateral position has been described in this circumstance.[84]

*Procedure-specific variations from ACLS.* Several contexts of intraoperative cardiac arrest require consideration of an approach to resuscitation that is in addition to ACLS guidelines.

*Hemorrhage.* If the cardiac arrest is due to exsanguination, then every effort is directed to volume, blood, platelet, and FFP replacement. Rapid administration of blood products containing citrate can exacerbate the problem through hypocalcemia such that periodic empiric $CaCl_2$ is appropriate and ionized calcium should be assessed periodically.[26] Aggressive therapy for hypothermia may be required.

*Anesthetic or surgical contributors.* Evaluation of correctable problems that may have arisen during surgery to cause the cardiac arrest must be considered and treated:

- ***Pneumothorax or hemothorax*** should be considered if a central line was placed or surgery is near the chest.
- ***Major vascular injury*** of the iliac vessels, vena cava, or aorta should be considered when cardiac arrest without apparent cause arises during spinal surgery.[104]
- ***VAE*** is a possibility any time the surgical site is above the heart or can occur as an error related to an open central catheter or air-filled IV administration system.[40,41]
- ***Retroperitoneal hematoma*** should be considered if there has been recent instrumentation of the femoral or iliac artery.[105]
- ***Hyperkalemia*** can arise due to endogenous medical problems, inadvertent potassium administration, succinylcholine, or blood products. Patients may be susceptible to succinylcholine-induced hyperkalemia if there is a preexisting condition such as rhabdomyolysis or one associated with increased postjunctional cholinergic receptor density. Such conditions include paralysis and prolonged bed rest.[106]
- ***Inadequate airway control*** may be causative. The airway must always be interrogated. Problems such as unrecognized ETT kinks or obstruction, or ETT dislodgement, must be considered. In the event that ventilation and oxygenation cannot be effected with mask or LMA, a surgical airway is indicated.[107] Needle cricothyrotomy has been shown to be a quick way to achieve oxygenation sufficient to attenuate an hypoxic asystolic cardiac arrest.[92]
- ***Anaphylaxis*** can be a contributing factor. Given the exposure to multiple drugs and latex that can arise during surgery, this is an important consideration in evaluating the potential causes of intraoperative cardiac arrest.[108]
- ***Excessive hypothermia.*** If the central temperature has fallen during surgery to <30°C, then there is an increased possibility of lethal arrhythmias leading to cardiac arrest.[109]

- ***Local anesthetic toxicity*** can cause a cardiac arrest. Cardiac arrest that is thought to be possibly related to bupivacaine toxicity will require infusion of Intralipid.[110]
- ***Malignant hyperthermia*** is a rare problem that can cause a cardiac arrest.

*Therapeutic hypothermia.* In the context of out-of-hospital cardiac arrest, data suggest a beneficial effect of hypothermia, although there continues to be debate regarding the depth of hypothermia and whether the neuroprotective effect is actually prevention of fever. The decision to implement this during or after surgery is not straightforward. Given that the patient is under the influence of anesthetics, one cannot reliably assess post-CPR mental status to determine whether there is a decrement in level of consciousness, which would support the use of hypothermia. Moreover, hypothermia may produce problematic coagulopathy, which may produce a postoperative hemorrhage. If intracranial or perispinal, this could negate any possible advantages of the hypothermia.

*Extracorporeal support.* Given that the patient sustaining an intraoperative cardiac arrest is in a surgical suite, often with equipment and expertise nearby, failure to respond to CPR makes it appropriate to consider the option of venoarterial bypass support of circulation and gas exchange. This is never straightforward because this maneuver typically includes anticoagulation, but if the clinical circumstances are acceptable, it should be considered. This may be particularly true in the situation of refractory bupivacaine toxicity,[111] hypothermia,[112] massive venous or thrombotic or air embolism,[113–115] or other potentially reversible causes.

## POSTOPERATIVE COMPLICATIONS

### Key Concepts

Therapy of anaphylaxis

- Remove inciting allergen; consider latex
- Epinephrine
- Bronchodilators
- H1 and H2 antagonists
- Glucocorticoids
- Coagulopathy monitoring and management

Postoperative management after an intraoperative cardiac arrest entails ongoing consideration of the intraoperative concerns regarding etiology.

*Ongoing hemorrhage* requires continuous vigilance and therapy for hemorrhage, coagulopathy, and thrombocytopenia.

*Post–anoxic ischemic encephalopathy* is an immediate postoperative concern and can be difficult to ascertain early after surgery. The previously noted concerns regarding application of hypothermic therapy continue into the postoperative period. Assessment of cognitive function is obfuscated by residual anesthetic effects, and assessments about

## Box 7.2  Managing a Malignant Hyperthermia Crisis

**During an MH Crisis**

**Health Care Professionals:**

**CALL the MH 24-hour Hotline (for emergencies only)**

- United States: 1+800–644–9737
- Outside the US: 00+1+209–417–3722

**Start Emergency Therapy for MH Acute Phase Treatment**

1. Discontinue volatile agents and succinylcholine; get help; get dantrolene; notify surgeon
2. Dantrolene sodium for injection 2.5 mg/kg rapidly IV through large-bore IV, if possible
3. Bicarbonate for metabolic acidosis
4. Cool the patient
5. Dysrhythmia: usually responds to treatment of acidosis and hyperkalemia
6. Hyperkalemia
7. Follow: end-tidal $CO_2$, electrolytes, blood gases, creatine kinase, serum myoglobin, core temperature, urine output and color, and coagulation studies

Adapted from MHAUS. If You Need To Manage an MH Crisis Right Now. 2014 [cited 2014 April 23, 2014]; Available from: http://www.mhaus.org/healthcare-professionals.

cognitive function require input from the anesthesia team. Consideration can be given to reversal of some anesthetic effects with naloxone or flumazenil, but with cautious consideration of potential side effects of hypertension[116] and/or seizure.[117]

*Temperature.* Dangerously low temperature needs to be treated because of risk of arrhythmias, central nervous system depression, and coagulopathy. Conversely these patients are prone to fever,[118] and this must be aggressively prevented or treated.[119]

*Infection.* Typically the patient will arrive with the surgical wound rapidly closed, packed with gauze or fabric, or simply covered with a drape. Attention to preventing infection of the surgical site is required. Administration of antibiotics seems appropriate, and as soon as feasible a return to the operating room may be needed to complete the surgery, complete hemostatic procedures, or simply provide for sterile wound closure.

*Anaphylaxis.* Ongoing management of anaphylaxis must continue into the postoperative period.

*Malignant hyperthermia (MH) is a rare complication of anesthesia.* The approach to management of MH during and after surgery is summarized in Box 7.2.

## Summary

Several catastrophic problems can arise during neurosurgery. They typically arise from a variety of commonly interacting factors related to patient anatomy and pathology; surgical position; experience of anesthesia and neurosurgery teams; and disparate hospital factors related to experience, protocols in place, and resource availability.

## References

1. Riha GA, Schreiber MA. Update and new developments in the management of the exsanguinating patient. *J Intensive Care Med.* 2013;28(1):46–57.
2. Couture DE, Ellegala DB, Dumont AS, Mintz PD, Kassell NF. Blood use in cerebrovascular neurosurgery. 2002:994–997.
3. Schaller B, Graf R, Wienhard K, Heiss WD. A new animal model of cerebral venous infarction: ligation of the posterior part of the superior sagittal sinus in the cat. *Swiss Med Weekly.* 2003;133(29–30):412–418.
4. Batjer H, Samson DS. Management of intraoperative aneurysm rupture. *Clin Neurosurg.* 1990;36:275–288.
5. Elijovich L, Higashida RT, Lawton MT, et al. Predictors and Outcomes of Intraprocedural Rupture in patients treated for ruptured intracranial aneurysms: the CARAT study. *Stroke.* 2008;39(5):1501–1506.
6. Dhandapani S, Pal S, Gupta S, Mohindra S, Chhabra R, Malhotra S. Does the impact of elective temporary clipping on intraoperative rupture really influence neurological outcome after surgery for ruptured anterior circulation aneurysms? A prospective multivariate study. *Acta Neurochir.* 2013;155(2):237–246.
7. Kumon Y, Sakaki S, Kohno K, Ohta S, Ohue S, Oka Y. Asymptomatic, unruptured carotid-ophthalmic artery aneurysms: angiographical differentiation of each type, operative results, and indications. *Surg Neurol.* 1997;48(5):465–472.
8. Ghatge SB, Modi DB. Treatment of ruptured ICA during transsphenoidal surgery: two different endovascular strategies in two cases. *Intervent Neuroradiol.* 2010;16(1):31–37.
9. Orozco LD, Buciuc RF, Parent AD. Endovascular embolization of prominent intercavernous sinuses for successful transsphenoidal resection of cushing microadenoma: case report. *Neurosurgery.* 2012;71(suppl 1):onsE204–onsE208.
10. Karadimov D, Binev K, Nachkov Y, Platikanov V. Use of activated recombinant factor vII (NovoSeven) during neurosurgery. *J Neurosurg Anesth.* 2003;15(4):330–332.
11. Cushing H. Original memoirs: the control of bleeding in operations for brain tumors: with the description of silver "clips" for the occlusion of vessels inaccessible to the ligature. 1911, *Yale J Biol Med.* 2001;74(6):399–412.
12. Bateman BT, Lin E, Pile-Spellman J. Definitive embolization of meningiomas. A review. *Intervent Neuroradiol.* 2005;11(2):179–186.
13. Manke C, Bretschneider T, Lenhart M, et al. Spinal metastases from renal cell carcinoma: effect of preoperative particle embolization on intraoperative blood loss. *American Journal of Neuroradiology.* 2001;22:997–1003.
14. Hu SS. Blood loss in adult spinal surgery. In: Szpalski M, Gunzburg R, Aebi M, Weiskop RB, eds. *Haemost Spine Surg.* Springer; 2005.
15. Elgafy H, Bransford RJ, McGuire RA, Dettori JR, Fischer D. Blood loss in major spine surgery: are there effective measures to decrease massive hemorrhage in major spine fusion surgery? *Spine.* 2010;35(suppl 9S):S47–S56.
16. Rigamonti A, Gemma M, Rocca A, Messina M, Bignami E, Beretta L. Prone versus knee-chest position for microdiscectomy: a prospective randomized study of intra-abdominal pressure and intraoperative bleeding. *Spine.* 2005;30(17):1918–1923.
17. Park CK. The effect of patient positioning on intraabdominal pressure and blood loss in spinal surgery. *Anes Analg.* 2000;91(3):552–557.
18. Gerlach R, Krause M, Seifert V, Goerlinger K. Hemostatic and hemorrhagic problems in neurosurgical patients. *Acta Neurochir.* 2009;151(8):873–900.
19. Barcelona SL, Vilich F, Cote CJ. A comparison of flow rates and warming capabilities of the Level 1 and rapid infusion system with various-size intravenous catheters. *Anesth Analg.* 2003;97(2):358–363.
20. Thornton JA. Estimation of blood loss during surgery. *Ann R Coll Surg Engl.* 1963;33:164–174.
21. Eerenberg ES, Kamphuisen PW, Sijpkens MK, Meijers JC, Buller HR, Levi M. Reversal of rivaroxaban and dabigatran by prothrombin complex concentrate: a randomized, placebo-controlled, crossover study in healthy subjects. *Circulation.* 2011;124(14):1573–1579.
22. Manke C, Bretschneider T, Lenhart M, et al. Spinal metastases from renal cell carcinoma: effect of preoperative particle embolization on intraoperative blood loss. *Am J Neuroradiol.* 2001;22(5):997–1003.

23. Lapierre F, D'Houtaud S, Wager M. Hemostatic agents in neurosurgery. In: Signorelli F, ed. *Explicative Cases of Controversial Issues in Neurosurgery*. InTech; 2012. http://www.intechopen.com/about-intech.html.

24. Block JE. Severe blood loss during spinal reconstructive procedures: the potential usefulness of topical hemostatic agents. *Med Hypotheses*. 2005;65(3):617–621.

25. Hartmann A, Stapf C, Hofmeister C, et al. Determinants of neurological outcome after surgery for brain arteriovenous malformation. *Stroke*. 2000;31(10):2361–2364.

26. Sihler KC, Napolitano LM. Complications of massive transfusion. *Chest*. 2010;137(1):209–220.

27. Watts DD, Trask A, Soeken K, Perdue P, Dols S, Kaufmann C. Hypothermic coagulopathy in trauma: effect of varying levels of hypothermia on enzyme speed, platelet function, and fibrinolytic activity. *Journal of Trauma - Injury, Infection and Critical Care*. 1998;44(5):846–854.

28. Levy JH. Massive transfusion coagulopathy. *Semin Hematol*. 2006;43(suppl 1):S59–S63.

29. Miller RD, Robbins TO, Tong MJ, et al. Coagulation defects associated with massive blood transfusions. *Ann Surg*. 1971;174(5):794–801.

30. Horlocker TT, Wedel DJ, Rowlingson JC, et al. Regional anesthesia in the patient receiving antithrombotic or thrombolytic therapy: American Society of Regional Anesthesia and Pain Medicine Evidence-Based Guidelines (third edition). *Reg Anesth Pain Med*. 2010;35(1):64–101.

31. Chan KH, Mann KS, Chan TK. The significance of thrombocytopenia in the development of postoperative intracranial hematoma. *J Neurosurg*. 1989;71(1):38–41.

32. Greer SE, Rhynhart KK, Gupta R, Corwin HL. New developments in massive transfusion in trauma. *Curr Opin Anaesthesiol*. 2010;23(2):246–250.

33. Johansson PI, Ostrowski SR, Secher NH. Management of major blood loss: an update. *Acta Anaesthesiol Scand*. 2010;54(9):1039–1049.

34. Ledgerwood AM, Blaisdell W. Coagulation challenges after severe injury with hemorrhagic shock. *J Trauma Acute Care Surg*. 2010;72(6):1714–1718.

35. Pathak A, Dutta S, Marwaha N, Singh D, Varma N, Mathuriya SN. Change in tissue thromboplastin content of brain following trauma. *Neurol India*. 2005;53(2):178–182.

36. Basali A, Mascha E, Kalfas I, Schubert A. Relation between perioperative hypertension and intracranial hemorrhage after craniotomy. *Anesthesiology*. 2000;93(1):48–54.

37. Glotzbecker MP, Bono CM, Wood KB, Harris MB. Postoperative spinal epidural hematoma: a systematic review. *Spine*. 2010;35(10):E413–E420.

38. Shere-Wolfe RF, Galvagno Jr SM, Grissom TE. Critical care considerations in the management of the trauma patient following initial resuscitation. *Scand J Trauma Resuscitation Emerg Med*. 2012; 20: 68.

39. Park PK, Cannon JW, Ye W, et al. Transfusion strategies and development of acute respiratory distress syndrome in combat casualty care. *J Trauma Acute Care Surg*. 2013;75(2 suppl 2):S238–S246.

40. Mirski MA, Lele AV, Fitzsimmons L, Toung TJK. Diagnosis and treatment of vascular air embolism. *Anesthesiology*. 2007;106(1):164–177.

41. Palmon SC, Moore LE, Lundberg J, Toung T. Venous air embolism: a review. *J Clin Anesth*. 1997;9(3):251–257.

42. Albin MS, Babinski M, Maroon JC, Jannetta PJ. Anesthetic management of posterior fossa surgery in the sitting position. *Acta Anaesthesiol Scand*. 1976;20(2):117–128.

43. Harris MM, Yemen TA, Davidson A, et al. Venous embolism during craniectomy in supine infants. *Anesthesiology*. 1987;67(5):816–819.

44. Gómez-Perals LF, Bayo R, Lorenzana-Honrado LM, Antona-Díaz M, Cabezudo JM. Severe intraoperative air embolism during convexity meningioma surgery in the supine position: case report. *Surg Neurol*. 2002;57(4):262–266.

45. Wilkins RH, Albin MS. An unusual entrance site of venous air embolism during operations in the sitting position. *Surg Neurol*. 1977;7(2):71–72.

46. Bunegin L, Albin MS, Helsel PE, Hoffman A, Hung TK. Positioning the right atrial catheter: a model for reappraisal. *Anesthesiology*. 1981;55(4):343–348.

47. Chang JL, Albin MS, Bunegin L, Hung TK. Analysis and comparison of venous air embolism detection methods. *Neurosurgery*. 1980;7(2):135–141.

48. Fathi AR, Eshtehardi P, Meier B. Patent foramen ovale and neurosurgery in sitting position: a systematic review. *Br J Anaesth*. 2009;102(5):588–596.

49. Imanishi M, Nishimura A, Tabuse H, Miyamoto S, Sakaki T, Iwasaki S. Intracranial gas on CT after cardiopulmonary resuscitation: 4 cases. *Neuroradiology*. 1998;40(3):154–157.

50. Benson J, Adkinson C, Collier R. Hyperbaric oxygen therapy of iatrogenic cerebral arterial gas embolism. *Undersea Hyperb Med*. 2003;30(2):117–126.

51. El-Sabbagh AM, Toomasian CJ, Toomasian JM, Ulysse G, Major T, Bartlett RH. Effect of air exposure and suction on blood cell activation and hemolysis in an in vitro cardiotomy suction model. *ASAIO J*. 2013;59(5):474–479.

52. Langfitt TW, Kassell NF. Acute brain swelling in neurosurgical patients. *J Neurosurg*. 1966;24(6):975–983.

53. Marshall W, Jackson J, Langfitt T. Brain swelling caused by trauma and arterial hypertension. Hemodynamic aspects. *Arch Neurol*. 1969;21:545.

54. Marshall W, Weinstein J, Langfitt T. The pathophysiology of brain swelling produced by mechanical trauma and hypertension. *Surg Forum*. 1968;19:431.

55. Salunke P, Sodhi HBS, Aggarwal A, et al. Is ligation and division of anterior third of superior sagittal sinus really safe? *Clin Neurol Neurosurg*. 2013;115(10):1998–2002.

56. Rasmussen M, Bundgaard H, Cold GE. Craniotomy for supratentorial brain tumors: risk factors for brain swelling after opening the dura mater. *J Neurosurg*. 2004;101(4):621–626.

57. Whittle IR, Viswanathan R. Acute intraoperative brain herniation during elective neurosurgery: pathophysiology and management considerations. *J Neurol Neurosurg Psychiatry*. 1996;61(6):584–590.

58. Fehr M, Anderson D. Incidence of progression or rebleeding in hypertensive intracerebral hemorrhage. *J Stroke Cerebrovasc Dis*. 1991;1:111.

59. Wise BL, Andrews RJ, Bringas JR. A review of brain retraction and recommendations for minimizing intraoperative brain injury. *Neurosurgery*. 1994;35(1):172–173.

60. Miller C, Mirski M. Anesthesia considerations and intraoperative monitoring during surgery for arteriovenous malformations and dural arteriovenous fistulas. *Neurosurg Clin North Am*. 2012;23(1):153–164.

61. Batjer H, Devous MS, Meyer Y, Purdy P, Samson D. Cerebrovascular hemodynamics in arteriovenous malformation complicated by normal perfusion pressure breakthrough. *Neurosurgery*. 1988;22:503.

62. Duke BJ, Ryu RK, Brega KE, Coldwell DM. Traumatic bilateral jugular vein thrombosis: case report and review of the literature. *Neurosurgery*. 1997;41(3):680–683.

63. Lang SS, Kofke WA, Stiefel MF. Monitoring and intraoperative management of elevated intracranial pressure and decompressive craniectomy. *Anesthesiol Clin*. 2012;30(2):289–310.

64. Paine JT, Batjer HH, Samson D. Intraoperative ventricular puncture. *Neurosurgery*. 1988;22(6 I):1107–1109.

65. Samadani U, Huang JH, Baranov D, et al. Intracranial hypotension after intraoperative lumbar cerebrospinal fluid drainage. *Neurosurgery*. 2003;52(1):148–151. discussion 51–52.

66. van Velthoven V, Auer LM. Practical application of intraoperative ultrasound imaging. *Acta Neurochir*. 1990;105(1–2):5–13.

67. Marshall LF, Hoi Sang U. Treatment of massive intraoperative brain swelling. *Neurosurgery*. 1983;13(4):412–414.

68. Suarez JI. Hypertonic saline for cerebral edema and elevated intracranial pressure. *Cleve Clin J Med*. 2004;71(suppl 1):S9–S13.

69. Simard JM, Kent TA, Chen M, Tarasov KV, Gerzanich V. Brain oedema in focal ischaemia: molecular pathophysiology and theoretical implications. *Lancet Neurol*. 2007;6(3):258–268.

70. Cho CW, Kim BG, Na HS, Choi ES, Jeon YT. Delayed emergence from anesthesia resulting from posterior cerebral artery infarction after Guglielmi detachable coil embolization. *Korean J Anesthesiol*. 2014;65(6 suppl):S113–S114.

71. Chen Z, Zhang X, Jiang Y, Wang S. Delayed emergence from anesthesia resulting from bilateral epidural hemorrhages during cervical spine surgery. *J Clin Anesth.* 2013;25(3):244–245.

72. Nakazawa K, Yamamoto M, Murai K, Ishikawa S, Uchida T, Makita K. Delayed emergence from anesthesia resulting from cerebellar hemorrhage during cervical spine surgery. *Anesth Analg.* 2005;100(5):1470–1471.

73. Kozasa Y, Takaseya H, Koga Y, et al. A case of delayed emergence from anesthesia caused by postoperative brain edema associated with unexpected cerebral venous sinus thrombosis. *J Anesth.* 2013;27(5):764–767.

74. Nimjee SM, Powers CJ, Kolls BJ, Smith T, Britz GW, Zomorodi AR. Endovascular treatment of venous sinus thrombosis: a case report and review of the literature. *J Neurointerv Surg.* 2011;3(1):30–33.

75. Liu EHC, Koh KF. A prospective audit of critical incidents in anaesthesia in a university teaching hospital. *Ann Acad Med Singapore.* 2003;32(6):814–820.

76. Irita K, Kawashima Y, Morita K, et al. Critical events in the operating room among 1,440,776 patients with ASA PS 1 for elective surgery. *Jpn J Anesthesiol.* 2005;54(8):939–948.

77. Irita K, Tsuzaki K, Sawa T, et al. Critical incidents due to drug administration error in the operating room: an analysis of 4,291,925 anesthetics over a 4 year period. *Jpn J Anesthesiol.* 2004;53(5):577–584.

78. Kelly WN. Potential risks and prevention, part 1: fatal adverse drug events. *Am J Health-System Pharm.* 2001;58(14):1317–1324.

79. Bedell SE, Deitz DC, Leeman D, Delbanco TL. Incidence and characteristics of preventable iatrogenic cardiac arrests. *JAMA.* 1991;265(21):2815–2820.

80. Aldridge J. Potential air embolus from a level 1 rapid infuser. *Anaesthesia.* 2005;60(12):1250–1251.

81. Biboulet P, Aubas P, Dubourdieu J, et al. Fatal and non fatal cardiac arrests related to anesthesia. *Can J Anaesth.* 2001;48(4):326–332.

82. McGrane S, Maziad J, Netterville JL, Saied NN. Therapeutic hypothermia after exsanguination. *Anesth Analg.* 2012;115(2):343–345.

83. Matjasko J, Petrozza P, Cohen M, Steinberg P. Anesthesia and surgery in the seated position: analysis of 554 cases. *Neurosurgery.* 1985;17(5):695–702.

84. Takei T, Nakazawa K, Ishikawa S, Uchida T, Makita K. Cardiac arrest in the left lateral decubitus position and extracorporeal cardiopulmonary resuscitation during neurosurgery: a case report. *J Anesth.* 2010;24(3):447–451.

85. Doyle DJ, Mark PWS. Reflex bradycardia during surgery. *Can J Anaesth.* 1990;37(2):219–222.

86. Dixit S. Bradycardia associated with high cervical spinal cord injury. *Surg Neurol.* 1995;43:514.

87. Luostarinen T, Takala RSK, Niemi TT, et al. Adenosine-induced cardiac arrest during intraoperative cerebral aneurysm rupture. *World Neurosurg.* 2010;73(2):79–83.

88. Cheitlin MD. Pathophysiology of valvular aortic stenosis in the elderly. *Am J Geriatr Cardiol.* 2003;12(3):173–177.

89. Cheney FW, Posner KL, Lee LA, et al. Trends in anesthesia-related death and brain damage: a closed claims analysis. *Anesthesiology.* 2006;105(6):1081–1086.

90. Domino KB, Posner KL, Caplan RA, Cheney FW. Airway injury during anesthesia: a closed claims analysis. *Anesthesiology.* 1999;91(6):1703–1711.

91. Dworacek H, Dworacek H. Larynx injury caused by intubation anesthesia. *Wien Klin Wochenschr.* 1958;70(37):680–681.

92. Kofke WA, Horak J, Stiefel M, Pascual J. Viable oxygenation with cannula-over-needle cricothyrotomy for asphyxial airway occlusion. *Br J Anaesth.* 2011;107(4):642–643.

93. Peterson GN, Domino KB, Caplan RA, Posner KL, Lee LA, Cheney FW. Management of the difficult airway: a closed claims analysis. *Anesthesiology.* 2005;103(1):33–39.

94. Cavallone LF, Vannucci A. Extubation of the difficult airway and extubation failure. *Anesth Analg.* 2013;116(2):368–383.

95. Ito J, Ohtsuka M, Kurahashi K. A case of laryngopharyngeal edema after a spinal tumor resection in prone position with extensive neck flexion. *Jpn J Anesthesiol.* 2012;61(2):189–192.

96. Miura Y, Mimatsu K, Iwata H. Massive tongue swelling as a complication after spinal surgery. *J Spinal Disord.* 1996;9(4):339–341.

97. Huehns TY, Yentis SM, Cumberworth V. Apparent massive tongue swelling. A complication of orotracheal intubation on the intensive care unit. *Anaesthesia.* 1994;49(5):414–416.

98. Sriram K, Khorasani A, Mbekeani KE, Patel S. Tongue necrosis and cleft after prolonged transesophageal echocardiography probe placement. *Anesthesiology.* 2006;105(3):635.

99. Gupta R. Unilateral transient sialadenopathy: another complication of oropharyngeal airway. *Anesthesiology.* 1998;88(2):551–552.

100. Abrishami A, Zilberman P, Chung F. Brief review: airway rescue with insertion of laryngeal mask airway devices with patients in the prone position. *Can J Anesth.* 2010;57(11):1014–1020.

101. Hung MH, Fan SZ, Lin CP, Hsu YC, Shih PY, Lee TS. Emergency airway management with fiberoptic intubation in the prone position with a fixed flexed neck. *Anesth Analg.* 2008;107(5):1704–1706.

102. Tobias JD, Mencio GA, Atwood R, Gurwitz GS. Intraoperative cardiopulmonary resuscitation in the prone position. *J Pediatr Surg.* 1994;29(12):1537–1538.

103. Cassorla L, Lee J-W. Patient positioning and anesthesia. In: Miller RD, ed. *Miller's Anesthesia.* Maryland Heights, MO: Churchill-Livingstone; 2009:1151–1170.

104. Fantini GA, Pappou IP, Girardi FP, Sandhu HS, Cammisa Jr FP. Major vascular injury during anterior lumbar spinal surgery: incidence, risk factors, and management. *Spine.* 2007;32(24):2751–2758.

105. Murai Y, Adachi K, Yoshida Y, Takei M, Teramoto A. Retroperitoneal hematoma as a serious complication of endovascular aneurysmal coiling. *J Korean Neurosurg Soc.* 2010;48(1):88–90.

106. Martyn JAJ, Richtsfeld M. Succinylcholine-induced hyperkalemia in acquired pathologic states: etiologic factors and molecular mechanisms. *Anesthesiology.* 2006;104(1):158–169.

107. Apfelbaum JL, Hagberg CA, Caplan RA, et al. Practice guidelines for management of the difficult airway: an updated report by the American Society of Anesthesiologists Task Force on Management of the Difficult Airway. *Anesthesiology.* 2013;118(2):251–270.

108. Hepner DL, Castells MC. Anaphylaxis during the perioperative period. *Anesth Analg.* 2003;97(5):1381–1395.

109. Trinkle JK, Franz JL, Furman RW, Mobin-Uddin K, Bryant LR. Circulatory arrest during deep hypothermia induced by peritoneal dialysis. *Arch Surg.* 1971;103(5):648–649.

110. Picard J, Ward SC, Zumpe R, Meek T, Barlow J, Harrop-Griffiths W. Guidelines and the adoption of 'lipid rescue' therapy for local anaesthetic toxicity. *Anaesthesia.* 2009;64(2):122–125.

111. Long WB, Rosenblum S, Grady IP. Successful resuscitation of bupivacaine-induced cardiac arrest using cardiopulmonary bypass. *Anesth Analg.* 1989;69(3):403–406.

112. Sepehripour AH, Gupta S, Lall KS. When should cardiopulmonary bypass be used in the setting of severe hypothermic cardiac arrest? *Interactive Cardiovascular and Thoracic Surgery.* 2013;564–569.

113. Cooley DA, Beall Jr AC. Surgical treatment of acute massive pulmonary embolism using temporary cardiopulmonary bypass. 1962. *Chest.* 2009;136(5 suppl):pp e30.

114. Frickey N, Kraincuk P, Zhilla I, Binder T, Plöchl W. Fulminant pulmonary embolism treated by extracorporeal membrane oxygenation in a patient with traumatic brain injury. *J Trauma Inj Infect Crit Care.* 2008;64(3):E41–E43.

115. Mohamed H, Zombolas T, Schultz J, et al. Massive carbon dioxide gas embolism: a near catastrophic situation averted by use of cardiopulmonary bypass. *J Extra-Corporeal Techn.* 2009;41(2):110–113.

116. Estilo AE, Cottrell JE. Naloxone, hypertension, and ruptured cerebral aneurysm. *Anesthesiology.* 1981;54(4):352.

117. Spivey WH. Flumazenil and seizures: analysis of 43 cases. *Clin Ther.* 1992;14(2):292–305.

118. Greer DM, Funk SE, Reaven NL, et al. Impact of fever on outcome in patients with stroke and neurologic injury: a comprehensive meta-analysis. *Stroke.* 2008;39(11):3029–3035.

119. Hypothermia After Cardiac Arrest Study Group. Mild therapeutic hypothermia to improve the neurologic outcome after cardiac arrest. *N Engl J Med.* 2002;346(8):549–556.

# Craniotomy

# 8 *Carotid Endarterectomy*

JOSHUA T. BILLINGSLEY, PEGGY WHITE, BRENDA G. FAHY, and BRIAN L. HOH

## Introduction

The impact of stroke on our country cannot be understated. Stroke is the most common lethal neurological disease: 795,000 people suffer a new or recurrent stroke each year, accounting for one death every 4 minutes from stroke.[1] In 2010 about 1 of every 19 deaths in the United States was the result of stroke. Over the next 20 years, the total direct medical stroke-related costs are projected to triple, from $71.6 billion to $184.1 billion.[2] About 87% of strokes are ischemic, with the rest being hemorrhagic of varying etiologies.[3] Most ischemic strokes are the result of cerebral arterial occlusion caused by embolism from the heart or extracranial arteries, with a frequent source of embolic material being the atherosclerotic, diseased cervical carotid artery. Carotid stenosis is responsible for one-fifth of all strokes, and carotid endarterectomy (CEA) is the most common surgical procedure to prevent stroke.[4,5] Consequently, much research, including multiple prospective randomized trials, have established a role for CEA in the prevention of stroke in patients with symptomatic and asymptomatic cervical carotid artery stenosis.

Several large prospective, randomized trials have validated CEA, establishing it as a vital surgical procedure in the prevention of stroke. The North American Symptomatic Carotid Endarterectomy Trial (NASCET) demonstrated that in patients with symptomatic high-grade carotid stenosis (70%–99%), the cumulative risk of ipsilateral stroke was reduced by 17% over 2 years when comparing medically managed patients with those who underwent CEA.[6] Furthermore, the risk of major or fatal stroke was reduced by nearly 11% over the same period. The effect was less robust for those with symptomatic moderate stenosis (50%–69%), but a significant 10.6% reduction in death or stroke at 30 days was observed for those who underwent CEA.[7] Although controversial, other well-cited studies such as Asymptomatic Carotid Atherosclerosis Study (ACAS)[8] and Asymptomatic Carotid Surgery Trial (ACST)[9] demonstrated a modest surgical benefit for patients with asymptomatic carotid stenosis greater than 60%. There was about a 6% risk reduction for any stroke,[8] as well as a 2.6% risk reduction of disabling or fatal strokes,[9] in patients who underwent CEA compared with those who were medically managed.

CEA is a mainstay in the surgical management of stroke. To assist in the management of stroke patients prior to and after CEA, the relevant anatomy and a description of the surgical procedure will be explained here. Perioperative considerations essential to reducing risk during the operative procedure will be described and, importantly, the rest of the chapter will be devoted to the recognition and management of postoperative complications.

## Neuroanatomy and Procedure

### Key Concepts

**Neuroanatomy and Procedure**

- Multiple prospective randomized trials have established a role for carotid endarterectomy in the prevention of stroke in patients with carotid artery stenosis.
- The location of the carotid bifurcation is important in the surgical planning of carotid endarterectomy. A bifurcation high in the neck, near the angle of the mandible, can make surgical access difficult and increase complications.
- Carotid endarterectomy can be performed under general anesthesia or using only local anesthetics, and each method has its benefits and drawbacks.

### CAROTID ARTERY ANATOMY

The human aortic arch most commonly gives rise to three branches. From right to left, these are the innominate artery, the left common carotid artery (CCA), and the left subclavian artery. The right CCA arises from the innominate artery, which is also the origin of the right subclavian artery. In contrast, the left CCA typically arises directly from the aorta. In the most common variant of aortic arch branching, often erroneously described as a bovine arch, the left CCA shares a common origin with the innominate artery (Fig. 8.1). In the next most common variant, the left CCA arises as a branch of the innominate artery.

Coursing cephalad, the arteries travel within the carotid sheath, together with the ansa cervicalis, the vagus nerve, and internal jugular vein. There are no normal branches from the CCA in the neck. The CCA bifurcates into the internal and external carotid arteries, and there is anatomical variation in the location at which this occurs (Fig. 8.2). About 80% of the time, the bifurcation is located between C3 and C5. The next most common location, in about 13% of the population, occurs at C5–6.[10] The location of the bifurcation is important in the surgical planning of CEA. A bifurcation high in the neck, near the angle of the mandible, can make surgical access difficult and increase complications. Distal to the bifurcation, the internal carotid artery courses posterolateral to the external carotid artery and then gradually turns medially to enter the skull base at the carotid canal.

### SURGICAL PLANNING

CEA can be performed under general anesthesia or using only local anesthetics (LAs) with a regional anesthetic

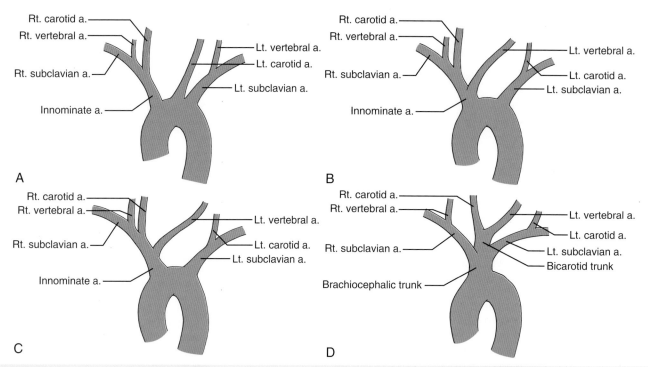

**Fig. 8.1** **(A)** The most common anatomy of the aortic arch in humans. The right CCA arises from the innominate artery, also the origin of the right subclavian artery. In contrast, the left CCA typically arises directly from the aorta. **(B)** The most common variant of the human aortic arch, often erroneously described as a bovine arch. The left CCA shares a common origin with the innominate artery. **(C)** The left CCA arises as a branch of the innominate artery in the next most common arch variant. **(D)** A true bovine arch with a single brachiocephalic trunk that trifurcates. This is rarely, if ever, seen in humans. (Courtesy of M.E. Robin Barry, MA.)

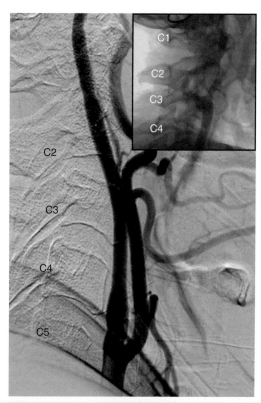

**Fig. 8.2** Digital subtraction angiography of a carotid bifurcation. Eighty percent of the time the carotid bifurcation is located between C3 and C5. The next most common location occurs at C5–6 in about 13% of the population. The bifurcation here appears at the superior endplate of C5, below the angle of the mandible. (Courtesy of M.E. Robin Barry, MA.)

technique. The decision to choose one technique over the other depends on patient factors, personal preference, the surgeon, and the technical skills of the anesthesiologist; each option has its benefits and drawbacks. Proponents of the LA technique emphasize improved hemodynamic stability, more reliable assessment of hemodynamically significant alterations in blood flow that may indicate the necessity for intervention—including a shunt or mean arterial pressure (MAP) augmentation, and immediate availability of postoperative neurological assessment. The drawback of this technique is that it requires the patient to lie still for the duration of the procedure, thereby requiring the surgeon to be efficient. An additional risk of this technique is increased patient anxiety and possible alteration in mental status, rendering the patient unable to remain still and/or unable to protect the airway; this may require emergent conversion to a general anesthetic (GA).

LA is performed with superficial and deep cervical plexus blocks by the anesthesiologist, with additional supplementation by the surgeon, who generally injects LA before carotid cross-clamping. In an attempt to preserve the postoperative neurological examination of the patient, typically, no additional sedation is given for the procedure. If necessary, for patient comfort, some anesthesiologists may use a low-dose remifentanil infusion or small doses of anxiolytic.

Complications can arise from a deep cervical plexus block. Serious complications include LA toxicity due to intravascular injection, respiratory distress as a result of phrenic nerve dysfunction (the phrenic nerve is innervated by the C3–5 nerve roots), seizures from LA infiltration into the epidural or subdural space, and, although less likely, an ipsilateral pneumothorax. Additionally, there is the risk of an incomplete or failed block, requiring conversion to a GA.

In contrast, those in support of the GA technique recognize that benefits include reduced patient anxiety, improved sedation/analgesia, a secure airway, optimal oxygenation and ventilation, and a blunted sympathetic response to surgery. General endotracheal anesthesia can be performed as a standalone technique or in combination with a superficial cervical plexus block. The authors' preference is to utilize a combination anesthetic of GA and LA, which secures the airway and creates fewer hemodynamic changes in the perioperative period.

When GA is administered, cerebral perfusion and cortical cellular integrity can be assessed throughout the procedure with intraoperative neuromonitoring. Modalities used in this setting include electroencephalogram and somatosensory evoked potentials, both requiring technical equipment and trained personnel to record and interpret tracings. Vascular integrity can be monitored by cerebral oximetry, carotid stump pressure, or transcranial Doppler ultrasound. The anesthesiologist's decision to augment MAP, to suggest placement of a shunt, or to induce cerebral protection through burst suppression is often based on changes noted with the use of these specialized modalities.

It is important to mention that the use of a shunt during CEA is controversial. Shunting is a process that utilizes a segment of silicone tubing to connect the common carotid artery to the internal carotid artery, effectively "bypassing" the diseased segment of artery. This maintains flow to the intracranial circulation during the surgery, avoiding potential hypoxic events.

Some surgeons use a shunt routinely, claiming it avoids ipsilateral cerebral hypoperfusion and allows the surgeon to work in an unhurried manner. Other surgeons contend that this is not necessary because cerebral hypoperfusion is a very uncommon cause of stroke during CEA and, furthermore, simply placing a shunt can dislodge microemboli, resulting in stroke. Finally, there are surgeons who reserve the use of a shunt for only those situations where intraoperative neuromonitoring is suggestive of cerebral hypoperfusion.

A recent study compared the neurological outcomes of patients undergoing CEA with or without shunting.[11] More than 3000 patients were included in the study, and they were matched for many critical patient- and procedure-related variables. The study found no significant difference in the incidence of postoperative stroke or transient ischemic attack (TIA) between the groups. Interestingly, when an analysis was restricted to only patients who had severe stenosis or occlusion of the contralateral carotid artery, the use of a shunt was associated with a twofold greater incidence of stroke/TIA.

Several large randomized controlled trials have evaluated the use of GA compared with LA for carotid surgery. The landmark study, General Anesthesia versus Local Anesthesia for carotid surgery (GALA), enrolled 3526 people from 95 centers and 24 countries.[12] The results revealed no statistically significant difference between LA and GA for all major endpoints, including stroke, myocardial infarction (MI), and death.

Another study evaluated anesthetic modality and followed perioperative variables including hospital length of stay, operative mortality, stroke, infection, hematoma, and cranial nerve injury.[13] The GA group had more episodes of perioperative hemodynamic instability requiring treatment with intravenous vasoactive medications or fluid boluses. There was no difference between the two groups for all other variables that were measured. Key markers of stress, such as adrenocorticotropic hormone, cortisol, prolactin, hemodynamics, and C-reactive protein were also monitored during and up to 3 days after the CEA procedure, with no statistically significant difference in the stress response of patients undergoing the procedure based on anesthetic technique.[14]

## Clinical Pearl

There is no clear evidence to support one anesthetic modality over the other. Therefore, choice of anesthetic should focus on patient factors, as well as anesthesiologist and surgeon preference.

## SURGICAL PROCEDURE

The patient is placed in the supine position with the head turned 30 degrees away from the side of the operation. The neck is slightly extended. Placing a rolled towel under the shoulders may facilitate this. Prior to making an incision, the anatomical location of the carotid bifurcation is localized under fluoroscopy to the appropriate cervical vertebral level and demarcated with a skin marker (Fig. 8.3A). An incision is then made along the medial border of the sternocleidomastoid muscle (SCM). The subcutaneous tissues are sharply divided down to the platysma muscle, and the muscle is then divided as well. Meticulous hemostasis must be achieved throughout the procedure because the patient will be administered heparin, and bleeding will obstruct the surgeon's view and impede the identification of anatomical structures. A self-retractor is placed in the wound to open the superficial tissues. If the retractor is placed deep in the wound, damage to the recurrent laryngeal nerve or superior laryngeal nerve can occur, so the retractor is placed to open only the skin and subcutaneous tissues. Dissection continues beneath the SCM to identify the internal jugular vein and a branch, the common facial vein. It is usually necessary to double-ligate and transect the common facial vein to facilitate further dissection. The internal jugular vein is then gently retracted laterally with the SCM to expose the carotid artery. Exposure of the carotid artery allows identification of the carotid sheath, and this can be opened, beginning inferiorly and extending upward to the level of the omohyoid muscle.

Next, the CCA and internal and external carotid arteries (ICA and ECA), with the superior thyroid artery, are dissected (Fig. 8.3B). At this point, the hypoglossal nerve must be identified and protected to avoid injury. It lies superficial to the ECA and ICA, below the digastric muscle. Additionally, as dissection continues to fully expose the carotid

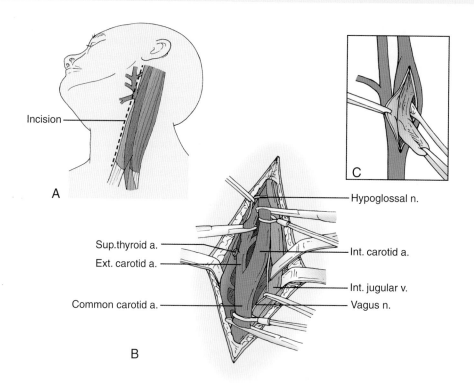

**Fig. 8.3** **(A)** The procedure begins with an incision along the medial border of the sternocleidomastoid muscle. The position and location of the incision should be appropriate for the anatomical location of the patient's carotid bifurcation. **(B)** The surgical field showing dissection of the CCA, ICA, ECA, and superior thyroid artery. Adequate exposure of the proximal CCA and ICA, well beyond the plaque, is imperative. **(C)** After clamping the vessels and making the arteriotomy, the plaque is carefully separated from the wall of the artery, starting in the CCA and working superiorly. (Courtesy of M.E. Robin Barry, MA)

system, injury to the vagus nerve must also be avoided. The vagus lies deep, between the carotid and internal jugular veins. If dissection in this region is necessary, one must be wary of the vagus and its superior laryngeal branch, because damage to this nerve can result in dysphagia and changes in voice pitch postoperatively.

The carotid bulb can be injected with 2 cc of 2% lidocaine to minimize the bradycardia and hypotension experienced with manipulation of the artery. Vessel loops are placed around the CCA, ICA, and ECA. At this stage, before proceeding, it is necessary to have adequate exposure of the proximal CCA for control, as well as distal ICA exposure beyond the level of the plaque.

Using a sterile marker, the arteriotomy incision site is drawn. Prior to vessel clamping, IV heparin is given at a dose of 100 U/kg. The vessels are clamped in order starting with the ICA, CCA, and then ECA. Clamping in this order is believed to reduce the risk of embolization. A #11 blade is used to make the arteriotomy, starting about 1 cm below the bifurcation. With the vessel open, beginning inferiorly in the CCA, the plaque is separated from the wall of the artery, extending proximally into the ICA. Last, the plaque is removed from the ECA as far proximally as possible (Fig. 8.3C). It is imperative to leave the wall of the artery smooth as the plaque is removed. Continuous irrigation with heparinized saline during and after the plaque is removed is used to wash out all debris.

After meticulous removal of all debris, the arteriotomy is closed with running 6-0 suture. The ICA clamp is removed prior to closure of the last few sutures to flush the vessel and assess patency. The vessel clamps are removed first from the ECA, then the CCA, and finally the ICA. The carotid sheath is reapproximated, the platysma is closed in a separate layer, and a running subcuticular stitch closes the skin.

## Perioperative Considerations

### Key Concepts

**Perioperative Considerations**

- Periprocedural MI is the leading cause of increased morbidity and mortality with carotid endarterectomy.
- Patients should undergo a preoperative workup appropriate to their level of estimated risk based on presentation, history, and comorbidities.
- Other risk factors contributing to increased surgical risk are age, gender, and history of congestive heart failure.

One of the most significant events contributing to increased morbidity and mortality after carotid revascularization is periprocedural myocardial infarction (PMI).[15,16] This most commonly occurs within 24 to 48 hours of the procedure and is often caused by stable coronary artery disease (CAD), resulting in a mismatch between myocardial oxygen supply and increased demand secondary to augmented stress from the procedure.[17]

The Carotid Revascularization Endarterectomy versus Stenting Trial (CREST) was one of the first studies to show on a large scale the significance of PMI on outcomes after CEA. PMI, for this study, consisted of CK-MB or troponin elevation exceeding the upper limit of normal, combined with chest pain or ischemic electrocardiogram (ECG) changes. PMI was independently associated with mortality, which continued to be an ongoing risk for up to 4 years when MI occurred with carotid revascularization.[17,18] Compared with a control group that did not experience any periprocedural events, PMI alone was a strong predictor of mortality.[18] Because the majority of patients undergoing carotid revascularization will also have CAD, preprocedural cardiac evaluation is imperative.[19]

Patients should undergo further preoperative workup appropriate to their level of estimated risk based on presentation, history, and comorbidities. This discussion will focus specifically on cardiac evaluation. Intermediate and high-risk patients should have noninvasive cardiac testing prior to the procedure, including ECG and resting ECG. Stress testing should be considered for these patients, but this is often controversial. A multinational study randomized 770 intermediate-risk patients undergoing vascular surgery to receive preoperative stress testing or receive no testing.[20] A small number of very high-risk patients were identified and referred for coronary revascularization prior to surgery. Thirty days after the procedure, the incidence of PMI or cardiac death was not significantly different between the groups (1.8% vs. 2.3%, p = 0.62). In another similar randomized trial, preoperative dobutamine stress testing did not improve outcomes in patients undergoing vascular surgery.[21] Current recommendations support additional noninvasive stress testing in patients with one or more perioperative cardiac risk factors and poor functional capacity.[22] In those with active unstable coronary disease that requires treatment, there is no consensus on whether to perform coronary revascularization before, after, or concomitant with CEA. Several studies have compared whether staging these procedures or performing them simultaneously is superior, with no clear result.[23,24]

Other risk factors found to contribute to increased surgical risk in this population are age, gender, and history of congestive heart failure (CHF). Postoperative stroke or death was more frequent in women age 75 years or greater and those with a history of CHF.[25–27] Women, compared with men, were three times more likely to suffer stroke or death after CEA.[25] Patients older than 75 years and those with a history of CHF were about fourfold more likely to suffer stroke or death.[25]

# Postoperative Complications

## Key Concepts

### Postoperative Complications

- Postoperative complications are often directly related to anesthetic technique, surgical technique, or the patient's coexisting diseases.
- The most common and critical postoperative complications from carotid endarterectomy are MI and stroke.
- Postoperative hypertension is the single most important modifiable factor contributing to morbidity and mortality after CEA.

---

**Box 8.1    Complications of CEA Ranked in Order of Severity**

1. Stroke
2. Myocardial infarction
3. Intracerebral hemorrhage
4. Hyperperfusion syndrome
5. Postoperative wound hematoma
6. Cranial nerve injury – hypoglossal/vagus nerve
7. Seizure
8. Cardiovascular – postoperative complications
   a. Hypertension
   b. Hypotension

---

Most postoperative complications are directly related to one of the following: anesthetic technique, surgical technique, or the patient's coexisting diseases. Complications include MI, stroke, hypertension, cerebral hyperemia, intracerebral hemorrhage (ICH), seizure, neck hematoma, and/or cranial nerve dysfunction (Box 8.1). Many of these complications occur within 24 to 48 hours of the operation but can manifest days to months after discharge. Those complications requiring immediate attention and having the potential for increasing morbidity and/or leading to death usually occur early in the postoperative period and thus will be the focus of this discussion on optimizing care during this acute period.

## MYOCARDIAL INFARCTION

Postprocedure hypotension can affect 5% to 10% of CEA patients.[28,29] Benign hypotension usually lasts only 24 to 48 hours and generally responds well to administration of phenylephrine and fluids. Hemodynamic fluctuations and arrhythmias, including bradycardia, can be attributed to carotid sinus or vagal nerve dysfunction. However, the physician needs to maintain a high index of suspicion for MI when hypotension is refractory to therapy. These patients require an ECG and serial cardiac enzyme studies.

MI is an independent predictor of mortality after CEA.[30] Most studies have defined MI as having cardiac biomarker elevation and ECG changes plus or minus chest pain; however, biomarker elevation *only* after CEA has been independently identified with increased mortality over 4 years.[31,32] In a more recent study, non-ST elevation MI, which was once considered a benign event after CEA, has been shown to be strongly associated with higher rates of in-hospital mortality.[33]

Periprocedural MI increases morbidity and mortality in patients undergoing carotid revascularization. In a subanalysis of the CREST study, the incidence of periprocedural MI as defined by this group was about twofold greater for patients undergoing CEA (2.3%) than for those undergoing carotid artery stenting (CAS) (1.1%; p = 0.03).[31] The Stenting and Angioplasty With Protection In Patients at High Risk for Endarterectomy study reported a postprocedure MI rate of 5.9% for CEA and 2.4% for CAS.[34] Both of these studies employed the routine collection of serial cardiac enzymes on patients in the postoperative period.

Importantly, the definition of MI consisted of positive troponin regardless of the CK total and CK-MB, likely leading to MI being overdiagnosed. These rates are higher than in other studies and can be attributed to the identification of asymptomatic patients through this liberal definition of MI based on biomarkers. In other studies such as Endarterectomy versus Angioplasty in Patients with Symptomatic Severe Carotid Stenosis (EVA-3S), International Carotid Stenting Study (ICSS), and Stent-Protected Angioplasty versus Carotid Endarterectomy (SPACE), the incidence of periprocedural MI was between 0.4% and 0.8%.[34–36] In these studies, the definition of MI was more conservative, was based on clinical symptomatology and cardiac workup, and did include positive biomarker elevation.

Further analysis of these studies has suggested that patients with preexisting cardiopulmonary disease or renal insufficiency are more prone to periprocedural MI. The use of high-dose statins, beta blockade, and dual antiplatelet therapy should be considered in this population. Any indication of myocardial ischemia should elicit a complete workup, especially in the setting of CEA. A heightened clinical suspicion and aggressive management should be employed for early recognition to further reduce the extent of myocardial injury.

## HYPERTENSION

Postoperative hypertension is the single most important modifiable factor contributing to periprocedural morbidity and mortality after CEA.[29] It can be seen in up to 73.5% of patients, with one of the strongest predictors being preexisting hypertension.[29] This condition can lead to a wound hematoma or hyperperfusion syndrome.[37] Optimal management of episodic hypertension within the first 48 hours after CEA includes the use of a short-acting intravenous antihypertensive agent. The optimal agent would provide peripheral vasodilatation with minimal effect on cerebral vasculature or myocardial conduction; these desired hemodynamic goals can usually be obtained with the use of a nicardipine infusion, but other drugs such as nitroglycerine or labetalol can also be efficacious. All decisions should be based on patient comorbidity for optimal selection of therapy.

Another cause of postprocedure hypertension—baroreflex failure syndrome—occurs when there is damage to the carotid sinus or vagus nerve. This is typically seen with bilateral carotid disease and is related to the dissection and plaque removal. Although this usually resolves in the first 24 to 48 hours, it can persist for up to 12 weeks after CEA.[38]

## HYPERPERFUSION SYNDROME

Hyperperfusion syndrome is a condition of dysfunctional cerebral autoregulation that usually occurs with high-grade stenosis, coexisting contralateral stenosis, and/or poorly controlled hypertension. It develops when the patient has lived with a stenotic carotid artery for an extended period, because this creates a distal low-flow state in the cerebral vasculature. The intracranial arteries/arterioles maximally dilate in this situation in an attempt to increase flow to deprived tissue. This prolonged vasodilation uncouples the intracerebral autoregulation in that territory, causing a more linear relationship between MAP and cerebral perfusion pressure. After normalization of flow

through the carotid artery, such as after CEA, sustained or episodic hypertension can potentially cause what is termed *normal perfusion pressure breakthrough.* This can result in complications that range from cerebral edema to ICH. After the carotid stenosis is corrected, the systolic blood pressure should be maintained between 110 and 150 mm Hg.[39]

ICH and cerebral edema are evident on neuroimaging and will likely be associated with increased velocities in transcranial Doppler ultrasound. Strict blood pressure control in the acute postoperative period can prevent these complications.

## INTRACRANIAL HEMORRHAGE

ICH occurs in less than 1% of CEAs and usually occurs after correction of high-grade stenosis. Conditions associated with ICH include hyperperfusion syndrome, anticoagulation, and perioperative ischemia. Postprocedure ICH is often devastating, with a significant increase in morbidity and mortality. In a retrospective case control study that assessed risk factors associated with ICH after CEA, 0.4% of patients undergoing a CEA during the time period studied developed an ipsilateral ICH. An ICH that develops within a previous stroke territory results from damage to the basal lamina of the endothelial cells after the infarct, weakening them and increasing the propensity for breakthrough bleeding. Preexisting hypertension and amyloidosis are also risk factors for ICH because they may predispose to microvasculature damage.

Interestingly, more recent studies that have reviewed large numbers of patients having undergone carotid revascularization suggested a significant sixfold to sevenfold increase in the frequency of ICH with CAS compared with CEA.[40] Furthermore, for these patients, ICH was predictive of a 30-fold increase in mortality prior to discharge. In another study that focused on ICH related to hyperperfusion syndrome in nearly 4500 patients after CEA or CAS, there was a greater frequency, although not of statistical significance, of ICH with CAS.[41] Failure to adhere to a strict blood pressure control regimen was significantly associated with the development of ICH in CEA patients exhibiting signs and symptoms of cerebral hyperperfusion.

> **Clinical Pearl**
>
> Postoperative hematoma formation can quickly become a life-threatening emergency. In the event of rapid hematoma formation immediate action is required, including suture release and securing airway.

## STROKE

The risk of perioperative stroke with CEA is about 5%.[42] Postoperative restenosis and stroke can be attributed to surgical technique, microemboli with shunting, the use of protamine sulfate for heparin reversal, and perfusion deficit during carotid cross-clamping.

In the Asymptomatic Carotid Surgery Trial-1 (ACST-1) trial, 2707 patients were randomized to medical management or immediate CEA and followed for a median of 80 months.[46] The primary endpoint included new occlusion of the carotid artery. Duplex ultrasound or angiography was used for evaluation and determination of the absence of internal carotid artery flow. New carotid artery occlusion, ipsilateral or contralateral, was found in 7.3% of patients. Median time to occlusion was 73 to 75 months, with an annual risk of occlusion of 1.1%. The risk of occlusion was lower in the immediate CEA group and higher in patients with high stenosis in the medical management arm. Risk factors associated with the development of occlusion included male gender, medical management alone, greater than 70% stenosis, diabetes mellitus, and hypertension. Gender and deferment of CEA were the only statistically significant factors associated with carotid artery occlusion. All factors were associated with the development of stroke, with 11% having a stroke during the follow-up period. This study characterized the risk of stroke with medical management alone versus CEA. The mechanisms for acute periprocedure stroke include graft occlusion, vessel kinking, insufficient perfusion with cross-clamp, or emboli.

## NECK HEMATOMA

The formation of a neck hematoma after CEA is a potentially life-threatening complication. Many factors can lead to hematoma formation, including perioperative antiplatelet medication use, intraoperative heparinization without reversal with protamine sulfate, surgical technique (eversion), reflexive coughing with endotracheal tube removal during GA emergence, or uncontrolled hypertensive episodes causing stress on the suture line. Although it is difficult to evaluate true hematoma incidence due to underreporting of minute hematomas and different interpretations of hematoma formation (i.e., only reporting hematomas requiring surgical reexploration), Baracchin et al. report an incidence ranging from 1.5% to 12%.[43] The NASCET study reported that 5.5% of patients undergoing CEA had documented wound hematomas[6] and most of these were managed conservatively with observation; 1.4% required surgical exploration.

The use of intraoperative protamine sulfate for heparin reversal at the end of the procedure can significantly reduce the incidence and severity of postoperative hemorrhage. It has been shown to significantly reduce the risk of postoperative hematoma formation[43] and causes minimal risk of thrombotic complications such as MI or ischemic stroke/carotid restenosis. In one group, Mazzalai et al. showed that no neck hematomas developed in a protamine reversal group versus 8.2% in a group where no heparin reversal was used.[43] Moreover, the incidence of stroke was not significant and was 0.5% in the protamine group versus 0% in the no-reversal arm.

In the NASCET trial, the risk of neck hematoma was 5.5% for patients who did not receive protamine sulfate and was 1.8% (p = 0.0004) for patients who received reversal.[6] In this population, the stroke rate was comparable but did not reach statistical significance. Similarly, a post hoc analysis of the GALA trial showed a statistically significant decrease in the risk of postoperative hematoma formation in the protamine group compared with a group who did not receive heparin reversal (7.4% versus 10.4%).[12] The stroke rate did not reach significance and was 2.9% for the protamine group and 4.4% for the nonprotamine group.

There is currently no consensus on the perioperative management of antiplatelet therapy. Some surgeons prefer to continue antiplatelet medications, citing a high risk for restenosis or coronary artery embolism. However, these patients are at higher risk for bleeding and must be carefully observed in the postoperative period, especially if heparin is not reversed after the procedure.

In the event postoperative hemorrhage does occur, caution should be taken in observing the patient. A large expanding neck hematoma can very rapidly cause airway obstruction and tissue distortion. This feared complication makes oral endotracheal intubation difficult and cricothyroidotomy or open tracheostomy extremely challenging. The initial management for an enlarging hematoma that is causing airway obstruction includes immediate decompression via wound opening. This is preferentially performed in the operating room, but if the hematoma is rapidly expanding and compromising the airway, opening the wound at the bedside should be performed immediately. Attention should also simultaneously be focused on securing the airway.

## SEIZURE

Postprocedure seizure is an uncommon event and is usually the result of hypertensive encephalopathy, cerebral edema, hyperperfusion syndrome, cerebral ischemia, or ICH. Despite its low incidence, seizure after CEA is associated with adverse outcomes. According to Nielsen et al., the incidence of seizure after CEA is about 3%.[44] All of these patients had ipsilateral high-grade stenosis of the internal carotid artery. In another large study that focused on the presentation management and outcome after seizure post-CEA, the incidence was about 1% in a 30-day period after CEA.[45] Seizure was not associated with age or gender, and nearly all of the patients had labile hypertension and severe bilateral carotid and/or vertebral disease. All eight patients had significantly elevated blood pressure at the onset of the seizure. Immediate computed tomography scans were performed on all patients, and three scans showed white-matter edema, one ICH, and one edema with diffuse hemorrhage. Three of the scans were normal. Seven of the patients had a postictal deficit. Two of the patients either died or had a severe disabling stroke. Although a direct cause-and-effect relationship cannot be made for seizure after CEA, this study strongly suggests that post-CEA hyperperfusion syndrome plays a large role in those who suffer seizures. Consequently, prompt treatment of hypertension concurrent with seizure treatment may be beneficial.

## Conclusion

Carotid endarterectomy is an essential surgical procedure in the management of patients with symptomatic and asymptomatic carotid stenosis. Multiple randomized, controlled trials have now established the benefit of this surgery in reducing the risk of stroke and improving patient survival. However, meticulous attention to detail is necessary to achieve good outcomes, and this includes not only in the surgical procedure, but in preoperative and postoperative care as well. The surgeon, anesthesiologist, and neurointensivist all provide key elements in a successful outcome.

## References

1. Go AS, Mozaffarian D, Roger VL, et al. Heart disease and stroke statistics—2014 update: a report from the american heart association. *Circulation.* 2014;129(3):e28–e292.
2. Ovbiagele B, Goldstein LB, Higashida RT, et al. Forecasting the future of stroke in the United States: a policy statement from the American Heart Association and American Stroke Association. *Stroke.* 2013;44 (8):2361–2375.
3. Woo D, Gebel J, Miller R, et al. Incidence rates of first-ever ischemic stroke subtypes among blacks: a population-based study. *Stroke.* 1999;30(12):2517–2522.
4. Go AS, Mozaffarian D, Roger VL. Heart disease and stroke statistics—2013 update: a report from the American Heart Association. *Circulation.* 2013;127(1):e6–e245.
5. Rajamani K, Chaturvedi S. Medical management of carotid artery disease. *Semin Neurol.* 2005;25(4):376–383.
6. North American Symptomatic Carotid Endarterectomy Trial C. Beneficial effect of carotid endarterectomy in symptomatic patients with high-grade carotid stenosis. *N Engl J Med.* 1991;325 (7):445–453.
7. Barnett HJ, Taylor DW, Eliasziw M, et al. Benefit of carotid endarterectomy in patients with symptomatic moderate or severe stenosis. North American Symptomatic Carotid Endarterectomy Trial Collaborators. *N Engl J Med.* 1998;399:1415–1425.
8. Endarterectomy for asymptomatic carotid artery stenosis. Executive Committee for the Asymptomatic Carotid Atherosclerosis Study. *JAMA.* 1995;273(18):1421–1428.
9. Halliday A, Mansfield A, Marro J, et al. Prevention of disabling and fatal strokes by successful carotid endarterectomy in patients without recent neurological symptoms: randomised controlled trial. *Lancet.* 2004;363(9420):1491–1502.
10. Thomas JB, Antiga L, Che SL, et al. Variation in the carotid bifurcation geometry of young versus older adults: implications for geometric risk of atherosclerosis. *Stroke.* 2005;36(11):2450–2456.
11. Bennett KM, Scarborough JE, Cox MW, Shortell CK. The impact of intraoperative shunting on early neurologic outcomes after carotid endarterectomy. *J Vasc Surg.* 2015;61(1):96–102.
12. Group GTC, Lewis SC, Warlow CP, et al. General anaesthesia versus local anaesthesia for carotid surgery (GALA): a multicentre, randomised controlled trial. *Lancet.* 2008;372(9656):2132–2142.
13. Watts K, Lin PH, Bush RL, et al. The impact of anesthetic modality on the outcome of carotid endarterectomy. *Am J Surg.* 2004;188 (6):741–747.
14. Marrocco-Trischitta MM, Tiezzi A, Svampa MG, et al. Perioperative stress response to carotid endarterectomy: the impact of anesthetic modality. *J Vasc Surg.* 2004;39(6):1295–1304.
15. Riles TS, Kopelman I, Imparato AM. Myocardial infarction following carotid endarterectomy: a review of 683 operations. *Surgery.* 1979;85 (3):249–252.
16. Hertzer NR, Lees CD. Fatal myocardial infarction following carotid endarterectomy: three hundred thirty-five patients followed 6-11 years after operation. *Ann Surg.* 1981;194(2):212–218.
17. Stilp E, Baird C, Gray WA, et al. An evidence-based review of the impact of periprocedural myocardial infarction in carotid revascularization. *Cathet Cardiovasc Intervent.* 2013;82(5):709–714.
18. Gray WA, Simonton CA, Verta P. Overview of the 2011 Food and Drug Administration Circulatory System Devices Panel meeting on the ACCULINK and ACCUNET Carotid Artery Stent System. *Circulation.* 2012;125(18):2256–2264.
19. Schouten O, Bax JJ, Poldermans D. Preoperative cardiac risk assessment in vascular surgery patients: seeing beyond the perioperative period. *Eur Heart J.* 2008;29(3):283–284.
20. Poldermans D, Bax JJ, Schouten O, et al. Should major vascular surgery be delayed because of preoperative cardiac testing in intermediate-risk patients receiving beta-blocker therapy with tight heart rate control? *J Am Coll Cardiol.* 2006;48(5):964–969.
21. Falcone RA, Nass C, Jermyn R, et al. The value of preoperative pharmacologic stress testing before vascular surgery using ACC/AHA guidelines: a prospective, randomized trial. *J Cardiothoracic Vasc Anest.* 2003;17(6):694–698.
22. Adams Jr HP, del Zoppo G, Alberts MJ, et al. Guidelines for the early management of adults with ischemic stroke: a guideline from the American Heart Association/American Stroke Association Stroke Council, Clinical Cardiology Council, Cardiovascular Radiology and Intervention Council, and the Atherosclerotic Peripheral Vascular Disease and Quality of Care Outcomes in Research Interdisciplinary Working Groups: the American Academy of Neurology affirms the value of this guideline as an educational tool for neurologists. *Stroke.* 2007;38 (5):1655–1711.
23. Naylor AR, Mehta Z, Rothwell PM. A systematic review and meta-analysis of 30-day outcomes following staged carotid artery stenting and coronary bypass. *Eur J Vascular Endovascular Surg.* 2009;37 (4):379–387.
24. Chiappini B, Dell'Amore A, Di Marco L, Di Bartolomeo R, Marinelli G. Simultaneous carotid and coronary arteries disease: staged or combined surgical approach? *J Cardiac Surg.* 2005;20 (3):234–240.
25. Goldstein LB, Samsa GP, Matchar DB, Oddone EZ. Multicenter review of preoperative risk factors for endarterectomy for asymptomatic carotid artery stenosis. *Stroke.* 1998;29(4):750–753.
26. Tu JV, Wang H, Bowyer B, et al. Risk factors for death or stroke after carotid endarterectomy: observations from the Ontario Carotid Endarterectomy Registry. *Stroke.* 2003;34(11):2568–2573.
27. Rothwell PM, Eliasziw M, Gutnikov SA, Warlow CP, Barnett HJ. Carotid Endarterectomy Trialists C. Endarterectomy for symptomatic carotid stenosis in relation to clinical subgroups and timing of surgery. *Lancet.* 2004;363(9413):915–924.
28. Tan TW, Eslami MH, Kalish JA, et al. The need for treatment of hemodynamic instability following carotid endarterectomy is associated with increased perioperative and 1-year morbidity and mortality. *J Vasc Surg.* 2014;59(1):16–24 e1–2.
29. Biller J, Feinberg WM, Castaldo JE, et al. Guidelines for carotid endarterectomy: a statement for healthcare professionals from a Special Writing Group of the Stroke Council, American Heart Association. *Circulation.* 1998;97(5):501–509.
30. Pini R, Faggioli G, Longhi M, et al. Impact of postoperative transient ischemic attack on survival after carotid revascularization. *J Vasc Surg.* 2014;59(6):1570–1576.
31. Mantese VA, Timaran CH, Chiu D, Begg RJ, Brott TG, Investigators C. The Carotid Revascularization Endarterectomy versus Stenting Trial (CREST): stenting versus carotid endarterectomy for carotid disease. *Stroke.* 2010;41(10 suppl):S31–S34.
32. Blackshear JL, Cutlip DE, Roubin GS, et al. Myocardial infarction after carotid stenting and endarterectomy: results from the carotid revascularization endarterectomy versus stenting trial. *Circulation.* 2011;123 (22):2571–2578.
33. Khan A, Adil MM, Qureshi AI. Non-ST-elevation myocardial infarction in patients undergoing carotid endarterectomy or carotid artery stent placement. *Stroke.* 2014;45(2):595–597.
34. Yadav JS, Wholey MH, Kuntz RE, et al. Protected carotid-artery stenting versus endarterectomy in high-risk patients. *N Engl J Med.* 2004;351(15):1493–1501.
35. Ederle J, Dobson J, Featherstone RL, et al. Carotid artery stenting compared with endarterectomy in patients with symptomatic carotid stenosis (International Carotid Stenting Study): an interim analysis of a randomised controlled trial. *Lancet.* 2010;375(9719):985–997.
36. Group SC, Ringleb PA, Allenberg J, et al. 30 day results from the SPACE trial of stent-protected angioplasty versus carotid endarterectomy in symptomatic patients: a randomised non-inferiority trial. *Lancet.* 2006;368(9543):1239–1247.
37. Schroeder T, Sillesen H, Sorensen O, Engell HC. Cerebral hyperperfusion following carotid endarterectomy. *J Neurosurg.* 1987;66 (6):824–829.
38. Robertson D, Hollister AS, Biaggioni I, Netterville JL, Mosqueda-Garcia R, Robertson RM. The diagnosis and treatment of baroreflex failure. *N Engl J Med.* 1993;329(20):1449–1455.
39. Naylor AR. Optimal medical therapy during carotid endarterectomy: a personal view. *Acta Chir Belg.* 2009;109:285–291.

40. McDonald RJ, Cloft HJ, Kallmes DF. Intracranial hemorrhage is much more common after carotid stenting than after endarterectomy: evidence from the National Inpatient Sample. *Stroke.* 2011;42 (10):2782–2787.

41. Ogasawara K, Sakai N, Kuroiwa T, et al. Intracranial hemorrhage associated with cerebral hyperperfusion syndrome following carotid endarterectomy and carotid artery stenting: retrospective review of 4494 patients. *J Neurosurg.* 2007;107 (6):1130–1136.

42. Heyer EJ, Mergeche JL, Anastasian ZH, Kim M, Mallon KA, Connolly ES. Arterial blood pressure management during carotid endarterectomy and early cognitive dysfunction. *Neurosurgery.* 2014;74 (3):245–253.

43. Baracchini C, Gruppo M, Mazzalai F, Lorenzetti R, Meneghetti G, Ballotta E. Predictors of neck bleeding after eversion carotid endarterectomy. *J Vasc Surg.* 2011;54(3):699–705.

44. Nielsen TG, Sillesen H, Schroeder TV. Seizures following carotid endarterectomy in patients with severely compromised cerebral circulation. *Eur J Vascular Endovascular Surg.* 1995;9(1):53–57.

45. Naylor AR, Evans J, Thompson MM, et al. Seizures after carotid endarterectomy: hyperperfusion, dysautoregulation or hypertensive encephalopathy? *Eur J Vascular Endovascular Surg.* 2003;26(1):39–44.

46. den Hartog AG, Halliday AW, Hayter E, et al. Risk of Stroke From New Carotid Artery Occlusion in the Asymptomatic Carotid Surgery Trial-1. *Stroke.* 2013;44:1652–1659.

# 9 *Aneurysm Surgery*

JUSTIN M. CAPLAN, NEERAJ NAVAL, JUDY HUANG, and RAFAEL J. TAMARGO

## Introduction

Microsurgical clipping of cerebral aneurysms was first introduced in 1937 by Walter E. Dandy at the Johns Hopkins Hospital.[1] In the ensuing three-quarters of a century, the underlying principle of obliterating an aneurysm from the intracranial circulation by applying a clip across the neck of the aneurysm has not changed. However, there has been a revolution in surgical approaches, perioperative management, and intraoperative management of patients undergoing surgery for aneurysms, which has dramatically improved the outcomes for these patients.[2] As the methods and technology have improved over the years, so have the complexity and knowledge base required to treat these patients.[3] A keen understanding of what happens in the operating room is critical to the postoperative care of these complex patients. This chapter aims to provide a comprehensive overview of aneurysm surgery to those who participate in the postoperative neurocritical care of these patients. The distinctions in surgical approach between ruptured and unruptured aneurysms are noted when relevant.

Aneurysmal subarachnoid hemorrhage (SAH) results in physiological derangements that affect essentially every system in the body, and the management of these patients is complex and is best handled in specialized units. However, this chapter is not intended to serve as a comprehensive guide of the neurological intensive care unit (Neuro ICU) management of SAH, but rather to review the management of issues related to the surgery itself. An overview of the Neuro ICU management of SAH is reviewed elsewhere.[3]

## Neuroanatomy and Procedure

### Key Concepts

- Proper padding of all pressure points is essential to minimize position-related injuries.
- Surgical approaches for aneurysm clipping are designed to maximize bony removal to minimize brain disturbance.
- Intraoperative neurophysiological monitoring is essential to reduce the risk of ischemia.

Aneurysm surgery takes place in the subarachnoid space. Aneurysms are approached through dissection of the arachnoid that allows adhered areas of brain to fall away from one another to open natural planes in which the cerebral vessels lie. For unruptured, uncomplicated aneurysms, the entire microsurgical portion of the case may be bloodless with no cortical pial violation. For larger or ruptured aneurysms, a more invasive dissection may be necessary. Bony removal may continue once the surgery progresses to the intradural space, to reveal otherwise hidden aneurysms. For example, an anterior or posterior clinoidectomy might be performed to facilitate access to the ophthalmic or basilar artery, respectively.

### MICROSURGERY

Aneurysms are approached using the principle tenets of all vascular surgery: first ensure proximal and distal control of the parent vessel and then expose the aneurysm. The goal of aneurysm surgery is to obliterate the aneurysm from the circulation by placing a microsurgical clip across the neck of the aneurysm while preserving all inflowing, outflowing, and perforating vessels to prevent a stroke. In the simplest of cases this will require a single aneurysm clip. However, in more complex cases an aneurysm may require the use of several clips and advanced clipping configurations.[4] In instances where this is not possible, vessel sacrifice with arterial bypasses may be necessary. When none of these options are available, wrapping of the aneurysm and reinforcement with fibrin glue may also be utilized. It is important for the providers to understand what occurred in each individual case because it may affect postoperative management, including elevated blood pressure goals in the case of concern for vessel stenosis from aneurysm clipping or the need for postoperative antiplatelet therapy in arterial bypasses.

### PATIENT POSITIONING AND SURGICAL APPROACHES

An understanding of patient positioning is required to recognize potential postoperative complications related to positioning, such as the development of a compartment or peripheral nerve entrapment syndromes. Patient positioning depends on the surgical approach. In general, there are two main approaches used for aneurysm surgery: 1) the frontosphenotemporal (pterional) craniotomy for anterior circulation aneurysms, basilar apex, and superior cerebellar artery aneurysms; and 2) the retrosigmoid craniotomy/craniectomy for posterior circulation aneurysms (i.e., PICA (posterior inferior cerebellar artery) and AICA (anterior inferior cerebellar artery) aneurysms). Each approach has modifications involving further bone removal to approach difficult aneurysms, including modified orbitozygomatic (MOZ) osteotomies for the pterional approach and C1 laminectomy and occipital condylectomy for the retrosigmoid ("far-lateral") approach.[5]

Pterional/MOZ craniotomies are performed with the patient supine and the ipsilateral shoulder elevated and

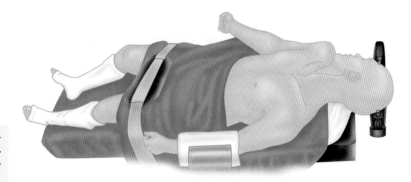

**Fig. 9.1** Patient positioning for pterional and orbitozygomatic craniotomies. (Reprinted from Jandial, R, et al., eds. *Core Techniques in Operative Neurosurgery.* Philadephia, Saunders, Elsevier; 2011: pp. 4–12.)

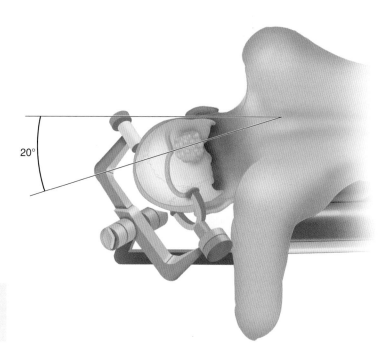

**Fig. 9.2** "Park bench" position for retrosigmoid and far-lateral craniotomies. (Reprinted from Jandial, R, et al., eds., *Core Techniques in Operative Neurosurgery.* Philadephia, Saunders, Elsevier; 2011: pp. 104–9.)

head turned (Fig. 9.1). Retrosigmoid/far-lateral craniotomies are performed in the "park bench" position with the patient lying on the side contralateral to the aneurysm (Fig. 9.2). Proper padding of all dependent areas is essential to prevent compressive and entrapment injuries. See Chapter 2 for a full description.

Each craniotomy is performed with rigid head fixation using metal pins affixed to the skull, such as the Mayfield Skull Clamp (Integra, Plainsboro, NJ). When the skull clamp is removed, small lacerations remain where the pins were located. These typically heal with conservative wound care and only require application of antibiotic ointment. Because scalp veins communicate with the diploic veins in the skull, which in turn communicate with the dural venous sinuses, rare instances of venous air emboli have been associated with removal of the Mayfield Skull Clamp.[6,7] Therefore in instances of circulatory collapse, especially those associated with a drop in the end-tidal $CO_2$, venous air emboli should be on the differential diagnosis. Use of a local anesthetic may mitigate hemodynamic changes associated with clamp placement.[8]

For patients with unruptured aneurysms, the pterional craniotomy is performed (i.e., the bone flap removed during surgery is replaced prior to wound closure). However, in surgery for SAH, sometimes the bone is not replaced (i.e., craniectomy) to allow for brain swelling. The bone is either cryopreserved (placed in a freezer) or surgically placed in an abdominal subcutaneous pocket. At a later date, once the brain swelling has resolved, the bone is replaced (i.e. cranioplasty). The method of storage is often determined by surgeon preference because data indicate there may be no difference in the risk of subsequent infections.[9] The retrosigmoid approach may be performed as a craniotomy or as a craniectomy. However, this approach is often performed as a craniectomy, even in unruptured cases, to better preserve the posterior fossa dura, which is more fragile compared with the supratentorial dura. In these instances, a cranioplasty using a metal mesh is often performed at the time of the initial surgery. It is important for the Neuro ICU practitioners to know whether cranial defects are present postoperatively to avoid unintended brain injury from patient positioning or ambulation (see later).

# Perioperative Considerations

## Key Concepts

- Communication with the anesthesia team throughout the case is critical.
- A thorough hand-off is necessary when transferring care from the operative team to the neurocritical care team.
- Any deviation in the expected improvement in the patient's neurological examination after emergence from anesthesia should prompt an immediate head computed tomography (CT).

## ANESTHESIA AND INTRAOPERATIVE MEDICATIONS

Operative management begins with the induction of general anesthesia. Typically, if not already present, a radial arterial line is placed for close hemodynamic monitoring. At our institution, we do not routinely obtain central venous access for unruptured aneurysms. When there is concern for intraoperative aneurysm rupture, large-bore venous access is obtained to allow for aggressive volume fluid resuscitation and rapid blood transfusion. Large-bore venous access should be secured when concern for air embolism is high (e.g., when operating near the venous sinuses).

Intraoperative administration of medications depends on aneurysm location and rupture status. For supratentorial craniotomies, we routinely administer a loading dose of an antiepileptic drug (AED): levetiracetam (Keppra) 500 to 1500 mg and/or fosphenytoin 15 to 20 mg/kg, regardless of rupture status. For posterior fossa craniotomies AEDs are not administered. To reduce brain volume, intravenous mannitol may be administered (0.25–1.0 g/kg), and end-tidal $CO_2$ is maintained at 25 to 30 mm Hg. Prophylactic antibiotics, such as cefazolin (2 g every 4 hours) or clindamycin (600 mg every 6 hours), may be given intravenously to prevent surgical site infections. Dexamethasone may also be administered to reduce vasogenic cerebral edema (Table 9.1).

After the induction of anesthesia, arterial and/or venous catheter placement, and review of operative medications with the anesthesia team, the patient is delivered to the surgical team. If intraoperative angiography is planned after aneurysm clip placement, then an arterial femoral sheath is placed prior to final patient positioning and draping.[10]

## INTRAOPERATIVE MONITORING AND TEMPORARY CLIPPING

Intraoperative neuromonitoring allows for feedback to the neurosurgeon about the electrophysiological consequences of surgical manipulation in real time. Changes in electroencephalography (EEG) and slowing or loss of somatosensory evoked potentials (SSEPs) and/or motor evoked potentials provide valuable information regarding possible postoperative deficits, as well as indicators that may direct postoperative management. In one report, for example, changes in SSEPs occurred in 4% of surgeries for unruptured aneurysms; reversible changes were associated with a 20%

**Table 9.1** Parameters/Medications to Review with Anesthesia Team in the Operating Room

| Medications | Dose/Route | Interval | Notes |
|---|---|---|---|
| Cefazolin | 2000 mg IV | q4h | Surgical site infection prophylaxis. To be given within 1 hour of skin incision |
| Clindamycin | 600 mg IV | q6h | Surgical site infection prophylaxis. To be given within 1 hour of skin incision. Used for patients allergic to cefazolin |
| Dexamethasone | 4–10 mg IV | q4h | For brain relaxation |
| Mannitol | 0.25–1.0 g/kg IV | Once | Given rapidly over 15 minutes at the beginning of the case for brain relaxation. Higher doses for SAH |
| Levetiracetam | 500–1500 mg IV | q12h | Seizure prophylaxis for supratentorial craniotomies |
| Fosphenytoin | 15–20 mg/kg IV | Once | Seizure prophylaxis for supratentorial craniotomies |
| Physiologic Parameters | | | Vary depending on case and patient |
| End-Tidal $CO_2$ | 25–30 | | To allow for brain relaxation |
| Blood Pressure Goals | Normotensive | | Maintain patient at least with normotension. Hypertension may be required if temporary clipping is being used. |

*SAH*, subarachnoid hemorrhage.

stroke rate, whereas irreversible changes were associated with an 80% stroke rate.[11]

Neuromonitoring is indispensable during temporary artery occlusion (also known as *temporary clipping*) during aneurysm surgery. During the temporary clipping maneuver, efferent and/or afferent vessels are briefly occluded to facilitate aneurysm dissection and clipping. Indications for temporary clipping include intraoperative aneurysm rupture, aneurysm manipulation that may result in release of emboli, high aneurysm turgor that precludes optimal clip placement, and the need to open the aneurysm for optimal clip placement.[12] Changes in neuromonitoring may prompt the neurosurgeon to remove the temporary clip sooner than would otherwise have been anticipated. The use of EEG to achieve burst suppression may also confer an advantage in protecting against ischemic infarcts.[13] Recent data suggest that temporary clipping is safe in surgery for both ruptured and unruptured aneurysms.[14,15]

## Clinical Pearl

Changes in intraoperative neurophysiological monitoring may help to predict postoperative deficits, particularly in patients undergoing surgery for unruptured aneurysms.

## INTRAOPERATIVE RUPTURE

Intraoperative rupture of an aneurysm during surgery represents one of the most challenging scenarios to the neurosurgeon. The incidence of intraoperative rupture is 7% to 19%; the wide variability is due to the initial rupture status of the aneurysm.[16–18] Patients who experience intraoperative rupture have an increased rate of periprocedural death or disability (31%) compared with those who do not (18%).[16] Greater surgical experience may lead to improved outcomes when intraoperative rupture does occur.[18] Interestingly, recent evidence suggests that intraoperative rupture does not increase the risk of vasospasm.[19]

Once an aneurysm ruptures, several neurosurgical techniques may be used to control bleeding, including application of direct pressure to the bleeding site with cotton, large-scale suction over the bleeding site, temporary clipping of the parent artery (see earlier), and adenosine-induced asystole for transient circulatory arrest.[20] In this latter technique, adenosine is given to induce asystole and hypotension for a brief period to enable the surgeon to clear the field of blood, visualize the bleeding site, and place a clip (either permanent or temporary). Khan and colleagues recently demonstrated the safety of this technique in relation to 30-day perioperative cardiac complications and mortality in patients with a low risk of coronary artery disease.[21] Adenosine-induced flow arrest may also be used to soften an aneurysm, especially for those along the skull base and for those with a broad neck.[22]

## INTRAOPERATIVE ASSESSMENT OF ANEURYSM OCCLUSION

Once the aneurysm has been occluded, various modalities may be employed to ensure that the aneurysm has been fully obliterated and that surrounding vessels and perforating arteries are patent. Intraoperative catheter angiography, used routinely at many institutions, is the gold standard.[10,23,24] Indocyanine green fluorescence videoangiography utilizes an intravenous fluorescent dye that can be visualized using the operative microscope.[25] However, this technique has a significant false-negative rate and thus caution must be exercised when used alone.[26,27]

## EMERGENCE FROM ANESTHESIA

At the conclusion of the case, after wound closure and dressing application, the patient is removed from the skull clamp and returned to the supine position (if the operating position was not supine) and then returned to the anesthesiology team for emergence from anesthesia. It is critical that the patient be allowed to wake up for a neurological examination prior to transfer to the Neuro ICU. The postoperative examination will vary depending on the patient's preoperative neurological status and intraoperative complications. Anesthetic choice may also affect emergence time.[28] A differential diagnosis should be determined for failure to emerge at the expected rate or with the expected examination. (For a more detailed discussion, please refer to Chapter 45.) When anesthetic/metabolic etiologies have been sufficiently excluded, emergent head CT should be obtained prior to intensive care unit (ICU) transfer to rule out acute pathologies that may require emergent reoperation (e.g., epidural or intracerebral hematoma).

## IMMEDIATE POSTOPERATIVE PERIOD

At the conclusion of the case, the patient should be directly transported to the Neuro ICU by the anesthesia and neurosurgical teams. A formal and thorough sign-out should be given by both the neurosurgical and anesthesia teams to the neurocritical care team to ensure all team members understand what occurred in the operating room and the resultant postoperative plan. This process should include the practitioner assuming care of the patient and the patient's bedside nurse, as well as a neurosurgeon and anesthesiologist directly involved in the operation. To ensure everyone's full attention, hand-off should not begin until all lines and monitors have been transferred and secured from the portable apparatus to the in-room apparatus. A comprehensive understanding of the nuances of the surgery should prompt the critical care practitioner to probe the neurosurgical and anesthesia teams to clarify any unanswered questions (Table 9.2).

## MANAGING SURGICAL DRAINS, DRESSINGS, AND WOUNDS

Postoperatively a patient may have one or more surgical drains. It is important to distinguish surgical drains, which are typically in the subgaleal space to drain postoperative blood and serous fluid that would otherwise accumulate, from ventriculostomy drains, which are inserted into the intraventricular space to drain cerebrospinal fluid (CSF). Surgical drains may be connected to a self-sustaining suction bulb to allow for a slow, continuous drainage of fluid. As the bulb fills, it will lose suction, indicating that the fluid should be emptied from the collection reservoir, measured and recorded, and suction reapplied. In the early postoperative period this may need to be done frequently, but further from surgery this frequency will decrease, although it should be performed at least every 8 hours. In the immediate postoperative period, the drainage is typically sanguineous with a near-blood appearance and evolves into a thin serous fluid over a couple of days. These drains are typically removed between the first and third postoperative day.

Surgical dressings typically consist of bacteriostatic gauze covered by a sterile dressing, which may be secured either with tape or by wrapping with a gauze roll. Head wraps are compressive and may be employed when the incision creates a scalp flap under which fluid can accumulate. Ideally dressings should remain until postoperative day two, but may be removed sooner if needed (e.g., to place scalp electrodes for an EEG if seizures are suspected). Head

**Table 9.2** Important Discussion Points for Hand-Off from Surgical Team to Neuro ICU Team

| Discussion Point | Notes |
|---|---|
| Patient Identification | |
| Aneurysm(s) Locations and Sizes | |
| Patient Positioning | Predict possible compartment or entrapment syndromes related to patient positioning |
| Surgical Approach | |
| Craniotomy vs. Craniectomy | |
| Status of Bone Flap | Does the patient need a helmet? |
| Use of Temporary Clipping | Predictor of ischemia |
| Changes in EEG/ SSEPs | Predictor of ischemia |
| Vessels Sacrificed | Predictor of ischemia (arterial or venous) |
| Status of Brain Edema | Define sodium goals |
| Drain Placement | Should drain be to suction or straight drainage? |
| Postop Medications Indicated | |
| Postop Imaging Indicated | |

*Neuro ICU,* neurological intensive care unit; *EEG,* electroencephalogram; *SSEP,* somatosensory evoked potential.

wraps may cause headache if applied too tightly. A wrap is considered tight if a finger cannot be inserted between the head wrap and scalp. Slits may be cut to relieve pressure and to treat headache.

Surgical wounds are typically closed with a combination of absorbable and/or nonabsorbable sutures for deep tissue layers. The skin is closed with either surgical staples or nonabsorbable sutures (such as nylon). Skin sutures or staples are left in place for 7 to 14 days postoperatively for initial operations, and longer for reoperations. The surgical dressing should be assessed frequently, particularly after craniotomy that involved the use of the cranial skull clamp. Occasionally a pin site can have significant bleeding postoperatively. This should be suspected if the dressing has more than minimal blood staining on it. In this instance, the head wrap should be removed and the surgical wound and pin sites assessed. Bleeding from a pin site will often stop with a couple minutes of manual compression; however, occasionally a suture or surgical staple may be necessary.

It is important that the ICU team is made aware of whether a craniotomy or a craniectomy was performed and whether a cranioplasty was performed to reconstruct any bony defects in the skull. In the event of craniectomy, a sign should be posted above the patient's bed to remind all caregivers and visitors that no bone flap is present on that side of the head. A helmet should be obtained and worn at

any point when the patient is out of bed until a cranioplasty has been performed. If the patient needs to be turned on to the side of the cranial defect, a "doughnut" pillow may be used to prevent pressure being placed on the site of the skull defect.

**Clinical Pearls**

- Surgical drains should be maintained to self-suction and emptied as needed.
- Surgical dressings may be removed earlier than expected if an EEG needs to be obtained.
- Patients with supratentorial craniectomies should wear a helmet when out of bed.

## Postoperative Complications

**Key Concepts**

- Seizures, hydrocephalus, and venous thromboembolism are infrequent but important complications associated with aneurysm surgery.
- Anatomy-specific complications such as frontal nerve palsy, frontal sinus violation, and optic neuropathy should be recognized and managed appropriately.
- Postoperative pain is frequently present and should be treated accordingly.

### DEATH

A recent study by Bekelis et al. examined a national sample of patients undergoing microsurgical clipping of aneurysms.[29] The study included 7651 patients, of which 48% had unruptured aneurysms and 52% had ruptured aneurysms (SAH). The mortality rate was 0.68% in patients with unruptured aneurysms and 11.5% in patients with SAH. For patients with unruptured aneurysms, preoperative age and stroke were risk factors for death in their multivariate analysis. For patients with SAH, coagulopathy, chronic obstructive pulmonary disease, stroke, and age were preoperative risk factors for death, whereas hypercholesterolemia and coronary artery disease decreased the risk of death in multivariate analysis.

### SEIZURES

The rate of in-hospital postoperative seizures after surgery for unruptured aneurysms is 2.7% in one recent large series of 3098 surgical clippings.[30] In this study, hemorrhagic complications were associated with higher seizure risk. In the International Subarachnoid Hemorrhage Trial (ISAT), in the period between treatment and discharge, the seizure rate was 3.1% (33 of 1070 patients in the neurosurgical arm).[31] Long-term follow-up from this trial demonstrates a 5.1% and 9.6% risk of a seizure at 1 and 5 years after discharge, respectively.[32] A recent review of the literature suggests a 2.3% incidence of early postoperative seizures and a 5.5% incidence of late postoperative seizures after SAH.[33]

Although practice varies, in the majority of patients with SAH (72.7%), AEDs are used for an average of 8.2 months.[33] A survey across 25 academic centers revealed a rate of 52%.[34] However, Raper, et al. reported no difference in early seizure occurrence between the cohort of patients who did and did not receive AEDs, nor between patients undergoing clipping compared with coiling.[33] In this study, the most commonly used AEDs were phenytoin and valproic acid. In patients with SAH, the indications for and duration of routine AED administration have not been clearly established. There is evidence that a short course of phenytoin (3 days) may be similar to a longer course (7 days).[35] Furthermore, there is evidence that the outcome in patients with SAH is worse in patients receiving AEDs, especially phenytoin.[36]

The American Heart Association SAH guidelines state that administration of prophylactic anticonvulsants may be considered in the immediate posthemorrhagic period, although routine long-term treatment is not recommended.[37] Patients with SAH who have associated intracerebral hemorrhage, age <40, middle cerebral artery aneurysms, poor clinical grade, and cocaine-positive toxicology have a high risk for seizures.[38] Neurosurgeons may consider additional AED administration in the operating room. Continuation and duration of AED for primary or secondary seizure prophylaxis are based on risk stratification.

For unruptured aneurysms, intraoperative seizure medications may be given and continued postoperatively, with discontinuation of the medications prior to hospital discharge.

## HYDROCEPHALUS, CEREBROSPINAL FLUID DIVERSION, AND FENESTRATION OF THE LAMINA TERMINALIS

Hydrocephalus after SAH was first described by Bagley in 1928 in an experimental model.[39] In SAH, hydrocephalus can be noncommunicating, communicating, or a combination of both. The rates of hydrocephalus in SAH vary across the literature but typically range from approximately 20% to 50%.[40-42] Patients undergoing elective microsurgical clipping of unruptured aneurysms typically do not experience hydrocephalus.

In the operating room, hydrocephalus is managed with CSF diversion, typically in one of three ways: 1) ventriculostomy placement, 2) lumbar drain placement, or 3) fenestration of the lamina terminalis. Several factors contribute to which approach is chosen, including the etiology of the hydrocephalus (noncommunicating vs. communicating), surgical approach (e.g., accessibility of the lamina terminalis), and surgeon preference. Ventriculostomies and lumbar drains may be placed preoperatively in the setting of acute hydrocephalus and a poor neurological status. Ventriculostomy placement is preferred to lumbar drainage because it is well tolerated, does not risk downward herniation, and allows for accurate measurement of intracranial pressure, which is particularly important in high-grade patients with a poor neurological examination. A ventriculostomy may be placed at the bedside or in the operating room.[43] Aggressive CSF drainage may be associated with a remote cerebellar hemorrhage (see later).[44]

Fenestration of the lamina terminalis is a surgical procedure to treat noncommunicating hydrocephalus. The lamina terminalis sits just superior to the optic chiasm and is easily accessed through the pterional approach. In our experience, fenestration of the lamina terminalis results in an 80% decrease in shunt dependence.[45] However, other studies have failed to demonstrate a benefit, and the current American Heart Association guidelines do not endorse its routine use.[46,47]

## POSTOPERATIVE IMAGING

After aneurysm surgery, routine postoperative imaging may not be necessary for all patients. To assess the adequacy of clip reconstruction, we perform intraoperative angiography.[10] With regard to cranial imaging, if the patient emerges from anesthesia at his or her preoperative neurological baseline, then routine brain imaging is deferred unless there is an examination change. If an intraoperative ventriculostomy was placed, a noncontrast head CT may be obtained to assess placement. Garrett, et al. demonstrated that routine postoperative head CTs or postventriculostomy CT scans revealed only a 4.7% and 6.5% probability of a positive finding, respectively.[48] The rates requiring an intervention based on these findings were even lower. However, there was a 30.3% rate of positive findings on head CTs obtained for a change in the patient's examination.

## VENOUS THROMBOEMBOLISM

The incidence of deep venous thrombosis (DVT) after SAH ranges widely in the literature, from 0% in unscreened populations to 24% in asymptomatic patients who undergo routine screening.[49-54] Risk factors for DVT include tobacco use, race, and length of stay.[49,53] After aneurysm surgery and/or SAH, the practitioner must decide when and whether to initiate chemical DVT prophylaxis in addition to mechanical prophylaxis. If the patient develops venous thromboembolism (VTE), then a decision must be made on treatment of the VTE that balances the risks of anticoagulation against the risks of VTE itself.

Several studies have suggested the safety of multiple DVT prophylaxis strategies. A metaanalysis of 30 studies, including 7770 neurosurgical patients, suggested that low-molecular-weight heparin (LMWH) vs. compression stockings and intermittent compression devices (ICDs) vs. placebo significantly reduced the rates of DVTs, without a difference in the incidence of intracranial hemorrhage (ICH) between LMWH and nonpharmacological methods of DVT prophylaxis.[55] There was no difference in VTE or ICH risk between LMWH vs. unfractionated heparin (UFH). However, this study included a mixed neurosurgical population and thus limits the generalizability to aneurysm patients specifically.

Data regarding DVT prophylaxis in aneurysm surgery specifically are limited. Recent guidelines for DVT prophylaxis in SAH suggest that ICDs should be used in all patients and that UFH should be considered for high-risk patients, with an understanding of the risk for increased hemorrhagic complications.[54] With regard to hemorrhagic complications following ventriculostomy placement in patients with early chemical prophylaxis, a recent study by Tanweer, et al. suggests there is no difference compared with patients receiving delayed prophylaxis.[56] However, the authors also did not find a difference in rates of VTE either.

Compression stockings should be worn by all patients at the time of admission (for SAH) or intraoperatively. We begin chemical prophylaxis 24 hours postoperative with 5000 units of UFH subcutaneous injection every 8 to 12 hours and continue this until the patient is discharged from the hospital. UFH may be preferred over LMWH given decreased bleeding risk and ease of reversibility. If a patient develops a VTE requiring therapeutic anticoagulation, there is evidence from a small retrospective study documenting its safety.[57] For patients who require therapeutic anticoagulation, we first obtain a baseline head CT to document any blood products. We then start intravenous UFH (no sooner than 24 hours postop) without a bolus to target a goal activated partial thromboplastin time (aPTT) of 50 to 65 seconds (or an aPTT ratio of 1.5–2.0). A follow-up head CT is obtained after the patient has reached the therapeutic range.

## REMOTE CEREBELLAR HEMORRHAGE

Remote cerebellar hemorrhage (RCH) is a rare complication associated with <5% of supratentorial craniotomies.[44] The pathophysiological mechanisms that cause RCH are incompletely understood, with CSF volume loss felt to be related.[44] Overall, patients recover well from an RCH (>50% with mild neurological symptoms or complete recovery) with death occurring in 10% to 15% of cases.[44] Treatment for RCH is largely supportive, although suboccipital decompression may be required.

## FRONTAL BRANCH OF FACIAL NERVE INJURY

Frontal branch nerve palsies of the facial nerve occur after pterional craniotomy for aneurysm surgery.[58] This injury is likely related to incisional, thermal, or stretch injury to the nerve associated with raising the scalp flap in which the frontal branch is at risk. Several dissection techniques are now routinely performed to protect the nerve, including an interfascial, subfascial, or submuscular dissection.[59,60] Despite these techniques, it is possible the patient may develop a frontal branch palsy, which manifests as unilateral upper face weakness (i.e., inability to raise the unilateral eyebrow). Unlike in a cortical etiology of facial weakness, this deficit will spare the lower face, whereas a cortical injury would be expected to have the opposite pattern (i.e., involve the lower face and spare the upper face). This is an important distinction for the practitioner to make to spare the patient an unnecessary ischemic workup for facial weakness after a pterional craniotomy, or to incorrectly assume that lower facial weakness is a complication of the surgical approach.

### Clinical Pearl

Unilateral facial weakness from a frontalis palsy may be distinguished from cortical injury by involvement of the upper face and sparing of the lower face.

## FRONTAL SINUS VIOLATION

During pterional/modified orbito-zygomatic and other anterior skull base approaches, the frontal sinus is at risk for violation, permitting communication with the intracranial space. The radiographic incidence of frontal sinus violation is estimated at 9.1%.[61] Repair of the sinus typically involves a combination of mucosal exenteration, cranialization of the sinus, occlusion of the space with a bone substitute, and overlay with a vascularized pericranial graft. Early complications from frontal sinus violation, such as tension pneumocephalus, are rare.[62] Delayed complications include CSF leak, formation of a mucocele, and infections.

## POSTOPERATIVE PAIN

Postoperative pain after intracranial surgery represents a significant challenge to the practitioner because most patients will experience moderate to severe pain.[63] In surgery for aneurysms, postoperative pain can be the result of the surgical intervention, but in patients with SAH, some pain may also be directly related to their hemorrhage. Pain management in these patients, as with all craniotomy patients, requires a balance of adequate analgesia with the dose-limiting side effects of the analgesic medications. For example, opiate narcotics typically play a role in postcraniotomy analgesia, but can be limited by nausea, vomiting, and respiratory and mental status depression. There is a growing literature regarding postoperative pain management after craniotomy, but recommendations are not universal. One recent randomized blinded study demonstrated the benefit of tramadol in combination with narcotic pain medication versus narcotics and acetaminophen.[64] However, another study comparing morphine, tramadol, and codeine after craniotomy revealed that morphine was superior to tramadol in producing analgesia and was associated with less vomiting and retching.[65] A more recent approach to postoperative pain management after craniotomies is the use of intravenous patient-controlled analgesia (PCA). The use of PCA after supratentorial intracranial surgery has been demonstrated in a randomized controlled trial (RCT) to be safe and more efficacious at treating pain compared with the use of fentanyl administered on an as-needed basis.[66] In addition, PCA use has been shown in an RCT to be effective compared with as-needed therapy for surgery in the posterior fossa, although larger trials are needed to establish the safety of this approach.[67]

For postoperative analgesia, a reasonable strategy might be administration of intravenous short-acting narcotics in the immediate postoperative period and then transitioning on postoperative day 1 to oral analgesic medications. In our experience, patients undergoing elective aneurysm surgery typically do not require narcotic analgesia for more than 1 to 2 weeks. Patients with SAH may have greater persistence of their pain, which is likely due to the SAH rather than to the craniotomy.

## INFECTIONS

The overall rate of infections after neurosurgical procedures is low. In one large study of 844 patients, the rate was 4.1%, of which 75.5% were due to *Staphylococcus aureus.*[68]

There are many risk factors associated with infections, including previous history of skin infections.[68-70] RCTs have demonstrated the benefit of perioperative antibiotics in reducing neurosurgical infections.[71,72] Preoperative antibiotics, such as cefazolin or clindamycin, may be considered. Postoperatively, antibiotics may be continued for 24 hours. There is a higher rate of postoperative bacteremia for those treated with intraoperative hypothermia compared with those maintained at normothermia.[73]

## OPTIC NEUROPATHY

Ophthalmic-region aneurysms present a unique challenge to the neurosurgeon. The optic nerve often lies over the dome of ophthalmic artery aneurysms. To uncover the aneurysm and to facilitate microsurgical clipping, the falciform ligament, a dural fold over the optic canal, must first be divided. The anterior clinoid process is then removed using either a high-speed drill or ultrasonic bone cutter. The optic nerve can then be more safely mobilized to permit visualization of the aneurysm neck and its relationship to the ophthalmic artery to permit clipping. Despite these adjunctive measures, there is a 27% rate of new visual loss after treatment of these aneurysms.[74] Given the propensity for microvascular ischemia of the optic nerve, some surgeons target a goal hemoglobin level of >11 g/dL. Postoperative administration of high-dose steroids may reduce nerve edema associated with the mass effect on the optic nerve from the aneurysm clip.

## Conclusions

The management of patients after aneurysm surgery is frequently challenging. However, a thorough understanding of the anatomy and surgical approaches to treating these lesions allows the neurocritical care team to anticipate, avoid, and appropriately manage complications associated with these surgeries (Table 9.3). As in all areas of medicine, frequent communication between the neurosurgical and neurocritical care teams is absolutely essential for optimal patient care.

**Table 9.3** Complications of Aneurysm Surgery

| Complication | Possible Avoidance Techniques |
| --- | --- |
| Pressure injuries/compartment syndromes from patient positioning | Ensure proper padding during positioning |
| Air embolism from pin removal | Risk is highest in sitting or semi-sitting position. Adequate volume status may limit risk. |
| Hemodynamic changes associated with skull clamp application | Use of local anesthetic/proper general anesthesia |
| Brain injury in patients with no bone flap | Sign over patients bed informing caregivers/visitors status of bone flap; use of protective helmet when out of bed |
| Seizures | AEDs |
| Hydrocephalus | Fenestration of lamina terminalis |
| Intracranial hemorrhage | Meticulous surgical hemostasis |
| DVT/PE | Mechanical and chemical prophylaxis |
| Frontal nerve injury | Interfascial, subfascial, or submuscular dissection techniques |
| Frontal sinus violation | Craniotomy planning based on preoperative imaging Appropriate repair if violated |
| Optic neuropathy | Postoperative steroids and avoid anemia |
| Postoperative pain | Multimodal analgesic therapy, PCA |
| Infection | Preincision antibiotics and postoperative antibiotics |
| Intraoperative aneurysm rupture | Temporary clipping |
| Intraoperative ischemia | Neuromonitoring |
| Postoperative ischemia | Appropriate hemodynamic parameters |
| Air embolus | Avoidance of dural sinus violation |
| Remote cerebellar hemorrhage | Minimize CSF drainage |

*AED*, antiepileptic drug; *DVT*, deep vein thrombosis; *PE*, pulmonary embolism; *PCA*, patient-controlled analgesia; *CSF*, cerebrospinal fluid.

### References

1. Dandy WE. Intracranial aneurysm of the internal carotid artery: cured by operation. *Ann Surg.* 1938;107(5):654–659.
2. Naval NS, Chang T, Caserta F, Kowalski RG, Carhuapoma JR, Tamargo RJ. Improved aneurysmal subarachnoid hemorrhage outcomes: a comparison of 2 decades at an academic center. *J Crit Care.* 2012;28(2):182–188.
3. Caplan JM, Colby GP, Coon AL, Huang J, Tamargo RJ. Managing subarachnoid hemorrhage in the neurocritical care unit. *Neurosurg Clin N Am.* 2013;24(3):321–337.
4. Clatterbuck RE, Galler RM, Tamargo RJ, Chalif DJ. Orthogonal interlocking tandem clipping technique for the reconstruction of complex middle cerebral artery aneurysms. *Neurosurgery.* 2006;59(4 Suppl 2):ONS347–ONS351. discussion ONS351–2.
5. Colby GP, Coon AL, Tamargo RJ. Surgical management of aneurysmal subarachnoid hemorrhage. *Neurosurg Clin N Am.* 2010;21(2):247–261.
6. El-Zenati H, Faraj J, Al-Rumaihi G. Air embolism related to removal of Mayfield head pins. *Asian J Neurosurg.* 2012;7(4):227.
7. Prabhakar H, Ali Z, Bhagat H. Venous air embolism arising after removal of Mayfield skull clamp. *J Neurosurg Anesthesiol.* 2008;20(2):158–159.
8. Arshad A, Shamim MS, Waqas M, Enam H, Enam SA. How effective is the local anesthetic infiltration of pin sites prior to application of head clamps: a prospective observational cohort study of hemodynamic response in patients undergoing elective craniotomy. *Surg Neurol Int.* 2013;4:93.
9. Inamasu J, Kuramae T, Nakatsukasa M. Does difference in the storage method of bone flaps after decompressive craniectomy affect the incidence of surgical site infection after cranioplasty? Comparison between subcutaneous pocket and cryopreservation. *J Trauma.* 2010;68(1):183–187.
10. Chiang VL, Gailloud P, Murphy KJ, Rigamonti D, Tamargo RJ. Routine intraoperative angiography during aneurysm surgery. *J Neurosurg.* 2002;96(6):988–992.
11. Wicks RT, Pradilla G, Raza SM, et al. Impact of changes in intraoperative somatosensory evoked potentials on stroke rates after clipping of intracranial aneurysms. *Neurosurgery.* 2012;70(5):1114–1124.
12. Eftekhar B, Morgan MK. Indications for the use of temporary arterial occlusion during aneurysm repair: an institutional experience. *J Clin Neurosci.* 2011;18(7):905–909.

13. Lavine SD, Masri LS, Levy ML, Giannotta SL. Temporary occlusion of the middle cerebral artery in intracranial aneurysm surgery: time limitation and advantage of brain protection. *J Neurosurg.* 1997;87 (6):817–824.

14. Griessenauer CJ, Poston TL, Shoja MM, et al. The impact of temporary artery occlusion during intracranial aneurysm surgery on long-term clinical outcome: part I. Patients with subarachnoid hemorrhage. *World Neurosurg.* 2014;82(1-2):140–148.

15. Griessenauer CJ, Poston TL, Shoja MM, et al. The impact of temporary artery occlusion during intracranial aneurysm surgery on long-term clinical outcome: part II. The patient who undergoes elective clipping. *World Neurosurg.* 2014;82(3-4):402–408.

16. Elijovich L, Higashida RT, Lawton MT, et al. Predictors and outcomes of intraprocedural rupture in patients treated for ruptured intracranial aneurysms: the CARAT study. *Stroke.* 2008;39(5):1501–1506.

17. Madhugiri VS, Ambekar S, Pandey P, et al. The pterional and suprabrow approaches for aneurysm surgery: a systematic review of intraoperative rupture rates in 9488 aneurysms. *World Neurosurg.* 2013;80 (6):836–844.

18. Lawton MT, Du R. Effect of the neurosurgeon's surgical experience on outcomes from intraoperative aneurysmal rupture. *Neurosurgery.* 2005;57(1):9–15 discussion. 9–15.

19. Sheth SA, Hausrath D, Numis AL, Lawton MT, Josephson SA. Intraoperative rerupture during surgical treatment of aneurysmal subarachnoid hemorrhage is not associated with an increased risk of vasospasm. *J Neurosurg.* 2014;120(2):409–414.

20. Groff MW, Adams DC, Kahn RA, Kumbar UM, Yang BY, Bederson JB. Adenosine-induced transient asystole for management of a basilar artery aneurysm. Case report. *J Neurosurg.* 1999;91(4):687–690.

21. Khan SA, McDonagh DL, Adogwa O, et al. Perioperative cardiac complications and 30-day mortality in patients undergoing intracranial aneurysmal surgery with adenosine-induced flow arrest: a retrospective comparative study. *Neurosurgery.* 2014;74(3):267–271. discussion, 271–2.

22. Bendok BR, Gupta DK, Rahme RJ, et al. Adenosine for temporary flow arrest during intracranial aneurysm surgery: a single-center retrospective review. *Neurosurgery.* 2011;69(4):815–820. discussion, 820–1.

23. Tang G, Cawley CM, Dion JE, Barrow DL. Intraoperative angiography during aneurysm surgery: a prospective evaluation of efficacy. *J Neurosurg.* 2002;96(6):993–999.

24. Klopfenstein JD, Spetzler RF, Kim LJ, et al. Comparison of routine and selective use of intraoperative angiography during aneurysm surgery: a prospective assessment. *J Neurosurg.* 2004;100(2):230–235.

25. Raabe A, Beck J, Seifert V. Technique and image quality of intraoperative indocyanine green angiography during aneurysm surgery using surgical microscope integrated near-infrared video technology. *Zentralbl Neurochir.* 2005;66(1):1–6. discussion, 7–8.

26. Washington CW, Zipfel GJ, Chicoine MR, et al. Comparing indocyanine green videoangiography to the gold standard of intraoperative digital subtraction angiography used in aneurysm surgery. *J Neurosurg.* 2013;118(2):420–427.

27. Caplan JM, Sankey E, Yang W, et al. Impact of indocyanine green videoangiography on rate of clip adjustments following intraoperative angiography. *Neurosurgery.* 2014;75(4):437–444.

28. Bhagat H, Dash HH, Bithal PK, Chouhan RS, Pandia MP. Planning for early emergence in neurosurgical patients: a randomized prospective trial of low-dose anesthetics. *Anesth Analg.* 2008;107 (4):1348–1355.

29. Bekelis K, Missios S, MacKenzie TA, et al. Predicting inpatient complications from cerebral aneurysm clipping: the Nationwide Inpatient Sample 2005–2009. *J Neurosurg.* 2014;120(3):591–598.

30. Lai LT, O'Donnell J, Morgan MK. The risk of seizures during the in-hospital admission for surgical or endovascular treatment of unruptured intracranial aneurysms. *J Clin Neurosci.* 2013;20(11): 1498–1502.

31. Molyneux AJ, Kerr RSC, Yu L-M, et al. International subarachnoid aneurysm trial (ISAT) of neurosurgical clipping versus endovascular coiling in 2143 patients with ruptured intracranial aneurysms: a randomised comparison of effects on survival, dependency, seizures, rebleeding, subgroups, and aneurysm occlusion. *Lancet.* 2005;366 (9488):809–817.

32. Hart Y, Sneade M, Birks J, Rischmiller J, Kerr R, Molyneux A. Epilepsy after subarachnoid hemorrhage: the frequency of seizures after clip occlusion or coil embolization of a ruptured cerebral aneurysm:

33. Raper DMS, Starke RM, Komotar RJ, Allan R, Connolly ES. Seizures after aneurysmal subarachnoid hemorrhage: a systematic review of outcomes. *World Neurosurg.* 2013;79(5-6):682–690.

34. Dewan MC, Mocco J. Current practice regarding seizure prophylaxis in aneurysmal subarachnoid hemorrhage across academic centers. *J Neurointerv Surg.* 2015;7(2):146–149.

35. Chumnanvej S, Dunn IF, Kim DH. Three-day phenytoin prophylaxis is adequate after subarachnoid hemorrhage. *Neurosurgery.* 2007;60(1):99–102. discussion, 102–3.

36. Rosengart AJ, Huo JD, Tolentino J, et al. Outcome in patients with subarachnoid hemorrhage treated with antiepileptic drugs. *J Neurosurg.* 2007;107(2):253–260.

37. Bederson JB, Connolly ES, Batjer HH, et al. Guidelines for the management of aneurysmal subarachnoid hemorrhage: a statement for healthcare professionals from a special writing group of the Stroke Council, American Heart Association. *Stroke.* 2009;40(3):994–1025.

38. Chang TR, Kowalski RG, Carhuapoma JR, Tamargo RJ, Naval NS. Cocaine use is an independent predictor of seizures after aneurysmal subarachnoid hemorrhage. *J Neurosurg.* 2016;124(3):730–735.

39. Bagley C. Blood in the cerebrospinal fluid: resultant functional and organic alterations in the central nervous system. A. Experimental data. *Arch Surg.* 1928;17(1):18–26.

40. van Gijn J, Hijdra A, Wijdicks EF, Vermeulen M, van Crevel H. Acute hydrocephalus after aneurysmal subarachnoid hemorrhage. *J Neurosurg.* 1985;63(3):355–362.

41. de Oliveira JG, Beck J, Setzer M, et al. Risk of shunt-dependent hydrocephalus after occlusion of ruptured intracranial aneurysms by surgical clipping or endovascular coiling: a single-institution series and meta-analysis. *Neurosurgery.* 2007;61(5):924–933. discussion, 933–4.

42. Dehdashti AR, Rilliet B, Rufenacht DA, de Tribolet N. Shunt-dependent hydrocephalus after rupture of intracranial aneurysms: a prospective study of the influence of treatment modality. *J Neurosurg.* 2004;101(3):402–407.

43. Paine JT, Batjer HH, Samson D. Intraoperative ventricular puncture. *Neurosurgery.* 1988;22(6 Pt 1):1107–1109.

44. Brockmann MA, Groden C. Remote cerebellar hemorrhage: a review. *Cerebellum.* 2006;5(1):64–68.

45. Komotar RJ, Olivi A, Rigamonti D, Tamargo RJ. Microsurgical fenestration of the lamina terminalis reduces the incidence of shunt-dependent hydrocephalus after aneurysmal subarachnoid hemorrhage. *Neurosurgery.* 2002;51(6):1403–1412. discussion, 1412–3.

46. Komotar RJ, Hahn DK, Kim GH, et al. Efficacy of lamina terminalis fenestration in reducing shunt-dependent hydrocephalus following aneurysmal subarachnoid hemorrhage: a systematic review. Clinical article. *J Neurosurg.* 2009;111(1):147–154.

47. Connolly ES, Rabinstein AA, Carhuapoma JR, et al. Guidelines for the management of aneurysmal subarachnoid hemorrhage: a guideline for healthcare professionals from the American Heart Association/American Stroke Association. *Stroke.* 2012;43(6):1711–1737.

48. Garrett MC, Bilgin-Freiert A, Bartels C, Everson R, Afsarmanesh N, Pouratian N. An evidence-based approach to the efficient use of computed tomography imaging in the neurosurgical patient. *Neurosurgery.* 2013;73(2):209–215. discussion, 215–6.

49. Ray WZ, Strom RG, Blackburn SL, Ashley WW, Sicard GA, Rich KM. Incidence of deep venous thrombosis after subarachnoid hemorrhage. *J Neurosurg.* 2009;110(5):1010–1014.

50. Mack WJ, Ducruet AF, Hickman ZL, et al. Doppler ultrasonography screening of poor-grade subarachnoid hemorrhage patients increases the diagnosis of deep venous thrombosis. *Neurol Res.* 2008;30(9): 889–892.

51. Kshettry VR, Rosenbaum BP, Seicean A, Kelly ML, Schiltz NK, Weil RJ. Incidence and risk factors associated with in-hospital venous thromboembolism after aneurysmal subarachnoid hemorrhage. *J Clin Neurosci.* 2014;21(2):282–286.

52. Tapaninaho A. Deep vein thrombosis after aneurysm surgery. *Acta Neurochir.* 1985;74(1-2):18–20.

53. Serrone JC, Wash EM, Hartings JA, Andaluz N, Zuccarello M. Venous thromboembolism in subarachnoid hemorrhage. *World Neurosurg.* 2013;80(6):859–863.

54. Vespa P. Participants in the International Multi-Disciplinary Consensus Conference on the Critical Care Management of Subarachnoid

Hemorrhage. Deep venous thrombosis prophylaxis. *Neurocrit Care.* 2011;15(2):295–297.

55. Collen JF, Jackson JL, Shorr AF, Moores LK. Prevention of venous thromboembolism in neurosurgery: a metaanalysis. *Chest.* 2008;134(2):237–249.

56. Tanweer O, Boah A, Huang PP. Risks for hemorrhagic complications after placement of external ventricular drains with early chemical prophylaxis against venous thromboembolisms. *J Neurosurg.* 2013;119(5):1309–1313.

57. Scheller C, Rachinger J, Strauss C, Alfieri A, Prell J, Koman G. Therapeutic anticoagulation after craniotomies: is the risk for secondary hemorrhage overestimated? *J Neurosurg.* 2014;75(01):2–6.

58. Aoki N. Incision of facial nerve branch at aneurysm surgery. *J Neurosurg.* 1987;66(3):482.

59. Yasargil MG, Reichman MV, Kubik S. Preservation of the frontotemporal branch of the facial nerve using the interfascial temporalis flap for pterional craniotomy. Technical article. *J Neurosurg.* 1987;67(3):463–466.

60. Coscarella E, Vishteh AG, Spetzler RF, Seoane E, Zabramski JM. Subfascial and submuscular methods of temporal muscle dissection and their relationship to the frontal branch of the facial nerve. Technical note. *J Neurosurg.* 2000;92(5):877–880.

61. Patel RS, Yousem DM, Maldjian JA, Zager EL. Incidence and clinical significance of frontal sinus or orbital entry during pterional (frontotemporal) craniotomy. *Am J Neurradiol.* 2000;21(7):1327–1330.

62. Alibai EA, Rahmanian AK, Razmkon A, Nabavizadeh SA. Tension pneumocephalus following pterional craniotomy for treatment of intracavernous internal carotid artery aneurysm. *Emerg Radiol.* 2008;15(6):441–444.

63. Gottschalk A, Berkow LC, Stevens RD, et al. Prospective evaluation of pain and analgesic use following major elective intracranial surgery. *J Neurosurg.* 2007;106(2):210–216.

64. Rahimi SY, Alleyne Jr CH, Vernier E, Witcher MR, Vender JR. Postoperative pain management with tramadol after craniotomy: evaluation and cost analysis. *J Neurosurg.* 2010;112(2):268–272.

65. Sudheer PS, Logan SW, Terblanche C, Ateleanu B, Hall JE. Comparison of the analgesic efficacy and respiratory effects of morphine, tramadol and codeine after craniotomy. *Anaesthesia.* 2007;62(6):555–560.

66. Morad AH, Winters BD, Yaster M, et al. Efficacy of intravenous patient-controlled analgesia after supratentorial intracranial surgery: a prospective randomized controlled trial. Clinical article. *J Neurosurg.* 2009;111(2):343–350.

67. Morad A, Winters B, Stevens R, et al. The efficacy of intravenous patient-controlled analgesia after intracranial surgery of the posterior fossa: a prospective, randomized controlled trial. *Anesth Analg.* 2012;114(2):416–423.

68. Lietard C, Thébaud V, Besson G, Lejeune B. Risk factors for neurosurgical site infections: an 18-month prospective survey. *J Neurosurg.* 2008;109(4):729–734.

69. Faraday N, Rock P, Lin EE, et al. Past history of skin infection and risk of surgical site infection after elective surgery. *Ann Surg.* 2013;257(1):150–154.

70. Chiang H-Y, Kamath AS, Pottinger JM, et al. Risk factors and outcomes associated with surgical site infections after craniotomy or craniectomy. *J Neurosurg.* 2014;120(2):509–521.

71. Young RF, Lawner PM. Perioperative antibiotic prophylaxis for prevention of postoperative neurosurgical infections. A randomized clinical trial. *J Neurosurg.* 1987;66(5):701–705.

72. Blomstedt GC, Kyttä J. Results of a randomized trial of vancomycin prophylaxis in craniotomy. *J Neurosurg.* 1988;69(2):216–220.

73. Todd MM, Hindman BJ, Clarke WR, Torner JC. Intraoperative Hypothermia for Aneurysm Surgery Trial (IHAST) Investigators. Mild intraoperative hypothermia during surgery for intracranial aneurysm. *N Engl J Med.* 2005;352(2):135–145.

74. Kanagalingam S, Gailloud P, Tamargo RJ, Subramanian PS, Miller NR. Visual sequelae after consensus-based treatment of ophthalmic artery segment aneurysms: the Johns Hopkins experience. *J Neuroophthalmol.* 2012;32(1):27–32.

# 10 *Intracranial Arteriovenous Malformations and Dural Arteriovenous Fistulas*

MARIO ZANATY, NOHRA CHALOUHI, STAVROPOULA TJOUMAKARIS, ROBERT H. ROSENWASSER, and PASCAL JABBOUR

## Introduction

Brain arteriovenous malformations (AVMs) are abnormal connections between arteries and veins, leading to arteriovenous shunting with an intervening network of vessels, or nidus (Fig. 10.1). The prevalence varies between 15 and 18 per 100,000 adults, although estimates of the prevalence are increasing due to improved imaging techniques.[1] Roughly half of patients with brain AVMs present with intracranial hemorrhage (ICH), resulting in a first-ever hemorrhage rate of 0.55 per 100,000 person-years.[2] Recent evidence suggests that medical management is superior to the combination of medical management and interventional therapy with regard to mortality or stroke in patients with unruptured AVMs.[3] However, knowledge of surgical treatment options, relevant neuroanatomy, and operative complications remains essential, especially for those patients who present with an AVM-related hemorrhage. The Spetzler Martin grading system is used to classify AVMs and stratify operative risk.[4]

Dural AVMs or arteriovenous fistulas (AVFs) are abnormal connections between an artery and a meningeal vein or dural sinus. These lesions are thought to be acquired, including from sinus thrombosis, trauma, and surgery. Although some of these lesions require surgery, many can be treated effectively with endovascular therapy. Dural AVFs can present with a variety of symptoms, including pain, tinnitus, bruits, and more serious symptoms related to hemorrhage or focal neurological deficit. The most important characteristic determining symptoms and treatment is the pattern of venous drainage[5,6] (Fig. 10.2).

## Neuroanatomy and Procedure

### Key Concepts

- AVMs are abnormal vascular shunts that present with hemorrhage, headaches, seizures, and focal deficits.
- The goal of treatment is complete eradication of the lesion because partial treatment may increase the chance of bleeding.
- AVMs may be treated with stereotactic radiosurgery or surgical resection. This is often preceded by endovascular treatment to reduce the size of the lesion. Occasionally all three modalities are utilized for the same lesion.

- Microsurgery allows for high rates of complete obliteration and durable results, but it may be limited by the patient's anatomy and the AVM location.
- Embolization is insufficient for curative treatment; it supplements radiosurgery or surgical resection.
- The aim of radiotherapy is to ablate the AVM to prevent future hemorrhage. This is a time-dependent effect.
- The vast majority of dural AVFs are treated endovascularly.

AVMs are high-flow connections between the arteries and the veins that bypass the capillary network. Although they are considered congenital, parenchymal AVMs may undergo significant angioarchitectural changes, such as the development of associated aneurysms. They can occur anywhere in the brain. AVMs have three components: (1) arterial feeders, (2) a central nidus, and (3) draining veins (Fig. 10.3). The central nidus is the network of dysplastic thin-walled vessels; the impedance of the nidus determines the degree of shunting. Nidal vessels are usually the source of hemorrhage, but aneurysms associated with the AVM can also hemorrhage. Cerebral AVMs are most often pyramidal in shape, with the apex pointing toward the ventricle and the base parallel to the cortical surface. Some classify AVMs as pial, parenchymal, paraventricular, or combined. Approximately 7% of patients with AVMs have an associated aneurysm, and 75% of these are located on a major feeding artery presumably because of increased flow. Aneurysms can also arise in the nidus or on draining veins.[7]

Brain AVMs commonly present with ICH that may be intraparenchymal, intraventricular, subarachnoid, or subdural in location. Patients may present with headaches, seizures, focal deficits, or altered mental status.[2] The diagnosis is usually made by computed tomography (CT) scan or magnetic resonance imaging (MRI). The MRI sequences most useful in the diagnosis include T1- and T2-weighted images and the gradient-echo sequence. Angiography is necessary for treatment planning. Combining images of digital subtraction angiography (DSA) and MRI for evaluation of AVMs shows greater visualization of the feeding artery and draining vein course in AVMs, as well as spatial relationships of these structures to surrounding parenchyma; this could not be determined as effectively with either technique in isolation. Addition of MRI to DSA in preoperative evaluation enhances the surgeon's ability to predict functional risks associated with unexpected vessel injuries[8–12] (Fig. 10.4).

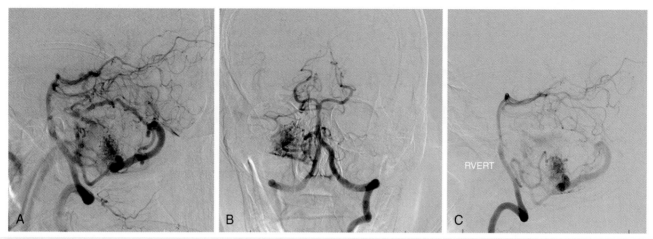

**Fig. 10.1 (A–C)** 12 × 21 mm right cerebellar arteriovenous malformation in a 63-year-old male, fed by distal posterior inferior cerebellar artery and superior cerebral artery branches.

The goal of the treatment is to cure the malformation and to eradicate the potential risk of hemorrhage.

The treatment modalities for brain AVMs include microvascular surgery, endovascular embolization, stereotactic radiosurgery, or a combination of the three. The Spetzler-Martin grading system, which estimates the risk of AVM surgery, is used to guide treatment decisions (Table 10.1). It assigns scores based on size, pattern of venous drainage, and association with eloquent cortex. Higher scores are associated with greater morbidity and mortality.[13] This chapter focuses on microvascular surgery because the other modalities mentioned are discussed in detail in other chapters (see Chapter 36 for a detailed description of endovascular treatment of AVMs and Chapter 25 for stereotactic radiosurgery). Treatment should be tailored to the individual patient based on patient anatomy; treatment risks; history of previous hemorrhage; and AVM morphology, including size, flow state, associated aneurysms, location, and natural history. A metaanalysis of 137 observational studies with 13,698 patients undergoing AVM treatment reported a decrease in case fatality and complication rate over time due to technical advances and experience. The treatment arms evaluated in the metaanalysis were microvascular neurosurgery, endovascular embolization, stereotactic radiosurgery, and fractionated radiotherapy. The authors concluded that AVM treatment remains associated with considerable adverse events and subtotal efficacy, justifying the need for randomized controlled trials comparing the different modalities.

There are advantages and disadvantages to the different treatments. Radiotherapy is usually reserved for small lesions (<3 cm nidus) and especially deep, surgically inaccessible lesions. Although it offers the advantage of being noninvasive, a latency period of 1 to 2 years[14] is needed before complete obliteration of the lesion. Endovascular therapy is minimally invasive but has a lower obliteration rate and decreased durability compared with surgery.[1] Small lesions can be completely obliterated, whereas large lesions may be reduced in size in preparation for surgery.[15] Endovascular therapy may be used as a palliative treatment to control refractory

seizure in patients when microsurgery or radiosurgery is not indicated.[16] The major drawback of endovascular treatment before surgical excision of the AVM is the risk of stroke from retrograde and anterograde embolization, as well as embolization from arterial feeders that still contribute to vital cerebral tissue. The use of a temporary balloon, which could be deflated if signs of clinical deterioration are observed, might mitigate this problem.[17]

AVMs that are near the basal ganglia or ventricles with deep drainage require significant dissection. Thus the authors prefer either radiosurgery when the size is <3 cm or staged embolization followed by radiosurgery for larger ones, knowing that deep AVMs have a more challenging angioarchitecture and consequently a higher risk associated with embolization. Lesions fed by lateral branches of lenticulostriate arteries are associated with a higher risk of internal capsule damage when approached surgically, making radiation therapy a more appealing intervention. For grade I and II cortical AVMs, microsurgery is indicated, whereas for grade III AVMs in an eloquent area, radiosurgery or staged embolization followed by radiosurgery is indicated. However, grade III in a noneloquent area can be treated by embolization followed by surgical resection. Finally, grade IV or more AVMs are managed conservatively except in two scenarios:

- If the AVM has produced one or more hemorrhages and the patient already has the deficit that is expected with resection.
- If the AVM has focal areas of high-steal or feeding vessel aneurysms, partial embolization could potentially decrease the risk of future hemorrhage.

Supratentorial deep AVMs are approached via interhemispheric transcallosal or transcortical routes; the deep infratentorial AVM approach is more complicated and outside the scope of this chapter. For infratentorial AVMs the most used approaches are suboccipital, retrosigmoid, subtemporal, and petrosal. The operation is planned depending on the location and angioarchitecture.[15,18–20]

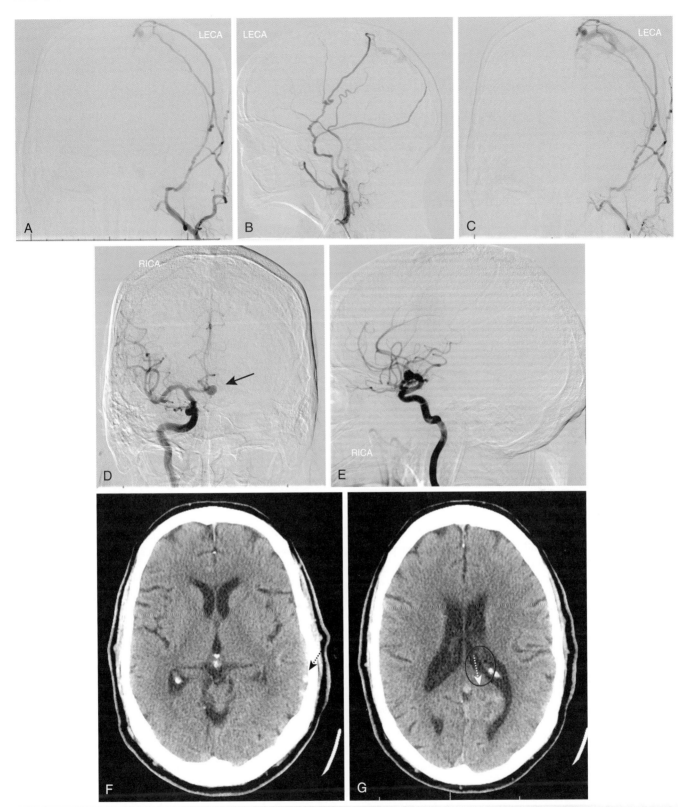

**Fig. 10.2 (A–E)** Angiography of a 72-year-old male with a dural arteriovenous fistula with cortical venous drainage fed by bilateral middle meningeal arteries draining into the superior sagittal sinus and an anterior communicating artery aneurysm 6.3 × 6.9 mm. **(F–G)** The CT shows dilated vessels, presumably veins, about the left cerebral hemisphere posteriorly. Findings are suggestive of a vascular malformation such as an arteriovenous fistula.

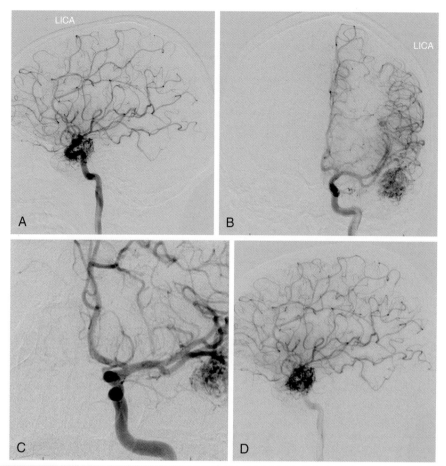

**Fig. 10.3 (A–D)** Angiography of a 21-year-old male with Spetzler-Martin grade 3 arteriovenous malformation, measuring 2.4 × 2 × 2.3 cm with superficial venous drainage.

## Microsurgery

Surgical positioning is similar to surgery for other lesions and is covered in other sections of this text. The goal of surgery is to completely eliminate the shunt. This may be achieved in four stages: 1) comparison of the AVM location/configuration with the preoperative angiogram; 2) preservation of all branches of the arterial-feeding vessels that supply normal brain tissue; 3) occlusion of the feeders as close as possible to the fistula; and 4) occlusion of the draining veins with complete excision of the lesion. First, the AVM should be localized and the relationship between the feeders and the normal brain supply evaluated. Feeders must be divided as close as possible to the AVM to ensure that blood supply to normal brain is preserved and to avoid retrograde venous/arterial thrombosis if future endovascular treatment is warranted. Draining veins must also be carefully identified. The last remaining draining vein can be divided after total collapse of the AVM when the vein no longer appears arterialized. Premature occlusion of the venous outflow or occlusion before securing all feeding vessels might lead to venous hypertension and intraoperative hemorrhage. Proper hemostasis with suction coagulators, vascular microclips, and minimal retraction may reduce the incidence of postop hematomas. After packing the surgical site, the anesthesiologist is asked to perform an induced Valsalva maneuver to assess the hemostasis before proceeding with the closure.

Resection of healthy brain tissue should be avoided whenever possible. Frameless stereotaxy or electrophysiological monitoring may be used to help localize the AVM. The surgical approach should be planned depending on the AVM nidus location so that the angle of approach is perpendicular to the major feeding arteries. A wide opening is necessary because it allows accommodation of brain swelling, allows complete identification of the anatomy, and offers immediate protection should bleeding occur.[18–20]

Depending on the eloquence of adjacent cortex, resection of cerebral AVMs can be associated with significant functional risk. When involving or adjacent to motor cortices, neuromonitoring of motor responses is frequently used by the surgeon. Reduction of motor evoked potentials of up to 15% of the initial values from direct brain stimulation during AVM resection was associated with good recovery of motor function postoperatively.[21] Conversely, disappearance of evoked potentials intraoperatively correlated with long-term motor function impairment via decreased modified Rankin score.[22]

Because the goal of surgical resection is complete obliteration of the AVM, various methods are utilized intraoperatively to assess extent of resection. Bilbao et al. compared indocyanine videoangiography (ICGV) to DSA intraoperatively in the assessment of residual cerebral AVM after resection and found that ICGV had a lower yield for detecting residual AVM nidus, especially with deeper-seated and

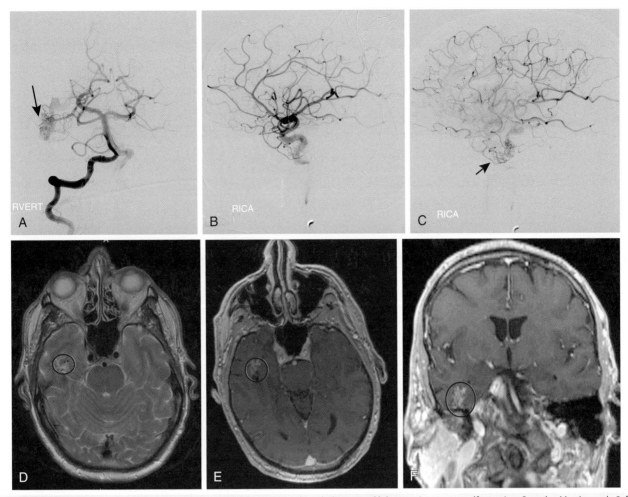

**Fig. 10.4 (A–C)** Cerebral angiogram of a 58-year-old male showing a right-sided temporal lobe arteriovenous malformation, Spetzler-Martin grade 2, fed by multiple feeders of the distal posterior cerebral artery on the right and posterior temporal arteries and draining deeply through two draining veins. **(D–F)** The MRI in the same patient shows a small cluster of abnormal vessels within the anterior right temporal lobe, measuring 1.8 cm in maximum dimension most compatible with an arteriovenous malformation. Venous drainage appears to be via the right basal vein of Rosenthal into the vein of Galen.

**Table 10.1** Spetzler-Martin Grading Scale for Arteriovenous Malformations

| Characteristics | Points |
| --- | --- |
| **Size** | |
| Small: <3 cm | 1 |
| Medium: 3–6 cm | 2 |
| Large: >6 cm | 3 |
| **Location** | |
| Noneloquent | 0 |
| Eloquent | 1 |
| **Pattern of venous drainage** | |
| Superficial only | 0 |
| Deep component | 1 |

higher-grade lesions.[23] False-negative rates of ICGV and DSA for dural AVF (DAVF) have been similarly reported at 8.7% and 10.5%, respectively.[23,24] A primary application of ultrasound intraoperatively is to confirm resection in the operating room without the use of angiography.[25] It has been used during the surgical treatment of AVMs.[25] It may allow for optimization of AVM removal without sacrifice of unnecessary veins. Transcranial Doppler has been shown to correlate well with cerebral angiography for detection of AVM and evaluation of size and location.[26]

Microsurgery is associated with a high rate of complete obliteration and durable results.[1] The risks of surgery include intraoperative rupture, retraction edema, and vessel thrombosis, as well as resection of normal brain tissue and normal perfusion pressure breakthrough (NPPB). Even with these risks, microsurgery yields high rates of favorable outcomes.[8] A metaanalysis of 2425 patients treated with microsurgical excision showed a postoperative mortality of 3.3% and a permanent morbidity of 8.6%.

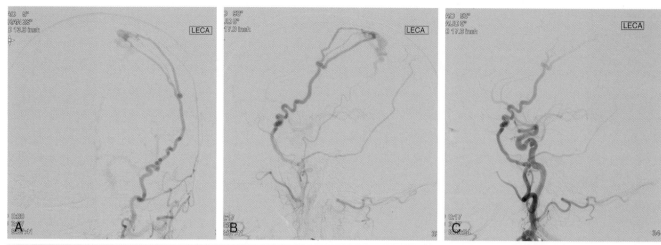

**Fig. 10.5 (A–C)** Angiogram of a 67-year-old female showing an arteriovenous fistula fed by bilateral feeders of the middle meningeal arteries with cortical venous drainage.

DAVFs are composed of a network of microvascular connections with thickened dural arteries and dilated draining veins in the wall of the dural sinus. In contrast to brain AVMs, DAVFs are generally acquired abnormalities, not congenital ones, and they rarely contain a discrete nidus.[5] (Fig. 10.5). These vascular lesions are generally thought to result from stenosis or occlusion of a dural venous sinus, often resulting from sinus thrombosis (chronic infection as from the mastoid), trauma, or surgery. The transverse sinus is a very common location, and the occipital artery is a common arterial feeder. Another common location is the cavernous sinus. They can be subclassified based on origin of the feeding artery and include pial, mixed pial and dural, and pure dural. Common clinical presentations include pulsatile tinnitus, occipital bruit, headache, visual impairment, and papilledema. The Borden and Cognard classification systems grade the fistulas based on their venous drainage pattern.[5] In both systems higher-grade lesions with antegrade flow into subarachnoid/cortical veins are associated with a higher hemorrhage rate and other neurological sequelae. DAVFs associated with the poor prognostication of cortical venous reflux tend to demonstrate leptomeningeal vessels without an identifiable nidus on MRI.[27,28] Preoperative planning requires adequate imaging for a better definition of the pathology. Catheter angiography also remains the definitive diagnostic technique for DAVF, especially when located in the spine—showing early pial vein or dural sinus filling during the arterial phase of contrast injection.[10,11]

The vast majority of DAVF can be treated effectively with endovascular techniques, especially with the newer embolization agents. Even with incomplete obliteration these lesions can be followed clinically and radiographically. The goal of surgical treatment includes ligation of the point of fistula. Partial resection does not protect against future hemorrhage risk and therefore intraoperative angiography is being used more frequently.[5]

Surgery for aggressive DAVFs has included complete excision of the lesion by coagulating the dura and the feeding artery, the venous sinus (if involved), and all arterialized leptomeningeal veins followed by skeletonization of the sinus when it is draining normal brain. This extensive resection is associated with significant complications, and hence staged embolization may be used or embolization alone can be used, especially when surgical access is challenging.[5,6]

## Perioperative Considerations

### Key Concepts

- Intraoperative rupture can result in massive and life-threatening hemorrhage.
- NPPB and obliteration hyperemia can cause significant perioperative challenges.
- Angiography is necessary to confirm successful treatment.

One of the main considerations with AVMs is whether they are ruptured or unruptured. We will focus on the ruptured AVM because the perioperative management is more complicated. In a patient presenting with hemorrhage, the first issue is whether this is someone with a known AVM and preexisting imaging versus initial presentation. Other important issues include the patient's neurological status, amount of intracranial blood, and associated shift. In a patient presenting with ICH concerning for vascular malformation after the initial CT, a computed tomographic angiography (CTA) will generally detect an AVM and give information about the size, location, drainage pattern, and associated aneurysms. Except for very small AVMs, trying to resect these lesions in someone with significant shift and neurological decline can be extremely challenging.[29,30] One strategy is to do a decompressive craniectomy without aggressive removal of ICH. This very often controls ICP and allows further workup including MRI, angiography, and possible embolization prior to further surgical treatment. With this strategy surgery is often delayed (approximately 3–4 weeks after initial hemorrhage), which permits liquefaction of clot and reduction of brain swelling, which facilitates resection.[29]

# Normal Perfusion Pressure Breakthrough and Occlusive Hyperemia

Spetzler initially suggested that hypoperfusion could induce local vessels surrounding the nidus to chronically dilate and predispose the vascular territory to vasomotor paralysis.[31] Upon restoration of normal perfusion after AVM resection, normal perfusion pressure breakthrough (NPPB) postulates that an impaired autoregulatory capacity may then be unable to compensate for increases in arterial flow and ultimately cause hyperemia, edema, or intracerebral hemorrhage. Patients are considered at high risk of NPPB if the AVM has a nidus >4 cm in diameter on angiography, there is evidence of rapid fistula flow preventing visualization of normal circulation, the arterial feeders are long and large, and focal deficits suggesting hemispheric ischemia are present. These features suggest a significant steal phenomenon and loss of autoregulation in the vascular bed. The approach to trying to avoid NPPB was a gradual increase in perfusion to the "ischemic" hemisphere by staged embolization, which is still advocated. The other recommendation included lowering blood pressure after resection. Other previously recommended strategies in addition to hypotension included mannitol, barbiturate coma, hyperventilation, and steroids. In general hypotension is avoided in the perioperative period because it is unclear if it affects the proposed mechanism of NPPB and may have potentially deleterious effects.[31–33]

Occlusive hyperemia (OH) is an alternative mechanism potentially explaining cerebral edema and hemorrhage after AVM resection. This theory suggests that venous outflow obstruction and stagnant arterial flow adjacent to the AVM are the primary causes of hyperperfusion injury after complete removal of the nidus. Recent evidence has contradicted some of the components of this theory. The underlying cause of edema and hemorrhage after AVM surgery remains controversial, and it may be that NPPB and occlusive hyperemia are related and complementary explanations for this phenomenon. Currently, the recommendations are for maintenance of normal blood pressure after resection and elimination of the possibility of residual AVM as a cause of postoperative hemorrhage because intraoperative imaging has a recognized false-negative rate.[32–34]

# Intraoperative/Postoperative Considerations

## Key Concepts

- Strict control of intracranial pressure (ICP), blood pressure, and volume status is mandatory.
- ICH is associated with increased morbidity and mortality.
- Postoperative hemorrhage must raise the question of residual AVM even with negative intraoperative imaging.
- There continues to be debate about the definition and contribution of NPPB and OH in AVM hemodynamics. Maintenance of normal blood pressure, however, has become the prevailing perioperative approach.

The best way of preventing complications is by anticipating their possible occurrence and planning strategies ahead to deal with them (Table 10.2). Intraoperative rupture can

**Table 10.2** Prevention and Management of Complications

| Complications | Prevention | Treatment |
|---|---|---|
| **INTRAOPERATIVE COMPLICATION** | | |
| Ischemic injury | Feeders should be divided as close as possible to the fistula | |
| Antegrade/retrograde embolization | Feeders should be divided as close as possible to the fistula | |
| Intraoperative hemorrhage | Volume reduction of the AVM<br>Occlusion of the venous outflow should take place only after occluding the feeders<br>Adequate fluid resuscitation | Temporary clipping<br>Reduction of the blood pressure<br>Suction<br>Cauterization |
| Intraoperative hydrocephalus | Avoidance of the ventricles during the surgery | Insertion of a ventricular catheter |
| **POSTOPERATIVE COMPLICATIONS** | | |
| Postoperative hematoma | Aggressive hemostasis<br>Minimal retraction<br>Adequate fluid resuscitation<br>Strict control of blood pressure<br>Correction of coagulopathy | Hyperventilation<br>Diuretics/osmotic agents treatment<br>Barbiturate infusions<br>Surgical evacuation<br>Craniectomy |
| Postoperative hydrocephalus | Avoidance of the ventricles during the surgery | Ventriculoperitoneal shunting |
| Normal perfusion pressure breakthrough bleeding | Strict control of blood pressure<br>Strict control of ICP | Adrenergic blockade<br>Surgery |
| Seizures | Anticonvulsant<br>Prevention of rebleeding<br>Prevention of ischemia | Anticonvulsant |

*AVM*, arteriovenous malformation; *ICP*, intracranial pressure.

lead to significant blood loss and necessitates adequate IV access with large-bore lines and/or a central venous line and arterial line monitoring. Some surgeons ask for induced hypotension to help control intraoperative bleeding, which obviously can have neurological sequelae.[30,34] With significant blood loss patients may require ongoing resuscitation in the Neuro ICU. Brain swelling, regardless of the mechanism (brain manipulation, ischemia, NPPB, OH), may require utilization of mannitol, which can also reduce volume status. With significant brain swelling, other interventions such as hyperventilation and induced burst suppression with agents such as pentobarbital or propofol may be utilized. Propofol and barbiturates can drop blood pressure precipitously, especially when patients are relatively hypovolemic secondary to blood loss/mannitol. The use of barbiturates can significantly delay being able to obtain a reliable neurological examination. Not infrequently the surgeon asks that the patient be maintained in burst suppression postoperatively, which obviously makes neurological assessment difficult and has an unclear role in the treatment or prevention of NPPB or OH. Even without induced burst suppression, utilization of neuromonitoring requires more of a dependence on IV agents for anesthesia. Again with long cases this will delay emergence from anesthesia.[30,34-39]

Hydrocephalus may occur as a result of intraventricular hemorrhage secondary to an AVM rupture. When this occurs, urgent insertion of ventricular drainage catheters may be necessary. These catheters can also be used to monitor the ICP in patients in the Neuro ICU setting.

If there are concerns intraoperatively about increased intracranial pressure (ICP), especially in the setting of intraoperative rupture or brain swelling, some consideration should be given to leaving the bone off and augmenting the dura at the end of the case (craniectomy). Also, in patients who may have delayed emergence from anesthesia, perhaps secondary to a desire to keep the patient sedated or in burst suppression, a ventriculostomy and or an intracranial monitor, perhaps with multimodality capability including brain oxygenation, should be considered. Continuous electroencephalograph monitoring is also a useful adjunct.[40-42]

The cornerstone of postoperative management is control of ICP and blood pressure, correction of coagulopathy, and maintenance of normovolemia (Table 10.3). The patient should be managed in the Neuro ICU for at least 24 hours.[43] Head-of-bed elevation to 30 to 40 degrees may optimize perfusion by balancing a reduction in ICP with a reduction in mean arterial pressure (compared with the supine state). Stool softeners are administered to decrease ICP during straining or Valsalva maneuvers. Other important aspects of postoperative management include pain control, pulmonary toilet, and prevention of deep venous thrombosis. Anticonvulsant medication administration should be continued to those patients who presented with seizure; a short course of anticonvulsant therapy may be administered to those who did not present with seizure.

If the patient had significant blood loss intraoperatively, an assessment of volume status and need for resuscitation to euvolemia is critical. Baseline and serial neurological

**Table 10.3**  The Utility and Target of Monitored Parameters in the Postoperative Period

| Parameters | Utility | Target point |
|---|---|---|
| ICP monitoring | Prognostic tool Guide management Strict control may be associated with favorable outcomes May be the only sign of neurological injury in a comatose patient | ICP < 20–25 mm Hg |
| Brain oxygen monitoring | May reflect tissue ischemia Allows for therapeutic measures to be implemented | Ischemia can be reflected by PbtO$_2$ < 20 mm Hg |
| Hemodynamic monitoring | Prevents bleeding Prevents hypoperfusion | Target SBP = 90–110 mm Hg CPP** >45–50 mm Hg Euvolemia Isoosmolarity |

*ICP*, intracranial pressure; *PbO$_2$*, Partial pressure of brain tissue O$_2$ tension; *SBP*, systolic blood pressure; *CPP*, cerebral perfusion pressure.

examinations are critical to detect future deterioration. A head CT is often obtained as a baseline, especially if the patient does not have a reliable examination. If there is a clinical deterioration or indications of increased ICP, a CT should be obtained to assess for new hemorrhage or increased brain swelling.

We have discussed the proposed mechanisms for these postoperative issues, including NPPB and OH, residual AVM, and routine postoperative hemorrhage. Because intraoperative imaging can have a false-positive result, consider postoperative imaging, including repeat angiography, especially if there is consideration of returning the patient to the operating room. New-onset hydrocephalus can also be addressed. New-onset seizure should also be in the differential for new neurological issues. New neurological deficits may also require an MRI to look for new areas of ischemia.

As discussed previously, there continues to be significant debate about the exact physiology of the postoperative hemorrhage, brain swelling, and ischemia previously attributed to NPPB and/or OH. Again, aside from preoperative embolization, there is no consensus about how to prevent or treat these entities. Adrenergic blockers have been used anecdotally in the prevention and treatment of NPPB.[44] Other prescribed treatments in addition to hypotension include mannitol, barbiturate coma, hyperventilation, and steroids. The current recommendations are to maintain euvolemia and normal blood pressure.[31-33]

As with all care of complex neurosurgical cases, management of vascular malformations requires seamless communication between anesthesia, the surgical team, and the neurocritical care team, such as when there is no uniformity or consensus with regard to issues such as NPPB.

# Conclusions

The resection of AVMs, although challenging, can have excellent outcomes. Staged surgery, preoperative embolization, and close follow-up in the perioperative and postoperative periods are recommended. Meticulous blood pressure and ICP control have been shown to improve the patient outcomes.

## References

1. Al-Shahi R, Fang JS, Lewis SC, Warlow CP. Prevalence of adults with brain arteriovenous malformations: a community based study in Scotland using capture-recapture analysis. *J Neurol Neurosurg Psychiatry.* 2002;73(5):547–551.
2. Hartmann A, Mohr JP. Acute management of brain arteriovenous malformations. *Curr Treat Options Neurol.* 2015;17(5):346. http://dx.doi.org/10.1007/s11940-015-0346-5.
3. Mohr JP, Parides MK, Stapf C, et al. Medical management with or without interventional therapy for unruptured brain arteriovenous malformations (ARUBA): a multicentre, non-blinded, randomised trial. *Lancet.* 2014;383:614–621.
4. Spetzler RF, Martin NA. A proposed grading system for arteriovenous malformations. *J Neurosurg.* 1986;65(4):476–483.
5. Signorelli F, Della Pepa GM, Sabatino G, et al. Diagnosis and management of dural arteriovenous fistulas: a 10 years single-center experience. *Clin Neurol Neurosurg.* 2015;128:123–129.
6. Zhao LB, Suh DC, Lee DG, et al. Association of pial venous reflux with hemorrhage or edema in dural arteriovenous fistula. *Neurology.* 2014;82(21):1897–1904.
7. Stapf C, Mohr JP, Pile-Spellman J, et al. Concurrent arterial aneurysms in brain arteriovenous malformations with haemorrhagic presentation. *J Neurol Neurosurg Psychiatry.* 2002;73(3):294–298.
8. Novakovic RL, Lazzaro MA, Castonguay AC, Zaidat OO. The diagnosis and management of brain arteriovenous malformations. *Neurol Clin.* 2013;31:749–763.
9. Josephson CB, White PM, Krishan A, Al-Shahi Salman R. Computed tomography angiography or magnetic resonance angiography for detection of intracranial vascular malformation in patients with intracerebral hemorrhage. *Cochrane Database Syst Rev.* 2014;9:CD009372.
10. Sharma A, Westesson P. Preoperative evaluation of spinal vascular malformation by mr angiography: how reliable is the technique: case report and review of literature. *Clin Neurol Neurosurg.* 2008;110:521–524.
11. Willems P, Brouwer P, Barfett J, terBrugge K, Krings T. Detection and classification of cranial dural arteriovenous fistulas using 4d-ct angiography: initial experience. *AJNR.* 2011;32:49–53.
12. Suzuki H, Maki H, Taki WE. Evaluation of cerebral arteriovenous malformations using image fusion combining three-dimensional digital subtraction angiography with magnetic resonance imaging. *Turkish Neurosurg.* 2012;22:341–345.
13. Castel JP, Kantor G. Postoperative morbidity and mortality after microsurgical exclusion of cerebral arteriovenous malformations. Current data and analysis of recent literature. *Neurochirurgie.* 2001;47:369–383.
14. Pollock BE, Lunsford LD, Kondziolka D, Maitz A, Flickinger JC. Patient outcomes after stereotactic radiosurgery for "operable" arteriovenous malformations. *Neurosurgery.* 1994;35(1):1–7.
15. Spetzler RF, Martin NA, Carter LP, Flom RA, Raudzens PA, Wilkinson E. Surgical management of large AVMs by staged embolization and operative excision. *J Neurosurg.* 1987;67(1):17–28.
16. Baranoski JF, Grant RA, Hirsch LJ, et al. Seizure control for intracranial arteriovenous malformations is directly related to treatment modality: a meta-analysis. *J Neurointerv Surg.* 2014;6(9):684–690.
17. Crowley RW, Ducruet AF, Kalani MY, Kim LJ, Albuquerque FC, McDougall CG. Neurological morbidity and mortality associated with the endovascular treatment of cerebral arteriovenous malformations before and during the Onyx era. *J Neurosurg.* 2015;122(6):1492–1497.
18. O'Shaughnessy BA, Getch CC, Bendok BR, Batjer HH. Microsurgical resection of infratentorial arteriovenous malformations. *Neurosurg Focus.* 2005;19(2):e5.
19. Pikus HJ, Beach ML, Harbaugh RE. Microsurgical treatment of arteriovenous malformations: Analysis and comparison with stereotactic radiosurgery. *J Neurosurg.* 1988;88(4):641–646.
20. Sisti MB, Kader A, Stein BM. Microsurgery for 67 intracranial arteriovenous malformations less than 3 cm in diameter. *J Neurosurg.* 1933;79(5):653–660.
21. Lepski G, Honegger J, Liebsch M, et al. Safe resection of arteriovenous malformation in eloquent motor areas aided by functional imaging and intraoperative monitoring. *Neurosurgery.* 2012;70:276–278.
22. Bilbao CJ, Bhalla T, Dalal S, Patel H, Dehdashti AR. Comparison of indocyanine green fluorescent angiography to digital subtraction angiography in brain arteriovenous malformation surgery. *Acta Neurochir (Wien).* 2015;157:351–359.
23. Thind H, Hardesty DA, Zabramski JM, Spetzler RF, Nakaji PT. The role of microscope-integrated near-infrared indocyanine green videoangiography in the surgical treatment of intracranial dural arteriovenous fistulas. *J Neurosurg.* 2015;122:876–882.
24. Zaidi HA, Abla AA, Nakaji P, Chowdhry SA, Albuquerque FC, Spetzler RF. Indocyanine green angiography in the surgical management of cerebral arteriovenous malformations: lessons learned in 130 consecutive cases. *Neurosurgery.* 2014;10:246–251.
25. Fu B, Zhao J, Yu L. The application of ultrasound in the management of cerebral arteriovenous malformation. *Neurosci Bull.* 2008;24:387–394.
26. Zuang L, Duan YY, Cao TS, Ruan LT. Potential of transcranial power doppled imaging on the diagnosis of cerebral arteriovenous malformation. *Chin J Ultrasonogr.* 2000;9:300–302.
27. Shin D, Park K, Yeul G, et al. The use of magnetic resonance imaging in predicting the clinical outcome of spinal arteriovenous fistula. *Yonsei Med J.* 2015;56:397–402.
28. Letourneau-Guillon L, Pablo Cruz J, Krings T. CT and MR imaging of non-cavernous dural arteriovenous fistulas: findings associated with cortical venous reflux. *Eur J Radiol.* 2015;84:1555–1563.
29. Jafar JJ, Rezai AR. Acute surgical management of intracranial arteriovenous malformations. *Neurosurgery.* 1994;34(1):8–12.
30. Hashimoto T, Young WL. Anesthesia-related considerations for cerebral arteriovenous malformations. *Neurosurg Focus.* 2001;11(5):e5.
31. Rangel-Castilla L, Spetzler RF, Nakaji P. Normal perfusion pressure breakthrough theory: a reappraisal after 35 years. *Neurosurg Rev.* 2015;38:399–405.
32. O'Connor TE, Fargen KM, Mocco J. Normal perfusion pressure breakthrough following AVM resection: a case report and review of the literature. *Open J Mod Neurosurg.* 2013;3:66–71.
33. Zacharia BE, Bruce S, Appelboom G, Connolly Jr S. Occlusive hyperemia versus normal perfusion pressure breakthrough after treatment of cranial arteriovenous malformations. *Neurosurg Clin N Am.* 2012;23:147–151.
34. Miller C, Mirski M. Anesthesia considerations and intraoperative monitoring during surgery for arteriovenous malformations and dural arteriovenous fistulas. *Neurosurg Clin N Am.* 2012;23:153–164.
35. Ravussin P, Tempelhoff R, Modica PA, Bayer-Berger MM. Propofol vs. thiopental-isoflurane for neurosurgical anesthesia: comparison of hemodynamics, CSF pressure, and recovery. *J Neurosurg Anesthesiol.* 1991;3(2):85–95.
36. Awad IA, Magdinec M, Schubert A. Intracranial hypertension after resection of cerebral arteriovenous malformations. Predisposing factors and management strategy. *Stroke.* 1994;25:611–620.
37. Batjer HH, Devous MD, Meyer YJ, Purdy PD, Samson DS. Cerebrovascular hemodynamics in arteriovenous malformation complicated by normal perfusion pressure breakthrough. *Neurosurgery.* 1988;22(3):503–509.
38. Leblanc R, Little JR. Hemodynamics of arteriovenous malformations. *Clin Neurosurg.* 1990;36:299–317.
39. Woodcock J, Ropper AH, Kennedy SK. High dose barbiturates in nontraumatic brain swelling: icp reduction and effect on outcome. *Stroke.* 1982;13(6):785–787.
40. Scheufler KM, Röhrborn HJ, Zentner J. Does tissue oxygen-tension reliably reflect cerebral oxygen delivery and consumption? *Anesth Analg.* 2002;95(4):1042–1048.
41. Scheufler KM, Lehnert A, Rohrborn HJ, Nadstawek J, Thees C. Individual value of brain tissue oxygen pressure, microvascular oxygen saturation, cytochrome redox level, and energy metabolites in detecting critically reduced cerebral energy state during acute changes in global cerebral perfusion. *J Neurosurg Anesthesiol.* 2004;16(3):210–219.

42. Menzel M, Soukup J, Henze D, et al. Brain tissue oxygen monitoring for assessment of autoregulation: preliminary results suggest a new hypothesis. *J Neurosurg Anesthesiol.* 2003;15(1):33–41.

43. Ogilvy CS, Stieg PE, Awad I, et al. Recommendations for the management of intracranial arteriovenous malformations : a statement for healthcare professionals from a special writing group of the stroke council, american stroke association. *Stroke.* 2001;32: 1458–1471.

44. Bloomfield EL, Porembka DT, Ebrahim ZY, et al. Analysis of catecholamine and vasoactive peptide release in intracranial arterial venous malformations. *J Neurosurg Anesthesiol.* 1996;8 (2):101–110.

# 11 *Cavernous Malformations*

YIN C. HU and MICHAEL F. STIEFEL

## Introduction

### Key Concepts

- Cavernoma resection should be considered in patients with recurrent hemorrhages, progressive neurological deterioration, or intractable epilepsy.
- Developmental venous anomalies are variants of normal venous drainage and must be preserved to reduce the risk of postoperative venous infarction.
- An inside-out technique with piecemeal resection is specific for resection of cavernous malformations located in eloquent cortex and brainstem.
- Gliotic tissue surrounding cavernous malformation is resected in noneloquent regions but is left untouched in eloquent areas.

Cavernous malformations (CMs), or cavernomas, account for 5% to 13% of all vascular lesions of the central nervous system. Most cranial CMs are supratentorial, whereas an approximately 9% to 35% are found in the infratentorial region.[1,2] The diagnosis of incidental cavernomas is rising, given the increased ease, frequency, and sensitivity of radiological imaging, specifically magnetic resonance imaging (MRI). Up to 40% of CMs are asymptomatic, which challenges the understanding of their epidemiology and natural history.[3]

Cavernomas are well circumscribed and contain no intervening brain tissue. Grossly, it has a mulberry appearance with a reddish or purplish coloration. Histologically, the walls consist of a single endothelial layer lacking muscular cells, a typical part of the arterial vessel wall. Hemorrhage, of varying age, either adjacent or within the lesion, is the defining characteristic of CMs. Gliotic tissue surrounding the lesion is stained yellow from residual hemosiderin of previous hemorrhages. Calcification may occur and is often mistaken for hemorrhage on computed tomography (CT) scan. Other vascular malformations may be associated with CMs, in particular, developmental venous anomalies (DVAs). These anomalies are variants of normal venous drainage and are often found associated with CMs, especially CMs of the brainstem.

### Clinical Pearl

Epileptogenic foci are caused by hemosiderin deposits and gliosis from the cavernous malformations. They may cause medical refractory epilepsy over time.

## Neuroanatomy and Procedure

Clinical symptoms depend on the location of the CMs in the nervous system. Lesional hemorrhages are typically low pressure and often do not cause clinically significant symptoms. However, in eloquent regions, such as the brainstem, patients may become symptomatic, and even debilitated, from small hemorrhages. The most common symptoms are seizures, headaches, and focal neurological deficits. Perilesional hemosiderin deposits and gliosis may be epileptogenic; seizures caused by cavernomas may become refractory to medical therapy over time.

Cavernoma resection should be considered in patients with recurrent hemorrhages, progressive neurological deterioration, or intractable epilepsy. The complexity of the microsurgical procedures is dictated by the locations of the CMs in relation to the eloquence of the surrounding neural tissue. The goal of the surgery is complete resection of the cavernoma, including the gliotic tissue. However, there are several surgical caveats. In eloquent locations, such as the brainstem or motor cortex, the gliotic tissue cannot be removed because it will cause worsening neurological deficits. Associated DVAs must also be meticulously preserved to maintain normal venous drainage and prevent venous infarctions. A thorough examination of the surgical cavity is crucial to ensure no residual cavernoma, because residual CMs may enlarge over time and rehemorrhage.

### Clinical Pearl

Developmental venous anomalies are often found in association with cavernous malformations, especially those in the brainstem. They are variants of normal venous drainage and must be preserved during surgery.

The surgical approach in extirpating a cavernoma is guided by the two-point method, used to describe resection of brainstem lesions.[4] The surgical route incorporates the shortest distance between the skull and the center of the cavernoma while traversing the least amount of neuronal tissue. Typically, this is assessed on the preoperative MRI. Optimal patient positioning, gravity retraction, appropriate approach, neuronavigation, maximal subarachnoid dissection, and minimal brain transgression are principles and tools that serve to minimize surgical trauma and injury to the surrounding neural tissue during removal of the cavernoma.

Supratentorial CMs may be subclassified based on location or eloquence. Noneloquent cortical cavernomas that abut the gyral surface are the most surgically accessible lesions given the least amount of neural tissue that must be transgressed (Fig. 11.1). Transsulcal dissection is used when a CM comes to a sulcal surface or when a sulcus avoids eloquent regions. Resection of CMs in eloquent cortex and/or subcortical regions (i.e., basal ganglia, thalamus) have been reported[5–10] but are less described because of significant surgical morbidity. Although good functional outcomes may result from surgical resection in this group, optimal patient selection remains the key.[5,11,12] Functional MRI, awake craniotomy, frameless stereotaxis, and intraoperative mapping are useful adjuncts to aid in the resection of CMs in eloquent and deep-seated locations.

Accessible lesions near the caudate head may be approached from a contralateral interhemispheric transcallosal approach, which optimizes the visualization of the lesions. Cavernomas that are situated in the anterior inferior basal ganglia superior to the hippocampus can be accessed through an anterior transsylvian dissection. A supracarotid-infrafrontal approach to the anterior inferior basal ganglia for resection of CMs has been recently described.[13] Those that are located in the posterior portion of the basal ganglia are approached via a transsulcal, transcortical, parietooccipital craniotomy. In addition, the technical aspects of a supracerebellar-supratrochlear approach to CMs located in the posterior inferior thalamus have been reported.[14] Insular or subinsular CMs can be resected from a distal transsylvian dissection followed by a transinsular corticotomy. Similar to resection of brainstem CMs, an inside-out technique is used to extirpate these lesions in eloquent regions. MRI navigation or ultrasound can be helpful to localize the lesions if they are hidden beneath the cortex. A small corticotomy and gentle parting of the tissue are performed to minimize disruption of neural tissue. Instead of circumferential dissection, the lesion is entered through its capsule and drained to shrink it. Electrocautery is used minimally at low current intensity or not at all. The CM is

then dissected from the surrounding tissue from the inside and pulled toward the center of the surgical cavity for piecemeal removal.

## Clinical Pearl

The surgical approach to cavernous malformations is highly dependent on the location of the lesion. Variations of the approach are surgeon dependent and often based on experience. In eloquent regions, an inside-out technique is recommended for extirpation of the CM.

Because of the eloquence of the brainstem, symptoms from infratentorial CM–related hemorrhages are often more debilitating than hemorrhages from supratentorial CMs. Optimal timing of surgical resection of symptomatic brainstem CMs is unclear. Both good and poor outcomes are reported when resection is performed in the acute or subacute setting after a hemorrhage.[15,16] Operations in the subacute period after hemorrhage may be preferable because of improved operative visualization of the lesion and stable neurological status of the patient.[17,18]

Surgical approaches for brainstem CMs are guided by the locations of the lesions. Variations of approaches have been described with successful outcomes but are also dependent on the surgeon's experience. CMs that are hidden from the brainstem surface mandate accurate frameless stereotaxis for localization. An inside-out technique for resection described earlier applies to resection of the brainstem CMs.

CMs of the midbrain can be resected anterolaterally by an orbitozygomatic-pterional craniotomy, laterally by a subtemporal craniotomy, or posteriorly by lateral supracerebellar-infratentorial (LSCIT) craniotomy (Fig. 11.2). For some surgeons, petrosal approaches have been replaced

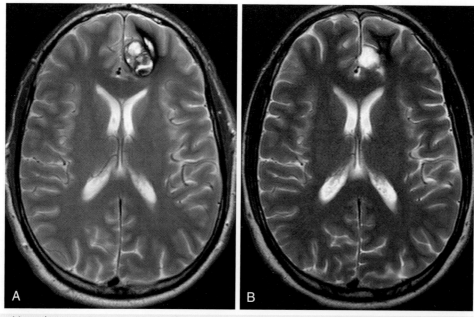

**Fig. 11.1** A 32-year-old gentleman with recurrent headaches and seizures secondary to a left frontal cavernoma. Preoperative MRI T2 sequence **(A)** showed a 2.5-cm left frontal cavernous malformation with hemosiderin ring. Postoperative MRI T2 sequence **(B)** at 3 months showed complete resection of the lesion.

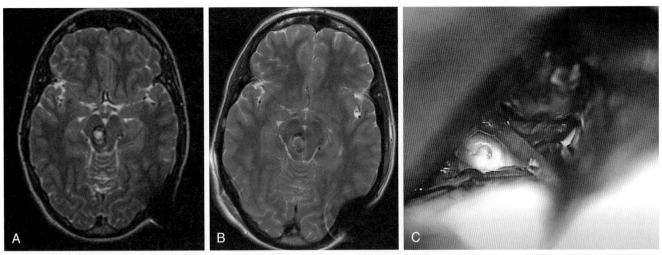

**Fig. 11.2** A 28-year-old with recurrent diplopia and left-sided numbness was found to have right midbrain cavernous malformation with evidence of previous hemorrhages. Preoperative MRI T2 sequence **(A)** showed a right posterolateral midbrain cavernoma. Postoperative MRI T2 sequence **(B)** showed complete resection. A lateral supracerebellar-infratentorial approach to the lesion was performed with intraoperative imaging **(C)** of the cavernous malformation.

by less invasive approaches because of the higher associated morbidity with petrosal surgeries.[19,20] However, the tenet of maximal bony exposure still applies with less invasive approaches to improve visualization and reduce brain retraction. When necessary, a combination of approaches is utilized, such as far lateral/retrosigmoid craniotomy for lesions of the anterolateral pontomedullary junction. Posterolateral pontine CMs that are located more inferiorly are approached via a retrosigmoid craniotomy with the surgical entry zone between the trigeminal and facial fibers. Similar pontine lesions that are more superiorly located can be removed with an LSCIT approach. Lesions that abut the pia of the fourth ventricle or posterior medulla can be accessed by a suboccipital approach. Addition of telovelar dissection enables access to CMs located in the inferomedial middle cerebral peduncles without splitting the vermis. A far-lateral approach usually suffices for CMs in the lateral and anterolateral medulla.

Rarely, CMs can occur on cranial nerves, including the optic nerve and chiasm, oculomotor, trochlear, facial, and vestibulocochlear nerves. Symptoms involve the specific cranial nerve affected. In some patients, the imaging is nondiagnostic and the lesion is only confirmed during surgery. Typically, postoperative functional recovery of the involved nerve does not occur, but there may be some improvement over time.

## Perioperative Considerations

### Key Concepts

- Frameless stereotaxis is necessary to accurately locate deep-seated supratentorial and infratentorial cavernomas.
- Antiepileptic drugs (AEDs) should be continued postoperatively in patients with epilepsy secondary to the CM.
- Advancements in neuroimaging and microsurgical tools have improved surgical outcomes in cavernomas previously believed to be unresectable.

Several advances in MRI resolution have allowed for better anatomical localization of CMs. This in turn has informed the surgical approach and treatment of CMs. Different MRI sequences (i.e., susceptibility weighted imaging) have improved identification of DVAs in relation to CM. Diffusion tensor imaging allows for fiber tracking of the white matter, and 3D reconstruction shows the relationship between the neural elements to the CMs perioperatively.[21] Intraoperatively, frameless stereotaxis (i.e., MRI guidance) has become a powerful tool in microvascular neurosurgery and significantly increases the accuracy of surgical trajectory for resection of these lesions, thus minimizing surgical morbidity.

Improvements in microsurgical technology have advanced the quality of microsurgery of CMs. Lighted suction catheters and bipolar cautery have improved operative visualization of deeper lesions (i.e., brainstem, basal ganglia) during resection. A $CO_2$ laser may be useful in selected cases (i.e., noncalcified cavernomas) to aid the resection of cavernomas in difficult regions.[22] Intraoperative mapping of the ventricular floor guides operative decision making, optimizes the surgical trajectory, and minimizes surgical morbidity.[23] In patients with multiple cavernomas and epilepsy, intracranial monitoring with subdural grids and strips may be helpful to determine an epileptogenic candidate lesion. Cortical mapping of motor and language regions may refine understanding of the relationship between eloquent structures and the lesion. Awake craniotomy may be useful for CMs situated in the eloquent cortex and resection of the epileptogenic gliotic tissue.

### Clinical Pearl

Advances in microsurgical skills, imaging, and instruments have reclassified nonoperable CMs to operable ones, often with good functional outcomes and acceptable morbidity.

Because refractory epilepsy secondary to CMs is an indication for surgery, patients who undergo surgical resection of cavernomas for this indication should continue their AEDs postoperatively. The likelihood of seizure freedom is >70% after surgery.[24,25] It is reasonable to wean AEDs to monotherapy by the first postoperative year if the patient remains seizure free or only has aura or simple partial seizures.

Complete resection of a CM does not guarantee a surgical cure. De novo cavernoma can occur after complete resection; this highlights the dynamic nature of these lesions.[26] Associated DVAs, venous hypertension, and alteration in regional blood flow may contribute to recurrence, especially in the brainstem. It is imperative to inform the patient of this possibility and to stress the importance of serial imaging surveillance postoperatively.

## Clinical Pearl

Cavernous malformations are dynamic lesions as evidenced by the de novo recurrence after complete resection.

## Postoperative Complications

### Key Concepts

- Venous infarctions occur when an associated DVA is disrupted during CM resection, interrupting the normal venous drainage of surrounding neural tissue.
- Patients with brainstem CM resections should not be extubated in the early postoperative period until they can demonstrate adequate cough and gag reflexes.
- Early rehemorrhage in the surgical cavity is highly suggestive of subtotal resection and the presence of residual CM.

For cerebral CMs, the complications associated with postoperative resection are related to the patient's overall health, location of the CMs, and individualized surgical approach and techniques. Wound infections and cerebrospinal fluid (CSF) leaks are not unique to the surgeries, and each surgeon should anticipate steps to avoid these complications as much as possible. Revision of the CSF leak and wound washout are often necessary to resolve these complications. Appropriate long-term antibiotics are needed to treat wound infections.

All patients are monitored in the intensive care unit after surgery to monitor for airway, respiratory, and cardiac abnormalities, particularly after brainstem CM resection. Normal blood pressure is maintained, and a neurological examination is obtained as soon as possible to evaluate clinical status. Early postoperative CT scan is routinely performed to rule out hemorrhage or other treatable conditions. The appropriate timing of postoperative MRI has not been established. It is often difficult to distinguish between blood products and residual CMs in the surgical cavity on immediate postoperative MRI. However, an enlarging surgical cavity or rehemorrhage is highly suggestive of residual CM. Return to the operating room for

removal of the hemorrhage and remaining cavernoma is warranted to protect from future hemorrhages.

## Clinical Pearl

Enlarging or new hemorrhages within the surgical cavity are highly suggestive of residual cavernous malformation. Reoperation is warranted to evacuate the hemorrhage, reduce mass effect, and remove residual CM.

Postoperative neurological deficits are highly specific for each approach. Venous infarction may occur when an associated DVA is disrupted during surgery. Significant mass effect may cause elevated and life-threatening intracranial pressure. Decompressive hemicraniectomy or suboccipital craniectomy may become necessary. External ventricular drains, hyperosmolar therapies, deep sedation, and possibly medically induced paralysis may be needed to control intracranial pressure. Hypoxia and hypotension should be avoided to minimize secondary cellular damage. In some centers, measurement of cerebral oxygen partial pressure and blood flow are available and monitored. Cerebral microdialysis may be used to monitor for cerebral metabolic crisis.

## Clinical Pearl

Venous infarction can occur if the associated DVA is disrupted during surgery. Depending on the size of the infarction and the location, craniectomy may be needed to control refractory elevated intracranial pressure.

Patients who undergo resection of brainstem CMs should not be extubated in the early postoperative period because of possible airway compromise. They should be extubated only when they can protect the airway and can generate an adequate cough. Furthermore, patients with dysfunction of the lower cranial nerves may require tracheostomy and percutaneous endoscopic gastrostomy (PEG). Postoperative morbidity in brainstem CM surgery may include an internuclear ophthalmoplegia, cranial nerve palsies, weakness, numbness, truncal and gait ataxia, and spasticity. These symptoms may or may not improve with time.

## Clinical Pearl

Early extubation in patients after brainstem cavernoma resection is ill advised because cough and gag reflexes may be affected. Tracheostomy and PEG placement may be needed in some patients as they recover over time.

## Conclusion

A CM is an abnormal cluster of capillaries and venules that periodically bleed and give rise to hemorrhages in the brain or spinal cord. Most CMs declare themselves by causing seizures, headaches, or bleeds. Cavernoma resection should be considered in patients with recurrent hemorrhages, progressive neurological deterioration, or intractable epilepsy. A variety of surgical techniques exists for the treatment of CM, with the goal of the surgery being complete resection of the cavernoma, including the gliotic tissue, if possible.

## References

1. Detwiler PW, Porter RW, Zabramski JM, Spetzler RF. De novo formation of a central nervous system cavernous malformation: implications for predicting risk of hemorrhage. Case report and review of the literature. *J Neurosurg.* 1997;87(4):629–632. Review. PubMed PMID: 9322853.
2. Labauge P, Brunereau L, Coubes P, et al. Appearance of new lesions in two nonfamilial cerebral cavernoma patients. *Eur Neurol.* 2001;45(2):83–88. PubMed PMID: 11244270.
3. Leblanc GG, Golanov E, Awad IA, Young WL. Biology of vascular malformations of the brain NWC. Biology of vascular malformations of the brain. *Stroke.* 2009;40(12):e694–e702. PubMed PMID: 19834013. Pubmed Central PMCID: 2810509.
4. Brown AP, Thompson BG, Spetzler RF. The two-point method: evaluating brain stem lesions. *BNI Q.* 1996;(12):20–24.
5. Chang EF, Gabriel RA, Potts MB, Berger MS, Lawton MT. Supratentorial cavernous malformations in eloquent and deep locations: surgical approaches and outcomes. Clinical article. *J Neurosurg.* 2011;114(3):814–827. PubMed PMID: 20597603.
6. Matsuda R, Coello AF, De Benedictis A, Martinoni M, Duffau H. Awake mapping for resection of cavernous angioma and surrounding gliosis in the left dominant hemisphere: surgical technique and functional results: clinical article. *J Neurosurg.* 2012;117(6):1076–1081. PubMed PMID: 23039148.
7. Wostrack M, Shiban E, Harmening K, et al. Surgical treatment of symptomatic cerebral cavernous malformations in eloquent brain regions. *Acta Neurochir.* 2012;154(8):1419–1430. PubMed PMID: 22739772.
8. Zhou H, Miller D, Schulte DM, et al. Transsulcal approach supported by navigation-guided neurophysiological monitoring for resection of paracentral cavernomas. *Clin Neurol Neurosurg.* 2009;111(1):69–78. PubMed PMID: 19022559.
9. Zotta D, Di Rienzo A, Scogna A, Ricci A, Ricci G, Galzio RJ. Supratentorial cavernomas in eloquent brain areas: application of neuronavigation and functional MRI in operative planning. *J Neurosurg Sci.* 2005;49(1):13–19. PubMed PMID: 15990714.
10. Li D, Zhang J, Hao S, et al. Surgical treatment and long-term outcomes of thalamic cavernous malformations. *World Neurosurg.* 2013;79(5-6):704–713. PubMed PMID: 22381871.
11. Zaidi HA, Chowdhry SA, Nakaji P, Abla AA, Spetzler RF. Contralateral interhemispheric approach to deep-seated cavernous malformations: surgical considerations and clinical outcomes in 31 consecutive cases. *Neurosurgery.* 2014;75(1):80–86. PubMed PMID: 24618803.
12. Pandey P, Westbroek EM, Gooderham PA, Steinberg GK. Cavernous malformation of brainstem, thalamus, and basal ganglia: a series of 176 patients. *Neurosurgery.* 2013;72(4):573–589. discussion 88–89. PubMed PMID: 23262564.
13. Waldron JS, Lawton MT. The supracarotid-infrafrontal approach: surgical technique and clinical application to cavernous malformations in the anteroinferior basal ganglia. *Neurosurgery.* 2009;64(3 Suppl):86–95; discussion 95. PubMed PMID: 19240576.
14. Sanai N, Mirzadeh Z, Lawton MT. Supracerebellar-supratrochlear and infratentorial-infratrochlear approaches: gravity-dependent variations of the lateral approach over the cerebellum. *Neurosurgery.* 2010;66(6 Suppl Operative):264–274. discussion 74. PubMed PMID: 20489515.
15. Samii M, Eghbal R, Carvalho GA, Matthies C. Surgical management of brainstem cavernomas. *J Neurosurg.* 2001;95(5):825–832. PubMed PMID: 11702873.
16. Mathiesen T, Edner G, Kihlstrom L. Deep and brainstem cavernomas: a consecutive 8-year series. *J Neurosurg.* 2003;99(1):31–37. PubMed PMID: 12854740.
17. Sandalcioglu IE, Wiedemayer H, Secer S, Asgari S, Stolke D. Surgical removal of brain stem cavernous malformations: surgical indications, technical considerations, and results. *J Neurol Neurosurg Psychiatry.* 2002;72(3):351–355. PubMed PMID: 11861694. Pubmed Central PMCID: 1737795.
18. Wang CC, Liu A, Zhang JT, Sun B, Zhao YL. Surgical management of brain-stem cavernous malformations: report of 137 cases. *Surg Neurol.* 2003;59(6):444–454. discussion 54. PubMed PMID: 12826334.
19. Abla AA, Turner JD, Mitha AP, Lekovic G, Spetzler RF. Surgical approaches to brainstem cavernous malformations. *Neurosurg Focus.* 2010;29(3):E8. PubMed PMID: 20809766.
20. Gross BA, Dunn IF, Du R, Al-Mefty O. Petrosal approaches to brainstem cavernous malformations. *Neurosurg Focus.* 2012;33(2):E10. PubMed PMID: 22853828.
21. Ulrich NH, Kockro RA, Bellut D, et al. Brainstem cavernoma surgery with the support of pre- and postoperative diffusion tensor imaging: initial experiences and clinical course of 23 patients. *Neurosurg Rev.* 2014;37(3):481–492. PubMed PMID: 24801720.
22. Consiglieri GD, Killory BD, Germain RS, Spetzler RF. Utility of the $CO_2$ laser in the microsurgical resection of cavernous malformations. *World Neurosurg.* 2013;79(5–6):714–718. PubMed PMID: 22381271.
23. Cohen-Gadol AA. Large pontine cavernous malformations: resection through the telovelar approach and mapping of the 4th ventricular floor. *Neurosurgery.* 2014;10(Suppl 4):655; discussion 655. PubMed PMID: 24932709.
24. Robinson JR, Awad IA, Little JR. Natural history of the cavernous angioma. *J Neurosurg.* 1991;75(5):709–714. PubMed PMID: 1919692.
25. Labauge P, Brunereau L, Levy C, Laberge S, Houtteville JP. The natural history of familial cerebral cavernomas: a retrospective MRI study of 40 patients. *Neuroradiology.* 2000;42(5):327–332. PubMed PMID: 10872151.
26. Pozzati E, Acciarri N, Tognetti F, Marliani F, Giangaspero F. Growth, subsequent bleeding, and de novo appearance of cerebral cavernous angiomas. *Neurosurgery.* 1996;38(4):662–669. discussion 9–70. PubMed PMID: 8692382.

# 12 Bypass Surgeries for Moyamoya Disease

CHITRA VENKATASUBRAMANIAN, SUNIL V. FURTADO, KYLE S. HOBBS, and GARY K. STEINBERG

## Introduction

Bypass surgeries result in revascularization of the brain by connecting a branch of the external carotid (EC) artery to a branch of the internal carotid (IC) artery (EC–IC bypass) either directly or via a vein graft. These procedures are performed most commonly for Moyamoya disease (MMD), but also when a parent vessel like the intracranial ICA, middle cerebral artery, or posterior inferior cerebellar artery needs to be deliberately occluded, or "trapped," in order to exclude a complex aneurysm or excise a tumor. In symptomatic carotid occlusions, EC–IC bypass was a treatment modality until the recent publication of the Carotid Occlusion Surgery Study (COSS), which failed to demonstrate clinical superiority of bypass over the best medical therapy.[1]

### Key Concepts

- MMD is a rare, idiopathic, progressive vasculopathy causing stenosis and occlusion of unilateral or bilateral distal internal carotid arteries (ICAs), the proximal middle cerebral arteries (MCAs), and anterior cerebral arteries (ACAs) with development of fine collaterals to maintain cerebral perfusion.
- MMD presents with transient ischemic attacks (TIAs), strokes, or brain hemorrhage.
- EC–IC bypass is performed to restore cerebral perfusion and decrease future strokes.

MMD is a rare, chronic, idiopathic, and progressive vasculopathy characterized by stenosis and occlusion of one or both distal ICAs, leading to decreased cerebral blood flow (CBF). It often involves the proximal MCAs and ACAs. Early in its course, cerebral perfusion is maintained by collateral networks of small vessels that develop in response to low CBF.[2] Later, it results in both cerebral ischemic and intraparenchymal hemorrhage. It can also present with headaches, seizures, or movement disorders. It most commonly affects patients of Asian descent but has been observed in all ethnic groups.[3,4] MMD has a bimodal age of onset with peaks at ages 5 and 40 years.[2]

The brain maintains optimal cerebral perfusion pressures (CPPs) between 50 and 150 mm Hg through reflex arteriolar vasodilation or vasoconstriction, that is, autoregulation. The vasodilatory ability of cerebral vessels to maintain CBF (normal range 45–55 mL/100 g/min)

despite decreased CPP is known as *cerebrovascular reserve (CVR)*, and this is markedly reduced in MMD. In MMD, stenosis of the terminal ICA can lead to reduction in CPP because the arterioles are maximally dilated and autoregulation is lost. This leads to an increase in regional oxygen extraction fraction (OEF) in the affected territory, which is temporarily able to avoid irreversible ischemic damage; however, if CPP remains low, permanent and continued ischemia may occur.

### Clinical Pearl

EC–IC bypass is most commonly performed for MMD to restore cerebral perfusion and decrease future strokes.

The treatment for MMD is revascularization surgery.[4–7] Surgical revascularization augments cerebral perfusion and replenishes blood flow to the ischemic areas by enhancing CBF. This increases CBF and CVR and decreases OEF,[4–6] thereby providing protection from oligemia during physiological stress, such as hypotension and hypoxemia. Concomitant with radiographic improvement, there is a reduction in TIAs and decreased risk of future ischemic and hemorrhagic strokes. Preoperative imaging, intraoperative management, and postoperative neurocritical care of a typical MMD patient are discussed in this chapter.

## Perioperative Considerations

### Key Concepts

- Preoperative evaluation includes magnetic resonance imaging (MRI) with perfusion to quantify stroke burden, Xenon-computed tomography (Xe-CT) (MRI or single-photon emission CT [SPECT]) without and with acetazolamide to evaluate CBF and CVR, and a cerebral angiogram to select a donor vessel for bypass.
- Patients are well hydrated and placed on aspirin leading up to surgery.
- In patients with bilateral MMD, surgery is performed initially on the side with worse CVR and larger infarct burden.

## PREOPERATIVE EVALUATION

### Clinical Pearl

Preoperative evaluation includes quantification of stroke burden, cerebral perfusion, cerebrovascular reserve, and selection of donor vessel for bypass.

Imaging for MMD focuses on evaluation of cerebrovascular reactivity, predictors of ischemic and hemorrhagic episodes, and predictors of postoperative ischemia and complications.[7] This includes:

a) *Quantification of tissue ischemia:* Chronic infarcts in the white matter and the side with the higher infarct load are determined with $T_2$ and fluid-attenuated inversion recovery sequences on brain MRI (Fig. 12.1), whereas diffusion weighted imaging (DWI) with apparent diffusion coefficient identifies acute infarcts.

b) *Quantification of tissue perfusion:* Perfusion weighted imaging (PWI) MRI using gadolinium bolus tracking techniques or CT perfusion (CTP) is used to generate quantitative maps of relative CBF, cerebral blood volume (CBV), mean transit time (MTT), and time to maximum of the residue function (Tmax).[4,6,8,9] Patients with MMD have an elevated rCBV, delayed MTT, delayed Tmax, and reduced rCBF. (Fig. 12.1)

c) *Evaluation of cerebrovascular reactivity:* Cerebrovascular reserve can be calculated by performing Xe-CT or SPECT or PWI scans at baseline and after administration of a vasodilator ($CO_2$ or acetazolamide [Diamox]).[8,9] In Xe-CT (Fig.12.2), patients inhale a mixture of $O_2$ and stable xenon gas. Xenon enters brain tissue by diffusion, and its accumulation correlates with regional CBF. After a baseline Xe-CT, acetazolamide is administered to derive the CVR. This technique can identify appropriate augmentation of blood flow (i.e., intact cerebral autoregulation), poor hemodynamic reserve, or a steal phenomenon.

d) *Anatomical imaging of cerebral vasculature:* The cerebral vasculature can be imaged noninvasively with MR angiography (MRA) or by a cerebral angiogram. The latter is used to stage the disease and to identify the extent of MMD (Fig. 12.3). The image derived from External Carotid Artery (ECA) injection is used to qualify the donor vessel for bypass. Quantitative MRA with NOVA software is a new technique that demonstrates blood flow in large ICAs and in the superficial temporal artery (STA) after revascularization.[7]

e) *Neuropsychological testing:* Neuropsychological testing and assessment are performed preoperatively and postoperatively.[10,11]

## Neuroanatomy and Procedure

### Key Concepts

- Direct bypass involves anastomosis between branches of the external carotid artery (ECA), usually the STA and distal branches of the MCA, providing immediate restoration of blood flow.

- Direct anastomosis of arteries less than 0.7 mm is technically challenging and carries a higher risk of occlusion.
- Indirect bypass includes laying a vascular tissue (artery, muscle, pericranium, omentum) on the brain surface to induce indirect revascularization: encephaloduroarteriosynangiosis (EDAS) and encephaloduroarteriomyosynangiosis (EDAMS). These procedures are mostly done in children.

## SURGICAL TREATMENT

### Preoperative Preparation

Antiplatelet agents (other than aspirin) and antihypertensive medications are discontinued at least 5 days and 2 days prior to surgery, respectively. Patients are asked to keep themselves well hydrated.

### Clinical Pearl

In bilateral MMD, surgery is initially performed on the side with worse cerebrovascular reserve and larger infarct burden.

Generally, in MMD affecting bilateral hemispheres, the hemisphere with the worse CVR and larger infarct burden is bypassed first. Patients with large acute infarcts or hemorrhage are allowed to recover from the insult. This minimizes the risk of further ischemia during the procedure and minimizes the chance of cerebral hyperperfusion syndrome (CHS), which results in intracerebral hemorrhage due to hyperemia from dysfunctional cerebral autoregulation.

## DIRECT REVASCULARIZATION

Direct revascularization methods reestablish blood flow by bypassing the ICA using a conduit vessel from the extracranial circulation anastomosed directly to a distal branch of the MCA (usually an M4 branch) in the affected hemisphere (Fig. 12.4).[7] The direct technique is preferred because blood flow is restored immediately. Branches of the STA most commonly serve as the donor vessel. If the STA is unavailable (e.g., due to prior trauma, craniotomy, or failed bypass), the occipital artery can be used. Its location makes it particularly useful for posterior MCA territory ischemia. A less common maneuver is to anastomose the cervical external carotid artery or proximal STA "stump" to an MCA branch using a saphenous interposition or radial artery graft as a conduit. These are larger-diameter grafts and carry higher flow leading to a greater risk of hyperemia and possibly CHS. Similarly, a mismatch between the diameter of donor and recipient vessel may increase occlusion risks associated with graft stenosis. A donor or recipient vessel less than 0.7 mm in diameter also makes the anastomosis technically more difficult.[12]

### STA-MCA Bypass

General anesthesia is induced carefully to avoid hypotension. Mean arterial pressure (MAP) goals are titrated based on the patient's baseline MAP. Generally, a MAP of 80 to 90 mm Hg is maintained in adult patients during the initial arterial dissection and increased to 90 to 100 mm Hg

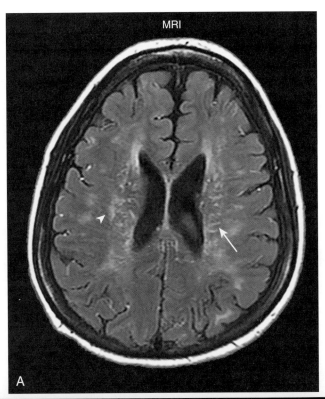

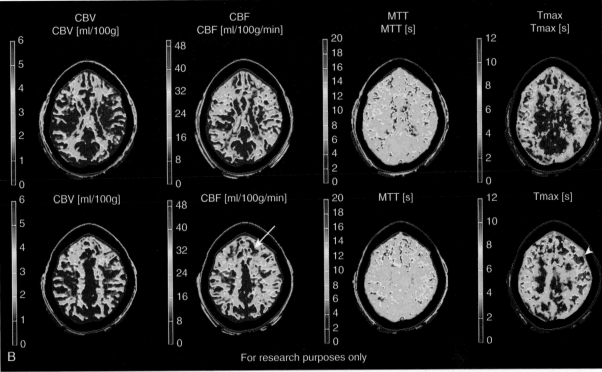

**Fig. 12.1** Preoperative imaging of tissue ischemia and baseline cerebral perfusion. **(A)** Preoperative MRI showing extensive chronic, watershed territory infarcts in bilateral white matter (*arrowhead*) and prominent leptomeningeal and lenticulostriate collaterals (*arrow*). **(B)** Preoperative CT perfusion showing deep white matter and bifrontal cortical hypoperfusion with low cerebral blood flow (CBF) (*blue areas* on CBF map, *arrow*), low cerebral blood volume (CBV), and prolonged time to maximum (Tmax). There is also increase in CBV and prolonged Tmax in the temporoparietal areas indicating collateral flow (*arrowhead*).

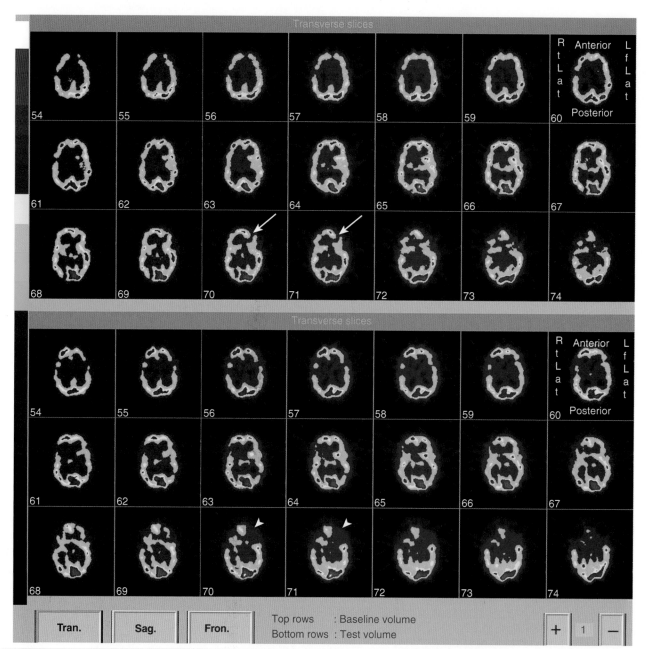

**Fig. 12.2** Preoperative assessment of cerebrovascular reactivity. On the baseline SPECT scan, there is hypoperfusion in the bifrontal regions, worse on the left (*arrow*). After acetazolamide, there is an enlargement of the hypoperfused area (*arrowhead*) indicating failure of augmentation of cerebral blood, poor cerebrovascular reserve, and steal phenomenon.

during the bypass. Mild hypothermia (33°C) is maintained until the anastomosis is completed.[13,14] The end-tidal pressure of $CO_2$ is maintained between 35 and 40 mm Hg to maintain adequate cerebral vasodilation (Fig. 12.5).

The STA is mapped preoperatively using Doppler ultrasound. The STA, including a cuff of vascular fascia around it, is dissected out from 1 cm above the zygomatic root to the distal end of the selected parietal or frontal branch. The temporalis is split and retracted, leaving the vessel intact. A circular frontotemporoparietal craniotomy about 6 cm in diameter with the base overlying the sylvian fissure is turned below the vessel. The recipient vessel (usually a frontal M4 branch arising from the sylvian fissure) is dissected from the arachnoid over a 7-mm length. A high-visibility background is placed behind the vessel. The recipient vessel is then covered with a cotton pledget containing papaverine or nicardipine while the donor vessel is prepared.

The donor vessel is prepared by first placing a temporary mini aneurysm clip on the proximal end and then occluding and transecting the distal end at the wound edge. The vessel is flushed with heparinized saline. Adventitia is dissected from the distal donor artery for 1 cm from the distal end. The diameter of the distal orifice of this vessel is matched to the recipient vessel by making an angular cut across the distal vessel to create a "fish mouth." Indigo carmine blue dye is used to highlight the vessel edges of both donor and recipient vessels.[12]

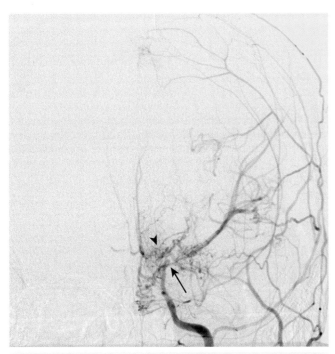

**Fig. 12.3** Preoperative evaluation of cerebral vessels. Cerebral angiogram of the left CCA injection (AP) view shows occlusion of the terminal ICA (*arrow*) with extensive moyamoya collaterals from the lenticulostriate arteries (*arrowhead*).

The recipient vessel is prepared by placing temporary aneurysm clips proximal and distal to the planned opening. Prior to temporary occlusion, hypothermia is confirmed, and the patient is placed in burst suppression using propofol and monitored using a frontal scalp electroencephalogram (EEG) grid. A diamond-shaped arteriotomy in the superficial vessel wall is performed. The recipient vessel is flushed with heparinized saline. The anastomosis is then undertaken by stitching the heel and toe (proximal and distal corners of the diamond opening) of the anastomosis using 10-0-monofilament interrupted stitches. Prior to the final stitch insertion the anastomosis is irrigated with heparinized saline.[15–17] Temporary clips are then removed from the recipient vessel followed by the donor vessel. Minor bleeding may be corrected by applying pressure with a small piece of cotton, surgicel, or gelfoam at the anastomosis site. Additional interrupted sutures may also be used, but care must be taken to avoid stenosis of the anastomosis. Doppler ultrasound and indocyanine green (ICG) fluorescence angiography are used to demonstrate flow and its directionality in the graft (Fig. 12.5). Rewarming is initiated before the actual target hypothermia temperature is reached, so that 33°C temperature usually coincides with midway through the bypass.

Perioperative quantitative blood flow information from the donor and recipient vessels are determined using devices such as Charbel Transonic Flow Probes (Transonic Systems, Inc.) and thermal diffusion probes (Bowman Perfusion

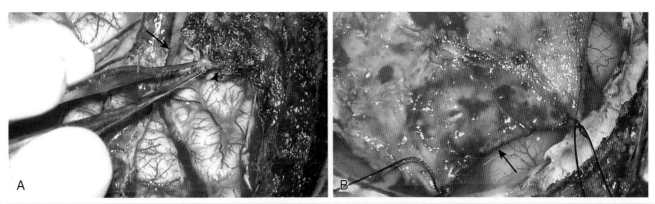

**Fig. 12.4** Operative imaging. Indirect anastomosis: Superficial temporal artery (STA) (*arrow*) laid on the pial surface with temporalis muscle (*arrowhead*) being mobilized. Then the temporalis muscle is sutured to dural margin (*arrow*).

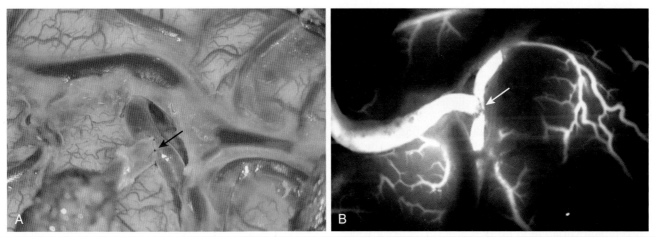

**Fig. 12.5** Direct STA–M4 bypass intraoperative image with good flow across the bypass anastomosis seen under direct vision and on intraoperative ICG angiogram (*arrows*).

Monitor, Hemedex, Inc.). This information is used to determine the likelihood of postoperative complications.[7,15–17] For example, a very high postanastomotic MCA flow is associated with postoperative ischemic infarcts, transient neurological events, and hemorrhage. In these patients, a tighter blood pressure is warranted postoperatively.

The proximal burr hole is enlarged to accommodate the entry of the STA graft with the cuff of adventitia, and the STA with a cuff of vascularized tissue is laid on the cortical surface, which provides additional indirect revascularization over time. The craniotomy is fastened with titanium plates, and the temporalis muscle and skin are closed. Graft patency can be checked intermittently by confirming proximal STA flow with the Doppler ultrasound.[15–17] Meticulous hemostasis is secured in order to prevent postoperative blood collection, especially when these patients are continued on aspirin postoperatively. Graft patency is also checked with a postoperative angiogram at 6 months.

## INDIRECT REVASCULARIZATION

Indirect methods apply vascularized tissue to the surface of the brain, thereby utilizing the inherent ability of the MMD ischemic brain to drive neoangiogenesis from the graft to the pial surface over months to years (a minimum of 3 months). Children have a greater likelihood of neoangiogenesis from donor tissue.[18] In MMD patients there is an increase in serum vascular endothelial growth factor, monocyte chemoattractant protein 1, matrix metalloproteinase 9 and platelet-derived growth factor, and, in spinal fluid, an increase in fibroblast growth factor, presumably secondary to upregulation from the ischemic brain. These are either markers of a proangiogenic state or directly contribute to angiogenesis.[19–21]

Donor tissues for indirect revascularization include the temporal artery and its surrounding adventitia and soft tissue, temporalis muscle, pericranium, galea, dura, and omentum.[20] Indirect procedures are usually shorter in time with less exposure to potential anesthesia risks such as hypotension, hypoxemia, and hypercarbia or hypocarbia. Another theoretical advantage is that no temporary vessel occlusion is required.[7] The disadvantage is that no immediate increase in blood flow occurs, and therefore the postoperative risk of a new ischemic stroke may increase.

The most common indirect revascularization technique is EDAS.[22] In this procedure the STA is exposed through an incision placed on top of the artery. The artery is carefully dissected with a cuff of soft tissue along an 8- to 10-cm length. The vessel is left in situ with blood flow proximally from the artery origin and out distally into the scalp. The vessel is retracted to the side, and a craniotomy is performed. The dura is opened under the length of the vessel, and the arachnoid and overlying fissures and cortical vessels are gently opened in multiple locations under the vessel.[22] The vessel is placed on the pial surface. The soft tissue cuff is sewn to the dural edges to secure the vessel in place. Pial synangiosis uses a similar technique, but opposes the vessel directly to the surface of the brain by suturing the STA to the edges of a linear opening in the pia using interrupted 10-0 monofilament.[7,22]

A common variation to EDAS is EDAMS, where a wider craniotomy is performed to maximize exposure of the brain.

The temporalis muscle is brought into the craniotomy anterior or posterior to the arterial entry.[22] The STA is laid over the surface of the brain as previously described; however, in EDAMS the muscle is laid over the STA and over the surface of the brain. The dural margins are resected maximally to allow the muscle to be sutured into place on the remaining dural edges, securing the muscle in place on the surface of the brain. The bone flap inner table is removed to allow for the bulk of muscle graft and then replaced over the muscle and arterial tissue by creating a slot-shaped orifice at the base of the craniotomy that can accommodate the additional tissue passing through the opening.

Combinations of indirect and direct techniques can be performed, and pial synangiosis can be added to EDAS, EDAMS, dural, pericranial, and galeal flap procedures to increase exposure of the brain to the STA or vessels within the donor tissue.[22–25] Similarly, multiple burr holes can be added during any indirect procedure adjacent to the craniotomy to increase the potential for indirect revascularization.[26] Vascularized pericranium can also be brought down into the burr hole to lie on the pia.

# Postoperative Complications

**Clinical Pearl**

Strict blood pressure control and adequate intravascular volume should be maintained in the immediate postoperative period to maintain adequate cerebral perfusion.

**Key Concepts**

- Tight control of MAP extends into the immediate postoperative period and is based on the patient's baseline MAP.
- Good intravascular volume is maintained to avoid hypoperfusion and postoperative ischemia.
- Aspirin is continued on postoperative day 1 and lifelong to maintain graft patency.
- Tight-fitting masks are to be avoided in order to prevent extrinsic compression of the bypass graft above the zygoma.

## POSTOPERATIVE CARE

Routine in-hospital cranial imaging is not performed unless warranted clinically, although we perform a routine postoperative MRI after discharge after the second or unilateral bypass surgery. Neurological examination is performed hourly on the first day of surgery. Aspirin is started on the day after surgery to maintain graft patency, to be continued indefinitely. Tight-fitting nasal masks or other assisted-breathing appliances that can potentially compress the donor side of the graft above the zygoma are avoided. Patients are encouraged to ambulate the day after surgery to reduce the risk of pulmonary atelectasis and deep vein thrombosis (DVT). Patients are scheduled for a routine post–hospital discharge visit and additional clinic visits at 6 months and 3 and 10 years after their bypass surgeries. A cerebral angiogram,

MRI of the brain with perfusion studies, and neuropsychology evaluation are performed at each visit.

## Postoperative Hemodynamic Monitoring and Maintenance of Intravascular Volume

Many of the complications observed after surgical revascularization are a result of the preexisting deranged CBF and CVR. In severe cases of MMD with impaired cerebral autoregulation, it requires a few weeks for the brain and the cerebral vasculature to adjust to a new robust blood flow. DWI positive hemispheric ischemic lesions at the time of surgery are a risk factor for postoperative ischemic deficits. Maintaining a MAP similar to or slightly higher than preoperative baseline is important. Typically, the postoperative MAP is kept at 90 to 110 for the first postoperative day in the intensive care unit. Maintenance of adequate intravascular volume is also essential to ensure good perfusion to the brain across the bypass graft and prevent postoperative infarcts. Indirect measures of the adequacy of intravascular volume are central venous pressure (CVP) and bedside echocardiographic assessment of inferior vena cava compressibility.

To mitigate or preempt ischemia, patients are empirically administered non-dextrose-containing intravenous fluids on the first postoperative day. The volume of fluid infusion is titrated to maintain a CVP of 6 to 8 cm of $H_2O$ in adult nonintubated patients, although there is no clear evidence to support this practice. Continuous and bolus administration of normal saline solution may be administered to meet this goal. Immediate postoperative MAPs are maintained within a tight range, which is determined by the patient's baseline MAP. Infusions of antihypertensives, such as esmolol, nitroprusside, and nicardipine, are used if the MAP is sustained above the determined goal. In the case of relative hypotension, intravenous fluid boluses and vasopressor agents, such as phenylephrine, are used. MAP goals are gradually relaxed to baseline levels on postoperative day 2. If the clinical status warrants, the MAP may be augmented for an extended period and oral agents, such as midodrine, may be used.

## POSTOPERATIVE COMPLICATIONS

### Clinical Pearl

A new focal neurological deficit in the postoperative period may be due to ischemia, cerebral hyperperfusion syndrome, focal hypoperfusion, extraaxial or intraaxial hemorrhage, or seizures. Prompt neuroimaging and/or EEG monitoring is indicated.

### Key Concepts (see Box 12.1)

- Sudden onset of a focal neurological deficit can be due to ischemia, CHS, hemorrhage, or seizures and must be promptly investigated with neuroimaging and EEG.
- CHS is characterized by hyperperfusion of previously ischemic brain with robust flow via the new graft and is heralded by onset of headache and focal neurological deficits.
- Postoperative ischemia can occur due to hemodynamic fluctuations, competing flow between the collaterals and the graft, and graft occlusion or compression.

### Box 12.1   Postoperative Complications

1. Cerebral ischemia causing transient neurological deficit or stroke
2. Cerebral hyperperfusion causing headaches or hemorrhage
3. Subdural hemorrhage, usually asymptomatic
4. Epidural hemorrhage
5. Seizures
6. Wound dehiscence
7. Graft compression or occlusion

A new focal neurological deficit in the postoperative period can be due to ischemia, CHS, extraaxial or intraaxial hemorrhage, or seizures. Urgent CT scan may be performed to rule out hemorrhage. MRI with DWI/PWI can assess for ischemia or hyperperfusion. An angiogram can also be performed to visualize graft patency and the status of the native anterior and posterior circulations. Continuous EEG may be performed to rule out seizures.

## POSTOPERATIVE ISCHEMIA

Postoperative ischemia is an infrequent but concerning complication of any bypass surgery and can occur from a number of different mechanisms, including failure of CVR, hypoperfusion from competition between the graft and native collateral flow, graft occlusion, and donor vessel compression.

### Ischemia Due to Failure of Cerebrovascular Reserve

In the COSS trial,[1] 15% of patients had a perioperative stroke, most of which occurred within 2 days of bypass. Twenty-one percent were thought to be due to complications of the bypass. However, strokes from graft occlusion were rare; graft patency was 98% at 30 days. The remaining strokes occurred in the cortical border zone or in a large MCA core region.[27] Similarly, focal hypoperfusion on SPECT has been shown in both adult and pediatric MMD patients treated with indirect or direct bypasses. These patients manifest clinically with temporary or sometimes permanent neurological deficits.[28,29] Risk factors for postoperative ischemia in adults include preoperative hypodensity on CT or positive DWI lesion on MRI and multiple preoperative ischemic episodes, indicating unstable CBF.[29] If new ischemic areas are identified on postoperative MRI, the MAP goal is raised using fluids and phenylephrine to increase cerebral perfusion. For prolonged hypoperfusion, oral midodrine is started.

### Ischemia Due to Graft Occlusion

Graft occlusion causing postoperative ischemia (Fig. 12.6) is uncommon, with bypass patency rates >97% in multiple series.[27] Contributing factors include prolonged hypotension, hypovolemia, or intraoperative difficulties creating the anastomosis, particularly when the diameter of the donor and recipient vessels are too small or mismatched.[30] Antiplatelet therapy with aspirin is started preoperatively

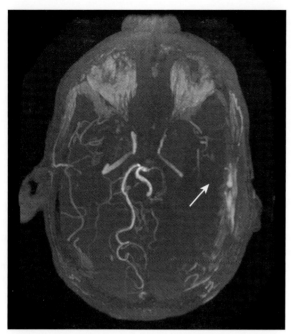

Fig. 12.6 Postoperative ischemia. MRA of the circle of Willis confirms nonvisualization of the left EC–IC bypass graft (*arrow*).

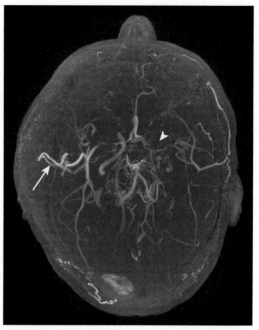

Fig. 12.7 Postoperative ischemia. Postoperative MRA of circle of Willis in another patient shows patent right STA–MCA bypass graft (*arrow*) with new nonvisualization of the contralateral (left) terminal ICA (*arrowhead*).

to help maintain graft patency, while acknowledging the small potential for increased risk of hemorrhage. Therapy with a single antiplatelet agent has been shown to improve neurological outcome after bypass; dual antiplatelet therapy may be associated with worse outcomes due to hemorrhage.[31] If neurological deficits occur that indicate anastomotic thrombosis has occurred, immediate vessel imaging (MRI/MRA, CTA, or cerebral angiogram) should be performed to assess graft patency and the need for anastomotic revision.

### Contralateral Ischemia

In rare instances, new strokes or extension of hypoperfused areas at risk of stroke occur in the hemisphere contralateral to the side of the graft (Fig. 12.7). A potential risk factor for this is very severe bilateral impaired CVR, which is worsened by blood pressure fluctuations intraoperatively and postoperatively. On MRA, CTA, or cerebral angiogram, the contralateral ICA or MCA can be newly occluded due to a drop in blood flow across the vessel from hemodynamic fluctuations on the backdrop of impaired autoregulation. This underscores the importance of tight MAP control in the perioperative period. When this occurs, the MAP is raised using fluids and pressors.

### Ischemia Due to Compression of Donor Vessel

Experimental compression of the STA after bypass has been shown to cause electrographic evidence of slow waves in the affected region, as well as causing an increase in central conduction time by somatosensory evoked potential, suggesting local ischemia.[32,33] A tight scalp closure can compress the graft and needs surgical revision. Tight-fitting oxygen masks are to be avoided. In the case of combined procedures, swelling of the temporalis muscle may compress the donor vessel. Vessel compression can also be due to extraaxial hemorrhage (i.e., epidural

or subdural) that needs prompt detection and surgical evacuation.

## CEREBRAL HYPERPERFUSION SYNDROME

This important complication has been extensively described after carotid endarterectomy,[7,34,35] but is also a known occurrence after EC–IC bypass surgery,[36,37] despite the relatively low-flow nature of the EC–IC bypass. Pathologically, it occurs due to a rapid increase in blood flow to chronically ischemic regions of the brain.

The exact incidence of CHS after EC–IC bypass is currently unclear and varies widely, possibly due to differences in definition[35] and inclusion of asymptomatic patients with only radiographic evidence of CHS. Estimates range from 18% in patients who underwent EC–IC bypass for atherosclerotic occlusive cerebrovascular disease[37] to as high as 28% to 38% in patients with adult-onset MMD.[36,38]

Risk factors for the development of CHS include reduced CVR,[39,40] adult-onset MMD, and hemorrhagic presentation of MMD.[36] Although the degree of intraoperative ischemia is a risk factor for CHS in carotid endarterectomy, this has not been definitively demonstrated in MMD.[36,40]

This syndrome is characterized clinically by nonspecific symptoms, including headache, facial pain, vomiting, confusion, visual disturbances, and focal motor seizures (often with secondary generalization). Other deficits, including aphasia, dysarthria, orofacial apraxia, or sensorimotor loss, have been reported to cause either transient or permanent deficits.[35] In its most severe form, intracerebral or subarachnoid hemorrhage may result from CHS. It is postulated to be due to increased blood flow in fragile collateral moyamoya vessels or into ischemic areas and can be fatal.[28,30,35]

Hyperperfusion syndrome should be suspected in any bypass patient who develops new-onset neurological deficits or seizures postoperatively. Advanced imaging modalities, such as SPECT, may allow preoperative and postoperative CBF assessment, which may identify those at risk of developing CHS. Quantitative CBF assessment may also distinguish CHS from ischemia; however, access to this modality may be limited.[41] Hemorrhage or infarct/diffusion lesions are not present on the MRI. Radiological descriptions of CHS have frequently been described as an increase in regional CBF of >100% of preoperative values around a patent bypass with diminished perfusion in watershed areas without evidence of infarct.[35]

Any patient with new neurological deficits should have urgent imaging either with CTP or PWI (Fig. 12.8) to assess for CHS versus ischemia. MRI may demonstrate areas of ischemia or edema and may be preferred. A cerebral angiogram may demonstrate brisk, robust, and hyperemic filling of the bypassed hemisphere with a widely patent graft.

There are two schools of thought regarding treatment strategies for patients with new postoperative neurological

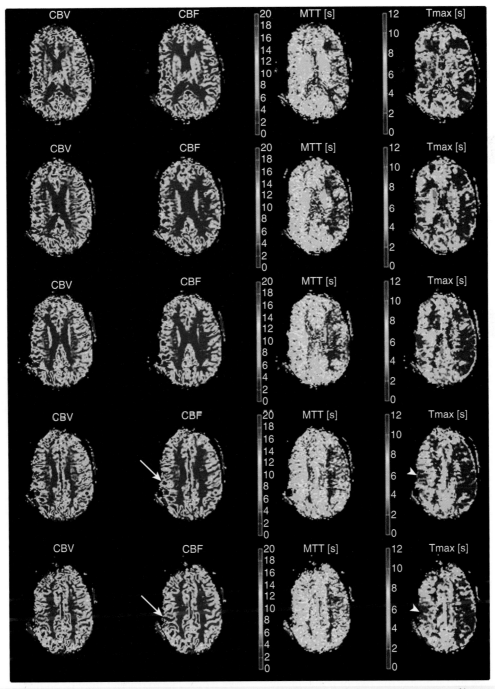

**Fig. 12.8** Postoperative hyperperfusion. Postoperative perfusion MRI after a direct STA–MCA graft demonstrating an area of hyperperfusion with high CBF (*arrow*) and low Tmax (*arrowhead*) in the right MCA territory supplied by the graft.

deficits. In one, it is believed that the deficits are due to CHS, and the mainstay treatment is primarily aimed at decreasing perfusion to the hyperperfused area.[7] It is thought that due to the altered cerebrovascular autoregulation in MMD after bypass, CBF in the area of the graft is reflective of systemic blood pressure, and thus treatment of CHS consists of decreasing blood pressure. In a series of 144 patients who underwent surgical revascularization, patients who experienced CHS trended toward higher postoperative MAP.[28] There are, however, no specific known MAP parameters to avoid CHS. Generally, systolic blood pressure (SBP) of 90 to 140 mm Hg is targeted.[42] Normotension is maintained using nicardipine, esmolol, and/or nitroprusside infusions as needed in the immediate postoperative period, transitioning to oral antihypertensives in the subsequent days, if needed. Blood pressure is lowered further if a patient has persistent clinical and imaging characteristics consistent with CHS, with the goal of avoiding intracranial hemorrhage (ICH). In rare instances, for persistent CHS refractory to blood pressure control, propofol coma has been used.[43] At the most extreme, STA ligation has been used for severe CHS.[36] For patients manifesting with seizure due to CHS, antiepileptic therapy is indicated, along with EEG monitoring if there is concern for subclinical status epilepticus. Significant edema or hemorrhage associated with CHS may require hyperosmolar therapy and/or surgical intervention.

The other school of thought is that patients with postoperative neurological deficits (transient or permanent) actually have decreased perfusion, and this can be demonstrated on MRI or Xe-CT in some areas (ipsilateral or contralateral to the direct bypass), raising the possibility of competing flows between native collaterals and the bypass. In these situations the MAP is raised to a higher range than normally required. It is believed that local hypoperfusion is the cause of the deficit on the backdrop of impaired autoregulation and a fluctuating blood flow, contrary to the traditional view that attributes these to hyperperfusion.[43,44]

Prognosis after CHS without ICH is usually good. The neurological deficits are often transient and usually resolve within ~2 weeks. Although the transient neurological deficits attributed to CHS usually completely resolve, it is unclear what the long-term effects are. Hirooka et al. showed that CHS after carotid endarterectomy was a predictor of cognitive dysfunction in patients 1 month after surgery.[43] Finally, in a series of patients with CHS after carotid endarterectomy or carotid stenting, the presence of ICH increased the mortality rate from 3% to 26%,[42] but similar data with MMD patients are lacking.

## SUBDURAL/EPIDURAL HEMATOMA

Subdural hematoma (SDH) is a rare complication, occurring anywhere from 2 weeks to 2 months postoperatively.[45] Risk factors include preoperative brain atrophy, as well as the presence of a postoperative subdural effusion from a cerebrospinal fluid leak. It has been suggested that postoperative anticoagulation or antiplatelet therapy also contributes to the development of SDH, particularly when dual antiplatelet agents are used. However, the incidence of SDH is low enough that the risk of postoperative aspirin is outweighed by the benefit of maintaining graft patency.

Epidural hematoma is another significant complication. In pediatric MMD patients who underwent indirect bypasses, epidural hematoma was detected in 12.8% of patients, requiring surgical intervention in 4.8%.[46] These hematomas consist of blood between the inserted galeal flap of the indirect bypass and the overlying skull flap and were felt to be due to injury of fine moyamoya collaterals in the brain periphery. Intraoperative insertion of a subcutaneous drain may decrease the likelihood of postoperative epidural hematoma.

Symptoms of epidural and subdural hematomas are often nonspecific and include alteration of mental status, nausea, vomiting, weakness, and dysarthria, which may also be seen with postoperative cerebral ischemia. Epidural and subdural hematomas can be easily identified by noncontrast CT and may require surgical drainage or craniotomy, depending on the size and clinical symptoms; however, as mentioned earlier, many of these hematomas are managed conservatively.

## WOUND DEHISCENCE

Scalp ischemia from diversion of blood flow in surgery is unlikely, but if present could lead to necrosis of scalp edges, wound dehiscence, and poor healing. This has not been extensively described and is a rare complication.

## SYSTEMIC COMPLICATIONS

Systemic postoperative complications are possible after any invasive surgery. Fevers >24 hours after surgery warrant a standard infectious workup, including blood and urine cultures, chest radiograph, and assessment of the wound. Wound infection should be considered for any prolonged postoperative fever and may ultimately require removal of an infected bone flap.[47] Myocardial infarction can occur, particularly in older MMD patients who may have coronary artery disease. Aspiration is a risk, particularly in patients whose baseline neurological disease may have caused swallowing difficulties. DVT or pulmonary emboli are a risk to any patient in the hospital and should be avoided by early ambulation, sequential compression devices, and prophylactic anticoagulation in nonambulatory patients as soon as deemed safe from a surgical perspective.

# Conclusion

Bypass procedures are the mainstay of treatment for MMD and may be considered in complex brain tumor or cerebral aneurysm cases. These surgeries may be done directly or indirectly, and each approach has its particular advantages and disadvantages. These procedures are complex and may require sophisticated neuroimaging and advanced neuromonitoring. Thorough understanding of CBF and autoregulation is compulsory to care best for these patients.

# Acknowledgments

We would like to thank Cindy H. Samos for help with preparation of the manuscript and Elizabeth E. Hoyte for help with preparation of the figures.

# Funding Disclosures

Josef Huber Family Moyamoya Fund, Stanley and Alexis Shin, Reddy Lee Moyamoya Fund, William Randolph Hearst Foundation, Bernard and Ronni Lacroute, Russell and Elizabeth Siegelman (to GKS).

## References

1. Powers WJ, Clarke WR, Grubb Jr RL, et al. Extracranial-intracranial bypass surgery for stroke prevention in hemodynamic cerebral ischemia: the Carotid Occlusion Surgery Study randomized trial. *JAMA.* 2011;306(18):1983–1992.
2. Ryan RW, Chowdhary A, Britz GW. Hemorrhage and risk of further hemorrhagic strokes following cerebral revascularization in Moyamoya disease: a review of the literature. *Surg Neurol Int.* 2012;3:72.
3. Achrol AS, Guzman R, Lee M, et al. Pathophysiology and genetic factors in moyamoya disease. *Neurosurg Focus.* 2009;26(4):E4. [Research Support, Non-U.S. Gov't Review].
4. Kuriyama S, Kusaka Y, Fujimura M, et al. Prevalence and clinicoepidemiological features of moyamoya disease in Japan: findings from a nationwide epidemiological survey. *Stroke.* 2008;39(1):42–47. [Comparative Study Research Support, Non-U.S. Gov't].
5. Kanamaru K, Araki T, Kawakita F, et al. STA-MCA bypass for the treatment of ischemic stroke. *Acta Neurochir Suppl.* 2011;112:55–57.
6. Kuroda S, Houkin K, Kamiyama H, et al. Regional cerebral hemodynamics in childhood moyamoya disease. *Childs Nerv Syst.* 1995;11(10):584–590.
7. Pandey P, Steinberg GK. Neurosurgical advances in the treatment of moyamoya disease. *Stroke.* 2011;42(11):3304–3310.
8. Lee M, Zaharchuk G, Guzman R, et al. Quantitative hemodynamic studies in moyamoya disease: a review. *Neurosurg Focus.* 2009;26(4):E5.
9. Touho H, Karasawa J, Ohnishi H. Preoperative and postoperative evaluation of cerebral perfusion and vasodilatory capacity with 99mTc-HMPAO SPECT and acetazolamide in childhood Moyamoya disease. *Stroke.* 1996;27(2):282–289.
10. Karzmark P, Zeifert PD, Tan S, et al. Effect of moyamoya disease on neuropsychological functioning in adults. *Neurosurgery.* 2008;62(5):1048–1051. discussion 51–52.
11. Mogensen MA, Karzmark P, Zeifert PD, et al. Neuroradiologic correlates of cognitive impairment in adult Moyamoya disease. *AJNR.* 2012;33(4):721–725.
12. Guzman R, Lee M, Achrol A, et al. Clinical outcome after 450 revascularization procedures for moyamoya disease. Clinical article. *J Neurosurg.* 2009;111(5):927–935. [Research Support, Non-U.S. Gov't].
13. Bernard S, Buist M, Monteiro O, et al. Induced hypothermia using large volume, ice-cold intravenous fluid in comatose survivors of out-of-hospital cardiac arrest: a preliminary report. *Resuscitation.* 2003;56(1):9–13.
14. Polderman KH, Rijnsburger ER, Peerdeman SM, et al. Induction of hypothermia in patients with various types of neurologic injury with use of large volumes of ice-cold intravenous fluid. *Crit Care Med.* 2005;33(12):2744–2751.
15. Amin-Hanjani S, Singh A, Rifai H, et al. Combined direct and indirect bypass for moyamoya: quantitative assessment of direct bypass flow over time. *Neurosurgery.* 2013;73(6):962–967. discussion 7–8.
16. Charbel FT, Meglio G, Amin-Hanjani S. Superficial temporal artery-to-middle cerebral artery bypass. *Neurosurgery.* 2005;56(1 Suppl):186–190. discussion 186–190.
17. Lee M, Guzman R, Bell-Stephens T, et al. Intraoperative blood flow analysis of direct revascularization procedures in patients with moyamoya disease. *J Cereb Blood Flow Metab.* 2011;31(1):262–274.
18. Mizoi K, Kayama T, Yoshimoto T, et al. Indirect revascularization for moyamoya disease: is there a beneficial effect for adult patients? *Surg Neurol.* 1996;45(6):541–548. discussion 8–9. [Comparative Study].
19. Kang HS, Kim JH, Phi JH, et al. Plasma matrix metalloproteinases, cytokines and angiogenic factors in moyamoya disease. *J Neurol Neurosurg Psychiatry.* 2010;81(6):673–678. [Research Support, Non-U.S. Gov't].
20. Lim M, Cheshier S, Steinberg GK. New vessel formation in the central nervous system during tumor growth, vascular malformations, and Moyamoya. *Curr Neurovasc Res.* 2006;3(3):237–245. [Research Support, Non-U.S. Gov't Review].
21. Yoshimoto T, Houkin K, Takahashi A, et al. Angiogenic factors in moyamoya disease. *Stroke.* 1996;27(12):2160–2165.
22. Patel NN, Mangano FT, Klimo Jr P. Indirect revascularization techniques for treating moyamoya disease. *Neurosurg Clin N Am.* 2010;21(3):553–563. [Review].
23. Kim CY, Wang KC, Kim SK, et al. Encephaloduroarteriosynangiosis with bifrontal encephalogaleo(periosteal)synangiosis in the pediatric moyamoya disease: the surgical technique and its outcomes. *Childs Nerv Syst.* 2003;19(5–6):316–324. [Research Support, Non-U.S. Gov't].
24. Kinugasa K, Mandai S, Tokunaga K, et al. Ribbon enchephalo-duro-arterio-myo-synangiosis for moyamoya disease. *Surg Neurol.* 1994;41(6):455–461. [Case Reports].
25. Scott RM, Smith JL, Robertson RL, et al. Long-term outcome in children with moyamoya syndrome after cranial revascularization by pial synangiosis. *J Neurosurg.* 2004;100(2 Suppl Pediatrics):142–149. [Research Support, Non-U.S. Gov't].
26. Navarro R, Chao K, Gooderham PA, et al. Less invasive pedicled omental-cranial transposition in pediatric patients with moyamoya disease and failed prior revascularization. *Neurosurgery.* 2014;10(Suppl 1):1–14.
27. Reynolds MR, Grubb Jr RL, Clarke WR, et al. Investigating the mechanisms of perioperative ischemic stroke in the Carotid Occlusion Surgery Study. *J Neurosurg.* 2013;119(4):988–995.
28. Hayashi T, Shirane R, Fujimura M, et al. Postoperative neurological deterioration in pediatric moyamoya disease: watershed shift and hyperperfusion. *J Neurosurg Pediatr.* 2010;6(1):73–81.
29. Hyun SJ, Kim JS, Hong SC. Prognostic factors associated with perioperative ischemic complications in adult-onset moyamoya disease. *Acta Neurochir.* 2010;152(7):1181–1188.
30. Mesiwala AH, Sviri G, Fatemi N, et al. Long-term outcome of superficial temporal artery-middle cerebral artery bypass for patients with moyamoya disease in the US. *Neurosurg Focus.* 2008;24(2):E15.
31. Schubert GA, Biermann P, Weiss C, et al. Risk Profile in extracranial/intracranial bypass surgery-the role of antiplatelet agents, disease pathology, and surgical technique in 168 direct revascularization procedures. *World Neurosurg.* 2013 Nov;82(5):672–677. http://dx.doi.org/10.1016/j.wneu.2013.06.010. Epub 2013 Jul 6.
32. Dorfmuller G, Sollmann WP, Lorenz M, et al. Hemodynamic and electrophysiological evaluation following extracranial/intracranial bypass surgery. *Neurosurg Rev.* 1992;15(3):165–169.
33. Nakamura T, Iwata Y. Postoperative evaluation of EC/IC bypass surgery—long-term follow up study by donor artery compression test. *No Shinkei Geka.* 2000;28(12):1057–1062.
34. Coutts SB, Hill MD, Hu WY. Hyperperfusion syndrome: toward a stricter definition. *Neurosurgery.* 2003;53(5):1053–1058. discussion 8–60.
35. van Mook WN, Rennenberg RJ, Schurink GW, et al. Cerebral hyperperfusion syndrome. *Lancet Neurol.* 2005;4(12):877–888.
36. Fujimura M, Mugikura S, Kaneta T, et al. Incidence and risk factors for symptomatic cerebral hyperperfusion after superficial temporal artery-middle cerebral artery anastomosis in patients with moyamoya disease. *Surg Neurol.* 2009;71(4):442–447.
37. Yamaguchi K, Kawamata T, Kawashima A, et al. Incidence and predictive factors of cerebral hyperperfusion after extracranial-intracranial bypass for occlusive cerebrovascular diseases. *Neurosurgery.* 2010;67(6):1548–1554. discussion 54.
38. Fujimura M, Shimizu H, Inoue T, et al. Significance of focal cerebral hyperperfusion as a cause of transient neurologic deterioration after extracranial-intracranial bypass for moyamoya disease: comparative study with non-moyamoya patients using N-isopropyl-p-[(123)I]iodoamphetamine single-photon emission computed tomography. *Neurosurgery.* 2011;68(4):957–964. discussion 64–65.
39. Hosoda K, Kawaguchi T, Ishii K, et al. Prediction of hyperperfusion after carotid endarterectomy by brain SPECT analysis with semiquantitative statistical mapping method. *Stroke.* 2003;34(5):1187–1193.
40. Komoribayashi N, Ogasawara K, Kobayashi M, et al. Cerebral hyperperfusion after carotid endarterectomy is associated with preoperative hemodynamic impairment and intraoperative cerebral ischemia. *J Cereb Blood Flow Metab.* 2006;26(7):878–884.
41. Zhao WG, Luo Q, Jia JB, et al. Cerebral hyperperfusion syndrome after revascularization surgery in patients with moyamoya disease. *Br J Neurosurg.* 2013;27(3):321–325.
42. Ogasawara K, Sakai N, Kuroiwa T, et al. Intracranial hemorrhage associated with cerebral hyperperfusion syndrome following carotid endarterectomy and carotid artery stenting: retrospective review of 4494 patients. *J Neurosurg.* 2007;107(6):1130–1136.

43. Hirooka R, Ogasawara K, Sasaki M, et al. Magnetic resonance imaging in patients with cerebral hyperperfusion and cognitive impairment after carotid endarterectomy. *J Neurosurg.* 2008;108(6):1178–1183.

44. Mukerji N, Cook DJ, Steinberg GK. Is local hypoperfusion the reason for transient neurological deficits after STA-MCA bypass for moyamoya disease? *J Neurosurg.* 2015;122(1):90–94.

45. Andoh T, Sakai N, Yamada H, et al. Chronic subdural hematoma following bypass surgery: report of three cases. *Neurol Med Chir.* 1992;32(9):684–689.

46. Choi H, Lee JY, Phi JH, et al. Postoperative epidural hematoma covering the galeal flap in pediatric patients with moyamoya disease: clinical manifestation, risk factors, and outcomes. *J Neurosurg Pediatr.* 2013;12(2):181–186.

47. Matsushima Y, Aoyagi M, Suzuki R, et al. Perioperative complications of encephalo-duro-arterio-synangiosis: prevention and treatment. *Surg Neurol.* 1991;36(5):343–353.

# 13 Evacuation of Intracerebral Hemorrhages

JAMES E. SIEGLER, PATRICIA ZADNIK, H. ISAAC CHEN, and SHIH-SHAN LANG

## Introduction

Intracerebral hemorrhage (ICH) is a devastating subtype of stroke with a high rate of morbidity and mortality. Multiple studies have established the need for careful blood pressure control[1] and dedicated neurocritical care; however, the role for surgical decompression and hematoma evacuation has been debated.[2–6] This is partially due to the inherent heterogeneity of the patient population, as well as the expanding use of oral anticoagulants. Furthermore, ICH may be associated with devastating neurological sequelae, and patient goals of care and quality of life should be considered prior to intervention.[7] In this chapter, we review the neurosurgical and neuromedical approaches for the various etiologies and locations of ICH, as well as literature guiding surgical decision making for patients with ICH.

## Neuroanatomy and Procedure

### Key Concepts

- ICH is found within the brain tissue (or ventricle for intraventricular hemorrhage [IVH]).
- ICH, from hypertensive vasculopathy, is typically found in the basal ganglia (putamen/caudate), thalamus, pons, cerebellum, and subcortical white matter.

### ANATOMY AND PATHOLOGY

ICH is found within the brain tissue, whereas epidural, subdural, and subarachnoid hemorrhages are found outside of brain tissue. Clinical presentation is variable depending on the location of the hemorrhage. Hematoma in the basal ganglia or thalamus may present with contralateral sensorimotor deficit. Pontine hemorrhage typically presents with coma and pinpoint pupils due to damage within the reticular activating system. Cerebellar hemorrhage manifests as vertigo/dizziness, ataxia, and nausea/vomiting and also may cause hydrocephalus due to compression of the fourth ventricle.[8]

Spontaneous ICH (sICH) is most commonly caused by hypertensive vasculopathy and cerebral amyloid angiopathy but may also be due to other etiologies (Table 13.1). Hypertensive vasculopathy is generally thought to be due to intimal hyperplasia and lipohyalinosis of penetrating arteries, which leads to focal necrosis and ultimately rupture of the vessel wall. This type of vasculopathy typically affects vessels supplying the thalamus, putamen, caudate, pons, midbrain, and cerebellum. Cerebral amyloid angiopathy is characterized by amyloid beta peptide deposits within small to medium-sized blood vessels. These deposits preferentially affect cortical vessels and thus predispose to lobar hemorrhages.[9,10]

The size, location, and intraventricular extension dictate surgical approach, and intraparenchymal hemorrhage often necessitates craniotomy for access to the lesion of interest. In sICH with associated intracranial hypertension, decompressive hemicraniectomy is a life-saving approach to improve cerebral perfusion and subsequent ischemia.[11]

Enlargement of the hematoma is associated with neurological deterioration and worse outcomes. These observations indicate that significant improvements in patient outcome from ICH may be achieved by minimizing both secondary brain ischemia and hematoma enlargement. Computed tomography angiography has been shown to identify the "spot sign," which is a focal area of enhancement within hematomas. Studies show that this sign is associated with expansion of the hematoma, which leads to worse clinical outcomes.[12,13]

Hematoma enlargement also commonly occurs in anticoagulant-related hemorrhages. Conventional anticoagulation (i.e., warfarin) increases the risk of any ICH up to 10 times.[14] Some studies show that reversing the anticoagulation effect improves the outcome of warfarin-related ICH in terms of preventing neurological deterioration and hematoma expansion.[15] However, other studies show the rate of hematoma expansion in ICH patients taking anticoagulation is similar to nonanticoagulated ICH patients.[16] As a standard of care for all patients with ICH, it is important to immediately reverse the anticoagulation effects to prevent hematoma enlargement.

Surgical intervention for spontaneous supratentorial ICH has been studied extensively in the literature, with a recent series of randomized controlled clinical trials comparing the efficacy of surgical intervention versus optimal medical management for patients with intracerebral hemorrhage.[5,6] The Surgical Trial in Intracerebral Haemorrhage (STICH) compared outcomes of patients with spontaneous supratentorial ICH who received conservative medical management in a neurocritical care unit with patients undergoing early surgical intervention (mostly craniotomy and evacuation) and concluded that there was no overall benefit for patients receiving early surgery compared with initial conservative treatment.[5] This study was the first to utilize rigorous, randomized controlled trial methods to evaluate ICH outcomes; however, there was a 26% crossover rate for patients originally randomized to the initial conservative management group. Despite the failure of randomization, the results suggested a potential

**Table 13.1** Anatomical Sites of ICH

| Etiology of ICH | Anatomical Predilection |
| --- | --- |
| *Hypertension* | Deep gray nuclei, brainstem, cerebellar, lobar |
| *Trauma* | Cortical/lobar |
| *Coagulopathy* | Lobar, cerebellar |
| *Vascular* | |
|   Conversion of ischemic infarction | Deep gray nuclei, brainstem, cerebellar, lobar |
|   Amyloid angiopathy | Lobar, deep gray nuclei |
|   AVM/cavernoma/AVF/aneurysm | Cortical/lobar, deep gray nuclei, cerebellar, brainstem |
|   Venous sinus thrombosis | Cortical/lobar, thalamic (straight sinus, vein of Galen) |
| *Neoplastic* | |
|   Secondary: lung carcinoma, breast, renal cell, melanoma, choriocarcinoma, papillary thyroid carcinoma | Juxtacortical/lobar, cerebellar |
|   Primary: glioblastoma multiforme, glioma | Lobar |
| *Infectious* | |
|   Septic emboli | Juxtacortical/lobar |
|   Herpes simplex virus encephalitis | Mesial temporal lobe(s) |
| *Toxicity* | |
|   Cocaine | Deep gray nuclei, brainstem, lobar |
|   Amphetamines | Deep gray nuclei, brainstem, lobar |

*ICH,* intracranial hemorrhage; *AVM,* arteriovenous malformation; *AVF,* arteriovenous fistula.

benefit for those patients with hemorrhagic lesions within 1 centimeter from the cortical surface. The high crossover rate and potential improvement for patients with lobar ICH led to STICH II. STICH II compared extended Glasgow Outcome Scale scores for patients undergoing early surgical evacuation within 12 hours plus medical therapy versus medical therapy alone.[6] The authors concluded that early surgery did not increase death or disability at 6 months and resulted in a small survival advantage for patients without IVH.[6]

## NEUROSURGICAL INTERVENTIONS

The primary surgical interventions for ICH are either cerebrospinal fluid (CSF) diversion with ventriculostomy, craniotomy with hematoma evacuation, or decompressive hemicraniectomy. Minimally invasive approaches to hematoma evacuation are alternative approaches to open surgical intervention and show promise as potential novel therapeutic options.

Craniotomy utilizes one or more burr holes connected via a high-speed air drill to create a bone flap. A burr hole involves drilling a single hole into the skull using a

pneumatic or handheld device at a region near the known hematoma. The bone flap is removed, and the hematoma is removed without opening the dura. The dura is typically reapproximated unless there is elevated intracranial pressure (ICP). The bone flap is replaced and secured in place with titanium or plastic plates and screws.

Decompressive craniectomy follows similar methods compared with the craniotomy described earlier, with creation of a bone flap by making several burr holes and connecting them with a pneumatic drill. The dura is subsequently incised in a cruciate or stellate fashion and left open or covered with a dural substitute such as Duragen (Integra LifeSciences, Plainsboro, NJ) to further reduce brain swelling and improve cerebral perfusion pressure (CPP). In contrast to craniotomy, the bone flap is then placed in the patient's abdomen or a bone bank for storage.[17] Studies suggest that a craniectomy at least 12 cm in diameter provides the greatest benefit for patients with elevated ICP.[18] In some cases, such as bilateral frontal lobe injury, bilateral frontal subdural hematoma, or diffuse injury, a bifrontal craniectomy may be performed.

In cases of ICH complicated by IVH, an external ventricular drain (EVD) is almost universally required for prevention or management of obstructive hydrocephalus. This device is coupled with an external pressure transducer for ICP monitoring. EVDs and other ICP monitors are also used to continuously illustrate ICP waveforms, which can be used to predict future alterations in ICP and even clinical deterioration in experienced hands.[19] EVDs are often preferred for ICP monitoring because they permit removal of CSF for the identification of its chemical contents and for the treatment of elevated ICP.[20]

Unfortunately, this device is limited largely by its risk of infections such as meningitis and ventriculitis, seen in up to 10% of patients, and this risk is greater for patients with ICH than other neurological conditions.[21] This device, as well as any other implantable ICP monitor, is also associated with a small risk of subdural and intraparenchymal hemorrhage during insertion.[22]

In ICH extending to the ventricular system, blood products can reduce CSF resorption, leading to obstructive hydrocephalus, and an EVD functions to divert CSF out of the brain. Further, hemorrhage size and initial Glasgow Coma Scale (GCS) correlate with 30-day mortality in patients with ICH[23]; thus efforts have been made to reduce hemorrhage size. Because an EVD offers direct access to the ventricular system, it can be used for the administration of therapeutic agents. In the CLEAR-IVH trial, authors studied the effect of intraventricular recombinant tissue plasminogen activator (rtPA) on clot lysis in patients with IVH.[24] Intraventricular rtPA, administered 12 to 24 hours after hemorrhage, was found to accelerate the radiographic resolution of IVH; however, the effectiveness varied by hemorrhage location, with greatest effectiveness on midline ventricles and with higher doses of rtPA.[25] Infusion of rtPA was least effective on hemorrhage clearance in the posterolateral ventricles.[25]

Minimally invasive methods of hematoma evacuation have been proposed as an alternative to open craniotomy. Stereotactic and endoscopic evacuation of hemorrhage, coupled with local administration of rtPA, have also been studied in the neurosurgical treatment of IVH.[26] In the Minimally Invasive Surgery plus rtPA for Intracerebral

Hemorrhage Evacuation (MISTIE) trial, patients received rtPA via EVD followed by endoscopic hematoma aspiration.[24] The investigators reported a reduction in mean clot size of 46% in the treatment group compared with 4% in the medical management group.[24] In MISTIE-II, investigators also found a reduction in perihemorrhage edema in patients undergoing surgical evacuation of IVH.[26] Although these results are encouraging, these trials have been powered to assess treatment safety and efficacy, and no survival benefit has been demonstrated to date.

## POSTERIOR FOSSA HEMORRHAGE

As in the case of supratentorial hemorrhage, posterior fossa hemorrhage (PFH) is caused by hypertension in 60% to 90% of cases.[27] PFH may also be related to traumatic injury or vascular malformations. Cerebellar hemorrhages are occasionally reported in patients after supratentorial surgery, spinal surgery, and in patients with spontaneous intracranial hypotension.[1,2] The mechanism is thought to be removal of large amounts of CSF or continuing CSF leak from a dural breach. The hemorrhage is remote from the surgical site or anatomical defect and may result from transient occlusion or rupture of superior cerebellar bridging veins. Rarely, cerebellar ICH may be related to metastases. Among metastatic tumors that produce ICH, lung adenocarcinoma and melanoma are the most common, accounting for over one-quarter of all intracranial metastases regardless of hemorrhage.[9] In contrast, metastatic lesions that carry a higher propensity of hemorrhage include choriocarcinoma, papillary thyroid carcinoma, and renal cell carcinoma; however, these lesions are less frequently encountered.[10]

Location of the hemorrhage (midline vs. hemispheric) is important in determining symptoms and clinical course. Location may be more important than absolute hematoma size for prognosis. Generally speaking, the more lateral the hemorrhage and the smaller the hematoma, the more likely the brainstem structures are spared and the better the prognosis.[27]

Surgical management for PFH involves bilateral suboccipital craniectomy (SOC) for decompression of the brainstem, with or without EVD placement, to treat obstructive hydrocephalus from fourth ventricle compression. Current evidence guiding surgical decision making comprises case series and clinical practice guidelines, as PFH are generally excluded from randomized controlled trials due to the lack of clinical equipoise.[4,5] Current literature supports aggressive surgical intervention for patients with grade III fourth ventricular compression with complete obliteration of the fourth ventricle or distortion of the brainstem,[28] or intracerebellar hemorrhage diameter greater than 40 mm and GCS $\leq$13.[4] In patients with flaccid tetraplegia and severe brainstem or ventricular compression, surgical intervention is unlikely to improve outcome.[4,28,3,22,29]

SOC is the approach of choice for PFH and proceeds via a midline incision at the posterior aspect of the neck. A bone flap typically extends from the foramen magnum upwards toward the torcula, and the posterior ring of C1 may be removed for greater exposure.[30] The dura is incised for access to the hematoma, which is then evacuated with irrigation and suctioning. Unlike supratentorial hematomas, the bone flap is typically not replaced at the time of surgery or later.

## Perioperative Considerations

### Key Concepts

- Initial management of ICH includes airway protection, hemodynamic stabilization, and consideration of advanced neurological monitoring and/or neurosurgical intervention.
- In cases of anticoagulant-associated ICH, the underlying coagulopathy should be rapidly reversed in order to facilitate surgical intervention, prevent hematoma expansion, and mitigate neurological deterioration.

Initial medical management of ICH relies on hemodynamic and ventilatory support to promote adequate organ perfusion and function.[22] Admission to a neurocritical care unit equipped with all necessary resources and manned with appropriately trained personnel improves mortality in this patient population.[31] Strict blood pressure goals must be set because elevation may cause ICH progression, herniation, or even death.[1] However, caution should be exercised because rapid reduction of arterial blood pressure may lead to cerebral ischemia. Invasive monitoring using an arterial catheter allows for continuous assessment of blood pressure changes. Fever is commonly observed in ICH and may be central in origin or due to medical complications of ICH (e.g., pneumonia, urinary tract infection, deep vein thrombosis; see Table 13.2). Although there are no randomized trials to support targeted temperature management or therapeutic cooling, maintenance of normothermia should be achieved in these patients because fever is significantly associated with greater mortality.[32]

### Clinical Pearl

Early admission to a Neuro ICU prevents mortality in cases of ICH.

Many patients with ICH may require intubation due to altered mentation, irregular respiratory patterns (e.g., Kussmaul's or Cheyne-Stoke respirations), and impaired clearance of secretions. In acute or chronic hypertension, evaluation for other signs of end organ damage, especially renal and cardiac injury, should be assessed using serological and electrocardiographic assessment. Hematologic parameters must also be checked to ensure normal platelet count and coagulation function, the alterations of which may increase the likelihood for rebleeding.

Hyperglycemia is associated with deleterious outcomes in ICH.[33] However, tight glucose control has not been proven effective in the neurocritical care of patients with ICH because it may precipitate systemic hypoglycemia. There are no guidelines for targeted glucose management in ICH, but in the authors' experience, a liberal blood glucose goal (160–180 mg/dL) is a safe and effective approach

**Table 13.2** Associated Medical and Neurological Complications

**Complications of ICH**

*Neurological*

Hemorrhagic expansion

Cerebral edema with/without herniation

Intracranial hypertension

Obstructive hydrocephalus

Hematoma after ICH clot evacuation

Stroke

*Medical*

Nosocomial infections

Ventilator-associated pneumonia

Indwelling urethral catheter–associated urinary tract infection

Central venous catheter–associated bacteremia

Ventriculitis/meningitis due to intracranial pressure monitoring

Cellulitis/wound infection due to EVD placement or craniotomy/craniectomy

Fever

Infection

Fever due to deep venous thrombosis

Central nervous system fever

Vasculitis

End organ dysfunction

Acute kidney injury

Ventilator-dependent respiratory failure

Congestive heart failure exacerbation

Delirium

Delirium due to metabolic abnormalities or infection

ICU delirium

Pharmacological delirium

Intoxication or withdrawal of substances of abuse

*ICH*, intracranial hemorrhage; *EVD*, external ventricular drain; *ICU*, intensive care unit.

to critically ill patients with ICH. The use of insulin infusions may be considered on a case-by-case basis but should not be routinely implemented.

## HEMOSTASIS

Correction of an underlying coagulopathy should be performed within the first several hours of ictus and is a standard of care.[22] Platelet counts less than 10,000/mL may contribute to spontaneous ICH in otherwise healthy individuals and ought to be treated with transfusion to prevent major bleeding.[34] The most common causes of platelet dysfunction are platelet inhibitors such as aspirin, and this warrants correction with platelet transfusion in ICH. Other causes of platelet dysfunction, such as uremia, do not have guidelines in place for cases of ICH. Desmopressin is not strongly supported in these instances but may be considered.[35]

Defects in the coagulation cascade (genetic or acquired hemophilia) should be corrected with specific factor replacement or treatment of the underlying cause of acquired hemophilia (e.g., plasma exchange or intravenous steroids may be considered in the setting of autoantibodies toward procoagulant factors).[36] Hepatic insufficiency may produce a mixed coagulopathy/thrombophilia. Although coagulation markers may be abnormal in patients with underlying liver failure and ICH, there are limited data to support the efficacy of treating these laboratory abnormalities. One in eight cases of ICH are attributed to oral anticoagulant use, and this may be rising with the use of newer oral anticoagulants, such as direct thrombin inhibitors.[37] It is imperative to recognize coagulopathies and correct them as rapidly as possible.

Vitamin K antagonists (VKAs), such as warfarin, have long been heralded as the number-one culprit for iatrogenic coagulopathic ICH. For patients on VKAs, the historical recommendation had been to correct the international normalized ratio (INR) to <1.3 within 2 hours using fresh frozen plasma (FFP) and IV vitamin K.[38] FFP is advantageous in that it contains all the human procoagulant factors, specifically those whose production are directly inhibited by VKAs. However, there are many limitations of FFP treatment, including transfusion reactions and infections. Additionally, the volume of FFP required to reverse coagulopathy may result in transfusion-associated circulatory overload or transfusion-related lung injury. Furthermore, because plasma is stored in a frozen state, it needs to be thawed prior to infusion, increasing the time to medication delivery, and thus reversal.

The current recommendation for reversal of life-threatening VKA-related hemorrhages is 4-factor PCC (prothrombin complex concentrate), which contains the four procoagulant factors inhibited by VKAs (II, VII, IX, X) in combination with 5 to 10 mg of IV vitamin K.[39] When reconstituted, the volume is quite small, which allows for rapid preparation and infusion. It also does not have effects on mean arterial pressure (MAP), as do large volumes of FFP. In comparison to FFP, which may take several hours to achieve INR normalization, 4 F-PCC has been shown to reverse VKAs in minutes.[40] Recombinant FVIIa is another alternative for reversing coagulopathic ICH; however, it is associated with a higher risk of thrombotic complications and confers no significant survival benefit to placebo.[41]

### Clinical Pearl

Prothrombin complex concentrate is the preferred reversal agent for warfarin or rivaroxaban-induced ICH.

Data regarding factor Xa inhibitors (rivaroxaban, apixaban, and edoxaban) have demonstrated a superiority to VKA in (1) the prevention of ischemic stroke in nonvalvular atrial fibrillation, (2) risk of anticoagulant-associated ICH, and (3) all-cause mortality.[42] The data regarding appropriate reversal agents in humans are scant; animal data demonstrate mixed results regarding the benefit of PCC over activated PCC, factor eight inhibitor bypassing agent.[43] Currently, there are no data to support reversal efficacy in apixaban-related ICH.

Reversal of unfractionated heparin is achieved with protamine sulfate at a dose of 1 mg protamine for every 100 U of IV heparin, with a maximum dose of 50 mg. Reversal of IV bolus or infusion is warranted; prophylactic doses do not require reversal. The goal of treatment is to normalize the partial thromboplastin time (PTT) per the institution's laboratory standards and stop bleeding. PTTs should be serially assessed over the first 6 hours of reversal given the half-life of heparin. Low-molecular-weight heparins are thought to be less responsive to protamine sulfate during reversal attempts.

Dabigatran is a direct thrombin inhibitor used in secondary stroke prevention in patients with nonvalvular atrial fibrillation.[44] Previously, the only option to reverse dabigatran was hemodialysis in the event of an emergency. This requires insertion of a large-bore dialysis catheter, which may take time and carries a high risk of secondary hemorrhage in the patient who is already coagulopathic. Recently idarucizumab has been approved by the Food and Drug Administration as a monoclonal antibody reversal agent for dabigatran and has been shown to effectively reverse the anticoagulant effect of dabigatran.[45,46]

> ### Clinical Pearl
>
> There is evidence for surgical intervention for a subset of patients with ICH; however, an open discussion regarding goals of care and patient quality of life is appropriate in all patients with ICH.

> ### Clinical Pearl
>
> In ICH patients receiving conservative management prior to planned surgical intervention, close monitoring in a Neuro ICU is important to improve clinical outcome.

When medical management has failed to prevent significant neurological deterioration in ICH, surgical management may be necessary. Hemorrhage increases ICP, which decreases cerebral perfusion, thus resulting in delayed ischemic changes in the penumbra surrounding the initial hematoma if it is not evacuated. Once identified, surgical management reduces ICP through removal of the hematoma, bone, or both to reduce compression on the brain parenchyma in an effort to reduce cerebral edema. Access to the hematoma may be through a burr hole, craniotomy, or craniectomy. Hematoma removal involves drainage or irrigation, with or without placement of a drain. Reversal of oral anticoagulation is recommended to slow hematoma

expansion and improve intraoperative hemostasis prior to surgical intervention.[22]

## Postoperative ICU Management

> ### Key Concepts
>
> - In facilities with appropriately trained personnel and adequate resources, invasive ICP monitoring and treatment are recommended for a goal ICP <20 cm H$_2$O.
> - ICP may be reduced via reduction in central nervous system metabolic demand (e.g., sedation), hyperventilation, osmotic therapy (e.g., mannitol or hypertonic saline), and neurosurgical decompression.

### ICP MONITORING

Although the neurocritical management of ICH is largely based on standard critical care practices as stated earlier, the neuromedical aspects focus on physiological principles behind ICP management. In adults, elevated ICP can be loosely defined as >15 to 20 cm H$_2$O when the patient is lying in the lateral decubitus position.[20] The current practice of invasive ICP monitoring as a means to determine management in ICH and other neurocritical care scenarios remains extensively debated. ICP is traditionally monitored using an EVD, as described earlier.[47] The use of a Licox Brain Oxygen Monitoring System (Integra LifeSciences, Plainsboro, NJ) may provide added insight into hypoxic injury after ICH,[48] but its ability to improve outcomes after ICH has not been fully explored in prospective trials. Currently, experts recommend invasive ICP monitoring at centers where this is performed on a routine basis and clinicians are experienced at the interpretation and management of alterations in ICP. In cases where subtle changes early in the course of a patient's care may alter emergent treatment decisions, these changes may be detected early by using invasive monitoring devices.

> ### Clinical Pearl
>
> In experienced hands, invasive ICP monitoring may improve outcome in ICH.

With few exceptions (e.g., infants whose cranial sutures have not yet closed), the calvarium can be considered a rigid container enclosing a fixed volume of contents. In comparison, fluid and other soft tissues within the cranial vault are somewhat more compliant and may be slightly compressible with rising pressure changes.[20] However, the compressibility of neural parenchyma and surrounding fluid is trivial, rendering the pressure/volume adaptability of these tissues clinically negligible.[20] These theoretically distensible and compressible intracranial contents include three main components: brain, arterial and venous blood, and CSF. The Monro-Kellie doctrine states that because the volume of the cranial vault remains constant, any change in ICP or volume of a single intracranial component will produce a change in volume of the remaining components.

$$CPP = MAP - ICP$$

When represented mathematically, ICP is equivalent to MAP minus the CPP.[20] This simple formula is of paramount importance in neurocritical care because it demonstrates the dynamic nature of CPP as it is affected by changes in ICP and systemic arterial pressure. Any increase in ICP or reduction in systemic blood pressure will effectively reduce cerebral perfusion. Conversely, any reduction in ICP or rise in blood pressure will increase cerebral perfusion.

The relationship between MAP and CPP is not linear. Autoregulatory mechanisms within the central nervous system permit a stable CPP while MAP fluctuates (Fig. 13.1), except in certain conditions of impaired autoregulation such as ICH. These mechanisms remain highly effective except in situations of extreme hypotension (MAP <50 mm Hg) or hypertension (MAP >150 mm Hg) and intracranial insult producing autonomic disruption.[49]

## MANAGEMENT OF INTRACRANIAL HYPERTENSION

In the event of elevated ICP, the CPP should be kept at a goal of 60 to 150 mm Hg in order to preserve susceptible neural parenchyma.[22] The artificial augmentation of CPP may only affect cerebral blood flow when (1) cerebral autoregulation has failed (e.g., acute ischemic stroke or ICH) or (2) CPP is too low for cerebral autoregulatory mechanisms to compensate (e.g., distributive shock in the setting of sepsis). Goal ICP should be <20 cm $H_2O$. The head of bed

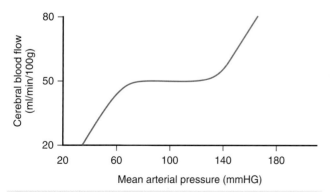

**Fig. 13.1** Logarithmic relationship between mean arterial pressure and cerebral blood flow with dynamic autoregulation. (Adapted from Peterson E, Chesnut RM. Static autoregulation is intact in majority of patients with severe traumatic brain injury. *J Trauma.* 2009;67:944–949.)

should be raised to >30 degrees, and the patient's neck should be midline in order to optimize jugular venous drainage. Metabolic demands of the central nervous system should be reduced—for example, fevers controlled, seizures treated with antiepileptic agents, etc. In patients who have indwelling EVDs that permit drainage of CSF, CSF removal should be considered.

For patients with elevated ICP, intubation and sedation should be considered first. Hypocarbia hyperventilation leads to cerebral vasoconstriction, which temporarily reduces cerebral blood flow and decreases ICP. This may be used as a bridge to more definitive therapy.[50] Deep sedation with propofol or barbiturates while intubated confers a secondary benefit of also reducing cerebral activity, which can reduce ICP.[22] The mainstay of treatments for intractable elevated ICP includes hyperosmolar therapy, namely mannitol or hypertonic saline (HTS) infusions. Mannitol is typically considered a first-line pharmacological agent for elevated ICP, except in the case of renal insufficiency, where it is relatively contraindicated. HTS may have neuroprotective effects; however, currently the literature suggests that these agents are equivalent in efficacy. Both mannitol and HTS increase the osmotic gradient across the blood–brain barrier and may effectively "draw out" osmoles from the brain parenchyma, thereby reducing ICP.[51]

As a final resort, patients with refractory ICH should be considered for EVD drainage first and then decompressive hemicraniectomy as described previously in this chapter. Fig. 13.2 outlines a recommended ICP management algorithm.

## RESUMPTION OF ANTICOAGULATION

One major difficulty in the treatment of anticoagulant-associated ICH is the timing of anticoagulant resumption. Current guidelines recommend *against* anticoagulation resumption in lobar ICH but may be considered in cases of other ICH; however, the level of evidence is moderate and further investigations are needed.[22] Data on resumption of antiplatelet therapies such as aspirin or clopidogrel are also lacking. Recommendations suggest there is utility in antiplatelet resumption after ICH as long as there are definite indications.[22] At our center, we resume antithrombotic therapy primarily in patients with a higher risk of recurrent thrombosis than of ICH. Special circumstances need to be addressed for patients on clopidogrel or other antiplatelet agents used to manage cardiovascular health. In patients with a recent coronary artery stent, clopidogrel is essential for reducing the risk of in-stent restenosis. The decision to resume antithrombotic therapy should be made on a case-by-case basis with the risks and benefits discussed with the patient and/or decision-making care provider.

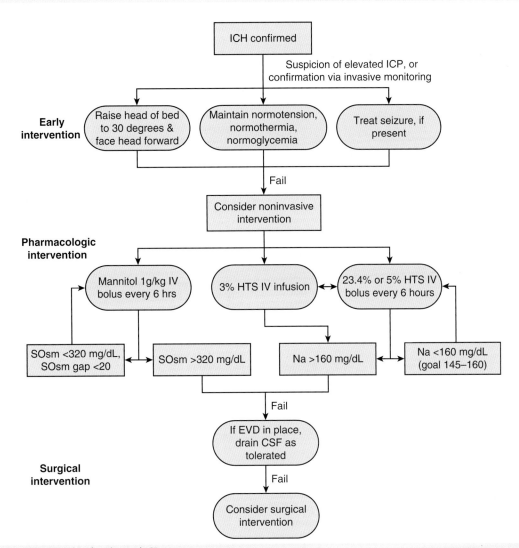

**Fig. 13.2** Management algorithm for elevated ICP.

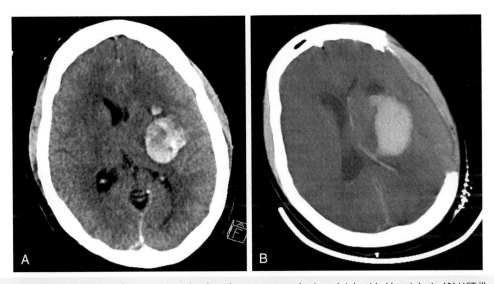

**Fig. 13.3** A 48-year-old female with history of hypertension developed acute-onset aphasia and right-sided hemiplegia. **(A)** HCT illustrated a left basal ganglia intraparenchymal hemorrhage. After developing signs of herniation, she underwent an emergent decompressive hemicraniectomy **(B)**.

**Table 13.3**  List of Variables for Scoring ICH

| ICH Score Item | Value |
|---|---|
| *Age* | |
| <80 years | 0 points |
| ≥80 years | 1 point |
| *Location* | |
| Supratentorial | 0 points |
| Infratentorial | 1 point |
| *Level of Consciousness* | |
| GCS 13–15 | 0 points |
| GCS 5–12 | 1 point |
| GCS 3–4 | 2 points |
| *ICH volume* | |
| <30 cc | 0 points |
| ≥30 cc | 1 point |
| *Intraventricular Extension* | |
| No | 0 points |
| Yes | 1 point |

*ICH*, intracranial hemorrhage; *GCS*, Glasgow Coma Scale.

## PROGNOSTICATION

Clinical classification of ICH based on severity and location is crucial in guiding surgical management, and rapidly acquired CT imaging is a necessary adjunct to the neurological examination when evaluating patients with suspected hemorrhage. Commonly, the validated ICH score is used to quantify the clinical severity of ICH, with higher scores associated with poorer outcomes (Table 13.3).[46] The Graeb score may be used to prognosticate for patients with significant IVH.[52] The Graeb score is calculated by adding together a score for each lateral ventricle separately (1 = trace blood, 2 = <50% ventricle filled with blood, 3 = >50% ventricle filled with blood, 4 = ventricle completely casted and expanded). The third and fourth ventricles, separately, are added to this total (1 = blood present, ventricle normal size; 2 = ventricle filled with blood and expanded) for a maximum score of 12. The Graeb scale is the most commonly reported scale in adults and correlates significantly with short-term outcome (Glasgow Outcome Score at 1 month).[12]

## Conclusions

ICH in the adult population is a common and important cause of neurological morbidity and mortality. Trauma, use of anticoagulation, and hypertension are the most frequent causes of ICH. In the appropriate setting, occult causes such as cerebral venous sinus thrombosis ought to be investigated given the dramatically different management (e.g., anticoagulation). There are limited studies in the literature discussing operative decision making and the type of operation to perform. Perioperative management of ICH requires a multidisciplinary team and dedicated neurocritical unit to optimize care.

## References

1. Anderson CS, Huang Y, Arima H, et al. Effects of early intensive blood pressure-lowering treatment on the growth of hematoma and perihematomal edema in acute intracerebral hemorrhage: the intensive blood pressure reduction in acute cerebral haemorrhage trial (interact). *Stroke.* 2010;41:307–312.
2. Bullock MR, Chesnut R, Ghajar J, et al. Surgical management of acute subdural hematomas. *Neurosurgery.* 2006;58:S16–S24. discussion Si–iv.
3. Chen SH, Chen Y, Fang WK, Huang DW, Huang KC, Tseng SH. Comparison of craniotomy and decompressive craniectomy in severely head-injured patients with acute subdural hematoma. *J Trauma.* 2011;71:1632–1636.
4. Kobayashi S, Sato A, Kageyama Y, Nakamura H, Watanabe Y, Yamaura A. Treatment of hypertensive cerebellar hemorrhage: surgical or conservative management? *Neurosurgery.* 1994;34:246–250. discussion 250–241.
5. Mendelow AD, Gregson BA, Fernandes HM, et al. Early surgery versus initial conservative treatment in patients with spontaneous supratentorial intracerebral haematomas in the international surgical trial in intracerebral haemorrhage (STICH): a randomised trial. *Lancet.* 2005;365:387–397.
6. Mendelow AD, Gregson BA, Rowan EN, et al. Early surgery versus initial conservative treatment in patients with spontaneous supratentorial lobar intracerebral haematomas (STICH II): a randomised trial. *Lancet.* 2013;382:397–408.
7. Honeybul S, Janzen C, Kruger K, Ho KM. Decompressive craniectomy for severe traumatic brain injury: is life worth living? *J Neurosurg.* 2013;119:1566–1575.
8. Hallevi H, Albright KC, Aronowski J, et al. Intraventricular hemorrhage: anatomic relationships and clinical implications. *Neurology.* 2008;70:848–852.
9. Barnholtz-Sloan JS, Sloan AE, Davis FG, Vigneau FD, Lai P, Sawaya RE. Incidence proportions of brain metastases in patients diagnosed (1973 to 2001) in the metropolitan detroit cancer surveillance system. *J Clin Oncol.* 2004;22:2865–2872.
10. Soffietti R, Ducati A, Ruda R. Brain metastases. *Handb Clin Neurol.* 2012;105:747–755.
11. Bullock MR, Chesnut R, Ghajar J, et al. Surgical management of traumatic parenchymal lesions. *Neurosurgery.* 2006;58:S25–S46. discussion Si–iv.
12. Demchuk AM, Dowlatshahi D, Rodriguez-Luna D, et al. Prediction of haematoma growth and outcome in patients with intracerebral haemorrhage using the ct-angiography spot sign (predict): a prospective observational study. *Lancet Neurol.* 2012;11:307–314.
13. Wada R, Aviv RI, Fox AJ, et al. CT angiography "spot sign" predicts hematoma expansion in acute intracerebral hemorrhage. *Stroke.* 2007;38:1257–1262.
14. Hart RG, Boop BS, Anderson DC. Oral anticoagulants and intracranial hemorrhage. Facts and hypotheses. *Stroke.* 1995;26:1471–1477.
15. Le Roux P, Pollack Jr CV, Milan M, Schaefer A. Race against the clock: overcoming challenges in the management of anticoagulant-associated intracerebral hemorrhage. *J Neurosurg.* 2014;121(Suppl):1–20.
16. Horstmann S, Rizos T, Lauseker M, et al. Intracerebral hemorrhage during anticoagulation with vitamin k antagonists: a consecutive observational study. *J Neurol.* 2013;260:2046–2051.
17. Iwama T, Yamada J, Imai S, Shinoda J, Funakoshi T, Sakai N. The use of frozen autogenous bone flaps in delayed cranioplasty revisited. *Neurosurgery.* 2003;52:591–596. discussion 595–596.
18. Bullock MR, Chesnut R, Ghajar J, et al. Surgical management of acute epidural hematomas. *Neurosurgery.* 2006;58:S7–S15. discussion Si–iv.
19. Chesnut R, Videtta W, Vespa P, Le Roux P. The Participants in the International Multidisciplinary Consensus Conference on Multimodality M. Intracranial pressure monitoring: fundamental considerations and rationale for monitoring. *Neurocrit Care.* 2014;21(2):64–84.
20. Steiner LA, Andrews PJ. Monitoring the injured brain: ICP and Cbf. *Br J Anaesth.* 2006;97:26–38.

21. Mayhall CG, Archer NH, Lamb VA, et al. Ventriculostomy-related infections. A prospective epidemiologic study. *N Engl J Med.* 1984;310:553–559.
22. Morgenstern LB, Hemphill 3rd JC, Anderson C, et al. Guidelines for the management of spontaneous intracerebral hemorrhage: a guideline for healthcare professionals from the American Heart Association/American Stroke Association. *Stroke.* 2010;41:2108–2129.
23. Broderick JP, Brott TG, Duldner JE, Tomsick T, Huster G. Volume of intracerebral hemorrhage. A powerful and easy-to-use predictor of 30-day mortality. *Stroke.* 1993;24:987–993.
24. Morgan T, Zuccarello M, Narayan R, Keyl P, Lane K, Hanley D. Preliminary findings of the minimally-invasive surgery plus rTPA for intracerebral hemorrhage evacuation (MISTIE) clinical trial. *Acta Neurochir.* 2008;105(Suppl):147–151.
25. Webb AJ, Ullman NL, Mann S, Muschelli J, Awad IA, Hanley DF. Resolution of intraventricular hemorrhage varies by ventricular region and dose of intraventricular thrombolytic: the clot lysis: evaluating accelerated resolution of IVH (clear IVH) program. *Stroke.* 2012;43:1666–1668.
26. Mould WA, Carhuapoma JR, Muschelli J, et al. Minimally invasive surgery plus recombinant tissue-type plasminogen activator for intracerebral hemorrhage evacuation decreases perihematomal edema. *Stroke.* 2013;44:627–634.
27. Amar AP. Controversies in the neurosurgical management of cerebellar hemorrhage and infarction. *Neurosurg Focus.* 2012;32:E1.
28. Kirollos RW, Tyagi AK, Ross SA, van Hille PT, Marks PV. Management of spontaneous cerebellar hematomas: A prospective treatment protocol. *Neurosurgery.* 2001;49:1378–1386. discussion 1386–1377.
29. Isla A, Alvarez F, Manrique M, Castro A, Amaya C, Blazquez MG. Posterior fossa subdural hematoma. *J Neurosurg Sci.* 1987;31:67–69.
30. Grover K, Sood S. Midline suboccipital burr hole for posterior fossa craniotomy. *Childs Nerv Syst.* 2010;26:953–955.
31. Diringer MN, Edwards DF. Admission to a neurologic/neurosurgical intensive care unit is associated with reduced mortality rate after intracerebral hemorrhage. *Crit Care Med.* 2001;29:635–640.
32. Schwarz S, Hafner K, Aschoff A, Schwab S. Incidence and prognostic significance of fever following intracerebral hemorrhage. *Neurology.* 2000;54:354–361.
33. Passero S, Ciacci G, Ulivelli M. The influence of diabetes and hyperglycemia on clinical course after intracerebral hemorrhage. *Neurology.* 2003;61:1351–1356.
34. Kaufman RM, Djulbegovic B, Gernsheimer T, et al. Platelet transfusion:a clinical practice guideline from the aabb. *Ann Intern Med.* 2015;162(3):205–213.
35. Hedges SJ, Dehoney SB, Hooper JS, Amanzadeh J, Busti AJ. Evidence-based treatment recommendations for uremic bleeding. *Nat Clin Pract Nephrol.* 2007;3:138–153.
36. Shander A, Walsh CE, Cromwell C. Acquired hemophilia: a rare but life-threatening potential cause of bleeding in the intensive care unit. *Intensive Care Med.* 2011;37:1240–1249.
37. Flaherty ML, Kissela B, Woo D, et al. The increasing incidence of anticoagulant-associated intracerebral hemorrhage. *Neurology.* 2007;68:116–121.
38. Huttner HB, Schellinger PD, Hartmann M, et al. Hematoma growth and outcome in treated neurocritical care patients with intracerebral hemorrhage related to oral anticoagulant therapy: comparison of acute treatment strategies using vitamin k, fresh frozen plasma, and prothrombin complex concentrates. *Stroke.* 2006;37:1465–1470.
39. Frontera JA, Lewin JJ 3rd, Rabinstein AA, et al. Guideline for reversal of antithrombotics in intracranial hemorrhage: A statement for healthcare professionals from the Neurocritical Care Society and Society of Critical Care Medicine. *Neurocrit Care.* 2016;24:6–46.
40. Leissinger CA, Blatt PM, Hoots WK, Ewenstein B. Role of prothrombin complex concentrates in reversing warfarin anticoagulation: a review of the literature. *Am J Hematol.* 2008;83:137–143.
41. Yuan ZH, Jiang JK, Huang WD, Pan J, Zhu JY, Wang JZ. A meta-analysis of the efficacy and safety of recombinant activated factor vii for patients with acute intracerebral hemorrhage without hemophilia. *J Clin Neurosci.* 2010;17:685–693.
42. Bruins Slot KM, Berge E. Factor xa inhibitors versus vitamin k antagonists for preventing cerebral or systemic embolism in patients with atrial fibrillation. *Cochrane Database Syst Rev.* 2013;8.
43. Eerenberg ES, Kamphuisen PW, Sijpkens MK, Meijers JC, Buller HR, Levi M. Reversal of rivaroxaban and dabigatran by prothrombin complex concentrate: A randomized, placebo-controlled, crossover study in healthy subjects. *Circulation.* 2011;124:1573–1579.
44. Connolly SJ, Ezekowitz MD, Yusuf S, et al. Dabigatran versus warfarin in patients with atrial fibrillation. *N Engl J Med.* 2009;361: 1139–1151.
45. Pollack Jr CV, Reilly PA, Eikelboom J, et al. Idarucizumab for dabigatran reversal. *N Engl J Med.* 2015;373:511–520.
46. Hemphill 3rd JC, Bonovich DC, Besmertis L, Manley GT, Johnston SC. The ICH score: a simple, reliable grading scale for intracerebral hemorrhage. *Stroke.* 2001;32:891–897.
47. Chesnut RM, Temkin N, Carney N, et al. A trial of intracranial-pressure monitoring in traumatic brain injury. *N Engl J Med.* 2012;367:2471–2481.
48. Ko SB, Choi HA, Parikh G, et al. Multimodality monitoring for cerebral perfusion pressure optimization in comatose patients with intracerebral hemorrhage. *Stroke.* 2011;42:3087–3092.
49. Paulson OB, Strandgaard S, Edvinsson L. Cerebral autoregulation. *Cerebrovasc Brain Metab Rev.* 1990;2:161–192.
50. Ropper AH. Hyperosmolar therapy for raised intracranial pressure. *N Engl J Med.* 2012;367:746–752.
51. Raichle ME, Plum F. Hyperventilation and cerebral blood flow. *Stroke.* 1972;3:566–575.
52. Morgan TC, Dawson J, Spengler D, et al. The modified graeb score: an enhanced tool for intraventricular hemorrhage measurement and prediction of functional outcome. *Stroke.* 2013;44:635–641.

# 14 *Pituitary Surgery*

ROBERT L. BAILEY, DEBBIE YI, and M. SEAN GRADY

## Introduction

Tumors involving the pituitary gland are commonly encountered within clinical neurosurgery, representing between 10% and 15% of all primary brain tumors and approximately 20% of surgically resected primary brain tumors.[1,2] Furthermore, a proportion of pituitary tumors are clinically silent based on the estimated incidence of these tumors in the population. Autopsy studies have revealed a prevalence ranging from 1.5% to 26.7% for pituitary adenomas less than 10 mm in diameter (microadenomas).[3] These data, in combination with additional epidemiological studies, suggest that pituitary tumors are in fact the third most common primary intracranial tumors, preceded only by gliomas and meningiomas, making this a diagnosis commonly encountered within the neurosurgery patient population.

## Neuroanatomy and Procedure

### Key Concepts

- Pituitary tumors are the third most common primary intracranial tumors.
- The majority of pituitary tumors are pituitary adenomas.
- Pituitary adenomas are classified as either microadenomas (<1 cm) or macroadenomas (>1 cm).

A variety of tumor types can involve the sella turcica. These include pituitary adenomas, craniopharyngiomas, meningiomas, primary and secondary carcinomas, and a number of additional pathologies. The overwhelming majority of these tumors are classified as pituitary adenomas. A number of clinical, pathological, and radiological classification systems are used to describe pituitary adenomas. The functional classification system is perhaps the most important for the clinician because it is based on the secretory activity of the tumor in vivo (Box 14.1).[4] Functional adenomas are those that secrete prolactin (PRL), growth hormone, thyroid-stimulating hormone (TSH), or adrenocorticotropic hormone (ACTH), thereby producing their respective clinical phenotypes of amenorrhea-galactorrhea syndrome, acromegaly or gigantism, secondary hyperthyroidism, and Cushing's disease or Nelson's syndrome.[5] Tumors not associated with a clinical hypersecretory state, including gonadotroph adenomas (secreting luteinizing hormone [LH] and/or follicle-stimulating hormone [FSH]) and various silent adenomas, are collectively classified as clinically nonfunctional adenomas.

Modern pathological classifications are based on sophisticated morphological techniques, with immunohistochemistry and electron microscopy representing the "gold standard" methods of classifying pituitary adenomas. Characterization on the basis of hormonal content, cellular morphology, and origin may permit conclusions on biological behavior, prognosis, and responsiveness to various treatment modalities.[2]

Radiologically, tumors are classified according to their size and growth characteristics (Box 14.2).[4] The most basic classification uses the term *microadenoma* for tumors <1 cm in diameter and *macroadenoma* for tumors >1 cm in diameter. Less commonly used classifications stratify tumors according to the degree and direction of suprasellar extension.

The clinical manifestation of pituitary adenomas is usually due to mass effect, hormonal hypersecretion, or pituitary insufficiency from compression of the pituitary stalk (Fig. 14.1). The most common objective feature is vision loss, with bitemporal hemianopsia being the classic finding due to compression of bilateral nasal visual fibers as they cross at the level of the optic chiasm. With further suprasellar extension, the tumors may begin to compress the hypothalamus and the numerous nuclei and pathways that traverse that vital structure. Although less common, extension into the third ventricle could cause obstruction of cerebrospinal fluid (CSF) flow and resultant hydrocephalus. Most of these symptoms develop slowly over time and therefore may go unnoticed.

In contrast, pituitary apoplexy leads to a more acute presentation. It is referred to as the abrupt and occasionally catastrophic acute hemorrhagic infarction of a pituitary adenoma and classically presents with an acute headache, meningismus, possible visual loss, ophthalmoplegia, and, occasionally, an alteration in consciousness. These patients often require a much more urgent workup and intervention for treatment of cranial nerve dysfunction and pituitary hormone crisis.

Some patients present to clinic with a pituitary mass found incidentally after routine brain imaging for nonspecific or unrelated reasons. This is becoming more common with increased utilization of magnetic resonance imaging (MRI), with a recent literature stating more than 10% of new patients have incidentally discovered lesions.[6] However, upon discovery of the lesion some patients will demonstrate an associated abnormality, with 5% exhibiting a visual field deficit and up to 15% showing evidence of pituitary dysfunction.[7]

## SURGICAL APPROACH

### Key Concepts

- Various factors must be taken into consideration when selecting the operative approach for the individual patient.
- For the majority of pituitary tumors, the endonasal transsphenoidal approach (TSA) is the preferred operative approach to resection because it represents a more minimally invasive technique.
- In an effort to achieve maximal resection of tumors with a more expansive intracranial extension, a transcranial approach may be required as either a replacement for or adjunct to the TSA.

The aims of pituitary surgery are to correct any pituitary hormonal oversecretion, reverse any hormonal undersecretion, eliminate mass effect, decompress visual pathways, and obtain tissue for a definitive histopathological diagnosis, while attempting to preserve normal pituitary function and minimize surgical morbidity.[8] The tumor size, extension, configuration, magnitude of hormonal oversecretion, and experience of the operating surgeon are essential factors that determine whether these goals can be achieved.[9,10]

The surgical treatment of pituitary surgery has undergone considerable evolution during the past century. Ever since the first publication of a successful pituitary surgery by Schloffer in 1907,[11] a variety of surgical techniques have been utilized for the surgical resection of pituitary tumors. Today the overwhelming majority of pituitary tumors can be accessed through a TSA. In fact, this approach is so widely used today that some authors report transsphenoidal surgery as the approach of choice for 90% to 95% of pituitary tumors.[12] The remainder of cases requires a transcranial approach, consisting of pterional or subfrontal craniotomy, or a skull base approach that may be transcranial, extracranial, or a combination of the two.

The surgeon must consider multiple factors when selecting the surgical approach. These include the size of the sella and degree of mineralization, the size and pneumatization of the sphenoid sinus, the position and tortuosity of the carotid arteries, the presence and direction of any intracranial tumor extension, the position of the pituitary gland in relation to the tumor, and whether prior surgical therapy or radiotherapy has been administered. Extension of the tumor laterally beyond the boundary of the carotid arteries and into the middle cranial fossa and/or with significant posterior extension may necessitate the use of the transcranial approach in an effort to obtain a more complete resection. In addition, in cases such as sphenoid sinusitis or ectatic midline ("kissing") carotid arteries, the TSA may be contraindicated.[13] However, for the majority of pituitary tumors, the TSA is still preferred.

Each surgical approach has various nuances, most of which are beyond the scope of this chapter. However, it is imperative for all clinicians to have an understanding of the fundamental aspects of each surgical procedure to more accurately assess a patient's preoperative and postoperative care.

## TRANSSPHENOIDAL APPROACH

The TSA (Fig. 14.2) itself has many variations, allowing the surgeon to tailor the surgery to the individual patient's tumor and symptomatology. All variations (e.g., endonasal versus sublabial, endoscopic versus microscopical, submucosal versus direct sphenoidotomy) are minimally invasive and informed by the surgeon's experience and preference. The TSA represents the most physiological and minimally traumatic corridor of surgical access to the sella, providing direct and superior visualization of the pituitary gland and adjacent pathology.[5] The sublabial TSA has been replaced by the endonasal approach, which is associated with less patient discomfort and avoids postoperative numbness of the anterior teeth. Either a microscope or an endoscope is utilized to perform the procedure, with endoscopic

Preop                                    Postop

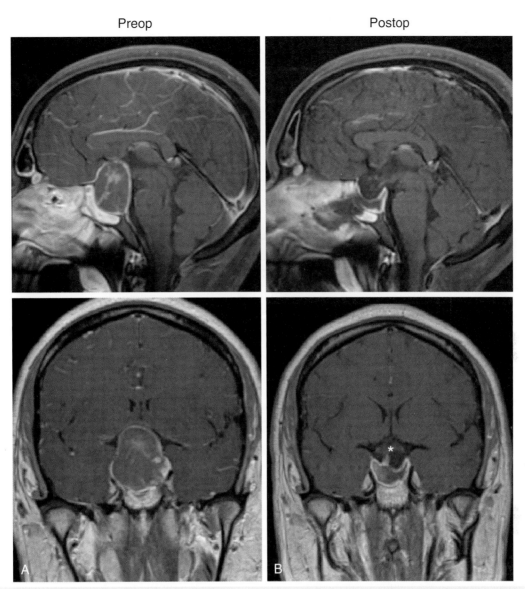

**Fig. 14.1 Pituitary apoplexy.** Preoperative and postoperative T1 weighted gadolinium-enhanced MRI images of patient with pituitary apoplexy **(A)** The large mass encompasses the entirety of the sella and extends into the suprasellar cistern, resulting in significant compression upon the optic chiasm as well as the hypothalamus. Bilateral carotid arteries are displaced laterally. The signal characteristics seen here as well as on other image series not shown are consistent with hemorrhage within the lesion and consistent with apoplexy. **(B)** After an endoscopic transsphenoidal resection of the mass, MRI demonstrates resolution of mass effect upon the optic chiasm (*) and hypothalamus, with a concave appearance of the diaphragm sella.

techniques becoming much more common in recent years due to the ability to use angled cameras and instruments to obtain improved visualization.

The patient is positioned supine with the head supported by a Mayfield headrest with an attached horseshoe pillow and elevated to approximately 15 degrees above the heart to encourage venous drainage. The thigh or lower abdomen is often prepared for a fat or fascia lata graft, should that be necessary. In the endoscopic approach, the turbinates are mobilized laterally to expose the sphenoid ostium. The ostia are then opened, and the posterior wall of the septum is resected to expose the face of the sella. A similar dissection may be used for the contralateral nasal passage to allow for a binostril approach. The decision to perform a binostril approach depends on the size of the tumor, the

need for extension of the sphenoidotomy, or surgeon preference. Although still a minimally invasive approach, a larger exposure trades the advantage of a wider surgical corridor and viewing window for distortion of the normal anatomy and nasal function.

Once the face of the sphenoid sinus is resected, the surrounding contents are exposed. The bone of the sella continues superiorly as the tuberculum sellae and then further on anterosuperiorly as the planum sphenoidale. Both the tuberculum sellae and the planum sphenoidale are often removed during an extended TSA. The carotid protuberance can be seen as a bony outpouching that serves to identify the underlying carotid artery as it runs vertically at the skull base on the lateral aspect of the sella. Intraoperative image guidance may assist with this anatomical

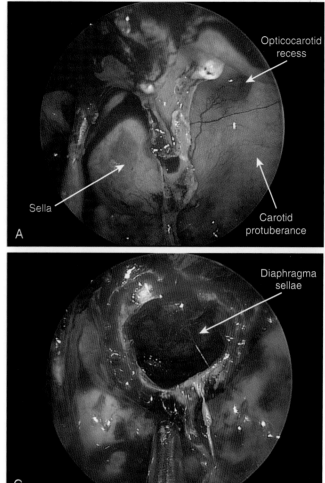

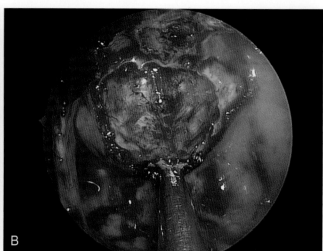

**Fig. 14.2** Intraoperative images from the endoscopic endonasal transsphenoidal approach. **(A)** View of the sella within the sphenoid sinus. Note the close relationship of the carotid to the lateral border of the sella. **(B)** Demonstration of the sella after removal of the bone and before opening of the dura. The adenoma is then exposed and removed by curettage. **(C)** After removal of the adenoma, the diaphragma sellae drops down into the sella cavity. Although the dura is opened to access the adenoma, the diaphragma is not violated and therefore no CSF leak is encountered.

localization. The sellar floor is then penetrated, and the opening is widened using a Kerrison punch. Adequate bony exposure is crucial to the success of the transsphenoidal surgery. The dura is incised, and an attempt is made to establish a definite cleavage plane between the pituitary gland or tumor and the underlying dura. It is worth noting that there are in fact two layers of dura in the sella. The potential for entering the cavernous sinus and encountering significant venous bleeding exists when dissecting between these two layers. The sellar pathology is then removed with ringed curettes and microinstruments. Internal debulking of the tumor allows for the capsule of the tumor to collapse down onto itself and become accessible to the surgeon. Finally, various angled endoscopes allow the surgeon to inspect the cavity for residual tumor.

Surgical closure proceeds uneventfully, as outlined later, in the absence of a CSF leak. However, if a tear in the arachnoid is observed, not only does it add to the complexity of the case, but further steps must be taken to close the communication between the sinonasal cavity and the intracranial compartment. Sellar reconstruction is performed by placing the autologous fascia lata and/or fat graft over the dural opening and packing it within the sphenoid sinus.

There are various methods for additional closure techniques, including the use of mesh, cartilage, bone, or tailored artificial grafts. However, at our institution, a nasoseptal flap, with its accompanying vascular supply from the nasoseptal branch of the sphenopalatine artery, is placed over the fat graft to provide an additional vascularized layer of protection.

For closure of the nasal portion of the procedure, the septal flaps are reapproximated and the nasal septum is returned to its midline insertion. Mucosal tears may be sutured closed. For cases in which the sphenoid sinus has been packed with a graft, small absorbable gelatin sponges may be placed in the sphenoethmoidal recess to buttress the sphenoid packing, and gauze packing is left in place within the nasal cavity. Otherwise, no nasal splints or packs are placed.

## TRANSCRANIAL APPROACH

A description of the techniques involved in a transcranial approach are beyond the scope of this chapter, except to say that indeed some pituitary cases may require utilization of the pterional or the anterior subfrontal approaches.

The major advantage of the craniotomy approach is that it affords the surgeon a complete view of the pituitary's effect on intracranial structures.[5] The optic nerves and chiasm, intracranial extensions into the anterior and middle cranial fossae, third ventricular extensions, and retrosellar clival extensions can be visualized and accessed. The major limitation of the transcranial approaches is that the intrasellar portion of the tumor can be more difficult to access. For this reason, some large macroadenomas with significant intracranial extension may require the use of both a transcranial approach and a TSA for complete tumor resection.

## Perioperative Considerations

### Key Concepts

- Prior to surgery, the size and type of pituitary tumor must be determined.
- An endocrinologist assesses the need for glucocorticoid and thyroid hormone replacement.
- The insulin tolerance test is the gold standard test for assessing hypothalamic-pituitary-adrenal (HPA) axis function prior to surgery.

There are important characteristics of a pituitary lesion that should be identified prior to surgery. Knowing the size of the lesion and type of lesion will help determine the surgical approach and then guide the preoperative, perioperative, and postoperative management for the patient. Typically, pituitary surgery is not emergent and can be done electively with careful endocrine management prior to surgery. Surgery becomes more urgent when vision becomes compromised.

A macroadenoma has a higher likelihood of compromising normal pituitary function, which can result in secondary adrenal insufficiency, growth hormone deficiency, hypothyroidism, and hypogonadism. Patients with a craniopharyngioma are much more likely to develop panhypopituitarism and diabetes insipidus after surgery.[14]

Prior to surgery, the combination of history, physical examination, and blood and urine tests aids in the diagnosis of pituitary dysfunction for an endocrinologist. Secondary adrenal insufficiency is suggested by symptoms of fatigue, weight loss, weakness, dizziness, and difficulty concentrating. Baseline endocrine studies include serum cortisol and ACTH, free thyroxine, TSH, PRL, LH, FSH, $\alpha$ subunit, insulinlike growth factor, and testosterone (in men). A less-than-normal morning cortisol with a normal ACTH level suggests secondary adrenal insufficiency and the need for glucocorticoid replacement. The most important assessments to be made preoperatively are the need for glucocorticoid and thyroid hormone replacement due to the stress of surgery. It is imperative to determine the need for glucocorticoid replacement before giving thyroid hormone replacement because giving thyroid hormone replacement to a patient with impaired ACTH reserve can precipitate an adrenal crisis.

If there is concern for Cushing's syndrome, the screening test is the 24-hour urine free cortisol (UFC) and creatinine concentrations. If the UFC concentration is elevated and the serum ACTH is normal or high, then dynamic tests will ensue. The definitive test is the inferior petrosal sinus sampling with Corticotroph Releasing Hormone administration and measurement of peripheral ACTH concentrations. This helps differentiate between an "incidentaloma" and a true functional microadenoma.

All patients with pituitary disease should receive diagnostic testing of HPA axis function prior to pituitary surgery. The insulin tolerance test is the gold standard test, but it is contraindicated in patients with coronary artery disease, seizure disorder, or general debility. Endocrinologists typically prefer the short ACTH 1-24 (Synacthen) test as the initial test of HPA axis function in a patient with a known pituitary tumor.

The decision regarding perioperative glucocorticoid coverage depends on the result of preoperative screening. If the ACTH 1-24 test is abnormal, a standard maintenance dose of glucocorticoid (based on age, sex, and body weight) should be started. The patient should receive 48 hours of perioperative supraphysiological glucocorticoid therapy, which can then be quickly reduced. A suggested regimen would be 50 mg hydrocortisone every 8 hours on day 0, 25 mg every 8 hours on day 1, and 25 mg in the morning on day 2. Patients with normal HPA axis function will have a return of baseline cortisol secretion within 48 hours of major surgery, and many patients have a rapid rise in secretion of pituitary hormones after pituitary adenomectomy. Barring any postoperative complications, glucocorticoid supplementation should be discontinued after 48 hours and depending on the daily morning plasma cortisol levels obtained between postop days 3 and 5. For patients with a normal ACTH 1-24 test, no perioperative glucocorticoid coverage is given. If the adenomectomy is surgically more extensive, glucocorticoid coverage for 48 hours should be provided as though the patient had an abnormal ACTH 1-24 test.

All patients with Cushing's disease require perioperative glucocorticoid coverage. A low plasma cortisol level after surgery is considered a surgical cure (although the actual level of cortisol is debated); therefore these patients require hydrocortisone replacement therapy with ongoing review of their HPA axis. If the cortisol level postoperatively is normal, this is an indication of ongoing ACTH secretion.

Identifying the type of secretory tumor has an implication on perioperative management. Intubation of a patient with acromegaly may be difficult and may necessitate an awake intubation. Postoperatively, patients with acromegaly may have difficulty breathing with nasal packing. Acromegalic patients commonly have obstructive sleep apnea requiring continuous positive airway pressure therapy, which is contraindicated after this surgery. The rare TSH-producing adenoma patient must be treated preoperatively for hyperthyroidism to decrease the risk of arrhythmia during surgery.[14] Prolactin-secreting tumors are almost always treated initially with cabergoline 0.5 mg twice weekly, even when causing mass effect on the optic chiasm.

As previously stated, hormonal status must be evaluated for each patient prior to surgical intervention. Prophylactic antibiotics are routinely administered in all cases just prior to incision. Both an arterial line and an indwelling urinary catheter are often used during these procedures for intraoperative and postoperative assessment. Depending on surgeon preference, some patients may undergo a preoperative high-resolution computed tomography (CT) or MRI scan for the specific purpose of providing intraoperative frameless stereotactic image guidance.

A potential adjunct to surgery is the placement of a lumbar drain to allow for CSF drainage during surgery. This may be of assistance in patients with a macroadenoma in an effort to potentially limit the amount of brain retraction that may be required during a craniotomy for resection or to divert CSF flow during a TSA in which a large dural defect may be encountered during the resection.

## Postoperative Complications

### Key Concepts

- Pituitary surgery is associated with a low rate of morbidity/mortality.
- Vascular injury has a low rate of occurrence but is associated with a high degree of morbidity.
- Given the significant vessels and cranial nerves surrounding the pituitary region, the surgeon and postoperative care providers must each be aware of potential complications from surgical resection.

With the advent of the TSA and the continued advancement in its technique, pituitary surgery has become safer and with a continued low rate of patient complications. A 2009 systematic review and metaanalysis specifically focused on endoscopic pituitary surgery outcomes within the literature.[15] They reported a 0.24% rate of mortality, similar compared with the <1% rate within a large series of traditional surgery.

Although relatively safe, TSA may be complicated by significant and occasionally fatal vascular injury.[16,17] Because the sella is in close proximity to the carotid artery, vascular injury remains a particular concern during pituitary surgery. The risk of vascular injury may be higher for the endoscopic endonasal TSA because the viewing window is small and dependent on a camera. It is extremely difficult to control brisk arterial blood flow when visualization of the operative field is obscured by blood and only limited instruments are available. Suction and tamponade can often provide the visual window necessary to control the situation. If adequate hemostasis is not obtained, the sphenoid sinus must be packed and alternative means must be pursued to achieve vascular repair, such as endovascular techniques.

Rhinological complications are unique to the endonasal approach and occur in approximately 1% to 2% of cases.[18] Although not considered a significant morbidity by clinicians, this complication may be troubling to affected patients. Hyposmia can also be seen in the postoperative period, but this is most often transient. Many of the rhinological complications can be avoided with meticulous and nondestructive surgical technique during the exposure.[5] Similarly, postoperative epistaxis is usually preventable

by careful coagulation of the branched vessels during dissection, most importantly the sphenopalatine artery.

Cavernous sinus injury may lead to cranial nerve deficits, with CN VI being affected more commonly than CN III and IV. The optic nerve and chiasm are particularly sensitive to injury, and damage may occur with even minimal amounts of retraction or even with overpacking the sella during sellar reconstruction. Case reports demonstrate that underpacking of the sella can lead to a secondary empty sella with late onset of vision loss due to chiasmatic prolapse, although this event has not been encountered by us. Additional complications, such as CSF leak and pituitary dysfunction, are discussed in greater detail in a separate portion of this chapter.

## Postoperative Management

### Key Concepts

- Diabetes insipidus occurs in 18% to 31% of patients undergoing pituitary surgery.
- There are three patterns of diabetes insipidus: transient, permanent, and triphasic.
- The management of a CSF leak depends on the degree of leak and time from surgery.

Patients undergoing pituitary surgery require intensive care unit (ICU) monitoring postoperatively. Central diabetes insipidus (cDI) causes hypotonic polyuria and occurs in 18% to 31% of patients postoperatively. There are three patterns of cDI: transient, permanent, and triphasic. Risk factors include young age, male gender, large intrasellar mass, and CSF leak. Specific characteristics of pituitary lesions, such as size and proximity to the pituitary stalk,[19] and certain pathological types, including craniopharyngiomas, Rathke's cleft cysts, and ACTH-secreting pituitary adenomas,[20] also increase the risk of postoperative cDI.

Transient cDI begins 24 to 48 hours after surgery and abates within several days. It resolves when the arginine vasopressin (AVP)–secreting neurons recover function. The triphasic pattern of cDI has three phases that physiologically can be explained by 1) partial or complete pituitary stalk section that severs the connection between cell bodies of AVP-secreting neurons in the hypothalamus and nerve terminals in the posterior pituitary gland and, as a result, there is no AVP secretion; 2) degenerating nerve terminals in the posterior pituitary lead to uncontrolled AVP release into the bloodstream and resultant antidiuresis; and finally 3) once all AVP stores have been released, if >80% to 90% of AVP-secreting neuronal cell bodies in the hypothalamus have degenerated, the result is permanent cDI. However, this triphasic pattern of cDI is uncommon and seen in only 3.4% of patients. The first phase typically lasts 5 to 7 days.[21] The second phase of syndrome of inappropriate antidiuretic hormone secretion (SIADH), in which urine becomes concentrated and urine output decreases markedly, lasts 2 to 14 days. It can last a short amount of time if the mass destroys the posterior pituitary with little residual AVP store. Some patients with limited damage to the neurohypophysis only have SIADH after surgery ("isolated" second phase). The third phase is related to the level of the lesion. If the lesion is closer to the AVP-secreting cell bodies within the hypothalamus, then the AVP stores will be depleted, causing permanent diabetes insipidus.

When confronted with diuresis after surgery, it should be assumed to be diabetes insipidus until proven otherwise. More commonly encountered than diabetes insipidus are postoperative diuresis and glucosuria. A central reason for ICU monitoring after pituitary surgery includes accurate measurements of input and output. Fluid intake from the operating room should be included in the total balance documented because fluid may have been administered intravenously during the operation. Because stress-dose glucocorticoids are routinely given intraoperatively and steroids induce insulin resistance, secondary hyperglycemia may ensue and cause an osmotic diuresis from glucosuria. To determine whether glucosuria is the cause of diuresis, monitor finger-stick glucose levels closely.

To diagnose diabetes insipidus (Fig. 14.3), the patient should have polyuria with volumes of 4 to 18 L/day that begin abruptly within 24 to 48 hours postoperatively. The urine will be hypotonic with a specific gravity <1.005 and urine osmolality <200. The patient will have polydipsia with a craving for ice-cold fluids. There will be a normal-to-increased serum osmolality and serum sodium greater than or equal to 145 mEq/L.[22]

The patient should have urine specific gravity or osmolality and serum sodium measured every 4 to 6 hours until stable. Fluid intake and output should be carefully monitored, and patients should be asked about thirst symptoms. Desmopressin (dDAVP) is the drug of choice for the acute and chronic treatment of central diabetes insipidus.[23] Desmopressin can be given in a dose of 1 to 2 micrograms subcutaneously, intramuscularly, or intravenously. It should be redosed when urine output reaches 200 to 250 mL per hour for greater than or equal to 2 hours with a specific gravity <1.005 (or urine osmolality less than 200 mOsm/kg $H_2O$).[24] All patients should drink according to thirst because this will be the best guide to water replacement.[19] In patients who cannot maintain a normal plasma osmolality (and serum sodium) through drinking fluids, hypotonic intravenous fluids may be administered.

Each dose of dDAVP should be given once polyuria recurs but prior to the patient becoming hyperosmolar. Desmopressin lasts 6 to 12 hours, but despite its administration, urine output, specific gravity or osmolality, and serum sodium should continue to be monitored every 4 to 6 hours. Side effects of dDAVP are uncommon but include headache, nausea, nasal congestion, flushing, and abdominal cramping.

Patients with postoperative diabetes insipidus, particularly those with a triphasic response, are likely having anterior pituitary dysfunction as well. Intravenous hydrocortisone in stress doses is typically administered before surgery and every 6 to 8 hours for 24 hours. This is typically tapered over 2 to 3 days and discontinued if postoperative serum cortisol levels are normal after stopping the hydrocortisone. The decision regarding ongoing glucocorticoid therapy is based on the level of the 0800 hour cortisol, which is obtained on days 1 to 3 in patients not treated with glucocorticoids and days 3 to 5 in patients covered with glucocorticoids for the initial 48 hours. A cortisol level of more than 450 nM postoperatively is considered low risk for adrenal insufficiency and should be considered as having normal HPA axis function. Patients with a level less than 100 nM are almost certainly ACTH deficient and should receive maintenance doses of glucocorticoid. Levels between 100 and 250 nM are possibly ACTH deficient and should be treated with a morning dose of hydrocortisone and instructed to increase the dose in times of illness. Levels between 250 and 450 nM are unlikely to be ACTH deficient and should be given hydrocortisone for times of illness only. A repeat 0800 hour plasma cortisol should be repeated at 4 to 6 weeks after surgery by an endocrinologist.

The management of patients with Cushing's disease varies by institution. These patients may not be given glucocorticoids at the time of surgery. Rather, a serum cortisol level may be acquired after surgery to guide medical management.

CSF leaks may occur days or even weeks after surgery. Persistent drainage of typically clear fluid from the nose suggests a CSF leak. This is potentially the most dangerous complication of transsphenoidal pituitary tumor resection. Concerning concomitant symptoms are fever and headache because they suggest meningitis. Those at greatest risk of a CSF leak include patients with large tumor removal and those who required a graft intraoperatively.

To diagnose a CSF leak, measuring glucose concentration in nasal fluid is helpful, but nondiagnostic. A more reliable method is measuring either alpha or beta transferrin, a protein within CSF. However, this test is not urgently available in most hospitals, limiting its utility. Therefore determination of a CSF leak is a clinical one, and it requires immediate neurosurgical evaluation. If the CSF leak is on postop day 0 or day 1, the patient will likely be taken back to the operating room for a repeat attempt at adequate sellar reconstruction. If the CSF leak is slightly later in the postoperative course, placement of a lumbar drain may provide resolution and closure of the CSF fistula. Typically lumbar drains are left in place for 3 to 4 days with 10 to 15 cc of CSF drained per hour until the decision is made

## DIAGNOSIS OF POSTOPERATIVE DIABETES INSIPIDUS

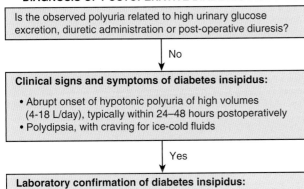

Is the observed polyuria related to high urinary glucose excretion, diuretic administration or post-operative diuresis?

No

**Clinical signs and symptoms of diabetes insipidus:**
- Abrupt onset of hypotonic polyuria of high volumes (4–18 L/day), typically within 24–48 hours postoperatively
- Polydipsia, with craving for ice-cold fluids

Yes

**Laboratory confirmation of diabetes insipidus:**
- Hypotonic urine (specific gravity <1.005 or urine osmolality <200 mOsm/kg $H_2O$)
- Serum [$Na^+$] ≥145 meq/L
- Normal to increased serum osmolality

Fig. 14.3 Diagnosis of postoperative diabetes insipidus.

to attempt a clamp trial for a day. If there is no evidence of CSF rhinorrhea after 24 hours of a clamp trial, the drain is removed. Patients who had a CSF leak are treated with a full course of antibiotic therapy targeting organisms common to the nasopharynx.

An unrecognized and/or prolonged postoperative CSF leak can potentially lead to intracranial hypotension, in which the patient first complains of a severe headache that can then quickly develop into ocular symptoms and a subsequent obtunded state. A CT scan of the brain may demonstrate pneumocephalus. MRI is much more sensitive, revealing widened extraaxial fluid spaces without a focal extraaxial fluid collection, as well as dural thickening and enhancement of the meninges. The brain is noted to sink downward in the cranium. Positioning the patient in the Trendelenburg position may assist in slowing down the progression of the brain herniation while a more permanent solution is pursued, such as an epidural blood patch if a lumbar drain was used, possible ventriculostomy, or definitive closure of the CSF fistula.

Visual field testing is a critical part of the postoperative neurological examination. In addition, inquiring about thirst, nasal drainage, fluid pooling, and a salty taste in the mouth are all mandatory parts of the patient evaluation. After transsphenoidal surgery, all patients are given sinus precautions, which include avoiding strenuous activity, coughing, or sneezing; avoiding the use of straws; and not blowing one's nose. Nausea and vomiting should be treated aggressively to avoid sinus pressure.

Oxygen therapy is delivered via a humidified oxygen mask or face tent rather than nasal cannula. Positive pressure ventilation is typically not recommended. Given that chronic glucocorticoid excess is thought to induce hypercoagulability, patients with Cushing's disease have a higher risk of developing a postoperative thromboembolism and should therefore engage in physical activity sooner.[25]

In the absence of surgical complications, such as diabetes insipidus or a profound CSF leak, the patient may be transitioned from an ICU to a regular inpatient unit on the first postoperative day. Patients without a leak can be out of bed on the day after surgery with sinus precautions and be discharged after 2 to 3 additional days with nasal saline. At our institution, the surgeon will have the patient perform a head dangle with the patient's chin tucked into chest on the third day after surgery to rule out an occult CSF leak. Patients with a CSF leak on head dangle must maintain bed rest, lie flat in bed, and undergo management as described earlier.

## Conclusion

Pituitary surgery is a common clinical scenario encountered within the neurocritical care setting. Over time, surgical resection of pituitary tumors has been demonstrated to be increasingly safer. However, as illustrated in this chapter, there are numerous potential complications to this surgery, and the postoperative management demands an attentive clinician (Table 14.1).

**Table 14.1** Complication Rates in Surgery

| Complication | Rate (%) |
| --- | --- |
| Mortality | 0–1.75 |
| Transient diabetes insipidus | 10–60 |
| Permanent diabetes insipidus | 0.5–5 |
| Anterior pituitary insufficiency | 1–10 |
| Cerebrospinal fluid leakage | 1–4 |
| Meningitis | 0–1.75 |
| Nasal septum perforation | 1–3 |
| Sinusitis | 1–4 |
| Epistaxis | 2–4 |
| Visual disturbances | 0.6–1.6 |

Adapted from Winn, HR, ed., *Youmans textbook of neurosurgery*, 6th ed. Philadelphia: Elsevier; 2011.

## References

1. Jane JA, Sulton LD, Laws ER. Surgery for primary brain tumors at United States academic training centers: results from the Residency Review Committee for neurological surgery. *J Neurosurg.* 2005;103 (5):789–793.
2. Kovacs K, Horvath E, Vidal S. Classification of pituitary adenomas. *J Neurooncol.* 2001;54(2):121–127.
3. Molitch ME, Russell EJ. The pituitary "incidentaloma." *Ann Intern Med.* 1990;112(12):925–931.
4. Kovacs K, Scheithauer BW, Horvath E, Lloyd RV. The World Health Organization classification of adenohypophysial neoplasms. A proposed five-tier scheme. *Cancer.* 1996;78(3):502–510.
5. Jane JA, Thapar K, Laws ER. Pituitary surgery. In: Winn HR, Berger MS, Dacey RG, eds. *Youman's Neurological Surgery.* 6th ed. Philadelphia, PA: Elsevier Saunders; 2011:1476–1510.
6. Scangas GA, Laws ER. Pituitary incidentalomas. *Pituitary.* 2014;17(5): 486–491.
7. Feldkamp J, Santen R, Harms E, Aulich A, Mödder U, Scherbaum WA. Incidentally discovered pituitary lesions: high frequency of macroadenomas and hormone-secreting adenomas - results of a prospective study. *Clin Endocrinol (Oxf).* 1999;51(1):109–113.
8. Vance ML. Perioperative management of patients undergoing pituitary surgery. *Endocrinol Metab Clin North Am.* 2003;32(2):355–365.
9. Joshi SM, Cudlip S. Transsphenoidal surgery. *Pituitary.* 2008;11 (4):353–360.
10. O'Malley BW, Grady MS, Gabel BC, et al. Comparison of endoscopic and microscopic removal of pituitary adenomas: single-surgeon experience and the learning curve. *Neurosurg Focus.* 2008;25(6):E10.
11. Loyo-Varela M, Herrada-Pineda T, Revilla-Pacheco F, Manrique-Guzman S. Pituitary tumor surgery: review of 3004 cases. *World Neurosurg.* 2013;79(2):331–336.
12. Schloffer H. Erfolgreiche Operation eines Hypophysentumors auf nasalem Wege. *Wien Klin Wochenschr.* 1907;20:621–624.
13. Buchfelder M, Schlaffer S. Surgical treatment of pituitary tumours. *Best Pract Res Clin Endocrinol Metab.* 2009;23(5):677–692.
14. Couldwell WT. Transsphenoidal and transcranial surgery for pituitary adenomas. *J Neurooncol.* 2004;69(1–3):237–256.
15. Tabaee A, Anand VK, Barrón Y, et al. Endoscopic pituitary surgery: a systematic review and meta-analysis. *J Neurosurg.* 2009;111(3): 545–554.
16. Jho HD. Endoscopic transsphenoidal surgery. *J Neurooncol.* 2001;54 (2):187–195.
17. Rudnik A, Zawadzki T, Wojtacha M, et al. Endoscopic transnasal transsphenoidal treatment of pathology of the sellar region. *Minim Invasive Neurosurg.* 2005;48(2):101–107.
18. Berker M, Hazer DB, Yücel T, et al. Complications of endoscopic surgery of the pituitary adenomas: analysis of 570 patients and review of the literature. *Pituitary.* 2012;15(3):288–300.

19. Lipsett MB, Maclean JP, West CD, Li MC, Pearson OH. An analysis of the polyuria induced by hypophysectomy in man. *J Clin Endocrinol Metab.* 1956;16(2):183–195.
20. Hensen J, Henig A, Fahlbusch R, Meyer M, Boehnert M, Buchfelder M. Prevalence, predictors and patterns of postoperative polyuria and hyponatraemia in the immediate course after transsphenoidal surgery for pituitary adenomas. *Clin Endocrinol (Oxf).* 1999;50 (4):431–439.
21. Hollinshead WH. The interphase of diabetes insipidus. *Mayo Clin Proc.* 1964 Feb;39(2):92–100.
22. Loh JA, Verbalis JG. Disorders of water and salt metabolism associated with pituitary disease. *Endocrinol Metab Clin North Am.* 2008; 37(1):213–234.
23. Richardson DW, Robinson AG. Desmopressin. *Ann Intern Med.* 1985;103(2):228–239.
24. Verbalis JG. Diabetes insipidus. *Rev Endocr Metab Disord.* 2003; 4(2):177–185.
25. Stuijver DJF, van Zaane B, Feelders RA, et al. Incidence of venous thromboembolism in patients with Cushing's syndrome: a multicenter cohort study. *J Clin Endocrinol Metab.* 2011;96(11):3525–3532.

# 15 *Meningiomas*

JORDINA RINCON-TORROELLA, NEERAJ NAVAL, and ALFREDO QUINONES-HINOJOSA

## Introduction

Meningiomas are common intracranial neoplasms classically characterized as slow-growing benign lesions that displace surrounding structures rather than invade them. However, meningiomas may be quite symptomatic. Treatment options include observation, radiosurgery, and surgical resection. Surgery is considered for symptomatic patients or those with marked enlargement, perilesional edema, and progressive symptoms related to the tumor. In cases with extensive involvement of nearby neurovascular structures, the goal may be debulking and decompression. Prevention of bleeding and preservation of the venous system are important points during the surgical resection of meningiomas. Recognized predictive factors of tumor recurrence and overall survival in meningiomas are age, comorbidities, extent of resection, histological grade, and proliferative markers. The extent of surgical resection is the most important factor in the prevention of tumor recurrence.

## Neuroanatomy and Procedure

### Key Concepts

- Conservative management and nonaggressive surgical treatment with close follow-up prevail over those interventions that can increase the risk of complications and postoperative deficits.
- Preoperative plan and intraoperative anesthesia management play a vital role in the surgery of meningiomas.
- The main goal in meningioma surgery is to achieve gross total resection of the lesion, its dural attachment, and the adjacent involved bone.

Meningiomas arise from the arachnoid cap cell.[1] They account for 15% to 20% of all intracranial neoplasms and 34% of all primary brain tumors; 90% are supratentorial, and there is an increased incidence in women. Meningiomas occur anywhere on the brain surface, skull base, and rarely in the ventricles. There are no typical symptoms that are unequivocally specific for meningiomas, and the clinical symptomatology mainly depends on their location, size, growth rate, and involvement of surrounding structures. They are classically characterized as noncancerous, slow-growing lesions that markedly displace the surrounding structures rather than invade them. However, meningiomas may be markedly symptomatic, have a high recurrence rate, or present with multiple foci (Fig. 15.1). Tumors growing near eloquent regions may lead to an early detection. Contrarily, tumors in silent areas may grow disproportionately before presenting any symptoms. More aggressive types have a high growth rate and can produce marked cerebral edema leading to seizures, confusion, and focal neurological symptoms (Table 15.1).[2]

Different treatment options, including observation, radiosurgery, and surgical resection, are available for meningiomas. Surgery for meningiomas is considered in symptomatic patients or those with marked enlargement of the lesion, perilesional edema, and progressive symptoms related to the tumor. With advances in medicine and neuroimaging, the incidence of incidental meningiomas is increasing (10%–15% of total meningiomas).

### Clinical Pearl

Conservative management is appropriate in calcified, slow-growing, asymptomatic meningiomas that are clinically and radiologically stable in follow-up MRI and can be considered in elderly patients with significant medical morbidities.

When surgery is considered for incidental meningiomas, the team needs to take into account age, expected survival, neurological status, and Karnofsky performance status (e.g., patients with considerable life expectancy with meningiomas in critical eloquent regions or growing meningiomas may benefit more from surgery than patients with limited life expectancy and multiple comorbidities).[3,4] In cases with extensive involvement of nearby neurovascular structures, the goal may be debulking and decompression.[5]

With the advances in management of these lesions, patients increasingly seek less invasive alternatives to surgery. During the past 2 decades, radiosurgery has emerged as a safe alternative to surgical removal. Although its use is typically reserved for lesions less than 3 cm in diameter, large clinical studies could potentially expand its indications in the near future. It is reasonable to treat selected meningiomas with radiosurgery alone, especially when the risk of surgery is too high. Selected meningiomas may be treated with fractionated radiotherapy instead of radiosurgery if there are contiguous critically radiosensible structures (optic nerves, brainstem) or if the tumor is too large for the radiosurgical approach. Moreover, radiotherapy may be useful as an adjuvant treatment for patients with atypical or malignant meningiomas and in subtotal or unresectable cases with evidence of growth. Multiple retrospective studies have reported improved progression-free survival after subtotal resections in those patients with postoperative fractionated proton beam therapy, compared with those not irradiated. In the case of World Health Organization (WHO) grade II and III meningiomas, the recurrence rates are high, and

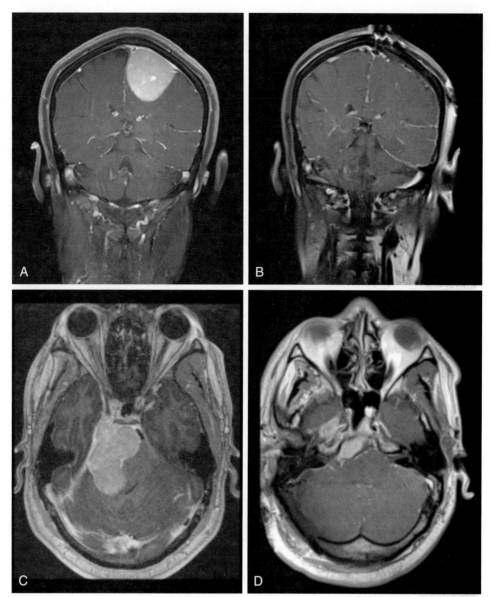

**Fig. 15.1** Imaging assessment in meningioma surgery. **(A, B)** Convexity meningioma before and after surgical resection. **(C, D)** Extensive petroclival meningioma with cavernous sinus invasion before and after surgical resection. Surgery is used for brainstem decompression and debulking; fractionated stereotactic radiation or additional surgery can be used for the management of the residual tumor in a second stage.

**Table 15.1**   The WHO Classification for Meningiomas

| WHO | Description | Recurrence |
| --- | --- | --- |
| Grade I | Well-differentiated meningioma | 9% |
| Grade II | Atypical meningioma | 29% |
| Grade III | Anaplastic meningioma | 50% |

Adapted from Louis DN, et al. The 2007 WHO classification of tumours of the central nervous system. *Acta Neuropathologica*. 2007;114(2):97–109.

postoperative adjuvant radiation therapy or radiosurgery for residual tumor is recommended. Chemotherapy has almost no role in the management of meningiomas.[6–12]

### Preoperative Planning

Magnetic resonance imaging (MRI) with contrast is the principal imaging study for meningiomas. The tumor is shown as a homogeneously enhancing lesion. The dural tail sign is typical for these lesions: a linear enhancement of the dura mater that continues within a few millimeters or centimeters and represents dural invasion or a hypervascular site where the tumor is attached (Fig. 15.1).[13–15] Thin MRI cuts in skull-base or posterior fossa meningiomas are required to study the anatomical relationship between the tumor and the surrounding neurovascular structures.

The computed tomography (CT) scan can be used to evaluate the presence of calcifications (sign of slow growth rate) and/or bone hyperostosis. Extensive encasement of vessels or nerves may compromise the extent of resection or the chances of recovery—especially if the tumor is highly calcified on the CT scan. In cases of extensive bone involvement, plastic surgery may be required during the same sitting or in a delayed fashion for extensive craniofacial reconstruction with the use of vascularized flaps, grafts, and/or customized bone flaps.

Preoperative embolization is still controversial and may be considered in selected cases of complex giant meningiomas, aggressive hypervascular meningiomas, or when profuse bleeding is anticipated and blood transfusion cannot be performed.[6,16–18]

Preoperative assessment includes a complete neurological examination to evaluate neurological deficits, level of consciousness, and presence or absence of elevated intracranial pressure (ICP). Associated medical disorders, such as diabetes, cardiac disease, or uncontrolled hypertension, increase the risk of surgery. These patients may have impaired autoregulation of cerebral perfusion and require careful monitoring in the perioperative period.

In the presence of marked cerebral edema, the use of steroids (e.g., dexamethasone 4 mg/8 hr) is recommended to reduce peritumoral edema. Preoperative anticonvulsive drugs may be indicated in patients with seizures, but in general are not recommended prophylactically. Platelet aggregation inhibitors and coumadin should be stopped or transitioned to bridge therapy a week before surgery to ensure normal hemostasis at the time of surgery, with a goal international normalized ratio (INR) <1.3.[19,20]

As will be described in this chapter, additional specific preoperative tests may be required depending on the planned surgical position and the region and neurovascular structures affected by the tumor. Skull-base meningiomas often involve cranial nerves and vessels and might furthermore compress the brainstem and/or the spinal cord. To avoid cranial nerve and/or spinal cord injury, monitoring of nerve and spinal cord function is essential. Intraoperative electromyography, visual, auditory, somatosensory, or motor evoked potentials may be recorded to monitor and avoid cranial nerves and spinal deficits. The efficiency of neuromonitoring may depend on the anesthesia management and may be technician dependent.

## SURGERY FOR MENINGIOMAS

Although the surgical management and the surgical approach depend on the tumor location, some steps are common in meningioma resection.[21–23]

- *Operative positioning:* The positioning is tailored to the selected approach. In meningioma surgery, head elevation is essential to favor cerebral venous drainage and decrease venous congestion. In general, for anterior tumors, the patient is placed in a supine or lateral position. For occipital and posterior fossa tumors, the patient may be placed in a prone or sitting position. In the latter, the team needs to be aware of the inherent complications related to the sitting position (discussed later in this chapter) (Fig. 15.2).
- *Pinning:* The patient's head is fixed with a three-pin skull clamp. Coordination between the anesthesia and surgical teams is necessary to assure that the patient is adequately anesthetized before the pinning. Local anesthetic may be applied to the region to avoid bleeding from the puncture site, reduce vital sign elevation secondary to pain, and decrease the postoperative pain. Hematoma or bleeding at the pinning site may occur. Some cases have reported small bone fractures in areas with thin bone (e.g., temporal squama). Soreness at the pinning site is common and can be present weeks after the procedure. The patient needs to be well informed because this pain can be located far from to the incision site and may worry the patient.
- The *skin incision* is carefully performed in order to preserve the pericranium for dural reconstruction during the closure.
- Once the bone is exposed the surgeon proceeds with the *craniotomy*. Burr holes and craniotomy are strategically placed for a tailored opening. Meningiomas alter the morphology and consistency of the dura mater and bone such that the underlying dura mater is often tightly attached to the bone and the two are sometimes removed together during the flap elevation. Depending on the tumor location, the craniotomy cuts are placed to avoid the venous pools and venous sinuses. The relation of the tumor to the surrounding venous structures must be evaluated preoperatively because damage to the venous system during the craniotomy can be extremely dangerous. Sometimes these tumors promote abnormal

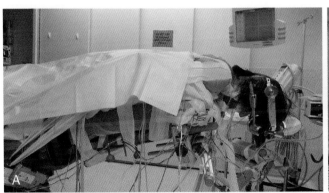 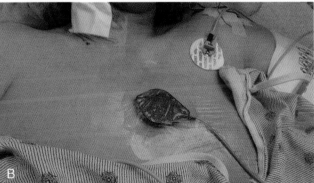

**Fig. 15.2 (A)** Prone position for a torcular meningioma. The prone position is preferred over the sitting position because it carries less risk of intraoperative air embolism. **(B)** Placement of intraoperative Doppler ultrasounds for early detection of air embolism.

venous drainage through the bone to be resected as part of the craniotomy. Sacrificing these plexus can lead to blood loss, air emboli, or both and lead to increased morbidity during the surgery. It is better to appreciate this before surgery in order to have a contingency plan for the resection of the tumor, which may include working around this segment of bone until the tumor is significantly debulked.

- If the tumor is tenaciously attached to the dura mater and prevents a standard dural opening, a round dural window is opened around the tumor, leaving the dura mater attached to it while preserving the underlying bridging veins. The affected dura will be removed together with the tumor. Pericranium or biosynthetic duraplasties can be used to substitute the dura during the closure (Fig. 15.3C).
- If the bone flap is hyperostotic, it can be undermined with a drill. If it is markedly affected and infiltrated by the tumor, it needs to be replaced (Fig. 15.3A).
- After tumor exposure, the tumor dura and/or surface are coagulated and feeding vessels are identified and coagulated. This eliminates some arterial supply to the tumor and decreases the bleeding during tumor resection. Meningiomas are mostly displacing rather invading tumors. The challenge is to identify the interface between the tumor and the surrounding structures and to dissect the tumor margins. In large meningiomas, central debulking of the tumor is performed first to facilitate tumor resection and limit brain retraction (Fig. 15.4A).

- The use of static brain retractors is minimized. Adequate positioning, opening of the arachnoid cisterns for cerebrospinal fluid (CSF) drainage, and promotion of diuresis is crucial to facilitate the tumor resection while avoiding excessive retraction and manipulation of the cerebral parenchyma. The use of cottonoid patties and/or long cotton strips can aid in the natural retraction of the brain without using brain retractors. When retractors are used, it is recommended to reposition them intermittently.
- Patient positioning is key. Ideally, the tumor is located at the highest point of the operative field. Head rotation is used strategically such that gravity favors retraction of the brain away from the tumor. Furthermore, positioning should allow meningeal structures (tent, falx, etc.) to serve as a natural point of retraction. Proper use of mannitol and controlled hypercapnia promote a relaxed brain, providing more space for retraction and maneuverability.
- Once the tumor margins have been identified, the surgeon carefully proceeds with dissection of major veins and arterial branches encased or displaced by the lesion. If involved, the cranial nerves are identified and dissected away from the tumor with delicate microsurgical technique. When the tumor is firmly attached to the neurovascular structures, it is preferable to leave minor residual portions of the tumor adherent to important neurovascular structures rather than sacrificing them (Fig. 15.4B).
- *Excision of the affected dura mater* is required to decrease the chances of recurrence. When complete resection of the dural attachment is not possible, the infiltrated dura mater is coagulated.[1]

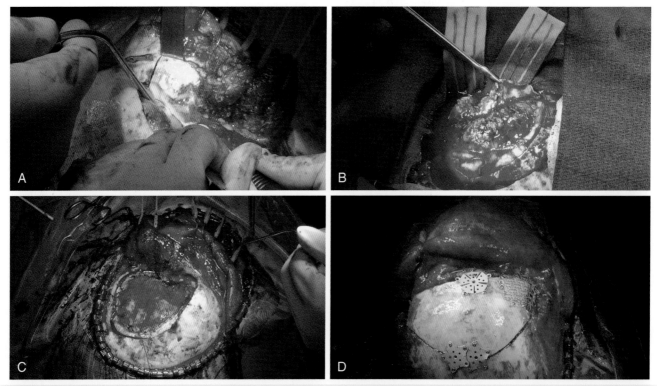

**Fig. 15.3** Intraoperative pictures. **(A)** Marked hyperostosis associated with a sphenoid wing meningioma prevents the use of a craniotome. An electric bone saw is used to cut the thick bone. **(B)** Notice the highly vascular nature of this giant convexity meningioma. The tumor is tightly attached to the dura mater that will be resected together with the mass. **(C)** Complex closure in meningioma surgery. The invaded dura mater had to be resected in the lateral surface of the brain. A piece of pericranium has been used as a dural substitute for a watertight closure. **(D)** Complex bone reconstruction after the removal of an anterior cranial fossa meningioma. *Hyperostotic bone.

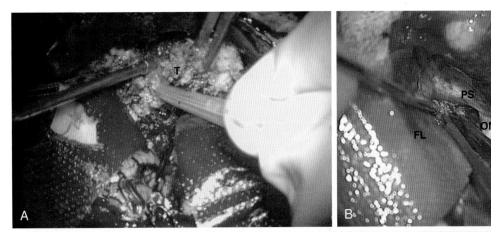

**Fig. 15.4** Intraoperative view of the surgical field under the magnification of the operative microscope. **(A)** Central debulking of a large convexity meningioma with an ultrasonic aspirator. **(B)** Notice the tight surgical corridor deep to the parasellar region and the close relationship in between this olfactory groove meningioma and the optic nerve and internal carotid artery. *FL,* frontal lobe; *ON,* optic nerve; *ICA,* internal carotid artery; *PS,* planum sphenoidale; *T,* tumor.

- Standard *closure* of dural, bone, and soft tissue is performed for the chosen approach. Bone cement and/or titanium mesh can be used to improve cosmesis when required (Fig. 15.3D).

## SPECIFIC CONSIDERATIONS

> ### Clinical Pearl
>
> Meningiomas occluding venous sinuses (falcine, parasagittal, torcular, tentorial) can produce venous congestion resulting in generalized edema and marked intracranial hypertension that can be the presenting symptom. Those patients may be first treated with steroids to decrease the edema.

- **Involvement of venous sinuses**: Surgical management of meningiomas arising from the venous sinuses or invading them is challenging. In most cases, preservation of the sinus prevails over complete resection of the tumor. Once the central part of the tumor has been debulked, the portion that is attached to the sinus is disconnected from the other margins to avoid pulling the sinus while maneuvering. As mentioned before, meningiomas are highly vascularized lesions, and tumor remnants increase the risk of postoperative hemorrhage. Standard management is coagulating the tumor remnants attached to the venous sinus with the goal of disconnecting possible feeders and achieving good hemostasis. Tumor recurrence may be managed with a "second look" surgery or radiation. In selected cases, the sinuses may be sacrificed. Only thrombosed sinuses with established collateral circulation will be amenable for disconnection. In those cases, the frontal part of the superior sagittal sinus (anterior third) and the transverse sinus (unilaterally) are relatively safe to sacrifice in order to attempt a total resection. Contrarily, the parietal segment of the sagittal sinus, the torcula, or a dominant transverse sinus is rarely sacrificed due to their extreme importance in venous outflow. There are some studies that advocate complete resection and sinus repair with reconstruction.[24] However, conservative management still prevails with good outcomes and fewer complications.[25–27]

- Current management of large skull-base meningiomas involving several neurovascular structures (e.g., cavernous sinus, petroclival, and cerebellopontine region) includes staged resection with combined approaches and partial resection with adjuvant radiotherapy.[28] Skull-base approaches to meningiomas often require interdisciplinary teamwork during surgery (ear/nose/throat, maxillofacial, plastic, and neuroophthalmology) and laborious reconstructions with specific techniques. The ability to safely follow tumor growth and the slow-growing progression and the displacing nature (rather than invading) of meningiomas favor the preservation of function and the patient's quality of life over a complete resection of the tumor.[29]

- **Optic sheath meningiomas**: Attempts at resection lead to marked postoperative deficits and visual impairment in almost all cases. Therefore surgical options are limited to the excision of the exophytic component and optic nerve decompression by unroofing the optic canal. Radiotherapy can stabilize the disease but may also produce visual impairment.

## Perioperative Considerations

### Key Concepts

- Securing good ventilation to avoid hypoxia and hypercarbia
- Maintaining controlled hypocarbia to help decrease the ICP
- Regulation of hydroionic balance and decreasing brain edema with osmotic agents (mannitol) while maintaining cerebral perfusion with fluids and inotropics
- Cerebral protection with choice of anesthetics and blood pressure management
- Awareness of potential complications when the patient is placed in the sitting position or the tumor involves the venous sinuses

The anesthesia team plays a key role during meningioma surgery. The intraoperative anesthetic management requirements are listed earlier. These goals are directed to provide adequate tissue perfusion to the brain while providing optimal surgical conditions (relaxed brain and low ICP). A slack brain facilitates maneuverability in deep and tiny corridors and may avoid the need of brain retractors, decreasing the total risk of postoperative deficits. This may be challenging because cerebral flow autoregulation may be altered as a consequence of parenchymal changes (edema, hypoxia, acidosis). The intraoperative hemodynamic management in meningioma surgery presents special challenges for the anesthesia team, especially with the concern of minimizing ICP. Patients may experience rapid changes in intravascular volume and cardiac filling pressures due to blood loss, aggressive diuresis, and anesthetic agents. Additionally, patients with preoperative nausea and vomiting due to cerebral edema and intraoperative mannitol administration may be hypovolemic. This requires continuous assessment of volume status.

Strict blood pressure control and respiratory management are essential during meningioma surgery, and coordination with the anesthesia team is highly recommended.

## INTRAOPERATIVE COMPLICATIONS

- **Bleeding from a highly vascularized tumor:** Meningiomas are highly vascularized lesions with peripheral feeding pedicles from local blood vessels. The feeding pedicle is cauterized early in the surgery whenever possible to avoid major blood loss during debulking. If induced hypotension is being used to decrease the bleeding, the pressure is normalized early after the tumor is resected and before the dura mater is closed to avoid inadvertent and incomplete hemostasis masked by the lowered blood pressure. The Valsalva maneuver can be used to evaluate the achievement of good hemostasis.

- **Bleeding from intracranial venous congestion:** Sagittal, parasagittal, and torcular meningiomas are often related to a complex network of normal and collateral veins. Especially when those tumors compress or block the venous sinuses, venous congestion may be present preoperatively. Because meningiomas are slow-growing tumors, collateral venous pools and veins may develop over time. Some of those veins drain extensive eloquent areas of the brain to the venous sinuses, and compromising them could lead to marked postoperative deficits. Sacrificing the surrounding veins to access the tumor or unexpected venous thrombosis may be harmless in some cases. However, excessive venous compromise or compromise from major veins may be devastating and lead to venous congestion, parenchymal edema, and even seizures, intracranial hypertension, and herniation in extreme cases. This may be accompanied by venous infarction with intraparenchymal hemorrhage.

- Preservation of the venous system is one of the most important points during the surgical resection of meningiomas. Preoperative MRI angiography and venography are essential for operative planning to decide which veins can be sacrificed and which are major draining veins that may be left intact. Indocyanine green (ICG) angiography allows intraoperative real-time evaluation of the intradural vessels related to the tumor. The use of intraoperative ICG can guide the surgeon in the identification and preservation of bridging veins as well as major sinuses[30] (Fig. 15.5). When the tumor is attached or arising from a major draining vein or sinus, there is a high risk of venous infarction associated with tumor removal. In those cases, complete resection is compromised, and the tumor remnant will be followed radiologically and clinically.

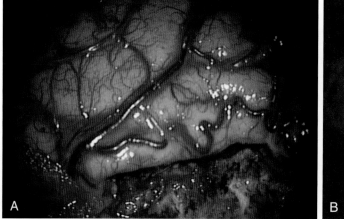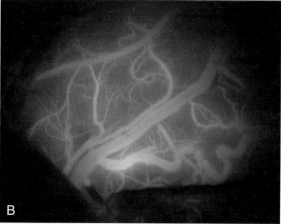

**Fig. 15.5** Recently intraoperative methods of venous flow recognition such as indocyanine green (ICG) videography have been studied to help identify and preserve potentially critical draining veins into the venous sinus during resection of meningiomas. The ICG is injected before the dural opening to evaluate the presence of underlying superficial veins. The tumor and surrounding veins are observed under the microscope with a fluorescent filter, and real-time flow assessment of the underlying veins can be done as the contrast reaches the tumor region. The veins can be marked on the dural surface with a pen. Dural opening and removal of the tumor are performed with preservation of the venous anatomy. After tumor resection, ICG videoangiography can be readministered to confirm vascular integrity. * and ** are used to point the same veins in the regular microscope and the fluorescent filter vision.

■ **Complications of venous sinus damage**: Damage to a venous sinus is one of the major risks during removal of meningiomas. It is associated with two important complications: air embolism and major venous bleeding. If a dural sinus lesion occurs, rapid control of the bleeding will reduce the chances of major complications, for example, air embolism. The negative pressure in a perforated venous sinus can aspirate air. Thus the risk of air embolism is markedly increased in the sitting position, where the level of the head is considerably above the level of the heart. If an air bolus reaches the heart, it can cause an air embolus in the pulmonary artery with potential pulmonary infarction or complete circulatory collapse. If there is a patent foramen ovale, air bubbles can enter the left ventricle with embolization to the coronary arteries, resulting in myocardial infarction, or to the cerebral vessels, causing a massive stroke. There are several techniques to prevent, detect, or limit an air embolism and their consequences. Special attention and coordination between the surgeons and anesthesia team are planned to react expeditiously.[31]

▪ PREVENT: All the patients placed in the sitting position require a preoperative cardiac Doppler/ultrasound. If a patent foramen ovale is demonstrated, the sitting position is contraindicated. The first maneuver to avoid or limit air emboli after a sinus lesion is applying copious irrigation/flooding the area and covering the sinus with cottonoids. At the same time, the anesthesia team immediately places the patient in the Trendelenburg position, moving the head down. Bleeding originating from the dural sinuses can be usually controlled with cotton balls, Surgicel, or Gelfoam. When bleeding continues despite those maneuvers, a piece of dura or a muscle graft can be sewn over the dural defect or the sinus can be repaired. If the attempts to repair the lesion don't succeed, ligation of the sinus may be performed to avoid life-threatening hemorrhages.

▪ DETECT: A large bolus of air in the heart will manifest with a constant "machinery" murmur by Doppler ultrasound. Thus the use of continuous intraoperative monitoring with Doppler ultrasound is recommended when the surgery takes place near a major venous sinus or if the patient is placed in the sitting position. Additionally, during the procedure the right atrial pressure is maintained and controlled with a central line (Fig. 15.2*B*).

▪ LIMIT: Left lateral decubitus and Trendelenburg positions can entrap the air bubble in the heart, avoiding further complications and allowing endovascular access to aspirate the air. The left lateral decubitus position can trap the air in the nondependent segment of the right ventricle and avoid its progression into the pulmonary artery, or to the left ventricle if a patent foramen ovale exists. The Trendelenburg position is intended to keep a left ventricular air bubble away from the coronary artery ostia, preventing occlusion of the coronary arteries.

■ **Neurocognitive or cranial nerve deficits**: Meticulous preoperative planning, delicate microsurgical technique, and intraoperative monitoring are used to avoid damage to the cerebral parenchyma or neurovascular structures.[32]

# Postoperative Complications

## Key Concepts

- Ease the recovery from anesthesia.
- Individualize care using specialized neuromonitoring.
- Optimize and balance hemodynamic and respiratory status.
- Observe vigilantly for postoperative complications and intervene early.
- Standardize and protocolize care to minimize the risk of medical complications.

The basic goals of postoperative neurosurgical care are listed earlier and major complications are listed below (Box 15.1). Minor postoperative complications include nausea/vomiting, shivering, agitation, and discomfort. Not a minor complication, postoperative pain often is underestimated and undertreated. No standardized pain protocols exist to assess and treat pain, and treatment usually consists of opiates.

CSF leak: Meningioma surgery often requires extensive dural resection. Skull-base and posterior fossa meningiomas may require extensive craniotomies and substantial bone drilling to access and remove the lesion. If hyperostosis is present, additional bone drilling may be required. Large bone and dural defects increase the risk of postoperative CSF leak and require complex reconstruction using duraplasties, cranioplasties, or titanium meshes (Fig. 15.3D). Once the dura mater has been closed, a Valsalva maneuver is helpful to determine the existence of an intraoperative CSF leak. Assuring watertight closure of the dura mater and careful reconstruction will decrease the risk of postoperative CSF leak and at the same time will help to achieve good postoperative cosmetic results.

Management: A clear discharge from the wound in the early postoperative period is suspicious of CSF leak. If there is no risk of herniation (hematoma, residual tumor, extensive pneumocephalus), a lumbar drain may be placed. If the discharge continues despite lumbar drain placement, surgical wound revision may be required.

Intracranial hemorrhage/intracranial hypertension: Intracranial hypertension and intracranial bleeding need to be detected and treated promptly. Because meningiomas are highly vascularized lesions, they are associated with an increased risk of postoperative hemorrhage, especially if there are tumor remnants and/or when venous outflow has been compromised in an attempt to remove the tumor. If significant blood loss has occurred, postoperative blood tests should include hematological and coagulation parameters.

## Box 15.1    Major Complications After Meningioma Resection

▪ CSF leak
▪ Intracranial hypertension with bleeding
▪ Hematoma
▪ Seizures
▪ Wound infection
▪ Hydrocephalus
▪ Pneumocephalus
▪ Systemic venous thromboembolism

Abnormal parameters are addressed promptly and treatments are initiated. This is especially important in those patients who cannot receive blood transfusion. Intracranial bleeding may require emergent surgery with revision of the surgical bed to locate and reduce tumor remnants.

Management of associated intracranial hypertension should be protocolized to ensure rapid and escalating treatment as needed. It should include management of an unsecured airway, optimization of mean arterial and cerebral perfusion pressure, short-term hyperventilation if deemed necessary, use of hyperosmolar therapy (mannitol and hypertonic saline), external ventricular drainage in select cases, and, in the most refractory cases, pharmacological coma and/or decompressive hemicraniectomy. Frequent monitoring of electrolytes to ensure normonatremia (and, when necessary, hypernatremia) is warranted.

Venous infarction: It is important to elucidate the underlying etiology of significant cerebral edema. In some cases, venous infarction may be responsible, reinforcing the need to preserve the integrity of venous structures as much as possible. Patients considered at highest risk for this complication include those requiring bifrontal craniotomies and superficial location (parasagittal/parafalcine), as well as those patients with lateral or medial sphenoid wing meningiomas, where the veins in the sylvian fissure are often sacrificed. Although anticoagulation is considered the standard of care in the setting of "spontaneous" cerebral venous sinus thrombosis, this intervention certainly carries a significantly higher risk of postoperative bleeding when used after neurosurgical manipulation and should be used cautiously, if considered at all. Avoidance of hypovolemia is strongly recommended postoperatively to prevent hyperviscosity in compromised or damaged venous structures.[33]

Seizures: There are no standardized protocols for seizure prophylaxis in meningioma surgery. The American Academy of Neurology, through a metaanalysis of four level I studies, does not recommend the prophylactic use of antiepileptic drugs (AEDs) in newly diagnosed brain tumors. Depending on the center, prophylactic anticonvulsants may be administered preoperatively and intraoperatively. Patients with meningiomas without a history of seizures are at a much lower risk for postoperative seizures than patients with uncontrolled preoperative seizures. In fact, meningioma surgery may serve to eradicate seizures in over half the patients who had preoperative seizures.[34] Supratentorial convexity, parasagittal or parafalcine location, or sphenoid wing meningiomas carry the highest risk of preoperative seizures, whereas the presence of increased cerebral edema is associated with a higher incidence of postoperative seizures.

In a systematic analysis of efficacy conducted by Komotar et al., prophylactic administration of anticonvulsants during resection of supratentorial meningiomas provides no benefit in the prevention of either early or late postoperative seizures.[35,36] In the setting of ongoing postoperative seizures, however, particular attention is paid to possible airway compromise, and an urgent CT scan may be ordered to rule out postoperative bleeding as a possible cause. A multitude of AEDs may be used, with benzodiazepines preferred for immediate cessation of seizure, and other antiseizure agents such as phenytoin, fosphenytoin, and levetiracetam useful in preventing generalization of seizures.

At our institution, patients without preoperative seizures were typically given AEDs for seizure prophylaxis immediately before surgery and weaned off. In patients with preoperative seizures, antiseizure medication can be continued typically for indication based of postoperative seizure recurrence. If a patient has recurrent seizures, obtaining a follow-up MRI is recommended. Additionally, anti-seizure medications may be prescribed indefinitely.[34]

Infection: Surgery of meningiomas often involves extensive openings and long surgeries that increase the risk of wound infection. Sometimes these surgeries may require opening the frontal sinus, which may require special care with sinus exenteration and the use of a vascularized pericranial flap to cover the defect. Preoperative and intraoperative antibiotic therapy may be used to prevent surgical site infection. Delayed postoperative wound discharge and fever may indicate infection of the surgical site. Superficial infections may be treated with local debridement of the wound edges and systemic antibiotics. Deeper infections may extend to the bone flap leading to osteomyelitis with increased risk of meningitis. Broad-spectrum antibiotics that target gram-positive (including methicillin-resistant *Staphylococcus aureus* [MRSA]), gram-negative, and anaerobic bacteria can be used (a combination of vancomycin, fourth-generation cephalosporin, and metronidazole is reasonable), with subsequent adjustment based on wound or CSF cultures. When the bone flap is affected, surgical wound revision with extraction of the bone flap may be required. Once the infection has been treated and is cleared, a reconstructive surgery is required to implant a cranioplasty (Fig. 15.6).

Other postoperative complications may be site specific. Intrasellar, suprasellar, and parasellar meningiomas (e.g., tuberculum sellae meningiomas) are monitored closely for diabetes insipidus (DI) and CSF leak. Patients with DI may be administered vasopressin in the setting of significant urinary output (UO >250 cc/h for >2 hours), excretion of maximally dilute urine (urinary specific gravity <1.005), and uncorrected free water deficit (Na >145). If able, the patient is encouraged to drink to suppress thirst, and the aforementioned parameters are closely monitored with hourly urine output and hourly electrolyte and urine specific gravity monitoring. Monitoring of endocrine parameters (thyroid-stimulating hormone [TSH], adrenocorticotropic hormone [ACTH], cortisol, etc.) may be considered with correction of observed imbalances.

Jugular foramen meningiomas are at high risk for postoperative cranial nerve palsies, especially in patients who presented with preexisting deficits. These deficits may be reversible in some, but not all, cases. Such patients may exhibit loss of protective airway reflexes due to bulbar palsies, and liberation from the ventilator may be attempted with extreme caution, with standby support from advanced airway experts, especially when vocal cord paralysis may render a patient with a "difficult airway." In selected cases, a planned tracheostomy and/or gastrostomy may be a reasonable option.

Resection of olfactory groove meningiomas may be associated with a high postoperative risk of anosmia. Resections in this location, however, are associated with a relatively low risk of permanent morbidity, with very low recurrence rates.

Medical complications: These include congestive heart failure/volume overload, pneumonia leading to compromised respiratory status, deep venous thrombosis/pulmonary

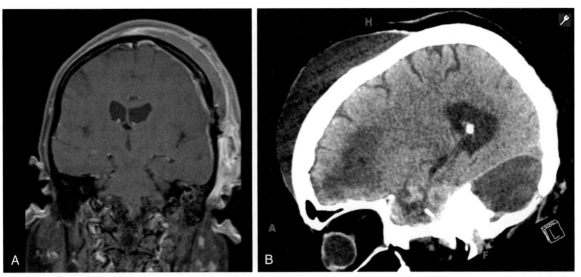

**Fig. 15.6** Postoperative complications. **(A)** Wound infection. **(B)** Venous infarct with subsequent brain edema.

embolism, cardiac ischemia, and cardiac arrhythmias such as postoperative atrial fibrillation. Elderly patients are at the highest risk for development of medical complications and require especially close monitoring after surgical resection of meningiomas. Additionally, patients with multiple medical comorbidities based on the Charlson comorbidity index, as well as poor preoperative functional status, are more likely to have a prolonged postsurgical hospital course. Preoperative counseling and education are essential, both for purposes of optimizing medical stability for surgery and for risk stratification.

## FOLLOW-UP AND PROGNOSIS

Recognized predictive factors of tumor recurrence and overall survival in meningiomas are age, comorbidities, extent of resection, histological grade, and proliferative markers. The extent of surgical resection is the most important factor in the prevention of tumor recurrence.[10,37] The Simpson grading system has been used for decades to predict the possibility of tumor recurrence (Table 15.2). Contemporary histopathological molecular and genetic markers (Ki-67 or MIB-1) help determine the proliferation index. Those cannot be the sole determinant for grading, but correlate with the risk of recurrence and can be of assistance for a tailored follow-up strategy and management.[1,38–41]

The use of radiosurgery alone for small to medium-sized meningiomas has been growing exponentially for the past 2 decades. The goals of radiosurgery are preventing further tumor growth while avoiding the risk of open surgery. Although there are no available Level I data with prospective randomized trials, a Level II cohort study for tumors <3.5 cm in diameter reported that the control rate after radiosurgery is at least equivalent to that after resection of meningiomas. Level II evidence in contemporary retrospective studies with a large series of cases have suggested that the tumor control rate for grade I tumors is greater than 90%.[42–45]

MRI is the preferred follow-up method. Follow-up assessments should be conducted every 6 months to a year; if

**Table 15.2** Simpson Grading System for Removal of Meningiomas

| Simpson Grade | Definition | Recurrence (Time to Recurrence) |
|---|---|---|
| 1 | Macroscopically complete removal of tumor, *with excision* of its dural attachment, and abnormal bone. Resection of venous sinus if involved. | 9% (62 months) |
| 2 | Macroscopically complete removal of tumor and its visible extensions *with coagulation* of its dural attachment. | 19% (59 months) |
| 3 | Macroscopically complete removal of the tumor, *without* resection or coagulation of its dural attachment or its extradural extensions. (e.g., hyperostosis) | 29% |
| 4 | *Partial* removal, leaving intradural tumor in situ | 40% |
| 5 | Simple decompression ± biopsy | |

Adapted from Simpson D. The recurrence of intracranial meningiomas after surgical treatment. *J Neurol Neurosurg Psychiatry.* 1957;20(1):22–39.

growth is not detected, it can be extended to every 2 years. Other tests such as ophthalmological assessment and audiograms may be useful in those meningiomas affecting the respective cranial nerves.

## Conclusions

Although the intraoperative and postoperative complications of intracranial surgery for meningiomas are challenging, they can be prevented by means of rigorous preoperative planning, methodical surgical skills, systematic periodical postoperative care, and thorough attention and quick responsiveness to early signs and symptoms.

# References

1. Simpson D. The recurrence of intracranial meningiomas after surgical treatment. *J Neurol Neurosurg Psychiatry.* 1957;20(1):22–39.
2. Louis DN, Ohgaki H, Wiestler OD, et al. The 2007 WHO classification of tumours of the central nervous system. *Acta Neuropathol.* 2007;114(2):97–109.
3. Zlotnick D, Kalkanis SN, Quinones-Hinojosa A, et al. FACT-MNG: tumor site specific web-based outcome instrument for meningioma patients. *J Neurooncol.* 2010;99(3):423–431.
4. Grossman R, Mukherjee D, Chang DC, et al. Preoperative Charlson comorbidity score predicts postoperative outcomes among older intracranial meningioma patients. *World Neurosurg.* 2011;75(2):279–285.
5. Quinones-Hinojosa A, Kaprealian T, Chaichana KL, et al. Preoperative factors affecting resectability of giant intracranial meningiomas. *Can J Neurol Sci.* 2009;36(5):623–630.
6. Quinones-Hinojosa A, Raza SM. *Controversies in Neuro-Oncology: Best Evidence Medicine for Brain Tumor Surgery.* New York: Thieme; 2013.
7. Adeberg S, Hartmann C, Welzel T, et al. Long-term outcome after radiotherapy in patients with atypical and malignant meningiomas—clinical results in 85 patients treated in a single institution leading to optimized guidelines for early radiation therapy. *Int J Radiat Oncol Biol Phys.* 2012;83(3):859–864.
8. Boskos C, Feuvret L, Noel G, et al. Combined proton and photon conformal radiotherapy for intracranial atypical and malignant meningioma. *Int J Radiat Oncol Biol Phys.* 2009;75(2):399–406.
9. Pasquier D, Bijmolt S, Veninga T, et al. Atypical and malignant meningioma: outcome and prognostic factors in 119 irradiated patients. A multicenter, retrospective study of the Rare Cancer Network. *Int J Radiat Oncol Biol Phys.* 2008;71(5):1388–1393.
10. Condra KS, Buatti JM, Mendenhall WM, Friedman WA, Marcus Jr RB, Rhoton AL. Benign meningiomas: primary treatment selection affects survival. *Int J Radiat Oncol Biol Phys.* 1997;39(2):427–436.
11. Starke RM, Williams BJ, Hiles C, Nguyen JH, Elsharkawy MY, Sheehan JP. Gamma knife surgery for skull base meningiomas. *J Neurosurg.* 2012;116(3):588–597.
12. Stafford SL, Pollock BE, Foote RL, et al. Meningioma radiosurgery: tumor control, outcomes, and complications among 190 consecutive patients. *Neurosurgery.* 2001;49(5):1029–1037. discussion 37–38.
13. Borovich B, Doron Y. Recurrence of intracranial meningiomas: the role played by regional multicentricity. *J Neurosurg.* 1986;64(1):58–63.
14. Borovich B, Doron Y, Braun J, et al. Recurrence of intracranial meningiomas: the role played by regional multicentricity. Part 2: clinical and radiological aspects. *J Neurosurg.* 1986;65(2):168–171.
15. Nagele T, Petersen D, Klose U, Grodd W, Opitz H, Voigt K. The "dural tail" adjacent to meningiomas studied by dynamic contrast-enhanced MRI: a comparison with histopathology. *Neuroradiology.* 1994;36(4):303–307.
16. Alberione F, Iturrieta P, Schulz J, et al. Preoperative embolisation with absorbable gelatine sponge in intracranial meningiomas. *Rev Neurol.* 2009;49(1):13–17.
17. Bendszus M, Rao G, Burger R, et al. Is there a benefit of preoperative meningioma embolization? *Neurosurgery.* 2000;47(6):1306–1311. discussion 11–12.
18. Dean BL, Flom RA, Wallace RC, et al. Efficacy of endovascular treatment of meningiomas: evaluation with matched samples. *Am J Neuroradiol.* 1994;15(9):1675–1680.
19. Jaffer AK. Perioperative management of warfarin and antiplatelet therapy. *Cleve Clin J Med.* 2009;76(Suppl 4):S37–S44.
20. White RH, McKittrick T, Hutchinson R, Twitchell J. Temporary discontinuation of warfarin therapy: changes in the international normalized ratio. *Ann Intern Med.* 1995;122(1):32–40.
21. DeMonte F, McDermott M. *Al-Mefty's meningiomas.* New York: Thieme; 2011.
22. Quinones-Hinojosa A. *Schmidek and Sweet: Operative Neurosurgical Techniques 2-Volume Set, Indications, Methods and Results (Expert Consult-Online and Print), 6: Schmidek and Sweet: Operative Neurosurgical Techniques 2-Volume Set.* London: Elsevier Health Sciences; 2012.
23. Yasargil MG. *Microneurosurgery. Vol IV, Microneurosurgery of CNS Tumors.* Stuttgart: Thieme Stratton; 1984.
24. Sindou M. Meningiomas involving major dural sinuses: should we attempt at radical removal and venous repair? *World Neurosurg.* 2014;81(1):46–47.
25. Raza SM, Gallia GL, Brem H, Weingart JD, Long DM, Olivi A. Perioperative and long-term outcomes from the management of parasagittal meningiomas invading the superior sagittal sinus. *Neurosurgery.* 2010;67(4):885–893. discussion 893.
26. Quinones-Hinojosa A, Chang EF, Chaichana KL, McDermott MW. Surgical considerations in the management of falcotentorial meningiomas: advantages of the bilateral occipital transtentorial/transfalcine craniotomy for large tumors. *Neurosurgery.* 2009;64(5 Suppl 2):260–268 discussion 268.
27. Quinones-Hinojosa A, Chang EF, McDermott MW. Falcotentorial meningiomas: clinical, neuroimaging, and surgical features in six patients. *Neurosurg Focus.* 2003;14(6):e11.
28. Park SH, Kano H, Niranjan A, Flickinger JC, Lunsford LD. Stereotactic radiosurgery for cerebellopontine angle meningiomas. *J Neurosurg.* 2014;120(3):708–715.
29. Kalkanis SN, Quinones-Hinojosa A, Buzney E, Ribaudo HJ, Black PM. Quality of life following surgery for intracranial meningiomas at Brigham and Women's Hospital: a study of 164 patients using a modification of the functional assessment of cancer therapy-brain questionnaire. *J Neurooncol.* 2000;48(3):233–241.
30. Jusue-Torres I, Navarro-Ramirez R, Gallego MP, Chaichana KL, Quinones-Hinojosa A. Indocyanine green for vessel identification and preservation before dural opening for parasagittal lesions. *Neurosurgery.* 2013;73(2 Suppl Operative):145. discussion.
31. Rozet I, Vavilala MS. Risks and benefits of patient positioning during neurosurgical care. *Anesthesiol Clin.* 2007;25(3):631–653. x.
32. Chaichana KL, Jackson C, Patel A, et al. Predictors of visual outcome following surgical resection of medial sphenoid wing meningiomas. *J Neurol Surg B Skull Base.* 2012;73(5):321–326.
33. Sughrue ME, Rutkowski MJ, Shangari G, et al. Incidence, risk factors, and outcome of venous infarction after meningioma surgery in 705 patients. *J Clin Neurosci.* 2011;18(5):628–632.
34. Chaichana KL, Pendleton C, Zaidi H, et al. Seizure control for patients undergoing meningioma surgery. *World Neurosurg.* 2013;79(3–4):515–524.
35. Komotar RJ, Raper DM, Starke RM, Iorgulescu JB, Gutin PH. Prophylactic antiepileptic drug therapy in patients undergoing supratentorial meningioma resection: a systematic analysis of efficacy. *J Neurosurg.* 2011;115(3):483–490.
36. Ngwenya LB, Chiocca EA. Do meningioma patients benefit from antiepileptic drug treatment? *World Neurosurg.* 2013;79(3-4):433–434.
37. Mendenhall WM, Friedman WA, Amdur RJ, Foote KD. Management of benign skull base meningiomas: a review. *Skull Base.* 2004;14(1):53–60. discussion 1.
38. Shibata T, Burger PC, Kleihues P. Ki-67 immunoperoxidase stain as marker for the histological grading of nervous system tumours. *Acta Neurochir Suppl.* 1988;43:103–106.
39. Kolles H, Niedermayer I, Schmitt C, et al. Triple approach for diagnosis and grading of meningiomas: histology, morphometry of Ki-67/Feulgen stainings, and cytogenetics. *Acta Neurochir.* 1995;137(3–4):174–181.
40. Bruna J, Brell M, Ferrer I, Gimenez-Bonafe P, Tortosa A. Ki-67 proliferative index predicts clinical outcome in patients with atypical or anaplastic meningioma. *Neuropathology.* 2007;27(2):114–120.
41. Perry A, Scheithauer BW, Stafford SL, Lohse CM, Wollan PC. "Malignancy" in meningiomas: a clinicopathologic study of 116 patients, with grading implications. *Cancer.* 1999;85(9):2046–2056.
42. Santacroce A, Walier M, Regis J, et al. Long-term tumor control of benign intracranial meningiomas after radiosurgery in a series of 4565 patients. *Neurosurgery.* 2012;70(1):32–39. discussion 9.
43. Kondziolka D, Levy EI, Niranjan A, Flickinger JC, Lunsford LD. Long-term outcomes after meningioma radiosurgery: physician and patient perspectives. *J Neurosurg.* 1999;91(1):44–50.
44. Zada G, Pagnini PG, Yu C, et al. Long-term outcomes and patterns of tumor progression after gamma knife radiosurgery for benign meningiomas. *Neurosurgery.* 2010;67(2):322–328. discussion 8–9.
45. Kreil W, Luggin J, Fuchs I, Weigl V, Eustacchio S, Papaefthymiou G. Long term experience of gamma knife radiosurgery for benign skull base meningiomas. *J Neurol Neurosurg Psychiatry.* 2005;76(10):1425–1430.

# 16 *Gliomas*

ANDREW S. VENTEICHER, JONATHAN ROSAND, and WILLIAM T. CURRY, JR.

## Introduction

The goals of tumor resection include obtaining a tissue diagnosis, improving neurological symptoms, and maximizing survival. The increasing repertoire of tools, including stereotactic guidance, advanced imaging, awake craniotomy, and intraoperative mapping, have enhanced our ability to maximize safe glioma resection.[1–3] This is of paramount importance because the extent of resection (EOR) correlates with improved survival. In this chapter, we outline the anatomical, perioperative, and postoperative considerations in modern glioma surgery.

## Neuroanatomy and Procedure

### Key Concepts

- Accurate localization of neurological and vascular structures includes the combined use of preoperative and intraoperative studies to maximize extent and safety of glioma resection.
- Knowledge of neuroanatomical structure–function relationships is necessary to anticipate the range of potential postoperative complications.
- Motor areas are identified with preoperative tractography, functional magnetic resonance imaging (MRI), central sulcus mapping, and cortical/subcortical stimulation.
- Language areas can be identified by preoperative tractography, functional MRI, and language mapping during awake craniotomy in cooperative patients with adequate language function.

Gliomas occur throughout the intracranial compartment, and thus resection requires a number of approaches, each with equally distinct anatomical considerations largely divided into functional zones and vascular structures relevant to a particular tumor location.

*Frontal/temporal gliomas.* Frontal lobe lesions are generally favorable for aggressive resection when anterior to the precentral gyrus. Two major functional zones of the frontal lobes relate to motor cortices bilaterally and language in the dominant hemisphere, such as Broca's area in the inferior frontal lobe. Motor regions include (from anterior to posterior) the prefrontal cortex, supplemental motor areas, and the motor cortex encoded in the precentral gyrus.

When gliomas involve the temporal lobes, at least three functional zones need to be considered: receptive language areas, optic pathways, and memory/limbic structures encoded medially. When the temporal lobe of the dominant hemisphere is affected, functional MRI (fMRI) may locate changes in cortical oxygen consumption during language activation, demonstrating the location of Wernicke's area. In addition, mapping language tracts around and from Wernicke's area can be accurately accomplished with preoperative diffusion-tensor imaging (DTI) and/or intraoperative speech mapping during awake craniotomy. Preoperative ophthalmological evaluation, as well as DTI, is helpful in delineating the optic radiations, both for preoperative patient counseling and to ensure their avoidance during surgical resection if possible. For tumors near the sylvian fissure and inferior anastomotic vein of Labbe, computed tomography (CT) angiogram is often helpful to map perforating vessels that frequently travel in or around the tumor.

We often combine fMRI and DTI to detect motor pathways, including primary motor cortex and corticospinal tracts, and language pathways, focusing on Broca's area, Wernicke's area, and the arcuate fasciculus that connects these two areas and is a component of a larger tract called the *superior longitudinal fasciculus* (Fig. 16.1). These preoperative studies set the stage and can help focus the use of intraoperative central sulcus mapping and direct cortical stimulation for intraoperative motor and speech mapping. Awake craniotomy is used for patients with satisfactory preoperative language function and patients who will tolerate the awake procedure psychologically. A seminal study mapping language areas during awake glioma surgery cautioned about the variability of language areas, emphasizing the utility of intraoperative speech mapping.[4]

### Clinical Pearl

Ultrasound, electrocorticography, and intraoperative MRI are adjunctive tools that should be considered when tissue manipulation during the procedure is anticipated to distort important anatomical landmarks that may render preoperatively obtained navigation studies inaccurate.

*Parietal gliomas.* Three classical functional zones are described for the parietal lobes: somatosensory processes, integrative motor functions, and visual-spatial recognition.

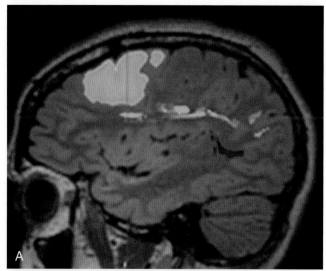

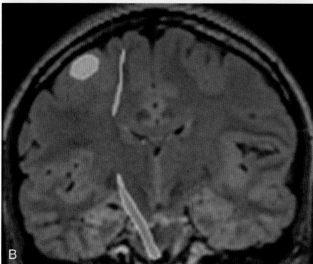

**Fig. 16.1** Diffusion-tensor imaging (DTI) to delineate the relationship between a left frontal glioma (*light blue*) and language and motor white-matter tracts. DTI of the superior longitudinal fasciculus (SLF) (*multicolor*) layered onto left lateral view of fluid-attenuated inversion recovery (FLAIR) MRI (**A**) shows the tumor lies superiorly and medially to the SLF. DTI of the corticospinal tract (*yellow*) layered onto anterior view of FLAIR MRI (**B**) shows the tumor lies anteriorly and laterally to the corticospinal tract. An awake craniotomy with speech and motor mapping was used in this case to confirm the tractography data and to identify Broca's area, given the location of this large glioma in the frontal lobe.

Preserving these functions has a significant effect on the quality of life for these patients postoperatively. Anatomically, somatosensory cortex (postcentral gyrus) is bordered by the central sulcus anteriorly and the postcentral sulcus posteriorly. Behind the postcentral sulcus lie the superior and inferior parietal lobules (Fig. 16.2), with the inferior parietal lobule comprising the supramarginal and angular gyri. The superior parietal lobule primarily involves visual guidance for limb and head movements, as well as imaginary movements for objects. The inferior parietal lobule controls visual-spatial cognition, calculation, and reading ability.

Patients with gliomas in the parietal lobe may present with contralateral constructional apraxia, which include visuospatial tasks such as the inability to copy facial gestures or to draw a picture. In addition, ocular ataxia (inability to reach for objects using visual guidance) may result on the contralateral side. Right parietal lesions tend to produce neglect or extinction to simultaneous stimulation toward the contralateral side of the body, as well as an inability to accurately detect spatial relationships between objects. Left-sided parietal lesions may produce ideomotor apraxia, deficits in arithmetic and reading, and difficulty differentiating left from right. Gerstmann's syndrome is a left parietal syndrome comprising left-right confusion, acalculia, agraphia without alexia, and finger agnosia.

Vascular structures in the parietal lobes include the middle cerebral artery branches supplying this area that originate from the sylvian fissure. Venous structures include the superficial draining veins leading either to the superior sagittal sinus or the middle cerebral vein. The major vein nearby is the superior anastomotic vein of Trolard, as it links the superior sagittal sinus to the middle cerebral vein.

A large cohort of patients undergoing resection for parietal lobe gliomas at University of California, San Francisco, demonstrated that those involving the supramarginal gyrus had the highest number of postoperative neurological deficits.[5] The most likely deficits were those involving language (13.4% at 1 month and 8.4% at 6 months) and vision (9.2% at 1 month and 6.7% at 6 months). Importantly and somewhat surprisingly, resection of right parietal tumors also carried a significant risk of language dysfunction (20% at 6 months).[5]

*Cingulate gliomas.* Gliomas involving the cingulate gyrus can be separated into four functional zones: perigenual/anterior (emotional control), midcingulate (motor control), posterior cingulate (visual-spatial function), and retrosplenial (memory access) (Fig. 16.3).[6] In many cases, gliomas extend into adjacent frontal and/or parietal regions. The two most common surgical approaches are transcortical and interhemispheric (Fig. 16.3B). The most common early postoperative finding is the supplementary motor area (SMA) syndrome, which refers to a constellation of impaired volitional movement without loss of muscle tone, hemineglect, and dyspraxia of the contralateral limbs. If the dominant SMA cortex is affected, then speech hesitancy or mutism can result. SMA syndrome after resection of cingulate cortex gliomas occurs in 20% to 34% of patients transiently, but only 2% at 6 months postoperatively, most often with anterior/midcingulate lesions involving the superior frontal gyrus.[6,7] Other less common transient postoperative neurological deficits include weakness (6%), sensory changes (2%), and memory disturbance (1%).[6]

## Clinical Pearl

After cingulate glioma resection, a common and usually temporary finding is SMA syndrome, which should be differentiated from true limb weakness.

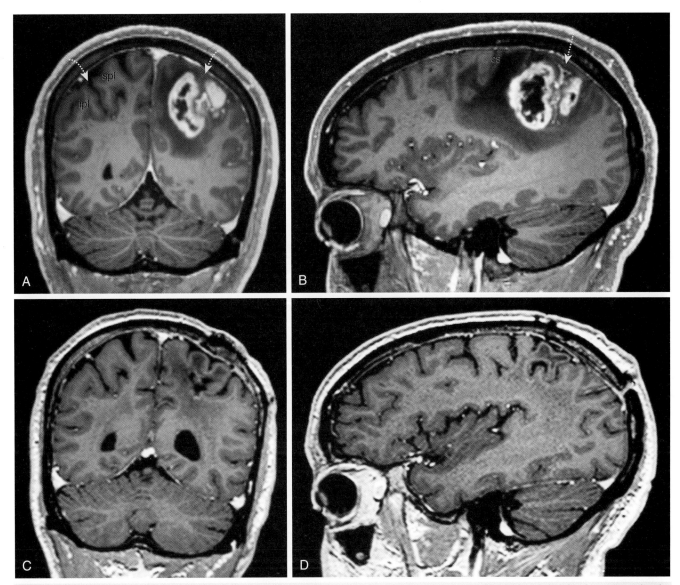

**Fig. 16.2** Left parietal lobe glioblastoma infiltrating the superior and inferior parietal lobules in a 61-year-old right-handed male who presented with apraxia and inability to operate his car. **(A, B)** Preoperative MRI reveals a 4-cm ring-enhancing lesion in the left superior parietal lobule (spl), tracking under the interparietal sulcus (*dashed yellow lines*) to the inferior parietal lobule (ipl). Patient underwent gross total resection followed by temozolomide and radiation per the Stupp protocol. Note that mapping was unnecessary because the tumor was behind the central sulcus (cs). Immediate postoperative MRI (not shown) and surveillance scan after 19 months **(C, D)** reveals no evidence of residual tumor. He is driving without further episodes of apraxia and is neurologically intact aside from mild acalculia.

*Insular gliomas.* Insular gliomas are among the most challenging lesions in all of neurosurgery because the insula incorporates and is surrounded by many eloquent white-matter tracts and critically important vascular structures.[8] About 11% of glioblastomas and 25% of low-grade gliomas involve the insula.[9] Anatomically, the insula typically comprises three short gyri and two long gyri that are delimited by periinsular sulci (Fig. 16.4), although anatomical variation is not uncommon. The insular cortex is shrouded by frontal, parietal, and temporal opercula. When involved, adjacent opercular regions may require extension of the resection zone to these areas. Two main approaches are used to access insular gliomas: a transsylvian approach that begins by splitting the sylvian fissure widely to separate the opercula and sylvian vessels,[8] and a transcortical approach that uses several frontal and/or temporal windows to access the tumor.[10]

Key functional tracts relevant for insular glioma resection include language, motor, and limbic tracts. More superficial language areas include Broca's area (inferior frontal gyrus) and Wernicke's area (posterior superior temporal gyrus). The arcuate fasciculus is a deeper tract that connects these language areas, which normally lies at the superior aspect of the insula, approximately at the level of the superior periinsular sulcus. Awake craniotomy with speech mapping is an important tool to identify and protect these areas.

Motor areas include superficial cortical structures, including the precentral gyrus and supplemental motor area more anteriorly. Deep structures surrounding the insula

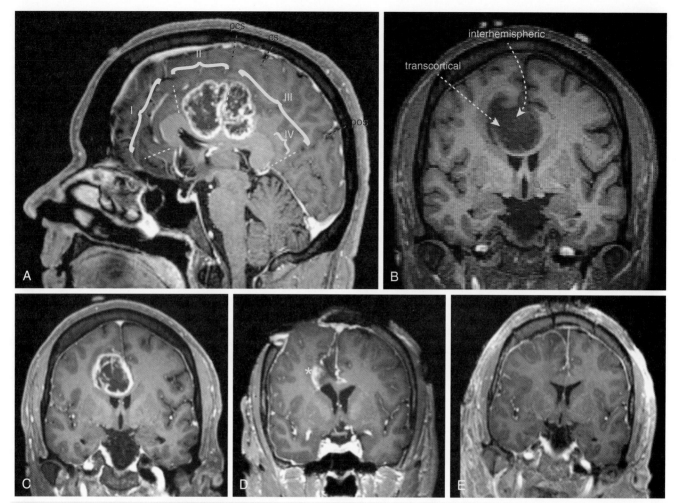

**Fig. 16.3** Right cingulate glioblastoma resected via interhemispheric approach with intraoperative MRI. **(A)** Cingulate gliomas may involve the anterior (I), middle (II), posterior (III), or retrosplenial (IV) cingulate cortex, with borders as defined in Ref. 6 and the precentral sulcus (pcs) demarcating II from III. The central sulcus (cs) and parieto-occipital sulcus (pos) as also shown. This tumor included the middle and posterior cingulate cortex (II + III). **(B)** Preoperative functional MRI shows the areas activated with left-foot motor tasks (*green*) and how an interhemispheric or transcortical approach could be planned to avoid this motor area. **(C)** Preoperative MRI shows the right cingulate glioblastoma from **(A)** in coronal view, which was resected using an interhemispheric approach. **(D)** Intraoperative MRI shows residual tumor (enhancing tumor just medial to the *asterisk*), which was then further resected with stereotactic navigation. **(E)** Postoperative MRI shows no residual tumor. The patient awoke postoperatively with SMA syndrome involving the left upper extremity, which completely resolved by 2 weeks after surgery.

include the corona radiata superiorly and internal capsule posteriorly. Cortical and subcortical motor mapping delineates these areas because they are often distorted from their normal location by mass effect by expansile gliomas.

White-matter tracts thought to be important for higher language and limbic functions include the uncinate fasciculus, which connects the orbitofrontal and temporal lobes, and the inferior occipitofrontal fasciculus (IFOF) (Fig. 16.4F). The uncinate fasciculus lies at the level of the inferior periinsular sulcus and is thought to be important in facial recognition, naming, emotion, and memory.[11] The IFOF runs close to the uncinate fasciculus and has two components: a dorsal pathway between frontal, superior parietal, and superior occipital gyri, and a ventral pathway between frontal, posterior temporal, and inferior occipital gyri.[12] IFOF is thought to have functions in semantic processing and is avoided when possible during glioma resection.

A rich vascular network lies both superficially and deep to the insula and is mapped preoperatively by CT angiography. Superficially, the middle cerebral artery (MCA) and vein with their perforators are protected while obtaining insular access. Deep vessels of the insula include the lateral lenticulostriate vessels that branch from the M1 segment of the MCA. The lateral lenticulostriate vessels mark the basal ganglia and the extent of the medial border for resection, because injury to these small perforators may cause devastating injury.[8]

Tools to identify critical neurophysiological white-matter tracts and vascular structures have pushed the boundaries for achieving >90% EOR, which is correlated with longer survival. For both high- and low-grade insular gliomas, EOR >90% is correlated with a statistically significant increase in overall survival and with longer interval until malignant progression.[10,13] Immediate postoperative deficit is reported at 33% overall (16.7% with motor deficits and 16.7% with speech disturbances); however, persistent motor or speech deficits at 3 to 6 months follow-up are only 3% to 6%.[10,13]

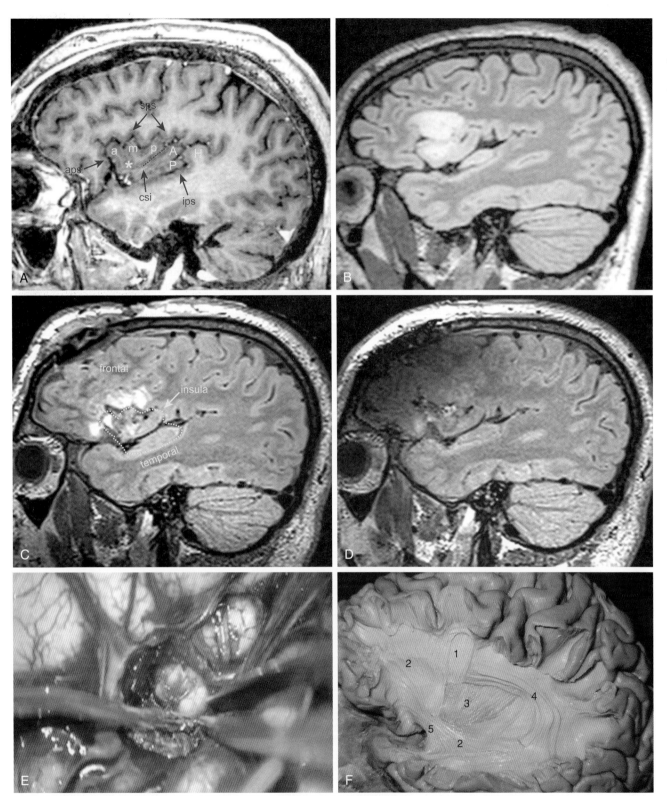

**Fig. 16.4** Right frontoinsular grade II oligodendroglioma in a 29-year-old right-handed male found incidentally after head trauma resected via transsylvian approach with guidance of intraoperative MRI. **(A)** Normal insular anatomy illustrated on a sagittal T1-weighted MRI in a different patient. The insula typically comprises three short gyri (*a*, anterior short insular gyrus; *m*, middle short insular gyrus; *p*, posterior short insular gyrus) and two long gyri (*A*, anterior long insular gyrus; *P*, posterior long insular gyrus) that are bordered by the three peri-insular sulci (*aps*, anterior periinsular sulcus; *sps*, superior periinsular sulcus; *ips*, inferior periinsular sulcus), although variation in the number of gyri is not uncommon. The short gyri meet at the apex (*asterisk*) and are separated from the long gyri by the central sulcus of the insula (csi). Primary auditory cortex (*H*, Heschl's gyrus) borders the posterior long insular gyrus. **(B)** Preoperative sagittal FLAIR MRI shows the oligodendroglioma involving the anterior insula and frontal operculum. **(C)** Intraoperative sagittal FLAIR MRI shows residual tumor in the frontal operculum wrapping around the lateral aspect of the insula, which was used to guide further resection. Frontal, temporal, and insular (*dashed yellow line*) regions are labeled. **(D)** Postoperative sagittal FLAIR MRI shows gross total resection. **(E)** Intraoperative photo showing the transsylvian approach and skeletonized middle cerebral vessels. **(F)** Fiber dissection of a gross anatomical specimen shows important white-matter tracts adjacent to the insula (*1*, corona radiata; *2*, inferior occipitofrontal fasciculus; *3*, putamen; *4*, superior longitudinal fasciculus; *5*, uncinate fasciculus). (Reprinted from Winn H. *Youmans Neurological Surgery*, 6th ed. New York: Saunders; 2011.)

*Cerebellar gliomas.* In adults, cerebellar gliomas are rarer than supratentorial gliomas and constitute approximately 0.6% to 1.5% of all gliomas. Prognosis is generally regarded as worse than that for supratentorial gliomas, and there are mixed data regarding whether EOR, chemoradiation, or lack of brainstem involvement is correlated with improved survival.[14–16] Medial cerebellar tumors are approached with the patient in the prone position through a midline suboccipital incision. Lateral cerebellar tumors may be approached with the patient in the supine or lateral position through a retrosigmoid incision. Initial dissection is carried out down to bone and then in a periosteal fashion in order to avoid injury to the vertebral artery inferolaterally. If the venous sinuses must be skeletonized (transverse sinus superiorly and sigmoid sinus laterally), then care is taken to prevent tearing of the sinuses or venous air embolism as the bone is drilled around the sinuses. The dura is opened in a fashion that allows for watertight closure at the end of the operation, because posterior fossa surgery is associated with a higher risk of cerebrospinal fluid (CSF) leak/fistula and pseudomeningocele. If primary closure of the dura is not possible, then the patient's own pericranium or a commercially available allograft is used as a dural substitute.

Because the numbers of cerebellar gliomas in adults are low, there is little reported in the literature regarding outcomes after cerebellar glioma surgery. However, postoperative deficits from any posterior fossa surgery may include appendicular ataxia and tremor for lateral cerebellar hemisphere lesions or truncal discoordination from medially located lesions. Flocculonodular involvement may disrupt equilibrium and gait. More commonly in children, cerebellar mutism may result from injury to the dentate nuclei outflow tracts (dentatothalamocortical tracts) and superior cerebellar peduncles.[17] Involvement of brainstem nuclei may cause cranial neuropathy or more devastating injury if areas governing wakefulness/attention are perturbed, such as the reticular activating system.

*Procedure.* Preoperative discussion between all operating room staff, including nursing, anesthesiology, neurology, and neurosurgery teams, should outline the operative plan, including positioning and administering anesthetic/paralytic medications, antiepileptic medications (particularly for intraoperative monitoring cases), and antibiotics. For cases involving general anesthesia, total intravenous anesthesia with propofol and a short-acting opiate is used in most cases. For awake craniotomy cases, an asleep-awake-asleep method is often planned, where dexmedetomidine is used for the awake portion of the case. The patient is usually positioned such that the lesion is positioned toward the highest point in the operative field. For most supratentorial lesions, a supine position with rotated and elevated head is used, often with padding to elevate the ipsilateral shoulder to make the lesion high in the operative field. For lateral suboccipital approaches, either a supine or lateral positioning strategy is employed. If a midline suboccipital craniotomy is planned, then a prone position with neck flexion is used.

We use a Mayfield clamp to achieve three-pin fixation around the cranium, which also allows for attachment to a stereotactic guidance system. In cases that require intraoperative MRI, a magnetic coil is placed underneath the head and attached to the Mayfield clamp. Hair is shaved in a strip demarcating the incision. The field is sterilized and draped, and antibiotics, antiepileptic drugs (AEDs), and dexamethasone are given. A preincision checklist is done to again confirm patient, procedure, equipment, anticipated steps, and potential complications. The skin is incised and bone is exposed of sufficient size to access the lesion and perform any cortical mapping that is necessary during the case. The bone flap is removed and dura is opened. If high intracranial pressure is anticipated, then brain relaxation, including mannitol and furosemide, are given prior to bone flap removal to help keep dura intact. The tumor is located and resected using knowledge of anatomical landmarks, stereotactic navigation systems, and cortical and subcortical mapping to minimize impact on normal brain tissue. When resection is complete, hemostasis to the resection cavity is achieved with a combination of bipolar cautery and hemostatic agents such as cellulose matrices (e.g., Surgicel). Dura is closed primarily with pericranium or with dural substitutes to prevent CSF leak and pneumocephalus. Watertight closure of dura is particularly important in posterior fossa approaches given the higher risk of CSF leak. Dural tenting sutures peripherally and centrally are attached to the bone to prevent epidural hematoma formation. The bone flap is replaced with small titanium plates, the galea and skin are closed in layers, and the incision is covered with a sterile dressing.

## Perioperative Considerations

Anticipating potential pitfalls in the perioperative period is an important component of operative planning, which may be categorized as preoperative, intraoperative, and postoperative considerations. Preoperative considerations include medical optimization and obtaining useful and relevant imaging studies. Patient optimization includes holding anticoagulation/antiplatelet agents when possible, avoiding recent chemoradiation such as vascular endothelial growth factor (VEGF)–pathway inhibitors, given that these may predispose to a higher risk of postoperative hemorrhage, cardiac assessment if patients have a significant cardiac history or recent cardiac stenting,[18] and pulmonary assessment if, for example, a long prone case is planned for a patient with lung disease. Imaging studies are obtained preoperatively in anticipation of localization and functional information that may be needed during the operation, including stereotactic navigation, fMRI, or diffusion tractography to assess white-matter tracts that may border the glioma. For glioma locations that may threaten language function, awake craniotomy is considered. Patients scheduled for awake craniotomy must be carefully selected. Contraindications include lack of cooperation, difficult airway, extreme anxiety, difficulty with communication, or inability to lie still for the 2- to 3-hour portion required for most awake craniotomy procedures. For awake craniotomy cases, the head position is fixed in a Mayfield head holder that can accommodate both surgical resection and intubation after the mapping component of the case is completed.

## Clinical Pearl

For awake craniotomy cases, there should be a strategy for resection under general anesthesia, if appropriate, in the case that the patient is unable to tolerate the procedure awake.

Intraoperative considerations include planning at every step of the operation to avoid complications. A frozen section is sent early to avoid an extensive resection for a chemosensitive or radiosensitive tumor that may mimic glioma radiographically, such as lymphoma. In addition, CSF diversion via external ventricular drain or lumbar drain placement may be required to obtain sufficient brain relaxation. In cases of acute intraoperative swelling, administration of mannitol or hypertonic saline may be necessary for relaxation. If the craniotomy requires exposure of major venous sinuses, then venous air embolism precautions may be necessary, including central venous access to the right atrium and precordial Doppler ultrasound and/or transesophageal echocardiography to detect air emboli. In cases utilizing electrocorticography and language/motor mapping, several techniques should be available to break a seizure should one develop, including ice-cold saline irrigation and a variety of escalating AED regimens. Bite blocks are placed on both sides to prevent tongue laceration. When cases may involve a risk of venous air embolism or intraoperative seizure, a rehearsal between the neurosurgery, anesthesia, neurophysiologists, and nursing staff is done on how to detect and manage these complications.

Postoperative considerations include careful monitoring in the acute phase, as well as anticipating pitfalls during the next phase of a patient's treatment for glioma. Postcraniotomy patients are typically monitored in the neurological intensive care unit or stepdown postprocedure unit, where serial neurological examinations are obtained and arterial lines are monitored to maintain blood pressure and brain perfusion in the normal range. Dexamethasone is typically given as a taper over 4 to 8 days, with attention to prevent hyperglycemia and gastrointestinal ulcer formation. Antibiotics are continued for 24 hours to reduce the risk of infection. Most high-grade glioma patients will go on to require chemoradiation, especially in cases of glioblastoma, per the Stupp protocol.[19] Especially in cases of repeat craniotomy for recurrent glioma, consideration for closure strategies may include local or free flap closures with the assistance of plastic surgery colleagues if the skin is particularly thin or will be under tension with a traditional closure.

## Postoperative Complications

### Key Concepts

- Up to one-third of postcraniotomy glioma patients will have at least one postoperative complication, and up to one-fourth will develop a neurological deficit that is most often transient.
- Workup for a postoperative neurological examination change starts with a head CT to detect hemorrhage or edema and, if negative, an electroencephalogram (EEG) to detect seizure activity, MRI to detect stroke, and toxic-metabolic workup to rule out a postoperative infectious, electrolyte, or pulmonary etiology.
- The use of antiepileptic drugs in the perioperative setting in glioma patients without a history of epilepsy is controversial and surgeon specific.
- Patients with glioma are at high risk for deep venous thrombosis (DVT) and pulmonary embolism (PE), especially in the postcraniotomy setting.

Surgical planning for glioma surgery is aimed toward achieving the maximal EOR possible while limiting complications. This requires an intimate knowledge of the relevant anatomy and mastery of adjunctive surgical tools, including preoperative tractography and/or fMRI, intraoperative MRI, stereotactic navigation, and intraoperative central sulcus and language mapping with awake craniotomy protocols. A useful framework put forth from the group at MD Anderson classifies complications in three categories: (1) neurological deficits (including motor/sensory, language, or visual changes); (2) regional complications (surgical site or intracranial-related conditions including edema, infection/abscess, and seizures); and (3) systemic complications (including myocardial infarction [MI], PE, urinary tract infections [UTI], pneumonia, and hyponatremia).[20] Some complications are anticipated—for example, transient weakness or neglect after a lesion is resected in the supplementary motor or nondominant parietal areas—whereas others are unexpected.

*Overall complication rates.* Incidence of complications after glioma surgery ranges from 19% to 33% in part due to different definitions of complications (Table 16.1).[21–23] Factors influencing complication rates include patient age, Karnofsky performance status, location of tumor, tumor proximity to eloquent cortex, primary resection versus reoperation, caseload of the medical center, and comorbidities. Work from our institution and others has documented clear correlation with decreasing incidence of complications with surgeons of increasing caseload.[24,24] Those with complications are less likely to receive chemotherapy and/or radiation therapy.[21] Locations such as deep midline gliomas or those that are located bilaterally have increased risk of medical or neurological complications.[22] In patients undergoing first resection for glioma, complications occurred in 24% relative to 33% in those undergoing reoperation.[23]

## Clinical Pearl

Intraoperative motor mapping may cause a postoperative contralateral limb weakness that improves over the course of hours to a few days.

*Neurological deficit.* Postoperative neurological injury usually results from direct mechanical injury to brain tissue, edema, seizures, reversible and irreversible ischemia, or hemorrhage. Neurological deterioration occurs in 8% to 26% of patients undergoing neurosurgical procedures (Table 16.1).[2,21–23] For patients undergoing

**Table 16.1** Neurological and Medical Complication Rates after Glioma Surgery

| Complication | Fadul et al. 1988 | Chang et al. 2003* | Gulati et al. 2011 | McGirt et al. 2009 |
|---|---|---|---|---|
| Neurological deterioration | 26% | 8.1%, 18% | 15.3% | 11% |
| — Minor deterioration | 6.5% | — | 2.6% | — |
| — Major deterioration | 19% | — | 16.8% | — |
| Brain herniation | 4.7% | — | — | — |
| Hemorrhage | — | 1.6%, 4.4% | 5.6% | — |
| Reoperation for bleed | 4.7% | — | 3.5% | — |
| Wound infection | 1.5% | 0.5%, 1.1% | 1.4% | 1% |
| CSF leak | — | — | 0.7% | — |
| Meningitis | — | — | 1.4% | — |
| Hydrocephalus | 1.5% | — | 0% | — |
| Seizure | — | 7.5%, 10% | 6.2% | — |
| Stroke | 1.5% | — | 1.4% | — |
| Deep venous thrombosis | 2.3% | 4.2%, 5.6% | 0% | 1% |
| Pulmonary embolism | 1.5% | 0.5%, 2.2% | 1.4% | 5% |
| Myocardial infarction | 0.9% | — | 0.7% | — |
| GI bleeding | 0.9% | — | — | — |
| Urinary tract infection | — | — | 4.2% | — |
| Pneumonia | 3.3% | — | 1.4% | — |
| Systemic infection | — | 0%, 4.4% | 0% | — |
| Depression | — | 11%, 20% | — | — |
| Drug reaction | — | 5.2%, 2.2% | — | — |
| Other | — | — | — | — |
| At least one complication | 31% | 24%, 33% | 19.4% | — |

*CSF*, cerebrospinal fluid; *GI*, gastrointestinal.
*Values indicate incidence in patients undergoing their first surgery and reoperation, respectively.

resection of glioblastoma, approximately 5% have surgically acquired language deficits, and 6% have surgically acquired motor deficits. These functional deficits affect glioblastoma patient longevity, as overall survival was lower by about 3 to 4 months in these patients.[2] Later we outline some of the key causes of neurological deficit in the postoperative neurosurgical patient, as well as management considerations.

A common algorithm to investigate etiology for an unexpected neurological deficit usually begins with immediate head CT to rule out a postoperative hemorrhage or edema. If that is negative, a spot EEG may be used to detect seizure activity and MRI can be obtained to detect ischemic stroke. Rarely, vasospasm may contribute to neurological deficit, particularly if arterial vessels are manipulated during surgery, for example, after transsylvian approach to an insular glioma. CT angiogram may be useful to detect vasospasm if clinical suspicion is high.

*Edema and herniation.* Brain edema is an increase in apparent brain volume from local excess of water, which may be vasogenic or cytotoxic in origin. Edema is a frequent contributor to morbidity and may affect cortex and white matter at a distance from the boundaries of the tumor itself. Edema from gliomas is largely vasogenic in the preoperative setting and may be treated with corticosteroids. Dexamethasone is the steroid of choice because it has limited mineralocorticoid activity. Preoperative dexamethasone is indicated to limit peritumoral edema when symptoms are significant and relief of symptoms in advance of surgery is desired.[26] Corticosteroids should be avoided preoperatively if a diagnosis of lymphoma is being considered because their use can lead to rapid lymphodepletive effect.[27]

Postoperatively, brain edema may result from direct brain tissue manipulation during surgical resection, effect of retraction, or subtotal resection of malignant glioma. In order to limit postoperative edema from brain tissue manipulation, dexamethasone is often initiated and typically tapered off over 4 to 8 days. It is important during surgical planning to design a resection strategy that will minimize or negate the need for retraction by using proper head positioning and stereotaxy to approach the tumor directly. If a subtotal resection is planned, then maximal debulking should be pursued because partial glioma resection can be associated with a higher risk of morbidity than total resection due to the effect of edema exerted from the residual tumor and necrosis on adjacent normal brain tissue.[28] This "wounded glioma syndrome" is rare but may evolve rapidly (Fig. 16.5).

A common starting dose for dexamethasone is 4 milligrams four times a day. Corticosteroids have significant side effects on all organ systems, including hyperglycemia, increased infection risk (particularly for pneumonia), gastrointestinal bleeding, mood alteration, insomnia, and impaired wound healing. We routinely keep these patients on ulcer prophylaxis with H2 or proton pump inhibitors and insulin coverage for hyperglycemia. Patients on long-term dexamethasone therapy are placed on prophylaxis for *Pneumocystis jirovecii* pneumonia such as trimethoprim-sulfamethoxazole.

When neurological examination changes are thought to be caused by increased intracranial pressure and impending herniation, then emergency measures must be taken. Positioning, including raising the head of bed and ensuring that the head is midline so that venous outflow through the internal jugular veins is preserved, can rapidly aid in lowering intracranial pressure. Hyperosmolar therapy, including mannitol and hypertonic saline, also is administered, although these can precipitate renal failure with extreme hyperosmolarity. Finally, neurosurgical

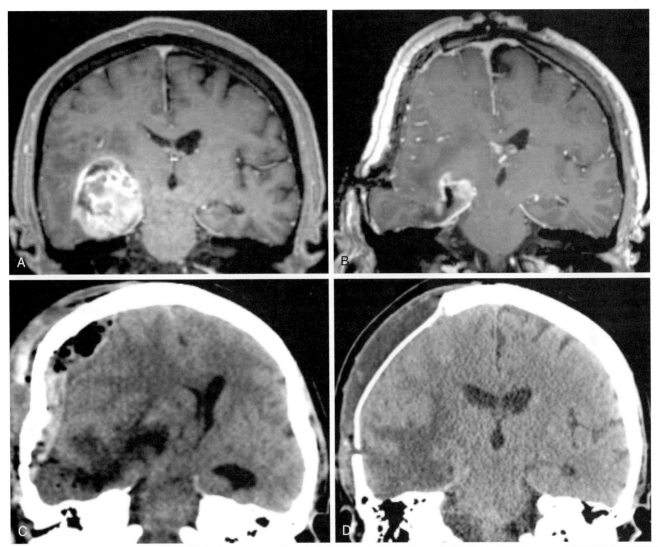

**Fig. 16.5** Dramatic example of wounded glioma syndrome after subtotal resection of a right temporoinsular glioblastoma via transcortical approach in a 60-year-old left-handed male presenting with left-hand clumsiness and mood lability. **(A)** Preoperative coronal T1 postcontrast MRI shows a large heterogenous enhancing lesion centered in the mesial temporal lobe. **(B)** Postoperative coronal T1 postcontrast MRI shows subtotal resection and early signs of edema. The patient was given dexamethasone and hypertonic saline supplementation for mild hyponatremia. **(C)** Emergent head CT in coronal view on postoperative day 2 after patient became obtunded shows peritumoral edema causing herniation, midline shift, and entrapment of the temporal horns. There is also an ipsilateral extraaxial collection of hematoma and pneumocephalus. Patient was taken for immediate craniectomy and resection of residual mesial temporal tumor. **(D)** Within 24 hours, the patient returned to his normal mental status and had full power in all extremities. Head CT showed resolution of the herniation and temporal horn entrapment.

procedures, including CSF diversion via external ventricular drain placement or craniectomy, can be used if nonoperative measures are insufficient.

*Hematomas.* Postoperative hematoma incidence is reported in the 1.6% to 5.6% range (Table 16.1)[20,22,29] Hematomas may form in the intraparenchymal, subdural, or epidural compartments. Intraparenchymal hematomas may develop when hemostasis is not complete within the tumor bed or when tumor is subtotally resected because residual tumor can recruit edema and is prone to hemorrhage, the so-called *wounded glioma syndrome.*[28] Bipolar coagulation is used to achieve complete hemostasis within the tumor bed, and the tumor cavity is normally lined with oxidized cellulose matrices that promote clotting such as Surgicel. Subdural hematomas may develop if bridging veins on the cortical surface are sheared, the risk of which is reduced by limiting retraction and limiting brain shifts,

such as those induced by giving excessive mannitol, or by entry into the ventricular system. Epidural hematomas can be prevented by using dural tenting sutures centrally and peripherally to bring the dura up to the bone inner table, using bone wax to tamponade bleeding from bone emissary veins and hemostatic agents over the dura. Note should be made if hemostatic gelatin sponges such as Gelfoam or collagen sponges such as Bicol are used over the dura, because these theoretically may swell and behave as a compressive epidural mass.

Postoperative hematoma may manifest as focal neurological changes, seizure, or decreased level of arousal. Immediate head CT should be obtained to detect postoperative hematoma if patients are slow to awaken from anesthesia or for any change in examination during the postoperative course as soon as it is clinically suspected (Fig. 16.6). Commonly, antiplatelet agents such as aspirin

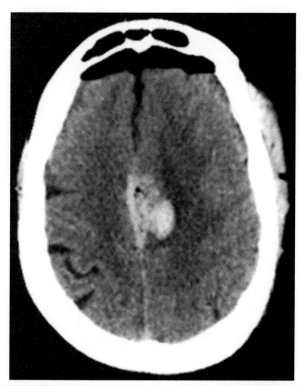

**Fig. 16.6** Left middle/posterior (zone II + III) cingulate grade III anaplastic oligoastrocytoma status post subtotal resection via interhemispheric approach in a 77-year-old right-handed female with history of diabetes and obesity who initially presented with right-sided numbness followed by a seizure. On postoperative day 1, she was noted with SMA syndrome of the right arm. On postoperative day 2, she developed new expressive aphasia and underwent a head CT that showed a moderate amount of intraparenchymal hemorrhage just posterior to the resection cavity that extended frontally, which was managed expectantly. Later that day, she developed a new oxygen requirement and, given her comorbidities, a chest CT was done that revealed segmental pulmonary emboli. Given her finding of hemorrhage on head CT, she was not a candidate for therapeutic anticoagulation and thus underwent inferior vena cava filter placement on postoperative day 3. She was given a longer 14-day dexamethasone taper due to edema. At her 1 month follow-up appointment, she had fluent speech and her SMA syndrome resolved. She subsequently underwent temozolomide chemotherapy, but she elected to not receive radiation. Three years after her operation, her MRI showed no evidence of tumor progression and her neurological examination was at her preoperative baseline.

and clopidogrel are held 7 days, and warfarin is held until international normalized ratio is less than 1.4 before elective cases. More recent use of antiplatelet agents preoperatively should raise suspicion for platelet dysfunction if bleeding diathesis is suspected postoperatively. Recent use of chemotherapy and AEDs and their effects on coagulation should be noted. For example, the use of bevacizumab is increasing for recurrent glioma, and there are data both for and against increased risk of intracranial hemorrhage in patients with intracranial tumors.[30–32] Bevacizumab is often held several weeks prior to elective craniotomy when possible. Myelosuppression and thrombocytopenia are side effects for chemotherapeutic agents, including temozolomide, as well as AEDs, including carbamazepine and valproic acid.

*Seizures.* The approach to seizure prevention in the perioperative setting for glioma surgery requires further standardization and often varies from surgeon to surgeon. The incidence of seizures in the postoperative period after craniotomy for glioma ranges from 6% to 25% (Table 16.1). By recent estimates, approximately 88% of patients with malignant glioma currently receive perioperative AEDs.[33]

Attention to preoperative characteristics and expected postoperative seizure outcomes for each patient is necessary to guide their management in the immediate postoperative setting. Preoperative characteristics that tend to influence management of seizures and seizure prevention include presence of preoperative seizures, involvement of the temporal lobe or sensorimotor cortex (if motor or language mapping techniques are used during the operation), and status of the patient's neurological examination. Importantly, 70% to 90% of patients with low-grade gliomas present with seizures,[34–36] whereas 54.5% of grade III gliomas[37] and 24% to 52% of patients with high-grade gliomas (grade III or IV) present with seizures.[34,37,39] Risk factors for seizures in glioma patients include low grade—especially oligodendroglioma and oligoastrocytoma subtypes, cortical location, temporal lobe or sensorimotor cortex involvement, simple partial ictal semiology, preoperative seizure history over 1 year, incomplete surgical resection, and glioma recurrence.[35,38,40] In patients with low-grade glioma and preoperative seizures, reported seizure outcomes scored by the Engel classification[41] at 12 months after surgery are Engel class I in 67% (seizure free), Engel class II in 17% (rare seizures), Engel class III in 8% (meaningful seizure improvement), and Engel class IV or V in 9% (no change or worsening).[35] Specifically for temporal lobe low-grade gliomas, a literature review incorporating nearly 1,200 patients in 41 studies showed that, whereas Engel class I was achieved in 43% of patients after subtotal resection, 79% were Engel class I after gross total resection with further improvements if concomitant hippocampectomy and/or anterior temporal corticectomy was employed.[42] In patients with high-grade glioma and preoperative seizures, reported seizure outcomes 12 months after surgery are Engel class I in 77%, Engel class II in 12%, Engel class III in 6%, and Engel class IV in 5%.[38]

Practice parameters set forth by the American Academy of Neurology concluded that there was no evidence for starting prophylactic AEDs in patients with a new diagnosis of brain tumor; however, it was acknowledged that more studies were necessary for those undergoing neurosurgical procedures in the perioperative period.[43] Two relevant cohorts have been studied with respect to administration of AEDs in the perioperative setting: patients undergoing craniotomy for any cause and patients undergoing craniotomy for brain tumors, which have traditionally included all tumor types such as gliomas, metastases, and meningiomas. For patients undergoing craniotomy for any cause (chiefly trauma, tumor, vascular lesions), a Cochrane systematic review[44] that included four randomized controlled trials comparing prophylactic AEDs with placebo showed that only one study showed a statistically significant reduction in early postoperative seizures with AED treatment. For patients with tumors undergoing craniotomy, there have been several studies, but they differ in study design, AED used, spectrum of tumors included, and measured outcomes. The bulk of the data, which include only two randomized controlled trials testing utility of an AED (phenytoin in these two trials) to no treatment,[45,46] indicate no evidence for use of AEDs.

Newer AEDs, including levetiracetam, are now first-line agents for glioma patients given their mild adverse effect profile and low potential for interaction with concomitantly given chemotherapeutic agents.[47] Because levetiracetam does not induce liver enzyme pathways and has a favorable profile, it has supplanted phenytoin as the AED of choice in patients undergoing any craniotomy,[48,49] craniotomy for any intracranial tumor,[50] and craniotomy for glioma specifically.[51] As levetiracetam and other next-generation AEDs are increasingly used, more data will be needed to test the benefit of these agents in glioma patients undergoing craniotomy.

Workup for suspected seizures should include head CT for epileptogenic causes, including hematoma and edema, and EEG monitoring (preferably continuous video EEG). Metabolic factors, including hyponatremia, other electrolyte/glucose abnormalities, and acidosis, can lower the seizure threshold. Urinary tract infections and other inflammatory conditions are well-known precipitants for seizures. Finally, screening medications such as antibiotics and hepatic enzyme inhibitors/inducers can reveal a potential etiology for the onset of seizures.

*Wound infections.* Craniotomy site infections span the spectrum from superficial scalp infections to deeper infections, including osteitis, meningitis/ventriculitis, or abscess/empyema. Overall, these occur in 0.8% to 4.7% of cases.[52-54] Risk factors for craniotomy site infections include preoperative length of stay of at least 1 day, emergency surgery, recent neurosurgery, nasal sinus involvement, operative time over 4 hours, and postoperative CSF leak.[53-57] Prior chemotherapeutics, such as VEGF inhibitors and radiation in patients with glioma, are linked with increasing risk of craniotomy site dehiscence.[58,59]

Wound infections may present with fever, erythema/tenderness, frank drainage, seizures, or changes in mental status. Whereas scalp infections and meningitis can present within 1 to 2 weeks from the date of surgery, bone flap infections and abscesses tend to present after 2 weeks typically.[57] Common organisms include *Staphylococcus aureus* and *S. epidermidis*, *Propionibacterium acnes*, gram-negative organisms (such as *Klebsiella*, *Enterobacter*, *Pseudomonas*, and *Serratia*), or polymicrobial involvement.[53,54,56] Prophylactic antibiotics given at the time of surgery reduce rates of surgical site infections including meningitis.[60,61] These are routinely continued for 24 hours postoperatively. Presence of a craniotomy site infection is correlated with increasing length of hospital stay and rates of readmission, reoperation, and mortality.[57]

Early recognition of potential infection is important to prevent deeper involvement. Clinical suspicion based on history and physical examination is most useful, and adjunctive CSF sampling may yield a culprit organism in microbial culture. MRI with diffusion-weighted imaging is often used but can be misleading in the setting of recent surgery because it may be associated with a high false-negative and false-positive rate.[62] Superficial infections, including suture abscesses and meningitis/ventriculitis, can be treated with good wound care and antibiotics alone. Organized infections of deeper cavities such as subgaleal, epidural, subdural, or intraparenchymal abscesses require debridement to allow penetration for parenteral antibiotics. In most cases, the bone flap is removed and discarded, although there are reports of treating native bone flaps, particularly if the bone appears noninvolved or minimally involved.[55,63]

*Systemic complications.* Patients with glioma are at higher than average risk for a range of systemic complications, including DVT, PE, MI, UTIs, pneumonia, gastrointestinal bleeding, and depression (Table 16.1). Incidence of DVT in glioma patients is as high as 20% to 30% and is highest in the postoperative period.[47] The hypercoagulable state attributed to glioma is exacerbated by relative immobility or extremity paresis, age over 60 years, length of surgery, higher glioma grade, and chemotherapy use.[64-66] Therefore in the perioperative setting, ambulation is encouraged early, mechanical DVT prophylaxis with compression boots is used during the hospital course (including preoperatively), and we typically start chemoprophylaxis with low-molecular-weight heparin on postoperative day one. If there is concern for higher-than-average bleeding risk from surgery, then standard heparin is preferred because it can be partially quenched with protamine. For extremity pain or swelling, there should be a low threshold to obtain Doppler ultrasound studies to detect DVT, and CT of the chest should be done for any respiratory symptoms or pleuritic pain suggestive of PE.

Patients with glioblastoma have a higher incidence of comorbid conditions, including heart failure, coronary artery disease, and MI.[67] Rate of MI after surgery for glioma is less than 1% (Table 16.1).[21,22] Postcraniotomy MI may be managed acutely in the traditional way, which includes oxygenation, pain control, and vasodilators. Antiplatelet agents can be considered if the benefits to such therapy are thought to outweigh the increased risk of intracranial hemorrhage. Interventional approaches, including percutaneous coronary intervention that require intraprocedural heparinization, are relatively contraindicated in the early postcraniotomy setting. Because there are no set guidelines regarding when heparinization may be safe, assessment of the risks and benefits on a case-by-case basis is necessary.

UTI and pneumonia are frequent causes of postcraniotomy fever, occurring at 1.4% to 4.2% (Table 16.1).[21,22] We routinely screen patients with preoperative urinalysis, the results of which should be reviewed to ensure that any antibiotic that is started will cover an organism that may have been previously treated. Urinary catheters are removed on postoperative day one or earlier when the patient is ambulatory. We encourage incentive spirometry and early ambulation to minimize atelectasis and pneumonia. Any antibiotics that lower seizure threshold are avoided.

*Readmission.* As medical care becomes increasingly cost conscious, readmission rates are being carefully studied in hopes of prevention and to maximize the quality of patient care. In California between 1995 and 2010, more than 18,000 patients underwent craniotomy for malignant glioma, of which 73% of patients were discharged home, 24% were transferred to another facility, and 2.2% died during the index surgical admission. The readmission rate within 30 days for patients discharged home was 13.2%.

The most common cause was seizures in 21%, infection in 14%, and new motor deficit in 13%. Readmission rates were higher if the patient's medical history included MI, if hydrocephalus developed, or when patients developed DVT/PE.[68] A similar study regarding patients undergoing surgery for glioblastoma specifically found a readmission rate within 30 days of 15.8%, of which neurological symptoms in 30%, thromboembolic complications in 20%, and infection in 18% were the most frequent causes.[69]

*Mortality.* Perioperative mortality is usually defined in the literature as death within 30 days of surgery, which may or may not be related to the surgical procedure. Prior to 1980, mortality rate after craniotomy for tumor surgery was 7.6%, but this has gradually decreased steadily by decade.[70] Modern studies have shown a mortality rate of 1.0% to 2.2%, with risk factors that include age over 70, poor histological grade, and multifocality.[2,70] In patients with age over 70, perioperative death occurred in 6.6% compared with only 1.1% in patients younger than 70.[70] Centers with lower volumes have mortality rates of 2.8% to 4.5%, whereas high-volume centers have mortality rates 1.1% to 1.5%.[24,25]

# Conclusions

Significant advances have been made to better understand the molecular mechanisms underlying glioma formation and growth; however, surgical resection remains the mainstay of treatment. Surgical planning for glioma surgery is aimed at achieving the maximal extent of resection possible while limiting complications. This requires an intimate knowledge of the relevant anatomy and mastery of adjunctive surgical tools, including preoperative tractography and/or fMRI, intraoperative MRI, stereotactic navigation, and intraoperative central sulcus and language mapping with awake craniotomy protocols.

## References

1. Sanai N, Berger MS. Glioma extent of resection and its impact on patient outcome. *Neurosurgery.* 2008;62(4):753–764. discussion 264–266.
2. McGirt MJ, Chaichana KL, Gathinji M, et al. Independent association of extent of resection with survival in patients with malignant brain astrocytoma. *J Neurosurg.* 2009;110(1):156–162.
3. Orringer D, Lau D, Khatri S, et al. Extent of resection in patients with glioblastoma: limiting factors, perception of resectability, and effect on survival. *J Neurosurg.* 2012;117(5):851–859.
4. Sanai N, Mirzadeh Z, Berger MS. Functional outcome after language mapping for glioma resection. *N Engl J Med.* 2008;358(1):18–27.
5. Sanai N, Martino J, Berger MS. Morbidity profile following aggressive resection of parietal lobe gliomas. *J Neurosurg.* 2012;116(6):1182–1186.
6. Tate MC, Kim CY, Chang EF, Polley MY, Berger MS. Assessment of morbidity following resection of cingulate gyrus gliomas. Clinical article. *J Neurosurg.* 2011;114(3):640–647.
7. von Lehe M, Schramm J. Gliomas of the cingulate gyrus: surgical management and functional outcome. *Neurosurg Focus.* 2009;27(2):E9.
8. Rey-Dios R, Cohen-Gadol AA. Technical nuances for surgery of insular gliomas: lessons learned. *Neurosurg Focus.* 2013;34(2):E6.
9. Duffau H, Capelle L. Preferential brain locations of low-grade gliomas. *Cancer.* 2004;100(12):2622–2626.
10. Sanai N, Polley MY, Berger MS. Insular glioma resection: assessment of patient morbidity, survival, and tumor progression. *J Neurosurg.* 2010;112(1):1–9.
11. Von Der Heide RJ, Skipper LM, Klobusicky E, Olson IR. Dissecting the uncinate fasciculus: disorders, controversies and a hypothesis. *Brain.* 2013;136(Pt 6):1692–1707.
12. Martino J, Brogna C, Robles SG, Vergani F, Duffau H. Anatomic dissection of the inferior fronto-occipital fasciculus revisited in the lights of brain stimulation data. *Cortex.* 2010;46(5):691–699.
13. Skrap M, Mondani M, Tomasino B, et al. Surgery of insular nonenhancing gliomas: volumetric analysis of tumoral resection, clinical outcome, and survival in a consecutive series of 66 cases. *Neurosurgery.* 2012;70(5):1081–1093. discussion 93–94.
14. Adams H, Chaichana KL, Avendaño J, Liu B, Raza SM. Quiñones-Hinojosa A. Adult cerebellar glioblastoma: understanding survival and prognostic factors using a population-based database from 1973 to 2009. *World Neurosurg.* 2013;80(6):e237–e243.
15. Babu R, Sharma R, Karikari IO, Owens TR, Friedman AH, Adamson C. Outcome and prognostic factors in adult cerebellar glioblastoma. *J Clin Neurosci.* 2013;20(8):1117–1121.
16. Jeswani S, Nuño M, Folkerts V, Mukherjee D, Black KL, Patil CG. Comparison of survival between cerebellar and supratentorial glioblastoma patients: surveillance, epidemiology, and end results (SEER) analysis. *Neurosurgery.* 2013;73(2):240–246. discussion 6; quiz 6.
17. Pitsika M, Tsitouras V. Cerebellar mutism. *J Neurosurg Pediatr.* 2013;12(6):604–614.
18. Fleisher LA, Beckman JA, Brown KA, et al. 2009 ACCF/AHA focused update on perioperative beta blockade incorporated into the ACC/AHA 2007 guidelines on perioperative cardiovascular evaluation and care for noncardiac surgery: a report of the American College of Cardiology Foundation/American Heart Association Task Force on practice guidelines. *Circulation.* 2009;120(21):e169–e276.
19. Stupp R, Mason WP, van den Bent MJ, et al. Radiotherapy plus concomitant and adjuvant temozolomide for glioblastoma. *N Engl J Med.* 2005;352(10):987–996.
20. Sawaya R, Hammoud M, Schoppa D, et al. Neurosurgical outcomes in a modern series of 400 craniotomies for treatment of parenchymal tumors. *Neurosurgery.* 1998;42(5):1044–1055. discussion 55–56.
21. Gulati S, Jakola AS, Nerland US, Weber C, Solheim O. The risk of getting worse: surgically acquired deficits, perioperative complications, and functional outcomes after primary resection of glioblastoma. *World Neurosurg.* 2011;76(6):572–579.
22. Fadul C, Wood J, Thaler H, Galicich J, Patterson RH, Posner JB. Morbidity and mortality of craniotomy for excision of supratentorial gliomas. *Neurology.* 1988;38(9):1374–1379.
23. Chang SM, Parney IF, McDermott M, et al. Perioperative complications and neurological outcomes of first and second craniotomies among patients enrolled in the Glioma Outcome Project. *J Neurosurg.* 2003;98(6):1175–1181.
24. Barker FG, Curry WT, Carter BS. Surgery for primary supratentorial brain tumors in the United States, 1988 to 2000: the effect of provider caseload and centralization of care. *Neuro Oncol.* 2005;7(1):49–63.
25. Nuño M, Mukherjee D, Carico C, et al. The effect of centralization of caseload for primary brain tumor surgeries: trends from 2001-2007. *Acta Neurochir (Wien).* 2012;154(8):1343–1350.
26. Lacy J, Saadati H, Yu JB. Complications of brain tumors and their treatment. *Hematol Oncol Clin North Am.* 2012;26(4):779–796.
27. Geppert M, Ostertag CB, Seitz G, Kiessling M. Glucocorticoid therapy obscures the diagnosis of cerebral lymphoma. *Acta Neuropathol.* 1990;80(6):629–634.
28. Ciric I, Ammirati M, Vick N, Mikhael M. Supratentorial gliomas: surgical considerations and immediate postoperative results. Gross total resection versus partial resection. *Neurosurgery.* 1987;21(1):21–26.
29. Cabantog AM, Bernstein M. Complications of first craniotomy for intra-axial brain tumour. *Can J Neurol Sci.* 1994;21(3):213–218.
30. Khasraw M, Holodny A, Goldlust SA, DeAngelis LM. Intracranial hemorrhage in patients with cancer treated with bevacizumab: the Memorial Sloan-Kettering experience. *Ann Oncol.* 2012;23(2):458–463.

31. Seet RC, Rabinstein AA, Lindell PE, Uhm JH, Wijdicks EF. Cerebrovascular events after bevacizumab treatment: an early and severe complication. *Neurocrit Care*. 2011;15(3):421–427.

32. Fraum TJ, Kreisl TN, Sul J, Fine HA, Iwamoto FM. Ischemic stroke and intracranial hemorrhage in glioma patients on antiangiogenic therapy. *J Neurooncol*. 2011;105(2):281–289.

33. Chang SM, Parney IF, Huang W, et al. Patterns of care for adults with newly diagnosed malignant glioma. *JAMA*. 2005;293(5):557–564.

34. van Breemen MS, Wilms EB, Vecht CJ. Epilepsy in patients with brain tumours: epidemiology, mechanisms, and management. *Lancet Neurol*. 2007;6(5):421–430.

35. Chang EF, Potts MB, Keles GE, et al. Seizure characteristics and control following resection in 332 patients with low-grade gliomas. *J Neurosurg*. 2008;108(2):227–235.

36. Pallud J, Audureau E, Blonski M, et al. Epileptic seizures in diffuse low-grade gliomas in adults. *Brain*. 2014;137(Pt 2):449–462.

37. Tandon PN, Mahapatra AK, Khosla A. Epileptic seizures in supratentorial gliomas. *Neurol India*. 2001;49(1):55–59.

38. Chaichana KL, Parker SL, Olivi A, Quiñones-Hinojosa A. Long-term seizure outcomes in adult patients undergoing primary resection of malignant brain astrocytomas. Clinical article. *J Neurosurg*. 2009;111(2):282–292.

39. Moots PL, Maciunas RJ, Eisert DR, Parker RA, Laporte K, Abou-Khalil B. The course of seizure disorders in patients with malignant gliomas. *Arch Neurol*. 1995;52(7):717–724.

40. Kim OJ, Yong Ahn J, Chung YS, et al. Significance of chronic epilepsy in glial tumors and correlation with surgical strategies. *J Clin Neurosci*. 2004;11(7):702–705.

41. Engel J. Surgical treatment of the epilepsies. 2nd ed. New York: Raven Press; 1993, 786pp.

42. Englot DJ, Han SJ, Berger MS, Barbaro NM, Chang EF. Extent of surgical resection predicts seizure freedom in low-grade temporal lobe brain tumors. *Neurosurgery*. 2012;70(4):921–928. discussion 8.

43. Glantz MJ, Cole BF, Forsyth PA, et al. Practice parameter: anticonvulsant prophylaxis in patients with newly diagnosed brain tumors. Report of the Quality Standards Subcommittee of the American Academy of Neurology. *Neurology*. 2000;54(10):1886–1893.

44. Pulman J, Greenhalgh J, Marson AG. Antiepileptic drugs as prophylaxis for post-craniotomy seizures. *Cochrane Database Syst Rev*. 2013;2:CD007286.

45. De Santis A, Villani R, Sinisi M, Stocchetti N, Perucca E. Add-on phenytoin fails to prevent early seizures after surgery for supratentorial brain tumors: a randomized controlled study. *Epilepsia*. 2002;43(2):175–182.

46. Wu AS, Trinh VT, Suki D, et al. A prospective randomized trial of perioperative seizure prophylaxis in patients with intraparenchymal brain tumors. *J Neurosurg*. 2013;118(4):873–883.

47. Omuro A, DeAngelis LM. Glioblastoma and other malignant gliomas: a clinical review. *JAMA*. 2013;310(17):1842–1850.

48. Fuller KL, Wang YY, Cook MJ, Murphy MA, D'Souza WJ. Tolerability, safety, and side effects of levetiracetam versus phenytoin in intravenous and total prophylactic regimen among craniotomy patients: a prospective randomized study. *Epilepsia*. 2013;54(1):45–57.

49. Milligan TA, Hurwitz S, Bromfield EB. Efficacy and tolerability of levetiracetam versus phenytoin after supratentorial neurosurgery. *Neurology*. 2008;71(9):665–669.

50. Kern K, Schebesch KM, Schlaier J, et al. Levetiracetam compared to phenytoin for the prevention of postoperative seizures after craniotomy for intracranial tumours in patients without epilepsy. *J Clin Neurosci*. 2012;19(1):99–100.

51. Lim DA, Tarapore P, Chang E, et al. Safety and feasibility of switching from phenytoin to levetiracetam monotherapy for glioma-related seizure control following craniotomy: a randomized phase II pilot study. *J Neurooncol*. 2009;93(3):349–354.

52. Edwards JR, Peterson KD, Mu Y, et al. National Healthcare Safety Network (NHSN) report: data summary for 2006 through 2008, issued December 2009. *Am J Infect Control*. 2009;37(10):783–805.

53. McClelland S, Hall WA. Postoperative central nervous system infection: incidence and associated factors in 2111 neurosurgical procedures. *Clin Infect Dis*. 2007;45(1):55–59.

54. Korinek AM. Risk factors for neurosurgical site infections after craniotomy: a prospective multicenter study of 2944 patients. The French Study Group of Neurosurgical Infections, the SEHP, and the C-CLIN Paris-Nord. Service Epidémiologie Hygiène et Prévention. *Neurosurgery*. 1997;41(5):1073–1079. discussion 9–81.

55. Bruce JN, Bruce SS. Preservation of bone flaps in patients with post-craniotomy infections. *J Neurosurg*. 2003;98(6):1203–1207.

56. Dashti SR, Baharvahdat H, Spetzler RF, et al. Operative intracranial infection following craniotomy. *Neurosurg Focus*. 2008;24(6):E10.

57. Chiang HY, Kamath AS, Pottinger JM, et al. Risk factors and outcomes associated with surgical site infections after craniotomy or craniectomy. *J Neurosurg*. 2014;120(2):509–521.

58. Clark AJ, Butowski NA, Chang SM, et al. Impact of bevacizumab chemotherapy on craniotomy wound healing. *J Neurosurg*. 2011;114(6):1609–1616.

59. Barami K, Fernandes R. Incidence, risk factors and management of delayed wound dehiscence after craniotomy for tumor resection. *J Clin Neurosci*. 2012;19(6):854–857.

60. Barker FG. Efficacy of prophylactic antibiotics for craniotomy: a meta-analysis. *Neurosurgery*. 1994;35(3):484–490. discussion 91–92.

61. Barker FG. Efficacy of prophylactic antibiotics against meningitis after craniotomy: a meta-analysis. *Neurosurgery*. 2007 May;60(5):887–894. discussion 894.

62. Farrell CJ, Hoh BL, Pisculli ML, Henson JW, Barker FG, Curry WT. Limitations of diffusion-weighted imaging in the diagnosis of postoperative infections. *Neurosurgery*. 2008;62(3):577–583. discussion 583.

63. Auguste KI, McDermott MW. Salvage of infected craniotomy bone flaps with the wash-in, wash-out indwelling antibiotic irrigation system. Technical note and case series of 12 patients. *J Neurosurg*. 2006;105(4):640–644.

64. Perry JR. Thromboembolic disease in patients with high-grade glioma. *Neuro Oncol*. 2012;14(Suppl 4):iv73–iv80.

65. Chaichana KL, Pendleton C, Jackson C, et al. Deep venous thrombosis and pulmonary embolisms in adult patients undergoing craniotomy for brain tumors. *Neurol Res*. 2013;35(2):206–211.

66. Semrad TJ, O'Donnell R, Wun T, et al. Epidemiology of venous thromboembolism in 9489 patients with malignant glioma. *J Neurosurg*. 2007;106(4):601–608.

67. Fisher JL, Palmisano S, Schwartzbaum JA, Svensson T, Lönn S. Comorbid conditions associated with glioblastoma. *J Neurooncol*. 2014;116(3):585–591.

68. Marcus LP, McCutcheon BA, Noorbakhsh A, et al. Incidence and predictors of 30-day readmission for patients discharged home after craniotomy for malignant supratentorial tumors in California (1995-2010). *J Neurosurg*. 2014 May;120(5):1201–1211.

69. Nuño M, Ly D, Ortega A, et al. Does 30-day readmission affect long-term outcome among glioblastoma patients? *Neurosurgery*. 2014;74(2):196–204. discussion 205.

70. Solheim O, Jakola AS, Gulati S, Johannesen TB. Incidence and causes of perioperative mortality after primary surgery for intracranial tumors: a national, population-based study. *J Neurosurg*. 2012;116(4):825–834.

# 17 Tumors of the Lateral Ventricle and the Pineal Region

TRACY S. MA, PREETHI RAMCHAND, R. ALEXANDER SCHLICHTER, and STEVEN BREM

## Introduction

This chapter will focus on tumors of the lateral ventricle and pineal region. The anatomy will be discussed in conjunction with surgical approaches unique to lateral ventricle and pineal tumors. Perioperative considerations as well as postoperative complications will be reviewed in detail. The goal of this chapter is to enrich the neurosurgeon's or neurointensivist's fund of knowledge in order to enhance patient care.

## Neuroanatomy and Procedure

### Key Concepts

- Plan a safe, precise corridor to the target tumor with knowledge of the regional and specific anatomy to employ neuronavigation.
- Maximize extent of resection whenever possible to achieve gross total or near-total removal.
- Obtain excellent local oncologic control and avoid cerebrospinal fluid (CSF) seeding.
- Maintain "physiologic neurosurgery" by avoiding extremes of intracranial hypertension and/or hypotension, that is, avoid hydrocephalus or overdrainage of CSF.
- Detect and control perioperative hydrocephalus.

### LATERAL VENTRICLE TUMORS

#### Frontal Horn

Tumors of the lateral ventricles are often low-grade or benign lesions that exhibit a relatively slow growth rate; as such, these lesions often reach several centimeters before presentation to a neurosurgeon.[1] These tumors also tend to displace, rather than invade, the brain. Thus symptoms are often that of hydrocephalus (headaches, nausea, vomiting, gait instability, and visual disturbances). A careful study by the neurosurgeon of the exact location, size, and extent of displacement of normal structures, as well as the experience of the surgeon, informs the best approach. Computer-based neuronavigation software is useful to plan the safest, most direct path.

### Clinical Pearl

Careful preoperative planning with particular emphasis on the tumor's proximity to vascular structures is essential.

The interhemispheric transcallosal approach is especially valuable for tumors of the frontal horn of the lateral ventricle.[1–3] This approach can also be used for tumors in the region of the third ventricle (Fig. 17.1). For a complete view of the interhemispheric fissure, a craniotomy that exposes the superior sagittal sinus is preferred. The bridging veins must be preserved, and a retractor, if necessary, can be slowly advanced along the interhemispheric fissure in order to allow the neurosurgeon to identify the cingulate gyrus and pericallosal arteries. The judicious use of mannitol and tilting of the table to use gravity may lessen the need for retraction, which has postoperative complications that the neurointensivist should be aware of as they pertain to swelling and mental status changes.

Below the inferior edge of the falx, small veins adherent to the cingulate gyrus can be sacrificed if they obstruct the surgical view, and the frontal lobe is then displaced laterally. The callosomarginal and pericallosal arteries are identified, allowing the neurosurgeon access to the lateral ventricle body via a callosotomy. The pericallosal artery demarcates the callosum midline, and injury to this artery has significant postoperative implications.[4] After the corpus callosotomy, it is necessary to identify the foramen of Monro and thalamostriate vein lateral to the choroid plexus.[5] When hydrocephalus is present, this approach may be used to reach the contralateral ventricle. Because lateral ventricular tumors are often quite large, initial internal debulking may be required, and the tumor margin is carefully dissected away from the surrounding ventricular structures.[4–8]

#### Medial/Lateral Atrium and Temporal Horn

Tumors of the atrium can be accessed via the posterior transcortical approach. The craniotomy should not cross midline, and dissection occurs along the interparietal sulcus to minimize brain retraction. The vascular pedicle of the tumor should be identified and coagulated as early as possible to avoid excessive bleeding.[1] Preoperative planning by studying the venous anatomy on a contrast-enhanced magnetic resonance image (MRI) or a specific magnetic resonance venogram is useful because the draining cortical veins to the superior sagittal sinus are a formidable challenge.[1,9]

For tumors of the lateral atrium, a middle temporal gyrus (T2) approach is favored (Fig. 17.2).[10] The patient is positioned so that the falx is parallel to the floor. This provides a straightforward and minimally invasive approach to the lateral ventricle. On the dominant side (usually the left), it is important to retract in a ventral, inferior direction to

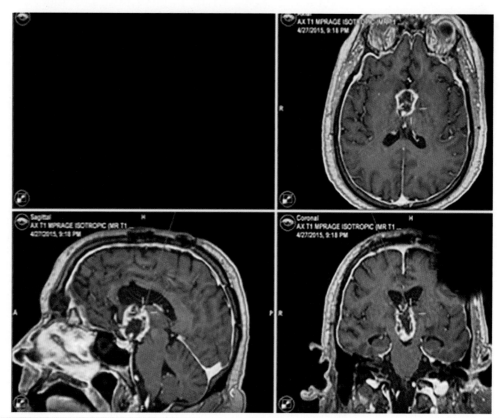

**Fig. 17.1** This is a view of the intraoperative navigation software utilized to resect this tumor of the third ventricle. The *green cross-hairs* indicates the anatomic target (top right). The *green line* marks the trajectory of the interhemispheric transcallosal approach to reach this tumor (bottom left), and the degree of retraction (bottom right).

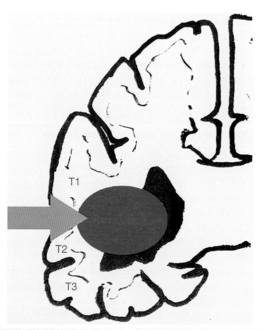

**Fig. 17.2** Schematic view of the middle temporal gyrus approach. (Reprinted from Juretschke FR, Guresir E, Marquardt G, et al. Trigonal and peritrigonal lesions of the lateral ventricle-surgical considerations and outcome analysis of 20 patients. *Neurosurg Rev.* 2010;33 (4):457–464.)

avoid injury to the white-matter tracts mediating language function (i.e., the arcuate fasciculus).

Tumors of the temporal horn are accessed via the middle temporal gyrus or inferior temporal gyrus, or through the temporal lobe tip. For the middle temporal gyrus approach, a horizontal cortical incision is made along the anterior portion because the temporal horn is approximately 3.5 cm posterior to the temporal tip and sphenoid ridge. This also ensures that the incision avoids the vein of Labbé and the optic radiations. Postoperatively, the neurointensivist should note visual field deficits that correlate with the surgical area of interest. The craniotomy in both cases should be sufficiently low in order to access the middle and inferior temporal gyri.[7]

### Occipital Horn

Tumors of the occipital horn can be removed via the superior parietal lobule; alternatively, the posterior transcallosal approach spares the speech and visual pathways within the parietal lobe. However, the latter trajectory interrupts the corpus callosum and is thus contraindicated in patients with preoperative homonymous hemianopsia; there is also the risk of postoperative alexia. The craniotomy should expose the superior sagittal sinus and extend laterally 3 to 4 cm. As with all tumors near the midline, care should be taken to preserve the large draining veins when reflecting the dura medially. Because the atrium of the ventricle is paramedian, the splenium should be incised lateral to the midline, revealing the internal cerebral veins.[1] Care must be taken during the division of the splenium to avoid injury to the splenial branches of the posterior cerebral artery.[11]

## PINEAL TUMORS

### Surgical Approach: An Overview

Oppenheim and Krause first reported the successful removal of a pineal region tumor in 1913 via an infratentorial supracerebellar approach.[12] Pineal tumors are excised via microsurgery using a variety of surgical approaches that have been refined frequently by neurosurgeons.[13] This section will discuss a few of these approaches and a paradigm shift toward endoscopic management.

### Infratentorial Supracerebellar Approach

The infratentorial supracerebellar and occipital transtentorial approaches are the most common surgical trajectories for pineal tumors.[14] The infratentorial supracerebellar approach is favored for its direct midline trajectory, minimizing intraoperative variation.[15] A sitting positioning has been traditionally used because of three benefits: 1) cerebellar retraction away from the tentorium by the gravitational field; 2) decreased pooling of blood and CSF into the surgical field; and 3) minimization of venous engorgement[13,16–18] (these advantages can also be realized using the Concorde position, discussed later in this chapter).

A midline incision above the external occipital protuberance in the region of the lambdoid suture is made to extend down to the C2 vertebrae. To maximize exposure during this approach, a bilateral symmetric craniotomy should be made above the foramen magnum and extending above the inferior margin of the lateral sinuses and torcula (Fig. 17.3). Semioval dural incisions can be placed below the lateral sinuses; stay sutures pulled cephalad and placed in the tentorium's inferior leaf (anterior to the transverse sinus) provide deeper illumination and minimize the need

for retractors.[14] The inferosuperior surgical corridor in the infratentorial supracerebellar approach allows for dissection without violating the Galenic system, the major veins located superior to the pineal tumor.[17–19] The patency of the sinus can be evaluated intraoperatively using a micro-Doppler probe.[20] The tumor is dissected after identification and coagulation of the precentral cerebellar vein and the superior vermian vein.[21] To avoid collateral venous circulation thrombosis, which could prove catastrophic or fatal, the precentral cerebellar veins should be coagulated as far as possible from the confluence of the basal veins of Rosenthal.[22,23]

### Occipital Transtentorial Approach

The occipital transtentorial approach for pineal region tumors offers the surgeon a wide view of the supratentorial and infratentorial domains (Fig. 17.4). This approach is favored for tumors with inferior involvement of the cerebellomesencephalic cistern.[21] The skin incision is linear or a horseshoe shape, and the neurosurgeon must identify the lambdoid suture as well as the upper insertions of the neck muscles.[14] The craniotomy must expose the posterior region of the superior sagittal sinus, above the edge of the torcula; this should be followed by a dural opening (C-shaped or a pair of triangular leaves) that allows for a surgical corridor between the occipital lobe and falx cerebri.[14,17] Gentle occipital lobe elevation laterally and superiorly off the tentorium is a safe tactic due to the anterolateral course of the occipitobasal vein toward the preoccipital notch and into the lateral tentorial sinus.[14,21,24]

### Neuroendoscopy

Intraventricular neuroendoscopy has dramatically affected the surgical treatment of pineal region tumors (Fig. 17.5). Simultaneous endoscopic third ventriculostomy

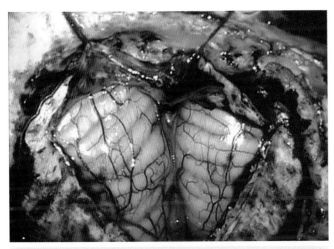

**Fig. 17.3** Infratentorial supracerebellar approach showing suboccipital craniotomy extension laterally toward transverse-sigmoid junction and extension inferiorly to cisterna magna. (Reprinted from Oliveira J, Cerejo A, Silva PS, et al. The infratentorial supracerebellar approach in surgery of lesions of the pineal region. *Surg Neurol Int*. 2013;4:154.)

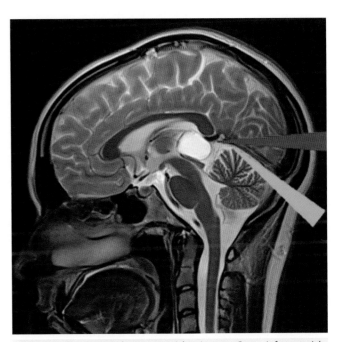

**Fig. 17.4** *Blue:* occipital transtentorial trajectory. *Green:* Infratentorial supracerebellar trajectory.

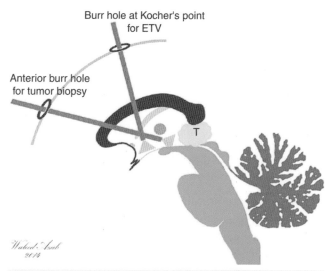

Burr hole at Kocher's point
for ETV

Anterior burr hole
for tumor biopsy

**Fig. 17.5** ETV and tumor biopsy burr holes. (Reprinted from Azab WA, Nasim K, Salaheddin W. An overview of the current surgical options for pineal region tumors. *Surg Neurol Int.* 2014;5:39.)

(ETV) and biopsy for pineal tumors offers diagnostic and therapeutic treatment for pineal tumor patients who often present with noncommunicating hydrocephalus.[25] CSF should be collected prior to ETV and tumor biopsy.[26] A burr hole can be placed at Kocher's point for ETV procedures. A single burr hole 2 to 3 cm anterior to Kocher's point can also be employed for tumor biopsy for lesions that are 1) anterior to the massa intermedia; 2) associated with a small massa intermedia; 3) to undergo biopsy without resection; or 4) associated with significant ventriculomegaly.[27,28] Two burr holes (Kocher's point and an additional anterior burr hole) are optimal for tumors that are 1) posterior to the massa intermedia; 2) associated with a large massa intermedia; 3) <2 cm (total removal is possible); or 4) associated with moderate or minimal ventriculomegaly.[29] When a single entry site is used, a 30-degree endoscope lens allows the neurosurgeon a posterior direction of view. When a separate anterior entry is used for biopsy, a 0-degree lens offers posterior third ventricle visualization.[30]

The superiority of rigid versus flexible endoscopes is a topic of much debate. Rigid endoscopes are perceived to improve diagnostic yield and allow for the use of wider biopsy forceps to allow for larger tumor specimens.[31] On the other hand, flexible endoscopes may overcome nonlinear trajectories, especially when a single burr hole is used.[31] Flexible endoscopes have a disadvantage of a smaller surgical corridor and therefore a decreased image definition.[29,30] For this reason, many neurosurgeons prefer rigid endoscopes for tumor resection.

With the addition of endoscopes to the neurosurgical repertoire, there have been reports of endoscopic infratentorial supracerebellar approaches for pineal tumors. A burr hole is placed 1.5 to 2.5 cm at the transverse sinus inferior margin and 1 to 2 cm lateral to the torcula. The endoscope is inserted via a paramedian corridor in order to avoid vermis obstruction. This approach is contraindicated in tumors with high vascularity or

tumors that have extended bilaterally or above the tentorium.[32]

## Perioperative Considerations

### Key Concepts

- Position the patient in the appropriate manner to maximize surgical safety and visibility of the tumor.
- Recognize the advantages and disadvantages of the sitting and prone positions.
- Utilize the Concorde position as an alternative to the sitting and prone positions.

The perioperative considerations for lateral ventricle and pineal region tumor surgeries are similar to other intracranial operations: brain volume and, rigorous control of blood pressure and intracranial pressure (ICP) via alteration of carbon dioxide tension, fluid management, etc. This section will briefly review patient positioning with regard to pineal tumor resections. The patient's position needs to allow the surgeon access to the tumor while minimizing bleeding and brain swelling, as well as encouraging adequate venous drainage. Historically the positions included sitting, prone, lateral, and the Concorde position.

The sitting position (both standard and "beach chair" modifications) has traditionally provided favorable conditions for pineal tumor resection (Fig. 17.6).[33] Advantages include minimal arterial bleeding and excellent venous drainage. For the anesthesiologist, the position provides improved pulmonary mechanics, access to the face and endotracheal tube, and access to lines in the upper extremities. However, the sitting position is not without its disadvantages. Due to the elevated position of the head high over the thorax, the risk of venous air embolism obligates the anesthesiologist to place additional monitors, including precordial Doppler, end-tidal nitrogen, and a right atrial catheter (an invasive procedure). Some centers use continuous intraoperative transesophageal echocardiogram, although this adds time and cost.[34] The serious consequences of a venous air embolism (VAE) can also be difficult to address while the patient is in a frame. The actions that must be taken when a VAE is diagnosed include lowering the head down to the level of the heart. In severe cases leading to cardiac compromise, it may be necessary to initiate chest compressions. Additionally, pneumocephalus was found in one study to be 100% in the sitting position compared with the lateral (72%) and prone (52%) positions.[35,36] The sitting position also increases the risk of orthostatic hypotension due to venous pooling in the lower extremities, which can lower cerebral, retinal, and spinal perfusion pressure, thereby increasing the risk of ischemia to the brain, eye, or spinal cord, respectively. Finally, failure

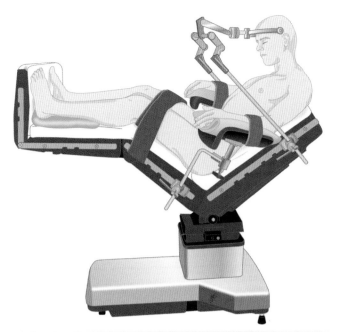

Fig. 17.6 Sitting position. (Reprinted from Cassorla L, Lee J. Patient positioning and associated risks. In: Miller RD, Eriksson LI, Fleisher LA, et al, eds. *Miller's Anesthesia* 8th ed. San Francisco: Elsevier Saunders; 2014: pp. 1240–1265.)

to pad the patient's extremities properly (especially in thin or elderly patients) can lead to abdominal compression syndrome, lower extremity injury, or sciatic and peroneal neuropathies. The risks associated with sitting-position craniotomies, as well as with the difficulty of positioning, padding, and monitoring these patients (as well as what is perceived as an awkward, fatiguing approach for certain surgeons), have led many neurosurgical centers to reduce or even abandon the sitting approach.

An alternative to the sitting position is the prone position (Fig. 17.7).[33] Although associated with lower incidence of VAE and pneumocephalus,[36,37] the head is still above the heart, so there remains a risk, albeit reduced. Positioning is straightforward compared with the sitting position but can still be challenging, especially in morbidly obese patients. Restrictive frames such as the Wilson (as opposed to the less restrictive Andrews and Jackson) can compress the abdomen and worsen pulmonary mechanics. Lines and monitors attached to the patient can be dislodged during pronation, leading to loss of access or masking of cardiovascular changes until monitoring is reestablished. Careful attention must be paid to securing the airway because oral and gastric secretions can undo adhesives; gravity can cause the endotracheal tube to become dislodged (resecuring the airway in the prone position is obviously difficult). Cases lasting more than a few hours are associated with considerable facial and airway edema: the risks of immediate extubation after surgery need to be measured against the loss of airway and difficult reintubation. Finally, optic arterial ischemia and venous thrombosis from hypotension can lead to postoperative visual loss, a well-known complication of surgery in the prone position.[38]

The simple prone procedure may not allow for optimal flexion of the neck for some posterior fossa surgical approaches, especially if the tumor is located in the pineal region, the anterior superior vermis, or any lesion near the tentorial notch. In 1983 Kobayashi first described what he referred to as the "Concorde position."[16] The surgeon operates from the left with the head flexed and positioned higher than the heart (Fig. 17.8).[39] Although the head is above the heart, the risk of VAE is lower than the risk in the sitting position; there is less surgical fatigue while maintaining a surgical field relatively free of blood.[16] Koyoshima described an arm-down or "modified" Concorde, where the arm nearest the primary surgeon is flexed below the bed on a special arm holder (Fig. 17.9).[39] This improves the surgical approach in patients with muscular shoulders, short necks, or the morbidly obese. The overall result allows for superior visualization and improved access to the surgical field.[39] In addition, the down arm is more accessible (for lines and monitors) to the anesthesiologist than when tucked at the sides (for prone and Concorde positions). However, care must be taken in positioning and padding the down arm: instability of the arm support can lead to

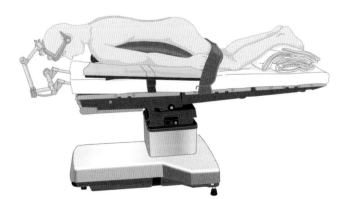

Fig. 17.7 Prone position. (Reprinted from Cassorla L, Lee J. Patient positioning and associated risks. In: Miller RD, Eriksson LI, Fleisher LA, et al, eds. *Miller's Anesthesia* 8th ed. San Francisco: Elsevier Saunders; 2014: pp. 1240–1265.).

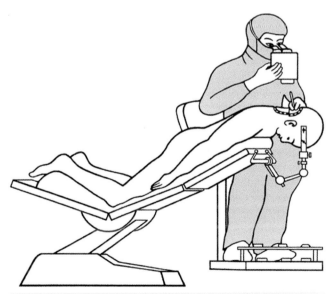

Fig. 17.8 Concorde position: The patient's head is flexed and elevated above the heart. The surgeon sits on the patient's left. (Reprinted from Kyoshima K. Arm-down Concorde position: a technical note. *Surg Neurol.* 2002;57(6):443–445.)

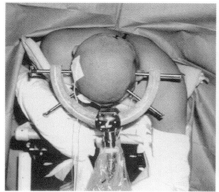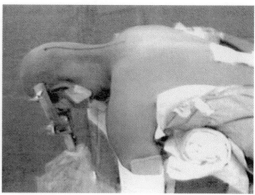

**Fig. 17.9** Modified Concorde position: The patient's left arm is flexed at the elbow with an arm holder used as support. The left arm is positioned over the operating table's end. (Reprinted from Kyoshima K. Arm-down Concorde position: a technical note. *Surg Neurol.* 2002;57(6):443–445.)

ulnar neuropathy; if the support fails, brachial plexopathies may result. The modified Concorde is technically more challenging to position than the simple prone position, but it carries less risk for VAE, as well as a superior view of the tentorial notch and pineal area.

### Clinical Pearl

The modified Concorde position improves the neurosurgeon's view of the surgical field while minimizing intraoperative anesthesia-related complications.

## Postoperative Complications

### Key Concepts

- Understand the neuroanatomy of common postoperative complications.
- Recognize postoperative neurologic deficits with regard to general surgical approaches.

Surgical resection is the primary treatment for tumors in the lateral ventricle and pineal region. Recent data have shown surgery for these tumors to be well tolerated and safe with a reported mortality of less than 3% and 5% for lateral ventricle and pineal region tumors, respectively.[1,40,41] The variety of surgical approaches employed by neurosurgeons to resect these lesions aims to traverse noneloquent brain parenchyma, but may result in a heterogeneous array of postoperative complications (Box 17.1). Anticipation and recognition of clinical deterioration in patients postoperatively is critical to the patient's overall care. Management of these patients in a dedicated neurological/neurosurgical intensive care unit (ICU) with continuous monitoring, including frequent neurologic examinations by nurses and physicians, contributes to optimal outcomes for these patients.

### Clinical Pearl

The neurosurgeon and the neurointensivist must work closely together to optimize patient care in the postoperative period.

---

### Box 17.1    Important Postoperative Complications

**Hemorrhage**
**Paresis**
Transient
Permanent
**Visual deficit**
Hemianopsia
Oculomotor dysfunction
**Language deficit**
**Seizures**
**Memory loss**
**Infections**
**Hydrocephalus**
**Venous ischemia or thrombosis**

---

Lethargy and drowsiness can be the first symptoms of early hydrocephalus, and therefore the use of narcotics to control postoperative headaches should be given sparingly and with caution. If needed, short-acting fentanyl in aliquots ranging from 25 mcg (elderly, thin patients) to 100 mcg can be given in the ICU.

Because patients with intraventricular tumors are at risk for developing hydrocephalus, a head computed tomography (CT) scan should be obtained to assess ventricular size if the patient becomes lethargic.

If an external ventricular drain (EVD) is already in place and the CSF becomes sanguineous, a head CT can detect intraventricular bleeding.

Anticoagulation for patients with an EVD after resection of an intraventricular bleed is problematic; it is important to balance the risk of a venous thromboembolism (from being confined to bed rest) against the risk of an intraventricular hemorrhage. Waiting for 48 hours or until the CSF drainage clears (if an EVD is in place) can be prudent.

### HEMORRHAGE

One of the more feared, potentially fatal complications of tumor resection is hemorrhage near or within the tumor cavity. A high index of suspicion, as well as early detection, is critical to avoid long-term morbidity. The most significant risk factor for postoperative bleeding is tumor histopathology, which determines tumor vascularity. Because angiogenesis is a hallmark of malignancy, these tumors tend to be vascular and have a higher risk of postoperative hemorrhage. For lateral ventricle tumors, intraventricular hemorrhage leads to significant postoperative hydrocephalus.[41] When this is suspected, urgent neurosurgical evaluation is required to determine whether an EVD or immediate surgery is necessary to relieve the increase in ICP. The ventricular system is less amenable to tamponade by adjacent tissue structures; thus pineal tumors are highly susceptible to persistent bleeding.[42] The pineal gland's proximity to the deep cerebral veins places lesions in this region at high risk for postoperative hemorrhage, ischemia, or infarction.[43,44] If hemorrhage is suspected due to new focal deficits, nausea, vomiting, or vital sign changes, an immediate noncontrast head CT should be obtained. If there are signs of bleeding, emergent neurosurgical engagement is required.

## WEAKNESS

Temporary or persistent paresis is an important postoperative complication in lateral ventricle and pineal tumor resection. Retraction of brain tissue or damage to venous supply can result in weakness or sensory deficits.[45,46] The duration of these deficits depends on the extent of the injury, the integrity of fiber tracts in the white matter, the age of the patient (neuroplasticity), collateral blood supply, and comorbidities. Early identification of any new deficits postoperatively via a thorough neurologic examination must be investigated with neuroimaging.

## VISUAL DEFICITS

Postoperative visual deficits are commonly associated with tumors of the lateral ventricle and pineal region. Specifically, trigone meningiomas often present with visual field dysfunction and have a 54% risk of new or worsened postoperative deficits.[46] This is largely due to the proximity of the geniculocalcarine fibers to the trigone lateral surface. Likewise, the transcortical approach through the superior parietal lobule is associated with a 20% to 70% incidence of new or worsened visual field defect.[47] Injury to the occipital lobe from mechanical retraction or vascular insult during a pineal tumor resection also often results in hemianopsia.[48]

Depending on the location and extent of perioperative injury, postoperative visual field loss may present in any number of ways, from homonymous hemianopsia with macular sparing to quandrantanopias or isolated scotomatous defects. Studies have shown that some patients with visual field deficits in the immediate postoperative period have also been associated with visual hallucinations, described as formed objects that are seen in the field of their deficits. For the neurointensivist, this is an important consideration because these hallucinations may contribute to postoperative delirium. Although hallucinations may be ictal in etiology, it is speculated that these are most likely the result of disruptions in visual circuitry that has been directly manipulated during the procedure.[49] Most patients recover from visual field deficits within weeks to months, although some may have persistent deficits several years after surgery.[50] Depending on the patient's level of arousal, visual field testing (formal field test or confrontation test) should be part of the routine postoperative examination. When detected, field cuts should prompt serial

ophthalmological examinations and possible outpatient neuroimaging if symptoms fail to improve.

For patients with pineal area tumors, particular emphasis must be placed on the oculomotor examination as part of Parinaud's, or superior aqueduct, syndrome. Ophthalmoplegias are primarily due to damage of the dorsal midbrain, specifically the tectum, Edinger-Westphal nucleus, or superior colliculus.[51] Upward-gaze palsy with compensatory backward head tilt and lid retraction is the most commonly noted oculomotor abnormality in this syndrome. Other features of Parinaud's syndrome include convergence/retraction nystagmus, pupillary light-near dissociation, exotropia, esotropia, and skew deviations.[52] Patients with normal preoperative ocular motility are generally less likely to develop these symptoms after surgery. However, because ophthalmoplegias are subtle and have significant functional implications, the neurointensivist must diligently discern postoperative visual field disturbances.

## SEIZURES

Transcortical surgical approaches for lateral ventricle or pineal tumors are associated with postoperative seizures. Prior to routine use of MRI for preoperative planning, the transcortical approach for tumor resection was associated with a 26% to 70% postoperative seizure rate.[47,53] Given this high incidence, some neurosurgeons historically advocated for the transcallosal over the transcortical approach.[54,55] In the MRI era, recent studies have reported an incidence of <7% with transcortical approaches.[56] However, a recent study, including multivariate analysis, found that the transcortical approach actually had a lower seizure incidence (8%) compared with the transcallosal approach (25%).[46] Therefore regardless of the surgical trajectory, the neurointensivist must have a high suspicion for seizures in the postoperative period and have a low threshold for initiation of electroencephalogram monitoring.

## MEMORY LOSS

The Papez memory circuit includes the hippocampal commissure, fornix, forniceal columns, mammillary bodies, anterior thalamic nucleus, and thalamocortical fibers. Surgery in and around the ventricles carries the risk of damage to this circuit with subsequent postoperative memory dysfunction. It has been reported that 12% of transcortical approaches and 23% of transcallosal approaches for lateral ventricle tumor resection result in new or worsened memory postoperatively.[46] In particular, substantial memory deficits occur with bilateral forniceal injury. Minor unilateral fornix injury may result in a significant decrease in performance intelligence quotient and temporary memory difficulties.[57] Therefore vigilant neurologic examinations that specifically interrogate the patient's capacity for memory are valuable postoperatively.

## MISCELLANEOUS

As with any surgical procedure, the neurointensivist should exclude common postoperative complications such as infections. Typical pathogens in postoperative central nervous system (CNS) infections include methicillin-sensitive and resistant *Staphylococcus aureus* as well as *S. epidermidis*, although regional variability exists in local pathogens.[58] When the index of suspicion is high for CNS infection, lumbar puncture or interrogation of CSF using an EVD should be pursued with antimicrobial therapy tailored toward the offending pathogen.

# Conclusion

Surgical approaches of lateral ventricle and pineal region tumors have significant hazards for the patient in the postoperative period. The neurointensivist must be broadly familiar with the anatomic trajectories of surgical resection, as well as with perioperative events, in order to anticipate postoperative complications. This multidisciplinary approach serves to enhance patient care and improve surgical outcomes.

## References

1. Danaila L. Primary tumors of the lateral ventricles of the brain. *Chirugia (Bucur)*. 2013;108(5):616–630.
2. Kawashima M, Li X, Rhoton AL, et al. Surgical approaches to the atrium of the lateral ventricle: microsurgical anatomy. *Surg Neurol*. 2006;65(5):436–445.
3. Piepmeier JM. Tumors and approaches to the lateral ventricles. Introduction and overview. *J Neurooncol*. 1996;30(3):267–274.
4. Fuji K, Lenkey C, Rhoton Jr AL. Microsurgical anatomy of the choroidal arteries: lateral and third ventricle. *J Neurosurg*. 1980;52(2):65–88.
5. Bellotti C, Pappada G, Sani R, et al. The transcallosal approach for lesions affecting the lateral and third ventricles. Surgical considerations and results in a series of 42 cases. *Acta Neurochir (Wien)*. 1991;111(3–4):103–107.
6. Shucart WA, Stein BM. Transcallosal approach to the anterior ventricular system. *Neurosurgery*. 1978;3(3):339–343.
7. Timurkaynak E, Rhoton Jr AL, Barry M. Microsurgical anatomy and operative approaches to the lateral ventricles. *Neurosurgery*. 1986;19(5):685–723.
8. Hellwig D, Bauer BL, Schulte M, et al. Neuroendoscopic treatment for colloid cysts of the third ventricle: the experience of a decade. *Neurosurgery*. 2003;52(3):525–533.
9. Bertalanffy H. Neuroendoscopic treatment for colloid cysts of the third ventricle: the experience of a decade. *Neurosurgery*. 2003;52(3):525–533.
10. Juretschke FR, Guresir E, Marquardt G, et al. Trigonal and peritrigonal lesions of the lateral ventricle-surgical considerations and outcome analysis of 20 patients. *Neurosurg Rev*. 2010;33(4):457–464.
11. Perlmutter D, Rhoton Jr AL. Microsurgical anatomy of the distal anterior cerebral artery. *J Neurosurg*. 1978;49(2):204–228.
12. Oppenheim H, Krause F. Operative Erfolge bei Geschwulsten der Sehhugel und Vierhugelgegend. *Berlin Klin Wschr*. 1913;50:2316–2322.
13. Radovanovic I, Dizdarevic K, de Tribolet N, et al. Pineal region tumors: neurosurgical review. *Med Arh*. 2009;63(3):171–173.
14. Konovalov AN, Pittskhelauri DI. Principles of treatment of the pineal region tumors. *Surg Neurol*. 2003;59(4):250–268.
15. Behari S, Garg P, Jaiswal S, et al. Major surgical approaches to the posterior third ventricular region: a pictorial review. *J Pediatr Neurosci*. 2010;5(2):97–101.
16. Kobayashi S, Sugita K, Tanaka Y, et al. Infratentorial approach to the pineal region in the prone position: concorde position. Technical note. *J Neurosurg*. 1983;58(1):141–143.
17. Lozier AP, Bruce JN. Surgical approaches to posterior third ventricular tumors. *Neurosurg Clin N Am*. 2003;14(4):527–545.
18. Little KM, Friedman AH, Fukushima T. Surgical approaches to pineal region tumors. *J Neurooncol*. 2001;54(3):287–299.
19. Oliveira J, Cerejo A, Silva PS, et al. The infratentorial supracerebellar approach in surgery of lesions of the pineal region. *Surg Neurol Int*. 2013;4:154.
20. Rey-Dios R, Cohen-Gadol AA. A surgical technique to expand the operative corridor for the supracerebellar infratentorial approaches: technical note. *Acta Neurochir (Wein)*. 2013;155(10):1895–1900.
21. Azab WA, Nasim K, Salaheddin W. An overview of the current surgical options for pineal region tumors. *Surg Neurol Int*. 2014;5:39.
22. Kanno T. Surgical pitfalls in pinealoma surgery. *Minim Invasive Neurosurg*. 1995;38(4):153–157.
23. Kodera T, Bozinov O, Surucu O, et al. Neurosurgical venous considerations for tumors of the pineal region resected using the infratentorial supracerebellar approach. *J Clin Neurosci*. 2011;18(11):1481–1485.
24. Rhoton A. The cerebral veins. *Neurosurgery*. 2002;51(4 Suppl):S159–S205.
25. Ellenbogen RG, Moores LE. Endoscopic management of a pineal and suprasellar germinoma with associated hydrocephalus: technical case report. *Minim Invasive Neurosurg*. 1997;40(1):13–15.
26. Al-Tamimi YZ, Bhargava D, Surash S, et al. Endoscopic biopsy during third ventriculostomy in pediatric pineal region tumours. *Childs Nerve Syst*. 2008;24(11):1323–1326.
27. Yurtseven T, Ersahin Y, Demirtas E, et al. Neuroendoscopic biopsy for intraventricular tumors. *Minim Invasiv Neurosurg*. 2003;46(5):293–299.
28. Morgenstern PF, Souweidane MM. Pineal region tumors: simultaneous endoscopic third ventriculostomy and tumor biopsy. *World Neurosurg*. 2013;79(2 Suppl):S18.e9–S18.e13.
29. Neuwelt EA, Glasbery M, Frenkel E, et al. Malignant pineal region tumors. a clinic-pathological study. *J Neurosurg*. 1979;51(5):597–607.
30. Mohanty A, Santosh V, Devi BI, Satish S, Biswas A. Efficacy of simultaneous single-trajectory endoscopic tumor biopsy and endoscopic cerebrospinal fluid diversion procedures in intra- and paraventricular tumors. *Neurosurg Focus*. 2011;30(4).
31. Endo H, Fujimura M, Kumabe T, et al. Application of high-definition flexible neuroendoscopic system to the treatment of primary pineal malignant B-cell lymphoma. *Surg Neurol*. 2009;71(3):344–348.
32. Uschold T, Abla AA, Fusco D, et al. Supracerebellar infratentorial endoscopically controlled resection of pineal lesions: case series and operative technique. *J Neurosurg Pediatr*. 2011;8(6):554–564.
33. Cassorla L, Lee J. Patient positioning and associated risks. In: Miller RD, Eriksson LI, Fleisher LA, Wiener-Kronish JP, et al. *Miller's Anesthesia* 8th ed. San Francisco: Elsevier Saunders; 2014:1240–1265.
34. Mammoto T, Hayashi Y, Ohnishi Y, et al. Incidence of venous and paradoxical air embolism in neurosurgical patients in the sitting position: detection by transesophageal echocardiography. *Acta Aneasth Scand*. 1988;42(6):643–647.
35. Di Lorenzo N, Caruso R, Floris R, et al. Pneumocephalus and tension pneumocephalus after posterior fossa surgery in the sitting position: a prospective study. *Acta Neurochir (Wien)*. 1986;83(3–4):112–115.
36. Toung TJ, McPherson RW, Ahn H, et al. Pneumocephalus: effects of patient position on the incidence and location of aerocele after posterior fossa and upper cervical cord surgery. *Anesth Analg*. 1986;65(1):65–70.
37. Black S, Ockert DB, Oliver Jr WC, et al. Outcome following posterior fossa craniectomy in patients in the sitting or horizontal positions. *Anesthesiology*. 1988;69(1):49–56.
38. Lee LA, Roth S, Posner KL, et al. The American Society of Anesthesiologists Postoperative Visual Loss Registry: analysis of 93 spine surgery cases with postoperative visual loss. *Anesthesiology*. 2006;105(4):652–659.
39. Kyoshima K. Arm-down Concorde position: a technical note. *Surg Neurol*. 2002;57(6):443–445.
40. Konovalov AN, Pitskhelauri DI. Principles of treatment of the pineal region tumors. *Surg Neurol*. 2003;59(4):250–268.
41. D'Angelo VA, Galarza M, Catapano D, et al. Lateral ventricle tumors: surgical strategies according to tumor origin and development – a series of 72 cases. *Neurosurgery*. 2008;62(Suppl3):1066–1075.
42. Allen JC, Bruce J, Kun LE, et al. Pineal region tumors. In: *Cancer in the Nervous System*. New York: Churchill Livingstone; 1996:171–185.
43. Little KM, Friedman AH, Fukushima T. Surgical approaches to pineal region tumors. *J Neurooncol*. 2001;54(3):287–299.
44. Yamamoto I. Pineal region tumor: surgical anatomy and approach. *J Neurooncol*. 2001;54(3):263–275.
45. Bruce JN, Ogden AT. Surgical strategies for treating patients with pineal region tumors. *J Neurooncol*. 2004;69(1–3):221–236.

46. Milligan BD, Meyer FB. Morbidity of transcallosal and transcortical approaches to lesions in and around the lateral and third ventricles: a single-institution experience. *Neurosurgery.* 2010;67(6):1483–1496.

47. Kobayashi S, Okazaki H, MacCarty CS. Intraventricular meningiomas. *Mayo Clin Proc.* 1971;46(11):735–741.

48. Qi S, Fan J, Zhang XA, et al. Radical resection of nongerminomatous pineal region tumors via the occipital transtentorial approach based on arachnoidal consideration: experience on a series of 143 patients. *Acta Neurochir (Wien).* 2014;156(12):2253–2262.

49. Yoshimoto K, Araki Y, Amano T, et al. Clinical features and pathophysiological mechanism of the hemianoptic complication after the occipital transtentorial approach. *Clin Neurol Neurosurg.* 2013;115(8):1250–1256.

50. Chi JH, Lawton MT. Posterior interhemispheric approach: surgical technique, application to vascular lesions, and benefits of gravity retraction. *Neurosurgery.* 2006;59(1 Suppl 1):ONS41–ONS49.

51. Nazzaro JM, Shults WT, Neuwelt EA. Neuro-ophthalmological function of patients with pineal region tumors approached transtentorially in the semisitting position. *J Neurosurg.* 1992;76(5):746–751.

52. Hart MG, Sarkies NJ, Santarius T, et al. Ophthalmological outcome after resection of tumors based on the pineal gland. *J Neurosurg.* 2013;119(2):420–426.

53. Fornari M, Savoiardo M, Morello G, et al. Meningiomas of the lateral ventricles: neuroradiological and surgical considerations in 18 cases. *J Neurosurg.* 1981;54(1):64–74.

54. Anderson RC, Ghatan S, Feldstein NA. Surgical approaches to tumors of the lateral ventricle. *Neurosurg Clin N Am.* 2003;14(4):509–525.

55. Kasowski H, Piepmeier JM. Transcallosal approach for tumors of the lateral and third ventricles. *Neurosurg Focus.* 2001;10(6).

56. Ellenbogen RG. Transcortical surgery for lateral ventricular tumors. *Neurosurg Focus.* 2001;10(6).

57. Geffen G, Walsh A, Simpson D, et al. Comparison of the effects of transcortical and transcallosal removal of intraventricular tumors. *Brain.* 1980;103(4):773–788.

58. Guanci MM. Ventriculitis of the central nervous system. *Crit Care Nurs Clin North Am.* 2013;25(3):399–406.

# 18 *Skull-Base Tumors*

MICHAEL E. IVAN, W. CALEB RUTLEDGE, VINCENT LEW, and MANISH K. AGHI

## Introduction

A variety of histological tumor types are present in the skull base. Primary tumors of this area may be derived from bone, paranasal sinuses, nasopharynx, dura, cranial nerves, pituitary gland, meninges, and brain. Mass effect causes the majority of symptoms, although aggressive tumors may manifest symptoms from local invasion. Selection of surgical approaches to the skull base is based on balancing risk reduction with maximizing extent of resection. Here we review the anatomy and spectrum of neoplastic entities found in the anterior and lateral skull base in adults and discuss the perioperative and postoperative management of these patients.

## Neuroanatomy and Procedure

### Key Concepts

- The most critical neurologic structures in the anterior skull base include the olfactory bulb and tracts, optic nerves, pituitary gland and stalk, and inferior frontal lobe.
- The most critical neurologic structures in the lateral skull base include the temporal lobe, trochlear, oculomotor, and abducens and facial nerves.

The base of the anterior cranial fossa is deeper medially than it is laterally and is formed by the orbital process of the frontal bone, ethmoid bone, and body and lesser wing of the sphenoid bone (Fig. 18.1). The superior surface of the sphenoid body articulates anteriorly with the cribriform plate of the ethmoid bone and contains a smooth central surface, the planum sphenoidale. Posteriorly within the sphenoid bone, the chiasmatic sulcus forms a slight depression and leads laterally to the optic canals. The tuberculum sellae, a bony elevation, is posterior to the chiasmatic sulcus, and the sella turcica is posterior to the tuberculum sellae and forms the posterior border of the anterior skull base. Key neural structures within the anterior skull base include the olfactory bulbs and tracts, inferior frontal lobe, optic nerves, and the pituitary gland and stalk. The middle fossa, or lateral skull base, is defined anteriorly by the lesser wings of the sphenoid bone and the anterior clinoid processes. The floor of the lateral skull base is formed by the body and greater wing of the sphenoid bone, as well as temporal and parietal bone. The middle fossa contains the temporal lobes and critical neurovascular structures. The lacrimal, frontal, trochlear, oculomotor, nasociliary, and abducent nerves all traverse the superior orbital fissure. The facial nerve travels through the temporal bone as well as the petrous portion of the carotid and must be carefully localized in a lateral skull-base approach.

## ANTERIOR AND LATERAL SKULL-BASE TUMOR PATHOLOGY

### Anterior skull base

Most of the malignant pathology located in the anterior skull base consists of rare tumors that present in an aggressive, invasive stage. The most common pathologies of the anterior skull base are pituitary adenomas, spontaneous cerebrospinal fluid (CSF) leaks, meningiomas, and craniopharyngiomas (Fig. 18.2).[1] These lesions are benign but often require surgical resection. Less common benign tumors in the anterior skull base include schwannomas and osteomas.[1] Meningiomas are the most common anterior skull-base tumors and are found at three specific locations of the anterior skull base, from anterior to posterior: olfactory groove, planum sphenoidale, and tuberculum sellae. Less common lesions of the anterior skull base include chordoma, Rathke's cleft cysts, and esthesioneuroblastoma. See Table 18.1 for examples of anterior skull-base pathology.

### Lateral skull base

Tumors of the middle cranial base are usually benign. Tumors in this location include pituitary adenomas, craniopharyngiomas, meningiomas, temporal bone tumors, trigeminal schwannomas, cholesteatomas, and chondrosarcomas. Meningiomas in the middle fossa can be classified by their origin as sphenoid wing (Fig. 18.3), cavernous sinus, clinoid, or middle fossa. Meningiomas of the cavernous sinus present a unique challenge because resection is likely to damage multiple cranial nerves, and therefore nonsurgical treatments are typically preferred. Trigeminal schwannomas are less common tumors and originate within the ganglion of the trigeminal nerve. About 50% of these tumors are limited to the middle fossa, whereas 30% extend into the posterior fossa and 20% are dumbbell-shaped and extend into both fossae.[2] Malignant tumors that involve the skull base are less common than their benign counterparts. Skull-base metastases usually arise from prostate, breast, lung, or head and neck primary tumors or from lymphoma. See Table 18.1 for examples of lateral skull-base pathology. The first sign of metastatic skull-base invasion is typically cranial neuropathy.

## SURGICAL APPROACHES

### Key Concepts

- Minimally invasive and open approaches are available to approach the anterior and lateral skull base surgically.
- Large reconstruction efforts are typically needed after skull-base surgery and are focused on prevention of CSF leakage.

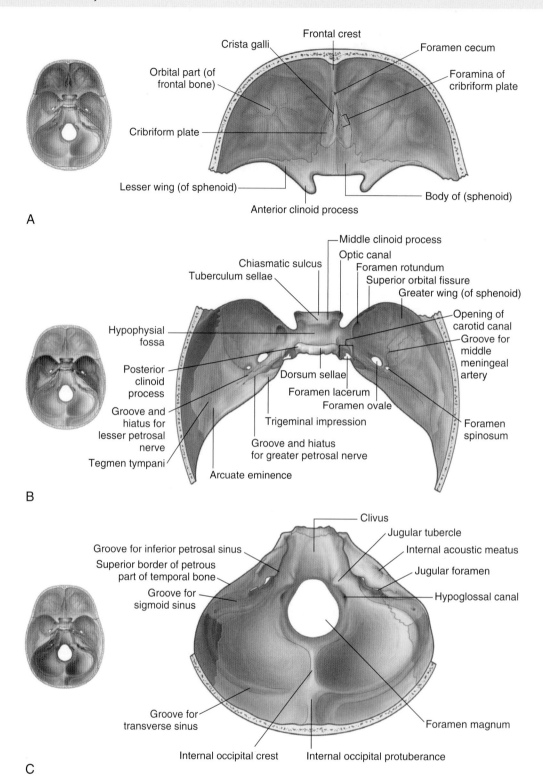

**Fig. 18.1** Floor of the cranial cavity, showing the cranial fossae. **(A)** Anterior cranial fossa. **(B)** Middle cranial fossa. **(C)** Posterior cranial fossa. (Reprinted from *Transport of the critical care patient*. Mosby/JEMS; 2011: pp. 169–223. Originally from Standring S. *Gray's Anatomy: The Anatomical Basis of Clinical Practice*, 40th ed. Philadelphia: Churchill Livingstone; 2008.)

Skull-base surgery requires using the most direct access with the least amount of risk and brain manipulation. Traditional open approaches to the anterior skull base include bifrontal craniotomies, extended bifrontal craniotomies, pterional craniotomies, and complex transfacial operations. These approaches require a large incision and significant brain exposure that places critical structures at risk and increases recovery time.[3] With the recent application of concepts from endonasal sinus surgery, neurosurgeons, working with otolaryngologists, can obtain access with a direct anatomical route to the lesion with a minimal opening that limits brain exposure and minimizes

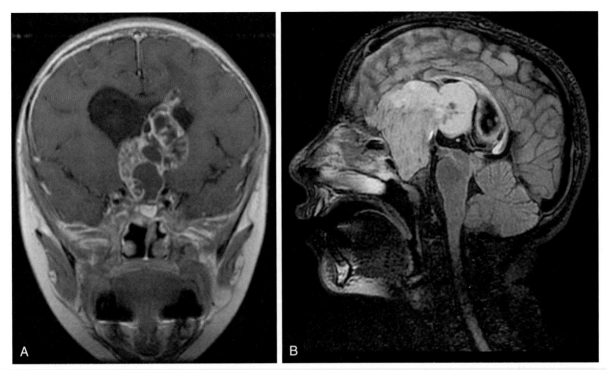

**Fig. 18.2** Coronal T1 + contrast MRI and sagittal T2 FLAIR MRI in an 11-year-old female with a large complex craniopharyngioma of the anterior skull base that extends superiorly into the third and lateral ventricles. This tumor required both transsphenoidal and transcranial approaches for resection.

**Table 18.1**   Anterior and Lateral Skull-Base Pathology

|  | **Anterior Skull Base** | **Lateral Skull Base** |
|---|---|---|
| Benign but aggressive | Meningiomas<br>▪ Olfactory groove<br>▪ Planum sphenoidale<br>▪ Tuberculum sellae<br>Pituitary adenoma<br>Suprasellar craniopharyngiomas<br>Infrasellar chordomas | Meningiomas<br>▪ Sphenoid wing<br>▪ Cavernous sinus<br>▪ Clinoid<br>▪ Middle fossa<br>Trigeminal schwannoma<br>Craniopharyngioma<br>Paraganglioma<br>Chordoma |
| Malignant | **Neuroendocrine sinonasal malignancies**<br>Esthesioneuroblastomas and nonesthesioneuroblastomas<br>▪ Neuroendocrine carcinomas<br>▪ Sinonasal undifferentiated carcinoma<br>▪ Small cell carcinomas<br><br>**Nonneuroendocrine sinonasopharyngeal tumors**<br>Adenoid cystic carcinoma<br>Squamous cell carcinoma<br>Adenocarcinoma<br>Nasopharyngeal carcinomas<br>Osteogenic sarcoma<br>Fibrous sarcoma<br>Melanoma metastases<br>Hemangiopericytoma<br>Rhabdomyosarcoma<br>Malignant salivary gland tumor<br><br>**Other malignancies**<br>Atypical/malignant meningioma<br>Pituitary carcinomas<br>Metastases | Hemangiopericytoma<br>Chondrosarcoma<br>Osteosarcoma<br>Plasmacytoma<br>Metastasis<br>Squamous cell carcinoma<br>Adenocarcinomas<br>Melanoma metastases |
| Nontumor | Vascular lesion (aneurysms, cavernous malformations)<br>Congenital lesions (Rathke's cleft cyst, meningoencephalocele)<br>Infectious lesions (abscess, fungal mass)<br>Inflammatory lesions (Langerhans cell histiocytosis). | Vascular lesion (aneurysms, cavernous malformations)<br>Infectious lesions (abscess, fungal mass) |

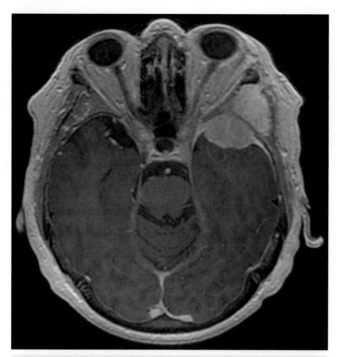

**Fig. 18.3** A 65-year-old male who presented with decreasing vision in his left eye. T1 postcontrast axial MRI scan showing an enhancing left sphenoid wing meningioma with extracranial extension. A left orbital-pterional craniotomy was performed for tumor resection.

iatrogenic trauma. Proponents argue that, in contrast to the various transcranial approaches, minimally invasive approaches avoid brain manipulation and retraction[4] and provide a better cosmetic result.[5] Typically, minimally invasive approaches forego skin incisions and use the natural apertures of the face to gain access. Many tumors require staged approaches, first transcranial and then transfacial. The selected approach is difficult to describe in an algorithmic manner, but instead reflects a combination of surgeon experience, tumor localization and pathology, and patient-specific considerations.

The approach to lateral skull-base lesions targets the floor of the middle fossa and the infratemporal fossa. For lesions lateral to the internal carotid artery (ICA), a pterional craniotomy with zygomatic osteotomy may be used. Lesions of the infratemporal fossa lying medial to the ICA are best exposed via mandibulotomy or via a minimally invasive endonasal approach through the maxillary sinus.

Typically any skull-base tumor surgery requires a complex reconstructive plan, including the possibility of free tissue flaps. Meticulous attention to closure of dura is needed to prevent CSF leak and subsequent infection.[6]

## SURGICAL TREATMENT

The decision regarding surgical intervention is made on a case-by-case basis and depends not only on extent of tumor growth and invasion but also on symptomatology, life expectancy, patient age, tumor type and grade, and involvement of surrounding critical anatomy. Surgical intervention may be performed to establish a diagnosis by biopsy or to achieve maximal safe resection. At a minimum, a tissue diagnosis is almost always necessary to guide

treatment and provide prognosis. Although tumor removal may lead to improvement in preoperative neurologic deficits, cranial neuropathies are frequently irreversible. Tumor locations such as the medial sphenoid wing, especially with cavernous sinus invasion, allow only subtotal resection because of the high risk of injury to adjacent structures such as the internal carotid artery and cranial nerves.

## Perioperative Considerations

### Key Concept

A team approach is necessary for skull-base surgery to assist with the major vascular structures, neurologic structures, reconstruction, pharyngeal components, and postoperative issues of tumor management.

The goal of surgical intervention is to maximize functional outcome while minimizing patient morbidity. Because these tumors expand over several vital systems, a team approach to treatment is often required. The following specialists are often involved in the treatment of skull-base lesions[7]:

- Anesthesia
- Oncology
- Radiation oncology
- Radiology
- Physical rehabilitation
- Neurology
- Neurophysiology
- Ophthalmology
- Oral/maxillofacial surgery
- Otolaryngology
- Plastic surgery
- Neurosurgery

### Key Concepts

- Preoperative imaging is required to allow a thorough understanding of involved bone, soft tissue, vasculature, and neurologic structures.
- Most anterior skull-base lesions involve the pituitary gland or stalk, and a full endocrine evaluation should be performed.
- A thorough neurologic evaluation of cranial nerves is needed preoperatively, with additional specialty tests if indicated.

Any patient with a skull-base lesion will need preoperative imaging consisting of magnetic resonance imaging (MRI) and computed tomography (CT) of the brain and skull base to provide a better understanding of the bony skull base and soft tissues. Special attention to the anatomy of the sinuses, especially with respect to septations, bony curvatures, hyperostosis, and prior surgical openings, is helpful in identifying midline structures during surgery. Careful attention to vascular and cranial nerves is required, and in some cases a dedicated CT angiogram or digital subtraction angiogram is useful when the petrous carotid artery is involved. For meningiomas and other vascular tumors, angiographic embolization of appropriate feeding vessels can reduce blood loss during tumor resection and facilitate tumor removal. In rare cases, a balloon test occlusion may be indicated if there is concern for large-vessel compromise due to tumor involvement and to inform the surgeon whether the patient might tolerate vessel sacrifice or if a bypass procedure is required.

Patients with anterior skull-base lesions often have concomitant endocrine disturbances. Those with pituitary lesions or craniopharyngiomas must be carefully evaluated for pituitary hypofunction and may need hormone replacement prior to surgery. Most critical is the need for "stress-dose" steroids in patients whose tumors have caused adrenal insufficiency from damage to the pituitary gland.

## Clinical Pearl

Thyroid and corticosteroid replacement must be performed for patients with pituitary hypofunction prior to surgery to prevent cardiopulmonary complications.

Preoperative testing should include evaluation of electrolytes and glucose. Finally, additional tests are used to formally evaluate cranial nerve function. Tests may include a formal ophthalmologic and visual field evaluation, audiography, or a swallow study.

## Key Concepts

- Preoperative antibiotics must cover skin and sinonasal flora for many skull-base procedures.
- Hemostasis is critical for skull-base procedures. Blood loss may be minimized by patient position and reducing positive end-expiratory pressure (PEEP).

Preoperative antibiotics are chosen to cover sinus bacteria and to prevent meningeal invasion. For transcranial approaches, antibiotics targeting skin flora (e.g., cefazolin) are sufficient unless the approach will open a corridor to the endonasal sinuses, in which case broader antibiotics (listed later) for the endonasal approaches should be used. Despite intracranial contamination with sinonasal flora during endoscopic endonasal skull-base surgery, the risk of central nervous system infection is low. However, in such cases, third or fourth generation cephalosporins is recommended. Vancomycin and aztreonam may be administered to beta-lactam–allergic patients.[8] If sinusitis is identified preoperatively, an intradural approach should not be undertaken until the infection has cleared.[9] If CSF is noticed during surgery and postoperative packing is used, postoperative antibiotics should be continued until the packing is removed.[8]

One challenging aspect of skull-base surgery is hemostasis.[10] All skull-base procedures are performed under general anesthesia to allow for strict control of blood pressure and intracranial pressure (ICP). Many structures of the skull base are highly vascularized, and therefore a low or normal systolic blood pressure is recommended. A preoperative

angiogram with embolization may improve hemostasis. Early ligation of the tumor's dural attachments and ethmoidal feeding arteries decreases heavy bleeding.[10]

## Clinical Pearl

For endonasal procedures, pretreatment with vasoconstricting agents to the mucosal layers can help in reducing bleeding in the corridors.

For endonasal procedures, monitoring blood pressure is imperative. Lowering venous pressure by elevating the head of the bed and reducing the PEEP may also improve hemostasis. Another recommendation is to use a diamond drill tip, which acts with more hemostatic effect when removing bone.[10] If major vascular injury does occur during surgery, packing or clipping is used to control bleeding while the patient is transferred to the neurovascular suite for angiogram and possible interventional repair.

## Clinical Pearl

If air embolism is suspected during surgery, first flood the surgical field and lower the head of the bed.

Massive bleeding may occur from injury to the cavernous sinus; this may lead to air embolism. Precautions against air embolism, including precordial Doppler and placement of a central line, are recommended for exposures expecting to cross the sagittal sinus. Finally, at the completion of the surgical case, the field should be inspected again for bleeding.

Anticonvulsants are typically not administered for extra-axial tumors because corticectomy is rarely needed. A lumbar drain is typically placed when brain relaxation is needed for transcranial approaches or when a CSF leak is planned or identified for endonasal approaches.

Motor and sensory evoked potentials are monitored if the lesion has a large intracranial component and/or significant vascular involvement/encasement. Cranial nerve monitoring is not performed on cranial nerves I and II. Cranial nerves III through XII may be monitored depending on the location of the lesion and the preoperative deficits.

After dural closure, a Valsalva maneuver is used to increase intrathoracic pressure to elicit a CSF leak if present.

## Postoperative Management

## Key Concepts

- Observe closely for neurologic deterioration; respond quickly to any neurologic event; respond quickly to any airway, breathing, or circulation dysfunction; and prevent further complications.
- Positive pressure devices are contraindicated after skull-base surgery.
- Fluid balance should be carefully monitored, especially in lesions that involve the pituitary axis where diabetes insipidus (DI) is likely.

Whether a patient needs postoperative intensive care unit (ICU)–level care requires consideration of the procedure performed, anesthetics, difficulty of airway, patient comorbidities, and training of staff with regard to the disease process. Nonfatal complications occur in 7% to 30% of supratentorial tumor resections and 8% to 18% of transsphenoidal resections.[11] Determination of the optimal postoperative environment is an important consideration to minimize complications. Patients with worse preoperative functional status have a higher risk of postoperative complications.[11] High-volume neurosurgery centers may have better outcomes in these complicated cases.[12]

After transcranial approaches, patients usually benefit from a brief ICU stay to monitor neurologic recovery and to assess for signs of intracranial hemorrhage or cerebral edema. After endonasal surgery, patients with intracranial extension of tumor may also benefit from a brief ICU stay, whereas patients with lesions that are entirely sinonasal do not require ICU-level monitoring unless there is concern, such as significant intraoperative blood loss. Strict blood pressure control and serial neurologic examinations should be performed.

## ABCs

Initial and continuous monitoring of airway, breathing, and circulation is of utmost importance after anterior and lateral skull-base surgery. Because the floor of the skull base is compromised either by tumor or by surgical approach, there is direct communication between the oral pharynx and the intracranial space. Therefore any positive pressure devices (e.g., continuous positive airway pressure [CPAP], bilevel positive airway pressure [BiPAP]) are contraindicated. This increased pressure could cause air to flow into the intracranial space and cause pneumocephalus or tension pneumocephalus. The "Mount Fuji" sign can be seen on CT scans showing air in the frontal lobes of the brain, resulting in a tented appearance (Fig. 18.4).[13] Treatment is removal of the offending positive pressure airflow, continuous 100% oxygen, and supine positioning of the patient. In cases of tension pneumocephalus, return to the operative room for urgent evacuation and repair of the intracranial communication are required. Pneumocephalus may result in delayed awakening from anesthesia after surgery, altered mental status, and occasionally headache. Pneumocephalus and tension pneumocephalus may also occur without positive pressure airflow, and therefore patients should be monitored carefully for symptoms. In cases of severe respiratory issues where positive pressure is necessary, a tracheostomy may be needed to bypass the oral pharynx.

Cardiopulmonary status and fluid balance should be monitored in all patients, but it is critical in lesions that involve the pituitary axis. Careful monitoring of intraoperative and postoperative fluid balance may identify development of DI postoperatively. After transsphenoidal surgery, DI occurs between 9% and 64% of cases.[14–16] Craniopharyngiomas and Rathke's cleft cysts, as well as intraoperative CSF leak, were associated with the highest incidence of postoperative DI in a series of 881 patients who underwent transsphenoidal microsurgery.[14] Indicators of DI include serum sodium >145 and urine excretion

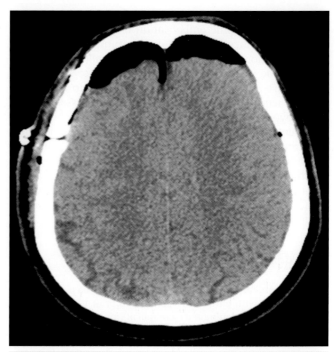

**Fig. 18.4** Mount Fuji sign/pneumocephalus. Noncontrast head CT showing bifrontal pneumocephalus after a right orbit-pterional craniotomy.

of 200 to 250 mL/h, with osmolality <200 mOsm/kg $H_2O$ or specific gravity <1.005. Patients in DI often require treatment with desmopressin.[17] Careful monitoring of the amount of fluid intake and output, recording of urine specific gravity every 4 to 6 hours, and frequent measurement of serum sodium is important postoperatively. If a patient is unable to drink or maintain a positive fluid balance, desmopressin given intravenously or subcutaneously at an initial dose of 1 to 2 mcg is recommended. Intranasal administration is not generally preferred early in the postoperative course due to altered absorption.

### Clinical Pearl

If a patient is awake, encouragement of fluid maintenance with oral intake is preferred over intravenous replacement during the management of DI.

Administration of desmopressin on an as-needed basis rather than scheduled is recommended due to the changing levels of antidiuretic hormone in the triphasic pattern if the posterior lobe of the pituitary is injured. Finally any patient with postoperative DI should be presumed to have anterior pituitary insufficiency as well. These patients should receive corticosteroid replacement therapy. In the immediate postoperative setting, hydrocortisone (25 to 50 mg intravenously every 8 hours) is generally used until anterior pituitary function can be definitively evaluated.

Early extubation of neurosurgical patients is preferred, unless there has been significant intraoperative bleeding, prolonged anesthesia, or if there are concerns regarding the airway and pulmonary function.

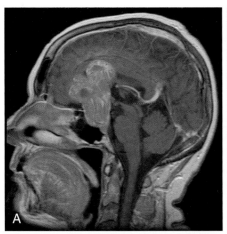
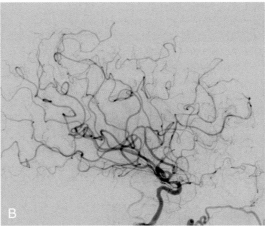
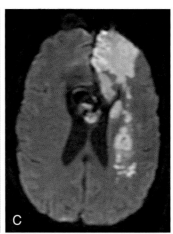

**Fig. 18.5** A 63-year-old female who presents with a large hemorrhagic pituitary adenoma who presented with headaches and weakness. (A) MRI T1 with contrast shows a large hemorrhagic sellar/suprasellar mass with extension into the third and lateral ventricles. Postoperatively the patient developed worsening mental status and weakness. (C) Axial MRI diffusion-weighted imaging showed left-sided infarcts in the anterior cerebral artery (ACA) and middle cerebral artery (MCA) territory. (B) Lateral angiogram demonstrated severe ACA vasospasm and mild MCA vasospasm.

## BLOOD PRESSURE CONTROL

Strict blood pressure control is warranted in all postoperative patients. Typically the blood pressure goal is for the patient to remain normotensive in the postoperative period. However, if a vascular bypass procedure has been performed, hypertension may be indicated to maintain adequate brain perfusion pressure.

Cerebral arterial vasospasm rarely occurs after skull-base surgery (Fig. 18.5). The development of vasospasm is associated with manipulation of skull vasculature and presence of subarachnoid blood. Quick diagnosis is important to prevent stroke and neurologic insult. Optimization of volume status should be ensured, and induced hypertension should be considered.

## NAUSEA/VOMITING AND DIET

Nausea and vomiting is a common postoperative symptom for the neurosurgical patient that occurs in 30% to 50% of patients.[11] After surgery via the endonasal approach, blood may enter the gastric system through the oral pharynx and cause irritation postoperatively. A nasogastric tube placed prior to the operation may assist in suctioning of blood at the conclusion of the case. However, insertion of gastric tubes after these approaches, either through the oral or nasal pharynx, is contraindicated unless the entire procedure can be performed under direct visualization or with the assistance of fluoroscopy due to concern for migration of the tube through the cranial floor defect.

### Clinical Pearl

Blind insertion of gastric tubes through the oral or nasal pharynx is contraindicated after skull-base surgery.

Nausea and vomiting may also result from postoperative hydrocephalus, intracranial hemorrhage, or metabolic issues, including hyponatremia, and should not be ignored.

After endonasal approaches, a diet may be resumed and advanced slowly several hours postoperatively once the patient has returned to his or her neurologic baseline. For larger anterior and lateral skull-base procedures, typically 24 hours of nothing per mouth is recommended to prevent aspiration. A swallow study should be performed if there is concern for aspiration.

## PAIN CONTROL

Narcotics in the postoperative patient must be used cautiously. Overuse can cause sedation or hypoventilation with an increased $PaCO_2$ and lead to increased ICP or aspiration. However, inadequate pain control may result in hypertension and tachycardia. Postoperative hypertension may cause bleeding into the resection cavity and should be avoided.

### Clinical Pearl

Benzodiazepines and other sedatives are typically avoided in the postoperative patient until they have returned to their neurologic baseline.

# Neurologic Complications

### Key Concepts

- Frequent neurologic examinations are required to identify and prevent permanent neurologic postoperative complications.
- Determination of the time of onset of any cranial nerve, focal neurologic, or global neurologic deficit will assist in determining the severity and urgency of the complication.
- A CSF leak should be diagnosed quickly and efficiently in order to prevent meningitis, pneumocephalus, and intracranial hypotension.

Skull-base surgery patients bring with them a unique set of risk factors that predispose them to complications that are best prevented by frequent and thorough neurologic examinations. Worsening neurologic status should be investigated quickly. Preoperative neurologic deficit will likely be present postoperatively, and therefore a thorough preoperative evaluation is critical. The timing, speed of onset, and severity of the neurologic deficit will all help with determining the cause. Evaluation should determine whether there is a cranial nerve deficit, focal neurologic deficit, or global neurologic deficit.

## CRANIAL NEUROLOGIC DEFICIT

Cranial nerve deficits may be expected after skull-base surgery; however, dissection around any of the intracranial or extracranial portions of a cranial nerve may result in unplanned cranial nerve deficit. The location of the tumor determines which cranial nerves are at risk. Anterior skull-base tumors most commonly affect cranial nerve I, and patients frequently suffer from anosmia. However, visual symptoms may also occur and warrant urgent evaluation. Cranial nerves II, IV, V1, and VI run through the cavernous sinus and may be transgressed during anterior and lateral approaches. Cranial nerve VII runs through the temporal bone and can be injured in temporal bone tumors or lateral approaches. Patients with facial nerve palsies and/or impaired corneal sensation because of injury of the first division of the trigeminal nerve require special eye protection and may require permanent tarsorrhaphy.

Loss of visual acuity or a new field cut postoperatively suggests a new mass lesion, such as a hematoma, ischemic event, or postoperative edema. Ophthalmoplegia may also be due to mass lesions or cavernous sinus thrombosis. A dilated and fixed pupil may indicate cerebral herniation. Worsening cranial nerve function may be devastating and irreversible if not addressed promptly. Emergent CT imaging and neurosurgical evaluation are required.

Cranial nerve deficits seen after skull-base surgery and the requisite neurologic examination to assess for them are described in Table 18.2.

## FOCAL NEUROLOGIC DEFICIT

New focal neurologic deficits in the postoperative period, such as numbness or weakness, are less common after skull-base surgery. Focal deficits signal ischemia, intracranial hemorrhage, vasospasm, or postoperative edema, and urgent neurosurgical evaluation and CT are warranted.

> **Clinical Pearl**
>
> For any worsening focal or cranial nerve postoperative deficit, emergent neurosurgical evaluation should be requested.

## GLOBAL NEUROLOGIC DEFICIT

Altered mental status or delayed emergence from anesthesia is common in neurosurgical patients. The differential is

**Table 18.2** A Skull-Base Cranial Nerve Neurologic Examination

| | Deficit | Examine |
|---|---|---|
| Olfactory nerve (I) | Anosmia | Smell |
| Optic nerve (II) | Optic atrophy<br>Papilledema<br>Loss of pupillary light reflex<br>Decreased visual acuity<br>Visual field deficit | Fundoscopy<br>Fundoscopy<br>Pupillary light reflex<br>Visual acuity<br>Visual fields |
| Oculomotor nerve (III) | Inhibition of medial and vertical gaze<br>Eye "down and out"<br>Drooping of the upper eyelid (ptosis)<br>Dilated pupil (mydriasis)<br>Absent pupillary light reflex<br>Absent accommodation reflex | Extraocular movements<br>Pupillary light reflex<br>Accommodation |
| Trochlear nerve (IV) | Eye "upward and inward" | Extraocular movements |
| Trigeminal nerve (V) | Weakness of masticator muscles<br>Loss of sensation in face<br>Loss of corneal reflex (bilateral forced eye closure in response to stimulation) | Contraction of masseter and temporal muscles<br>Facial sensation<br>Corneal reflex |
| Abducens nerve (VI) | Medial deviation of the eye | Extraocular movements<br>Vestibuloocular reflex (cold caloric test) |
| Facial nerve (VII) | Facial paralysis<br>Loss of taste | Facial symmetry<br>Taste in anterior two-thirds of tongue |
| Vestibulocochlear nerve (VIII) | Hearing loss<br>Imbalance | Hearing<br>Weber and Rinne test<br>Balance and gait<br>Vestibuloocular reflex (cold caloric test) |
| Glossopharyngeal nerve (IX) | Hoarseness<br>Dysphagia<br>Impaired gag reflex | Gag response<br>Palatal articulation<br>Guttural articulation |
| Vagus nerve (X) | Hoarseness<br>Dysphagia<br>Impaired gag reflex | Gag response<br>Palatal articulation<br>Guttural articulation |
| Accessory nerve (XI) | Weakness of sternocleidomastoid and trapezius muscles | Shrug shoulders<br>Turn head side to side |
| Hypoglossal nerve (XII) | Dysphagia and dysarthria<br>Deviation of tongue | Tongue protrusion test |

broad and includes seizure, hydrocephalus, cerebral edema, pneumocephalus, stroke, metabolic abnormalities (such as electrolyte disturbances), and intracranial hemorrhage, or sedation from narcotics. When a postoperative intracranial hemorrhage occurs, 50% of patients deteriorate within 6 hours.[11] Neurosurgical evaluation along with radiographic evaluation is typically indicated. Electroencephalogram, ICP measurements, and other laboratory studies may be required.

## CEREBROSPINAL FLUID LEAK

One of the greatest challenges of skull-base surgery is prevention of postoperative CSF leaks, pneumocephalus, and infection with tight dural closure. There are several types of closures available, but these are limited due to the availability of local vascularized flaps. Options for repair include microvascular free flaps, pericranial scalp flaps, synthetic dural substitute, suturable dural substitute, fat graft packing of the sphenoid sinus, and nasal packing with balloon catheters. In one large series of 800 cases using a variety of methods to close dura, the rate of postoperative CSF leak after endoscopic endonasal skull-base surgery was 16%. Others report postoperative CSF leaks in up to 30% to 58% of their patients. The advantage of large craniofacial open techniques is the use of vascular pedicle flaps and suturing techniques that provide a watertight seal and result in a low postoperative CSF leak rate of below 2%.[18] With minimally invasive approaches, the use of a nasoseptal flap (NSF) (Fig. 18.6) has been reported to significantly decrease postoperative CSF leak rates from 20% to less than 5% in multiple series,[19–21] results closer to those achieved with open approaches. The NSF is based on a large posterior pedicle, which includes the nasoseptal artery, a branch of the posterior septal artery.[20]

Certain patient populations may be at higher risk of development of postoperative CSF leak than others. Obese, middle-aged females with elevated CSF pressures after repair have an increased risk of postoperative CSF leak.[9] Patients who cough, gag, or retch during emergence from anesthesia and those with obstructive sleep apnea, morbid obesity, and excessive nose blowing may also be at increased risk of CSF leak.[9] Despite initial success, such patients remain at risk for recurrent CSF leaks months to years after repair. One helpful adjunct in patients who are at risk for CSF leak is to place a subarachnoid lumbar drain to allow CSF diversion, lower ICP, and improve healing of the nasal flap.[9] Usually the CSF removal is done at a rate of 10 to 15 mL every hour. Overdrainage should be avoided because it may create negative ICP (i.e., suction effect) that may result in headache, nausea/vomiting, and even coma from paradoxical, or low ICP, herniation. Pneumocephalus, tension pneumocephalus, remote hemorrhage, and meningitis are other potential complications from lumbar CSF drainage.[22]

Diagnosis of CSF leak in the postoperative patient can be challenging but important. The risk of meningitis is 20% to 30% in the presence of a CSF leak.[23] One should start by examining the patient for a CSF leak by asking him or her to lean forward for a period of time to elicit a leak.

### Clinical Pearl

A postoperative CSF leak may be confirmed with a beta-2 transferrin test.

In some cases, a leak will be noticed by large amount of clear or pink drainage from a surgical wound drain. Subsequently, identifying where the leak is coming from is needed to plan the repair. A thorough endoscopic examination of the nasal cavity may reveal the site of the leak. In addition, a high-resolution CT scan of the sinuses with contrast may prove useful.[22] If a sizeable defect is noted, a follow-up MRI may be indicated to investigate a possible meningocele or encephalocele. Finally, a last resort would include intrathecal injection of contrast materials and radioactive tracers to confirm a CSF leak and identify the site of origin.[22] Typically, a CSF leak from a defect in the primary closure should be repaired in the operating room.

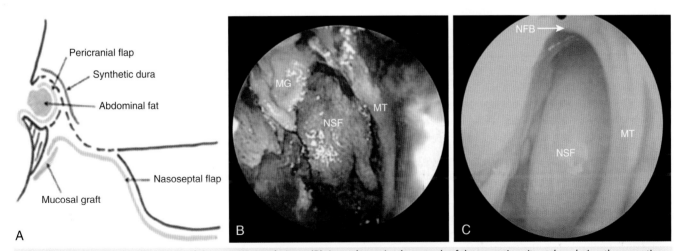

**Fig. 18.6 (A)** A schematic illustration of the operative technique. **(B)** An endoscopic photograph of the operation sites taken during the operation. **(C)** An endoscopic picture taken at postoperative 12 months. The nasoseptal flap is well adapted on the wound, and the mucosal graft has been reabsorbed. *MG*, mucosal graft; *NFB*, nasofrontal beak; *NSF*, nasoseptal flap; *MT*, middle turbinate. (Reprinted from Versatility of the pedicled nasoseptal flap in the complicated basal skull fractures. *Auris Nasus Larynx.* 2013 Jun;40(3):334–337. Fig. 2.)

## SEIZURES

Seizures are uncommon in skull-base tumors because many are extraaxial lesions. Seizure prophylaxis is recommended only for tumors that invade into brain parenchyma.

## CEREBRAL EDEMA

Postoperative cerebral edema or traction-related cerebritis usually does not produce focal signs but does delay recovery. Brain manipulation should be avoided to prevent edema. Restriction of fluids intraoperatively and postoperatively, as well as the use of hyperventilation, diuretics, and steroid therapy, are also indicated. A short course of steroids in the postoperative period may be useful to prevent cerebral edema.

# Nonneurologic Complications

## Key Concepts

- Most common medical complications are pneumonia, renal dysfunction, arrhythmia, deep vein thrombosis/pulmonary embolism (DVT/PE), and urinary tract infection (UTI) with bacteremia.
- The strongest predictor of a medical complication is a new or worsened neurological deficit postoperatively.

Despite the complexity, duration, and risk of neurologic injury in surgery for tumors of the skull base, the risk of major medical complications postoperatively is relatively low. In a large series of meningioma patients undergoing resection, only 7% experienced a serious medical complication.[24] The most common complications were pneumonia, renal dysfunction, arrhythmia, DVT/PE, and UTI with bacteremia, each occurring in only about 1% of patients. The strongest predictor of a medical complication was a new or worsened neurologic deficit postoperatively.[24] Patients with altered consciousness or cranial neuropathies are at increased risk of aspiration, whereas paretic patients are at increased risk of DVT and pneumonia.[25]

DVT prophylaxis should be initiated early. Risk factors for venous thromboembolism include advanced age, male gender, and nonambulatory status.[26] There is no evidence that early initiation of low-dose enoxaparin increases the risk of intracranial hemorrhage.[27]

## INFECTION

Anterior skull-base approaches include the nasal mucosa, and therefore monitoring for postoperative infection is important. Wound complications include the following: cellulitis, infected cranial bone flap, oronasal fistula, mucocele, and encephalocele. Because the nasal cavity may be included in the wound, chronic sinusitis from infection, loss of sinus mucociliary transport, and stenosis of the sinus ostia can occur. In addition, nasal airway stenosis may occur. Postoperative infections, including bacterial meningitis, have a low incidence of 1% to 2%.[8,9,19] This has been attributed to the use of perioperative antibiotics, frequent irrigation

**Table 18.3** Complications of Skull-Base Surgery

| | Neurologic | Nonneurologic |
|---|---|---|
| Transsphenoidal Surgery | Carotid injury<br>Stroke<br>Intracranial hemorrhage<br>Vasospasm<br>Bitemporal visual field loss<br>Vision loss<br>Meningitis<br>CSF leak (rhinorrhea)<br>Diabetes Insipidus | Pulmonary embolism<br>Panhypopituitarism<br>Hypothyroidism<br>Adrenal insufficiency<br>Renal dysfunction<br>Sinusitis<br>Arrhythmia<br>Urinary tract infection<br>Cerebral salt wasting |
| Transcranial Surgery | Intracranial hemorrhage<br>Stroke<br>Tension pneumocephalus<br>Cerebral edema<br>Seizure<br>Vasospasm<br>Epidural abscess<br>Vision loss<br>Hydrocephalus<br>Meningitis<br>Opthalmoplegia<br>CSF leak (rhinorrhea or otorrhea)<br>Diabetes insipidus<br>Pneumocephalus<br>Cerebral edema<br>Enophthalmos | Pulmonary embolism<br>Panhypopituitarism<br>Wound infection<br>Pulmonary infection<br>Renal dysfunction<br>Arrhythmia<br>Urinary tract infection<br>Deep venous thrombosis<br>Cerebral salt wasting<br>Mucocele<br>Chemosis<br>Periortibal edema |

*CSF,* cerebrospinal fluid.

intraoperatively, careful reconstruction with vascularized flaps, and absence of nonbiodegradable materials at the completion of surgery.[9] Risk factors for infection include male sex, complex tumors, presence of an external ventricular drain or shunt, and postoperative CSF leak.[8]

## ORBITAL EDEMA

With large anterior or lateral skull-base approaches, manipulation of the orbit and ocular contents may be necessary, leading to periorbital edema and chemosis, which can be minimized by raising the head of the bed to reduce swelling. In severe cases, especially when the eye cannot completely close, ophthalmology may be consulted to measure intraocular pressures.

Table 18.3 identifies the most common neurologic and nonneurologic complications of skull-base surgery in order of severity.

# Conclusion

Anterior and lateral skull-base surgery involves difficult anesthesia, often with complex tumor resections involving the head and neck and requiring an experienced multidisciplinary team, meticulous closure and reconstruction, and neurocritical care in the postoperative period. There is potential for devastating patient outcomes if complications occur. Although surgical resection remains the mainstay of treatment for these tumors, patients often require additional therapies. There are many reports of excellent outcomes after skull-base surgery that are the product of an experienced medical team exercising proper patient and case selection with a high level of perioperative neurocritical care.

## References

1. Schwartz TH, Fraser JF, Brown S, et al. Endoscopic cranial base surgery: classification of operative approaches. *Neurosurgery.* 2008;62 (5):991–1002. discussion 1005.
2. Wanibuchi M, Fukushima T, Zomordi AR, et al. Trigeminal schwannomas: skull base approaches and operative results in 105 patients. *Neurosurgery.* 2012;70(1 Suppl Operative):132–143. discussion 43–44.
3. Park HS, Park SK, Han YM. Microsurgical experience with supraorbital keyhole operations on anterior circulation aneurysms. *J Korean Neurosurg Soc.* 2009;46(2):103–108.
4. Ceylan S, Koc K, Anik I. Extended endoscopic transphenoidal approach for tuberculum sellae meningiomas. *Acta Neurochir (Wien).* 2011;153(1):1–9.
5. Wang Q, Lu XJ, Ji WY, et al. Visual outcome after extended endoscopic endonasal transphenoidal surgery for tuberculum sellae meningiomas. *World Neurosurg.* 2010;73(6):694–700.
6. Kryzanski JT, Annino Jr DJ, Heilman CB. Complication avoidance in the treatment of malignant tumors of the skull base. *Neurosurg Focus.* 2002;12(5).
7. Deschler DG, Gutin PH, Mamelak AN, et al. Complications of anterior skull base surgery. *Skull Base Surg.* 1996;6(2):113–118.
8. Kono Y, Prevedello DM, Snyderman CH, et al. One thousand endoscopic skull base surgical procedures demystifying the infection potential: incidence and description of postoperative meningitis and brain abscesses. *Infect Control Hosp Epidemiol.* 2011;32(1):77–83.
9. Snyderman CH, Kassam AB, Carrau R, et al. Endoscopic reconstruction of cranial base defects following endonasal skull base surgery. *Skull Base.* 2007;17(1):73–78.
10. Snyderman CH, Pant H, Carrau RL, et al. What are the limits of endoscopic sinus surgery?: the expanded endonasal approach to the skull base. *Keio J Med.* 2009;58(3):152–160.
11. Bhardwaj A, Mirski MAZ. *Handbook of Neurocritical Care.* 2nd ed. New York: Springer; 2011: xix, 554.
12. Barker 2nd FG, Klibanski A, Swearingen B. Transsphenoidal surgery for pituitary tumors in the United States, 1996-2000: mortality, morbidity, and the effects of hospital and surgeon volume. *J Clin Endocrin Metab.* 2003;88(10):4709–4719.
13. Sadeghian H. Mount Fuji sign in tension pneumocephalus. *Arch Neurol.* 2000;57(9):1366.
14. Nemergut EC, Zuo Z, Jane Jr JA, et al. Predictors of diabetes insipidus after transsphenoidal surgery: a review of 881 patients. *J Neurosurg.* 2005;103(3):448–454.
15. Schreckinger M, Walker B, Knepper J, et al. Post-operative diabetes insipidus after endoscopic transsphenoidal surgery. *Pituitary.* 2013;16(4):445–451.
16. Pratheesh R, Swallow DM, Rajaratnam S, et al. Incidence, predictors and early post-operative course of diabetes insipidus in paediatric craniopharygioma: a comparison with adults. *Childs Nerv Syst.* 2013;29(6):941–949.
17. Verbalis JG. Diabetes insipidus. *Rev Endocrin Metab Disord.* 2003; 4(2):177–185.
18. Zimmer LA, Theodosopoulos PV. Anterior skull base surgery: open versus endoscopic. *Curr Opin Otolaryngol Head Neck Surg.* 2009;17(2):75–78.
19. Kassam AB, Prevedello DM, Carrau RL, et al. Endoscopic endonasal skull base surgery: analysis of complications in the authors' initial 800 patients. *J Neurosurg.* 2011;114(6):1544–1568.
20. El-Sayed IH, Roediger FC, Goldberg AN, et al. Endoscopic reconstruction of skull base defects with the nasal septal flap. *Skull Base.* 2008;18(6):385–394.
21. Kassam AB, Thomas A, Carrau RL, et al. Endoscopic reconstruction of the cranial base using a pedicled nasoseptal flap. *Neurosurgery.* 2008;63(1 Suppl 1):ONS44–ONS52. discussion ONS–53.
22. Carrau RL, Snyderman CH, Kassam AB. The management of cerebrospinal fluid leaks in patients at risk for high-pressure hydrocephalus. *Laryngoscope.* 2005;115(2):205–212.
23. Solero CL, DiMeco F, Sampath P, et al. Combined anterior craniofacial resection for tumors involving the cribriform plate: early postoperative complications and technical considerations. *Neurosurgery.* 2000;47(6):1296–1304. discussion 304–305.
24. Sughrue ME, Rutkowski MJ, Shangari G, et al. Risk factors for the development of serious medical complications after resection of meningiomas. Clinical article. *J Neurosurg.* 2011;114(3):697–704.
25. Danish SF, Burnett MG, Ong JG, et al. Prophylaxis for deep venous thrombosis in craniotomy patients: a decision analysis. *Neurosurgery.* 2005;56(6):1286–1292. discussion 92–94.
26. Gerber DE, Segal JB, Salhotra A, et al. Venous thromboembolism occurs infrequently in meningioma patients receiving combined modality prophylaxis. *Cancer.* 2007;109(2):300–305.
27. Cage TA, Lamborn KR, Ware ML, et al. Adjuvant enoxaparin therapy may decrease the incidence of postoperative thrombotic events though does not increase the incidence of postoperative intracranial hemorrhage in patients with meningiomas. *J Neurooncol.* 2009;93(1):151–156.

# 19 *Cerebellopontine Angle Tumors*

GEOFFREY P. STRICSEK, JAMES J. EVANS, and CHRISTOPHER J. FARRELL

## Introduction

The cerebellopontine angle (CPA) is a wedge-shaped cisternal space within the posterior fossa bounded by the petrous temporal bone laterally, the cerebellum and brainstem medially, and the lower cranial nerves (CN IX, X, and XI) inferiorly. The CPA is the most common site of tumor formation within the posterior fossa and the location of approximately 5% to 10% of all intracranial tumors.[1] Acoustic neuromas arising from the vestibulocochlear nerve (CN VIII) account for nearly 80% of tumors within the CPA, although a variety of lesions may originate within this space, including meningiomas, epidermoid and dermoid cysts, and nonacoustic schwannomas. Additionally, adjacent tumors derived from the tentorium, foramen magnum, jugular foramen, and petroclival region may frequently extend into the CPA and cause compressive symptoms related to the cranial nerves and brainstem. Despite the relatively common occurrence of tumors within the CPA, surgical resection in this region remains a challenge for even the most experienced surgeons due to the critical neurovascular structures traversing the CPA and limited surgical access, with reported complication rates significantly higher than those for supratentorial surgery.[2]

From a historical perspective, the earliest attempts at surgery within the CPA were associated with astonishingly high rates of mortality, although these surgical pioneers were typically operating on extremely large tumors in patients with advanced neurologic symptoms. In 1917, Harvey Cushing described the "cerebellopontine angle syndrome" as the constellation of progressive neurologic findings associated with lesions of this region, consisting of ipsilateral hearing loss followed by onset of facial hypesthesia, hydrocephalus, and brainstem compression leading to death.[3] Sir Charles Ballance is frequently credited with the first successful resection of a CPA tumor, describing his surgical technique in which a "finger had to be insinuated between the pons and tumor to get it away."[4,5] Not surprisingly, reported mortality rates for surgery in the CPA reached as high as 84%.[6] Technical advances, including introduction of the operating microscope and neurophysiologic monitoring, along with the cooperative efforts of neurosurgeons and neurootologists to modify and refine the surgical approaches to the CPA, have made this complex area more accessible and dramatically improved outcomes. Despite these advances, however, the majority of complications experienced by patients with CPA tumors are related to the difficulties in surgically removing tumors from this region. In this chapter, we will describe the microsurgical anatomy of the CPA, along with the most common surgical procedures performed, followed by a discussion of the various complications that may be encountered as well as their surgical and neurocritical care management.

## Neuroanatomy and Procedure

### Key Concepts

- The CPA is the most common site of tumor location within the posterior fossa.
- The CPA is most commonly accessed surgically by the retrosigmoid, translabyrinthine, or middle fossa approaches. Extensions of these approaches may be necessary for tumors extending beyond the CPA to the petroclival, foramen magnum, or jugular foramen regions.
- Morbidity associated with the surgical removal of CPA tumors is most commonly due to vascular, cranial nerve, or brainstem injury.

A variety of skull-base approaches to the CPA have been described, with each approach affording relative advantages and limitations in terms of anatomic access and functional preservation. Choice of surgical approach is determined by the presumed pathology based on imaging characteristics, size of the lesion, extension into adjacent neuroanatomic regions, neurologic manifestations, and surgeon preference. The relevant surgical anatomy of the CPA is depicted in Fig. 19.1, revealing the course of the cranial nerves and vasculature through the cistern. Because acoustic neuromas account for the overwhelming majority of tumors located within the CPA, we will focus our discussion of surgical approaches on this tumor while describing the various modifications that may be utilized to reach lesions extending into adjacent areas such as the petroclival region and foramen magnum.

Acoustic neuromas arise from the vestibular component of CN VIII near the porus acoustic. The tumor may extend laterally within the internal auditory canal (IAC) toward the cochlea or medially within the CPA cistern, resulting in compressive symptoms. Patients with acoustic neuromas most frequently present with sensorineural hearing loss, tinnitus, and disequilibrium. Large tumors may cause additional cranial neuropathies, including trigeminal symptoms, dysphonia, and dysphagia, whereas cerebellar and brainstem compression may result in ataxia, weakness, and obstructive hydrocephalus (Fig. 19.2A). Despite the adjacent course of the facial nerve within the IAC, facial weakness is infrequently encountered with acoustic neuromas, and its presentation may suggest a nonacoustic lesion such as a facial nerve schwannoma or malignancy. The most common surgical approaches to the CPA used for

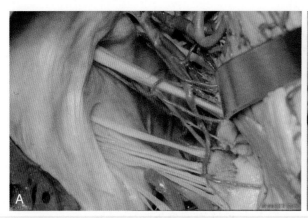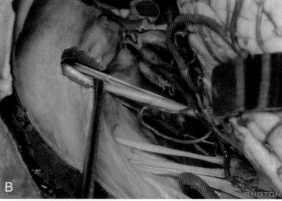

**Fig. 19.1** Anatomy of the cerebellopontine angle (CPA). **(A)** CPA as viewed posteriorly by the retrosigmoid approach demonstrating the relevant cranial nerve and vascular anatomy. **(B)** The vestibulocochlear nerve (CN VIII) has been retracted to expose the facial nerve (CN VII) entering the internal auditory canal, which has been partially drilled. (Images courtesy of Dr. Albert Rhoton – The Rhoton Collection.)

resection of acoustic neuromas are the retrosigmoid, translabyrinthine, and subtemporal middle fossa approaches. Extensions of these approaches involve additional bony removal of the petrous bone and occipital condyles and may be performed to provide improved access and minimize brain retraction.

The retrosigmoid approach (Fig. 19.2B) is an extremely common and versatile approach to the lateral posterior fossa and may be used for the microsurgical treatment of extraaxial neoplastic and vascular lesions of the CPA, including microvascular decompression of the trigeminal and facial nerves, as well as removal of intraaxial cerebellar lesions such as hemangioblastomas, gliomas, and metastases. This approach provides a nearly parallel trajectory to the CPA along the posterior petrous bone and lateral cerebellar surface. A suboccipital craniotomy or craniectomy is performed with skeletonization of the transverse and sigmoid sinuses in order to maximize lateral exposure and minimize cerebellar retraction. Direct injury to the venous sinuses at the time of bony removal or from overaggressive hemostasis may lead to partial or complete venous thrombosis, resulting in cerebellar edema as described later in this chapter. Additionally, failure to appropriately occlude any mastoid air cells exposed during the craniotomy may lead to postoperative cerebrospinal fluid (CSF) rhinorrhea or otorrhea. Upon opening of the dura, cerebellar relaxation is achieved either by CSF drainage using a lumbar drain or by fenestration of the cisterna magna arachnoid. Access to the CPA may require sacrifice of the petrosal vein, although careful attention to this maneuver is necessary to avoid inadvertent injury to the superior cerebellar artery (SCA) as it courses along the tentorium. In the setting of acoustic neuroma removal, the posterior tumor capsule is exposed (Fig. 19.2C) and an intracapsular debulking performed, followed by careful dissection of the capsule away from the facial, trigeminal, and lower cranial nerves using neurophysiologic adjuncts such as facial nerve electromyography (EMG) to assess the functional integrity of these structures during their dissection. The facial nerve is typically densely adherent to the tumor capsule, with the rates of facial nerve preservation directly correlated to tumor

size.[7] The lateral portion of the tumor is accessed by drilling the posterior aspect of the IAC. Potential complications associated with drilling of the IAC include inadvertent entry into the posterior semicircular canal, resulting in hearing loss, or failure to address air cells within the IAC, leading to CSF leakage. After resection of the tumor, the dura is closed in a watertight fashion using either a synthetic dural substitute or an autologous tissue such as pericranium or fascia. Reconstruction of the bony defect has been shown to reduce the incidence of headaches after the retrosigmoid approach and is typically performed unless the surgeon is concerned about the potential for postoperative cerebellar edema due to excessive retraction, incomplete tumor resection, or vascular injury.[8] An inferior extension of the suboccipital craniotomy termed the *far-lateral approach* provides improved access to the foramen magnum and ventral medulla and is most frequently performed for the management of foramen magnum meningiomas and distal posterior inferior cerebellar (PICA) or vertebral artery (VA) aneurysms. To avoid manipulation of the upper cervical spinal cord and lower brainstem, the occipital condyle can be partially or completely removed, with the extent of bony removal depending on the access needed. If more than half of the condyle is removed, craniocervical stabilization is necessary. Tumors of the foramen magnum often displace or encompass the vertebral artery, increasing the potential for vascular injury and the need for possible arterial sacrifice in order to achieve complete resection. Preoperative temporary balloon-occlusion testing is utilized to assess the ability of the collateral circulation to support VA sacrifice.

Otologists specializing in the surgical treatment of temporal bone disorders commonly perform the translabyrinthine approach (Fig. 19.2B), which involves sequential drilling of the mastoid and petrous portions of the temporal bone to access the posterior fossa and IAC. After mastoidectomy, the ossicles, semicircular canals, and facial canal are defined. In order to gain access to the IAC, the vestibule representing the junction of the lateral and posterior semicircular canals must be opened, resulting in sacrifice of any preexisting hearing. As such, the translabyrinthine approach is typically

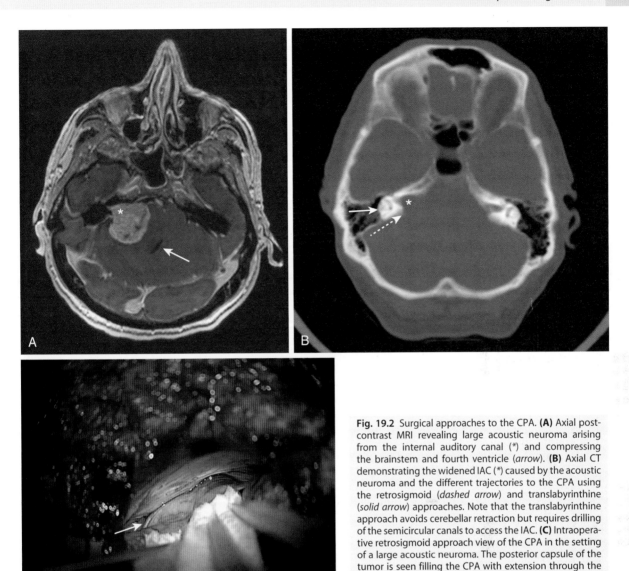

**Fig. 19.2** Surgical approaches to the CPA. **(A)** Axial post-contrast MRI revealing large acoustic neuroma arising from the internal auditory canal (*) and compressing the brainstem and fourth ventricle (*arrow*). **(B)** Axial CT demonstrating the widened IAC (*) caused by the acoustic neuroma and the different trajectories to the CPA using the retrosigmoid (*dashed arrow*) and translabyrinthine (*solid arrow*) approaches. Note that the translabyrinthine approach avoids cerebellar retraction but requires drilling of the semicircular canals to access the IAC. **(C)** Intraoperative retrosigmoid approach view of the CPA in the setting of a large acoustic neuroma. The posterior capsule of the tumor is seen filling the CPA with extension through the IAC (*) and displacement of the lower cranial nerves (*arrow*).

avoided in patients with acoustic neuromas and serviceable hearing, unless the tumor is large enough (>2 cm) that hearing preservation is unlikely to be achieved by any microsurgical approach.[9] Once the posterior fossa dura has been opened, tumor removal proceeds as described for the retrosigmoid approach. A watertight dural closure, however, is not possible via the translabyrinthine approach, and prevention of CSF leakage is reliant on abdominal fat graft packing, external pressure dressings, and often lumbar drainage. Modification of the translabyrinthine approach includes the transcochlear approach, which involves more anterior drilling of the cochlea and petrous bone to access the petroclival and prepontine regions. Access to the cochlea, however, often requires transposition of the facial nerve and sacrifice of the greater superficial petrosal nerve, which may result in facial paresis and decreased ipsilateral lacrimation, respectively.

The middle fossa approach is primarily used for resection of intracanalicular acoustic neuromas in patients with serviceable preoperative hearing, although the approach may be modified (anterior transpetrosal approach) to access the petrous apex, petrous carotid artery, and petroclival area. In the middle fossa approach, a subtemporal craniotomy is performed, followed by gentle retraction of the temporal lobe in an extradural fashion to expose the superior surface of the petrous bone. Temporal lobe retraction may lead to direct injury, resulting in aphasia (in the dominant hemisphere) or seizures, as well as traction injury to the vein of Labbé with subsequent venous infarction and temporal lobe edema. The location of the IAC is identified on the basis of anatomic landmarks and carefully unroofed, avoiding injury to the cochlea and petrous carotid artery. The anterior petrosal approach involves additional drilling of the petrous apex.[10]

# Perioperative Considerations

## Key Concepts

- Vascular complications in the form of hematoma and infarction are the most serious postoperative complications of CPA surgery.
- CPA hemorrhages typically occur in the immediate postoperative period and may result in rapid development of brainstem compression and obstructive hydrocephalus.
- Lateral sinus thrombosis may complicate CPA surgery and result in headaches, visual loss, seizures, and aphasia.
- Facial nerve paresis is the most common cranial nerve morbidity associated with CPA surgery, and appropriate eye care is necessary to prevent corneal injury and visual impairment.
- Lower cranial nerve dysfunction is common after CPA surgery and may cause swallowing problems and aspiration.

Considerable advances have been made over the last several decades in microsurgical technique, neuroanesthesia, and neurophysiologic monitoring that have reduced the overall mortality rates for CPA surgery to less than 1%.[11,12] Although surgery in this precarious region has certainly become increasingly safer, surgical morbidity (Table 19.1) remains commonplace, with overall complication rates typically ranging from 21% to 32% in the recent literature.[2,11] These rates may be even higher for tumors originating in adjacent areas such as petroclival and jugular foramen meningiomas extending into the CPA.[13,14] Vascular complications, primarily in the form of hemorrhage, represent the most common cause of postoperative mortality, with additional complications, including ischemic vascular events, cranial neuropathy, cerebellar edema, CSF leakage, and meningitis, all potentially having devastating consequences and requiring appropriate neurocritical care.

## Postoperative Complications

### VASCULAR COMPLICATIONS

Vascular complications in the form of hematoma or infarction are the most serious postoperative complication after CPA tumor resection and may result from direct arterial or venous injury or as a consequence of inadequate cavity hemostasis, presence of residual vascular neoplasm, or cerebellar retraction.[2] Within the confined posterior fossa, there is little compensatory area to tolerate space-occupying lesions and life-threatening brainstem compression, and obstructive hydrocephalus may develop rapidly.[15] The literature on the incidence, management, and outcomes for vascular complications of CPA surgery is sparse, but treatment recommendations are generally similar to those for other cerebellar disorders such as embolic stroke. Venous injury and lateral sinus thrombosis represent specific concerns with CPA surgery and will be more extensively discussed.

The highest rates of symptomatic postoperative hemorrhage have been reported to occur within the CPA cisternal space (Fig. 19.3) and are associated with mortality rates ranging between 25% and 100%.[12,16,17] Vigilant attention

**Table 19.1** Postoperative Complications of Cerebellopontine Angle Tumor Removal

| | |
|---|---|
| Vascular Complications | ▪ Postoperative hemorrhage typically occurs immediately after surgery.<br>▪ The AICA is the most commonly injured artery in CPA surgery.<br>▪ Lateral sinus thrombosis occurs in approximately 5% of patients after CPA tumor removal. |
| Cranial Nerve Complications | ▪ Facial nerve paresis is more common with larger tumors, and the severity of injury is measured using the House-Brackmann scale (Table 19.2).<br>▪ Lower cranial nerve injury may result in speech and swallowing dysfunction. |
| Cerebrospinal Fluid Complications | ▪ Obstructive hydrocephalus may result from tumor enlargement or cerebellar edema after surgical resection. Overaggressive CSF drainage may lead to upward transtentorial herniation.<br>▪ Postoperative CSF leakage after CPA surgery is common and may lead to meningitis. |

*AICA,* anterior inferior cerebellar artery; *CPA,* cerebellopontine angle; *CSF,* cerebrospinal fluid.

to intraoperative surgical hemostasis and postoperative blood pressure control are imperative to prevent these avoidable complications. Although hemorrhage from the anterior inferior cerebellar artery (AICA) has been shown to be the most frequent cause of mortality after acoustic neuroma surgery, the exact source of postoperative CPA hematoma is rarely conclusively identified during surgical reexploration.[11] These hemorrhages tend to occur within

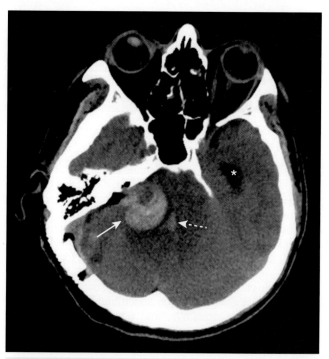

**Fig. 19.3** Postoperative hemorrhage after resection of an acoustic neuroma. Axial noncontrast CT revealing hemorrhage (*solid arrow*) within the resection cavity of a large acoustic neuroma with associated brainstem compression. There is hemorrhage within the fourth ventricle (*dashed arrow*) and associated hydrocephalus with enlargement of the temporal horn of the lateral ventricle (*).

the immediate postoperative period and present with progressive signs of headache, vomiting, cranial nerve deficits, and altered mental status.[16] With the increasing application of stereotactic radiosurgery for the treatment of small- and medium-sized tumors of the CPA, a general trend toward resection of larger tumors has emerged, as has a tendency to perform subtotal tumor resection to minimize cranial nerve complications. These trends, however, are likely to increase the risk of surgical hemorrhagic complications due to the presence of residual vascular neoplasm or vessels adherent to the wall of the tumor that are not completely visualized. Epidural, brainstem, and cerebellar hemorrhages may also occur postoperatively, with the latter usually resulting from venous congestion and retraction injury. Cerebellar edema and hemorrhage tend to develop in a more delayed and insidious pattern and may be more responsive to surgical and medical management.

Arterial ischemic complications are fortunately rarely encountered after CPA surgery, accounting for only 13% of reported postoperative vascular events.[11] This is likely a reflection of the preserved arachnoid plane separating arterial structures from the tumor capsule of acoustic neuromas, enabling meticulous microsurgical dissection in most instances. Conversely, meningiomas may invade the arterial adventitia, resulting in dissection injury and necessitating subsequent arterial sacrifice.[18] Although the AICA is the vessel most at risk during CPA surgery due to its location within the cistern, the PICA, SCA, and vertebrobasilar system may also be inadvertently injured. As discussed earlier, meningiomas originating from the foramen magnum and extending into the CPA often compress or completely encompass the vertebral artery. In these instances, preoperative temporary balloon test occlusion (TBO) should be performed to identify patients at risk for ischemic complication after parent artery occlusion. Unfortunately, the accuracy of TBO has imperfect predictive value, and hypoperfusion complications have been observed in 2% to 16% of patients who successfully passed TBO.[19,20] In the event of a failed TBO, subtotal resection or cerebral revascularization may be necessary.

The neurocritical care management of hematomas or cerebellar edema after CPA surgery, as with other space-occupying lesions of the posterior fossa, is directed at relieving mass effect upon the brainstem and treatment of associated hydrocephalus. Upward transtentorial herniation and downward herniation of the cerebellar tonsils through the foramen magnum are the most common causes of death in the acute setting, resulting from elevated posterior fossa intracranial pressure (ICP).[15,21] The most reliable sign of life-threatening mass effect is decreased level of consciousness.[22,23] New cranial nerve deficits may result from ischemic brainstem injury or direct compression by hematoma formation. In addition, pontine compression may lead to ophthalmoparesis, pupillary miosis, breathing irregularities, and cardiac dysrhythmias.[22] Initial management should focus on airway protection, adequate oxygenation, and diagnosis of the underlying cause of clinical deterioration by computed tomography (CT) imaging. For patients with hemorrhage or edema without significant mass effect or who are unable to undergo surgical decompression, initial conservative management may be appropriate, including intensive care unit (ICU) monitoring, blood pressure control, and escalation of ICP control measures as necessary. The utility of osmotic therapies, hyperventilation, and induced coma have not been well validated for the treatment of posterior fossa edema but are likely to be less effective than when employed to treat supratentorial swelling due to the reduced volume of cerebellar tissue. In patients with clinical deterioration and imaging evidence of mass effect upon the brainstem or fourth ventricle with obstructive hydrocephalus, emergent surgical decompression with placement of an external ventricular drain (EVD) should be performed. The existing bone flap or titanium mesh is removed, and the craniectomy extended across the foramen magnum and toward the midline occiput to provide bony decompression, along with evacuation of the hematoma and establishment of meticulous hemostasis. If concern for persistent cerebellar edema exists, removal of necrotic cerebellum and/or the lateral aspect of the cerebellum may be necessary. Ventriculostomy is most commonly performed by insertion of an EVD into the lateral ventricle in either the frontal or occipital horns. Although an occipital horn EVD may be placed using the same surgical position and exposure as the suboccipital decompression, accurate placement in the absence of image guidance is somewhat more difficult than for the frontal horn location. Overzealous supratentorial CSF drainage via the EVD prior to suboccipital decompression should be avoided because this may aggravate the potential for upward herniation, resulting in iatrogenic injury to the midbrain and diencephalon.[24]

## Clinical Pearl

Although CSF drainage via an EVD may be lifesaving in the setting of fourth ventricular compression and obstructive hydrocephalus, overdrainage may result in upward herniation unless the suboccipital area has been adequately decompressed.

Lateral (transverse) sinus thrombosis and cerebellar venous complications may also occur with CPA surgery and require neurocritical care intervention. Both the translabyrinthine and retrosigmoid approaches to the CPA, as well as their extensions, require some degree of exposure of the sigmoid and transverse sinuses. Although the true incidence of lateral sinus thrombosis after CPA surgery is uncertain because isolated thrombosis appears to be well compensated in the majority of patients, Keiper et al. identified sinus thrombosis in approximately 5% of patients after these procedures.[25] Thrombosis may occur as the result of prolonged retraction, inadvertent venous sinus entry during the craniotomy, and overexposure of the sinuses, leading to their drying and shrinkage during the course of prolonged surgical procedures under the heat of the operative microscope.[16,25] Development of symptoms depends primarily on the venous anatomy and the extent of the thrombosis. In the setting of an atretic or hypoplastic transverse sinus, compromise of the dominant sinus may lead to venous outflow obstruction with elevated ICP, visual loss secondary to papilledema, and possibly venous infarction and hemorrhages. Injury to a hypoplastic or codominant transverse sinus is frequently asymptomatic, although extension of the thrombosis to the vein of Labbé or torcula may cause temporal lobe edema, seizures, or other severe consequences.

The most common presentation of symptomatic lateral sinus thrombosis is headache and visual obscuration.[26] Focal neurologic deficits related to temporal or occipital lobe edema, including seizures, aphasia, and hemianopsia, have been reported in 31% of patients.[26] Hemorrhagic complications occur in nearly 50% of patients with venous infarction after sinus thrombosis, with temporal lobe involvement the most common site of bleeding with CPA-related sinus occlusion.[16,27] New-onset cranial neuropathy has also been reported, including a case of Collet-Sicard syndrome with CN IX–XII dysfunction related to thrombosis of the jugular bulb.[28] Early diagnosis of lateral sinus thrombosis prior to onset of complications requires a high degree of clinical suspicion, and confirmation is usually obtained by neuroimaging. Importantly, initial noncontrast CT scanning failed to show any abnormalities in 40% of patients with symptomatic sinus thrombosis, with the remainder of studies demonstrating hyperdensity within the venous sinuses and/or hemorrhagic or nonhemorrhagic parenchymal lesions, primarily within the temporal lobe.[26] Magnetic resonance (MR) (Fig. 19.4) or CT venography should be pursued if lateral sinus thrombosis is suspected, with these studies documenting the presence and extent of thrombosis, as well as the anatomy of the functioning venous collaterals. Treatment of isolated lateral venous thrombosis should be initiated cautiously and individualized based on clinical severity and extent of thrombosis. Although poor levels of evidence exist to guide optimal management of venous sinus thrombosis, including lateral sinus thrombosis, current guidelines recommend initiation of anticoagulation with heparin in the absence of contraindications for anticoagulation in order to arrest the thrombotic process, restore venous patency, and decrease the likelihood of venous infarction and embolism.[28] Unfortunately, the majority of lateral sinus thromboses present within several weeks of initial intracranial surgery, increasing the risks associated with anticoagulation. If thrombosis is confined to the sigmoid sinus or asymptomatic, some authors advocate withholding anticoagulation to avoid the associated risks and following the extent of thrombosis carefully with serial imaging studies to assess for progression.[29]

### Clinical Pearl

The presence of cortical neurologic dysfunction after CPA surgery, including seizures, aphasia, or visual changes, should prompt investigation for lateral sinus thrombosis.

## CRANIAL NERVE MORBIDITY

Cranial nerves III–XII may be at risk for injury during the surgical treatment of CPA tumors, with the likelihood of injury heavily influenced by the tumor pathology, size, consistency, and location.

### Facial Nerve Morbidity

The most common complication after acoustic neuroma resection is facial nerve paresis. This nerve is densely adherent to the tumor capsule, requiring careful and skillful manipulation to achieve complete tumor resection. As tumor size increases, the facial nerve becomes increasingly thinned and susceptible to injury. Facial nerve outcomes are reported using the House-Brackmann grading scale (Table 19.2), with the rate of clinically significant permanent facial nerve injury (HB ≥3) ranging from 3% for small tumors <1.5 cm to 45% for large tumors >3 cm.[7,30] Facial

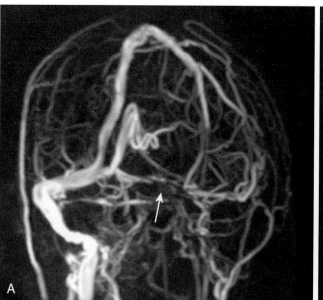
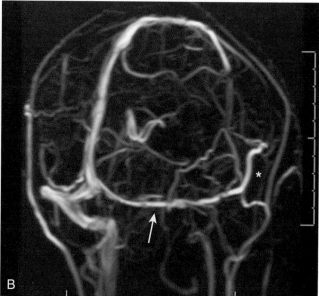

**Fig. 19.4** Lateral sinus thrombosis after removal of an acoustic neuroma. **(A)** MR venogram performed in a patient who presented with a seizure one week after acoustic neuroma removal, demonstrating sinus thrombosis with absent filling of the transverse (*solid arrow*) and sigmoid venous sinuses. **(B)** Follow-up MR venogram performed six weeks after institution of anticoagulation therapy revealing partial filling of the transverse (*solid arrow*) and sigmoid venous sinuses and reconstitution of the vein of Labbé (*).

**Table 19.2**  House-Brackmann Facial Nerve Palsy Score

| Grade | Definition |
|---|---|
| I | Normal symmetric function |
| II | Gross: Slight weakness identified on close inspection<br>At rest: Normal symmetry and tone<br>Motion: Complete eye closure with minimal effort; mouth: slight asymmetry; forehead: moderate to good function |
| III | Gross: Obvious weakness, but not disfiguring<br>At rest: Normal symmetry and tone<br>Motion: Forehead: slight to moderate movement; eye: complete closure with effort; mouth: slightly weak with maximal effort |
| IV | Gross: Obvious weakness and/or disfiguring asymmetry<br>At rest: Normal symmetry and tone<br>Motion: Forehead: none; eye: incomplete closure; mouth: asymmetric with maximum effort |
| V | Gross: Barely perceptible motion<br>Asymmetry at rest |
| VI | Complete absence of movement |

nerve monitoring is routinely used during acoustic neuroma surgery and microsurgical resection of other CPA lesions to help identify the location of the facial nerve and assess nerve function during dissection. Most facial nerve monitoring systems are EMG based, and lower facial nerve distal and proximal stimulation thresholds are correlated with improved postoperative CN VII outcomes.[31] In addition to cosmetic disfigurement, facial nerve weakness may lead to swallowing dysfunction and corneal injury related to exposure keratopathy. Appropriate and vigilant eye care is required in the ICU for patients with incomplete eye closure. Failure to provide this care may result in corneal ulceration, infectious keratitis, and visual loss. Corneal damage typically presents as eye pain in the awake patient with infection manifesting as conjunctival swelling and discharge or crusting of the lid margins.[32] The most effective means to prevent corneal damage remains somewhat controversial. Options including adherence to a strict eye care algorithm consisting of natural tear administration during the day and application of an ophthalmic lubricant such as Lacrilube (artificial tear ointment, Allergan, Inc., Irvine, CA) at night, along with taping of the eye closed. Alternatively, occlusive moisture chambers may be applied, which provide a means of corneal protection even when the eye is open. Several prospective studies comparing the rates of exposure keratopathy in the ICU setting demonstrate a decreased incidence using moisture chambers compared with lubricating ointments.[33,34] Although trigeminal neuropathy after acoustic surgery is generally well tolerated, a particularly dangerous condition exists when there is synchronous facial nerve palsy and CN $V_1$ deficit with diminished corneal sensation. Due to the extremely high risk for corneal injury in this setting, early tarsorrhaphy is frequently performed and maintained until there is sufficient cranial nerve recovery.

### Lower Cranial Nerve Morbidity

In a 2012 survey conducted by the Acoustic Neuroma Association of patients who had undergone surgical resection of an acoustic neuroma, 31% self-reported postoperative swallowing problems. In a retrospective review of patients who had undergone surgery for a CPA lesion at Johns Hopkins University, Starmer et al. revealed an identical rate of immediate postoperative dysphagia.[35] The majority of patients had oral stage deficits due to facial nerve weakness; however, pharyngeal swallowing deficits were noted in 49% of dysphagic patients, indicating some degree of lower cranial nerve dysfunction. In this study, 65% of patients with swallowing problems were managed with diet alterations, but 9% required feeding tube placement for safe nutrition. Lower cranial nerve injury after CPA surgery is directly related to tumor size and origin. Lower cranial nerve palsy may be observed preoperatively in patients with large acoustic neuromas as the tumor extends inferiorly within the CPA, causing a compressive neuropathy. Similarly, these nerves are at increased risk for injury at the time of surgery in the setting of large tumors due to the need for more extensive manipulation. Although glossopharyngeal palsy may cause diminished pharyngeal sensation, unilateral injury is unlikely to result in significant swallowing dysfunction. Conversely, patients with concurrent unilateral glossopharyngeal and vagal palsies are at high risk for aspiration with severe voice and swallowing dysfunction. Best et al. reported an overall 10% rate of postoperative vagal palsy after CPA surgery, with clinically significant rates of aspiration occurring in 67% of patients.[36] The risk for lower cranial nerve palsy is even greater in patients with tumors originating from the jugular foramen such as meningiomas and glomus jugulare paragangliomas.[14,37] Screening for swallowing dysfunction is extremely important after CPA surgery to prevent complications and assess aspiration risk. Videofluoroscopic swallowing assessment or direct laryngoscopy may be necessary for swallowing evaluation in the setting of suspected vagal palsy. If incomplete glottic closure is identified, most patients will benefit from temporary vocal cord medialization by injection of Gelfoam (Pharmacia Upjohn, Kalamazoo, MI), Teflon (DuPont, USA), or collagen with regard to their airway protection and dysphonia.[38] If persistent aspiration occurs, tracheotomy and gastrostomy should be pursued as early as possible.[37]

## CEREBROSPINAL FLUID LEAKAGE

CSF leakage is one of the most frequent complications of CPA surgery, with reported rates ranging from 2% to 31%.[17,39–41] The most serious sequelae of postoperative CSF leakage is development of meningitis, with Selesnick et al. demonstrating that the presence of CSF leakage increased the incidence of meningitis from 3% to 14%.[40] Leaks may present as either direct CSF drainage from the surgical wound or as rhinorrhea/otorrhea depending upon whether the tympanic membrane is incompetent, and occur as the result of nonwatertight dural closure, failure to obliterate air cell tracts within the temporal bone, or increased ICP. Appropriate management of CSF leaks should be initiated in a timely fashion to prevent meningitis because delays in treatment may be associated with mortality rates ranging from 5% to 41%.[42–44] The presence of altered mental status, decreased CSF glucose concentration, and gram-negative etiology are associated with more severe infection and increased morbidity and mortality.

Approximately 90% of CSF leaks occurring at the surgical wound site can be managed conservatively with oversewing of the incision, acetazolamide therapy, or lumbar drainage. Conversely, Mangus et al. found that 41% of patients with CSF rhinorrhea failed initial conservative management and ultimately required surgical intervention in the form of direct dural repair, mastoid and Eustachian tube obliteration, or CSF shunting.[39] CSF diversion using lumbar drain catheters is a commonly practiced neurosurgical intervention for both the treatment of postoperative CSF leaks and their prevention. Although complications of lumbar drainage are fortunately rare, iatrogenic intracranial hypotension may occur, with symptoms ranging from mild positional headaches to obtundation and coma. Imaging studies typically display evidence of downward displacement of the brainstem and cerebellum, tonsillar herniation, and engorged venous sinuses. The presence of bilateral subdural hygromas may also suggest intracranial hypotension, as well as diffuse meningeal enhancement, although this finding is of diminished diagnostic utility in the postoperative setting. In a review of the literature, Loya et al. noted the presence of cranial nerve palsies in 34% of reported cases of severe intracranial hypotension, with bilateral pupillary dilation and CN VI palsies potentially resulting from traction injury rather than brainstem compression.[45] The most challenging aspect of intracranial hypotension management is its timely recognition. Once the diagnosis of downward herniation has been made, treatment options should include cessation of lumbar drainage and transitioning the patient to the flat or Trendelenburg position until neurologic improvement is observed. Additionally, the patient should be adequately intravascularly rehydrated. Several reports have also noted rapid improvement in mental status after intrathecal saline administration through the lumbar drain.[46,47] Failure to recognize this condition and initiate treatment may lead to excessive posterior fossa crowding with brainstem compression and ischemia.

### Clinical Pearl

Prompt recognition and treatment of intracranial hypotension is associated with improved cranial nerve recovery.

## Summary

In summary, the cerebellopontine area is a frequent site of intracranial tumor formation. The difficulty in adequately accessing this region and the multitude of critical neurovascular structures within its confines create a significant challenge for the multidisciplinary team of neurosurgeons, otologists, and neurointensivists caring for patients with these tumors. A thorough understanding of the anatomy of the CPA, as well as the various surgical approaches used to remove tumors from this region, is critical to anticipate and recognize the complications that may ensue and respond appropriately to increase the likelihood of favorable outcomes.

## References

1. Patel N, Wilkinson J, Gianaris N, Cohen-Gadol AA. Diagnostic and surgical challenges in resection of cerebellar angle tumors and acoustic neuromas. *Surg Neurol Int.* 2012;3(17).
2. Dubey A, Sung WS, Shaya M, et al. Complications of posterior cranial fossa surgery - an institutional experience of 500 patients. *Surg Neurol.* 2009;72(4):369–375.
3. Cushing H. *Tumors of the nervus acusticus and the syndrome of the cerebellopontine angle (Reprint of the 1917 edition).* New York: Hafner; 1963.
4. Ballance CA. *Some points in the surgery of the brain and its membranes.* London: MacMillan and Co.; 1907.
5. Bambakadis NC, Megerian CA, Spetzler RF. *Surgery of the cerebellopontine angle.* Shelton, CT: People's Medical Publishing House; 2009.
6. Krause F. Zur Freilegung der hinteren Felsenbeinflache und des Kleinhirns. *Beitr Klin Chir.* 1903;37:728–764.
7. Ansari SF, Terry C, Cohen-Gadol AA. Surgery for vestibular schwannomas: a systematic review of complications by approach. *Neurosurg Focus.* 2012;33(3):E14.
8. Schessel DA, Nedzelski JM, Rowed D, Feghali JG. Pain after surgery for acoustic neuroma. *Otolaryngol Head Neck Surg.* 1992;107(3): 424–429.
9. Jian BJ, Sughrue ME, Kaur R, et al. Implications of cystic features in vestibular schwannomas of patients undergoing microsurgical resection. *Neurosurgery.* 2011;68(4):874–880.
10. Day JD, Fukushima T, Giannotta SL. Microanatomical study of the extradural middle fossa approach to the petroclival and posterior cavernous sinus region: description of the rhomboid construct. *Neurosurgery.* 1994;34(6):1009–1016.
11. Sughrue ME, Yang I, Aranda D, et al. Beyond audiofacial morbidity after vestibular schwannoma surgery. *J Neurosurg.* 2011;114(2): 367–374.
12. Mahboubi H, Ahmed OH, Yau AY, Ahmed YC, Djalilian HR. Complications of surgery for sporadic vestibular schwannoma. *Otolaryngol Head Neck Surg.* 2014;150(2):275–281.
13. Little KM, Friedman AH, Sampson JH, Wanibuchi M, Fukushima T. Surgical management of petroclival meningiomas: defining resection goals based on risk of neurological morbidity and tumor recurrence rates in 137 patients. *Neurosurgery.* 2005;56(3):546–559.
14. Bakar B. Jugular foramen meningiomas: review of the major surgical series. *Neurol Med Chir (Toyko).* 2010;50(2):89–96.
15. Neugebaur H, Witsch J, Zweckberger K, Jüttler E. Space-occupying cerebellar infarction: complications, treatment, and outcome. *Neurosurg Focus.* 2013;34(5).
16. Sade B, Mohr G, Dufour JJ. Vascular complications of vestibular schwannoma surgery: a comparison of the suboccipital retrosigmoid and translabyrinthine approaches. *J Neurosurg.* 2006;105(2): 200–204.
17. Sanna M, Taibah A, Russo A, Falcioni M, Agarwal M. Perioperative complications in acoustic neuroma (vestibular schwannoma) surgery. *Otol Neurotol.* 2004;25(3):379–386.
18. Kotapka MJ, Kalia KK, Martinez AJ, Sekhar LN. Infiltration of the carotid artery by cavernous sinus meningioma. *J Neurosurg.* 1994;81(2):252–255.
19. Graves VB, Perl 2nd J, Strother CM, Wallace RC, Kesava PP, Masaryk TJ. Endovascular occlusoin of the carotid or vertebral artery with temporary proximal flow arrest and microcoils: clinical results. *Am J Neuroradiol.* 1997;18(7):1201–1206.
20. Eskridge JM. The challenge of carotid occlusion. *Am J Neuroradiol.* 1991 Nov–Dec;12(6):1053–1054.
21. Heros RC. Surgical treatment of cerebellar infarction. *Stroke.* 1992;23(7):937–938.
22. Wijdicks EF, Sheth KN, Carter BS, et al. Recommendations for the management of cerebral and cerebellar infarction with swelling: a statement for healthcare professionals from the American Heart Association/American Stroke Association. *Stroke.* 2014;45 (4):1222–1238.
23. Hornig CR, Rust DS, Busse O, Jauss M, Laun A. Space-occupying cerebellar infarction. Clinical course and prognosis. *Stroke.* 1994;25 (2):372–374.
24. Yadav G, Sisodia R, Khuba S, Mishra L. Anesthetic management of a case of transtentorial upward herniation: an uncommon emergency situation. *J Anaesthesiol Clin Pharmacol.* 2012;28 (3):413–415.

25. Keiper Jr GL, Sherman JD, Tomsick TA, Tew Jr JM. Dural sinus thrombosis and pseudotumor cerebri: unexpected complications of suboccipital craniotomy and translabyrinthine craniectomy. *J Neurosurg.* 1999;91(2):192–197.

26. Damak M, Crassard I, Wolff V, Bousser MG. Isolated lateral sinus thrombosis: a series of 62 patients. *Stroke.* 2009;40(2):476–481.

27. Inamasu JSR, Kawase T, Kanzaki J. Haemorrhagic venous infarction following the posterior petrosal approach for acoustic neurinoma surgery: a report of two cases. *Eur Arch Otorhinolaryngol.* 2002;259 (3):162–165.

28. Handley TP, Miah MS, Majumdar S, Hussain SS. Collet-Sicard syndrome from thrombosis of the sigmoid-jugular complex: a case report and review of the literature. *Int J Otolaryngol.* 2010.

29. Bradley DT, Hashisaki GT, Mason JC. Otogenic sigmoid sinus thrombosis: what is the role of anticoagulation? *Laryngoscope.* 2002;112 (10):1726–1729.

30. House JW, Brackmann DE. Facial nerve grading system. *Otolaryngol Head Neck Surg.* 1985 Aug;93(2):146–147.

31. Hong RS, Kartush JM. Acoustic neuroma neurophysiologic correlates: facial and recurrent laryngeal nerves before, during, and after surgery. *Otolaryngol Clin North Am.* 2012 Apr;45(2):291–306.

32. Rosenberg JB. EisenLA. Eye care in the intensive care unit: narrative review and meta-analysis. *Crit Care Med.* 2008 Dec;36 (12):3151–3155.

33. Cortese D, Capp L, McKinley S. Moisture chamber versus lubrication for the prevention of corneal epithelial breakdown. *Am J Crit Care.* 1995 Nov;4(6):425–428.

34. Koroloff N, Boots R, Lipman J, Thomas P, Rickard C, Coyer F. A randomised controlled study of the efficacy of hypromellose and Lacri-Lube combination versus polyethylene/Cling wrap to prevent corneal epithelial breakdown in the semiconscious intensive care patient. *Intensive Care Med.* 2004 Jun;30(6):1122–1126.

35. Starmer HM, Best SR, Agrawal Y, et al. Prevalence, characteristics, and management of swallowing disorders following cerebellopontine angle surgery. *Otolaryngol Head Neck Surg.* 2012 Mar;146(3): 419–425.

36. Best SR, Stramer HM, Agrawal Y, et al. Risk factors for vagal palsy following cerebellopontine angle surgery. *Otolaryngol Head Neck Surg.* 2012 Aug;147(2):364–368.

37. Ramina R, Neto MC, Fernandes YB, Aguiar PH, de Meneses MS, Torres LF. Meningiomas of the jugular foramen. *Neurosurg Rev.* 2006 Jan;29(1):55–60.

38. Peterson KL, Fenn J. Treatment of dysphagia and dysphonia following skull base surgery. *Otolaryngol Clin North Am.* 2005 Aug;38 (4):809–817.

39. Mangus BD, Rivas A, Yoo MJ, et al. Management of cerebrospinal fluid leaks after vestibular schwannoma surgery. *Otol Neurotol.* 2011 Dec;32(9):1525–1529.

40. Selesnick SH, Liu JC, Jen A, Newman J. The incidence of cerebrospinal fluid leak after vestibular schwannoma surgery. *Otol Neurotol.* 2004 May;25(3):387–393.

41. Becker SS, Jackler RK, Pitts LH. Cerebrospinal fluid leak after acoustic neuroma surgery: a comparison of the translabyrinthine, middle fossa, and retrosigmoid approaches. *Otol Neurotol.* 2003 Jan; 24(1):107–112.

42. Srinivas D, Veena Kumari HB, Somanna S, Bhagavatula I, Anandappa CB. The incidence of postoperative meningitis in neurosurgery: an institutional experience. *Neurol India.* 2011 Mar–Apr;59(2):195–198.

43. Erdem I, Hakan T, Ceran N, et al. Clinical features, laboratory data, management and the risk factors that affect the mortality in patients with postoperative meningitis. *Neurol India.* 2008;56(4):433–437.

44. Federico G, Tumbarello M, Spanu T, et al. Risk factors and prognostic indicators of bacterial meningitis in a cohort of 3580 postneurosurgical patients. *Scand J Infect Dis.* 2001;33(7):533–537.

45. Loya JJ, Mindea SA, Yu H, Venkatasubramanian C, Chang SD, Burns TC. Intracranial hypotension producing reversible coma: a systematic review, including three new cases. *J Neurosurg.* 2012;117 (3):615–628.

46. Aghaei Lasboo A, Hurley MC, Walker MT, et al. Emergent image-guided treatment of a large CSF leak to reverse "in-extremis" signs of intracranial hypotension. *Am J Neuroradiol.* 2008;29(9): 1627–1629.

47. Akkawi N, Locatelli P, Borroni B, et al. A complicated case of intracranial hypotension: diagnostic and management strategies. *Neurol Sci.* 2006;27(1):63–66.

# 20 *Infratentorial and Cerebellar Tumors*

ALFRED POKMENG SEE, E. ANTONIO CHIOCCA, and WILLIAM B. GORMLEY

## Introduction

This chapter focuses on intraaxial lesions of the posterior fossa, because primary central nervous system extraaxial lesions and metastatic lesions are extensively discussed in the chapters on skull-base tumors and on metastases, respectively. The most common intraaxial pathologies following metastases in the posterior fossa include hemangioblastoma (Fig. 20.1), ependymoma, and subependymoma, as well as tumors that are more prevalent in the pediatric population but also appear in the adult population, such as medulloblastoma, diffuse intrinsic pontine glioma, exophytic medullary glioma, and tectal glioma. Astrocytic tumors of the posterior fossa, and more specifically of the cerebellum, span the full gamut from juvenile pilocytic astrocytomas to glioblastomas (Fig. 20.2). Low-grade cerebellar tumors may occur in adults, but higher-grade lesions are somewhat more frequent.[1]

Tumors in this region may come to clinical attention via direct impact on local neurological structures, obstruction of cerebrospinal fluid (CSF) flow through the cerebral aqueduct and fourth ventricle, or incidentally during evaluation for unrelated pathologies or symptoms. For a number of these lesions, including hemangioblastomas and ependymomas, a complete surgical resection is possible and should be the goal of surgery, if this can be done with low morbidity. In diffusely infiltrative pathologies, operative cure may not be possible. However, resolution of symptomatic hydrocephalus from obstruction of the fourth ventricle and decompression of cranial nerves and of white-matter tracts may provide significant clinical improvement in cases where posterior fossa mass effect causes reversible neurological deficits. Invasive pathology may directly infiltrate the cranial nerves or nuclei and induce neurological deficits, which would be less likely to improve from operative intervention.

## Neuroanatomy and Procedure

### Key Concepts

The anatomical determinants of the surgical approach are:

- the relationship to vascular structures
- the medial-to-lateral position
- the relationship of the mass to the cerebellar cortex
- the proximity to the 4th ventricle
- the association with cranial nerves and brainstem nuclei

Tumors of the posterior fossa typically derive vascular supply from the posterior inferior cerebellar artery (PICA), anterior inferior cerebellar artery (AICA), or the superior cerebellar artery (SCA).

Although tumors within the posterior fossa comprise a diverse group of pathologies, the surgical approach to these lesions is largely determined by the location within the posterior fossa. The primary anatomical determinants of a lesion relating to its surgical approach will be the relationship with vascular structures such as the sinuses and the arterial supply, the medial-to-lateral position, and the relationship of the lesion to the cortical cerebellar surface: petrosal, tentorial, or posterior. The shortest cortical trajectory to the lesion should be a strong consideration in selecting the surgical approach. Other considerations include involvement of the fourth ventricle, relation to and geometry of the tentorium, and relationship with cranial nerves or cerebellar and brainstem nuclei.

The trajectory of the approach can be limited by cranial nerves, major arteries or veins, and anatomical borders of the posterior fossa. The angle of the tentorium can limit the superior aspect of the reach and may necessitate specific positioning to capitalize on the effect of gravity. Further exposure can be achieved by CSF drainage, which, given the anatomy of the CSF cisterns, is always easily accessible to the surgeon early in the surgical approach. This anatomical fact obviates the need for lumbar drainage.

### VASCULAR ANATOMY

The vascular supply to the tumor is of vital importance for intraoperative control. Most typically, tumors of the posterior fossa will derive vascular supply from the PICA, AICA, or the SCA.

The PICA originates at the distal segment of the vertebral arteries to supply the medulla and the inferoposterior aspect of the cerebellum. The origin of the PICA may actually be extradural, arising immediately proximal to the site where the vertebral artery enters the dura.[2] The PICA courses from anterior to the medulla laterally at the level of the superior aspect of the cerebellar tonsils. Along this path, it variably interacts with the origins of the ninth, tenth, or eleventh cranial nerves. It then divides into medial and lateral branches to supply the vermis or the tonsils and hemisphere, respectively.[3]

The AICA branches at the proximal segment of the basilar artery to supply the anterior pons and lateral pons and lateral medulla, the inferior cerebellum, and the seventh and eighth cranial nerves. It commonly arises as a duplicated or even triplicated vessel. Originating in close proximity to and generally inferior to the internal auditory meatus, it often abuts the seventh and eighth cranial nerve complex.[4] The AICA perfuses the seventh and eighth nerves and nuclei, as well as the nuclei of the trigeminal nerve.

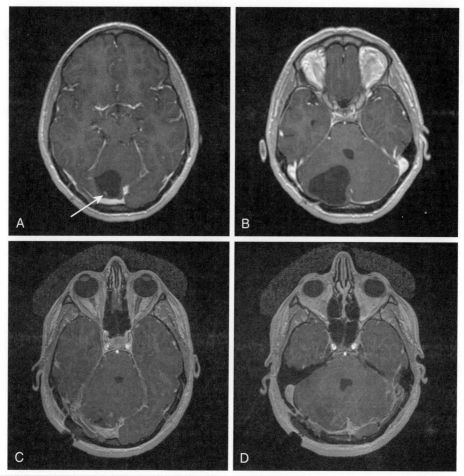

**Fig. 20.1  Hemangioblastoma. (A)** T1 magnetic resonance image (MRI) with gadolinium shows a hypointense cerebellar lesion with a small enhancing mural nodule (*arrow*). **(B)** The lesion is primarily cystic, with minimal fourth ventricular effacement. **(C, D)** Postoperative T1 MRI with gadolinium demonstrates gross total resection, including resection of the mural nodule. (Reprinted from Quinones-Hinojosa, A (Ed.). *Schmidek and Sweet: Operative Neurosurgical Techniques* 6th ed. New York: Elsevier Saunders; 2012.)

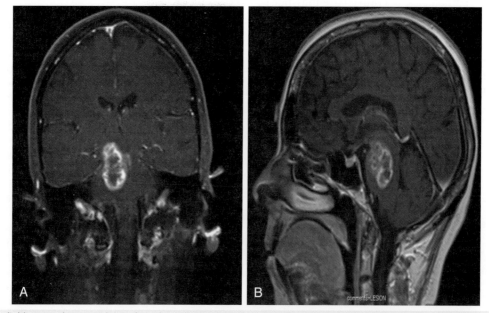

**Fig. 20.2**  Pontine glioblastoma that extends into the right midbrain and thalamus. (A) Postcontrast coronal MRI demonstrating the ring-enhancing cystic lesion. **(B)** Postcontrast sagittal MRI.  (Reprinted from Quinones-Hinojosa, A (Ed.). *Schmidek and Sweet: Operative Neurosurgical Techniques* 6th ed. New York: Elsevier Saunders; 2012.)

The most superior region of the posterior fossa is typically supplied by the SCA. This includes the cerebellar cortex and cerebellar nuclei and, by proxy, tumors within these regions. The SCA typically arises from the basilar artery, although it may also arise from the proximal posterior cerebral artery. It is not infrequently duplicated, with two branches arising directly from the basilar artery. It curves around the pons, inferior to the third, fourth, and fifth cranial nerves. It divides into two branches supplying the cerebellar cortex. Along its course, perforators supply the superior and middle cerebellar peduncles and the colliculi.[5] Because the tumor vasculature may not be independent of the vascular supply to normal tissue, there is also a risk of infarct in the distribution of shared vasculature.

The venous drainage is also prominent in the posterior fossa, with brainstem, bridging, superficial, and deep veins. Superficial veins drain the cerebellar cortex. These veins drain into the superior petrosal sinus, the transverse sinus, and the sigmoid sinus. The deep veins are along the roof and walls of the fourth ventricle; they serve as periventricular structures. The veins of the brainstem are on the anterior surface and drain into the petrosal and jugular sinuses and sometimes the sigmoid sinus. The transverse and sigmoid sinuses are typically the common final drainage outlet for the sagittal sinus, petrosal sinuses, and deep venous drainage pathways.[6] Although classically portrayed as a symmetrically redundant system, the transverse sinus is asymmetrical two-thirds of time.[7] The transverse and sigmoid sinus form the superior and anterior borders of many of the conventional approaches in this region. Skull-base approaches, including petrosal bone resection, alter these limitations by providing alternative angles to posterior fossa lesions, particularly those located in the anterolateral posterior fossa.[8–10]

Further nuances require a detailed understanding of the individual tumor vascular supply. Early access to vascular structures during the initial dissection is important to minimize hemorrhage and to avoid the complications of both blood loss and replacement, including anemia, coagulopathy, and transfusion reactions. Furthermore, although mannitol and dexamethasone during induction and surgery may aid in controlling edema, securing arterial access provides definitive control of edema in the lesion and surrounding tissue, which may become acutely worsened in the setting of venous compromise. In certain cases deep supply or supply derived from multiple distributions can complicate surgery. In the postoperative setting it is important to be aware of vascular compromise in cases that may merit particular vigilance for hypoperfusion or venous congestion and venous infarction.

Venous structures are critical in posterior fossa surgery, and constant awareness of their location is critical from the initial tumor approach to avoid venous injury. The junction between the transverse and sigmoid sinuses is commonly quoted to lie at the asterion, where the parietal, occipital, and temporal bone meet with three sutures.[11] It is reliable in delineating the anteroposterior location of the junction, but in up to 40% of cases, this landmark may mislead the operator in the inferosuperior axis and result in sinus injury.[12] A common technique described is the Frankfurt horizontal plane.[11] Alternatively, the axis between the asterion and the mastoid tip may approximate the sigmoid sinus trajectory, and the axis between the root of the zygoma and the inion may approximate the superoinferior level of the transverse sinus.[12]

## BONY ANATOMY

Image guidance for positioning and operative planning is less accurate and more difficult to register, because the posterior fossa is distant to the facial features, which are commonly used in registration.[13] Therefore image guidance may provide only limited improvement upon cutaneous and osseous landmarks in operative planning, determination of the operative site, and positioning, making deep knowledge of bony anatomy critical to successful surgery.

# Perioperative Considerations

### Key Concepts

- The clinical examination, cerebrovascular perfusion, radiographic imaging, and echocardiographic results guide intraoperative monitoring requirements.
- For all operative patient positions, areas exposed to pressure, such as the orbit, ankles, heels, knees, iliac crests, pelvis, breasts, axilla, elbow, wrist, and vascular access sites, require padding.
- Relative to the other positions, the sitting position is associated with venous air embolism (VAE) due to the relative elevation of the head compared with the heart.

The baseline history and physical examination of the patient evaluates the state of consciousness, cranial nerve function, intracranial pressure (ICP), blood pressure, and vascular perfusion, including risk factors such as carotid artery disease or systemic vascular insufficiency and vascular drainage. Patients should also be evaluated for abnormal communications between the venous and arterial circulation with echocardiography, because the size of patent foramen ovale and the degree of right-to-left shunting may increase the risk of VAE.[14] Patients deemed high risk for VAE may require additional monitoring including: electrocardiography, pulse oximetry, end-tidal $CO_2$ monitoring, echocardiography, invasive arterial blood pressure monitoring, central venous pressure monitoring, bispectral index monitoring, cranial nerve monitoring, motor evoked potentials (MEPs), and somatosensory evoked potentials (SSEPs).

VAE is most worrisome in the sitting position but can occur in any posterior fossa surgery if large venous structures are violated. There is no agreed-upon standard to monitor for VAE; techniques range from precordial Doppler to intraoperative transesophageal echocardiography.[15] Use of positive end-expiratory pressure (PEEP) may reduce the likelihood of clinically significant VAE by reducing the tendency for air to enter the central venous vasculature. Surgical vigilance is the most vital tool in avoidance of VAE when operating in the posterior fossa near large venous structures.

**Table 20.1** Operative Positioning[16,17,28,40,41]

| Position | Benefits | Disadvantages |
|---|---|---|
| Prone | Preserved midline relationships<br>Ease of positioning | Difficulty with access to superior regions of the posterior fossa<br>Position can impair venous drainage |
| Lateral | Gravitational tendency for lateral retraction for nonmidline structures<br>Bony landmarks for surgical guidance | Potential for altered anatomical relationships with rotated positioning<br>More complex positioning |
| Sitting/ modified recumbent | Gravitational tendency for inferior retraction and limited cerebellar retraction<br>Decreased edema with improved venous drainage | Operator comfort may be more difficult to obtain<br>Potential for increased venous air embolism<br>Lack of familiarity for surgeons and operating room team |

Intraoperative neurophysiological monitoring, including motor evoked potentials, SSEPs, and auditory evoked potentials, have become essential adjuncts to surgery in this region. Although clinically significant changes may be undetected on intraoperative monitoring, these techniques may often provide useful additional information to guide the aggressiveness of operative goals.

The patient position is critical in obtaining access and avoiding complications. Common operative positions include prone, lateral, or sitting.[16,17] Each position comes with different risks and nuances of preparation (Table 20.1). For all positions, areas exposed to pressure require padding, such as the orbit, ankles, heels, knees, iliac crests, pelvis, breasts, axilla, elbow, wrist, and vascular access sites. During any surgical positioning, the neck is susceptible to structural injury, and avoidance of this requires close attention to detail in the process. The prone position keeps the head in the neutral position with slight flexion to preserve standard anatomical distances and ease of orientation. The lateral position may involve turning of the head and can be accomplished in a lateral body position or with the patient supine with significant angulation. The sitting position involves head flexion and ideally keeps the head and heart in the same plane in order to minimize the possibility of VAE. It is imperative to assess both structural neck strain and preservation of cerebral venous return. One gauge is the chin-to-chest distance of about 3 cm.

Further specific concerns for the prone position include the turning technique, thoracic pressure, and retinal injury. Turning of the patient can result in injury, particularly to the neck or extremities. All extremities and the neck should be maintained in a neutral position during turning, which may require additional staff during the turn. Once in the prone position with standard cushioning issues addressed, the thoracic pressure also needs to be addressed because the prone position may limit ventilation as well as venous return, leading to hypoventilation and hypotension.

Relative to the other positions, the sitting position is associated with VAE due to relative elevation of the head compared with the heart. In the case of suspected VAE, the head should be lowered below the level of the heart as quickly as is safe. This should be discussed before the beginning of the case so that the team is appropriately prepared for such a maneuver. Although PEEP may increase the cerebral venous pressure and reduce the risk of VAE, it may also increase ICP. PEEP to prevent VAE remains controversial, particularly because most VAE are asymptomatic.[18]

Wound closure is particularly critical in the posterior fossa because of the close proximity of large CSF cisterns. This anatomical relationship makes the risk of postoperative CSF leaks high and increases the need for technical proficiency during closure. At the dural layer, primary closure can occasionally be achieved. However, anatomical changes, edema, dural retraction, and dural shrinkage (even in the setting of frequent irrigation) may result in insufficient material for closure. Dural substitutes include cadaveric skin processed into tissue matrix, cadaveric tensor fasciae latae, or pericranium. The suture closure of the dural opening can be further reinforced with synthetic agents, which vary in availability at each institution. These agents, which include different biological and chemical glues and bonding material, can be challenging to apply in the operative field, leading to irregular bonding and inconsistent layering, and can also be cost prohibitive. However, given the potential severity of a CSF leak or pseudomeningocele, use of these agents should still be considered if the reliability of the closure is in question, particularly in cases with irradiated tissue, reoperations, or cases with preexisting arachnoid scarring or hydrocephalus.

---

### Clinical Pearl

Clinical risk factors for poor wound healing include diabetes, prior irradiation, upcoming irradiation, corticosteroid usage, smoking, and malnutrition. Some of these are modifiable and represent an opportunity to improve outcomes.

---

The bony layer is often left uncovered in posterior fossa procedures, but replacing the bone may reduce the frequency of pseudomeningocele, CSF and wound infection, and postoperative headaches.[19–22] The midline keel may increase the risk of unintentional durotomy in a single-piece craniotomy. Although not yet evaluated, a heterologous source such as a lyophilized bone, plastic implant, or mesh with cement or bone fragments may be used in place of bone flap replacement. Soft tissue closure should emphasize reducing potential spaces and achieving a watertight closure.

## Postoperative Complications

Complications may become apparent either during the operation or after an otherwise successful operation

## Box 20.1 Intraoperative and Postoperative Complications[16,28]

**Complications Presenting Intraoperatively**

- Venous air embolism
- Injury to arteries
- Laceration of bridging veins
- Sinus injury
- Dural injury during exposure
- Insufficient hemostasis with overlooked hemorrhage

**Complications Presenting Postoperatively**

- Perioperative cranial nerve injury
- Perioperative cardiopulmonary instability
- Stroke syndromes
- Vision loss
- Faulty positioning resulting in spinal cord injury
- Faulty positioning resulting in neural compression injury, entrapment neuropathy
- Injury to cerebral arteries
- Subtle injury to bridging veins, deep cerebral veins resulting in venous infarct and edema
- CSF leak or pseudomeningocele
- Hydrocephalus
- Venous thromboembolism
- Hematoma
- Anemia due to overlooked intraoperative hemorrhage
- Pneumocephalus

(Box 20.1). Therefore many institutional and operator-specific policies may dictate the need for an intensive care unit for at least the initial postoperative period. Although intraoperative complications would generally have been stabilized before exiting the operating room, they may have continued monitoring requirements or ongoing impact on clinical status.

Arterial injury during the operation, whether due to unintended vessel injury and need to sacrifice the artery for hemostasis or intentional sacrifice to control tumor perfusion, may lead to infarct of healthy tissue. Posterior fossa infarction with cytotoxic edema may lead to mass effect, obstructive hydrocephalus, and compression of the brainstem, with catastrophic results. This edema may progress over the course of hours, and hemorrhagic conversion can hasten this process and make clinical deterioration precipitous.

Venous injury, whether from bridging veins or sinuses, causes a particularly fulminant edema, with venous congestion often accompanied by hemorrhagic conversion. Delayed development of focal neurological deficits localizing to the posterior fossa, such as deficits of the lower cranial nerves, ataxia, or nystagmus, may indicate a delayed injury to neurological structures via a congestive process. Injury to larger venous structures may result in a wider territory of congestion with symptoms of diffuse cerebral edema such as increased ICP, altered sensorium, headache, nausea, vomiting, paresis, or late signs of severe mass effect such as posturing or irregular respirations or heart rate.[23] Development of intracranial hypertension can be initially and temporarily managed with elevation of the head of the bed, hyperosmolar therapy, and respiratory control.

However, recovery from venous infarction is extended in duration and associated with cerebral edema, which dominates the direct mass effect of the hemorrhage. Therefore venous infarction may necessitate aggressive medical or surgical control of edema, CSF diversion, or posterior fossa decompressive operation.[24]

### Clinical Pearl

The timing of postoperative complications provides valuable information on the etiology of the complication. Whereas direct injury to neurological structures typically manifests on initial examination, the effects of edema, such as from venous injury and subsequent congestion, often have a delayed onset. Therefore early postoperative neurological examination is critical to establish a first time point.

Edema and mass effect from hemorrhage may also result in obstructive hydrocephalus.[25] Steroids may provide sufficient resolution of the edema to resolve the obstruction[26] if the underlying tumor lesion had significant associated edema. Edema from vascular compromise will not, however, respond to steroid therapy. Hydrocephalus may persist, and the supratentorial manifestations of hydrocephalus may necessitate an external ventricular drain (EVD).[23] However, EVDs that terminate in the lateral or third ventricle and parenchymal intracerebral pressure monitors may not provide adequate reflection of infratentorial pressures. Furthermore, overdrainage of supratentorial spinal fluid through an EVD leads to upward herniation, which may compress mesencephalic and diencephalic structures, including the midbrain and thalamus. In the absence of hydrocephalus, the clinical examination and serial radiographic imaging may provide the only reliable means of monitoring infratentorial pressure, such as demonstration of upward herniation or tonsilar herniation through the foramen magnum.

### Clinical Pearl

Hydrocephalus may not be synonymous with ventriculomegaly, particularly in operations of the posterior fossa where the dural opening lies in a dependent position. Development of pseudomeningocele is an alternative presentation of deranged CSF reabsorption and may also necessitate CSF diversion for definitive treatment and prevention of wound complications.

Even in the absence of venous infarct, edema of the resection cavity may result in sufficient mass effect to obstruct CSF flow and cause temporary hydrocephalus.[26] An EVD may provide a bridge for management of ICP and CSF bulk dynamics until the resolution of the obstructive pathology. Blood from the operation may also enter the ventricular spaces, which is associated with a communicating hydrocephalus. However, current understanding of hydrocephalus, the causes of ventriculomegaly, and increased ICP is surprisingly limited. As such, even after resolution of the apparent hydrocephalus etiology, permanent CSF diversion may still be required in 10% to 25% of patients. Some centers consider a preoperative shunt, resulting in 35% shunt usage, suggesting that in this group there is likely a higher utilization of shunting than may be needed. This demonstrates that we do not have a reliable means of predicting who will require a shunt, making preemptive shunt or EVD placement seem unwarranted in most circumstances. The most common permanent diversion would be a ventriculoperitoneal shunt. Although a frontal or occipital shunt of the nondominant hemisphere is most common, nontraditional shunts may be required if the hydrocephalus is not panventricular.

Postoperative hematomas can occur within the resection cavity, in the extradural compartment, or in the subcutaneous compartment. In the absence of clinically significant mass effect, observation of the spontaneously resolving hematoma may offer the best risk–benefit balance. The intradural hematoma is at highest risk of necessitating operative intervention, because the other compartments present a barrier between the hematoma and the neurological compartment and, with a craniectomy, there is increased compliance of the extradural compartment. An extradural hematoma may also necessitate evacuation, but may be a distinct entity from the epidural hematoma in the setting of an intact calvarium.[27]

CSF leaks and pseudomeningoceles are the most common surgical complications in the posterior fossa.[28] The mechanisms leading to CSF leaks and pseudomeningocele formation are unclear, but probably include inadequate dural and wound closures. Optimal dural closure is achieved when using native dura or harvested autologous material. A dural substitute should only be considered when a watertight closure cannot otherwise be obtained, because dural substitutes may increase complication rates. Small pseudomeningoceles may respond well to pressure bandages, needle aspiration, and lumbar CSF drainage. In some cases, CSF diversion may be required.

Rare but severe complications include perioperative cranial nerve injury with the complications these imply, such as corneal abrasions from facial weakness or aspiration pneumonia from lower cranial nerve injury. Deficits in lower cranial nerves may result in difficulty swallowing and inability to protect the airway. In many cases, patients may require feeding tube placement and a tracheostomy to prevent aspiration pneumonia until they sufficiently recover function. A formal approach to determine extubation readiness and swallowing function is optimal. Intraoperative monitoring may serve as a useful adjunct in the assessment of swallowing or airway compromise. These complications are more common for surgery for extraaxial lesions but can be seen occasionally from any approach in the posterior fossa.

A rare and perplexing complication of posterior fossa surgery is that of vision loss. It is poorly understood, and neither prediction nor prophylaxis is well described.[29] Prone cases have occasionally been associated with blindness (0.03%–1.3% perioperative visual loss [POVL]), thought to be from retinal ischemia with orbital compression, low perfusion pressure, and venous congestion resulting in ischemic optic neuropathy (Box 20.2).[30] There are also cases of central retinal artery occlusion, cortical infarction,

**Box 20.2   Causes of Perioperative Vision Loss in Descending Frequency[30]**

Ischemic optic neuropathy
Central retinal artery occlusion
Cortical infarction
External ocular injury

or ocular injury, although ischemic optic neuropathy contributes to nearly nine out of every ten cases.[31] Some cases are observed to be associated with ecchymosis or other local trauma, but even with proper positioning, cushioning, and absence of pressure, the prone position may often result in corneal edema. There are some suggestions that a neutral or head-up position may reduce the likelihood of POVL. Ultimately, this is a risk that needs to be discussed with the patient because proper screening for preoperative risk factors; proper positioning; and proper control of surgical time, blood pressure, and anemia have not been shown to associate with changes in frequency of POVL.[32]

Complications of positioning may be identified on the awake postoperative examination when the patient's extremity strength and sensation can be thoroughly evaluated. Prophylaxis of peripheral compression pathology is the most effective intervention. Therapy with physiatrists may aid in the recovery of strength resulting from peripheral motor deficits. Spinal cord injury from extremes of positioning may necessitate operative intervention. Again, the most effective intervention is prophylactic identification of patients at risk for cervical injury and judicious positioning. The use of SSEPs and brainstem auditory evoked responses prior to positioning can often alert the surgeon to compromise of neural structures during positioning. Treatment of an established spinal cord injury is complex and mostly ineffective; the use of steroids to treat traumatic spinal cord injury shows unclear benefit.[33] Prone positioning is also known to risk nipple necrosis, pressure injuries at the iliac crests and knees, and brachial plexus injury.[34]

Intensive care monitoring, including telemetry, maintenance of an arterial line, and a central venous catheter, allows early detection of rapidly evolving, potentially fatal complications (Table 20.1). Clinically significant VAE requires continued evaluation of cardiac function. Cardiac strain may lead to ischemic damage, which should be followed with serial electrocardiography and serum markers of cardiac ischemia and infarct. In cases of demonstrable cardiac dysfunction, further evaluation with echocardiography and a cardiologist may be merited. The presence of a right-to-left shunt increases the risk of significant cardiac injury from VAE, because coronary air embolus can be a direct cause of cardiac injury as well. Cardiac injury may be exacerbated by postoperative anemia. In the setting of known cardiac injury, a more generous hematocrit or hemoglobin goal may benefit cardiac function, and treatment of a symptomatic anemia is always warranted.[35–38]

Oncologic patients are generally at increased risk of venous thromboembolism (VTE). Mechanical and pharmacological prophylaxis has been shown as an effective means of reducing the occurrence of VTE even with consideration for the risk of postoperative hemorrhage.[39] Metaanalysis of randomized controlled trials estimate 91 cases of VTE prevented for every 1000 patients treated, with 35 cases of operative site hemorrhage. Although patients at high risk of intracranial hemorrhage are sometimes considered candidates for single mechanical-agent prophylaxis, there is neither consensus on the definition of a high-risk patient nor quantifiable means of measuring such risk. The decision to provide or to withhold prophylaxis is made on a case-by-case basis.

## Conclusion

The potential for postoperative complications in surgery of the posterior fossa is not only high, but the clinical significance of these complications is so large that it is imperative that all posterior fossa cases receive care in an intensive care setting. In addition, awareness by the critical care team of the potential problems and their solutions is imperative if poor outcomes are to be avoided.

### References

1. Packer RJ, Hoffman HJ, Friedman HS, Kun LE, Fuller GN. Presentation and chemotherapy of primitive neuroectodermal tumors. In: Levin VA, ed. *Cancer in the Nervous System.* Churchill Livingstone, New York; 1996:153–170.
2. Fine AD, Cardoso A, Rhoton Jr AL. Microsurgical anatomy of the extracranial-extradural origin of the posterior inferior cerebellar artery. *J Neurosurg.* 1999;91(4):645–652.
3. Lister JR, Rhoton Jr AL, Matsushima T, Peace DA. Microsurgical anatomy of the posterior inferior cerebellar artery. *Neurosurgery.* 1982;10(2):170–199.
4. Martin RG, Grant JL, Peace D, Theiss C, Rhoton Jr AL. Microsurgical relationships of the anterior inferior cerebellar artery and the facial-vestibulocochlear nerve complex. *Neurosurgery.* 1980;6(5):483–507.
5. Hardy DG, Peace DA, Rhoton Jr AL. Microsurgical anatomy of the superior cerebellar artery. *Neurosurgery.* 1980;6(1):10–28.
6. Rhoton Jr AL. The posterior fossa veins. *Neurosurgery.* 2000;47(3 Suppl):S69–S92.
7. Gokce E, Pinarbasili T, Acu B, Firat MM, Erkorkmaz U. Torcular Herophili classification and evaluation of dural venous sinus variations using digital subtraction angiography and magnetic resonance venographies. *Surg Radiol Anat.* 2014 Aug;36(6):527–536.
8. Gross BA, Tavanaiepour D, Du R, Al-Mefty O, Dunn IF. Evolution of the posterior petrosal approach. *Neurosurg Focus.* 2012;33(2).
9. Hafez A, Nader R, Al-Mefty O. Preservation of the superior petrosal sinus during the petrosal approach. *J Neurosurg.* 2011;114(5):1294–1298.
10. Sakata K, Al-Mefty O, Yamamoto I. Venous consideration in petrosal approach: microsurgical anatomy of the temporal bridging vein. *Neurosurgery.* 2000;47(1):153–160. discussion 60–1.
11. Lang Jr J, Samii A. Retrosigmoidal approach to the posterior cranial fossa. An anatomical study. *Acta Neurochir.* 1991;111(3–4):147–153.
12. Day JD, Kellogg JX, Tschabitscher M, Fukushima T. Surface and superficial surgical anatomy of the posterolateral cranial base: significance for surgical planning and approach. *Neurosurgery.* 1996;38(6):1079–1083. discussion 83–4.
13. da Silva Jr EB, Leal AG, Milano JB, da Silva Jr LF, Clemente RS, Ramina R. Image-guided surgical planning using anatomical landmarks in the retrosigmoid approach. *Acta Neurochir.* 2010;152(5):905–910.
14. Ammirati M, Lamki TT, Shaw AB, Forde B, Nakano I, Mani M. A streamlined protocol for the use of the semi-sitting position in neurosurgery: a report on 48 consecutive procedures. *J Clin Neurosci.* 2013;20(1):32–34.
15. Jadik S, Wissing H, Friedrich K, Beck J, Seifert V, Raabe A. A standardized protocol for the prevention of clinically relevant venous air embolism during neurosurgical interventions in the semisitting position. *Neurosurgery.* 2009;64(3):533–538 discussion 8–9.
16. Rajpal S, Iskandar BJ. Surgical approaches to pediatric midline posterior fossa tumors. In: Badie B, ed. *Neurosurgical Operative Atlas.* 2nd ed. New York, NY: Thieme Medical Publishers Inc; 2007:214.
17. Ogden AT, Bruce JN. Surgical approaches to pineal region tumors. In: Badie B, ed. *Neurosurgical Operative Atlas.* 2nd ed. New York, NY: Thieme Medical Publishers Inc; 2007:206.
18. Ganslandt O, Merkel A, Schmitt H, et al. The sitting position in neurosurgery: indications, complications and results. a single institution experience of 600 cases. *Acta Neurochir.* 2013;155(10):1887–1893.
19. Legnani FG, Saladino A, Casali C, et al. Craniotomy vs. craniectomy for posterior fossa tumors: a prospective study to evaluate complications after surgery. *Acta Neurochir.* 2013;155(12):2281–2286.
20. Dora B, Nikolaos B, Stylianos G, Damianos S. Intracranial hypotension syndrome in a patient due to suboccipital craniectomy secondary to Chiari type malformation. *World J Clin Cases.* 2013;1(9):295–297.
21. Parker SL, Godil SS, Zuckerman SL, Mendenhall SK, Tulipan NB, McGirt MJ. Effect of symptomatic pseudomeningocele on improvement in pain, disability, and quality of life following suboccipital decompression for adult Chiari malformation type I. *J Neurosurg.* 2013;119(5):1159–1165.
22. Lovely TJ. The treatment of chronic incisional pain and headache after retromastoid craniectomy. *Surg Neurol Int.* 2012;3:92.
23. Koh MS, Goh KY, Tung MY, Chan C. Is decompressive craniectomy for acute cerebral infarction of any benefit? *Surgical Neurol.* 2000;53(3):225–230.
24. Hornig CR, Rust DS, Busse O, Jauss M, Laun A. Space-occupying cerebellar infarction. Clinical course and prognosis. *Stroke.* 1994;25(2):372–374.
25. Schijman E, Peter JC, Rekate HL, Sgouros S, Wong TT. Management of hydrocephalus in posterior fossa tumors: how, what, when? *Childs Nerv Sys.* 2004;20(3):192–194.
26. Taylor WA, Todd NV, Leighton SE. CSF drainage in patients with posterior fossa tumours. *Acta Neurochir.* 1992;117(1-2):1–6.
27. Kawakami Y, Tamiya T, Tanimoto T, et al. Nonsurgical treatment of posterior fossa epidural hematoma. *Pediatr Neurol.* 1990;6(2):112–118.
28. Dubey A, Sung WS, Shaya M, et al. Complications of posterior cranial fossa surgery—an institutional experience of 500 patients. *Surg Neurol.* 2009;72(4):369.
29. Reed-Berendt R, Phillips B, Picton S, et al. Cause and outcome of cerebellar mutism: evidence from a systematic review. *Childs Nerv Sys.* 2014;30(3):375–385.
30. Roth S. Perioperative visual loss: what do we know, what can we do? *Br J Anaesth.* 2009;103(Suppl 1):i31–i40.
31. Uribe AA, Baig MN, Puente EG, Viloria A, Mendel E, Bergese SD. Current intraoperative devices to reduce visual loss after spine surgery. *Neurosurg Focus.* 2012;33(2).
32. Myers MA, Hamilton SR, Bogosian AJ, Smith CH, Wagner TA. Visual loss as a complication of spine surgery. A review of 37 cases. *Spine.* 1997;22(12):1325–1329.
33. Bracken MB. Steroids for acute spinal cord injury. *Cochrane Database Systematic Rev.* 2012;1.
34. Akhavan A, Gainsburg DM, Stock JA. Complications associated with patient positioning in urologic surgery. *Urology.* 2010;76(6):1309–1316.
35. Bae MH, Lee JH, Yang DH, Park HS, Cho Y, Chae SC. Usefulness of surgical parameters as predictors of postoperative cardiac events in patients undergoing non-cardiac surgery. *Circ J.* 2014;78(3):718–723.
36. Hare GM, Tsui AK, McLaren AT, Ragoonanan TE, Yu J, Mazer CD. Anemia and cerebral outcomes: many questions, fewer answers. *Anesth Analg.* 2008;107(4):1356–1370.
37. Hogue Jr CW, Goodnough LT, Monk TG. Perioperative myocardial ischemic episodes are related to hematocrit level in patients undergoing radical prostatectomy. *Transfusion.* 1998;38(10):924–931.
38. Nelson AH, Fleisher LA, Rosenbaum SH. Relationship between postoperative anemia and cardiac morbidity in high-risk vascular patients in the intensive care unit. *Crit Care Med.* 1993;21(6):860–866.
39. Hamilton MG, Yee WH, Hull RD, Ghali WA. Venous thromboembolism prophylaxis in patients undergoing cranial neurosurgery: a systematic review and meta-analysis. *Neurosurgery.* 2011;68(3):571–581.
40. Kikuta KI, Miyamoto S, Kataoka H, Satow T, Yamada K, Hashimoto N. Use of the prone oblique position in surgery for posterior fossa lesions. *Acta Neurochir.* 2004;146(10):1119.
41. Mottolese C, Szathmari A, Ricci-Franchi AC, Beuriat PA, Grassiot B. The sub-occipital transtentorial approach revisited base on our own experience. *Neuro-Chirurgie.* 2015 Apr-Jun;61(2-3):168–175.

# 21 Postoperative Management Following Craniotomy for Resection of Metastatic Lesions

GANESH M. SHANKAR, PATRICIA L. MUSOLINO, and DANIEL P. CAHILL

## Introduction

Brain metastases are common in patients with metastatic systemic cancers, and with recent advances in systemic treatments, they are becoming an increasingly prevalent clinical management issue in the care of these patients. There continues to be debate about the optimal way to manage brain metastasis with regard to surgery versus radiation.[1–3] Many brain metastases are managed with radiation therapy techniques such as whole-brain irradiation or stereotactic radiosurgery; however, larger symptomatic lesions, especially those in the posterior fossa, often necessitate surgical intervention and postoperative intensive care management.

## Neuroanatomy

The vast majority of brain metastasis are thought to arise from hematogenous spread and can therefore arise anywhere in the brain. The presenting signs and symptoms depend on the location in the brain, with possible compression of eloquent cortex, symptoms of increased intracranial pressure (ICP) from the mass and associated surrounding edema, and compression of cerebrospinal fluid (CSF) pathways leading to hydrocephalus. Even small cortical lesions can cause seizures, which may be an early indicator of metastatic disease. Magnetic resonance imaging (MRI) has a limit of resolution, and there are always concerns about micrometastasis not visible on standard MRI. It is not uncommon when patients are referred for radiation therapy for brain metastasis that when the patients have their planning MRI (which can be delayed by several weeks) more metastases are identified and may require alterations in planning. This is especially common in tumors such as lung cancer and melanoma. Finally, patients can have carcinomatous involvement of the meninges in addition to parenchymal lesions, which is a very poor prognostic sign. Careful attention should be given to examining the meninges for involvement by contrasted MRI scans. Finally, in general the metastases do not invade brain like primary tumors, but generally displace surrounding brain, which has an implication in the surgical approach.

> ### Key Concept
>
> Patients with metastatic disease often have had previous radiation and systemic chemotherapy, putting them at higher risk for wound complications.

The overall surgical approaches to metastatic brain tumors are not substantially different from approaches to primary tumors, with a few exceptions. Because these tumors do not invade brain, there often is a well-defined plane between the tumor and surrounding brain. The morbidity associated with these procedures is therefore related to the approach and trajectory to these tumors, including damage to surrounding brain and vessels.[4] Neuronavigation is very useful in planning the shortest distance through brain with the least likelihood of disrupting vital structures.[5] Once the capsule of the tumor is identified, the plane with normal brain can be circumferentially developed with or without internally debulking or piecemeal removal.

Issues somewhat unique to metastatic tumors include the approach to simultaneous removal of multiple lesions, which requires careful planning with regard to positioning and incision design. Less commonly, lesions are taken out through two separate surgical approaches—for instance, symptomatic lesions simultaneously in the cerebral cortex and posterior fossa that require staged approaches under the same anesthesia event. One other issue not necessarily unique to metastatic disease is that many of these patients have had previous radiation, have had recent chemotherapy, and may have immunological compromise and poor nutritional status, which can factor heavily into wound healing and should be considered when planning surgical incisions.

# Perioperative Considerations

## Key Concept

The decision regarding optimal treatment for brain metastasis must take into account the tumor type; number, size, and location of lesions; patient symptoms; previous therapy; and patient suitability for surgery.

## Clinical Pearl

Clinicians must remain attentive to neurological decline in patients who have undergone resections of metastases in the posterior fossa because these clinical changes may herald development of obstructive hydrocephalus.

The treatment options for patients with posterior fossa metastasis should be carefully considered even in patients with minimal symptoms because tumor swelling with radiation therapy can potentially cause patients to decompensate.

There continues to be debate about the optimal way to manage brain metastasis with regard to surgery versus radiation. There is also discussion about the appropriate type of radiation, that is, stereotactic radiosurgery versus whole-brain radiation.[6-8] There are many factors that need to be taken into account, including the type of cancer and its inherent radiosensitivity; the number of lesions (one versus multiple); the size and anatomical location, which factors into surgical accessibility; the patient's presenting symptoms; his or her previous history of treatment, especially previous radiation; his or her systemic cancer load and possible life expectancy; the patient's overall medical fitness to tolerate a craniotomy; and the patient's/family's wishes.

The simplest scenario is someone presenting with a solitary brain metastasis from a known cancer. Again, there are many factors that need to be considered when counseling patients with regard to surgery followed by radiotherapy and systemic therapy versus primary treatment with radiotherapy.[9-11] Among the first considerations are the size of the lesion, the surrounding edema, the anatomical location, and the patient's presenting symptoms. In a patient with a large surgically accessible lesion with significant mass effect and related symptoms who is surgically fit, primary resection is often the best choice, followed by radiation if indicated. With smaller lesions, especially with fewer symptoms of mass effect, in deep or eloquent cortex, with radioresponsive tumors, radiation therapy is a very reasonable option. This is especially true in patients who are overall poor surgical candidates. There is a trend toward stereotactic radiosurgery instead of whole-brain radiation due to the known cognitive and functional effects of whole-brain radiation.[6] The one brain region where the decision can be more difficult is a moderate-sized lesion in the posterior fossa even with a paucity of symptoms, because possible postradiation tumor swelling can sometimes lead to acute neurological decline.[12]

When there is more than one lesion, the surgical decision making is even more difficult—for example, if there are multiple lesions but perhaps only one or possibly a few that are truly symptomatic, especially in a patient who has had previous radiation or in radioresistant tumors such as melanoma. This is especially true when the alternative may be whole-brain or complex planning of multiple stereotactic radiosurgery targets. The question always arises about the utility of resecting multiple lesions with regard to increased life expectancy.[13-16]

# Postoperative Management

## COMMUNICATING EXPECTED CLINICAL TRAJECTORY

### Key Concept

Postoperative focal neurological deficits are normally referable to the location of the resected brain metastasis and may be a result of focal seizure or hemorrhage.

Postoperative management of the patient who has just undergone resection of intracranial metastatic lesions begins with clear communication between the surgical team, anesthesia and intensive care unit (ICU) physicians, and nursing staff. Most postoperative complications manifest within the first 6 hours, and accordingly observation of patients in an ICU for the first day postoperatively is recommended.[17-19] Typical etiologies of complications are postoperative hemorrhage, seizure, hydrocephalus, and, less commonly, mass effect from pneumocephalus.

The location of the lesion and operative approach guide the potential expected neurological deficits.[4] For example, metastases resected from the temporal lobe may increase the likelihood of postoperative seizure, whereas lesions resected from the posterior fossa would make deficits related to obstructive hydrocephalus more likely. Residual focal motor or sensory deficits may be initially observed postoperatively in patients who underwent resection of lesions adjacent to the motor strip, even with intraoperative mapping by electrocorticography. These are usually transient and resolve within the first 24 hours[20]; otherwise, concern for epilepsia partialis continua in the region surrounding the resection cavity, or more permanent cortical injury, should be a consideration. The specific neurological deficits attributable to resection of metastatic lesions are highlighted in Table 21.1 and Figs. 21.1 to 21.3.

These concerns regarding postoperative deficits and the expected time course of evolution need to form the basis of communication between the surgical team and the ICU team of physicians and nurses. Should the patient's postoperative clinical trajectory not meet the predicted outcome, further evaluation should involve expeditious head imaging with computed tomography or MRI to evaluate for hemorrhage or hydrocephalus, both of which can be intervened upon surgically.

**Table 21.1**   Expected Focal Neurological Impairments after Craniotomy for Resection of Metastatic Intracranial Lesion

| Location | Expected immediate deficits | Vascular considerations | Possible complications |
|---|---|---|---|
| Frontal lobe | Altered behavior, slowed executive functioning, depression, apraxia, contralateral weakness, motor aphasia, abulia | Sagittal sinus, convexity cortical veins | Edema, CVST, bleeding, seizures |
| Temporal lobe | Auditory hallucinations, memory deficits, contralateral superior homonymous quadrantanopsia, receptive aphasia | Vein of Labbe, transverse sinus | Seizures, edema with effacement of ambient cistern and uncal herniation, CVST |
| Parietal lobe | Contralateral sensory dysfunction, neglect syndrome with nondominant parietal lobe, Gerstmann syndrome (agraphia, acalculia, finger agnosia) with dominant parietal lobe, contralateral inferior homonymous hemianopsia | Sagittal sinus, convexity cortical veins | Edema, CVST, seizures, bleeding |
| Occipital lobe | Contralateral homonymous hemianopsia, cortical blindness, visual hallucinations, prosopagnosia | Torcula, sagittal, and transverse sinus | Seizures, bleeding, CVST |
| Cerebellum | Nystagmus, ipsilateral limb ataxia with lateral lesions, truncal ataxia with midline lesions | Transverse sinus | Edema, obstructive hydrocephalus from fourth ventricle compression, CVST |

*CVST,* cerebral venous sinus thrombosis.

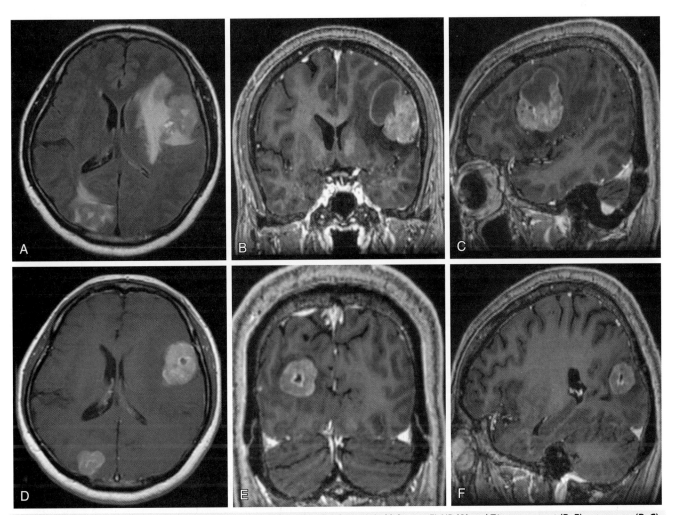

**Fig. 21.1** MRI images showing metastatic lesions in the left frontal and right occipital lobes on FLAIR **(A)** and T1 postcontrast **(B–F)** sequences. **(B–C)** Frontal lobe lesion affecting Broca's area, premotor, and supplementary motor cortex. **(E–F)** Occipital lesion compressing mostly the superior bank of the calcarine fissure, which corresponded to the patient's left inferior homonymous quadrantanopia.

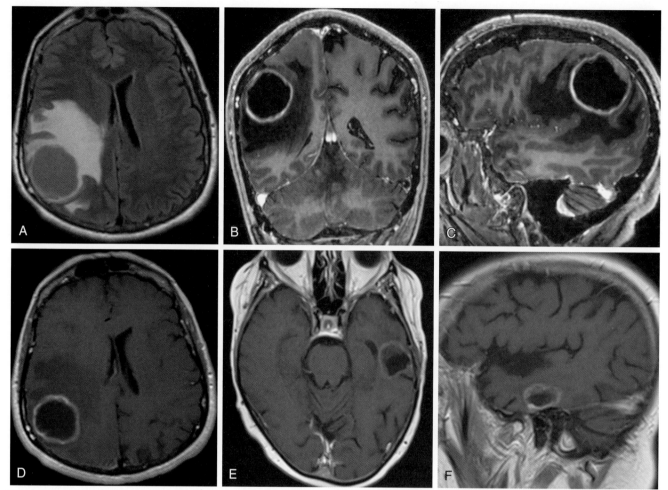

**Fig. 21.2** MRI images showing metastatic lesions in the right parietal and left temporal lobes on FLAIR **(A)** and T1 postcontrast **(B–F)** sequences. **(B–C)** Parietal lesion lobe lesion affecting predominantly the somatosensory cortex with edema extending into the superior parietal lobule. **(E–F)** Anterolateral temporal lobe lesion sparing receptive language areas of the superior temporal lobe gyrus.

## VENTRICULOSTOMY

### Key Concept

Preoperative ventriculostomy is utilized in patients with metastases in the posterior fossa to facilitate brain relaxation through intraoperative CSF drainage and to reduce the rate of pseudomeningocele formation.

Patients undergoing suboccipital craniotomy for resection of cerebellar metastases may require ventriculostomy placement. This aids safe resection by allowing for brain relaxation with intraoperative CSF diversion, but also may reduce rates of postoperative pseudomeningocele or CSF leak. If there is no concern for hydrocephalus or elevated ICP, the ventriculostomy may be weaned rapidly over 24 to 48 hours and removed prior to transitioning the patient from the ICU. Although not all posterior fossa craniotomies require prophylactic ventriculostomy, patients who will likely benefit from intraoperative drain placement are those with larger cerebellar lesions resulting in effacement of the fourth ventricle or descent of

the cerebellar tonsils with crowding at the foramen magnum. Importantly, vigilance for hydrocephalus should remain high in patients who have undergone posterior fossa metastasis resection who have a decline in neurological examination in the postoperative period. Most common symptoms of development of obstructive hydrocephalus are headache (with or without nausea or vomiting), blurred or double vision (secondary to cranial nerve VI paresis), sun setting of the eyes (or upgaze limitation), urinary incontinence, lethargy, drowsiness, irritability, and, if the patient is ambulating, gait difficulties. Timely imaging, ventriculostomy placement, and/or reexploration of the posterior fossa resection cavity can be critical for these patients.

### Clinical Pearl

Patients with posterior fossa metastasis are at risk for the development of hydrocephalus and pseudomeningocele that may require ventriculostomy and sometimes permanent CSF diversion (shunt) to treat.

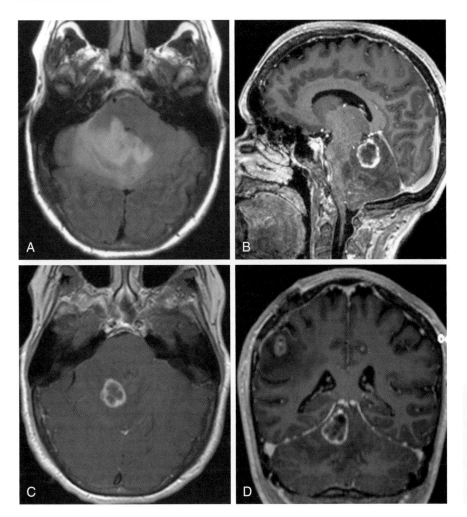

**Fig. 21.3** MRI images showing superior cerebellar metastasis on FLAIR **(A)** and T1 postcontrast **(B–D)** sequences. The fourth ventricle is effaced from mass effect produced by the surrounding edema. In coronal sections there is a second metastasis in the right parietal lobe **(D)**. Patient underwent ventriculoperitoneal shunt after resection due to persistent hydrocephalus (not shown).

## SEIZURE PROPHYLAXIS AND POSTOPERATIVE STEROIDS

### Key Concept

Patients are maintained on antiepileptics and steroids postoperatively, and these agents are tapered as allowed by the patient's clinical trajectory.

Routine prophylactic use of anticonvulsants is not recommended for patients with newly diagnosed brain metastases.[21] However, patients are often started on anticonvulsants preoperatively for supratentorial lesions and continued postoperatively, given concern for neocortical irritation after resection.[22] The choice of neuroleptic and the duration of treatment afterward in patients with no history of seizure can be individual surgeon and institution specific. In the absence of presenting seizures, some clinicians choose to use no neuroleptic prophylaxis. As mentioned earlier, fluctuating focal neurological examination changes corresponding to the site of surgery should raise concern for partial epilepsy phenomena, the diagnosis and treatment of which should be pursued aggressively.

Current guidelines recommend that asymptomatic patients with brain metastases do not need to be initiated on steroids, but symptomatic patients can be started on Decadron 4 to 8 mg/day, with up-titration to 16 mg/day.[23] Given that many patients who undergo craniotomy for metastasis resection normally present while on some level of steroid dosing, postoperatively patients can be tapered down on steroids in 4 to 14 days depending on the extent of decompression, residual intracranial disease, and concern for adrenal suppression. While patients are receiving exogenous steroids, it is important to supplement with an agent for gastrointestinal ulcer prophylaxis, such as a histamine antagonist or proton pump inhibitor.

## BLOOD PRESSURE MANAGEMENT

Patients undergoing craniotomy for tumor resection will usually have an arterial line placed perioperatively. This assists with titration of vasoactive agents during the procedure. Continued attention to blood pressure management postoperatively is important, especially in the first 24 hours after resection of a metastatic lesion. Perioperative hypertension increases risk of hemorrhage into the resection cavity by (1) disrupting hemostatic platelet plugs, (2) impairing cerebrovascular autoregulation, and (3) exploiting the disrupted blood–brain barrier in the resection cavity.[24] Basali et al. found that the median time for intracranial hemorrhage was 21 hours postoperatively. In this study, the odds ratio for postoperative hemorrhage was 4.6 for patients with systolic blood pressure (SBP) greater than 160 mm Hg.[25] Consequently, the SBP goal for the first postoperative day is 100 to 160 mm Hg or, more conservatively, 100 to 140 mm Hg. In patients with coronary artery disease or congestive heart failure, lower levels may be necessary. Titratable agents for hypertension include nicardipine and labetalol, whereas norepinephrine and Neo-Synephrine are the first-choice agents for pressors. Short-acting antihypertensive drugs (either IV infusion or orally administered), such as angiotensin-converting enzyme inhibitors, beta-blockers, and calcium channel blockers, are preferred given that blood pressure will usually return to baseline during the first 24 to 48 hours postcraniotomy.

## PAIN CONTROL

Pain management in the postoperative neurosurgical patient can be challenging because sedating agents can affect neurological assessments and lead to unnecessary imaging studies. Whereas the alert patient can be assessed directly for pain severity, the sedated patient may only declare inadequate analgesia by alterations in vital signs. However, tachycardia and hypertension may herald other underlying medical issues that merit evaluation prior to ascribing untreated pain as the etiology. These can be important considerations in this patient population because they typically will have other sites of systemic cancer and are thus at risk of systemic complications.

Narcotic pain medications such as morphine are often used with pain management given the ability to titrate dosing easily. Hydromorphone is synthesized as a hydrogenated ketone of morphine, and this lipophilicity allows for greater central nervous system penetration. Consequently, hydromorphone is 8 to 10 times more potent than morphine and is more difficult to titrate. An alternative strategy would be to provide patient-controlled analgesia with fentanyl, which has demonstrated improved efficacy compared with conventional as-needed therapy.[26] Nonsteroidal antiinflammatory agents are generally not used for pain control given the concern for impairing platelet function.

## MAINTAINING EUNATREMIA

Serum sodium concentration and osmotic gradient play a critical role in maintaining ICP and nervous system physiology. Neurosurgical patients are prone to fluctuations in serum sodium and will need to be monitored closely for these derangements because severe shifts in either direction can result in seizures, altered mental status, or coma. Hyponatremia in the setting of posterior fossa edema can precipitate a rapid downward cycle of localized swelling, obstructive hydrocephalus, and declining neurological examination.

The most common cause for hyponatremia in this population of patients is the syndrome of inappropriate release of antidiuretic hormone (SIADH), which results in retention of free water by renal collecting ducts. This represents a euvolemic state that can be noted by high urine osmolarity relative to serum osmolarity. The treatment of SIADH is fluid restriction and, in refractory cases, sodium supplementation through oral tablets or peripheral hypertonic saline infusions. Importantly, the correction of sodium should not be more rapid than 0.5 mEq/hour due to concern for central pontine myelinolysis. Cerebral salt wasting (CSW) also manifests as hyponatremia that can be difficult to distinguish from SIADH. CSW is a hypovolemic state that responds to fluid resuscitation. Hypernatremia can be a result of central diabetes insipidus from diminished antidiuretic hormone (ADH) release. This can be a consequence of manipulations of the hypothalamus or pituitary gland. The clinical syndrome is marked by high output of dilute urine, which requires repletion with isotonic normal saline. Desmopressin, a synthetic vasopressin analog, can be administered intranasally, orally, intravenously, or subcutaneously to augment this impaired endogenous secretion of ADH.

## VENOUS THROMBOEMBOLISM PROPHYLAXIS

Venous thromboembolism prophylaxis can be safely started 24 to 48 hours after elective craniotomy.[27,28] Prophylaxis is provided in the form of low-molecular-weight heparin and pneumatic compression boots worn continuously, with or without compression stockings. Patients with metastatic cancer are at increased risk of deep venous thrombosis (DVT)/pulmonary embolism, and without chemical prophylaxis, the incidence of DVT in neurosurgical patients has been quoted as high as 32%.[28]

## ANTIBIOTICS AND PREVENTION OF WOUND INFECTION

A metaanalysis of eight prospective trials confirmed that prophylactic antibiotics reduced postoperative wound infections by more than fourfold.[29] This effect was not dependent on coverage of gram-negative organisms or multiple dosings. The practice that is generally followed is administration of the initial dose within 30 to 60 minutes of incision followed by 24 hours of continued coverage. Gram-positive coverage with first-generation cephalosporin, or with vancomycin in patients with penicillin allergy, suffices for most cases. For resections of lesions where sinus mucosa may be encountered, gram-negative coverage is added with either third-generation or fourth-generation cephalosporin or aminoglycoside.

## TRANSITION FROM THE INTENSIVE CARE UNIT

Once patients undergoing elective craniotomy for tumor resection have been observed in the ICU for at least 6 hours and have been able to regain their preoperative neurological functioning, it would be reasonable to transfer care to the neurosurgical ward. Early mobilization of the patient has been shown to decrease postoperative complications. Depending on the patient's neurological status, early recruitment of physical therapists, occupational therapists, and case managers will also facilitate a shorter length of stay.

## References

1. Kimmell KT, LaSota E, Weil RJ, Marko NF. Comparative effectiveness analysis of treatment options for single brain metastasis. *World Neurosurg.* 2015;84(5):1316–1332.
2. Bertolini F, Spallanzani A, Fontana A, Depenni R, Luppi G. Brain metastases: an overview. *CNS Oncol.* 2015;4(1):37–46.
3. Patel AJ, Suki D, Hatiboglu MA, Rao VY, Fox BD, Sawaya R. Comparison between surgical resection and stereotactic radiosurgery in patients with a single brain metastasis from non-small cell lung cancer. *World Neurosurg.* 2015;83(6):900–906.
4. Buglione M, Pedretti S, Gipponi S, et al. Impact of surgical methodology on the complication rate and functional outcome of patients with a single brain metastasis. *J Neurosurg.* 2015;122(5):1132–1143.
5. Mert A, Buehler K, Sutherland GR, et al. Brain tumor surgery with 3-dimensional surface navigation. *Neurosurgery.* 2012;71(2 Suppl Operative):286–294.
6. Rava P, Ebner DK, Tybor DJ, et al. Predictors for long-term survival free from whole brain radiation therapy in patients treated with radiosurgery for limited brain metastases. *Front Oncol.* 2015;5:110.
7. Gorovets D, Rava P, Ebner DK, et al. The treatment of patients with 1-3 brain metastases: is there a place for whole brain radiotherapy alone, yet? A retrospective analysis. *Radiol Med.* 2015;120 (12):1146–1152.
8. Bowden G, Kano H, Caparosa E, et al. Gamma knife radiosurgery for the management of cerebral metastases from non-small cell lung cancer. *J Neurosurg.* 2015;122(4):766–772.
9. Kalkanis SN, Kondziolka D, Gaspar LE, et al. The role of surgical resection in the management of newly diagnosed brain metastases: a systematic review and evidence-based clinical practice guideline. *J Neurooncol.* 2010;96(1):33–43.
10. Lang FF, Sawaya R. Surgical treatment of metastatic brain tumors. *Semin Surg Oncol.* 1998;14(1):53–63.
11. Koyfman SA, Tendulkar RD, Chao ST, et al. Stereotactic radiosurgery for single brainstem metastases: the Cleveland Clinic experience. *Int J Radiat Oncol Biol Phys.* 2010;78(2):409–414.
12. Chaichana KL, Rao K, Gadkaree S, et al. Factors associated with survival and recurrence for patients undergoing surgery of cerebellar metastases. *Neurol Res.* 2014;36(1):13–25.
13. Hong N, Yoo H, Gwak HS, Shin SH, Lee SH. Outcome of surgical resection of symptomatic cerebral lesions in non-small cell lung cancer patients with multiple brain metastases. *Brain Tumor Res Treat.* 2013;1(2):64–70.
14. Schackert G, Lindner C, Petschke S, Leimert M, Kirsch M. Retrospective study of 127 surgically treated patients with multiple brain metastases: indication, prognostic factors, and outcome. *Acta Neurochir (Wien).* 2013;155(3):379–387.
15. Smith TR, Lall RR, Lall RR, et al. Survival after surgery and stereotactic radiosurgery for patients with multiple intracranial metastases: results of a single-center retrospective study. *J Neurosurg.* 2014;121 (4):839–845.
16. Nichol A, Ma R, Hsu F, et al. Volumetric radiosurgery for 1 to 10 brain metastases: a multicenter, single-arm, phase 2 study. *Int J Radiat Oncol Biol Phys.* 2016;94(2):312–321.
17. Bui JQH, Mendis RL, van Gelder JM, Sheridan MMP, Wright KM, Jaeger M. Is postoperative intensive care unit admission a prerequisite for elective craniotomy? *J Neurosurg.* 2011;115(6):1236–1241.
18. Hanak BW, Walcott BP, Nahed BV, et al. Postoperative intensive care unit requirements after elective craniotomy. *World Neurosurg.* 2014;81(1):165–172.
19. Taylor WA, Thomas NW, Wellings JA, Bell BA. Timing of postoperative intracranial hematoma development and implications for the best use of neurosurgical intensive care. *J Neurosurg.* 1995;82 (1):48–50.
20. Low D, Ng I, Ng W-H. Awake craniotomy under local anaesthesia and monitored conscious sedation for resection of brain tumours in eloquent cortex—outcomes in 20 patients. *Ann Acad Med Singapore.* 2007;36(5):326–331.
21. Mikkelsen T, Paleologos NA, Robinson PD, et al. The role of prophylactic anticonvulsants in the management of brain metastases: a systematic review and evidence-based clinical practice guideline. *J Neurooncol.* 2010;96(1):97–102.
22. Schwartz TH, Bazil CW, Forgione M, Bruce JN, Goodman RR. Do reactive post-resection "injury" spikes exist? *Epilepsia.* 2000; 41(11):1463–1468.
23. Ryken TC, McDermott M, Robinson PD, et al. The role of steroids in the management of brain metastases: a systematic review and evidence-based clinical practice guideline. *J Neurooncol.* 2010;96 (1):103–114.
24. Seifman MA, Lewis PM, Rosenfeld JV, Hwang PYK. Postoperative intracranial haemorrhage: a review. *Neurosurg Rev.* 2011; 34(4):393–407.
25. Basali A, Mascha EJ, Kalfas I, Schubert A. Relation between perioperative hypertension and intracranial hemorrhage after craniotomy. *Anesthesiology.* 2000;93(1):48–54.
26. Morad AH, Winters BD, Yaster M, et al. Efficacy of intravenous patient-controlled analgesia after supratentorial intracranial surgery: a prospective randomized controlled trial. Clinical article. *J Neurosurg.* 2009;111(2):343–350.
27. Cerrato D, Ariano C, Fiacchino F. Deep vein thrombosis and low-dose heparin prophylaxis in neurosurgical patients. *J Neurosurg.* 1978; 49(3):378–381.
28. Agnelli G, Piovella F, Buoncristiani P, et al. Enoxaparin plus compression stockings compared with compression stockings alone in the prevention of venous thromboembolism after elective neurosurgery. *N Engl J Med.* 1998;339(2):80–85.
29. Barker 2nd FG. Efficacy of prophylactic antibiotics for craniotomy: a meta-analysis. *Neurosurgery.* 1994;35(3):484–490. discussion 491–92.

# EPILEPSY SURGERY

# 22 *Standard Temporal Lobectomy*

MARK ATTIAH, PAULOMI BHALLA, VIVEK BUCH, and TIMOTHY LUCAS

## Introduction

### Key Concepts

- 2.3 million adults in United States have epilepsy, with one third resistant to medical treatment.
- Seventy-five percent to 80% of these patients who undergo resective surgery obtain seizure control.
- Preoperative and postoperative care of these patients present unique challenges and difficulties.

An estimated 2.3 million adults in the United States have epilepsy, and approximately one third have seizures that are resistant to medical therapy. In patients with a well-defined seizure focus, 75% to 80% of patients who undergo open surgical resection can obtain effective control of their seizures, an effect that has been shown to be durable up to 2 years by randomized control trials.[1,2]

Preoperative and postoperative care of the patient undergoing epilepsy surgery presents a unique set of challenges to both the neurosurgeon and the neurointensivist. Unlike other neurosurgical patients, epilepsy patients undergo extensive implantation of electrode arrays that reside in the subdural space or within the brain itself. Patients are, by definition, recalcitrant to antiepileptic medications and have frequent seizures that are difficult to control. Even before electrode implantation, these seizures often result in substantial personal injury. Patients also commonly suffer cognitive sequelae, both from their seizures and the near-toxic levels of antiseizure medications, clouding their baseline neurological examination. These factors make the care of the epilepsy surgery patient nuanced and beyond the scope of standardized intensive care unit (ICU) protocols developed for patients with head trauma or brain tumors. As such, this chapter aims to identify some of the core issues pertinent to the surgical and critical care team seeking to optimize care for this patient population.

### Clinical Pearl

Medically intractable epilepsy is a very difficult disease for patients and families to endure. Surgical therapy has been shown to be extremely safe and effective for controlling these seizures and can dramatically improve the quality of life for patients and their families. Once the diagnosis is made, early referral to a neurosurgeon is recommended to maximize the chance of gaining long-term seizure freedom.

## Neuroanatomy and Procedure

### Key Concepts

- Preoperative phase I identification of seizure foci includes imaging, neuropsychological assessments, and electrophysiological studies.
- Phase II studies consist of invasive electrophysiological recording from surgically implanted "grids and strips," which provide better resolution.
- Resection techniques, the most common being anterior temporal lobectomy, aim to maximize epileptogenic focus resection while minimizing potential damage to functional brain tissue and vital structures.
- Awake craniotomy for resection allows for better preservation of language, sensory, and motor functions, as well as immediate neurological examination postoperatively.
- New techniques, including laser-induced thermal therapy are currently being developed for minimally invasive ablation of seizure foci.

The overarching goal of epilepsy surgery, as with any neurological surgery, is to resect only the required amount of tissue necessary to achieve seizure control while preserving vital cognitive and neurological functions. This, of course, is dependent on the ability to identify an epileptogenic focus. The hunt for the focus requires characterization of the clinical seizure semiology, scalp electroencephalography (EEG), and specialized magnetic resonance imaging (MRI) (Fig. 22.1). In some instances, phase I evaluations include positron emission tomography (PET), ictal single photon-emission computed tomography, and magnetoencephalography. Neuropsychological assessments are performed during this phase of the workup. Psychiatric evaluation prior to surgery is often conducted because numerous studies have shown a lifetime prevalence of psychiatric disorders of up to 50% in patients with epilepsy.[3,4] Although data regarding the increased risk of postoperative seizures in this population are controversial, psychiatric evaluation can aid in the management of patients at highest risk of developing anxiety, depression, or aggressive behavior in the postoperative period.[5] If all of the previously mentioned data are concordant—that is, suggestive of the same seizure focus—patients may move directly to resective surgery.

Approximately 25% of patients[6] possess discordant or equivocal phase I evaluations. For these, "phase II" monitoring is indicated. Phase II monitoring consists of invasive EEG recordings. The use of subdural electrode arrays, or "grids," arose from the development of intraoperative electrocorticography (ECoG) techniques introduced by Foerster in the 1930s and further advanced by Penfield and Jasper

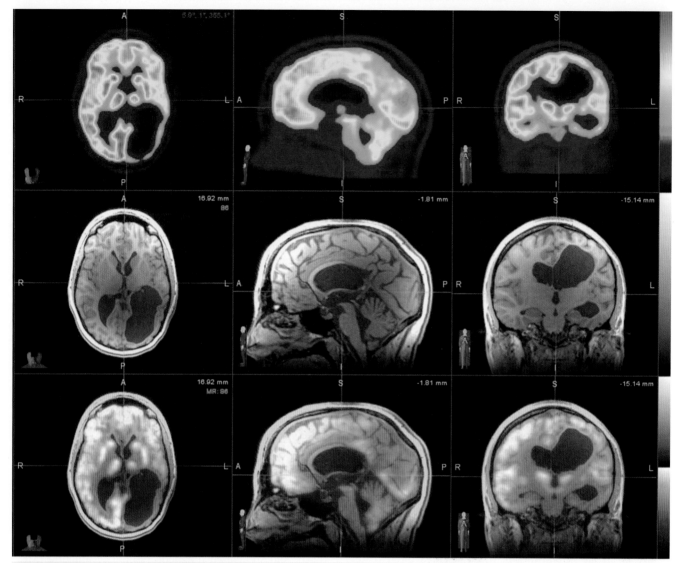

**Fig. 22.1** Epilepsy protocol MR-PET fusion. Specialized MR-PET fusion in a patient with seizures originating in the left posterior quadrant. Interictal Radiolabeled[18F]-2-fluoro-2-deoxy-D-glucose (FDG) PET shown in top row illustrates hypometabolism in the left parietal, temporal, and occipital regions. Middle row illustrates T1 weighted MR in the same planes as top column. Bottom row illustrates PET-MR fusion to highlight correspondence between hypometabolism and volumetric MR.

in the 1950s.[7] Using this type of technique, Talairach and Bancaud suggested that the so-called *epileptogenic zone* could be demarcated by recording the activity of neural populations during spontaneous seizures.[8-10]

The advantages to intracranial electrodes are numerous. First, the signal-to-noise ratio is superior to scalp electrodes because the skin, subcutaneous fat, muscle, bone, and dura act as an insulator to the neural signals. ECoG is therefore less susceptible to muscle artifact during tonic-clonic activity. The spatial resolution of the surface grids is finer as well, with interelectrode distances ranging between 5 mm and 1 cm. Finally, ECoG electrodes permit recordings from locations inaccessible from scalp EEG, such as the interhemispheric fissure, the depths of the hippocampus and amygdala, and the orbitofrontal cortex.

To complement cortical recording, depth electrodes may be implanted stereotactically to record activity in subcortical regions. This technique was initially developed as a tool to elucidate the role of basal nuclei in petit-mal and centrencephalic seizures.[11-13] Precise preoperative planning of array placement and depth electrode trajectory using computed tomography (CT) and MRI is crucial to avoid vascular structures, maneuver around eloquent cortical and subcortical regions, and provide the highest yield for possible seizure localization.

## Operative Procedure

Implantation of grid electrodes involves an initial operation where a wide craniotomy and durotomy expose the epileptogenic cortex (Fig. 22.2). Subdural grids are then laid across the area of interest with careful attention to the surface vasculature. Depth electrodes are penetrating electrodes that are advanced with the assistance of a semirigid stylet. These may be positioned stereotactically or on the basis of anatomical landmarks. The stylet is removed after implantation, and the depth electrode

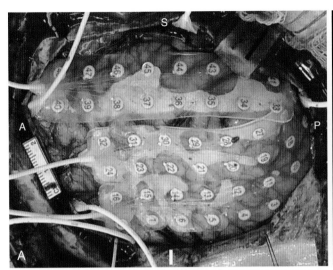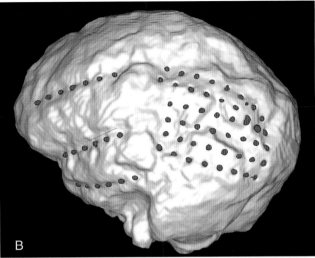

**Fig. 22.2** Intracranial electrodes. **(A)** Patient with posterior quadrant seizures undergoing grid and strip electrode implantation. Intraoperative photograph illustrating placement of electrodes relative to cerebral vasculature. **(B)** A surface render of the same patient using postoperative MR illustrates electrode positions (*red*) on a mask of the brain. *A*, anterior; *P*, posterior; *S*, superior; *I*, inferior.

remains within the brain parenchyma. Hybrid electrodes may be included. These have both macroelectrodes and microelectrodes ranging in size from 70 microns to 5 mm in diameter. At present, all Food and Drug Administration–approved arrays require the electrode tails to be tunneled out of the wound so that the electrodes may be connected to data acquisition systems. Several companies are testing wireless systems that aim to stream broadband neural recordings to wireless hubs located at the bedside. These devices will likely be available in the coming years.

Once the epileptogenic zone is identified, a number of approaches can be taken to resect it. The most common finding is mesial temporal lobe epilepsy, for which the most widely used resective procedure is the anterior temporal lobectomy (ATL) introduced by Falconer and Taylor in the 1960s.[14] For nondominant hemisphere surgery, ATL is performed asleep. For dominant hemisphere surgery, ATL is performed after intraoperative speech mapping. At our center, the neocortical portion of the anterior temporal lobe is removed en bloc to preserve the tissue architecture. The medial structures, including the amygdala and hippocampus, are then removed as separate specimens. At the conclusion of the dissection, the lateral midbrain, cerebral peduncle, posterior cerebral artery, and third cranial nerve are visible through the intact pia.

Awake craniotomy is indicated when the epileptogenic zone is near eloquent cortices such as the motor, sensory, or language cortex. Performing functional mapping ensures preservation of vital functions while optimizing the extent of resection.[15–18] Awake craniotomy allows for better preservation of language function, reduced permanent deficits, shorter length of stay in the hospital, fewer anesthesia-related complications, and reduced overall costs.[19–25] Further, seizure freedom rate is comparable to procedures under general anesthesia.[26] Successful mapping requires careful patient selection because patient cooperation is important for accurate mapping.[27,28] An added benefit of awake craniotomy is the ability to follow the neurological examination throughout the procedure and

immediately afterward. This avoids the difficult situation of ascertaining whether a slow return to neurological baseline after craniotomy is due to residual effects of anesthesia, neurological injury from surgery, or complications that developed after surgery. Awake patients are immediately examinable.

Beyond traditional craniotomy techniques, new techniques for treating intractable seizures are currently under investigation. Laser-induced thermal therapy promises to ablate epileptogenic zones by inducing focal tissue damage with radiant heat created by a laser.[29] This technique permits access to deep brain regions through small cranial burr holes. The reduced exposure may translate into shorter recovery times and lower morbidity profiles, although these hypotheses remain to be tested. As this treatment is developed, novel postoperative ICU protocols will need to be developed.

## Postoperative Complications

### Key Concepts

- Epilepsy surgery may result in complications including hematoma; stroke; cognitive, motor, and visual field deficits; cerebrospinal fluid (CSF) leak; infection; status epilepticus; and death.
- Visual field deficits are the most common postoperative complication and are due to disruption of the optic radiations.
- A dedicated ICU with well-trained nurses and health care practitioners is necessary to recognize and deal with potentially devastating postoperative complications.
- With vigilant care, epilepsy surgery is safe and effective.

Epilepsy surgery is highly successful in terms of seizure control.[1] Despite the marked success of epilepsy surgery, craniotomy for electrode implantation or brain resection is not without risk. Complications include hematoma, stroke,

---

**Box 22.1  Important Postoperative Complications**

Death
Hemorrhage/hematoma
Status epilepticus
Stroke/hemiparesis (anterior choroidal artery spasm or damage)
Visual field deficit
Cognitive deficit
Infection
Cerebrospinal fluid leak

---

cognitive deficit, cranial nerve deficit, visual field deficit, CSF leak, infection, status epilepticus, and death (Box 22.1). Appropriate postoperative care requires specific attention to the procedure performed. Patients must be carefully monitored in a neurological ICU in which the nursing staff is trained in detailed neurological examinations.

Neurological deficits in the perioperative period may have devastating consequences. Among the described deficits after epilepsy surgery are hemiparesis, cranial neuropathy, and visual field deficits. Hemiparesis may occur even in the most experienced hands. This complication is felt to be related to traction or spasm of the anterior choroidal artery during temporal lobe dissection.[30] Diplopia, a consequence of cranial nerve injury, is relatively common after epilepsy surgery. As many as 19% of patients experience at least transient double vision.[31,32] Traction or manipulation of the pia adjacent to the oculomotor or trochlear nerves is considered the likely etiology.[31] Importantly, oculomotor palsy is also an early sign of brain herniation. Critical care nurses and providers need to remain vigilant for these findings after surgery given these overlapping presentations.

Visual field deficits are the most common complication associated with temporal lobe resections, occurring in 55% to 75% of cases.[1,33] In a large number of patients, the extent of visual field loss is sufficient to prevent them from obtaining a driver's license.[34] Visual field loss is related to disruption of the optic radiations. Minimally invasive techniques have recently been developed to minimize the loss of vision after surgery.[35] Ongoing clinical trials will assess the degree to which minimally invasive techniques improve outcome.

Intracranial hemorrhage after electrode implantation is a recognized risk and estimated to be 0.5% to 4%.[36,37] Hematomas may arise in the epidural, subdural, and intracerebral locations. Hemorrhage is especially important to recognize because hematoma formation may lead to brain shift and herniation. It is our practice to perform a CT scan immediately after electrode implantation for this reason. As illustrated in the figure, epidural hematoma formation may be detected (Fig. 22.3) even in asymptomatic patients. Patients taking valproic acid are at higher risk of hemorrhage and must be observed very closely after surgery.[38] Patients should also be monitored for CSF leak at the site of lead placement and cerebral edema, because these have been associated with the use of multiple adjacent strips.[39] CT and MRI are obtained postoperatively. The complementing modalities permit coregistration of the electrode positions within the brain and permit evaluation of hemorrhagic complications.

Infection is another potential cause of morbidity in implanted patients. Meningitis, cerebritis, and abscess have the potential to cause lasting neurological deficits. A recent metaanalysis estimates incidence of pyogenic neurological infections at 2.3%, superficial infections at 3%, and positive CSF cultures at 7%.[40] Attempts to minimize infections vary with practice patterns across epilepsy centers. Surgeons often tunnel electrode tails away from the cranial incision to minimize the exchange of bacteria from the skin during monitoring. Attempts are made to minimize the duration of monitoring because duration is correlated with infection rate. One 17-year study noted that infection rates dropped from 18% to 6% from 1980 to 1997, which correlated with a shorter monitoring period with a median of 13 days to 9 days.[41] Some centers also employ prophylactic antibiotics throughout the monitoring phase, although this is not universal.

By definition, epilepsy patients suffer from intractable seizures. Postoperative seizures may be exacerbated by the physical and psychological stress of surgery. Thankfully, prolonged seizures, or status epilepticus, is relatively rare in this population,[42] in part due to the fact that they are under strict seizure observations. The management of seizures and antiepileptics should be guided in conjunction with an epileptologist. Established management protocols should be used to standardize "status" definitions and treatment algorithms in the ICU. Our policy is to administer benzodiazepines after two complex partial seizures within 1 hour, one generalized tonic-clonic seizure, or any seizure lasting longer than 3 minutes. Prior to admission, we also arrange a wean protocol on the patient's antiepileptic medications tailored to the individual's response to medications.

Postictal psychosis is a well-known psychiatric complication of temporal lobe epilepsy, generally presenting after a cluster of complex partial seizures or generalized tonic-clonic seizures[43] and often developing after a symptom-free period at 12 to 72 hours.[44] Current guidelines recommend treatment with antipsychotics, with treatment duration of 5 days for short episodes and up to 2 months for longer episodes.[45] Nonepileptic seizures, sometimes called *pseudoseizures*, can complicate care by being confused with electrographic events. Untrained personnel may inadvertently treat prolonged pseudoseizures as status, thus underscoring the need to have specific expertise in differentiating these two types of spells.

After an uneventful stay in the ICU, patients are moved to a dedicated epilepsy monitoring unit. Seizures are facilitated by the slow taper of antiepileptics and in some instances exposure to provocative measures like photic stimulation, hyperventilation, and sleep deprivation until a sufficient number of seizures is captured.

---

**Clinical Pearl**

The preoperative and postoperative care of epilepsy patients requires a highly dedicated, skilled, and knowledgeable ensemble of neurointensivists, neurosurgeons, and nursing staff. Standardized protocols at these various management levels should be implemented to help mediate some of the potential risks and complications of epilepsy surgery.

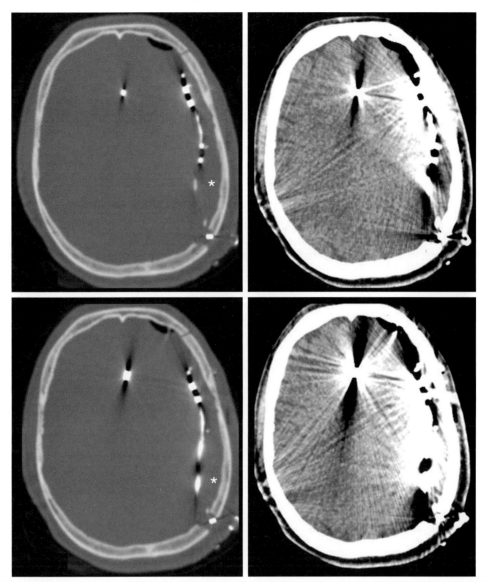

**Fig. 22.3** Postoperative epidural hematoma. Close postoperative surveillance is critical in epilepsy patients. This patient received a routine postoperative CT with bone windows illustrated on the left and brain windows illustrated on the right for two consecutive axial cuts. Electrode positions are best visualized on the bone windowing. As the top and bottom row illustrate, surface electrodes are pushed away from the bone surface (*), indicating epidural hematoma formation. Although the patient was asymptomatic, it was elected to return to the operating room for clot evacuation.

## Conclusions

The care of the epilepsy patient is nuanced and requires careful attention to problems unique to this patient group. Close relationships between the surgical and intensive care teams facilitate patient care. In controlled environments with well-trained teams, epilepsy surgery is safe and highly effective.

### References

1. Wiebe S, Blume WT, Girvin JP, Eliasziw M. Effectiveness and efficiency of surgery for temporal lobe epilepsy study group. A randomized, controlled trial of surgery for temporal-lobe epilepsy. *N Engl J Med*. 2001;345(5):311–318.
2. Téllez-Zenteno JF, Hernández Ronquillo L, Moien-Afshari F, Wiebe S. Surgical outcomes in lesional and non-lesional epilepsy: a systematic review and meta-analysis. *Epilepsy Res*. 2010;89(2-3):310–318.
3. Glosser G, Zwil AS, Glosser DS, O'Connor MJ, Sperling MR. Psychiatric aspects of temporal lobe epilepsy before and after anterior temporal lobectomy. *J Neurol Neurosurg Psychiatr*. 2000;68 (1):53–58.
4. Jones JE, Hermann BP, Barry JJ, Gilliam F, Kanner AM, Meador KJ. Clinical assessment of Axis I psychiatric morbidity in chronic epilepsy: a multicenter investigation. *J Neuropsychiatry Clin Neurosci*. 2005;17 (2):172–179.
5. Foong J, Flügel D. Psychiatric outcome of surgery for temporal lobe epilepsy and presurgical considerations. *Epilepsy Res*. 2007;75(2-3): 84–96.
6. Yuan J, Chen Y, Hirsch E. Intracranial electrodes in the presurgical evaluation of epilepsy. *Neurol Sci*. 2012;33(4):723–729.
7. Penfield W, Jasper H. *Epilepsy and the Functional Anatomy of the Human Brain*. Boston, Brown & Co: Little; 1954.
8. Rosenow F, Lüders H. Presurgical evaluation of epilepsy. *Brain*. 2001;124(Pt 9):1683–1700.
9. Centeno RS, Yacubian EMT, Caboclo LOSF, Júnior HC, Cavalheiro S. Intracranial depth electrodes implantation in the era of image-guided surgery. *Arq Neuropsiquiatr*. 2011;69(4):693–698.

10. Bancaud J, Talairach J. L'electroencephalographie de profondeur (S.E.E.G.) dans l'epilepsie. In: *Modern Problems of Pharmacopsychiatry-Epilepsy*. Basel: S. Karger. 1973;4:29–41.

11. Spiegel EA, Wycis HT, Reyes V. Diencephalic mechanisms in petit mal epilepsy. *Electroencephalogr Clin Neurophysiol*. 1951;3(4):473–475.

12. Jung R, Riechert T, Heines KD. Technique and value of operative electrocorticography and subcortical deduction of brain potentials. *Nervenarzt*. 1951;22(11):433–436.

13. Williams D, Parsons-Smith G. The spontaneous electrical activity of the human thalamus. *Brain*. 1949;72(3):450–482.

14. Falconer MA, Taylor DC. Surgical treatment of drug-resistant epilepsy due to mesial temporal sclerosis. Etiology and significance. *Arch Neurol*. 1968;19(4):353–361.

15. De Benedictis A, Moritz-Gasser S, Duffau H. Awake mapping optimizes the extent of resection for low-grade gliomas in eloquent areas. *Neurosurgery*. 2010;66(6):1074–1084. discussion 1084.

16. Reithmeier T, Krammer M, Gumprecht H, Gerstner W, Lumenta CB. Neuronavigation combined with electrophysiological monitoring for surgery of lesions in eloquent brain areas in 42 cases: a retrospective comparison of the neurological outcome and the quality of resection with a control group with similar lesions. *Minim Invasive Neurosurg*. 2003;46(2):65–71.

17. Duffau H, Lopes M, Arthuis F, et al. Contribution of intraoperative electrical stimulations in surgery of low grade gliomas: a comparative study between two series without (1985-96) and with (1996-2003) functional mapping in the same institution. *J Neurol Neurosurg Psychiatr*. 2005;76(6):845–851.

18. Sahjpaul RL. Awake craniotomy: controversies, indications and techniques in the surgical treatment of temporal lobe epilepsy. *Can J Neurol Sci*. 2000;27(Suppl 1):S55–S63. discussion S92–6.

19. Blanshard HJ, Chung F, Manninen PH, Taylor MD, Bernstein M. Awake craniotomy for removal of intracranial tumor: considerations for early discharge. *Anesth Analg*. 2001;92(1):89–94.

20. Danks RA, Rogers M, Aglio LS, Gugino LD, Black PM. Patient tolerance of craniotomy performed with the patient under local anesthesia and monitored conscious sedation. *Neurosurgery*. 1998;42(1):28–34. discussion 34–6.

21. Skucas AP, Artru AA. Anesthetic complications of awake craniotomies for epilepsy surgery. *Anesth Analg*. 2006;102(3):882–887.

22. Manninen PH, Tan TK. Postoperative nausea and vomiting after craniotomy for tumor surgery: a comparison between awake craniotomy and general anesthesia. *J Clin Anesth*. 2002;14(4):279–283.

23. Duffau H, Peggy Gatignol ST, Mandonnet E, Capelle L, Taillandier L. Intraoperative subcortical stimulation mapping of language pathways in a consecutive series of 115 patients with Grade II glioma in the left dominant hemisphere. *J Neurosurg*. 2008;109(3):461–471.

24. Serletis D, Bernstein M. Prospective study of awake craniotomy used routinely and nonselectively for supratentorial tumors. *J Neurosurg*. 2007;107(1):1–6.

25. Sanai N, Mirzadeh Z, Berger MS. Functional outcome after language mapping for glioma resection. *N Engl J Med*. 2008;358(1):18–27.

26. Kim CH, Chung CK, Lee SK. Longitudinal change in outcome of frontal lobe epilepsy surgery. *Neurosurgery*. 2010;67(5):1222–1229. discussion 1229.

27. Piccioni F, Fanzio M. Management of anesthesia in awake craniotomy. *Minerva Anestesiol*. 2008;74(7-8):393–408.

28. Sarang A, Dinsmore J. Anaesthesia for awake craniotomy—evolution of a technique that facilitates awake neurological testing. *Br J Anaesth*. 2003;90(2):161–165.

29. Tovar-Spinoza Z, Carter D, Ferrone D, Eksioglu Y, Huckins S. The use of MRI-guided laser-induced thermal ablation for epilepsy. *Childs Nerv Syst*. 2013;29(11):2089–2094.

30. Sasaki-Adams D, Hader EJ. Temporal lobe epilepsy surgery: surgical complications. In: *Textbook of epilepsy surgery*. London: Informa UK; 2008:1288–1298.

31. Cohen-Gadol AA, Leavitt JA, Lynch JJ, Marsh WR, Cascino GD. Prospective analysis of diplopia after anterior temporal lobectomy for mesial temporal lobe sclerosis. *J Neurosurg*. 2003;99(3):496–499.

32. Sindou M, Guenot M, Isnard J, Ryvlin P, Fischer C, Mauguière F. Temporo-mesial epilepsy surgery: outcome and complications in 100 consecutive adult patients. *Acta Neurochir (Wien)*. 2006;148(1):39–45.

33. Egan RA, Shults WT, So N, Burchiel K, Kellogg JX, Salinsky M. Visual field deficits in conventional anterior temporal lobectomy versus amygdalohippocampectomy. *Neurology*. 2000;55(12):1818–1822.

34. Manji H. Epilepsy surgery, visual fields, and driving: a study of the visual field criteria for driving in patients after temporal lobe epilepsy surgery with a comparison of goldmann and esterman perimetry. *Am J Ophthalmol*. 2000;129(5):704.

35. Chen HI, Bohman LE, Loevner LA, Lucas TH. Transorbital endoscopic amygdalohippocampectomy: a feasibility investigation. *J Neurosurg*. 2014;120(6):1428–1436.

36. McGonigal A, Bartolomei F, Regis J, et al. Stereoelectroencephalography in presurgical assessment of MRI-negative epilepsy. *Brain*. 2007;130(Pt 12):3169–3183.

37. Cossu M, Cardinale F, Castana L, et al. Stereoelectroencephalography in the presurgical evaluation of focal epilepsy: a retrospective analysis of 215 procedures. *Neurosurgery*. 2005;57(4):706–718. discussion 706–18.

38. Arya R, Mangano FT, Horn PS, Holland KD, Rose DF, Glauser TA. Adverse events related to extraoperative invasive EEG monitoring with subdural grid electrodes: a systematic review and meta-analysis. *Epilepsia*. 2013;54(5):828–839.

39. Winter SL, Kriel RL, Novacheck TF, Luxenberg MG, Leutgeb VJ, Erickson PA. Perioperative blood loss: the effect of valproate. *Pediatr Neurol*. 1996;15(1):19–22. Review.

40. Weinand ME, Oommen KJ. Lumbar cerebral spinal fluid drainage during long-term electrocorticographic monitoring with subdural strip electrodes: elimination of cerebral spinal fluid leak. *Seizure*. 1993;2(2):133–136.

41. Hamer HM, Morris HH, Mascha EJ, et al. Complications of invasive video-EEG monitoring with subdural grid electrodes. *Neurology*. 2002;58(1):97–103.

42. Hader WJ, Tellez-Zenteno J, Metcalfe A, et al. Complications of epilepsy surgery: a systematic review of focal surgical resections and invasive EEG monitoring. *Epilepsia*. 2013;54(5):840–847.

43. Logsdail SJ, Toone BK. Post-ictal psychoses. A clinical and phenomenological description. *Br J Psychiatry*. 1988;152:246–252.

44. Kanner AM, Stagno S, Kotagal P, Morris HH. Postictal psychiatric events during prolonged video-electroencephalographic monitoring studies. *Arch Neurol*. 1996;53(3):258–263.

45. Kerr MP, Mensah S, Besag F, de Toffol B, Ettinger A, Kanemoto K, et al. International consensus clinical practice statements for the treatment of neuropsychiatric conditions associated with epilepsy. *Epilepsia*. 2011;52(11):2133–2138.

# 23 Postoperative Care of the Epilepsy Patient with Invasive Monitoring

DANIEL J. DILORENZO, RICHARD W. BYRNE, and THOMAS P. BLECK

## Introduction

### Key Concept

Epilepsy is a relatively common disease with a high proportion of patients with seizures refractory to medical therapy. Seizure surgery may be a viable option for these patients and invasive monitoring may help identify these potential patients.

Epilepsy afflicts approximately 0.5% of the adult population,[1] with an estimated incidence of 150,000 new patients each year in the United States.[2] Approximately 40% of patients with epilepsy remain refractory to medical therapy.[3] From this population, a subset may be identified for whom surgical intervention holds the potential for improved quality of life and seizure freedom.[4,5]

The identification and localization of the seizure focus are not always readily determined by noninvasive workup comprising clinical presentation, imaging, and electroencephalogram studies. Therefore craniotomy with subacute placement of and recording from stereotactically placed depth electrodes and subdural strip and grid electrodes may be required. Depth electrodes may concurrently be placed through a craniotomy or through a burr hole.

Localization of seizure foci using these invasive electrode recording techniques facilitates good surgical and clinical outcomes from resective surgery.[6–11] With appropriate patient selection, outcomes exceeding 70% to 80% rates of seizure freedom can be achieved in temporal lobe epilepsy treated with temporal lobe resection,[12] greater than 50% in extratemporal resective surgery,[13] and up to 80% in completely resected cortical dysplasia. Fig. 23.1 depicts a sample of subdural and depth electrodes used for this purpose.

Patients undergoing these procedures endure the risk of surgical complications, including infection, intracranial hemorrhage (ICH), extraaxial fluid collections, cerebrospinal fluid (CSF) leaks, and others. Furthermore, patients are at risk for secondary medical complications due to immobility in the postoperative period, including deep venous thrombosis (DVT) and possible pulmonary embolus (PE). Although the reported complication rates vary significantly, data suggest 1) improvement over time and with cumulative experience and 2) a dependency on surgical technique and perioperative care.[14] Data regarding surgical technique and perioperative management protocols from other institutions, as well as from a recent review

and technical analysis from ours, are integrated in this chapter with the objective of presenting a protocol in which management is optimized to minimize complication rates.

By strict adherence to meticulous operative technique and diligent perioperative care, low complication rates may be achieved.[14] In this chapter, we attempt to outline the salient protocols for achievement of low complication rates and for proper management of complications when they do occur.

## Neuroanatomy and Procedure

### Key Concept

Electrodes are implanted superficially via craniotomy into the subdural space ipsilateral to the seizure focus. Strips represent a single row of electrodes whereas a grid represents multiple rows of electrodes. Depth electrodes are placed deep into parenchymal structures thought to be the culprit epileptic focus.

### NEUROANATOMY

Electrode grids and strips are usually implanted in the subdural space; this provides the optimal signal-to-noise and signal frequency characteristics for surface signal recording. These electrodes facilitate mapping of cortical activity and are helpful in the preoperative assessment of the location of the seizure source and in planning the extent of resection.

Depth electrodes are usually placed into deep structures suspected of being involved in the seizure source. Bancaud, Talairach, and colleagues first described the stereotactic technique for the placement of depth electrodes.[15,16] Common locations include the hippocampus and the adjacent white-matter tracts. Depth electrodes may also be placed into regions of cortical dysplasia or other suspected foci.

### OVERVIEW OF SURGICAL PROCEDURE

A multiplicity of surgical procedures and variations thereof may be used for implantation of subdural electrodes. The preferred technique used at our institution is summarized next.

Implantation of subdural grids and usually that of subdural strips requires the use of a craniotomy to provide sufficient exposure for safe implantation. For temporal lobe monitoring, a modified Yasargil incision is made in the

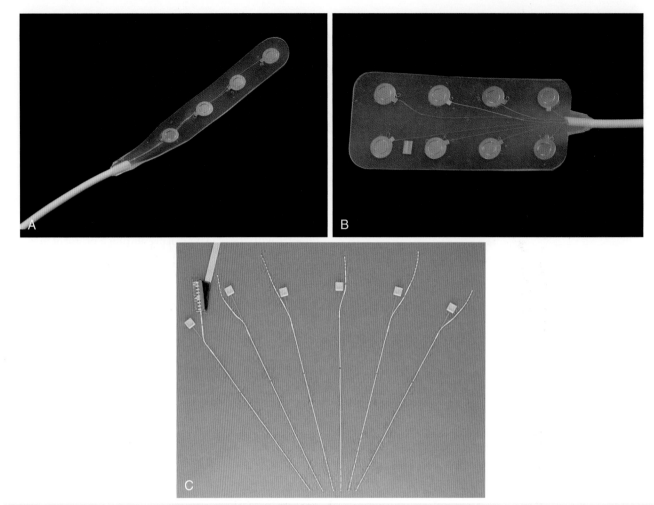

Fig. 23.1 Sets of commercially available subdural grid, subdural strips, and depth electrodes. **(A)** subdural strip electrode (4 × 1 configuration shown). **(B)** Subdural grid electrode (4 × 2 configuration shown). **(C)** Depth electrodes attached to stylets with the leftmost electrode array connected to monitoring connector and cable. (Courtesy of Ad-Tech Medical Instrument Corporation, Racine, WI, USA.)

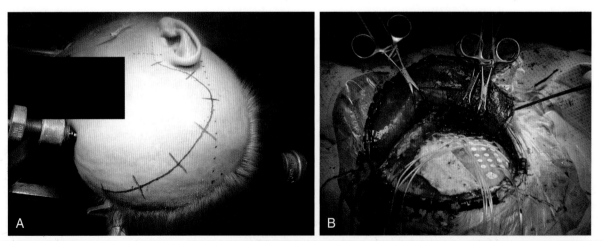

Fig. 23.2 Surgical exposure and electrode positioning. **(A)** Immediately prior to prepping and draping, the skin marking indicating the path of the planned scalp incision, beginning above the tragus to minimize risk to the superficial temporal artery (STA) and extending superiorly and anteriorly to terminate between the superior temporal line and the midline and behind the hairline. **(B)** Electrodes are positioned in their appropriate locations on the surface of the brain, and the emanating electrical cables are arranged to course in an approximately straight trajectory to the percutaneous exit sites in order to minimize torque applied to the electrodes and consequent angular movement against the brain surface.

scalp, as shown in Fig. 23.2A. A frontotemporal craniotomy is performed to expose the lateral temporal lobe and inferior portions of the posterior frontal lobe and anterior parietal lobe.

Subdural electrodes are carefully placed on the surface of the cortex of interest as shown in Fig. 23.2B. At our institution, for temporal lobe epilepsy, this generally involves an anterior and posterior laterobasal subdural strip and a subdural grid placed over the lateral temporal lobe and extending across the sylvian fissure to include at least one row of suprasylvian electrodes covering the inferior posterior frontal lobe and inferior anterior parietal lobe.

Implantation of depth electrodes may be performed concurrently with that of subdural electrodes, making use of the exposure afforded by the craniotomy; or they may be placed separately through burr holes using stereotactic technique. In the former, the depth electrodes are inserted through the exposed cortex, often through the lateral temporal convexity through a portion of the insular cortex carefully exposed for this purpose, and directed anteriorly to the hippocampus or immediately adjacent white matter. Alternately, depth electrodes may be inserted through an occipital burr hole and directed anteriorly to the hippocampus using fluoroscopic or stereotactic navigation.

Subdural electrodes are mechanically secured to the overlying dura, minimizing the likelihood of subsequent movement during closure and the perioperative and subsequent inpatient monitoring periods. The wires are kept grouped together and positioned in a loop, which is then sutured to the skin surface, and a subgaleal drain is then placed. In Fig. 23.3, the emanating electrical wires and drain are seen in the subgaleal space prior to closure with percutaneous passage through the scalp. Fig. 23.4 shows the scalp after closure with wires and drain secured to the scalp with sutures.

After being transported to the neurology intensive care unit (Neuro ICU), the patient is taken for a routine noncontrast head computed tomograph (CT) to confirm intracranial electrode location as well as absence of hematoma. A typical such imaging study is shown in Fig. 23.5, demonstrating some mass effect from the grid electrodes and surrounding extraaxial fluid. The patient is continued on perioperative antibiotics beyond the standard 24-hour duration and kept on these antibiotics for the duration, during which these percutaneous wires and implanted electrodes remain.

The method of stereoelectroencephalography (SEEG), originally developed by Talairach and Bancaud, has evolved with advances in stereotactic technique and neuroradiological imaging modalities.[17,18] The technique varies as a function of whether a craniotomy is performed concurrently for placement of subdural electrodes and as a function of the target location. Preoperative stereotactic magnetic resonance imaging (MRI) is performed, and preoperative angiography may also be performed. These images are either performed with a stereotactic frame in place, or they are registered to the patient intraoperatively using fiducial markers or skin surface registration techniques.[17,18] Trajectories are planned using three-dimensional surgical navigation planning software to reach the desired target while avoiding arterial and venous structures. The patient is positioned with the head rigidly fixed, either directly to the operating room (OR) table using a Mayfield frame and pins or using

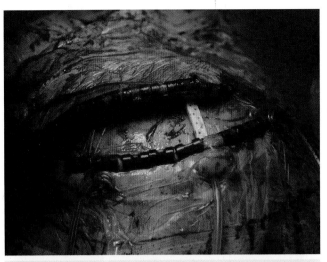

**Fig. 23.3** Intraoperative photograph after placement and suturing of electrode cable and placement of drain prior to closing of scalp. The subgaleal location of the extracranial segments of the wire and of the subgaleal drain is appreciated.

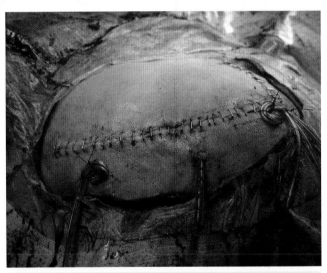

**Fig. 23.4** The scalp has been closed in two layers with a galeal stitch and staples, and the two electrical cables and the subgaleal drain are seen secured to the scalp with sutures.

a stereotactic frame, which is then rigidly attached to the OR table. The skin overlying the planned entry site is incised, and a burr hole is made using a twist drill or a powered drill with a cranial perforator bit. The dura is then opened with a surgical blade or with monopolar electrocautery. The cortical surface and overlying pia are then coagulated at the planned entry site with electrocautery. The depth electrode is affixed to a stereotactic insertion cannula and advanced to the target depth. Either fluoroscopy or optical tracking with 3D navigation may be used to monitor the trajectory and depth. Once the depth electrode has been confirmed to be at target, the depth electrode stylet is removed, leaving the depth electrode in place. The skin is closed, and the extracranial portion of the depth electrode is sutured to the scalp. Postoperative CT is performed to confirm positioning of the depth electrodes.[17–19]

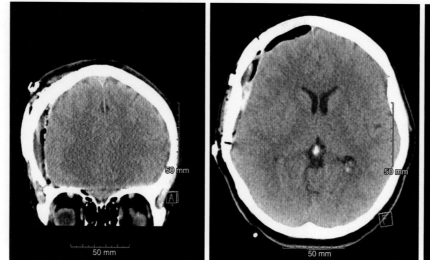
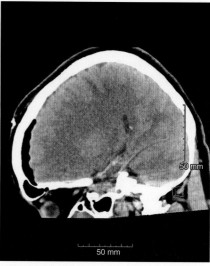

**Fig. 23.5** Postoperative CT taken on postoperative day #0 shortly after arrival to the neurosurgical ICU from the OR. Small extraaxial fluid collection with asymptomatic local mass effect and some midline shift is seen.

Placement of intracranial monitoring electrodes presently comprises the implantation and subsequent removal of subdural or epidural grid electrodes and strip electrodes, intraparenchymal depth electrodes, transsphenoidal foramen ovale electrodes, and epidural peg electrodes. Newer approaches recently reported involve the use of chronically implanted stimulation and recording systems for long-term characterization of neural activity and seizure source localization.[20] The NeuroPace Responsive Neurostimulation System system[21,22] (approved by Food and Drug Administration in November 2013) performs long-term monitoring and seizure detection and termination. The NeuroVista Seizure Advisory System (under development,[23] FIM (first in man) published 2013[24]) performs chronic monitoring and seizure likelihood warning or prediction.[25,26] Each of these and others in development may be used for chronic monitoring.

## Perioperative Considerations

### Key Concept

Adequate hemostasis is critical to strips and grids placement, as bleeding may be a complication of the surgery. Initial postoperative CT does not correlate with bleeding and may thus be obviated. Clinical symptoms (e.g. headache) are more suggestive of bleeding and warrant neuroimaging. Impeccable care of the head wrap and electrode wires are mandatory to avoid dislodgement in the post-operative period.

Meticulous operative technique is employed to ensure excellent hemostasis intraoperatively and during closure, and placement of a subgaleal drain provides some protection should oozing from the scalp develop during suturing or after closure. In a series of 127 patients, 1 (0.5%) developed a postoperative hemorrhage, and this presented as severe headache and speech difficulty on postoperative day (POD) #3 and was promptly confirmed that same day on head CT and prompted evacuation of subdural hematoma and removal of electrodes.[14] The delayed presentation of postoperative

hemorrhages was similarly described in a series of 40 children (average age 11.4 years).[27] Their findings suggested that the initial postoperative CT is not predictive of postoperative hemorrhage or significant midline shift, a mean of 4 mm of which was seen and usually without sequelae. In their series, two (5%) patients required surgery for evacuation of hematoma, and this was demonstrated on CT on POD #2 and #4.[27] MRI is not used in this capacity because it is slower, limited by susceptibility artifact, and was shown in a small series to demonstrate multiple clinically silent abnormalities, including small subdural hematomas (35%), cortical contusions (25%), local edema (25%), transburr hole cortical herniation (25%), and subdural hygromas (10%).[28]

Operative dressing includes a head wrap, which provides some mechanical protection of the percutaneous electrical wires. Strict attention to detail by the treating physicians and nurses is critical to ensure that patient movement and transfers (such as for imaging studies and activities of daily living while in the hospital) do not dislodge the wires. Dressing changes are most safely performed by the neurosurgical team, preferably one of the members present during surgery. Cables are best secured to the patient with tape or a harness, if available, to minimize tension on the percutaneous portions of the wires. Use of safety mittens and arm restraints on the patient may be used to reduce the likelihood of inadvertent dislodgment or removal of the electrodes by the patient. Seizure safety precautions, including the use of bed padding, are routinely used. Monitoring with video electroencephalography with telemetry is also used.

In the immediate postoperative period, the most threatening complication is hemorrhage, which could comprise a rapidly expanding space-occupying lesion. For this reason and to confirm electrode placement, a postoperative head CT is routinely performed once the patient has returned to the NICU. If a subsequent decline in clinical examination is detected, a head CT is repeated to detect or to rule out delayed hemorrhage or edema.

Postoperative reduction of hemorrhage risk is achieved through tight blood pressure control with systolic blood pressure usually maintained below 140 to 160 mm Hg depending on the surgeon or institution.

## Clinical Pearls

- Careful attention should be paid to the tension placed on the monitoring cables to avoid breakage and intracranial electrode movement.
- Surgical team members should perform all dressing changes.
- Serial monitoring should be performed to assess for neurological changes reflective of hemorrhage, which are most noticed several days after surgery.

## Postoperative Complications

The first systematic study of the use of subdural strip electrodes was published by Wyler et al. in 1984,[6] and the reported overall complication rate was 0.85%.[7] Subsequent literature has reported variable complication rates ranging from 0.85%[7] to as high as 26.3%.[10,29] In 2000 Hamer et al. reported one of the highest overall complication rates based upon an analysis of cases performed over a 17-year span (1980–1997) at a single institution.[10] This comprehensive study, which includes cases performed over 30 years ago, demonstrated a dramatic improvement in complication rates over this time span, beginning with an initial complication rate of 33% (1980–1991 cases), which improved to 19% (1992–1997 cases), and which continued to improve to 13.5% (1994–1997).[10] This improvement was attributed to the combination of improvements in grid technology, surgical technique, and postoperative care.[10] A metaanalysis published in 2013 by Arya et al. reviewed 21 studies totaling 2542 patients and demonstrated significant complication rates for the majority of a set of specific adverse events that were studied.[30] Pooled prevalence rates of the major complications included pyogenic infections 2.3% (with 95% confidence interval [CI] of 1.5%–3.1%), superficial infections 3.0% (with 95% CI of 1.9%–4.1%), hemorrhage 4.0% (with 95% CI of 3.2%–4.8%), hemorrhage requiring surgery for evacuation 3.5% (with 95% CI of 2.8%–4.2%), elevated intracranial pressure (ICP) 2.4% (with 95% CI of 1.5%–3.3%), and CSF leaks 12.1% (with 95% CI of 9.3%–14.9%).[30] Our institution published a series of 127 patients in which the technique described herein was utilized and which demonstrates a lower complication rate.[14]

Major complications include infection (superficial and neurological), hemorrhage (ICH, subdural hemorrhage [SDH], and epidural hematoma [EDH]), edema and elevated ICP, CSF leak, and hardware failure. Rates for these complications are shown in Table 23.1, and sections describing their prevention, early detection, and treatment are presented separately later. Whether transient neurological deficits should be considered complications is controversial. Transient neurological deficits are anticipated when performing surgery on or near eloquent neurological structures and may be inconsequential or clinically silent when near less eloquent areas.[14,31] Such expected transient side effects may be analogous to postoperative ileus and third spacing after general surgical procedures.

Complication rates from subdural electrode placement correlate strongly with increased duration of monitoring,[32]

number of grids,[32] number of electrodes,[33] size of grids,[33] left-sided grids,[32] implantation of electrodes over the left or the right central convexity surface,[33] presence of burr holes in addition to craniotomy,[32] and earlier chronological year of monitoring.[32] Complications may increase with electrode counts in excess of 60,[32] and in patients who have previously received high dose radiation therapy to the brain.[34] Complication rates increase approximately linearly with monitoring time, with the sharpest rise between 8 and 10 days.[32]

Depth electrodes have lower complication rates than subdural electrodes (0 serious complications in 68 patients with 136 electrodes in Behrens et al. 1997).[31] Strip electrodes have lower complication rates than grid electrodes or grid and strip combinations, and this is attributed to the greater tendency of grids to fold and buckle resulting in mass effect.[35] Complication rates for interhemispheric grid electrodes are less well characterized; Bekelis et al. reported an infection rate of 4% (2 of 50 patients).[36] Reported complication rates with depth electrodes vary from zero (0/100 infections and 1/100 asymptomatic hemorrhage)[37] to 2.4%.[18]

### Infection

Infectious complications span the spectrum from minor superficial ones to pyogenic abscesses and deep infections. Superficial infections may require treatments such as debridement of scalp infections and cranioplasty for osteomyelitis.[32,38–41] Pyogenic infections encountered in invasive epilepsy monitoring include bacterial meningitis, implantation-site abscesses, brain abscesses, subdural empyemas, and cerebritis.[14,29,32,41–46] These infections require craniotomy for wash-out and debridement or craniectomy for cerebral edema and intracranial hypertension.

Rates of infection of superficial tissues average 3% (95% CI 1.9%–4.1%, including 31 of 1342 patients), and rates of infection of neurological tissue average 2.3% (95% CI 1.5%–3.1%, including 31 of 1342 patients).[30] Rates of infection decrease with surgical experience. Wellmer et al. noted a lower infection rate of 1.12%, with three infections involving neural tissue (two cases of meningitis and one case of empyema) among 260 patients,[46] representing a substantial reduction in infection rate from 1.4% (in 4 of 279 electrode implantation cases) in a previous series from the same institution.[31,47]

Risk factors for infection include duration of operative case, duration of percutaneous intracranial monitoring, and number of electrodes. Implantation of more than 100 electrodes,[48] size of grid,[33] presence of more than 10 percutaneous cables,[48] placement of more than one cable exit site,[48] and study duration exceeding 14 days[48] have been shown to be risk factors for a positive epidural culture.[48] In a series of 429 cases (including diagnostic and therapeutic procedures) infectious complication rates were found to decline substantially over time, decreasing from 13.2% in 1987–1998 to 0% in 1993–1994 amid accumulating experience and growing clinical volumes (38 and 109, respectively).[31,47] Compromise of the superior temporal artery is believed to also be a risk factor and to contribute to scalp breakdown and consequent

**Table 23.1** Complication Rates from Subdural Electrode Placement

| | METAANALYSIS[30] | | | | | | RUMC 2014 SERIES[30] | | |
| | | | | | 95% CI | | | | |
| Complications | N | n | Incidence Mean % | σ | Low | High | N | n | Incidence % |
|---|---|---|---|---|---|---|---|---|---|
| **Infection** | | | | | | | | | |
| Superficial infection | 1010 | 30 | 3.0% | 0.56% | 1.9% | 4.1% | 127 | 1 | 0.8% |
| Neurological tissue infection | 1342 | 31 | 2.3% | 0.41% | 1.5% | 3.1% | 127 | 0 | 0.0% |
| **Hemorrhage (with neurological deficit requiring surgery)** | | | | | | | | | |
| Symptomatic and/or requiring surgery | 2356 | 34 | 1.4% | | | | 127 | 1 | 0.8% |
| Requiring surgery for evacuation (with focal neurological deficit) | 794 | 28 | 3.5% | 0.36% | 2.8% | 4.2% | 127 | 1 | 0.8% |
| Total | 2356 | 94 | 4.0% | 0.41% | 3.2% | 4.8% | 127 | 1 | 0.8% |
| CSF leak | 514 | 62 | 12.1% | 1.43% | 9.3% | 14.9% | 127 | 0 | 0.0% |
| Elevated ICP | 1090 | 26 | 2.4% | 0.46% | 1.5% | 3.3% | 127 | 0 | 0.0% |
| Permanent sequelae | 189 | 3 | | | | | 127 | 0 | 0.0% |
| Mortality | 2542 | 5 | | | | | 127 | 0 | 0.0% |
| **Deep venous thrombosis (DVT)** | | | | | | | | | |
| Among studies in which DVT was specifically reported | 447 | 5 | 1.1% | | | | 127 | 1 | 0.8% |
| Among all studies (may not fully represent the DVT incidence) | 1245 | 5 | 0.4% | | | | | | |
| **Pulmonary embolus (PE)** | | | | | | | | | |
| Among studies in which DVT was specifically reported | 447 | 2 | 0.4% | | | | 127 | 2 | 1.6% |
| Among all studies (may not fully represent the DVT incidence) | 1245 | 2 | 0.2% | | | | | | |

infection.[14] Nonsurgical factors, including extremes of age, presence of diabetes, immunocompromised state, and other medical conditions, also contribute to increased infection risk. Early diagnosis requires close monitoring of temperature for fever, sampling or following of white blood cells (WBCs) when indicated, examination of the incision sites for erythema or drainage, and close inspection of the electrodes during intraoperative removal.

The prevention of CSF leak through the incision site or through the percutaneous electrical cable passage sites is one of the most important technical approaches to reduce infection rates. CSF leaks are associated with elevated infection rates in skull-base neurosurgery,[49] and others have postulated the association between CSF leak and infection during invasive monitoring.[50] At our center, surgical technique is specifically tailored to minimize CSF leak by closing the dura, replacing the craniotomy flap, using a head dress to apply pressure to the scalp, and placement of a subgaleal percutaneous drain to provide a CSF diversion, virtually eliminating the risk of CSF flow through the scalp craniotomy or percutaneous cable incisions.[14] We also uniformly administer intravenous antibiotics for the full duration of percutaneous monitoring and for the 24-hour postoperative period after their removal.

For patients in whom no infection is clinically apparent at the time of electrode removal, successful resection at that time without sequelae has been reported even in patients in whom routine intraoperative epidural culture results subsequently came back positive.[48] In patients with evidence of infection at the time of electrode removal, treatment with intravenous antibiotics and delayed epileptic focus resection has produced successful clinical outcomes.[48]

## Hemorrhage

Hemorrhagic complications include SDH, EDH, ICH, and subgaleal hemorrhages. Overall rates of hemorrhage requiring surgery average 4.0% (95% CI 3.2%–4.8%).[30] Johnston reported higher rates of hemorrhage requiring decompression of 16% and 14%, respectively, during time intervals of 1985 to 1993 and of 2002 to 2008; notably no significant improvement in this complication rate was observed.[39] In a series of 127 patients from our institution, hemorrhage requiring surgery occurred in 1 (0.8%) patient.[14] Delayed hemorrhage after SEEG attributed to the development and rupture of a pseudoaneurysm related to electrode implantation has been reported.[51]

Perioperative risk factors for hemorrhage include baseline hypertension and perioperative hypertension. Comorbidities, including coagulopathies, functional or quantitative thrombocytopenia, and the use of antithrombotic agents (aspirin, clopidogrel, warfarin, and newer oral anticoagulants, such as dabigatran, rivaroxaban, and apixaban), are risk factors and should be treated and avoided. A detailed history regarding the use of herbal medications with antithrombotic properties should be specifically obtained; these medications should be discontinued at least 1 to 2 weeks in advance if used.

Clinically significant hemorrhage is usually first detected with a change in mental status or in the neurological examination. This is an important justification for the routinely close monitoring of patients in the epilepsy monitoring unit (EMU). At our institution, we perform a postoperative CT on POD #0, usually within an hour of arrival to the NICU from the OR. This is performed to confirm placement and to detect acute hemorrhage. In the absence of clinical change, no further imaging is performed. If a clinical change is detected, a head CT is immediately performed.

Postoperative imaging often demonstrates extraaxial fluid collections of unclear significance.[52] Interpretation of routine postoperative imaging is complicated by significant streak artifact from the metal electrodes. This may be improved with the use of bone windows rather than brain windows, although this may not definitively characterize the type of fluid or adequately localize the source of the collection.[52] MRI imaging has been shown to provide better visualization due to the more focally constrained susceptibility artifacts from the electrodes in comparison to the streak artifact from CT; however, MRI is more time consuming, expensive, and has been shown to commonly demonstrate findings (such as subdural hematomas, cortical contusions, local edema, transburr hole cortical herniation, subdural hygroma, and pneumocranium) that are not of clinical significance.[28]

Careful intraoperative technique and meticulous attention to hemostasis are crucial to reduce the risk of hemorrhage. Blood pressure should be monitored and aggressively treated if elevated. Avoidance of antiplatelet and anticoagulant medications is paramount. When hemorrhage is detected in the context of a clinical change, usually of a decrease in mental status or the development of a focal neurological deficit, prompt operative decompression is indicated and should be performed.

## Elevated Intracranial Pressure and Cerebral Edema

Symptomatic elevations in ICP occur in approximately 2.5% (26/1090) of patients.[30] At our institution, intracranial hypertension after strip and grid placement is extremely rare (0%) and may be attributed to the use of several techniques described later.[14] Elevated ICP may be associated with transtentorial or subfalcine herniation.[41]

Risk factors for elevated ICP and edema include use of large grids and more electrodes. Of the 2 fatalities (among 71 patients) reported by Wong et al., both had more than 100 electrodes (112 and 128 subdural electrodes, over the right and left frontoparietal regions, respectively, each over regions of encephalomalacia).[33] Seizures also increase the risk of cerebral edema and elevated ICP. However, antiseizure medications are intentionally decreased in these patients to induce seizures in the EMU, potentially promoting the development of cerebral edema and elevated ICP.[35]

Seizures result in transient increases in cerebral blood flow, thereby increasing blood volume and consequently increasing ICP. Transient elevations in ICP have been demonstrated after generalized tonic-clonic seizures.[35]

In a pediatric series, baseline ICP after subdural electrode placement has been shown to increase with the age of a child (approximately from 5–20 mm Hg as age increases from approximately 1–16).[35] The magnitude of ICP elevation during a seizure is related to the extent of seizure spread.[35] Risk factors include frequent seizures, presence of secondarily generalized tonic-clonic seizures, and older children within the pediatric population.[35]

### Clinical Pearls

- Complication rates are lower with shorter duration of monitoring, fewer number of electrodes, and fewer number/smaller size of grids.
- Infection rates are lower for shorter duration of percutaneous intracranial monitoring, fewer number of electrodes, smaller size of grid, presence of 10 or fewer percutaneous cables, placement of one cable exit site, and duration of study of 14 or fewer days.
- Rates for developing elevated ICP or cerebral edema are lower for smaller grids and fewer electrodes.
- Transient neurological deficits from edema and elevated ICP may develop within the first 24 hours and persist for more than a week.

Clinically significant elevation of ICP or cerebral edema manifests as a change in mental status or in the neurological examination and is a reason for routinely close monitoring of patients in the EMU. If a clinical change is detected, a head CT is immediately performed. Cases of fatal progression of elevated ICP resulting in death within 48 hours and unresponsive to decompressive surgery with electrode removal have been reported.[33] Similarly, a report has been published of a 26 year old man with implantation of 94 subdural electrodes who subsequently developed a stroke complicated by intracranial hypertension, transtentorial herniation, coma and death.[34] Therefore, careful attention to the preoperative examination and to serial examinations may prevent erroneous misinterpretation of deficits as being postictal in nature, which could otherwise lead to delayed detection of a progressive neurological deficit and larger impending problem.[33] Careful neurological examination of the postictal patient is warranted because mild preictal elevations in ICP may be exacerbated by seizures[35] or by periictal apnea, leading to a progressive decline, which may be partially masked by the postictal state.

The sensitivity and specificity of routine postoperative imaging is a poor predictor of clinical course. In a study of 22 patients, no difference in midline shift or thickness of extraaxial fluid collection was found between asymptomatic and symptomatic patient groups.[53] A statistically significant difference in volume of extraaxial fluid collection (7.7% versus 5.7% of total cranial volume) was shown in these groups, and two of the eight symptomatic patients required surgical evacuation of the fluid collection.[53] Routine intraoperative use of mannitol (given by protocol at time of incision) has been shown to increase midline shift on postoperative examination,[54] a finding consistent with the global reduction in brain volume and the effective increase in compliance (i.e., reduced spring constant) of midline displacement in response to a perturbing force or displacement applied at the lateral surface. In a study of 46 patients undergoing subdural electrode placement, all developed extraaxial fluid collections; the presence of midline shift, but not the degree, and of ventricular asymmetry were associated with the need for decompressive surgery.[52]

The use of a subgaleal drain, which involves intraoperative placement of a 7-mm silicone flat drain connected to a bag to provide drainage to "gravity" without suction, may virtually eliminate postoperative intracranial hypertension and edema.[14] One study recommended adoption of routine external ventricular drain (EVD) placement after a death arising from elevated ICP.[33]

Continuous ICP monitoring has been proposed and regularly used by some,[33,35] Wong described the routine use of a subdural ICP monitor for 24 hours postimplantation with removal at 24 hours if ICP and a postoperative MRI at 24 hours were both normal. Wong also advocated to include a 1:1 nursing ratio, hourly observations for the first 48 hours postoperatively, continuous monitoring of vitals (heart rate, blood pressure, oxygen saturation), and continuous ICP monitoring for the duration of the invasive monitoring session[33] given two fatalities at one institution. Routine use of ICP monitoring in patients with subdural grids has also been reported after a complication and mortality arising from elevation in ICP.[35]

When elevated ICP or edema is detected, usually presenting as a decrease in mental status or the development of a focal neurological deficit, prompt surgical treatment is warranted. Surgical treatment commonly involves evacuation of the fluid with early removal of some or all of the subdural grids, and this may also involve earlier-than-planned resection.[37,43,45]

## Cerebrospinal Fluid Leak

Whether a CSF leak represents an expected occurrence or surgical complication after subdural grid implantation remains controversial. Among studies that do characterize this as a complication, it was found to occur in an average of 12.1% (95% CI 9.3%–14.9%) in 62 of 514 patients,[30] although the rate at our institution was 0%. The low leak rate at our institution is attributed primarily to the use of a subgaleal drain described in the surgical technique section earlier and detailed next.[14]

Placement of percutaneous leads into the subdural space with the requisite durotomy, imperfect closure permitting passage of electrical cables, persistence of percutaneous sites, and propensity for elevated ICP due to subdural electrode mass effect create a situation in which a CSF leak is inherently likely. Further, the extravasation of CSF serves the beneficial function of acting as a pressure release valve. For these reasons, we advocate the routine use of CSF diversion and perform this with a subgaleal drain to gravity. This provides a low-resistance CSF pathway, thereby obviating the forces that would otherwise drive an undesirable and nonsterile percutaneous CSF leak, and therefore serves the multiple purposes of controlling ICP, preventing CSF leak, and reducing the consequent risk of infection.

Preoperative hydrocephalus may further increase the likelihood of a CSF leak, particularly if a CSF-diverting drain is not used.

Serial clinical examination of the dressing and pillow for signs of leak is mandatory and facilitates prompt detection of a CSF leak. If a leak is not detected and addressed, it poses a risk of infection as has been observed for other neurosurgical procedures.[49]

The use of a subgaleal drain, as described earlier, has been associated with a 0% incidence of both CSF leak and infection in a series of 127 patients at our institution.[14] In patients in whom a drain is placed, proper functioning of the drain should be verified. The head of the bed may be elevated to reduce ICP and thereby decrease the force driving CSF efflux. Acetazolamide may be given to reduce the rate of CSF production; however, the magnitude of this effect is limited, and the onset is not immediate. If these measures are ineffective, the site of the leak may be reinforced with staples or stitches. If the leak persists, a lumbar drain or an EVD may be placed to provide an alternative path of low resistance and to lower ICP.

---

### Clinical Pearls

- After the occurrence of a seizure, risk of developing elevated ICP and edema is increased, and vigilant neurological examination is warranted. Persistence of a neurological deficit beyond a typical postictal period should prompt a workup to evaluate for edema.
- Use of a percutaneous drain or EVD may reduce the risk of elevated ICP and of a CSF leak, thus reducing risk of infection.
- CSF leaks may be treated with head-of-the-bed elevation, administration of acetazolamide, and reinforcement of the site of the CSF leak with staples or stitches. If the leak persists, a lumbar drain or an EVD may be placed.
- Risk of DVT is reduced by mechanical prophylaxis with sequential compression devices and graduated elastic stockings, begun upon admission and continued for the duration of monitoring and augmented with pharmacoprophylaxis.

## Conclusions

Close perioperative clinical monitoring is imperative for the safe management of patients undergoing intracranial electrode monitoring. Clinical interrogation and examination for early detection and management of (1) mental status and focal neurological deficits reflective of elevated ICP, intracranial mass effect, or vascular compromise due to the presence of implanted electrodes or extraaxial fluid collections or intracranial hemorrhage; (2) calf pain or tenderness or elevations in WBC or temperature suggestive of DVT; (3) shortness of breath, pleuritic chest pain, tachycardia, or changes in oxygen requirements suggestive of a PE; and (4) presence of CSF leak, erythema, or elevation in WBC or temperature indicative of a risk for or development of an infection. With proper surgical technique, perioperative care, and postoperative management, subdural and depth electrode monitoring is an effective and relatively safe technique for seizure source localization.

## References

1. Tellez-Zenteno JF, et al. National and regional prevalence of self-reported epilepsy in Canada. *Epilepsia.* 2004;45(12):1623 [Series 4].
2. NIH Consensus Conference. National Institutes of Health Consensus Conference. Surgery for epilepsy. *JAMA.* 1990;264(6):729–733.
3. Brodie MJ, Kwan P. Staged approach to epilepsy management. *Neurology.* 2002;58(8 suppl 5):S2–S8.
4. Gagliardi IC, et al. Quality of life and epilepsy surgery in childhood and adolescence. *Arq Neuropsiquiatr.* 2011;69(1):23–26.
5. Donadio M, et al. Epilepsy surgery in Argentina: long-term results in a comprehensive epilepsy centre. *Seizure.* 2011;20(6):442–445.
6. Wyler AR, et al. Subdural strip electrodes for localizing epileptogenic foci. *J Neurosurg.* 1984;60(6):1195–1200.
7. Wyler AR, Walker G, Somes G. The morbidity of long-term seizure monitoring using subdural strip electrodes. *J Neurosurg.* 1991;74(5):734–737.
8. MacDougall KW, et al. Outcome of epilepsy surgery in patients investigated with subdural electrodes. *Epilepsy Res.* 2009;85(2–3):235–242.
9. Fountas KN, Smith JR. Subdural electrode-associated complications: a 20-year experience. *Stereotact Funct Neurosurg.* 2007;85(6):264–272.
10. Hamer HM, et al. Complications of invasive video-EEG monitoring with subdural grid electrodes. *Neurology.* 2002;58(1):97–103.
11. Lüders H, et al. Subdural electrodes in the presurgical evaluation for surgery of epilepsy. *Epilepsy Res Suppl.* 1992;5:147–156.
12. Sperling MR, et al. Temporal lobectomy for refractory epilepsy. *JAMA.* 1996;276(6):470–475.
13. Englot DJ, et al. Seizure outcomes after resective surgery for extratemporal lobe epilepsy in pediatric patients. *J Neurosurg Pediatr.* 2013;12(2):126–133.
14. Falowski SM, et al. Optimizations and nuances in neurosurgical technique for the minimization of complications in subdural electrode placement for epilepsy surgery. *World Neurosurg.* 2015;84(4):989–997. http://dx.doi.org/10.1016/j.wneu.2015.01.018. Epub 2015 Feb 11.
15. Bancaud J, et al. Functional stereotaxic exploration (SEEG) of epilepsy. *Electroencephalogr Clin Neurophysiol.* 1970;28(1):85–86.
16. Talairach J, et al. New approach to the neurosurgery of epilepsy. Stereotaxic methodology and therapeutic results. 1. Introduction and history. *Neurochirurgie.* 1974;(20 suppl 1):1–240.
17. Cossu M, et al. Stereoelectroencephalography in the presurgical evaluation of focal epilepsy: a retrospective analysis of 215 procedures. *Neurosurgery.* 2005;57(4):706–718. discussion 706–718.
18. Cardinale F, et al. Stereoelectroencephalography: surgical methodology, safety, and stereotactic application accuracy in 500 procedures. *Neurosurgery.* 2013;72(3):353–366. discussion 366.
19. Darcey TM, Roberts DW. Technique for the localization of intracranially implanted electrodes. *J Neurosurg.* 2010;113(6):1182–1185.
20. DiLorenzo DJ, et al. Chronic unlimited recording electrocorticography-guided resective epilepsy surgery: technology-enabled enhanced fidelity in seizure focus localization with improved surgical efficacy. *J Neurosurg.* 2014;120(6):1402–1414.
21. Fischell RE, Fischell DR, Upton ARM. *System for Treatment of Neurological Disorders, in U.S. Patent and Trademark Office.* NeuroPace; 2000.
22. Morrell MJ, RNSSiES Group, Morrell MJ. Responsive cortical stimulation for the treatment of medically intractable partial epilepsy. *Neurology.* 2011;77(13):1295–1304.
23. DiLorenzo DJ. *Apparatus and Method for Closed-Loop Intracranial Stimulation for Optimal Control of Neurological Disease.* [U.S. Patent Office, Ed.] USA: Daniel J. DiLorenzo; 2002.
24. Cook MJ, et al. Prediction of seizure likelihood with a long-term, implanted seizure advisory system in patients with drug-resistant epilepsy: a first-in-man study. *Lancet Neurol.* 2013;12(6):563.
25. DiLorenzo DJ. *Extracranial monitoring of brain activity.* USA: NeuroVista Corp; 2012.
26. DiLorenzo DJ, Gross RE. History and overview of neural engineering. In: DiLorenzo DJ, Bronzino JD, eds. *Neuroengineering.* Boca Raton, FL: CRC Press/Taylor and Francis Books; 2007:1-1–1-19.
27. Giussani C, et al. Is postoperative CT scanning predictive of subdural electrode placement complications in pediatric epileptic patients? *Pediatr Neurosurg.* 2009;45(5):345–349.
28. Al-Otaibi FA, et al. Clinically silent magnetic resonance imaging findings after subdural strip electrode implantation. *J Neurosurg.* 2010;112(2):461–466.
29. Behrens E, et al. Subdural and depth electrodes in the presurgical evaluation of epilepsy. *Acta Neurochir.* 1994;128(1–4):84–87.
30. Arya R, et al. Adverse events related to extraoperative invasive EEG monitoring with subdural grid electrodes: a systematic review and meta-analysis. *Epilepsia.* 2013;54(5):828–839.
31. Behrens EMD, et al. Surgical and neurological complications in a series of 708 epilepsy surgery procedures. *Neurosurgery.* 1997;41(1):1–10.
32. Hamer HM, et al. Complications of invasive video-EEG monitoring with subdural grid electrodes. *Neurology.* 2002;58(1):97–103.
33. Wong CH, et al. Risk factors for complications during intracranial electrode recording in presurgical evaluation of drug resistant partial epilepsy. *Acta Neurochir.* 2009;151(1):37–50.
34. Jobst BC, et al. An unusual complication of intracranial electrodes. *Epilepsia.* 2000;41(7):898–902.
35. Shah AK, et al. Seizures lead to elevation of intracranial pressure in children undergoing invasive EEG monitoring. *Epilepsia.* 2007;48(6):1097–1103.
36. Bekelis K, et al. Subdural interhemispheric grid electrodes for intracranial epilepsy monitoring: feasibility, safety, and utility. Clinical article. *J Neurosurg.* 2012;117(6):1182–1188.
37. Bekelis K, et al. Occipitotemporal hippocampal depth electrodes in intracranial epilepsy monitoring: safety and utility. *J Neurosurg.* 2013;118(2):345–352.
38. Wyllie E, et al. Subdural electrodes in the evaluation for epilepsy surgery in children and adults. *Neuropediatrics.* 1988;19(2):80–86.
39. Johnston JM, et al. Complications of invasive subdural electrode monitoring at St. Louis Children's Hospital, 1994–2005. *J Neurosurg Pediatr.* 2006;105(5):343–347.
40. Musleh W, et al. Low incidence of subdural grid-related complications in prolonged pediatric EEG monitoring. *Pediatr Neurosurg.* 2006;42(5):284–287.
41. Tanriverdi T, et al. Morbidity in epilepsy surgery: an experience based on 2449 epilepsy surgery procedures from a single institution. *J Neurosurg.* 2009;110(6):1111–1123.
42. Silberbusch MA, et al. Subdural grid implantation for intracranial EEG recording: CT and MR appearance. *AJNR Am J Neuroradiol.* 1998;19(6):1089–1093.
43. Lee W-S, et al. Complications and results of subdural grid electrode implantation in epilepsy surgery. *Surg Neurol.* 2000;54(5):346.
44. Burneo JG, et al. Morbidity associated with the use of intracranial electrodes for epilepsy surgery. *Can J Neurol Sci.* 2006;33(2):223–227.
45. Van Gompel JJ, et al. Intracranial electroencephalography with subdural grid electrodes: techniques, complications, and outcomes. *Neurosurgery.* 2008;63(3):498–505. discussion 505–506.
46. Ozlen F, et al. Surgical morbidity of invasive monitoring in epilepsy surgery: an experience from a single institution. *Turk Neurosurg.* 2010;20(3):364–372.
47. Wellmer J, et al. Risks and benefits of invasive epilepsy surgery workup with implanted subdural and depth electrodes. *Epilepsia.* 2012;53(8):1322.
48. Wiggins GC, Elisevich K, Smith BJ. Morbidity and infection in combined subdural grid and strip electrode investigation for intractable epilepsy. *Epilepsy Res.* 1999;37(1):73–80.
49. Horowitz G, et al. Association between cerebrospinal fluid leak and meningitis after skull base surgery. *Otolaryngol Head Neck Surg.* 2011;145(4):689–693.
50. Luders H, et al. Basal temporal subdural electrodes in the evaluation of patients with intractable epilepsy. *Epilepsia.* 1989;30(2):131–142.

51. Derrey SP, et al. Delayed intracranial hematoma following stereoelec-troencephalography for intractable epilepsy. *J Neurosurg Pediatr.* 2012;10(6):525–528.

52. Albert GW, et al. Postoperative radiographic findings in patients undergoing intracranial electrode monitoring for medically refractory epilepsy. *J Neurosurg.* 2009;112(2):449–454.

53. Mocco JMD, et al. Radiographic characteristics fail to predict clinical course after subdural electrode placement. *Neurosurgery.* 2006;58(1):120–125.

54. Etame AB, et al. Osmotic diuresis paradoxically worsens brain shift after subdural grid placement. *Acta Neurochir.* 2011;153(3): 633–637.

# 24 *Deep Brain Stimulation*

TODD M. HERRINGTON and EMAD N. ESKANDAR

## Introduction

Deep brain stimulation (DBS) induces electrical stimulation of specific brain structures to improve the symptoms of neurological and psychiatric illness. DBS has supplanted pallidotomy and thalamotomy in the treatment of Parkinson's disease and is approved for the treatment of medication-refractory epilepsy in Europe and Canada. Other indications are being actively explored and include depression, addiction, obesity, pain, and Alzheimer's dementia, to name a few. DBS lead implantation is typically done awake or with minimal sedation to facilitate microelectrode recording and stimulation, and to allow for clinical testing of the implanted lead. Complications do occur, and long-term outcomes depend on appropriate patient selection, meticulous surgical technique, and sophisticated perioperative care.

## Neuroanatomy and Procedure

### Key Concepts

- A DBS system consists of intracranial leads (electrodes) connected to an extracranial implantable pulse generator (IPG) that is typically placed in the subclavicular space.
- The most common indications for DBS are movement disorders, including Parkinson's disease, essential tremor, and dystonia, although many other indications in neurology and psychiatry are being actively explored.
- Intraoperative microelectrode recording to map the target nuclei likely confers a small additional risk of intracranial hemorrhage, but remains the most accepted method for accurate placement of DBS leads.
- DBS lead trajectories are chosen to avoid eloquent cortex, visualized vessels, and vessel-rich regions, including the depths of sulci and ventricles.

DBS involves chronic, therapeutic electrical stimulation of specific brain targets in order to ameliorate the symptoms of neurological and psychiatric illness (Fig. 24.1). The immediate forebears to DBS were stereotactically placed lesions of the thalamus (thalamotomy) and globus pallidus (pallidotomy) for the treatment of tremor and parkinsonism. Although chronic therapeutic stimulation for treatment of pain began in the 1950s, the modern era of DBS was pioneered by Dr. Alim-Louis Benabid, who in 1987 published a landmark study demonstrating suppression of tremor by high-frequency stimulation of the thalamus.[1] Today, stimulation has largely supplanted lesion therapy in the treatment of movement disorders due to its reversibility, greater or comparable efficacy, and lower frequency of side effects.[2]

DBS is approved in the United States for the treatment of motor symptoms of Parkinson's disease and essential tremor and has been granted a humanitarian device exemption for the treatment of medication-refractory primary dystonia and obsessive-compulsive disorder (OCD). DBS is additionally approved for the treatment of medication-refractory epilepsy in Europe and Canada, and a form of seizure-triggered neurostimulation is approved for use in the United States. A growing list of other indications are being actively explored, including chorea, Tourette's syndrome, chronic pain, depression, addiction, schizophrenia, obesity, anorexia, cluster headache, tinnitus, impairments of consciousness, and Alzheimer's dementia. The most widely accepted indications and targets at present include the subthalamic nucleus (STN) and the globus pallidus internus (GPi) for Parkinson's disease, the GPi for primary dystonia, the ventral intermediate (Vim) nucleus of the thalamus for essential tremor, and the anterior limb of the internal capsule for OCD. For the treatment of refractory epilepsy, stimulation can be applied chronically to the anterior thalamus or triggered by seizure onset and applied near the site of seizure onset.

A DBS system consists of a lead (electrode) with four to eight electrical contacts that are stereotactically inserted in the target and connected via a subcutaneously tunneled extension cable to an implantable pulse generator (IPG) typically placed in the subclavicular space (Fig 24.2). Leads may be placed unilaterally or bilaterally as guided by patient symptoms. Motor symptoms in Parkinson's disease and essential tremor respond primarily to contralateral stimulation, although a modest ipsilateral benefit may be seen.[3,4] Dual-channel IPGs are available that can deliver stimulation to two leads. IPG capabilities differ by manufacturer and model. Presently, three companies have DBS systems approved for human clinical use: Medtronic, St. Jude Medical, and Boston Scientific, although only the Medtronic devices are approved in the United States. These DBS systems operate by applying continuous electrical stimulation without sensing capability (so-called *open loop* stimulation). In addition, a *closed loop*, sensing-stimulating brain stimulation system is available for the treatment of refractory epilepsy (NeuroPace), and similar closed-loop stimulation strategies and technologies are being actively developed for other indications.

### Stereotactic Placement of Deep Brain Stimulation Leads

Effective DBS depends on accurate placement of the stimulating leads. There are several surgical approaches in current use. Most commonly subjects are imaged with a head-mounted, arc-radius stereotactic frame with fiducial markers that allow alignment of the brain target with the frame's coordinate system (Fig. 24.3). Leksell and

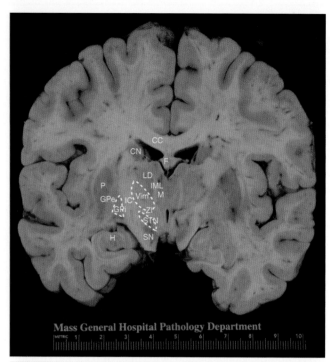

**Fig. 24.1** Most common DBS targets. Coronal section through normal, fixed brain with common DBS targets for movement disorders encircled. Although depicted on a single coronal section here, in practice the optimal targets are at different anterior-posterior coordinates relative to the midpoint of the AC-PC line: STN, 3 mm anterior; GPe, 3 mm posterior; Vim, 5 mm posterior. *CC*, corpus callosum; *CN*, caudate nucleus; *F*, fornix; *GPe*, globus pallidus externus; *GPi*, globus pallidus internus; *H*, hippocampus; *IC*, internal capsule; *IML*, internal medullary lamina; *LD*, lateral dorsal thalamus; *M*, medial thalamic group; *OT*, optic tract; *P*, putamen; *SN*, substantia nigra; *STN*, subthalamic nucleus; *Vim*, ventral intermediate nucleus of the thalamus; *ZI*, zona incerta. (Courtesy of Matthew Frosch, Massachusetts General Hospital.)

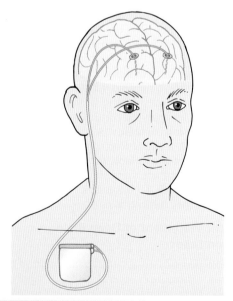

**Fig. 24.2** DBS system. The most commonly used DBS system consists of an intracranial lead (electrode) with four electrical contacts connected via a subcutaneously tunneled extension cable to a subclavicular implantable pulse generator (IPG).

Cosman-Roberts-Wells frames are commonly used. The imaging modality is either a perioperative magnetic resonance imaging (MRI) scan or a perioperative computed tomography (CT) scan that is fused to a preoperative MRI. A microdrive is mounted to the frame and allows for precise advancement of recording microelectrodes and the therapeutic macroelectrodes. As an alternative to frame-based stereotaxy, two frameless stereotactic systems are available in which bone-implanted fiducials are initially placed in the skull in an outpatient procedure, followed by preoperative MRI and CT imaging. A skull-mounted platform is then used to advance the electrodes intraoperatively. The platform is aligned with the preoperative imaging in one of two ways. In the Nexframe (Medtronic) system (Fig. 24.3D), a reusable platform is aligned intraoperatively with the skull fiducials using an optical tracking system. In the STarFix (FHC) system (Fig. 24.3E), a custom-designed platform is manufactured for each patient based on the surgeon's preoperative planning; the platform mounts to the bone-implanted fiducials, which double as anchoring points. Lastly, ClearPoint (MRI Interventions) is an intraoperative MRI-guided system that allows real-time MRI-guided lead placement under general anesthesia. This system is generally not compatible with intraoperative electrophysiological mapping secondary to limitations of the MR scanner and the reduced utility of microelectrode mapping under general anesthesia.

The arc-radius frame design has the advantage of being more flexible in the operating room and allowing for greater intraoperative adjustment of the lead entry point. The disadvantage of this design is that the frames are cumbersome, uncomfortable, and require the patient's head to be fixed in place for the duration of the surgery. The frameless systems do not similarly restrict the patient's head movements and allow for more of the stereotactic planning to be conducted preoperatively, improving operating room efficiency. However, frameless systems are less flexible intraoperatively, affording a narrower range of lead entry points and limited capacity to adjust lead trajectories if initial planning was suboptimal. Lastly, targeting based on MRI imaging alone is a novel alternative approach and is suitable for implantation under general anesthesia. To date there has been no head-to-head comparison of the safety and efficacy of these different approaches to stereotactic lead placement.

## Surgical Procedure

The skin incision and burr holes are made under local anesthesia or light sedation, and the bone sealed with bone wax to reduce the risk of venous air embolism through exposed skull veins. A durotomy and pial incision are performed to accommodate the electrode guide tubes, and hemostasis is assured. It is our practice to fill the burr hole with fibrin glue to reduce pneumocephalus, to reduce cerebrospinal fluid (CSF) leak and brain sag, and to mitigate the risk of venous air embolus through dural veins.

The target is identified on MRI with reference to standardized brain structures, most commonly the plane passing through the anterior and posterior commissures (AC-PC plane). In planning the trajectory, the goal is to place the lead precisely at the target location while avoiding eloquent tissue and vasculature. To minimize the risk of

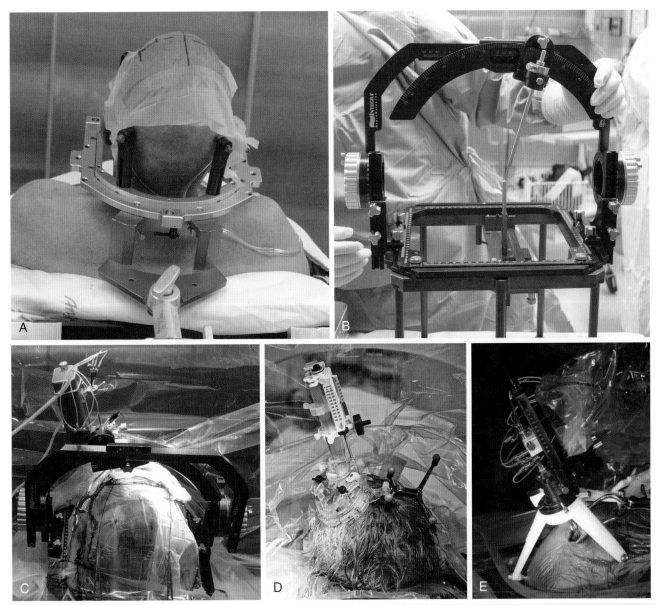

**Fig. 24.3** Stereotactic DBS lead implantation. **(A)** Patient with stereotactic head frame in place. An intraoperative CT is taken and fused to a preoperative MR for planning of the stereotactic lead trajectory. **(B)** A typical arc-radius design head frame is shown. **(C)** A microdrive attaches to the headframe and allows for advancement of microelectrodes for physiology mapping and for placement of the therapeutic DBS lead. **(D, E)** Alternative frameless systems are available including Medtronic NexFrame. (**D**, Courtesy of Kathryn Holloway, MD, Medical College of Virginia Hospital of Virginia Commonwealth University and FHC StarFix. **E**, Courtesy of FHC, Inc.)

hemorrhage, the surgeon should avoid traversing venous sinuses, depths of sulci, and the ventricles. At most centers, the target is further refined through microelectrode recording, although physiology protocols vary substantially among surgeons. A cannula is inserted first, terminating ~25 mm above the intended target. A smaller recording microelectrode is advanced through the cannula to the target, recording along the way to confirm characteristic physiological transitions between gray and white matter along the trajectory and characteristic neural responses to movement and sensory stimulation. Multiple electrode passes may be used sequentially or simultaneously until the optimal target is identified. Microstimulation can also be applied through the mapping electrode (or a separate stimulating sheath) to assess for clinical effects of

stimulation. Once the target has been identified, the chronic stimulating electrode is placed through the same cannula, which minimizes brain shift between the physiology mapping and electrode placement. After placement of the leads, macrostimulation is applied to each of the lead contacts in turn to assess for the voltages at which clinical benefits and side effects are seen. If the stimulation results in insufficient clinical benefit or intolerable side effects at low voltages, the surgeon can move the lead and retest.

Microelectrode recording is the historic gold standard for defining the optimal stimulation target, although no randomized head-to-head comparison has established its benefits relative to stereotactic placement without microelectrode recording, and the relative risks and benefits are intensely debated.[5-7] An older literature on pallidotomy suggests that rates of hemorrhage were higher at centers using microelectrode recording compared with macroelectrode mapping alone.[8,9] In DBS implantation, the number of microelectrode passes has been associated with an increased risk of hemorrhage,[10,11] although not all studies have confirmed this association.[12-15] We have adopted a modified microelectrode design in which the microelectrode is advanced over the last ~2.5 cm independently from its protective sheath, reducing the diameter of this final electrode segment from 0.56 mm to 0.25 mm. We observed a reduced rate of hemorrhage after implementing this design[12]; however, this configuration no longer allows microstimulation through the outer protective sheath. It remains to be seen if newer MRI-guided or CT-guided approaches designed to forgo microelectrode recording will achieve equal outcomes while reducing the rate of hemorrhage.[16,17]

After final lead placement, the lead is secured in place. Affixing the lead only with bone cement (methyl methacrylate) is insufficient and can result in subsequent lead migration. The lead can be secured using proprietary hardware such as Medtronic's Stimloc or using a combination of bone cement, suture, and/or a bone miniplate. Our practice is to secure the lead with bone cement, a silk ligature fixed to a small hole drilled in the medial edge of the burr hole, and a titanium miniplate. When using a titanium plate, care is taken to not overtighten the plate, which can result in fracture of the lead. The lead is tunneled into a subgaleal pocket in the parietal area, and several loops of lead are introduced as strain relief such that, once the extension cabling is connected to the IPG, tension is not transmitted to the lead anchor point.

## Placement of the Implantable Pulse Generator and Initiation of Stimulation

The IPG is placed in the subclavicular space, and extension wires are tunneled subcutaneously to connect the intracranial leads and IPG. The IPG implantation is done under general anesthesia and can be staged as a separate procedure. Many patients experience an immediate clinical benefit from the microelectrode implantation itself, termed the *microlesion effect*, that is likely related to local tissue disruption of the target nucleus analogous to the effect of lesion therapy. This benefit fades over days to a few weeks. During this period lead position may also migrate slightly as postoperative pneumocephalus resolves. For these reasons, therapeutic electrical stimulation is typically initiated 2 to 4 weeks after lead implantation.

---

### Clinical Pearl

After DBS lead placement, patients often experience a transient improvement in their symptoms, usually lasting a few days, termed the *microlesion effect.*

---

The IPG must be replaced as the battery capacity is exhausted. Replacement of the IPG is an outpatient procedure and can sometimes be performed under local anesthesia. The battery life depends on the specific model and the patient's stimulation settings, and typically varies between 2 and 5 years for patients with Parkinson's disease and essential tremor, and 1 and 3 years for patients treated for OCD, major depression, and dystonia who generally require greater stimulation intensity.[18] Rechargeable IPGs are also available but must also be replaced at intervals (9 years for Medtronic's Activa RC) and require greater patient attention.

## Perioperative Considerations

---

### Key Concepts

- DBS lead implantation is typically done awake or with minimal sedation to facilitate microelectrode recording and stimulation and to allow for clinical testing of the implanted lead.
- In Parkinson's disease, DBS lead implantation is done after withdrawal of dopamine replacement therapy in order to facilitate intraoperative testing of stimulation effects.

---

### ANESTHESIA

Lead implantation is usually performed while the patient is awake to optimize microelectrode mapping and macroelectrode testing. However, some patients will not tolerate an awake procedure, including children, those with extreme anxiety, and those in whom dystonic posturing or other movement disorders preclude proper intraoperative positioning. General anesthesia with propofol, dexmedetomidine, or inhalational anesthetics may alter the characteristic electrophysiology of the STN[19,20] and GPi,[21-23] although judicious use of anesthesia may mitigate this.[24] With the patient under general anesthesia, one can only perform very basic macrostimulation testing—for example, to assess for tonic muscle contractions that occur with stimulation of the internal capsule, but not more detailed assessments of clinical benefit or potential visual, somatosensory, motor, autonomic, or cognitive side effects.

### Withdrawal of Dopamine Replacement Therapy in Patients with Parkinson's Disease

Patients with Parkinson's disease typically undergo lead implantation after a 12- to 24-hour withdrawal of dopamine replacement therapy. Although this increases patient discomfort, it substantially aids implantation targeting as the effects of intraoperative macrostimulation are more evident when off medication. After DBS surgery, every effort should be made to resume the patient's oral dopamine replacement therapy. If a patient is unable to take oral medication secondary to dysphagia, for example, enteral access via nasogastric tube can be used to administer most medications. When enteral access cannot be obtained, the dopamine agonist rotigotine is available via transdermal patch. Lastly, intravenous formulations of the dopamine agonist, apomorphine, are available but should be used in consultation with a neurologist who has experience with these medications, their side effects, and titration.

There are case reports of neuroleptic malignant syndrome (also called *parkinsonism-hyperpyrexia syndrome* in this context) after overnight withdrawal of dopaminergic therapy.[25] The syndrome is characterized by fever, autonomic instability, rigidity, rhabdomyolysis, and altered mental status. Although rare, the surgical team should be aware of the possibility because the outcome depends on prompt treatment with supportive care for fever and autonomic instability, resumption of dopaminergic therapy ($\pm$ addition of bromocriptine), and the addition of the skeletal muscle relaxant dantrolene.[26]

# Perioperative and Postoperative Complications

## Key Concepts

- Symptomatic intracranial hemorrhage occurs in 1.5% of DBS lead implants and results in lasting neurological disability in 0.8% of cases.
- Infection occurs in 3.4% of cases and requires hardware removal in 1.8% of cases.
- Symptomatic, intraoperative venous air embolism occurs in ~1.3% of DBS cases and can be detected by a decrease in end-tidal $CO_2$ or through precordial Doppler ultrasound. The most common initial symptom is cough.
- DBS therapy requires long-term surgical care to perform IPG replacements as well as manage device-related complications, including lead fractures, lead migrations, and skin erosions.

Complications of DBS therapy can be divided into surgical complications, hardware complications, and complications related to stimulation. Here we will focus on surgical and hardware complications, addressing only those

medication-related and stimulation-related complications that affect perioperative care.

Table 24.1 summarizes the most common and serious complications and provides detailed references for each. The majority of deep brain stimulation implants are conducted for Parkinson's disease and other movement disorders, and consequently data regarding complications—especially infrequent complications—are primarily from this patient population. Complications have generally been noted to increase with increasing age,[27,28] and advanced age >70 is a relative contraindication to DBS. One may expect that DBS target would also influence perioperative complications, but data on this question are limited. In two randomized, head-to-head studies of STN and GPi DBS for Parkinson's disease, there was no difference in perioperative complication rates between the two targets, although these studies were not powered to detect differences in infrequent complications.[29,30] Although serious complications are infrequent, the rate of death from all causes within 3 months of DBS surgery is ~0.4% (Table 24.1).

### Intracranial Hemorrhage

The overall rate of intracranial hemorrhage after lead implantation is 3.3% (0.8%–6.4%) per case (Table 24.1). Differences in the reported rate of hemorrhage between studies are in part related to the frequency, modality, and quality of postoperative imaging with the ability to detect smaller asymptomatic hemorrhages. In centers that perform routine postoperative imaging, asymptomatic hemorrhage has been reported after 3.0% (1.6%–4.2%) of cases. Symptomatic hemorrhage has been documented in 1.5% (0.8%–2.3%) of cases. Rates of hemorrhage resulting in long-term neurological deficits lasting longer than 30 days are 0.7% to 0.8%.[13,27] Expressed on a per-lead basis, mean

**Table 24.1** Acute Procedure and Hardware-Related Complications of DBS Surgery

| Complication | Frequency | Range | References |
|---|---|---|---|
| Death within 3 month of surgery | 0.4% | 0%–2.6% | (11,27,60–62) |
| Intracranial hemorrhage – all | 3.3% (2.2%)[†] | 0.8%–6.4% | (11,12,27–31,44,54,60–65) |
| Intracranial hemorrhage – symptomatic | 1.5% (0.9%)[†] | 0.8%–2.3% | (12,27,31,44,54,61) |
| Intracranial hemorrhage – asymptomatic | 3.0% (2.1%)[†] | 1.6%–4.2% | (12,27,31,54) |
| Subdural hemorrhage | 0.8% | 0.8% | (33) |
| Ischemic stroke (symptomatic) | 0.5% | 0%–1.0% | (29–31,54) |
| Transient postoperative confusion or psychosis | 8.6% | 1.6%–25.1% | (29,30,54,60,61,64) |
| Seizures | 1.1% | 0.4%–4.7% | (11,27,28,30,31,44,54,60,64) |
| Venous air embolism (symptomatic) | 1.3% | 1.3% | (43) |
| Intraoperative respiratory compromise | 1.9% | 1.6%–2.2% | (28,44) |
| Infection (skin and hardware) | 3.4% | 2.8%–9.9% | (11,27,29–31,49,54,60,61,63,64) |
| Infection requiring hardware removal | 1.8% | 0.4%–9.9% | Same as above |
| Poor wound healing, skin erosion | 1.0% | 0.5%–3.2% | (11,49,54,63,64) |
| CSF leak | 0.3% | 0.3%–0.7% | (27,44,64) |
| Lead misplaced | 1.9% | 1.2%–3.2% | (11,31,54,63,64) |

The mean complication rate per patient and range of complication rate from individual series with at least 100 subjects are shown. See text for a full discussion of each complication.
[†]For intraparenchymal hemorrhage, complication rates per lead implanted are shown in parentheses.

hemorrhage rates were 2.2%, 0.9%, and 2.1% for all hemorrhages, symptomatic hemorrhages, and asymptomatic hemorrhages, respectively.

Most hemorrhages occur subcortically along the lead trajectory or intraventricularly when the lead traverses the ventricle (Figs. 24.4A and 24.4B). The transition point between the electrode and the guide-tube sheath, usually situated 2 to 3 cm above the target, may be a particularly frequent site of hemorrhage.[31] Hemorrhage may occur as a result of direct disruption of an intracranial vessel or sinus, or may arise secondary to venous congestion, infarction, and subsequent hemorrhage. Venous infarction was seen in 1.3% of patients (0.8% of 500 leads) in one series and may occur days after the lead implantation (Fig. 24.4D).[32] Hemorrhage may also occur in the epidural, subdural, or subarachnoid spaces.

One study of 500 lead insertions documented subdural hemorrhage in four (0.8%) cases (Fig.24.4C).[33]

## Clinical Pearl

Venous congestion and infarction can arise days after the DBS lead placement and should be considered if there is late neurological decline.

Hemorrhage may also occur with removal of DBS leads. In one series of DBS lead explants, 10/78 (12%) exhibited hemorrhage on postoperative imaging.[34] All hemorrhages in this series were asymptomatic.

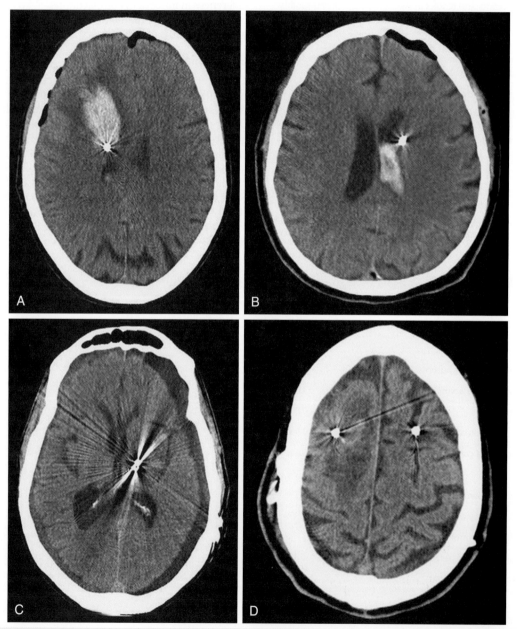

**Fig. 24.4** Intracranial hemorrhage. Axial CT scan images of various locations of hemorrhage that can occur after DBS lead implantation: intraparenchymal **(A)**, intraventricular **(B)**, subdural **(C)**, and secondary to venous infarction **(D)**. (Courtesy of Morishita T et al. Identification and management of deep brain stimulation intra- and postoperative urgencies and emergencies. *Parkinsonism Relat Disord.* 2010;Mar;16(3):153–62.)

Risk factors for hemorrhage include advanced age,[12,13] hypertension,[10,13,27] and a transventricular trajectory.[12] The use of multiple microelectrode passes has also been associated with an increased risk of hemorrhage,[10,11] although not all studies have confirmed this association.[12-15]

To reduce the risk of hemorrhage, one should avoid intraoperative hypertension (maintain systolic blood pressure <140, mean arterial pressure <90); plan trajectories to avoid visualized blood vessels, including cortical veins, depths of sulci, and ventricles; and to reduce the risk of venous thrombosis, minimize pneumocephalus using Gelfoam to seal the burr hole. When targeting the GPi, some surgeons record from the optic tract, which typically lies ~2 mm inferior to the inferior GPi. Our practice is to stop recording once the microelectrodes have clearly exited the pallidum to avoid injury to the optic tracts and vessel-rich choroid fissure.

In many cases of subdural hemorrhage, conservative management with nonoperative or limited burr hole drainage is sufficient, and clinically effective DBS can be achieved after a recovery period that may last up to several months.[33] Similarly, in most instances intraparenchymal and intraventricular hemorrhage can be managed conservatively. However, hemorrhage causing symptomatic mass effect or hydrocephalus may warrant therapeutic craniotomy or placement of an extraventricular drain.

## Ischemic Stroke

Symptomatic ischemic infarction is an infrequent complication of DBS, occurring in 0.5% (0%–1.0%)[35] of cases (see Table 24.1). Ischemia secondary to DBS lead implantation may result from surgical rupture of microvasculature, vasospasm along the lead trajectory, or venous infarction. Management is generally supportive with attention to a workup to identify and manage other etiologies of stroke, including hypoperfusion, intracranial or carotid stenosis, or cardioemboli.

## Neurological Deficits Not Due to Hemorrhage or Ischemia

New postoperative neurological deficits are sometimes noted after DBS lead implantation in the absence of hemorrhage or stroke on postoperative imaging. These symptoms may result from direct tissue injury from lead insertion and postoperative edema. Overall rates of such imaging-negative complications are not well estimated in the literature. A diversity of symptoms have been documented, including aphasia, mutism, visual field deficits, oculomotor palsies, facial palsies, dysphagia, dysarthria, eyelid opening apraxia, paresis, ballism, imbalance, and sensory loss.[30,35] Cognitive decline can occur after DBS in Parkinson's disease, variably affecting tests of global cognitive function, executive function, verbal fluency, and memory.[36] This decline appears to be more prominent after STN than GPi DBS. Psychiatric symptoms including depression, mania, psychosis, impulse control disorders, anxiety, and suicidality can also emerge or worsen,[37] some of which may be stimulation dependent.

## Delirium

In the immediate postoperative period after DBS lead implantation, acute confusion and psychosis are relatively common, documented in 8.6% (1.6%–25.1%) of cases and is likely underreported in most clinical series (Table 24.1). Delirium may be more common after STN than GPi lead implantation.[35] In patients with Parkinson's disease, these acute changes are exacerbated by preexisting cognitive deficits and perioperative withdrawal of medications. Management consists of identifying and treating reversible hemodynamic, metabolic, and infectious etiologies; judicious use of opiates, benzodiazepines, anticholinergics, and other deliriogenic medications; and nonpharmacologic interventions including encouraging normal sleep–wake cycles and minimizing overnight awakenings.[38] Dopaminergic and anticholinergic Parkinson's medications can exacerbate delirium, as can withdrawal from these medications, and inpatient adjustment should involve consultation with a neurologist familiar with their use. Judicious use of antipsychotics may also be helpful, and in Parkinson's disease the limited evidence generally favors quetiapine because it does not substantially worsen motor symptoms.[39]

## Seizure

Perioperative seizure after DBS lead implantation has been documented in 1.1% (0.4%–4.7%) of patients, most occurring within 48 hours of implantation (Table 24.1). Seizures may occur secondary to tissue disruption and edema from lead insertion and cortical irritant effects of pneumocephalus or intracranial hemorrhage. In one series, the presence of hemorrhage, edema, or ischemia on postoperative imaging was associated with a 50-fold increased risk of seizure; these findings were more common in patients older than 60 years of age and those for whom the lead trajectory was transventricular.[40] Meningitis and cerebral abscess are very rare etiologies of seizures, but critical to recognize because management is distinct. Seizures should be evaluated with a head CT to assess for hemorrhage, and if there is not rapid return to baseline, a more extensive evaluation targeting other potential etiologies. A short course of anticonvulsant therapy is reasonable, but long-term anticonvulsant therapy is generally not warranted.

## Venous Air Embolus

If monitored by continuous transthoracic or transesophageal echocardiography, transvenous air embolism has been documented to occur during 7% to 76% of neurosurgical procedures performed in the sitting position.[41] DBS, which represents a comparatively minor exposure of dura and bone, probably has overall lower rates of air embolism compared with more extensive craniotomies. One prospective study using precordial ultrasound monitoring identified air embolism in 1 of 21 patients (5%).[42] The rates of air embolism resulting in cardiorespiratory symptoms is less still, amounting to 6/467 (1.3%) in one series.[43] Two principle factors increase the risk of venous air embolus in DBS implantation: 1) the craniotomy is typically performed with the patient in the semireclined position, with head elevated above the level of the right atrium, and 2) awake patients not on mechanical ventilation generate negative intrathoracic pressure during inspiration, which increases the pressure gradient driving transvenous air entry. To reduce the risk of air embolism, one should maintain the patient's hydration, promptly apply bone wax to the craniotomy edges, and avoid dural venous sinuses.

Venous air emboli may manifest clinically as coughing, hypoxemia, and, if sufficient to impede pulmonary circulation, hypotension and cardiac arrest. Routine monitoring for air embolism should include, at a minimum, the use of continuous end-tidal $CO_2$ monitoring because this is the first detectable monitoring parameter to reflect the event. If an air embolism is suspected, one should immediately lower the head of the bed to at or below the level of the right atrium and flood the surgical field with saline. If symptoms are persistent and there is concern for ongoing air embolism, the jugular veins can be compressed while the incision is closed.

## Other Respiratory Complications

Intraoperative airway management for patients with Parkinson's disease and generalized dystonia may be complicated by poor respiratory reserve, diminished cough reflex, and sleep apnea. Perioperative respiratory complications, including airway obstruction, aspiration, and nosocomial pneumonia, are reported to occur in 1.6% to 2.2% of cases.[28,44] Careful preoperative evaluation and anticipation of potential airway compromise is essential because the stereotactic head frame may impede immediate access to the patient's airway. It is imperative that the surgical and anesthesia teams are familiar with the stereotactic frame and have the necessary tools on hand to manipulate it in case of an airway emergency.

## Infection

Infection originates at the site of surgical incisions and can extend to involve the IPG, extension cable, and intracranial lead. Infection has been reported in 3.4% (2.8%–9.9%) of cases (Table 24.1). Infections that require removal of the IPG, extension cable, or intracranial lead occur in 1.8% of patients (Table 24.1[45–47]). Intracranial spread of infection is an uncommon but serious complication. Poor wound healing, with or without active infection, occurs in 1.0% (0.5%–3.2%) of cases.

Sterile CSF leakage occurs in 0.3% of cases and can be mistaken for infection. CSF can also track along the lead extension to the IPG, resulting in a sterile fluid collection around the IPG. In such cases, if the collection is not warm, erythematous, or tender and the patient shows no systemic signs of infection, it can be managed with a pressure dressing and careful observation. Hemorrhage into the IPG pocket is a rare complication and usually managed nonoperatively.

Reported risk factors for infection after DBS include performing the procedure in an interventional MRI suite (although advances in MRI-suite surgical technique and instrumentation may mitigate this),[48] the use of semichronically externalized leads for postoperative testing,[49] and use of incisions that cross the burr hole site.[49]

Poorly healing wounds or superficial infections that do not directly involve implanted hardware can be treated initially with oral or intravenous antibiotics, wound care, and careful monitoring. Antibiotic choice should be guided by the local surgical-site infection pathogens and sensitivities. Infections that directly involve hardware are difficult to treat medically and usually require hardware explantation.[45,46,50] When infection involves the IPG and lead extension but has not tracked cranially, the intracranial

lead can often be preserved. Infected intracranial leads should always be immediately removed. After explantation, subjects should be treated with intravenous antibiotics and monitored for signs of persistent infection for at least 2 months before hardware is reimplanted.

## Misplaced Leads and Lead Migration

Leads are misplaced requiring surgical revision in 1.9% (1.2%–3.2%) of cases (Table 24.1). This may occur secondary to an error in initial stereotactic and physiological targeting or due to movement of the lead after implantation, such as retraction prior to securing it to the skull (Fig 24.5A). In addition, patients with prominent cervical dystonia, tics, or tremor may dislodge the stereotactic frame if it is not adequately secured.

Lead migration may also occur as a late complication if the lead is not firmly affixed to the skull. In most cases leads migrate superficially due to external tension on the lead. Less commonly, a lead may migrate deep into tissue with the potential to induce hemorrhage or cause neurological symptoms from mechanical disruption or stimulation of unintended targets (Fig. 24.5B).

### Clinical Pearl

DBS leads can migrate, resulting in loss of therapeutic benefit and emergence of new side effects due to stimulation of unintended targets.

## Long-Term Hardware Complications: Lead Fracture, Device Erosion, and Premature IPG Failure

Failure of the DBS system can result in a rapid and dramatic return of symptoms, and effective stimulation can wane in advance of overt battery depletion, necessitating battery replacement.[18] The lead may be unable to deliver therapeutic stimulation either due to an open circuit (due to a lead fracture or loose connection at the IPG or between the brain lead and extension cable) or a short circuit (current path that bypasses the brain). In general, the lead extension connector is typically placed retroauricularly under the scalp and should generally not be placed in the neck due to the greater stresses that result from neck movement. Anchoring the brain lead to the skull with titanium miniplates may cause lead fracture if the plate is secured too tightly. If a damaged lead is suspected, the entire system from brain lead to IPG should be imaged with serial x-rays (Fig. 24.6). If a site of fracture is not directly identified, the system can be tested intraoperatively and the dysfunctional components identified and replaced.

Two case series from the 1990s estimated rates of lead fracture, short circuit, migration, or erosion at 4% to 6% per lead-year.[51,52] Subsequent series in the 2000s reported somewhat lower failure rates, perhaps due to refinements of the technology. Starr et al. reported an 8-year experience in which 50/358 (14%) of patients required an unexpected return to the operating room for management of a complication, most commonly due to problems with the subcutaneous rather than intracranial hardware, and 5.9% of

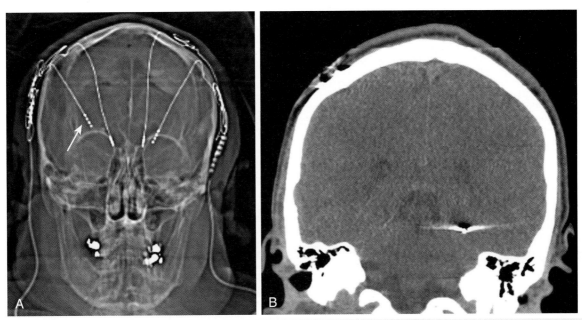

**Fig. 24.5** Lead migration. **(A)** Postoperative CT localizer image from patient with prior STN DBS leads who underwent placement of bilateral GPi leads. Intended right GPi lead (*white arrow*) has been retracted from its target and terminates in the putamen. **(B)** Seven years after lead implantation, a patient presented with seizures that ceased when DBS stimulation was halted. The left-sided GPi DBS lead had migrated into the patient's mesial temporal lobe. (Reprinted from Morishita T, Foote KD, Burdick AP, et al. Identification and management of deep brain stimulation intra- and postoperative urgencies and emergencies. *Parkinsonism Relat Disord.* 2010;Mar;16(3):153–62. Figure 1.)

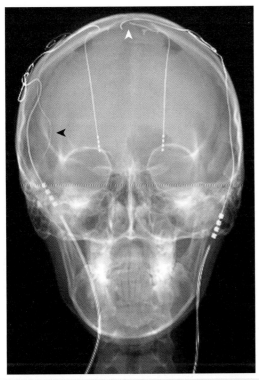

**Fig. 24.6** Lead fracture. Fracture of the left DBS lead as it exits the skull (*white arrowhead*). There is also a fragment of a prior DBS lead present on the right (*black arrowhead*).

patients required revision of the intracranial lead due to malfunction, misplacement, migration, or infection.[31] Allert et al. observed lead dysfunction in 4.6% of leads over 5 years and noted that 12% of leads had a new malfunction

after IPG replacement.[53] However, in most cases the dysfunctional leads still provided clinical benefit, and only 8% of the dysfunctional leads were surgically replaced. Fenoy et al. reported a 9-year experience in which 1.8% of patients had lead fracture, 0.5% had lead migration, and 0.1% had premature IPG failure.[54]

### Thermal Lesion

Magnetic and radiofrequency fields in MRI scanners can induce currents in DBS leads resulting in heating of the lead, can alter settings, or can turn the device on or off. There are established safety guidelines that are DBS device specific and generally limited to 1.5 Tesla, transmit-receive–type radiofrequency head coils (allowing for head imaging only) and specific absorption rates less than 0.1 W/kg at the head.[55,56] However, these guidelines are evolving and approaches are being explored to facilitate the broader use of modern MRI technology. In addition, patients should avoid other sources of electrical stimulation, including diathermy and elective cardioversion.[57,58]

## Conclusions

Successful DBS requires careful patient selection, exacting surgical technique, and sophisticated perioperative care to manage patients with multiple medical, neurological, and psychiatric conditions. Even in the most experienced centers, complications occur, and long-term outcomes depend on effective acute and chronic management best provided in multidisciplinary centers where neurology, neurosurgery, physical therapy, and rehabilitation providers can readily collaborate. Multidisciplinary expertise will likely become even more critical as the technology and indications for DBS advance.

## References

1. Benabid AL, Pollak P, Louveau A, Henry S, de Rougemont J. Combined (thalamotomy and stimulation) stereotactic surgery of the VIM thalamic nucleus for bilateral Parkinson disease. *Appl Neurophysiol.* 1987;50(1–6):344–346.
2. Hariz MI, Hariz G-M. Therapeutic stimulation versus ablation. *Handb Clin Neurol.* 2013;116:63–71.
3. Peng-Chen Z, Morishita T, Vaillancourt D, et al. Unilateral thalamic deep brain stimulation in essential tremor demonstrates long-term ipsilateral effects. *Parkinsonism Relat Disord.* 2013;19(12):1113–1117.
4. Shemisa K, Hass CJ, Foote KD, et al. Unilateral deep brain stimulation surgery in Parkinson's disease improves ipsilateral symptoms regardless of laterality. *Parkinsonism Relat Disord.* 2011;17(10):745–748.
5. Alterman RL, Weisz D. Microelectrode recording during deep brain stimulation and ablative procedures. *Mov Disord.* 2012;27(11):1347–1349.
6. Montgomery EB. Microelectrode targeting of the subthalamic nucleus for deep brain stimulation surgery. *Mov Disord.* 2012;27(11):1387–1391.
7. Zrinzo L, Foltynie T, Limousin P, Hariz MI. Reducing hemorrhagic complications in functional neurosurgery: a large case series and systematic literature review. *J Neurosurg.* 2012;116(1):84–94.
8. Palur RS, Berk C, Schulzer M, Honey CR. A metaanalysis comparing the results of pallidotomy performed using microelectrode recording or macroelectrode stimulation. *J Neurosurg.* 2002;96(6):1058–1062.
9. Alkhani A, Lozano AM. Pallidotomy for parkinson disease: a review of contemporary literature. *J Neurosurg.* 2001;94(1):43–49.
10. Gorgulho A, De Salles AAF, Frighetto L, Behnke E. Incidence of hemorrhage associated with electrophysiological studies performed using macroelectrodes and microelectrodes in functional neurosurgery. *J Neurosurg.* 2005;102(5):888–896.
11. Deep-Brain Stimulation for Parkinson's Disease Study Group. Deep-brain stimulation of the subthalamic nucleus or the pars interna of the globus pallidus in Parkinson's disease. *N Engl J Med.* 2001;345(13):956–963.
12. Ben-Haim S, Asaad WF, Gale JT, Eskandar EN. Risk factors for hemorrhage during microelectrode-guided deep brain stimulation and the introduction of an improved microelectrode design. *Neurosurgery.* 2009;64(4):754–762. discussion 762–763.
13. Sansur CA, Frysinger RC, Pouratian N, et al. Incidence of symptomatic hemorrhage after stereotactic electrode placement. *J Neurosurg.* 2007;107(5):998–1003.
14. Seijo FJ, Alvarez-Vega MA, Gutierrez JC, Fdez-Glez F, Lozano B. Complications in subthalamic nucleus stimulation surgery for treatment of Parkinson's disease. Review of 272 procedures. *Acta Neurochir (Wien).* 2007;149(9):867–875. discussion 876.
15. Elias WJ, Sansur CA, Frysinger RC. Sulcal and ventricular trajectories in stereotactic surgery. *J Neurosurg.* 2009;110(2):201–207.
16. Burchiel KJ, McCartney S, Lee A, Raslan AM. Accuracy of deep brain stimulation electrode placement using intraoperative computed tomography without microelectrode recording. *J Neurosurg.* 2013;119(2):301–306.
17. Larson PS, Starr PA, Bates G, Tansey L, Richardson RM, Martin AJ. An optimized system for interventional magnetic resonance imaging-guided stereotactic surgery: preliminary evaluation of targeting accuracy. *Neurosurgery.* 2012;70(1 Suppl Operative):95–103. discussion103.
18. Fakhar K, Hastings E, Butson CR, Foote KD, Zeilman P, Okun MS. Management of deep brain stimulator battery failure: battery estimators, charge density, and importance of clinical symptoms. *PLoS One.* 2013;8(3):e58665.
19. Hertel F, Züchner M, Weimar I, et al. Implantation of electrodes for deep brain stimulation of the subthalamic nucleus in advanced Parkinson's disease with the aid of intraoperative microrecording under general anesthesia. *Neurosurgery.* 2006;59(5):E1138. discussion E1138.
20. Elias WJ, Durieux ME, Huss D, Frysinger RC. Dexmedetomidine and arousal affect subthalamic neurons. *Mov Disord.* 2008;23(9):1317–1320.
21. Hutchison WD, Lang AE, Dostrovsky JO, Lozano AM. Pallidal neuronal activity: implications for models of dystonia. *Ann Neurol.* 2003;53(4):480–488.
22. Steigerwald F, Hinz L, Pinsker MO, et al. Effect of propofol anesthesia on pallidal neuronal discharges in generalized dystonia. *Neurosci Lett.* 2005;386(3):156–159.
23. Sanghera MK, Grossman RG, Kalhorn CG, Hamilton WJ, Ondo WG, Jankovic J. Basal ganglia neuronal discharge in primary and secondary dystonia in patients undergoing pallidotomy. *Neurosurgery.* 2003;52(6):1358–1370. discussion 1370–1373.
24. Fluchere F, Witjas T, Eusebio A, et al. Controlled general anaesthesia for subthalamic nucleus stimulation in Parkinson's disease. *J Neurol Neurosurg Psychiatr.* 2014;Oct;85(10):1167–1173.
25. Themistocleous MS, Boviatsis EJ, Stavrinou LC, Stathis P, Sakas DE. Malignant neuroleptic syndrome following deep brain stimulation surgery: a case report. *J Med Case Rep.* 2011;5:255.
26. Newman EJ, Grosset DG, Kennedy PGE. The parkinsonism-hyperpyrexia syndrome. *Neurocrit Care.* 2008;10(1):136–140.
27. Voges J, Hilker R, Bötzel K, et al. Thirty days complication rate following surgery performed for deep-brain-stimulation. *Mov Disord.* 2007;22(10):1486–1489.
28. Khatib R, Ebrahim Z, Rezai A, et al. Perioperative events during deep brain stimulation: the experience at Cleveland Clinic. *J Neurosurg Anesthesiol.* 2008;20(1):36–40.
29. Follett KA, Weaver FM, Stern M, et al. Pallidal versus subthalamic deep-brain stimulation for Parkinson's disease. *N Engl J Med.* 2010;362(22):2077–2091.
30. Odekerken VJJ, van Laar T, Staal MJ, et al. Subthalamic nucleus versus globus pallidus bilateral deep brain stimulation for advanced Parkinson's disease (NSTAPS study): a randomised controlled trial. *Lancet Neurol.* 2013;12(1):37–44.
31. Starr PA, Sillay K. Complication avoidance and management in deep brain stimulation surgery. In: Tarsy D, Vitek JL, Starr P, Okun M, eds. *Deep Brain Stimulation in Neurological and Psychiatric Disorders.* Totowa, NJ: Humana Press; 2008.
32. Morishita T, Okun MS, Burdick A, Jacobson CE, Foote KD. Cerebral venous infarction: a potentially avoidable complication of deep brain stimulation surgery. *Neuromodulation.* 2013;16(5):407–413. discussion 413.
33. Oyama G, Okun MS, Zesiewicz TA, et al. Delayed clinical improvement after deep brain stimulation-related subdural hematoma. Report of 4 cases. *J Neurosurg.* 2011;115(2):289–294.
34. Liu JKC, Soliman H, Machado A, Deogaonkar M, Rezai AR. Intracranial hemorrhage after removal of deep brain stimulation electrodes. *J Neurosurg.* 2012;116(3):525–528.
35. Videnovic A, Metman LV. Deep brain stimulation for Parkinson's disease: prevalence of adverse events and need for standardized reporting. *Mov Disord.* 2008;23(3):343–349.
36. Massano J, Garrett C. Deep brain stimulation and cognitive decline in Parkinson's disease: a clinical review. *Front Neurol.* 2012;3:66.
37. Voon V, Howell NA, Krack P. Psychiatric considerations in deep brain stimulation for Parkinson's disease. *Handb Clin Neurol.* 2013;116:147–154.
38. Bourgeois JA, Seritan A. Diagnosis and management of delirium. *Continuum.* 2006;12(5):15.
39. Friedman JH. Atypical antipsychotic drugs in the treatment of Parkinson's disease. *J Pharm Pract.* 2011;24(6):534–540.
40. Pouratian N, Reames DL, Frysinger R, Elias WJ. Comprehensive analysis of risk factors for seizures after deep brain stimulation surgery. Clinical article. *J Neurosurg.* 2011;115(2):310–315.
41. Leslie K, Hui R, Kaye AH. Venous air embolism and the sitting position: a case series. *J Clin Neurosci.* 2006;13(4):419–422.
42. Hooper AK, Okun MS, Foote KD, et al. Venous air embolism in deep brain stimulation. *Stereotact Funct Neurosurg.* 2009;87(1):25–30.
43. Chang EF, Cheng JS, Richardson RM, Lee C, Starr PA, Larson PS. Incidence and management of venous air embolisms during awake deep brain stimulation surgery in a large clinical series. *Stereotact Funct Neurosurg.* 2011;89(2):76–82.
44. Venkatraghavan L, Manninen P, Mak P, Lukitto K, Hodaie M, Lozano A. Anesthesia for functional neurosurgery: review of complications. *J Neurosurg Anesthesiol.* 2006;18(1):64–67.
45. Fenoy AJ, Simpson RK. Management of device-related wound complications in deep brain stimulation surgery. *J Neurosurg.* 2012;116(6):1324–1332.
46. Sillay KA, Larson PS, Starr PA. Deep brain stimulator hardware-related infections: incidence and management in a large series. *Neurosurgery.* 2008;62(2):360–366. discussion 366–367.

47. Fily F, Haegelen C, Tattevin P, et al. Deep brain stimulation hardware-related infections: a report of 12 cases and review of the literature. *Clin Infect Dis.* 2011;52(8):1020–1023.

48. Starr PA, Martin AJ, Ostrem JL, Talke P, Levesque N, Larson PS. Subthalamic nucleus deep brain stimulator placement using high-field interventional magnetic resonance imaging and a skull-mounted aiming device: technique and application accuracy. *J Neurosurg.* 2010;112(3):479–490.

49. Constantoyannis C, Berk C, Honey CR, Mendez I, Brownstone RM. Reducing hardware-related complications of deep brain stimulation. *Can J Neurol Sci.* 2005;32(2):194–200.

50. Temel Y, Ackermans L, Celik H, et al. Management of hardware infections following deep brain stimulation. *Acta Neurochir (Wien).* 2004;146(4):355–361. discussion 361.

51. Oh MY, Abosch A, Kim SH, Lang AE, Lozano AM. Long-term hardware-related complications of deep brain stimulation. *Neurosurgery.* 2002;50(6):1268–1274. discussion 1274–1276.

52. Blomstedt P, Hariz MI. Hardware-related complications of deep brain stimulation: a ten year experience. *Acta Neurochir (Wien).* 2005;147 (10):1061–1064. discussion 1064.

53. Allert N, Markou M, Miskiewicz AA, Nolden L, Karbe H. Electrode dysfunctions in patients with deep brain stimulation: a clinical retrospective study. *Acta Neurochir (Wien).* 2011;153(12):2343–2349.

54. Fenoy AJ, Simpson RK. Risks of common complications in deep brain stimulation surgery: management and avoidance. *J Neurosurg.* 2014;120(1):132–139.

55. Medtronic, Inc. *MRI Guidelines for Medtronic Deep Brain Stimulation Systems [Internet];* 2010. Available from: http://manuals.medtronic.com/manuals/search?region=US&cfn=37602&manualType=MRI+Technical+Manual.

56. Oluigbo CO, Rezai AR. Magnetic resonance imaging safety of deep brain stimulator devices. *Handb Clin Neurol.* 2013;116:73–76.

57. Yamamoto T, Katayama Y, Fukaya C, Kurihara J, Oshima H, Kasai M. Thalamotomy caused by cardioversion in a patient treated with deep brain stimulation. *Stereotact Funct Neurosurg.* 2000;74(2):73–82.

58. Baura GD. *Deep Brain Stimulators. Medical Device Technologies.* Academic Press; 2012297–314.

59. Morishita T, Foote KD, Burdick AP, et al. Identification and management of deep brain stimulation intra- and postoperative urgencies and emergencies. *Parkinsonism Relat Disord.* 2010;16(3):153–162.

60. Williams A, Gill S, Varma T, et al. Deep brain stimulation plus best medical therapy versus best medical therapy alone for advanced Parkinson's disease (PD SURG trial): a randomised, open-label trial. *Lancet Neurol.* 2010;9(6):581–591.

61. Weaver FM, Follett K, Stern M, et al. Bilateral deep brain stimulation vs best medical therapy for patients with advanced Parkinson disease: a randomized controlled trial. *JAMA.* 2009;301(1):63–73.

62. Erola T, Heikkinen ER, Haapaniemi T, Tuominen J, Juolasmaa A, Myllylä VV. Efficacy of bilateral subthalamic nucleus (STN) stimulation in Parkinson's disease. *Acta Neurochir (Wien).* 2005;148(4):389–394.

63. Schuepbach WMM, Rau J, Knudsen K, et al. Neurostimulation for Parkinson's disease with early motor complications. *N Engl J Med.* 2013;368(7):610–622.

64. Okun MS, Gallo BV, Mandybur G, et al. Subthalamic deep brain stimulation with a constant-current device in Parkinson's disease: an open-label randomised controlled trial. *Lancet Neurol.* 2012;11 (2):140–149.

65. Ford B. Subthalamic nucleus stimulation in advanced Parkinson's disease: blinded assessments at one year follow up. *J Neurol Neurosurg Psychiatr.* 2004;75(9):1255–1259.

# 25 *Stereotactic Radiosurgery*

NAVJOT CHAUDHARY, ANNA K. FINLEY CAULFIELD, and STEVEN D. CHANG

## Neuroanatomy and Procedure

### Key Concepts

- The gross target volume (GTV) is the contrast-enhancing portion of the lesion.
- The clinical target volume (CTV) accounts for micrometastases and typically includes a 2-mm margin around an intracranial tumor, or the vertebral body in the case of spine metastases.
- The planning target volume (PTV) takes uncertainties of the radiation delivery process into consideration and often includes 2-mm margins, accounting for patient motion and technical factors.

The term *radiosurgery* was first coined by Swedish neurosurgeon, Dr. Lars Leksell, in 1951. He defined radiosurgery as delivering a single high dose of radiation with a high degree of accuracy to a target of interest.[1] The appeal of this technique over conventional radiation therapy is that a high dose of radiation can precisely be delivered to the target lesion while tissue adjacent to the lesion receives a significantly lower dose. The initial application of radiosurgery included the treatment of trigeminal neuralgia by targeting the trigeminal ganglion and sparing adjacent tissue. Before the advent of computed tomography (CT) and magnetic resonance imaging (MRI), lesions treated with radiosurgery were limited to those that could be targeted with cisternography, ventriculography, and angiography. Contrast injection during cisternography was used to visualize the trigeminal nerve ganglion in Meckel's cave or vestibular schwannomas in the cerebellopontine angle.[2] Similarly, angiography was used to visualize arteriovenous malformations.[3] Currently, treatment plans include fusion of thin-slice CT and MRIs to contour lesions (Figs. 25.1–3).

The first dedicated stereotactic radiosurgery devices were gamma knife units, which include 179 to 201 Cobalt-60 (gamma radiation) sources. Later, the linear accelerator (LINAC) was developed to make radiosurgery possible in every center capable of using conventional x-ray beam therapy, making LINAC the most common form of radiosurgery.[4,5] LINAC uses multiple arcs of radiation that converge on a target within a millimeter of accuracy. The CyberKnife is a frameless image-guided radiosurgery system (Accuray, Sunnyvale, CA, USA), which was originally developed by Dr. John Adler at Stanford University.[6] The CyberKnife is a LINAC mounted on a movable industrial robot. The

maneuverability of the robot arm allows for submillimeter accuracy in detecting changes in the target position. The advantages of CyberKnife technology include the ability to treat both intracranial and extracranial targets, including the spine and visceral organs; to fractionate treatments to treat large lesions or those occurring in eloquent cortex; and to treat moving targets while preserving tight dosimetry around the lesion. When a fractionation schedule is used, the radiation dose is administered in one to five fractions, with a single dose being delivered on consecutive days. Structures outside the central nervous system (CNS) that have been treated include prostate and lung malignancies. Therefore CyberKnife takes radiosurgery outside the confines of neurosurgery and allows for the treatment of other organs.[7–12]

Several volumes have been described for treatment planning. The GTV is the contrast-enhancing portion of the lesion. For metastases or malignant lesions, a CTV is included to account for micrometastases. This typically includes a 2-mm margin around an intracranial tumor. When planning a CTV for bony metastases to the spine, considerations include the histology of the tumor, the goal of the treatment (i.e., palliative vs. oncologic), and integrity of the bone (i.e., preexisting vertebral body fractures). In the case of bony metastases to the spine, it is likely that tumor cells spread throughout the trabeculae of the bone, and therefore the entire vertebral body is often included in the target volume. The PTV takes uncertainties of the radiation delivery process into consideration and often includes 2-mm margins. The PTV accounts for patient motion and technical factors. In functional radiosurgery, the concepts of CTV and PTV do not apply because the dose is prescribed to a point.[13] The dose falloff in radiosurgery is steep, allowing for a high radiation dose to the target, with a very fast radiation dose falloff in the adjacent normal brain.[13] Critical structures adjacent to the target have maximum dose allowances in the planning process.[14]

### Clinical Pearl

In the brain, radiation-sensitive structures include the optic apparatus, brainstem, and pituitary gland. Among the cranial nerves, the special sensory nerves, including the optic and vestibulocochlear nerves, are the most radiosensitive. Somatic trigeminal afferents, visceral facial efferents, and somatic oculomotor and hypoglossal efferents are the next most radiosensitive.

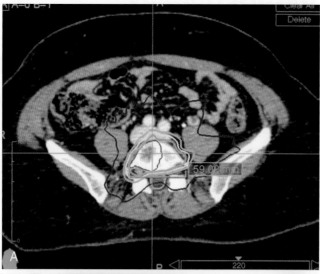

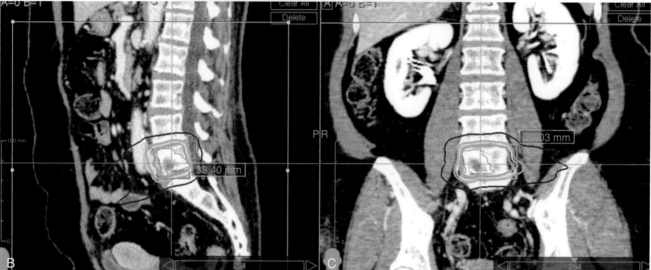

**Fig. 25.1** An axial, sagittal, and coronal CT scan of the lumbar spine demonstrates an osteolytic metastasis in the right anterior inferior L5 vertebral body (*red*). The GTV consists of the lesion (*red*), the CTV includes the entire vertebral body (*gold*), and the cauda equina (*light blue*) is contoured as a critical structure.

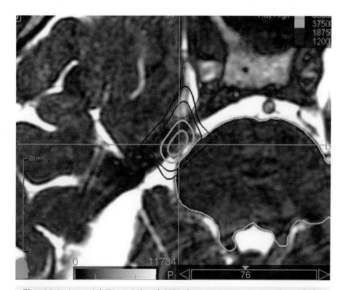

**Fig. 25.2** An axial T2-weighted MRI demonstrates contouring of the right trigeminal nerve (*red*) at the dorsal root entry zone. Meckel's cave (*purple*) and the brainstem (*light blue*) are contoured as critical structures. The cranial nerve VII and VIII complex (not visible on this slice) is also contoured in the case of vestibular schwannomas.

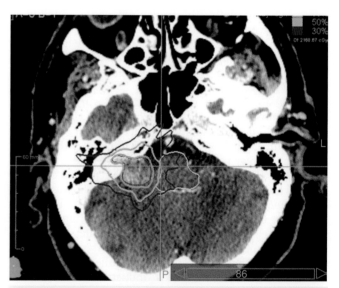

**Fig. 25.3** An axial CT scan demonstrates a right vestibular schwannoma (*red*) in the right cerebellopontine angle and internal auditory canal. The brainstem (*orange*) and cochlea (*purple*) are contoured as critical structures.

# Preoperative and Perioperative Management Considerations

## Key Concepts

- Stereotactic radiosurgery is generally a well-tolerated outpatient procedure.
- Factors that increase the likelihood of complications are large lesions, high radiation doses, whether the lesion is located in eloquent cortex, extremes of patient age, and whether patient is receiving concurrent or sequential chemotherapy.
- Perioperative complications include worsening cerebral edema, nausea/vomiting, and seizures.
- Patients are often treated with corticosteroids and antiemetics on the day of the procedure.
- Benzodiazepines and intravenous phenytoin or fosphenytoin should be readily available in the event of a seizure.

## Clinical Pearl

A multidisciplinary team consisting of a neurosurgeon, radiation oncologist, radiation therapist, physicist, and nurse is essential during the perioperative period.

Factors that increase the likelihood of complications include a large lesion, high radiation dose, whether the lesion is located in eloquent cortex, extremes of patient age, and whether the patient is receiving concurrent or sequential chemotherapy. Although side effects are uncommon in radiosurgery, the most common acute side effects include transient cerebral edema, which may manifest in headache, nausea, vomiting, and seizures. Transient mild cerebral edema secondary to radiation-induced disruption of the blood–brain barrier (BBB) can also lead to a transient worsening of pretreatment neurological deficits. At Stanford University, dexamethasone and ondansetron are routinely administered before every treatment to minimize these potential side effects. Patients with gastroesophageal reflux disease should be pretreated with proton pump inhibitors or H2 blockers, because lying supine for treatment may exacerbate their symptoms. In addition, it is important to manage pain and anxiety during the treatment. In cases where opiates or benzodiazepines are required, pulse oximetry should be implemented to assist in monitoring respiratory status. Although some patients are treated for preexisting seizure disorders, there is concern that the administration of radiosurgery can induce seizures. Therefore benzodiazepines and intravenous phenytoin or fosphenytoin should readily be available in the event of a seizure. For treatment planning imaging, creatinine should be checked prior to administering contrast dye, particularly patients who are elderly or have a history of renal dysfunction. Patients with cancer are at increased risk of hypercoagulation complications, and therefore any symptoms or signs on physical examination suggestive of thromboembolism warrant immediate investigation with a Doppler ultrasound and/or CT angiogram to look for deep venous thrombosis or pulmonary embolism. A number of patients receive radiosurgery after surgical resection.

Because radiation may adversely affect wound healing, it is important to assess wound healing at each visit and alert the neurosurgeon if there are any concerns of infection or cerebrospinal fluid leak. In the case of gamma knife treatment, the neurosurgeon performs a block of the scalp nerves before applying the stereotactic frame. Treatments for children or claustrophobic patients may rarely require the assistance of an anesthesiologist. Finally, any change in cognitive status should prompt a full neurological examination and an urgent CT scan of the brain. In the immediate perioperative period, the main concerns would be to rule out cerebral edema, hemorrhage, or hydrocephalus. An electroencephalogram might also be indicated to rule out a seizure, particularly if there is a preexisting history of seizures (Table 25.1).

# Management of Intraoperative and Postoperative Complications

## Key Concepts

- Stereotactic radiosurgery is generally a well-tolerated outpatient procedure.
- Complications may occur in an acute (0–90 days) and/or late (>90 days) time frames.
- Acute complications include cerebral edema, nausea/vomiting, and seizures.
- Early delayed complications include pseudoprogression, an abnormal area of enhancement in the treatment region that is difficult to distinguish from tumor recurrence.
- Late complications include radiation necrosis and, rarely, secondary malignancies.

## ACUTE COMPLICATIONS

## Clinical Pearl

Severe acute toxicities, including nausea, vomiting, seizures, and cerebral edema, are quite rare in radiosurgery.

A retrospective analysis examining 835 consecutive gamma knife procedures revealed that 18 patients (2.2%) had new neurological events, including focal neurological deficits or seizures, whereas 3 patients (0.4%) died (two deaths related to seizures and neurological deterioration) within 7 days of treatment.[15] Further, location of the tumor appears to affect the incidence of seizures after radiosurgery, with seizures occurring more frequently in lesions involving the motor cortex.[16] More commonly, transient cerebral edema occurring 12 to 48 hours after radiosurgery results in mild neurological symptoms. In one study examining 78 patients, one third of patients developed mild side effects of nausea, dizziness or vertigo, seizures, or new persistent headaches within 2 weeks of treatment.[17] Only two patients required hospitalization for seizures or new neurological deficits. Interestingly, acute toxicity was not predictive of the development of late toxicity.

**Table 25.1**    Radiation Complications and Management

| Acute (≤90 days) | Management |
| --- | --- |
| Cerebral edema | Corticosteroids (dexamethasone) |
| Nausea and vomiting | Antiemetics (ondansetron) |
| Pain, headache | Opioids and acetaminophen |
| Seizure | Acute treatment: benzodiazepine (lorazepam, midazolam, diazepam) and antiepileptic drugs (AEDs) (fosphenytoin or phenytoin, other IV AED: levetiracetam, valproic acid, phenobarbital) Chronic treatment: daily AED therapy; levetiracetam commonly used due to limited drug–drug interactions |
| Anxiety | Benzodiazepine |
| New neurological deficit | Head CT, MRI with contrast |
| Gastric reflux | Proton pump inhibitor or H2 blockers |
| **Early Delayed (60–120 days)** | **Management** |
| Pseudoprogression | Asymptomatic patients: serial monitoring Symptomatic patients: corticosteroids (dexamethasone), bevacizumab for high-grade gliomas in patients refractory to corticosteroids |
| **Late (>90 days)** | **Management** |
| Headache | Pain management strategies depending on severity and frequency: analgesic medications, trial of corticosteroids, headache prophylactic meds |
| Seizure | Benzodiazepines and AED (see earlier) |
| Radiation necrosis | Multimodal imaging for diagnostic assistance Asymptomatic patients: observation and serial imaging Symptomatic patients: Corticosteroids Bevacizumab Surgical biopsy if unclear diagnosis Consider: Trial of anticoagulation or antiplatelet for 3–6 months (felt to limit small-vessel vascular injury) Consider trial of hyperbaric oxygen therapy Rarely, surgical resection in lesions with mass effect and refractory to medical therapy |
| Secondary malignancy | Neurosurgical and oncological evaluation |

A number of case reports have documented significant complications on the day of radiosurgery. One study reported a patient who developed acute hydrocephalus secondary to cerebellar edema compressing the fourth ventricle during treatment of five posterior fossa metastases.[18] In another report, a patient developed acute onset of facial paralysis, vertigo, and hearing loss within 24 hours of radiosurgery treatment of a vestibular schwannoma.[19] In this case, imaging revealed an acute intracochlear hemorrhage, and the patient did not regain hearing during long-term follow-up, although the facial palsy completely resolved by 3 months.

## EARLY DELAYED COMPLICATIONS

### Clinical Pearl

Postradiosurgery MRI may occasionally demonstrate transient contrast enhancement at the site of therapy, approximately 2 to 3 months after radiosurgery. This enhancement may be difficult to distinguish from tumor progression and requires thorough investigation.

Pseudoprogression was first documented by Hoffman et al. in a study of 51 patients with high-grade gliomas, in which 12% had transient increased enhancement on CT scan.[20] The underlying pathophysiology remains unknown, but a combination of tumor necrosis, edema, and secondary inflammation leading to vessel permeability has been implicated. Several studies reveal pseudoprogression in 13% to 32% of patients with high-grade gliomas, in which biopsy did not demonstrate evidence of tumor progression.[21–26] Kaplan-Meir analysis found that patients with pseudoprogression after radiosurgery had improved survival compared with patients who did not show pseudoprogression.[27] In terms of diagnosis, a single imaging study is inadequate to distinguish between pseudoprogression and tumor progression. Serial imaging is recommended to make this distinction because their management differs greatly. Incorrectly treating pseudoprogression with further radiation therapy can lead to devastating effects, including acute encephalopathy and radiation necrosis. Further, surgery would subject patients to inherent risks of the procedure. The general management of suspected pseudoprogression in asymptomatic patients is serial monitoring. Therapeutic options for symptomatic patients may include administration of corticosteroids or, rarely in severe cases, surgery to alleviate mass effect. In cases involving high-grade gliomas, bevacizumab may be of benefit (see section on radiation necrosis) in a patient with limited response to corticosteroids.[28]

## LATE COMPLICATIONS

### Clinical Pearl

Radiation necrosis and secondary malignancies are serious, yet rare, long-term adverse effects of radiation treatment. Early diagnosis and treatment are crucial to achieving long-term quality of life for patients.

### Radiation Necrosis

If radiation necrosis develops, it typically occurs 1 to 3 years after radiation therapy. In the case of brain metastases, the actuarial incidence of radiation necrosis was found to be 5%, 8%, and 11% at 6, 12, and 24 months in the Radiation Therapy Oncology Group (RTOG) study.[29] A more recent publication using fluorodeoxygenase (FDG) positron emission tomography (PET) criteria indicates the risk of radiation necrosis after radiosurgery for brain metastases is approximately 10%.[30] The incidence of radiation necrosis is related to the dose of radiation. Using conventional fractionated radiotherapy, the dose that causes a 5% risk of focal radionecrosis is 55 to 60 Gy.[31]

The underlying pathophysiology of radiation necrosis is thought to be secondary to vascular endothelial damage, resulting in fibrinoid necrosis of small arterial vessels.[32] Disruption of the BBB may be partially mediated by vascular endothelial growth factor that is released in response to hypoxia.

Multimodal imaging can facilitate differentiation of recurrent tumor from radiation necrosis. Increased cerebral blood volume on perfusion imaging and increased uptake with FDG, methionine, or thallium chloride-201 PET are all suggestive of recurrent tumor rather than radiation necrosis.[33,34] A high lipid peak on magnetic resonance spectroscopy is consistent with radiation necrosis. Definitive diagnosis is only achieved with a biopsy.

Many cases of radiation necrosis are self-limited and require no treatment, particularly if patients are asymptomatic. For symptomatic patients, administration of corticosteroids may be beneficial. In cases that are refractory to corticosteroid administration, treatment options that have demonstrated some benefit in small case series include therapeutic anticoagulation, antiplatelet therapy, and hyperbaric oxygen therapy.[35,36] Surgical decompression and biopsy can be helpful in cases where there is diagnostic uncertainty or when there are progressive and refractory symptoms resulting from mass effect.[37]

Studies suggest that bevacizumab may be helpful in the treatment of radiation necrosis.[38–43] In a double blind trial, 14 patients with biopsy or radiologically confirmed cerebral radiation necrosis were randomly assigned to bevacizumab (7.5 mg/kg for four cycles at 3-week intervals) or a saline placebo.[41] All patients in the treatment group demonstrated a favorable clinical and radiological response. In contrast, no patient in the placebo group showed a favorable response. All patients who progressed while on the placebo did respond to bevacizumab during treatment crossover. Other series have found slightly less favorable symptom response rates of 75% to 90%, and there has been at least one case of worsening neurological status with bevacizumab treatment.[42,44]

## Secondary Malignancy

Radiation-induced tumors are defined by Cahan's criteria.[45] These criteria define a secondary neoplasm as follows: 1) the second tumor must occur within the original radiation field, but must not have been present on imaging at the time of initial irradiation; 2) there must be a latency period between the radiation exposure and the development of the second tumor; 3) the second tumor must be histologically unique to the original tumor; and 4) the patient cannot have a genetic syndrome that predisposes to cancer. Many tumors do not meet the third criterion because one reason for administering radiosurgery is to avoid open surgery. Therefore the primary diagnosis is often presumptive based on imaging appearance.

Studies indicate that few patients develop secondary neoplasms from radiosurgery. One study documented only six reported cases of malignant tumors in over 80,000 radiosurgery treatments for benign lesions, with an incidence of less than 1 in 1000.[46] A recent review of the literature by Patel and Chiang identified 36 cases of radiosurgery-induced CNS neoplasms.[47] The initial diagnosis in more than half of the cases included vestibular schwannomas. Arteriovenous malformations, pituitary tumors, meningiomas, cavernomas, and metastases made up the remainder of cases. The most common secondary neoplasms were malignant gliomas (36%) and malignant peripheral nerve sheath tumors (36%), followed by sarcomas, meningiomas, and vestibular schwannomas. The mean latency to develop a radiosurgery-induced neoplasm was 7.9 years (ranging from 0.7–19 years). Subanalysis demonstrates that malignant radiosurgery-induced neoplasms have a shorter mean latency (7.1 years, range 0.7–19 years) than benign radiosurgery-induced neoplasms (14.25 years, 10–19 years). These analyses estimated that the risk of radiosurgery-induced neoplasm was 0.04% at 15 years. This rate is lower than the rate of 1% to 3% that has been cited in the literature for traditional fractionated therapy.[48–50] One possible explanation for this discrepancy hinges on the concept of cytotoxicity versus mutagenesis.[47] To produce a secondary neoplasm, the radiation delivered must be mutagenic, but not cytotoxic. In other words, if the delivered radiation dose is too high, the normal cells will die and not have the chance to become neoplastic. Therefore the single high dose delivered during radiosurgery is thought to preferentially lead to cytotoxicity over mutagenicity. Animal and clinical studies have demonstrated that there is an increasing rate of secondary neoplasm development up to a maximum dose between 3 and 10 Gy, followed by a decrease in the risk at dose increases beyond this range. This may also explain why vestibular schwannomas, which are traditionally treated with lower doses, are associated with disproportionately higher rates of secondary neoplasms than expected.

## Conclusion

Radiosurgery delivers a single high dose of radiation to a target of interest. Gamma knife and LINAC are two early radiosurgery methods using frames to precisely treat lesions. CyberKnife is a frameless LINAC mounted on a movable industrial robot. The maneuverability of the robot arm allows for submillimeter accuracy in detecting changes in the target position. The advantages of CyberKnife technology include the ability to treat both intracranial and extracranial targets, including the spine and visceral organs; to fractionate treatments to treat large lesions or those occurring in eloquent cortex; and to treat moving targets while preserving tight dosimetry around the lesion. The most common acute radiosurgery side effects include cerebral edema, nausea, vomiting, and seizures; early delayed effects include pseudoprogression; and late effects include radiation necrosis and, rarely, secondary malignancies. With close monitoring, perioperative and long-term complications can be identified and managed to minimize their effects.

## References

1. Leksell L. The stereotaxic method and radiosurgery of the brain. *Acta Chir Scand.* 1951;102(4):316–319. PubMed PMID: 14914373. Epub 1951/12/13. eng.

2. Leksell L. A note on the treatment of acoustic tumours. *Acta Chir Scand.* 1971;137(8):763–765. PubMed PMID: 4948233. Epub 1971/01/01. eng.

3. Steiner L, Leksell L, Greitz T, Forster DM, Backlund EO. Stereotaxic radiosurgery for cerebral arteriovenous malformations. Report of a case. *Acta Chir Scand.* 1972;138(5):459–464. PubMed PMID: 4560250. Epub 1972/01/01. eng.

4. De Salles AA, Gorgulho AA, Selch M, De Marco J, Agazaryan N. Radiosurgery from the brain to the spine: 20 years experience. *Acta Neurochir Suppl.* 2008;101:163–168. PubMed PMID: 18642653. Epub 2008/07/23. eng.

5. Agazaryan N, Tenn SE, Desalles AA, Selch MT. Image-guided radiosurgery for spinal tumors: methods, accuracy and patient intrafraction motion. *Phys Med Biol.* 2008;53(6):1715–1727. PubMed PMID: 18367799. Epub 2008/03/28. eng.

6. Adler JR. Frameless radiosurgery. In: De Salles AAF, Goetsch SJ, ed. *Stereotactic Surgery and Radiosurgery.* Wisconsin: Medical Physics Publishing, 1993;17:237–248.

7. Chang SD, Main W, Martin DP, Gibbs IC, Heilbrun MP. An analysis of the accuracy of the CyberKnife: a robotic frameless stereotactic radiosurgical system. *Neurosurgery.* 2003;52(1):140–146. discussion 6–7. PubMed PMID: 12493111. Epub 2002/12/21. eng.

8. Ho AK, Fu D, Cotrutz C, et al. A study of the accuracy of cyberknife spinal radiosurgery using skeletal structure tracking. *Neurosurgery.* 2007;60(2 Suppl 1):ONS147–ONS156. discussion ONS56. PubMed PMID: 17297377. Epub 2007/02/14. eng.

9. Muacevic A, Staehler M, Drexler C, Wowra B, Reiser M, Tonn JC. Technical description, phantom accuracy, and clinical feasibility for fiducial-free frameless real-time image-guided spinal radiosurgery. *J Neurosurg Spine.* 2006;5(4):303–312. PubMed PMID: 17048766. Epub 2006/10/20. eng.

10. Yu C, Main W, Taylor D, Kuduvalli G, Apuzzo ML, Adler Jr JR. An anthropomorphic phantom study of the accuracy of Cyberknife spinal radiosurgery. *Neurosurgery.* 2004;55(5):1138–1149. PubMed PMID: 15509320. Epub 2004/10/29. eng.

11. Adler Jr JR, Gibbs IC, Puatawepong P, Chang SD. Visual field preservation after multisession cyberknife radiosurgery for perioptic lesions. *Neurosurgery.* 2006;59(2):244–254. discussion 254. PubMed PMID: 16883165. Epub 2006/08/03. eng.

12. Chang SD, Gibbs IC, Sakamoto GT, Lee E, Oyelese A, Adler Jr JR. Staged stereotactic irradiation for acoustic neuroma. *Neurosurgery.* 2005;56(6):1254–1261. discussion 61–3. PubMed PMID: 15918941. Epub 2005/05/28. eng.

13. De Salles AAF, Gorgulho AA, Agazaryan N. Linear accelerator radiosurgery: technical aspects. In: Winn, ed. *Youmans Neurological Surgery.* 6th ed. Philadelphia, PA: WB, Saunders; 2011:2622–2632.

14. Tishler RB, Loeffler JS, Lunsford LD, et al. Tolerance of cranial nerves of the cavernous sinus to radiosurgery. *Int J Radiat Oncol Biol Phys.* 1993;27(2):215–221. PubMed PMID: 8407394. Epub 1993/09/30. eng.

15. Chin LS, Lazio BE, Biggins T, Amin P. Acute complications following gamma knife radiosurgery are rare. *Surg Neurol.* 2000;53(5):498–502. discussion PubMed PMID: 10874151. Epub 2000/06/30. eng.

16. Gelblum DY, Lee H, Bilsky M, Pinola C, Longford S, Wallner K. Radiographic findings and morbidity in patients treated with stereotactic radiosurgery. *Int J Radiat Oncol Biol Phys.* 1998;42(2):391–395. PubMed PMID: 9788421. Epub 1998/10/27. eng.

17. Werner-Wasik M, Rudoler S, Preston PE, et al. Immediate side effects of stereotactic radiotherapy and radiosurgery. *Int J Radiat Oncol Biol Phys.* 1999;43(2):299–304. PubMed PMID: 10030253. Epub 1999/02/25. eng.

18. Wolff R, Karlsson B, Dettmann E, Bottcher HD, Seifert V. Pretreatment radiation induced oedema causing acute hydrocephalus after radiosurgery for multiple cerebellar metastases. *Acta Neurochir.* 2003;145(8):691–696. discussion 696. PubMed PMID: 14520550. Epub 2003/10/02. eng.

19. Franco-Vidal V, Songu M, Blanchet H, Barreau X, Darrouzet V. Intracochlear hemorrhage after gamma knife radiosurgery. *Otol Neurotol.* 2007;28(2):240–244. PubMed PMID: 17159493. Epub 2006/12/13. eng.

20. Hoffman WF, Levin VA, Wilson CB. Evaluation of malignant glioma patients during the postirradiation period. *J Neurosurg.* 1979;50(5):624–628. PubMed PMID: 430157. Epub 1979/05/01. eng.

21. Brandes AA, Franceschi E, Tosoni A, et al. MGMT promoter methylation status can predict the incidence and outcome of pseudoprogression after concomitant radiochemotherapy in newly diagnosed glioblastoma patients. *J Clin Oncol.* 2008;26(13):2192–2197. PubMed PMID: 18445844. Epub 2008/05/01. eng.

22. Chamberlain MC, Glantz MJ, Chalmers L, Van Horn A, Sloan AE. Early necrosis following concurrent Temodar and radiotherapy in patients with glioblastoma. *J Neurooncol.* 2007;82(1):81–83. PubMed PMID: 16944309. Epub 2006/09/01. eng.

23. Gunjur A, Lau E, Taouk Y, Ryan G. Early post-treatment pseudoprogression amongst glioblastoma multiforme patients treated with radiotherapy and temozolomide: a retrospective analysis. *J Med Imaging Radiat Oncol.* 2011;55(6):603–610. PubMed PMID: 22141608. Epub 2011/12/07. eng.

24. Hasegawa T, Kida Y, Yoshimoto M, Koike J, Goto K. Evaluation of tumor expansion after stereotactic radiosurgery in patients harboring vestibular schwannomas. *Neurosurgery.* 2006;58(6):1119–1128. discussion 1128. PubMed PMID: 16723891. Epub 2006/05/26. eng.

25. Sanghera P, Perry J, Sahgal A, et al. Pseudoprogression following chemoradiotherapy for glioblastoma multiforme. *Can J Neurol Sci.* 2010;37(1):36–42. PubMed PMID: 20169771. Epub 2010/02/23. eng.

26. Taal W, Brandsma D, de Bruin HG, et al. Incidence of early pseudoprogression in a cohort of malignant glioma patients treated with chemoirradiation with temozolomide. *Cancer.* 2008;113(2):405–410. PubMed PMID: 18484594. Epub 2008/05/20. eng.

27. Patel TR, McHugh BJ, Bi WL, Minja FJ, Knisely JP, Chiang VL. A comprehensive review of MR imaging changes following radiosurgery to 500 brain metastases. *AJNR.* 2011;32(10):1885–1892. PubMed PMID: 21920854. Epub 2011/09/17. eng.

28. Fink J, Born D, Chamberlain MC. Pseudoprogression: relevance with respect to treatment of high-grade gliomas. *Curr Treat Options Oncol.* 2011;12(3):240–252. PubMed PMID: 21594589. Epub 2011/05/20. eng.

29. Shaw E, Scott C, Souhami L, et al. Single dose radiosurgical treatment of recurrent previously irradiated primary brain tumors and brain metastases: final report of RTOG protocol 90-05. *Int J Radiat Oncol Biol Phys.* 2000;47(2):291–298. PubMed PMID: 10802351. Epub 2000/05/10. eng.

30. Chao ST, Ahluwalia MS, Barnett GH, et al. Challenges with the diagnosis and treatment of cerebral radiation necrosis. *Int J Radiat Oncol Biol Phys.* 2013;87(3):449–457. PubMed PMID: 23790775. Epub 2013/06/25. eng.

31. Emami B, Lyman J, Brown A, et al. Tolerance of normal tissue to therapeutic irradiation. *Int J Radiat Oncol Biol Phys.* 1991;21(1):109–122. PubMed PMID: 2032882. Epub 1991/05/15. eng.

32. Burger PC, Mahley Jr MS, Dudka L, Vogel FS. The morphologic effects of radiation administered therapeutically for intracranial gliomas: a postmortem study of 25 cases. *Cancer.* 1979;44(4):1256–1272. PubMed PMID: 387205. Epub 1979/10/01. eng.

33. Sugahara T, Korogi Y, Tomiguchi S, et al. Posttherapeutic intraaxial brain tumor: the value of perfusion-sensitive contrast-enhanced MR imaging for differentiating tumor recurrence from nonneoplastic contrast-enhancing tissue. *AJNR.* 2000;21(5):901–909. PubMed PMID: 10815666. Epub 2000/05/18. eng.

34. Valk PE, Budinger TF, Levin VA, Silver P, Gutin PH, Doyle WK. PET of malignant cerebral tumors after interstitial brachytherapy. Demonstration of metabolic activity and correlation with clinical outcome. *J Neurosurg.* 1988;69(6):830–838. PubMed PMID: 2848111. Epub 1988/12/01. eng.

35. Glantz MJ, Burger PC, Friedman AH, Radtke RA, Massey EW, Schold Jr SC. Treatment of radiation-induced nervous system injury with heparin and warfarin. *Neurology.* 1994;44(11):2020–2027. PubMed PMID: 7969953. Epub 1994/11/01. eng.

36. Chuba PJ, Aronin P, Bhambhani K, et al. Hyperbaric oxygen therapy for radiation-induced brain injury in children. *Cancer.* 1997;80(10):2005–2012. PubMed PMID: 9366305. Epub 1997/11/20. eng.

37. McPherson CM, Warnick RE. Results of contemporary surgical management of radiation necrosis using frameless stereotaxis and intraoperative magnetic resonance imaging. *J Neurooncol.* 2004;68(1):41–47. PubMed PMID: 15174520. Epub 2004/06/04. eng.

38. Gonzalez J, Kumar AJ, Conrad CA, Levin VA. Effect of bevacizumab on radiation necrosis of the brain. *Int J Radiat Oncol Biol Phys.*

2007;67(2):323–326. PubMed PMID: 17236958. Epub 2007/01/24. eng.

39. Torcuator R, Zuniga R, Mohan YS, et al. Initial experience with bevacizumab treatment for biopsy confirmed cerebral radiation necrosis. *J Neurooncol.* 2009;94(1):63–68. PubMed PMID: 19189055. Epub 2009/02/04. eng.

40. Liu AK, Macy ME, Foreman NK. Bevacizumab as therapy for radiation necrosis in four children with pontine gliomas. *Int J Radiat Oncol Biol Phys.* 2009;75(4):1148–1154. PubMed PMID: 19857784. Epub 2009/10/28. eng.

41. Levin VA, Bidaut L, Hou P, et al. Randomized double-blind placebo-controlled trial of bevacizumab therapy for radiation necrosis of the central nervous system. *Int J Radiat Oncol Biol Phys.* 2011;79 (5):1487–1495. PubMed PMID: 20399573. Pubmed Central PMCID: PMC2908725. Epub 2010/04/20. eng.

42. Boothe D, Young R, Yamada Y, Prager A, Chan T, Beal K. Bevacizumab as a treatment for radiation necrosis of brain metastases post stereotactic radiosurgery. *Neuro Oncol.* 2013;15(9):1257–1263. PubMed PMID: 23814264. Pubmed Central PMCID: PMC3748921. Epub 2013/07/03. eng.

43. Deibert CP, Ahluwalia MS, Sheehan JP, et al. Bevacizumab for refractory adverse radiation effects after stereotactic radiosurgery. *J Neurooncol.* 2013;115(2):217–223. PubMed PMID: 23929592. Epub 2013/08/10. eng.

44. Jeyaretna DS, Curry Jr WT, Batchelor TT, Stemmer-Rachamimov A, Plotkin SR. Exacerbation of cerebral radiation necrosis by bevacizumab. *J Clin Oncol.* 2011;29(7):e159–e162. PubMed PMID: 21149667. Epub 2010/12/15. eng.

45. Cahan WG, Woodard HQ, Higinbotham NL, Stewart FW, Coley BL. Sarcoma arising in irradiated bone: report of eleven cases.1948. *Cancer.* 1998;82(1):8–34. PubMed PMID: 9428476. Epub 1998/01/15. eng.

46. Loeffler JS, Niemierko A, Chapman PH. Second tumors after radiosurgery: tip of the iceberg or a bump in the road? *Neurosurgery.* 2003;52 (6):1436–1440. PubMed PMID: 12762888. Epub 2003/05/24. eng.

47. Patel TR, Chiang VL. Secondary neoplasms after stereotactic radiosurgery. *World Neurosurg.* 2013;81:594–599. PubMed PMID: 24148883. Epub 2013/10/24. Eng.

48. Armstrong GT, Liu Q, Yasui Y, et al. Long-term outcomes among adult survivors of childhood central nervous system malignancies in the Childhood Cancer Survivor Study. *J Natl Cancer Inst.* 2009;101(13):946–958. PubMed PMID: 19535780. Pubmed Central PMCID: PMC2704230. Epub 2009/06/19. eng.

49. Neglia JP, Robison LL, Stovall M, et al. New primary neoplasms of the central nervous system in survivors of childhood cancer: a report from the Childhood Cancer Survivor Study. *J Natl Cancer Inst.* 2006;98 (21):1528–1537. PubMed PMID: 17077355. Epub 2006/11/02. eng.

50. Salvati M, Frati A, Russo N, et al. Radiation-induced gliomas: report of 10 cases and review of the literature. *Surg Neurol.* 2003;60 (1):60–67. discussion 67. PubMed PMID: 12865017. Epub 2003/07/17. eng.

# 26 *Hemorrhagic Mass Lesions*

STEPHEN T. MAGILL, W. CALEB RUTLEDGE, J. CLAUDE HEMPHILL III, and GEOFFREY T. MANLEY

## Introduction

Traumatic brain injury (TBI) is a significant cause of death and disability. In the United States alone, there are 1.7 million TBIs each year, resulting in more than 53,000 deaths.[1,2] Treating these injuries, and their sequelae, cost society an estimated $60 billion each year.

TBI occurs when a mechanical force causes abrupt head movement, whether applied directly to the head or applied to the body causing secondary head movement. This abrupt motion leads to a spectrum of neurological injury ranging from mild concussion to severe axonal injury or hemorrhagic lesions that can cause swelling, herniation, and death. Injury to the brain parenchyma and the cerebral vasculature can cause elevations in intracranial pressure (ICP) due to swelling in response to axonal injury, contusion, hematoma, hypoxia, or ischemia. The location and severity of the lesion produced after head trauma is determined by the mechanism of injury, the magnitude of the applied force, and the motion of the brain and cerebral vasculature within the skull.

Severity of TBI is often frequently classified by clinical presentation and pathoanatomical findings.[3] The most widely used clinical scale is the Glasgow Coma Scale (GCS), which classifies mild TBI as GCS 13 to 15, moderate TBI as GCS 9 to 13, and severe TBI as GCS <8. The Marshall and Rotterdam computed tomography (CT) classification systems are the most widely used pathoanatomical classifications. The Marshall CT grading system is a 6-point scale with grades 1 to 4 indicating progressively worse diffuse injury, grade 5 an evacuated mass lesion, and grade 6 a nonevacuated mass lesion. The Rotterdam CT classification is a newer 6-point scale that scores for mass effect on the basal cisterns, midline shift, epidural hematoma (EDH), and intraventricular hemorrhage or traumatic subarachnoid hemorrhage (SAH). The Rotterdam score is an independent predictor of unfavorable outcomes after TBI.[4]

## Neuroanatomy and Procedure

### Key Concepts

- The mechanism of injury influences the location and source of bleeding (arterial vs. venous).
- Surgical intervention is determined by radiographic pathology (size of bleed, mass effect/midline shift), clinical condition (GCS score), and examination trajectory.
- The primary surgical interventions are hematoma evacuation via craniotomy or decompressive hemicraniectomy (DC).
- Placement of an external ventricular drain (EVD) or ICP monitor and brain tissue oxygenation monitor is indicated in patients with evidence of increased ICP and abnormal physiology who are not surgical candidates or do not require immediate surgery.

### Neuroanatomy of Traumatic Hemorrhagic Mass Lesions

During TBI, the motion of the brain in response to external force is determined by the location of the impact and the cerebral anatomy. The healthy brain is suspended within the skull by the cerebral spinal fluid, the buoyancy of which reduces its effective weight from 1500 g to 50 g. The meninges surround the brain and are made up of the dura, arachnoid, and pia. Together with the cerebral vasculature, they limit the brain's motion within the skull in response to external forces. The meninges and vasculature also limit volumetric distortion of the brain, causing it to be primarily susceptible to shear strain in response to external forces. Rotational injuries cause higher shearing forces than translational injuries (Fig. 26.1).[5] These properties lead to classic patterns of injury with axonal lesions and hemorrhages occurring most frequently at locations of maximal strain.

Brain movement within the skull leads to the coup-contrecoup phenomena where injuries occur directly below points of impact (coup) as well as on the surface of the brain opposite to the point of injury (contrecoup). Impacts with oblique components to their trajectory exert rotational forces on the brain, causing injury at high shear strain points in addition to the coup-contrecoup locations. The anterior frontal and inferior temporal poles are the most common locations of injury. These locations have high shear strains and are adjacent to irregular internal skull anatomy, increasing the risk of both parenchymal and vascular injury. Brain motion maximal relative to the skull at the vertex in the sagittal plane,[6] which leads to traumatic tearing of bridging veins and subdural hematoma (SDH). Occipital impacts typically cause contrecoup injuries to the frontal lobe with little coup injury. In contrast, lateral impacts typically cause both a coup and contrecoup injury.

In addition to injury mechanism, the unique anatomy and physiology of the cerebral vasculature influence the type of lesions that occur after TBI. There are two different intracranial vascular sources important to consider in TBI. The dura is supplied by the middle meningeal artery, whereas the brain is supplied by the internal carotid and vertebral arteries, which come together at the circle of Willis before branching out to supply the cerebrum. The distal arteries and arterioles travel along the surface of the brain before turning into the parenchyma. There is a rich capillary network with many anastomoses in the parenchyma, which provides a rich and redundant vascular supply to the neurons and glia. Blood exits the capillary bed and enters the cerebral veins, which converge and drain into the deep venous sinuses via bridging veins that are often injured during TBI. The sinuses converge and drain the cranium via the internal jugular veins. All the

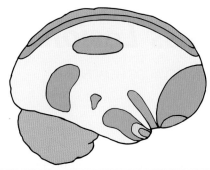

**Fig. 26.1** Maximal points of shear strain on a gelatin brain model. Points of maximal shear strain correlate with the classic anatomical locations for traumatic hemorrhagic or axonal injuries. (Reprinted from Holbourn A. Mechanics of head injuries. *Lancet.* 1943;242(6267):438–41.)

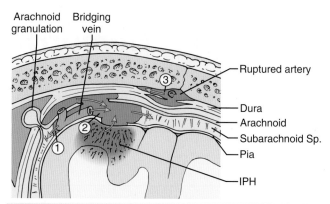

**Fig. 26.2** Sources of traumatic hemorrhagic mass lesions. EDHs *(3)* form between the skull and the dura, often after skull fracture with arterial injury. SDHs *(1)* form between dura and arachnoid, often after damage to bridging veins. Traumatic SAH hemorrhages *(2)* form between arachnoid and pia, often after damage to cortical arteries and veins. IPH/contusions occur after parenchymal injury. (Adapted from Freeman WD, Aguilar MI. Intracranial hemorrhage: diagnosis and management. *Neurol Clin.* 2012 Feb;30(1):211–40.[9])

major arteries and arterioles are covered by pia mater until they reach the depth of the capillary, where astrocyte end feet and tight junctions between endothelial cells make up the blood–brain barrier. When this barrier is disrupted, blood can escape into the surrounding spaces, where it sets off a chain of biochemically toxic actions. Extravascular blood can lead to parenchymal swelling, whereas subarachnoid blood can cause arterial vasospasm and subsequent downstream ischemia.

Arteries and veins respond differently during TBI due to differences in their mechanical properties.[7] The abrupt acceleration and deceleration in TBI cause axial stress on blood vessels. Cerebral arteries are much stiffer than cerebral veins. Consistent with this, the arteries can withstand twice as much axial strain as veins prior to rupturing. However, arteries can only stretch half as much as veins, making them susceptible to rupture when stretched.

Elderly individuals are at increased risk for hemorrhagic mass lesions after TBI. The brain atrophies during normal aging and even more so in dementia. This stretches the already thin-walled bridging veins, making them particularly suspect to injury during even mild TBI, which can lead to SDH formation. The aged vasculature is also at higher risk for compromise due to hypertension, amyloid deposition, and decreased compliance.[8]

Five distinct hemorrhagic lesions are found after TBI and originate from different sources (Fig. 26.2): EDH, SDH, SAH, intraparenchymal hemorrhages (IPHs)/contusion, and microhemorrhages associated with diffuse axonal injury (DAI).

**Epidural Hematoma.** Epidural hematomas (Fig. 26.3) form when bleeding occurs in the potential space between the skull and the dura. Classically, these lesions arise after impact to the temporal bone causing rupture of the middle meningeal artery. They are often accompanied by a lucid interval of several hours prior to neurological deterioration. EDHs respect the sutures, giving them their biconvex shape. They are often associated with temporal bone fractures, although they can form in its absence. Although typically associated with arterial injury, up to 10% of EDHs can form after venous injury.[10] Venous EDHs are found at the anterior pole of the middle cranial fossa and likely arise after injury to the sphenoparietal sinus. They typically do not require surgical intervention.

**Subdural Hematoma.** SDHs form when bleeding occurs in the potential space between the dura and the arachnoid membrane. SDHs can be acute, acute-on-chronic, or chronic (Fig. 26.4). In TBI, the primary concern is acute or acute-on-chronic SDH causing acute mass effect. The arachnoid is avascular, and the only vessels that cross between the arachnoid and dura are the bridging veins, which traverse the potential subdural space between the cortex and venous sinuses. Head trauma causes translation of the brain and arachnoid relative to the dura, stretching, and subsequently rupturing, the bridging veins. Although most SDH are venous in origin, they can arise from arteria sources that produce lacerations in the arachnoid, including ruptured cortical arteries, ruptured aneurysms, ruptured vascular malformations, hypertensive hemorrhages, and neoplasms, among others.[11] SDHs are most common over the anterior portion of the brain, particularly after occipital skull fractures. They also often occur along the falx cerebri. SDHs are more common in elderly individuals, likely due to cortical atrophy and stretching of bridging veins.

**Subarachnoid Hemorrhage.** SAH is common in TBI (Figs. 26.4C and 26.5). Rupture of small cortical arteries or veins can cause bleeding into the subarachnoid space. Traumatic SAHs (tSAH) are often seen in the gyri and are frequently the only radiographic finding on CT after mild TBI.[12] They occur diffusely after severe TBI and confer a twofold increase in mortality. In contrast, in mild TBI and isolated tSAH in patients younger than 40, patients often recover similar to a concussion.

**Contusion and Intraparenchymal Hemorrhage.** Cerebral contusions (Fig. 26.5) form after injury to brain parenchyma and vasculature and are often associated with IPH. They occur primarily at the crowns of gyri as well as at locations with high shear strain described earlier, notably the anterior temporal poles and inferior frontal lobes. Repeat imaging typically shows expansion of the contusions and development of surrounding edema that peaks

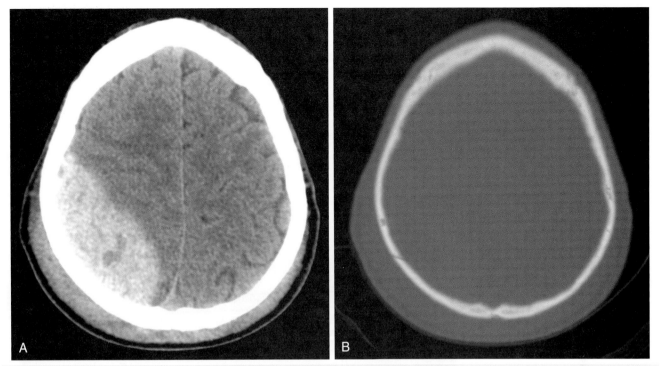

**Fig. 26.3** EDH. Large EDH **(A)** with hypodense components suggestive of hyperacute blood. The EDH formed after skull fracture **(B)**.

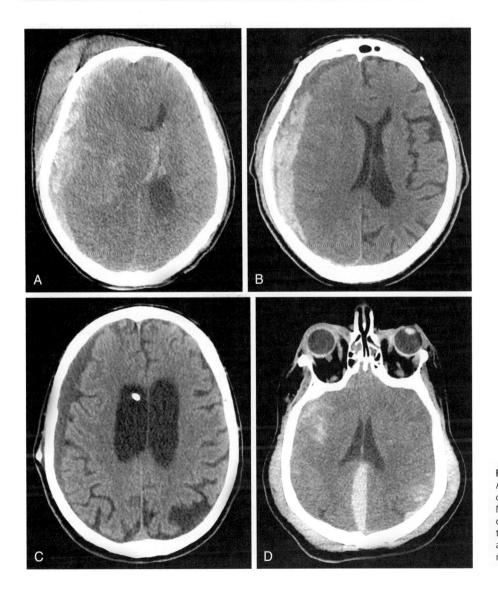

**Fig. 26.4** SDH at different timepoints. Acute SDH **(A)** after frontal TBI. Acute on chronic SDH **(B)**. Chronic SDH **(C)**. Notice how the degree of midline shift decreases with increasing chronicity of the bleed. Para-falcine SDH **(D)** with coup and contrecoup contusions and traumatic SAH seen after left occipital impact.

Presentation                          72 hrs Post-Injury

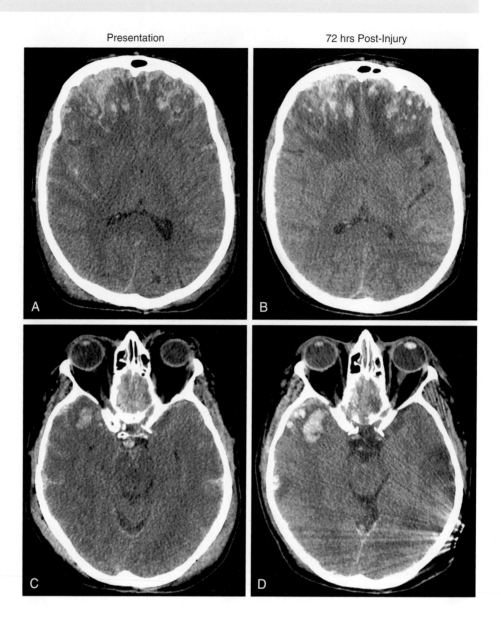

**Fig. 26.5** IPH/hemorrhagic contusions. After occipital impact, this patient developed frontal and temporal contusions. CT at presentation **(A, C)**. CT showing typical evolution of contusion with IPH enlargement and increase in surrounding edema after 72 hours **(B, D)**.

around 48 to 72 hours. In addition to supratentorial IPH, posterior fossa IPH can lead to rapid deterioration with acute compression of the brainstem and fourth ventricle.

**Microhemorrhages and Diffuse Axonal Injury.** DAI is one of the most common injuries after TBI and is associated with microhemorrhages. It occurs after high-speed deceleration injuries, which commonly happen during motor vehicle collisions. Initial head CT can be negative for acute hemorrhage, but subsequent magnetic resonance imaging, particularly susceptibility weighted imaging, will show hemosiderin deposits reflective of microhemorrhages in addition to the axonal damage on diffusion sequences.[13]

### Procedure

The primary surgical interventions for traumatic hemorrhagic mass lesions are either intracranial monitoring or surgical decompression. Intracranial monitoring can be done via placement of an ICP monitor or EVD. These can be augmented with a brain tissue oxygenation monitor.

Decompression can be achieved either with craniotomy and hematoma evacuation or with a hemicraniectomy. The indications for ICP monitoring and surgical decompression of hemorrhagic lesions are jointly published by the Brain Trauma Foundation and the American Association of Neurological Surgeons.

**External Ventricular Drain/Intracranial Pressure and Oxygenation Monitors.** There is level 2 evidence that an ICP monitor should be placed in salvageable patients with severe TBI (GCS 3–8) and an abnormal CT scan, defined as the presence of hematoma, contusion, swelling, herniation, or compressed basilar cisterns.[14] There is level 3 evidence that an ICP monitor should be placed for patients with a normal CT scan and two of the following: age greater than 40 years, motor posturing, or systolic blood pressure (SBP) <90 mm Hg. The choice of whether to monitor ICP with a standard intraparenchymal ICP monitor, or "bolt," versus an EVD is guided by the need for volume drainage to control ICP, such as evidence of swelling, mass effect, or midline shift. Knowledge of the patient's ICP allows treatment to be guided by cerebral perfusion pressure (CPP), rather than prophylactically treating presumed ICP elevations.

In addition to ICP monitoring, there is an emerging role for brain tissue oxygenation monitoring in the intensive care unit (ICU).[14,15] Current level 3 recommendations include treating jugular venous saturation of less than 50% or brain tissue oxygen levels less than 15 mm Hg. Primary damage to brain tissue occurs at the time of impact; however, secondary injury also occurs due to tissue hypoxia after the primary insult and can contribute to long-term morbidity. Monitoring brain tissue oxygenation allows the neurointensivist to titrate therapy to maintain brain oxygenation, rather than simply CPP. Brain desaturations are correlated with worse recovery and increased mortality and, interestingly, do not always correlate with high ICP or low CPP. Low brain oxygenation can be treated with multiple modalities, including head repositioning, fluid administration, airway suctioning, decreasing ICP, increasing CPP, and increasing $Fio_2$, among others.

PROCEDURE. Placement of an EVD, ICP monitor, or brain tissue oxygenation monitor all begin with shaving and sterilely prepping the head around Kocher's point (11–12 cm posterior to the nasion, 3 cm off midline). A skin incision is made with a scalpel, and a twist drill is used to drill through the skull. The dura is incised, and the monitor/drain can then be placed. For EVDs, the catheter is passed into the ventricle, tunneled under the skin, and sewn to the head. For ICP monitors/brain tissue oxygen monitors, the mount, or "bolt," is screwed into the skull and then the intraparenchymal probe is passed through the probe and placed into the brain.

**Craniotomy and Hemicraniectomy.** Indications for surgical decompression with craniotomy or hemicraniectomy are based primarily on radiographic and clinical criteria as follows:[16]

*EDH*: Urgent surgical evacuation should be performed for EDH with volume >30 cm³ or midline shift >5 mm. Nonoperative monitoring can be considered for EDH with <5 mm midline shift (MLS) and <1.5 cm thick and GCS >8 without focal neurological deficit, or anterior temporal EDH without deficit.

*Acute SDH*: Urgent surgical evacuation should be performed for acute SDH >1 cm or causing midline shift >5 mm regardless of GCS score. Urgent surgical evacuation should also be performed for acute SDH <1 cm with <5 mm midline shift, but GCS <9 with a worsening examination, any pupillary dilation/anisocoria, or ICP >20 mm Hg. ICP monitors should be placed in any patient with acute SDH and GCS <9.

*IPH/contusion*: Surgical decompression should be performed for patients with IPH/contusion who have progressive neurological signs attributable to the lesion, medically refractory elevated ICP, or radiographic signs of mass effect. Surgical decompression should also be performed in patients with GCS 6 to 8 and frontal or temporal contusions who show midline shift >5 mm and evidence of cistern compression. ICP monitoring and close observation are indicated in patients with IPH and no significant signs of mass effect.

*Posterior fossa hemorrhage*: Urgent surgical evacuation of hemorrhagic mass lesions in the posterior fossa with suboccipital craniectomy should be performed for patients with neurological signs attributable to the lesion and fourth ventricle compression, basal cistern compression, or obstructive hydrocephalus.

For evacuation of supratentorial hemorrhagic mass lesions, there is significant controversy about the optimal surgical procedure to perform. Historically, the primary options were a craniotomy and hematoma evacuation, a DC, or a bifrontal craniectomy. The Decompressive Craniectomy in Patients with Severe Traumatic Brain Injury trial recently showed that bifrontal craniectomy resulted in worse outcomes for patients with diffuse intracranial hypertension, which has led to that operation falling out of favor in most centers.[17] Currently, the choice between craniotomy and hemicraniectomy is determined by the neurosurgeon based on the radiographic characteristics of the lesion, the likelihood of progression, and the operative findings such as degree of brain swelling.

*Procedure*: For either DC or craniotomy with hematoma evacuation, an incision is made anterior to the tragus and extended over the ear posteriorly before turning superiorly and progressing anteriorly ipsilateral to midline. The scalp flap is raised with the temporalis muscle and reflected anteriorly. Burr holes are drilled in the skull and connected with a side-cutting drill, allowing elevation of the bone flap. Dural tack-up sutures are placed around the edges of the flap to keep the peripheral dura closely apposed to the skull, preventing epidural hematoma. The temporal bone is removed laterally until reaching the floor of the middle fossa. The dura is then opened in a starlike pattern, allowing broad decompression (Fig. 26.6). The hematoma is evacuated, and any sources of bleeding are identified and controlled. If there is limited brain swelling and low likelihood of progressive swelling, the bone flap can be replaced. If the swelling is significant, the bone is sent to a tissue bank until cranioplasty can be performed—typically at least 3 months postoperatively. After the decompression, a contralateral EVD is placed to allow for ICP monitoring and volume drainage as needed. (For a detailed discussion, please see Chapter 29).

## PERIOPERATIVE CONSIDERATIONS

### Key Concepts

- Control airway and breathing, and achieve hemodynamic stability.
- Temporary stabilization with hyperosmotic therapies should be initiated as soon as intracranial hypertension is suspected.
- Acute, short-term hyperventilation can be used as a temporizing measure while the patient is transported to the operating room.
- Traumatic or iatrogenic coagulopathy must be reversed.
- Seizure prophylaxis should be administered.
- Rapid transport to operating room reduces mortality.

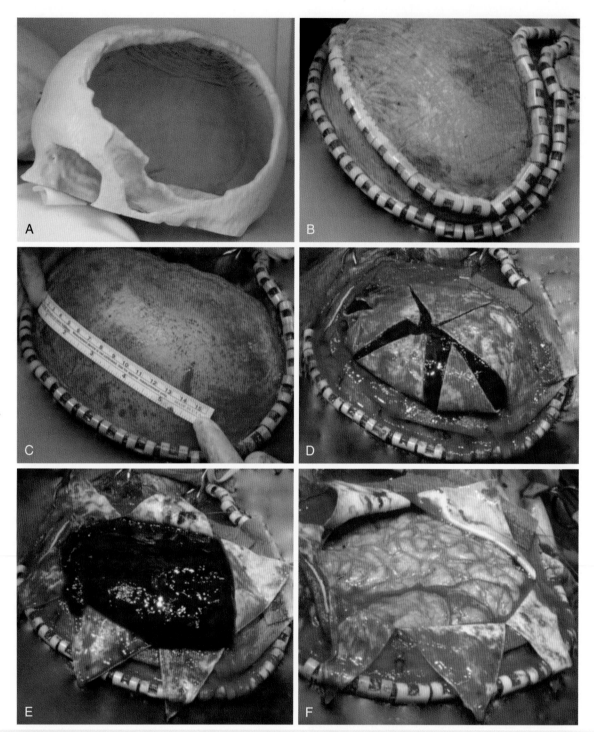

**Fig. 26.6** Decompressive hemicraniectomy. Skull model with bone flap removed **(A)**. Skin incision **(B)**. Skull exposed **(C)**. Bone flap removed and dura incised showing large SDH **(D)**. Dura reflected to allow clot evacuation **(E)**. Brain beneath clot prior to closure **(F)**.

## Initial Management from Trauma bay to Scanner to Operating Room

As with all traumas, control of airway, breathing, and hemodynamic stability must be achieved first. If possible, it is ideal to get an initial neurological examination prior to intubation. If intracranial hemorrhage is suspected as evidenced by pupil dilation, loss of pupil reactivity, or loss of brainstem reflexes, then hyperosmolar therapy can be initiated. Once stable, the patient should be transported to the CT scanner rapidly. If any vascular injury is suspected due to fractures or penetrating injury, a CT angiogram should be performed to rule out additional vascular pathology. If venous sinus injury is suspected, as with penetrating trauma or skull fracture, a delayed postcontrast scan can assess sinus patency. If surgically amenable hematoma is identified, the patient should be rapidly transported to the operating room. Operating within the first 4 hours of injury reduces mortality after acute SDH from 90% to 30%.[18]

## Immediate Interventions to Manage Intracranial Pressure

If neurological signs of elevated ICP and impending or active herniation are present in the trauma bay, hyperosmolar therapy should be initiated. If the patient is hemodynamically stable, 1 g/kg intravenous mannitol should be started. In the hypotensive patient who cannot tolerate mannitol, hypertonic saline solutions (such as 23% sodium chloride) can be administered. In addition to hyperosmolar therapy, short-term hyperventilation can induce vasoconstriction, decreasing intracranial blood volume and lowering ICP.

## Management of Coagulopathy

Initial laboratory studies should include coagulation studies because traumatic coagulopathy occurs in 30% of patients with isolated TBI.[19] In addition to traumatic coagulopathy, many elderly TBI patients are on anticoagulation medication for stroke prevention. The coagulopathies should be reversed as soon as they are identified. Prothrombin complex concentrate should be given for patients on warfarin. In addition, recombinant factors and concentrated cryoprecipitate can be administered for severe coagulopathy. The new-generation factor IIa and Xa inhibitors present a particularly difficult challenge because no direct antidote is available to them.[20] Typical strategies include administering concentrated cryoprecipitate, although the efficacy is variable.

## Seizure Prophylaxis

After moderate to severe TBI with EDH/SDH/ICH/contusion, there is a 15% risk of seizure in untreated patients.[21] These patients should receive a fosphenytoin load or, if contraindicated, levetiracetam.

# POSTOPERATIVE COMPLICATIONS

## Key Concepts

- All postsurgical traumatic patients require ICU monitoring and frequent and accurate neurological assessment.
- Postoperative head CT is necessary to assess for rebleed or contralateral bleed.
- Advanced neuromonitoring in conjunction with traditional ICU monitoring is useful for trending data and guiding optimal management.

Postsurgical severe TBI patients are critically ill and face a myriad of potential complications that require close monitoring and management. Common complications are listed in order of severity in Table 26.1 and will be discussed individually next. In addition to the specific neurosurgical complications, these patients have similar needs as other critically ill patients, including nutritional support, ventilator support, and long-term care planning, including rehabilitation, tracheostomy, and percutaneous gastrostomy tube placement. These patients are also susceptible to the general ICU risks, including ventilator-associated pneumonias, nosocomial infections, central line infections, urinary tract infections, and pressure ulcers; however, these have been well addressed in other texts and will not be discussed here.

**Table 26.1** Postoperative Complications in Order of Severity

| Complication | Incidence | References |
|---|---|---|
| Herniation/withdrawal of care/death | 14%–60% | (24–27) |
| Contralateral bleed | 1.3%–24% | (29,30,38) |
| Expansion of IPH | 58% | (31) |
| Hypotension | 32% | (50) |
| Seizure | 9%–15% | (14) |
| Hydrocephalus | 9%–45% | (33,38,44) |
| Hyponatremia | 27% | (36) |
| Hypernatremia | 16%–40% | (37) |
| External cerebral herniation | 27% | (38) |
| DVT/pulmonary embolism | 1%–2% | (27) |
| Wound infection | 3%–12% | (27,38,41,42) |
| Anemia requiring transfusion | 68% | (43) |
| Trephination syndrome | 13% | (38) |
| Hemorrhage around EVD/ICP monitor | 0.5% | (46) |
| Subdural hygroma formation | 21%–50% | (38,49) |

*IPH*, intraparenchymal hemorrhage; *DVT*, deep venous thrombosis; *EVD*, external ventricular drain; *ICP*, intracranial pressure.

Intensive monitoring of neurosurgical TBI patients is essential to guiding treatment, but is a complex undertaking. Postcraniotomy/postcraniectomy patients will have an ICP monitor or EVD and a brain tissue oxygenation monitor. ICP monitoring allows calculation of CPP to guide blood pressure parameters. Brain tissue oxygenation monitoring allows titration of $Fio_2$ to ensure adequate tissue oxygenation. Some centers also place microdialysis catheters, which allows assessment of metabolites whose levels can reflect local metabolism. These metabolites include glucose, lactate, pyruvate, and glycerol, molecules whose levels are altered during hypoperfusion or ischemia.[22] In addition, TBI patients often undergo an electroencephalogram during their postoperative care. New multimodal neuromonitoring units allow trending of these variables simultaneously over time and facilitate optimal visualization of data trends, allowing the intensivist to appreciate correlations between individual parameters, which can be used to guide therapy for each patient.[23]

# HERNIATION/WITHDRAWAL OF CARE/DEATH

The overall mortality rate after TBI is 19 per 100,000 in the United States, resulting in roughly 50,000 deaths/year. For patients who make it to the operating room and undergo DC after TBI, mortality is 28% at 6 months postop, reflecting the severity of these injuries and the attempted lifesaving nature of the operation.[24] Among patients who do survive, 63% have favorable outcomes, with Glasgow Outcomes Scale (GOS) scores of 4 or 5. Individual outcomes correlate with the severity of injury, age, initial GCS score, and preoperative pupil examination. Increased age and injury severity are correlated with poor outcomes.

Historically, mortality for patients with acute SDH was reported at 40% to 60%.[25,26] However, a recent large retrospective study reported a mortality rate of 14%, regardless of whether or not they underwent evacuation of the SDH.[27] In this cohort, 88% of evacuated acute SDH had a GCS of 13 to 15 at discharge. Functional assessment at discharge showed that 82% of patients were independent in expression, 66% were independent in feeding, and 29% were independent in locomotion.

Many of the deaths after TBI are due to withdrawal of life-sustaining care, particularly within the first 3 days after injury.[28] The decision to withdrawal care is based primarily on the perception of the patient's long-term prognosis by the medical team caring for the patient. Interestingly, recent data looking at trends of withdrawal of care between multiple centers observed that the rate of withdrawal of care varied significantly between centers.[28] This raises the possibility that some physicians are overly nihilistic about the patient's chances of survival and may be too pessimistic early in the hospital course after TBI, despite the knowledge that most survivors will have a reasonable quality of life.

## CONTRALATERAL BLEED

ICP increases rapidly after TBI, which can tamponade injured vessels. However, after hematoma evacuation and intracranial decompression, these injured vessels can begin hemorrhaging. Oftentimes they are contralateral to the side of decompression at the site of contrecoup injury. In one series, contralateral EDH formation after SDH evacuation occurred in 1.3% of patients.[29] In contrast, a different group reported results on 112 patients after evacuation of acute traumatic SDH where they observed contralateral bleed in 24% of their patients.[30] Contralateral bleed is typically observed on immediate postoperative CT, but can also be diagnosed intraoperatively with ultrasonography. Postoperative reaccumulation of SDH or contralateral bleed should be suspected in any patients whose neurological examination declines postoperatively.

## EXPANSION OF INTRAPARENCHYMAL HEMORRHAGE

In addition to allowing contralateral hematoma formation, reduced ICP after DC is frequently associated with enlargement of IPHs.[31] Interestingly, the degree of expansion correlates with mortality, with expansion greater than 20 cc after decompression significantly associated with mortality and worse GOS.

## HYPOTENSION

Multiple studies have shown that hypotension, defined as SBP <90 mm Hg, is an independent predictor of mortality after TBI. For review see Ref. 14. A single episode of hypotension in the absence of hypoxia increased the odds of mortality, and multiple episodes of hypotension had an odds ratio of 8.1 for mortality. Hypoxia ($PaO_2 < 60$), which often is associated with hypotension, also increases the risk of mortality and should be avoided at all costs.

Interestingly, prehospital administration of hypertonic saline, which can temporize patients with hemorrhagic mass lesions until surgical evacuation, also increased blood pressure. Finally, data are emerging that the degree of hypotension that correlates with increased mortality may vary by age and may actually be higher than the previously held SBP threshold of 90 mm Hg.[32] Looking at a population of more than 15,000 moderate and severe TBI patients, Berry et al. observed increases in mortality with SBP <110 mm Hg in patients 15 to 49 years old, SBP <100 mm Hg in patients 50 to 69 years old, and SBP <110 mm Hg in patients older than 70 years.

## SEIZURE

Seizure rates are high after TBI. In untreated patients, they range from 9% to 40%.[14] The landmark study by Temkin et al. demonstrated in a randomized, double-blinded, placebo-controlled trial enrolling more than 400 patients that phenytoin for 7 days at therapeutic levels reduced the rate of seizure during the first week postinjury from 14.2% to 3.6%.[21] In addition to seizures around the time of injury, 15% to 24% of patients with moderate-severe TBI will develop late-onset seizures. Unfortunately, at 2 years there was no reduction in the rate of late-onset seizures, regardless of early 7-day courses of phenytoin or valproate or 6 months of valproate therapy.[33] It is thought the sequelae of TBI can form small kindling foci that eventually generate seizures. It is important to counsel patients and families about this high risk.

## HYDROCEPHALUS

Another common complication of DC after TBI is hydrocephalus that requires implantation of a ventriculoperitoneal shunt (VPS). Honeybul et al. found that in a cohort of 156 patients with severe TBI who survived at least 6 months after surgery, 45% developed radiographic evidence of ventriculomegaly and 36% required a VPS.[34] It is unclear whether decompressive craniectomy is responsible for delayed hydrocephalus, because TBI itself is an independent risk factor for the development of hydrocephalus. Choi et al. showed that in a large cohort of 693 patients with severe TBI, 4% developed hydrocephalus.[35] In a subset of 55 patients undergoing decompressive craniectomy, 24% developed hydrocephalus. A number of risk factors for development of hydrocephalus have been reported, including size of the craniectomy, with large craniectomy carrying a higher risk of hydrocephalus.

## HYPONATREMIA AND HYPERNATREMIA

Disorders of salt and water balance are very common after TBI and a significant source of morbidity. These imbalances follow the triphasic response thought to arise after injury to the pituitary stalk. Axons from the hypothalamus project in the pituitary stalk through the diaphragm and into the posterior pituitary gland in the sella turcica. There they release antidiuretic hormone (ADH) and oxytocin into the blood. Under normal conditions ADH is released in response to increases in osmolality or angiotensin II, as well as decreases in plasma volume. During head trauma, the rapid acceleration and deceleration of the brain within the skull can stretch and damage the stalk. This damage blocks action potentials from reaching the posterior pituitary, decreasing ADH release during the first 3 to 7 days after injury. This manifests clinically with increasing urine output, increasing serum osmolality, low specific gravity, and hypernatremia. However, as the axons degenerate down to the synaptic terminals in the posterior pituitary, the ADH stored in the pituitary is released in an uncontrolled fashion, initiating the second phase of the response reflective of high ADH levels. Clinically this presents with hyponatremia and fluid retention, commonly seen from days 5 to 12 after injury. In the third and final phase of the response, patients can develop permanent diabetes insipidus (DI) if there has been permanent damage to the pituitary.

Lohani and Devkota reported hyponatremia in 9 of 40 moderate to severe TBI patients.[36] Five of these patients were volume overloaded, consistent with syndrome of inappropriate antidiuretic hormone secretion, whereas the rest appeared to have more of a cerebral salt-wasting phenotype. A recent extensive review of the literature reflecting more than 5000 severe TBI patients reported the incidence of DI ranging from 16% to 40%.[37] Both these conditions are very common and must be managed aggressively with strict ins and outs, frequent serum sodium and osmolality checks, and close monitoring of urine specific gravity. Initial management of DI involves fluid replacement with hypotonic crystalloid solutions. When refractory to fluid replacement, IV or intranasal DDAVP is administered. Patients with hyponatremia are managed with fluid restriction, salt tabs, and hypertonic saline. Because the management of the two conditions is directly opposite to one another, close attention must be paid when patients are experiencing this phenomenon, and the three phases should be anticipated to optimize management.

## EXTERNAL CEREBRAL HERNIATION

After decompression, the brain can continue to swell and herniate out through the defect in the skull. One study reported this in 27% of patients.[38] As the brain swells, it can cause compression of cortical arteries and veins on the surface of the brain against the bone at the edge of the decompression. To prevent this, a small window of decompression is avoided during surgery and the craniectomy is made as large as safely possible.

## DEEP VENOUS THROMBOSIS/PULMONARY EMBOLISM

TBI patients are at increased risk for deep venous thrombosis (DVT) if untreated, and a small number of those who develop DVT will go on to develop pulmonary embolism, which can be catastrophic. TBI is an independent risk factor in the trauma patient, with an odds ratio of 1.24.[39] Nevertheless, the rates of DVT and pulmonary embolism (PE) are both quite low in the modern era. After acute SDH, Ryan et al. identified 23 (2%) DVTs and 16 PEs (1%) in a recent series of 1427 patients with acute SDH.[27] There was no difference in incidence of DVT or PE between patients who have SDH evacuated and those treated conservatively. The latest Brain Trauma Foundation Guidelines provide a level 3 recommendation for use of mechanical and pharmacological prophylaxis.[14] The timing of when to initiate anticoagulation after a hemorrhagic intracranial lesion has remained an issue of debate. A recent review by Hawryluk et al. suggested that initiating anticoagulation 72 hours after a TBI provided the best balance between the risk of intracranial hemorrhage and risk of thromboembolic event.[40]

## WOUND INFECTION

As with any surgical procedure, craniotomy or craniectomy for hemorrhagic mass lesions carries the risk of infection. The risk is around 3% to 12%, depending on the study, although some studies report much higher rates.[27,38,41,42] In postcraniotomy/postcraniectomy patients, however, this is a significant complication because of the open channels to the brain and meninges, increasing the risk for meningitis or cerebritis. In addition, breakdown or dehiscence of the wound is difficult treat and can require additional surgeries, even occasionally requiring a free flap for closure.

## ANEMIA REQUIRING TRANSFUSION

Although a hemoglobin threshold of 7.0 g/dL is commonly practiced for ICU patients, this may be inappropriate for TBI patients. Anemia-induced cerebral arteriolar dilatation can result in increased blood flow, worsened cerebral edema, and intracranial hypertension in patients with TBI. Impaired brain tissue oxygenation can occur secondary to an insufficient systemic hemoglobin level. Sekhon et al. found that a mean 7-day hemoglobin concentration of <90 g/L was associated with increased mortality in 273 patients with severe TBI.[43] In their study, the incidence of transfusion was 68%, with the average transfusion hemoglobin of 78 g/L. However, in a systematic review, which included 537 patients from four studies of TBI, Desjardins et al. found no association between hemoglobin levels or transfusions and mortality, duration of mechanical ventilation, multiple organ failure, and length of stay.[44] The optimal hemoglobin level and transfusion threshold for patients with TBI remain unknown.

## TREPHINATION SYNDROME

Trephination syndrome occurs in up to 13% of patients undergoing DC. It is characterized by sinking of the flap that occurs in the late stage after hemicraniectomy. Symptomatically, patients can present with acute neurological deficits, such as motor impairment.[45] Interestingly, these symptoms resolve rapidly after cranioplasty and replacement of the skull or placement of a prosthesis. It is thought that the syndrome is caused by alterations in cerebrospinal fluid (CSF) flow caused by changes in the pattern of CSF drainage after injury, as well as reduced cerebral blood flow as the brain sags inward.

## HEMORRHAGE AROUND EXTERNAL VENTRICULAR DRAIN AND INTRACRANIAL PRESSURE MONITOR

There is a risk of hemorrhage anytime a monitor is placed in the brain. For EVD placement, the risk of hemorrhage is 5% to 9% in adults and children; however, only 0.5% of those are symptomatic.[46,47] ICP monitor placement is also very safe. In 140 placements there were 10 punctate hemorrhages, none of which caused a neurological deficit.[48]

## SUBDURAL HYGROMA FORMATION

Subdural hygroma formation is a common complication after DC for severe TBI.[38,49] These are benign lesions that typically resolve on their own and should not be cause for concern.

# Conclusions

TBI is a considerable cause of death and disability in the United States, affecting nearly 2 million people annually. Neurosurgical intervention focuses on the treatment of primary injury, whereas ICU management centers on preempting and mitigating secondary injury that occurs as a result of the primary injury. Although historically mortality has been very high for moderate-severe TBI, with early surgical intervention, dedicated ICU care, advanced neuromonitoring, and improved understanding of cerebrovascular physiology, outcomes continue to improve.

## References

1. Coronado VG, Xu L, Basavaraju SV, et al. Surveillance for traumatic brain injury-related deaths—United States, 1997-2007. *MMWR Surveill Summ.* 2011;60(5):1–32.
2. Faul MD, Xu L, Wald MM, Coronado VG. *Traumatic Brain Injury in the United States: Emergency Department Visits, Hospitalizations, and Deaths 2002—2006.* CDC; 2010. www.cdc.gov/TraumaticBrainInjury.
3. Saatman KE, Duhaime A-C, Bullock R, Maas AIR, Valadka A, Manley GT. Classification of traumatic brain injury for targeted therapies. *J Neurotrauma.* 2008;25(7):719–738.
4. Huang Y-H, Deng Y-H, Lee T-C, Chen W-F. Rotterdam computed tomography score as a prognosticator in head-injured patients undergoing decompressive craniectomy. *Neurosurgery.* 2012;71(1):80–85.
5. Holbourn A. Mechanics of head injuries. *Lancet.* 1943;242 (6267):438–441.
6. Shelden C, Pudenz R, Restarski J, Craig W. The lucite calvarium: a method for direct observation of the brain. *J Neurosurg.* 1944;1:67–75.
7. Monson KL, Goldsmith W, Barbaro NM, Manley GT. Axial mechanical properties of fresh human cerebral blood vessels. *J Biomech Eng.* 2003;125(2):288–294.
8. Mitchell GF, van Buchem MA, Sigurdsson S, et al. Arterial stiffness, pressure and flow pulsatility and brain structure and function: the age, gene/environment susceptibility—Reykjavik study. *Brain.* 2011;134(Pt 11):3398–3407.
9. Freeman WD, Aguilar MI. Intracranial hemorrhage: diagnosis and management. *Neurol Clin.* 2012;30(1):211–240. ix.
10. Gean AD, Fischbein NJ, Purcell DD, Aiken AH, Manley GT, Stiver SI. Benign anterior temporal epidural hematoma: indolent lesion with a characteristic CT imaging appearance after blunt head trauma. *Radiology.* 2010;257(1):212–218.
11. Matsuyama T, Shimomura T, Okumura Y, Sakaki T. Acute subdural hematomas due to rupture of cortical arteries: a study of the points of rupture in 19 cases. *Surg Neurol.* 1997;47(5):423–427.
12. Levy AS, Orlando A, Hawkes AP, Salottolo K, Mains CW, Bar-Or D. Should the management of isolated traumatic subarachnoid hemorrhage differ from concussion in the setting of mild traumatic brain injury? *J Trauma.* 2011;71(5):1199–1204.
13. Benson RR, Gattu R, Sewick B, et al. Detection of hemorrhagic and axonal pathology in mild traumatic brain injury using advanced MRI: implications for neurorehabilitation. *Neurorehabilitation.* 2012;31(3):261–279.
14. Author Group, Brain Trauma Foundation. Guidelines for the management of severe traumatic brain injury. *J Neurotrauma.* 2007;24(Suppl 1):S1–S106.
15. Beynon C, Kiening KL, Orakcioglu B, Unterberg AW, Sakowitz OW. Brain tissue oxygen monitoring and hyperoxic treatment in patients with traumatic brain injury. *J Neurotrauma.* 2012;29 (12):2109–2123.
16. Bullock MR, Chesnut R, Ghajar J, et al. Guidelines for the surgical management of traumatic brain injury. *Neurosurgery.* 2006;58(3 Suppl):S1–S62.
17. Cooper DJ, Rosenfeld JV, Murray L, et al. Decompressive craniectomy in diffuse traumatic brain injury. *N Engl J Med.* 2011;364 (16):1493–1502.
18. Seelig JM, Becker DP, Miller JD, Greenberg RP, Ward JD, Choi SC. Traumatic acute subdural hematoma: major mortality reduction in comatose patients treated within four hours. *N Engl J Med.* 1981;304(25):1511–1518.
19. Epstein DS, Mitra B, O'Reilly G, Rosenfeld JV, Cameron PA. Acute traumatic coagulopathy in the setting of isolated traumatic brain injury: a systematic review and meta-analysis. *Injury.* 2014;45 (5):819–824.
20. Straznitskas A, Giarratano M. Emergent reversal of oral anticoagulation: review of current treatment strategies. *AACN Adv Crit Care.* 25 (1):5–12; quiz 13–4.
21. Temkin NR, Dikmen SS, Wilensky AJ, Keihm J, Chabal S, Winn HR. A randomized, double-blind study of phenytoin for the prevention of post-traumatic seizures. *N Engl J Med.* 1990;323(8):497–502.
22. Cecil S, Chen PM, Callaway SE, Rowland SM, Adler DE, Chen JW. Traumatic brain injury: advanced multimodal neuromonitoring from theory to clinical practice. *Crit Care Nurse.* 2011;31 (2):25–36.
23. Feyen BFE, Sener S, Jorens PG, Menovsky T, Maas AIR. Neuromonitoring in traumatic brain injury. *Minerva Anestesiol.* 2012;78 (8):949–958.
24. Danish SF, Barone D, Lega BC, Stein SC. Quality of life after hemicraniectomy for traumatic brain injury in adults. A review of the literature. *Neurosurg Focus.* 2009;26(6).
25. Fell DA, Fitzgerald S, Moiel RH, Caram P. Acute subdural hematomas. Review of 144 cases. *J Neurosurg.* 1975;42(1):37–42.
26. Haselsberger K, Pucher R, Auer LM. Prognosis after acute subdural or epidural haemorrhage. *Acta Neurochir (Wien).* 1988;90 (3-4):111–116.
27. Ryan CG, Thompson RE, Temkin NR, Crane PK, Ellenbogen RG, Elmore JG. Acute traumatic subdural hematoma: current mortality and functional outcomes in adult patients at a level I trauma center. *J Trauma Acute Care Surg.* 2012;73(5):1348–1354.
28. Côte N, Turgeon AF, Lauzier F, et al. Factors associated with the withdrawal of life-sustaining therapies in patients with severe traumatic brain injury: a multicenter cohort study. *Neurocrit Care.* 2013;18 (1):154–160.
29. Shen J, Pan JW, Fan ZX, Zhou YQ, Chen Z, Zhan RY. Surgery for contralateral acute epidural hematoma following acute subdural hematoma evacuation: five new cases and a short literature review. *Acta Neurochir (Wien).* 2013;155(2):335–341.
30. Huang AP-H, Chen Y-C, Hu C-K, et al. Intraoperative sonography for detection of contralateral acute epidural or subdural hematoma after decompressive surgery. *J Trauma.* 2011;70(6):1578–1579.
31. Flint AC, Manley GT, Gean AD, Hemphill JC, Rosenthal G. Postoperative expansion of hemorrhagic contusions after unilateral decompressive hemicraniectomy in severe traumatic brain injury. *J Neurotrauma.* 2008;25(5):503–512.
32. Berry C, Ley EJ, Bukur M, et al. Redefining hypotension in traumatic brain injury. *Injury.* 2012;43(11):1833–1837.
33. Temkin NR, Dikmen SS, Anderson GD, et al. Valproate therapy for prevention of posttraumatic seizures: a randomized trial. *J Neurosurg.* 1999;91(4):593–600.

34. Honeybul S, Ho KM. Incidence and risk factors for post-traumatic hydrocephalus following decompressive craniectomy for intractable intracranial hypertension and evacuation of mass lesions. *J Neurotrauma*. 2012;29(10):1872–1878.

35. Choi I, Park H-K, Chang J-C, Cho S-J, Choi S-K, Byun B-J. Clinical factors for the development of posttraumatic hydrocephalus after decompressive craniectomy. *J Korean Neurosurg Soc*. 2008;43 (5):227–231.

36. Lohani S, Devkota UP. Hyponatremia in patients with traumatic brain injury: etiology, incidence, and severity correlation. *World Neurosurg*. 76(3-4):355–60.

37. Kolmodin L, Sekhon MS, Henderson WR, Turgeon AF, Griesdale DE. Hypernatremia in patients with severe traumatic brain injury: a systematic review. *Ann Intensive Care*. 2013;3(1):35.

38. Yang XF, Wen L, Shen F, et al. Surgical complications secondary to decompressive craniectomy in patients with a head injury: a series of 108 consecutive cases. *Acta Neurochir (Wien)*. 2008;150 (12):1241–1247. discussion 1248.

39. Knudson MM, Ikossi DG, Khaw L, Morabito D, Speetzen LS. Thromboembolism after trauma: an analysis of 1602 episodes from the American College of Surgeons National Trauma Data Bank. *Ann Surg*. 2004;240(3):490–496. discussion 496–8.

40. Hawryluk GWJ, Austin JW, Furlan JC, Lee JB, O'Kelly C, Fehlings MG. Management of anticoagulation following central nervous system hemorrhage in patients with high thromboembolic risk. *J Thromb Haemost*. 2010;8(7):1500–1508.

41. Sughrue ME, Bloch OG, Manley GT, Stiver SI. Marked reduction in wound complication rates following decompressive hemicraniectomy with an improved operative closure technique. *J Clin Neurosci*. 2011;18(9):1201–1205.

42. Huang AP-H, Tu Y-K, Tsai Y-H, et al. Decompressive craniectomy as the primary surgical intervention for hemorrhagic contusion. *J Neurotrauma*. 2008;25(11):1347–1354.

43. Sekhon MS, McLean N, Henderson WR, Chittock DR, Griesdale DE. Association of hemoglobin concentration and mortality in critically ill patients with severe traumatic brain injury. *Crit Care*. 2012;16 (4):R128.

44. Desjardins P, Turgeon AF, Tremblay M-H, et al. Hemoglobin levels and transfusions in neurocritically ill patients: a systematic review of comparative studies. *Crit Care*. 2012;16(2):R54.

45. Stiver SI, Wintermark M, Manley GT. Reversible monoparesis following decompressive hemicraniectomy for traumatic brain injury. *J Neurosurg*. 2008;109(2):245–254.

46. Wiesmann M, Mayer TE. Intracranial bleeding rates associated with two methods of external ventricular drainage. *J Clin Neurosci*. 2001;8(2):126–128.

47. Ngo QN, Ranger A, Singh RN, Kornecki A, Seabrook JA, Fraser DD. External ventricular drains in pediatric patients. *Pediatr Crit Care Med*. 2009;10(3):346–351.

48. Blaha M, Lazar D. Traumatic brain injury and haemorrhagic complications after intracranial pressure monitoring. *J Neurol Neurosurg Psychiatry*. 2005;76(1):147.

49. Aarabi B, Hesdorffer DC, Ahn ES, Aresco C, Scalea TM, Eisenberg HM. Outcome following decompressive craniectomy for malignant swelling due to severe head injury. *J Neurosurg*. 2006;104 (4):469–479.

50. Chesnut RM, Marshall SB, Piek J, Blunt BA, Klauber MR, Marshall LF. Early and late systemic hypotension as a frequent and fundamental source of cerebral ischemia following severe brain injury in the Traumatic Coma Data Bank. *Acta Neurochir Suppl (Wien)*. 1993;59:121–125.

# 27 *Penetrating Traumatic Brain Injury*

PETER LE ROUX and MONISHA KUMAR

## Introduction

Head injury is a major public health issue worldwide and may be classified as penetrating or nonpenetrating (blunt). Penetrating head injury, defined as a wound in which the cranium is breached by a projectile that is either missile (usually gun related) or nonmissile (most typically knife related), is less prevalent than closed or blunt head injury. However, more than 35,000 civilians die each year in the United States from penetrating head injury, particularly from gunshot wounds (GSWs), and firearms account for the largest proportion of deaths from traumatic brain injury (TBI) in the United States.[1,2] The victim of a GSW to the head is 35 times more likely to die than is a patient with a blunt TBI.[3,4] The outcome from nonmissile penetrating injuries (e.g., knife wounds) is better because the skull provides a protective barrier. However, these nonmissile injuries pose similar challenges in care to GSWs. As many as 75% of civilian GSWs in an urban setting die at the scene and another 10% to 15% die within 3 hours of injury.[5] The mortality associated with stab wounds is much less. Because mortality is high in cranial GSWs, aggressive management is often withheld in patients who arrive at the trauma center with a low Glasgow Coma Scale (GCS) score or with bihemispheric brain injuries.[6–9] However, over the last 20 years, advances in surgical techniques, hemodynamic resuscitation, and critical care have decreased mortality and morbidity in TBI patients, even for those patients with penetrating TBI (pTBI) traditionally thought unsurvivable.[10–14] This chapter will discuss the pathophysiological mechanisms, neuroanatomical structures, surgical techniques, and postoperative complications encountered in the management of pTBI.

## Neuroanatomy

### Key Concepts

- Outcomes from GSW to the head are substantially worse in general than other TBIs.
- The pathophysiology of penetrating injury is distinct from blunt TBI and helps explain the poor outcome.
- The most important prognostic factor is initial neurological examination.

Most nonmilitary GSWs involve low-velocity projectiles; brain injury is secondary to the crushing effect of the pressure wave following the projectile through the brain tissue. There are two major mechanisms of tissue damage: tissue crushing (or permanent cavitation) and temporary cavitation (or tissue stretching). Civilian bullets are not required to have (and frequently do not have) a full metal jacket, for example, hollow-point and soft-point bullets, and so are more likely to fragment or deform in tissue, particularly on striking bone; this can influence tissue damage. For example, hunting bullets by law are manufactured to deform ("mushroom") to increase the extent of tissue damage and the likelihood of a quick death to the animal. Perforating injuries are through-and-through injuries in which the bullet enters and exits the skull, that is, there are both entry and exit wounds. In penetrating and superficial injuries, the bullet remains in the victim. Greater than 80% of cranial GSWs are penetrating or perforating, but it is important to differentiate between the two because mortality is nearly threefold greater in perforating than penetrating injuries.[15–20]

### Clinical Pearl

The wounding potential of a bullet is determined by the equation $KE = 1/2MV^2$, where KE is kinetic energy, M is the mass of the bullet, and V is the impact velocity of the bullet; the impact velocity is by far the most important determinant of a bullet's wounding potential.

As with blunt TBI, primary and secondary brain injury occurs with pTBI. The primary insult occurs at the time of the penetration and causes immediate neuronal destruction associated with cutting, tearing, and stretching of brain tissue and the disruption of cerebral blood vessels. The extent of brain injury varies from a GSW to stab wound: GSWs also may cause petechial and linear hemorrhages and shear injuries distant from the missile path, whereas stab wounds tend to cause local injury.

Unlike blunt injury, pTBI may cause hypovolemic hypotension, hemorrhagic shock, or cardiopulmonary arrest associated with blood loss. Indeed, the most common cause of death in cranial stab wounds is blood loss.[21] This may be from the scalp, which is very vascular, or from an intracranial source with an open wound from the meningeal, parenchymal vessels, or the venous sinuses. In addition, with penetrating head injury, particularly craniofacial injury to the lower face, bleeding and edema may cause airway obstruction.

*Scalp:* All five layers of the scalp (skin, subcutaneous tissue, galea aponeurotica, underlying loose areolar tissue, and the skull periosteum) are injured even in superficial and tangential injuries. Hemorrhage may accumulate in the potential spaces of the scalp. Subperiosteal hematomas can occur in children,whereas subgaleal hematomas, that is, not confined by sutures, are more common in adults. In young children the scalp hematoma may be of sufficient size to cause shock.

*Bone:* The angle of impact and regional differences in skull thickness influence the severity of the fracture and brain injury. Fracture pattern and bone beveling may distinguish entry and exit sites, which have both clinical and medical-legal implications. Irregular stellate fractures that radiate from the point of impact are seen at the entry site; the inner table is usually more comminuted than the outer table. Where there is an exit wound, there are shorter fracture lines and the outer table may be more comminuted than the inner table.[19] Depressed skull fractures, usually comminuted, may occur with missile and nonmissile pTBI. These in-driven bony fragments may cause additional injury and pose management challenges when near a venous sinus.

*Intracranial contents:* When the pia and arachnoid are torn, cerebral laceration occurs. This usually results in a conical lesion with the base at the entrance and the laceration tapering inwards along the projectile tract. Several different pathologies are observed: pneumocephalus, extraaxial hemorrhage (extradural or subdural), and subarachnoid hemorrhage (SAH). These pathologies may predispose to cerebral vasospasm, intraventricular hemorrhage, and hemorrhagic contusion that may function as a nidus for intracerebral hemorrhage (ICH), cerebral edema, and obstructive hydrocephalus.[20] Mass lesions observed in stab wounds are usually hematomas; cerebral edema is inevitable with GSWs. Both can contribute to reduced cerebral perfusion pressure and infarction with or without herniation.

# Perioperative Considerations

## EVALUATION AND RESUSCITATION

Patients with pTBI should be resuscitated according to the Advanced Trauma Life Support and Emergency Neurological Life Support guidelines. Hemodynamic support is provided to maintain a systolic blood pressure (BP) of at least 90 mm Hg with fluids and vasopressors.[22,23] Hypotension can aggravate outcome, and low BP is a poor prognostic sign if from the brain injury alone.

A neurological examination, including the level of consciousness and GCS, particularly the motor score and pupillary reaction, is important to decide on triage and care. The patient's postresuscitative GCS should be documented. The wound requires careful examination because the scalp is highly vascular and significant blood loss may occur. A complete physical examination is recommended to evaluate for other injuries.[23] GSW to the face can damage ocular structures, making it difficult or impossible to assess the pupils. Pharmacological paralysis should be avoided and reversed if necessary to obtain an examination. Entry and exit wounds should be assessed, including the presence of contact burns, which may be important in determining trajectory and proximity of gun to the cranium. The cervical spine should be immobilized, but if there is no evidence for injury, further immobilization is not necessary.[24]

## Laboratory Studies

Routine laboratory tests, including electrolytes, glucose, and arterial blood gas, should be obtained at admission. Many patients have lost large amounts of blood before reaching the emergency department or may present with acute coagulopathy of trauma/shock. Consequently, determining the hemoglobin concentration, coagulation profile and platelet count, and a type and cross-match is important. In addition, a toxicology screen, including alcohol levels, is appropriate.

## Preoperative Imaging

After resuscitation, the next step is imaging. The scout views performed during the computed tomography (CT) examination have largely replaced the need for skull x-rays. CT is the primary technique used to image pTBI and always should include brain and bone windows. Coronal and sagittal views are helpful for patients with skull base or craniofacial involvement or high convexity injuries. Features that should be evaluated include 1) identification of in-driven bone and missile fragments; 2) characterization of the missile trajectory and its relationship to vessels and air-containing skull-base structures; 3) definition of exit and entry sites; 4) evaluation of the extent of brain injury, for example, does the track cross the midline or involve multiple lobes or the brainstem; and 5) detection of intracranial hematomas and mass effect, including edema and basal cistern effacement (Fig. 27.1). Metallic streak artifact may degrade CT image quality. Magnetic resonance imaging (MRI) may be useful for imaging of nonmetallic objects (e.g., wood, pencils, or glass).

Vascular studies are not necessary in the acute phase unless the CT scan suggests injury to large vascular structures or surgery is planned. Vascular imaging is warranted to plan surgical removal of a nonmissile object (e.g., a knife). A computed tomography angiogram (CTA) is generally the study of choice in the acute setting. Endovascular treatment of exsanguinating hemorrhage is sometimes required for injuries to major extracranial and/or intracranial vessels. However, vascular imaging is indicated in all pTBI patients within 7 to 10 days after injury to exclude delayed vascular complications (e.g., traumatic fistula or aneurysms). CT findings associated with an increased risk of vascular injury include where the wound trajectory is through or near 1) the sylvian fissure, that is, M1 and M2 segments of the middle cerebral artery; 2) the supraclinoid carotid artery (and cavernous sinus); 3) the vertebrobasilar vessels; or 4) there are bony fractures associated with or overlying dural venous sinuses.

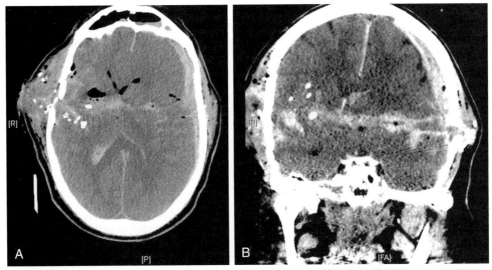

**Fig. 27.1** Axial CT **(A)** and coronal CT **(B)** showing nonsurvivable self-inflicted gunshot wound with deep bihemispheric trajectory with in-driven bullet/bone fragments and left-sided subdural hematoma.

# Procedure

## Key Concepts

- The primary goal of surgery is to eliminate mass effect and preserve remaining viable tissue.
- Secondary goals are to remove bone and missile fragments and close the dura and scalp.

There are three broad indications for surgery: 1) hematoma evacuation; 2) control of mass effect; and 3) restoration of dural, craniofacial, and scalp integrity for infection control. A large ICH on CT (ICH >3 cm, > 1 cm thick if extraaxial) requires emergency surgical evacuation. However, factors such as the patient's age and clinical condition and the hematoma location also influence a decision to perform emergency surgery. Hematomas and contusions in the temporal region or posterior fossa require more aggressive treatment because they tend to cause herniation more frequently than similar lesions elsewhere. Where there is

greater than 5-mm midline shift or refractory intracranial hypertension, a decompressive craniectomy is an option. In wounds with visible brain herniation (open depressed fractures), wound debridement and dural repair are indicated even in the fully conscious patient.

Once the decision is made to surgically intervene, the planned surgery must take into account several factors, including 1) entry and exit wounds, 2) bullet trajectory, and 3) intracranial fragments. Generally, cranial entry and exit wounds need to be prepped in the field so that they can be debrided and closed. Bullet tracks through the air sinuses may require debridement and isolation from the cranial contents. Trajectories suspicious for vascular injury require intraoperative preparation to deal with vascular injuries. Care must be taken when there is concern for venous sinus injury because loss of tamponade effect can result in life-threatening exsanguination. Given the likelihood of significant postoperative brain swelling, decompressive craniectomy is a common approach to cranial GSW (Fig. 27.2).[25,26]

There are several important technical considerations to operative intervention. First, head draping should cover

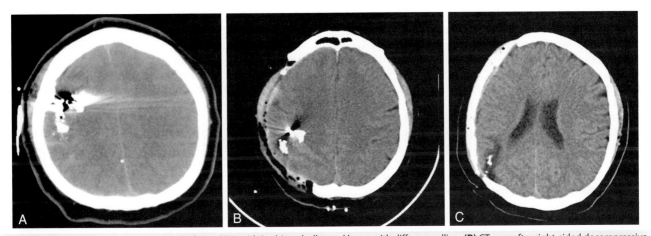

**Fig. 27.2 (A)** Axial CT showing right hemispheric GSW with in-driven bullet and bone with diffuse swelling. **(B)** CT scan after right-sided decompressive hemicraniectomy with debridement of entrance wound. Deeply in-driven bone and bullet fragments are not removed as to not cause further brain injury. **(C)** Postoperative scan after methacrylate cranioplasty (bone flap with positive cultures at time of initial surgery). Patient recovered with mild left-sided hemiparesis.

the entire available surface of the scalp to allow extension of the surgical incision beyond the wound's confines or to allow possible scalp rotation flaps to facilitate wound closure. Second, the skin incision is planned so that the blood supply to the scalp is not compromised. Third, a large craniotomy around the entry wound often is needed to permit visualization of the pathology and facilitate repair. Fourth, gentle debridement of devitalized brain is performed using suction and irrigation. When the trajectory or debrided cavity stays open with gentle irrigation, this suggests that sufficient debridement has been performed to limit subsequent cerebral swelling. Fifth, the surgeon should be prepared to manage potential vascular injuries that may be encountered. Traumatic aneurysms often are not suitable for direct clipping and so require vascular reconstruction or trapping.

Before consideration of decompressive craniectomy (DC), several technical considerations must be considered. First, there is no role for DC in patients where the bullet/projectile track penetrates the zona fatalis (midline skull base, thalamus, brainstem).[27–29] However, if there is an adequate GCS, transventricular injury does not preclude DC. Second, intracranial pressure (ICP) measurement (in the absence of large hematomas) before DC can be helpful when monitoring is feasible. Third, it is important to plan for future surgeries. Fourth, the decompression (i.e., size of the bone removal) should be as large as possible, at a minimum, 14 cm (anteroposterior) by 12 cm (superoinferior) for a unilateral or frontotemporoparietal craniectomy. Bifrontal decompression is indicated when there is bifrontal injury, transventricular trajectories, or extensive anterior cranial fossa disruption. This decompression should extend from the supraorbital ridge to the coronal suture. In these patients every effort should be made to repair the skull base with vascularized tissue, for example, a pericranial flap at the time of the initial surgery, because a cerebrospinal fluid (CSF) leak is associated with meningitis. Fifth, the removed bone should be cultured and ideally stored in a bone bank because those placed in the abdominal subcutaneous tissue frequently become infected and need to be discarded.

## VASCULAR INJURY

Vascular injury is common after pTBI and ranges between 5% and 40%.[30–34] The reported incidence may depend on management and diagnostic techniques. For example, during recent U.S. military involvement, Operation Iraqi Freedom (OIF), where there was improved diagnostic techniques (digital subtraction angiography [DSA] with 3D reconstruction), the incidence of cerebrovascular pathology was 30%. The cumulative incidence of traumatic intracranial aneurysms (TICAs) was 6% in the Iran–Iraq conflict.[33] Dural sinus injury, TICAs, traumatic extracalvarial aneurysms (TECAs), arterial dissections, and arteriovenous fistulae are the characteristic vascular injuries after pTBI.

*Dural venous sinus:* The major sinuses are superficial and therefore vulnerable to pTBI. The projectile can directly tear or lacerate the sinus, or injury can occur from the resulting skull fracture. Dural venous sinus injuries can be potentially life threatening and result in hemorrhage: epidural, subdural, or when the scalp is open, external hemorrhage that can be massive. Venous sinus thrombosis, both acute and delayed, also can result and contribute to increased ICP.

In a pTBI patient and ongoing bleeding with suspected sinus injury, the head of the bed is elevated to slow but not stop the bleeding to reduce the risk of air embolus. The bleeding may then be controlled with packing and external pressure. Injuries that involve the anterior third of the superior sagittal sinus allow sacrifice of the sinus, but injuries in other locations require sinus preservation. If near the transverse or sigmoid sinus and the patient is stable, angiography is advisable to determine whether there is sinus occlusion or one sinus is dominant. In some patients it may be best to leave alone a fracture that potentially involves a sinus. Surgery, however, needs to include strategies to manage massive blood loss (e.g., a cell saver and rapid infuser), and the planned scalp incision and craniotomy need to be large enough to gain early and wide proximal and distal control of the sinus. A variety of strategies to prevent blood loss, including direct suture, muscle plugs, pericranial patch grafts, and autologous vein grafts (e.g., saphenous vein with or without bypass), are available.

*Craniofacial injury:* The incidence of hematoma formation, direct vascular injury, contamination from the sinus, CSF fistula, and infection is high with craniofacial pTBI. Additional CTs to image craniofacial structures should be obtained before any surgery, and at the time of surgery closure of any dural defect with vascularized flaps augmented with fat grafts is essential. In patients with anterior skull-base fractures, nasogastric tubes should be avoided.

*Transorbital injury:* Objects will often penetrate the orbital roof because the frontal bone over the orbital roof is very thin. Frontal lobe injury is common in this type of orbital injury. Injury also occurs through the superior orbital fissure (SOF) when the bony shape of the orbit directs low-velocity objects that enter the orbit toward it. The bony anatomy tends to direct an object that penetrates the SOF lateral to the cavernous sinus, beneath the frontal lobe, medial to the temporal lobe, above the petrous ridge, and lateral to the brainstem. The least common route of penetration is the optic canal. Here the projectile is directed into the suprasellar cistern, toward the optic nerve and internal carotid artery. Although GSWs and knife wounds are frequent causes of transorbital injury, other unusual implements (e.g., pencils) also may be seen.

Transorbital injuries are best managed by a multidisciplinary team with input from neurosurgery, ophthalmology, otolaryngology, maxillofacial surgery, anesthesiology, and critical care. Patients with transorbital injury require dedicated maxillofacial, orbital, and head CT scanning. Angiography should be performed in patients with suspected vascular injury. Treatment varies, depending on the mechanism and extent of the injury, the path of penetration, and whether the foreign body remains in situ at the time of presentation[35]

*Stab wounds.* A narrow elongated defect, or so-called *slot fracture*, is produced by a stab wound and is diagnostic when identified. However, in some cases in which skull penetration is proven, no radiological abnormality can be identified. If vital areas are spared, objects can be removed through the same entrance wound, but when close to vascular structures, there is greater concern. In these patients the protruding object can be cut off but left in situ to facilitate transport. Comprehensive imaging, including vascular imaging, is necessary to know the depth, location, and type of object (e.g., does it have barbs?). The penetrating object then is removed once the dura is opened in the operating room, and the procedure can be performed under direct vision. Endovascular techniques can help facilitate removal, that is, to gain proximal vascular control. This may be performed in the interventional suite before surgery or in a hybrid operating room (OR). When the object is in or close to a major venous sinus, the OR needs to be set up to repair the sinus and deal with potential massive blood loss.[21]

## Postoperative Complications

### Key Concepts

- For survivors of pTBI, vascular injury, central nervous system infection, and CSF leaks are common.
- Common vascular injuries after pTBI include dural sinus injury, traumatic intracranial aneurysms, traumatic extracalvarial aneurysms, arterial dissections, and arteriovenous fistulae.

After surgery, patients with pTBI are managed in the neurocritical care unit. In general, critical care management is similar to patients with blunt TBI. However, there are several specific complications after a pTBI, including cerebral swelling, CSF leak, infection (e.g., meningitis and brain abscess), vascular injury, and posttraumatic seizures, that are further reviewed here.

### CEREBRAL SWELLING AND INTRACRANIAL PRESSURE

Limited clinical data are available on the specific indications and applications of ICP monitoring in pTBI patients, and so guidelines for TBI in general apply.[36–39] Fiber-optic parenchymal ICP monitors may be preferable when multiple lobes are involved and there is midline shift, because the ventricle may be difficult to assess. A ventriculostomy also may allow CSF diversion to manage a CSF leak. Published studies suggest a higher frequency of raised ICP in pTBI than blunt TBI patients, and when present, is associated with worse outcome.[36–39] The management of increased ICP is covered in Chapter 47.

### CEREBROSPINAL FLUID LEAK

A CSF fistula is common after pTBI; up to a third of patients may have a CSF leak,[40,41] and its presence is highly predictive of infectious complications. Risk factors include a bony breach and fractures of the anterior skull base with involvement of the paranasal sinuses or of the lateral skull base with involvement of the middle ear cavity and mastoid or after an orbitocranial-penetrating injury. In addition a CSF leak may develop when dural repair and scalp wound closure are inadequate or compromised (e.g., from hydrocephalus). When leaking fluid is collected on a sponge, CSF, unlike other nasal fluids, forms a halo sign. The diagnosis can be confirmed with fluid analysis for beta-2 transferrin.[41] Management may involve altered head position or temporary CSF diversion.

### INFECTION

There is a high risk of intracranial infection in patients with pTBIs associated with contaminated foreign bodies (e.g., metal fragments, skin, hair, bone fragments) that penetrate the skull and enter brain tissue along the projectile trajectory. Infections include scalp infection, meningitis, cranial osteitis, epidural abscess, subdural empyema, cerebritis, brain abscess, or ventriculitis. Risk factors of infection include CSF leaks, involvement of the paranasal or other air sinuses, orbitofacial injury, and transventricular injuries that cross the midline, that is, they involve multiple lobes and dehiscence of the traumatic or surgical wound. Other factors that increase the infection risk include age, sex, urban vs. rural origin, comorbidities that affect the immune response (e.g., diabetes, drug addiction, malnutrition), prolonged hospitalization, and the severity of neurological injury. The most important determinant of infection is a CSF leak, and hence early surgical closure is important in reducing the risk of infection. The number of retained bone or metal fragments may also be associated with infection.[42–44]

The role of prophylactic antibiotics after pTBI is debated. Indeed, infection prophylaxis may depend more on early surgical treatment of the wound and prevention of CSF leak than on antibiotic use. In addition, there is a considerable variation in the antibiotic regimen for prophylaxis in pTBI patients. Cephalosporins, however, are most frequently used, although these agents penetrate the noninflamed meninges poorly. When used, the duration of antibiotic therapy also remains controversial and often is based on the experience of the surgeon.[43]

The infections that are commonly encountered include meningitis, subdural empyemas, and brain abscesses. Meningitis typically presents with headache, fever, and neck stiffness. A subdural empyema may result from meningitis or as a complication of the initial wound, surgical intervention, or craniofacial injury. The collection can compress the brain and cause neurological deficits, headache, and decreased consciousness. Gram-positive cocci are common, but when there is paranasal involvement, gram-negative organisms are frequent. Mass effect should be alleviated through burr holes, craniotomy, or craniectomy. Source control with surgery may be required. Mortality remains high (up to 20%) if the diagnosis not appreciated, and 20% of survivors have neurological deficits.[42]

Brain abscesses that complicate pTBI are typically caused by skin-related bacterial pathogens. Gram-positive cocci, for example, *Staphylococcus* and *Streptococcus* species, are the most common organisms. Other organisms after pTBI include *Clostridium* and *Enterobacteriaceae*. Brain abscesses after pTBI are often associated with a retained foreign body. This has prompted debate about the extent of debridement at the initial surgery and whether retained bone or metal fragments should be removed.[45,46]

Precontrast and postcontrast CT or MRI should be obtained when an abscess is suspected, although MRI may not be possible due to retained metal fragments. Contrast-enhanced MRI is more sensitive than CT, especially with the addition of MR spectroscopy (MRS). Abscesses are ring enhancing on MRI and surrounded by edema (T1 low intensity and T2/FLAIR high intensity).

## Box 27.1   Indications for Surgical Excision of a Brain Abscess

Multiloculated large abscess
Fungal or gas-forming organism
Resistant bacteria
Abscess contains foreign body
Fistulous communication
Increased ICP and mass effect
Failure to respond to aspiration and antibiotics

The central cavity is hyperintense to CSF on T1 and hypointense to CSF on T2 images. On diffusion-weighted imaging images there is central restricted diffusion and hypointense signal on apparent diffusion coefficient images.[47,48] On MRS there is a high lactate peak and reduced Cho/Cr and N-acetyl aspartate (NAA) peaks. An elevated succinate peak is relatively specific but not frequently found.

Deep abscesses can be drained using frame-based stereotactic techniques. Indications for surgical excision as the initial choice of procedure are listed in Box 27.1. Antimicrobial monotherapy may be used, but generally is successful only if the abscess is small (<1.5 cm). If there is no response to antibiotics treatment, then repeat aspiration, surgical excision, intracavity antimicrobials, or placement of a closed drainage catheter become necessary. The role of intrathecal antibiotics is poorly defined. Adjuvant corticosteroids may help reduce edema.[49,50] Seizures are a frequent complication, so anticonvulsants should be administered.[51,52] Previously outcome after brain abscess was poor, but improved imaging, antibiotics, and surgical techniques (stereotaxy) have improved mortality and morbidity.[45,46]

## VASCULAR INJURY

Vascular injury is common after pTBI and ranges between 5% and 40%. (During OIF, improved diagnostic techniques [DS angiography with 3D reconstruction] demonstrated a 30% incidence of cerebrovascular pathology in pTBI patients.)[30–34] The cumulative incidence of TICAs was 6% in the Iran–Iraq conflict.[33] Dural sinus injury, TICAs, TECAs, arterial dissections, and arteriovenous fistulae are the characteristic vascular injuries after pTBI. Risk factors for vascular injuries in missile wounds include orbitofacial or pterional penetrating injury, ICH, SAH, and injuries with fragments crossing two or more dural compartments.

The major sinuses are superficial and thus vulnerable to pTBI. The projectile can directly tear or lacerate the sinus, or injury can occur from the resulting skull fracture. Dural venous sinus injuries can be potentially life threatening and result in hemorrhage: epidural, subdural, or when the scalp is open, external hemorrhage that can be massive. Venous sinus thrombosis, both acute and delayed, also can result and contribute to increased ICP.

### Traumatic Intracranial Aneurysms

Overall, TICAs comprise 1% of all forms of intracranial aneurysms. The incidence of TICA formation after pTBI ranges between 3% and 20%, but can be up to 50% in some populations. Of the penetrating injuries, stab wounds appear to have the highest probability of producing TICAs with a threefold to fourfold greater risk than GSWs.[31] Factors associated with a high risk of TICA formation include 1) penetrating trauma through the frontobasal or pterional window, 2) ICH or SAH along the trajectory of the penetrating object, 3) large vessels in proximity to the injury site, 4) bullet or bone fragments that pass through the areas where the vasculature is crowded (e.g., Sylvian fissure), and 5) delayed hemorrhage identified on CT scan.[33,34] In a study of 109 stab wounds to the head, TICAs were observed in 11 (14.9%) of the 74 patients who underwent angiography (Figs. 27.3 and 27.4).[31] By contrast, Aarabi et al.,[30] in a series of 223 patients who suffered high-velocity missile injuries and underwent angiography, found only eight (3.6%) traumatic aneurysms.

TICAs are unstable and have a high rate of rupture; approximately 50% may do so within the first 7 to 10 days after injury and up to 90% within 3 weeks of injury.[33] It is important then to perform a short-term follow-up angiogram (1–2 weeks) if a small aneurysm (2 mm) is identified and unable to be treated.

Conventional digital subtraction angiography (DSA) is the current diagnostic gold standard to detect TICAs. MR angiography (MRA), although sensitive for cervical and intracranial vascular injury, may be difficult to obtain in unstable patients and contraindicated when there are retained metal fragments. CTA is an excellent technique for rapid screening for neurovascular injury, but images may be degraded by metallic streak artifact, and both MRA and CTA may miss small TICAs with devastating consequences.

The unpredictable and early rupture rate of TICAs makes early treatment important. Prompt diagnosis based on arteriography and exclusion of the aneurysm from the circulation by surgical or endovascular methods is associated with better outcome than conservative treatment. Similarly, if an aneurysm is identified at the time of initial surgery, it should be occluded. Because most TICAs are false aneurysms, endovascular techniques are not considered a permanent solution, although recent military experience suggests otherwise.[33,34] The mortality rate for patients with ruptured TICAs may be as high as 50% and should they survive, neurological disability is frequent from secondary neurological injury.[30–34]

### Vasospasm

Vasospasm is defined as a reduction in the caliber of a blood vessel, usually in response to an external stimulus. After pTBI, the exact incidence may depend on how patients are investigated, but can be as high as 40% to 50%.[53,54] For example, during OIF, Armonda et al.[54] developed specific criteria for diagnostic cerebral angiography (Box 27.2); angiographically documented vasospasm was observed in 47.4% of patients. This incidence was significantly greater than that observed during the Iran–Iraq war of the 1980s. Factors associated with vasospasm included 1) an initial low GCS, 2) intracranial blood of any type but in particular SAH, 3) the number of lobes injured, and 4) a TICA. Vasospasm is more frequent in victims of blast injury and is observed in vessels remote from the site of penetration.

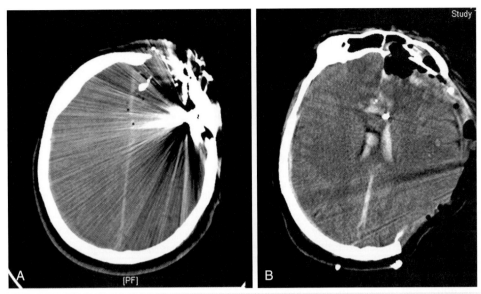

**Fig. 27.3 (A)** Patient with left frontal GSW with bullet fragments near anterior cerebral artery complex. **(B)** CT scan after decompressive craniectomy.

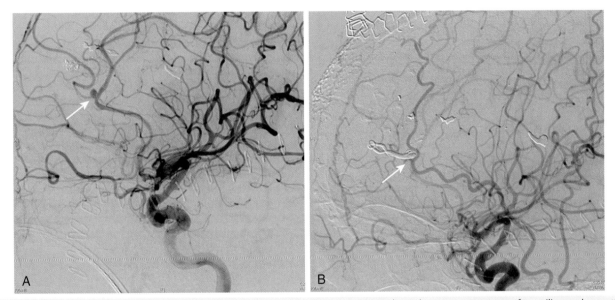

**Fig. 27.4 (A)** Lateral angiogram showing pseudoaneurysm (*arrow*). **(B)** Follow-up imaging showed recurrent aneurysm after coiling and so patient subsequently underwent clip occlusion (*arrow*).

**Box 27.2  Indications for Diagnostic Cerebral Angiography Following Military pTBI**

Penetrating injury: pterional, transorbital, posterior fossa
CT evidence for tSAH
Known cerebral vessel injury (observed at initial surgery)
Blast injury and GCS <8
TCD evidence for vasospasm
Known TICA
Decrease in pbtO₂ or CBF
Lack of improvement in GCS without clear explanation

Reprinted from Armonda RA, et al. Wartime traumatic cerebral vasospasm: recent review of combat casualties. *Neurosurgery.* 2006 Dec;59(6):1215–25; discussion 1225.

Patients with traumatic cerebral vasospasm (TCV) fare worse than those without[53,54]; however, evidence-based treatments remain scant. Transcranial Doppler (TCD) ultrasonography can detect TCV, with greatest sensitivity in the anterior circulation.[53,54] Diagnosis and management of TCV is similar to nontraumatic vasospasm and includes medical management and endovascular techniques (intraarterial pharmacological treatment, for example, nicardipine).

### Arterial Dissections

Arterial dissections occur when injury through the intima and occasionally the media allows entry of blood and separation of the inner and outer vascular layers. This compromises the vessel lumen and contributes to ischemia that may be transient, or a stroke. Management may require endovascular or surgical techniques, but frequently non-surgical treatment with antiplatelet agents is effective.[30,34]

## Arteriovenous Fistula

Fistulas develop when a focal arterial disruption develops a communication with the venous system. After pTBI, these lesions may involve vessels of the scalp or dura mater or cortical vessels. Dural fistulae can recruit cortical venous drainage or increase pressure in major sinuses, thus contributing to neurological symptoms, increased ICP, SAH, or ICH. Simple dural fistulae can be excised, but preoperative embolization or occlusion by endovascular means may be required when a dural sinus is involved. A carotid-cavernous sinus fistula, the most recognized posttraumatic fistula, is characterized by a clinical syndrome that consists of pulsating exophthalmos, chemosis, and a bruit. Therapy is directed at saving vision and eye movement. Carotid-cavernous fistulae are best diagnosed by cerebral angiography and treated by endovascular occlusion, often with great result.[30,33,34]

## POSTTRAUMATIC EPILEPSY

Moderate TBI increases the risk of seizures 3-fold, whereas severe TBI is associated with about a 17-fold increase in seizure risk. However, the exact incidence of seizures after pTBI is unclear, but the overall risk is likely between 20% and 30%.[50–52] Risk factors for long-term seizures after pTBI include low GCS, mode of injury, dural penetration (missile), ICH, transventricular injury, and early-onset seizures.[50–52] The heterogeneity of pTBI injuries, however, makes it difficult to reliably interpret data on seizure risk and in particular whether retained fragments are independent risk factors or not.

The type of seizures that occur in closed or penetrating TBI is similar. However, seizure frequency may be more frequent and first unprovoked seizures occur at earlier time in pTBI.[51] Data on prevention of posttraumatic seizures are not specific to pTBI. Phenytoin, valproate, and carbamazepine significantly reduce the incidence of provoked (early) seizures. However, none of the studied drugs (phenytoin, phenobarbital, their combination, carbamazepine, valproate, or magnesium) prevent long-term seizures.[55–57] In addition, newer antiepileptic drugs have not been rigorously tested in TBI. Consequently, seizure prophylaxis and treatment of long-term seizures in pTBI should be managed in a similar manner as TBI.[51,52]

## OUTCOME

Outcome and mortality from pTBI depends on several variables including whether in the military or civilian setting or whether a GSW or other penetrating injury e.g. knife wound. In addition outcome data are influenced by whether initial GCS or post resuscitation GCS is used in the study, pre-hospital care and decisions about treatment and futility.

In the civilian environment GSWs to the head have traditionally been associated with up to 90% mortality, three quarters of which occurs at the scene of the accident.[2,3,5–9] In part this may be affected by decisions about futility since management often was withheld in those with a GCS of 3-5. However in more recent series in which

## Box 27.3   Factors associated with worse outcome after cranial GSWs

Advanced age
Suicide attempt
Mode of injury: perforating injury > penetrating > tangenital
Hypotension (SBP <90 mmHg)
Respiratory distress
Coagulopathy
Low GCS (may differ in military and civilian)
Dilated, non-reactive pupils
Increased ICP
CT findings
    Bihemispheric transventricular lesions
    multilobar injuries
    intraventricular hemorrhage
    uncal herniation
    subarachnoid hemorrhage

aggressive management starting with pre-hospital resuscitation is used 50-70% of GSWs can be expected to survive, including survival rates of 23% in those with a GCS of 3-5.[12,13,27] Factors associated with poor outcome are listed in Box 27.3.

Injuries from military-grade weaponry differ significantly from those that occur in the civilian population. Several additional factors, including protective equipment (helmet, body armor), systemic injury burden, available resources in a war zone, immediacy of neurosurgical intervention, and field and overseas transport also affect outcome also limit conclusions about civilian GSWs based on military data. Up to one half of all combat related deaths result from head injury and 40-50% of patients die after a pTBI. However overall outcome has improved over time. Outcome also varies with the type of pTBI and is worse in patients with a GSW rather than injury form a blast fragment. Most patients with a GCS >5 are expected to survive.[58] Recent military experience also demonstrates favorable outcomes in select patients with a GCS of 3-5 who traditionally did not receive treatment.[58,59]

# Conclusions

Although the initial assessment and resuscitation of patients with penetrating head injuries may be similar to those with closed head injuries, prompt and aggressive cardiopulmonary resuscitation is critical because acute blood loss from cranial bleeding or concomitant penetrating injuries (e.g., to the abdomen) may complicate treatment. Knives or other low-velocity missiles protruding from the head should never be removed in the field or emergency department because they may serve to tamponade a damaged intracranial vessel. Operative intervention is often required for those deemed likely to survive. For gunshot wounds to the head, the surgeon should perform a limited débridement of the scalp and skull wound, removing scalp, bone, and bullet fragments penetrating the brain only if they lie near the surface. Easily accessible necrotic brain should be débrided and meticulous hemostasis achieved. Vascular structures should be evaluated. Dural closure is important because it reduces the risk of CSF leak and infection.

# References

1. Zafonte RD, Wood DL, Harrison-Felix C, et al. Severe penetrating head injury: a study of outcomes. *Arch Phys Med Rehabil.* 2001;82: 306–310.
2. Thurman DJ, Alverson C, Browne D, et al. *Traumatic Brain Injury in the United States: A Report to Congress. Atlanta: Centers for Disease Control and Prevention.* National Center for Injury Prevention and Control; 1999.
3. Levy ML, Masri LS, Lavine S, Apuzzo ML. Outcome prediction after penetrating craniocerebral injury in a civilian population: aggressive surgical management in patients with admission Glasgow Coma Scale scores of 3, 4, or 5. *Neurosurgery.* 1994;35(1):77–84. discussion 84–5.
4. Levy ML, Rezai A, Masri LS, et al. The significance of subarachnoid hemorrhage after penetrating craniocerebral injury: correlations with angiography and outcome in a civilian population. *Neurosurgery.* 1993;32:532–540.
5. Siccardi D, Cavaliere R, Pau A, Lubinu F, Turtas S, Viale GL. Penetrating craniocerebral missile injuries in civilians: a retrospective analysis of 314 cases. *Surg Neurol.* 1991;35(6):455–460.
6. Kaufman H, Levy M, Stone J, et al. Patients with Glasgow Coma Scale scores 3, 4, 5 after gunshot wounds to the brain. *Neurosurg Clin North Am.* 1995;6:701e714.
7. Aldrich EF, Eisenberg HM, Saydjari C, et al. Predictors of mortality in severely head-injured patients with civilian gunshot wounds: a report from the NIH Traumatic Coma Data Bank. *Surg Neurol.* 1992;38:418e423.
8. Martins RS, Siqueira MG, Santos MT, Zanon-Collange N, Moraes OJ. Prognostic factors and treatment of penetrating gunshot wounds to the head. *Surg Neurol.* 2003;60:98–104.
9. Rosenfeld JV. Gunshot injury to the head and spine. *J Clin Neurosci.* 2002;9:9e16.
10. Lin D, Lam F, Siracuse J, et al. Time is brain" the Gifford factor: Why do some civilian gunshot wounds to the head do unexpectedly well? A case series with outcomes analysis and a management guide. *Surg Neurol Int.* 2012;3:98.
11. Russell RJ, Hodgetts TJ, Mcleod J, et al. The role of trauma scoring in developing trauma clinical governance in the Defence Medical Services. *Philos Trans R Soc B.* 2011;366:171–191.
12. Joseph B, Aziz H, Pandit V, et al. Improving survival rates after civilian gunshot wounds to the brain. *J Am Coll Surg.* 2014;218(1): 58–65.
13. Dubose JJ, Barmparas G, Inaba K, et al. Isolated severe traumatic brain injuries sustained during combat operations: demographics, mortality outcomes, and lessons to be learned from contrasts to civilian counterparts. *J Trauma.* 2011;70:11–18.
14. Sinauer N, Annest JL, Mercy JA. Unintentional, nonfatal firearm-related injuries. A preventable public health burden. *JAMA.* 1996;275(22):1740–1743.
15. Jandial R, Reichwage B, Levy M, Duenas V, Sturdivan L. Ballistics for the neurosurgeon. *Neurosurgery.* 2008;62(2):472–480. discussion 480.
16. Hollerman JJ, Fackler ML, Coldwell DM, et al. Gunshot wounds: 1. Bullets, ballistics and mechanisms of injury. *Am J Roentgenol.* 1990;155(685):e90.
17. Crockard HA. Early intracranial pressure studies in gunshot wounds of the brain. *J Trauma.* 1975;15:339–347.
18. Crockard HA, Brown FD, Johns LM, Mullan S. An experimental cerebral missile injury model in primates. *J Neurosurg.* 1977;46(6): 776–783.
19. Quatrehomme G, Iscan MY. Characteristics of gunshot wounds in the skull. *J Forensic Sci.* 1999;44:568e76.
20. Campbell GA. The pathology of penetrating wounds of the brain and its enclosures. In: Aarabi B, Kaufman HH, eds. *Missile Wounds of the Head and Neck;* vol. I:Park Ridge, IL: American Association of Neurological Surgeons; 1999:73–89.
21. Pallett JR, Sutherland E, Glucksman E, Tunnicliff M, Keep JW. A cross-sectional study of knife injuries at a London major trauma centre. *Ann R Coll Surg Engl.* 2014;96(1):23–26.
22. Swadron SP, Le Roux P, Smith WS, Weingart SD. Emergency neurological life support: traumatic brain injury. *Neurocrit Care.* 2012;17 (Suppl 1):112–121.
23. Eckstein M. The pre-hospital and emergency department management of penetrating wound injuries. *Neurosurg Clin North Am.* 1995;6:741–751.
24. Como JJ, Diaz JJ, Dunham CM, Chiu WC, Duane TM. Practice management guidelines for identification of cervical spine injuries following trauma: update from the eastern association for the surgery of trauma practice management guidelines committee. *J Trauma.* 2009;67(3): 651–659.
25. Levy ML. Outcome prediction following penetrating craniocerebral injury in a civilian population: aggressive surgical management in patients with admission Glasgow Coma Scale scores of 6 to 15. *Neurosurg Focus.* 2000;8(1):e2.
26. Bell RS, Mossop CM, Dirks MS, et al. Early decompressive craniectomy for severe penetrating and closed head injury during wartime. *Neurosurg Focus.* 2010;28(5):E1.
27. Gressot LV, Chamoun RB, Patel AJ, et al. Predictors of outcome in civilians with gunshot wounds to the head upon presentation. *J Neurosurg.* 2014;121(3):645–652.
28. Kim KA, Wang MY, McNatt SA, et al. Vector analysis correlating bullet trajectory to outcome after civilian through-and-through gunshot wound to the head: using imaging cues to predict fatal outcome. *Neurosurgery.* 2005;57:737–747.
29. Amirjamshidi A, Abbassioun K, Rahmat H. Minimal debridement or simple wound closure as the only surgical treatment in war victims with low-velocity penetrating head injuries. Indications and management protocol based upon more than 8 years follow-up of 99 cases from Iran-Iraq conflict. *Surg Neurol.* 2003;60:105–110. discussion 110–1.
30. Aarabi B, Alden T, Chestnut R, et al. Vascular complications of penetrating brain injury. *J Trauma.* 2001;51(2 suppl):S26–S28.
31. du Trevou MD, van Dellen JR. Penetrating stab wounds to the brain: the timing of angiography in patients presenting with the weapon already removed. *Neurosurgery.* 1992;31:905–911. discussion 911–2.
32. Kieck CF, de Villiers JC. Vascular lesions due to transcranial stab wounds. *J Neurosurg.* 1984;60:42–46.
33. Amirjamshidi A, Rahmat H, Abbassioun K. Traumatic aneurysms and arteriovenous fistulas of intracranial vessels associated with penetrating head injuries occurring during war: principles and pitfalls in diagnosis and management. A survey of 31 cases and review of the literature. *J Neurosurg.* 1996;84:769–780.
34. Bell RS, Ecker RD, Severson 3rd MA, Wanebo JE, Crandall B, Armonda RA. The evolution of the treatment of traumatic cerebrovascular injury during wartime. *Neurosurg Focus.* 2010;28(5):E5.
35. Gonul E, Erdogan E, Tasar M, et al. Penetrating orbitocranial gunshot injuries. *Surg Neurol.* 2005;63:24e31.
36. Chesnut R, Videtta W, Vespa P, Le Roux P. The Participants in the International Multidisciplinary Consensus Conference on Multimodality Monitoring. Intracranial pressure monitoring: fundamental considerations and rationale for monitoring. *Neurocrit Care.* 2014;21 (Suppl 2):64–84.
37. Nagib MG, Rockswold GL, Sherman RS, Lagaard MW. Civilian gunshot wounds to the brain: prognosis and management. *Neurosurgery.* 1986;18:533–537.
38. Sarnaik AP, Kopec J, Moylan P, Alvarez D, Canady A. Role of aggressive intracranial pressure control in management of pediatric craniocerebral gunshot wounds with unfavorable features. *J Trauma.* 1989;29:1434–1437.
39. Le Roux P. Intracranial pressure after the BEST TRIP trial: a call for more monitoring. *Curr Opin Crit Care.* 2014;20(2):141–147.
40. Jimenez CM, Polo J, España JA. Risk factors for intracranial infection secondary to penetrating craniocerebral gunshot wounds in civilian practice. *World Neurosurg.* 2013;79(5–6):749–755. Epub 2012 Jun 19.
41. Ryall RG, Peacock MK, Simpson DA. Usefulness of beta 2-transferrin assay in the detection of cerebrospinal fluid leaks following head injury. *J Neurosurg.* 1992;77(5):737–739.
42. Aarabi B, Taghipour M, Alibaii E, Kamgarpour A. Central nervous system infections after military missile head wounds. *Neurosurgery.* 1998;42:500–507. discussion 507–9.
43. Bayston R, de LJ, Brown EM, Johnston RA, Lees P, Pople IK. Use of antibiotics in penetrating craniocerebral injuries. Infection in Neurosurgery Working Party of British Society for Antimicrobial Chemotherapy. *Lancet.* 2000;355:1813–1817.
44. Korinek AM, Golmard JL, Elcheick A, et al. Risk factors for neurosurgical site infections after craniotomy: a critical reappraisal of antibiotic prophylaxis on 4,578 patients. *Br J Neurosurg.* 2005;19(2): 155–162.
45. Nathoo N, Nadvi SS, Narotam PK, van Dellen JR. Brain abscess: management and outcome analysis of a computed tomography era experience with 973 patients. *World Neurosurg.* 2011;75(5–6):716–726. discussion 612–7.

46. Brouwer MC, Coutinho JM, van de Beek D. Clinical characteristics and outcome of brain abscess: systematic review and meta-analysis. *Neurology*. 2014;82(9):806–813. Epub 2014 Jan 29.

47. Xu XX, Li B, Yang HF, et al. Can diffusion-weighted imaging be used to differentiate brain abscess from other ring-enhancing brain lesions? A meta-analysis. *Clin Radiol*. 2014;69(9):909–915.

48. Rath TJ, Hughes M, Arabi M, et al. Imaging of cerebritis, encephalitis, and brain abscess. *Neuroimaging Clin N Am*. 2012;22:585e607.

49. Brouwer MC, McIntyre P, Prasad K, van de Beek D. Corticosteroids for acute bacterial meningitis. *Cochrane Database Syst Rev*. 2013;6.

50. van de Beek D, Farrar JJ, de Gans J, et al. Adjunctive dexamethasone in bacterial meningitis: a meta-analysis of individual patient data. *Lancet Neurol*. 2010;9(3):254–263.

51. Aarabi B, Taghipour M, Haghnegahdar A, Farokhi M, Mobley L. Prognostic factors in the occurrence of posttraumatic epilepsy after penetrating head injury suffered during military service. *Neurosurg Focus*. 2000;8:e1.

52. Eftekhar B, Sahraian MA, Nouralishahi B, et al. Prognostic factors in the persistence of posttraumatic epilepsy after penetrating head injuries sustained in war. *J Neurosurg*. 2009;110:319–326.

53. Kordestani RK, Counelis GJ, McBride DQ, Martin NA. Cerebral arterial spasm after penetrating craniocerebral gunshot wounds: transcranial Doppler and cerebral blood flow findings. *Neurosurgery*. 1997;41: 351–359.

54. Armonda RA, Bell RS, Vo AH, et al. Wartime traumatic cerebral vasospasm: recent review of combat casualties. *Neurosurgery*. 2006;59(6): 1215–1225. discussion 1225.

55. Temkin NR, Anderson GD, Winn HR, et al. Magnesium sulfate for neuroprotection after traumatic brain injury: a randomised controlled trial. *Lancet Neurol*. 2007;6:29–38.

56. Temkin NR, Dikmen SS, Anderson GD, et al. Valproate therapy for prevention of posttraumatic seizures: a randomized trial. *J Neurosurg*. 1999;91:593–600.

57. Temkin NR, Dikmen SS, Wilensky AJ, Keihm J, Chabal S, Winn HR. A randomized, double-blind study of phenytoin for the prevention of post-traumatic seizures. *N Engl J Med*. 1990;323:497–502.

58. Smith JE, Kehoe A, Harrisson SE, Russell R, Midwinter M. Outcome of penetrating intracranial injuries in a military setting. *Injury*. 2014; 45(5):874–878.

59. Weisbrod AB, Rodriguez C, Bell R, Neal C, Armonda R, Dorlac W, et al. Longterm outcomes of combat casualties sustaining penetrating traumatic brain injury. *J Trauma*. 2012;73:1525–1530.

# 28 Depressed Skull and Facial Fractures

ALEXANDER J. GAMBLE, GREGORY KAPINOS, NICHOLAS BASTIDAS, and RAJ K. NARAYAN

## Introduction

Traumatic head injury is responsible for a disproportionally large share of the morbidity and mortality associated with trauma. Closed head injury typically occurs when the head is struck, abruptly decelerates, or is shaken violently.[1] To fracture the skull typically requires tremendous forces and, not surprisingly, such fractures are often associated with significant injury to the underlying brain and vasculature. The mere presence of a cranial fracture is a strong risk factor for hemorrhagic intracranial lesions that may need surgery.[2] Depressed fractures of the skull and facial fractures occur in less than 10% of all head injuries, but should therefore tip off the clinician to look out for intracranial damage.[3–6]

In this chapter, we outline the significance of fractures of the skull and facial bones and the associated problems of which one must be cognizant. The specific management of mass lesions and neurovascular injuries related to these fractures is discussed in other chapters. The team caring for the patient with a skull fracture should be familiar with the common perioperative complications and secondary injuries listed in Table 28.1.

## Neuroanatomy and Procedure

The skull can be most simply divided into two portions: the vault and the base. Embryologically, the vault is formed by intramembranous ossification and structurally consists of two layers of hard cortical bone that sandwiches cancellous bone containing diploe and marrow. This structure of the frontoparietal parts of the temporal and occipital bones, and their synchondrosal fusion to one another at suture lines, is actually somewhat flexible and can undergo significant deformation before failure.[1,7] Bones comprising the base are formed largely by endochondral ossification and have many foramina for traversing nerves and vessels. Thus the ethmoid, sphenoid, and basal portions of the temporal and occipital bones are mechanically more brittle than those of the vault. The many foramina tend to concentrate energy with fractures commonly extending toward them.[1,7]

### BIOMECHANICS OF TRAUMATIC SKULL FRACTURES

#### Key Concepts

- Intracranial bleeding, seizures, and underlying brain damage are the most common complications associated with cranial fractures.

- Comminuted, depressed, and open fractures are more likely to be problematic. Linear, nondisplaced, and closed fractures usually have a more benign clinical course.

Impact upon the cranium causes shock waves to travel from the point of contact through the skull. Focal deformation, or in-bending, begins at the site of impact, and out-bending of the adjacent bone occurs as the stress wave propagates. If the area of in-bending after impact rebounds without fracturing locally, a linear fracture will form at the transition from in-bending to out-bending, extending both toward the point of impact and away. With greater energies, secondary and tertiary fractures will occur, leading to a stellate fracture.[7,8] There is clear evidence that the presence of any skull fracture significantly increases the risk of intracranial hemorrhage[2,5,8,9] and, in combination with an altered level of consciousness, raises the risk of an intracranial hematoma from 1 in 7900 to 1 in 4.[9] The relative velocity of the offending object is the most important determinant of depression or perforation.[1] If the area of in-bending at the impact site is great enough, a depressed skull fracture is created (Figs. 28.1 and 28.2).[10] Local failure of bone around the site of impact implies that much of the energy that would have been spread and dissipated through bone is now transferred to the intracranial contents, which is reflected in the increased incidence of hematoma, neurological deficit, and epilepsy compared with linear or comminuted fractures.[2,5,8–11]

### PERIPROCEDURAL AND ANESTHETIC CONSIDERATIONS

Anesthetic considerations for craniofacial fracture repair are consistent with general neurosurgical anesthetic recommendations.[12,13] Ideally anesthetic agents help to lower intracranial pressure (ICP) and cerebral metabolic rate, while avoiding hypotension, hypertension, and hypoxemia.[13] Prophylactic antibiotics and anticonvulsants are often used, despite limited evidence of their efficacy.[14] Volume repletion and hydration with IV fluids are recommended in trauma patients, and hypotonic IV fluids are to be avoided. The hematocrit and coagulation status are monitored to decide on the need for transfusion.[1,13] Intraoperative seizures are managed by loading antiepileptic medications along with propofol. Ketamine may also be a useful agent.[15,16] Adequate intravenous access is paramount because massive hemorrhage from a venous sinus, large vein, or arterial laceration can be a challenging complication during surgery.

**Table 28.1** Incidence of Complications Associated with Skull Fractures

| Complication | Incidence |
| --- | --- |
| Seizures[11,44,45] | 10% (convulsive) 25% (nonconvulsive) |
| Meningitis with DSF[17–20] | 5%–11% |
| Cranial Nerve Palsies [24,25,27,28] | 0%–25% |
| Facial palsy in temporal bone fracture [27,28] | 7%–10% |
| Traumatic CSF fistula [23,37–39] | 1%–5% |
| Meningitis due to CSF fistula, during the first 2 weeks [38] | 1.3% per day |
| Occipital condylar fractures [4,26] | 30% (of cervical spine fractures) |
| Carotid-cavernous fistula [40] | 4% (of basilar fractures) |
| Carotid or vertebral artery dissection[4] | n/a |
| Permanent neurological deficits [2,3,6,8–10,19,20] | 0%–10% |
| Death [2,3,6,8–10,19,20] | 0%–20% |

*DSF*, depressed skull fracture; *CSF*, cerebrospinal fluid.

## INFECTIOUS RISK

### Key Concepts

- Open depressed skull fractures (DSFs) with dural penetration are at a higher risk for central nervous system infection.
- Skull fractures with pneumocephalus probably have a dural tear, and although most resolve, these patients are at an increased risk of meningitis.

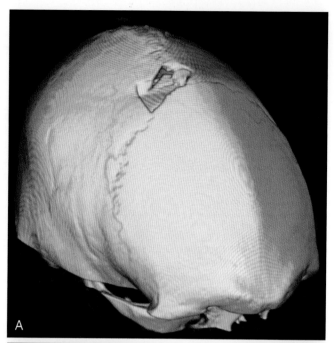

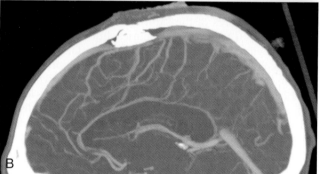

**Fig. 28.2** Depressed skull fracture involving the right parietal bone seen on CT (**A**) and compressing the superior sagittal sinus, as seen on CT venogram sagittal view (**B**).

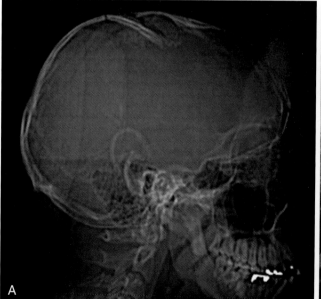

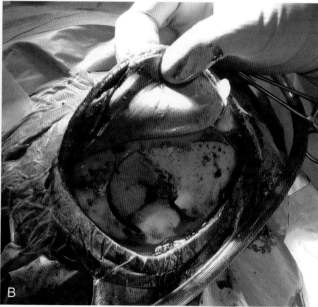

**Fig. 28.1** Depressed skull fracture involving the right parietal bone, seen on lateral skull x-ray (**A**) and before elevation (**B**).

Operative goals in the treatment of a DSF are appropriate exposure, copious irrigation, aggressive debridement, elevation of the fracture, evacuation of any mass lesion, and dural repair. In the past, the bone was often discarded because surgeons believed it a nidus for infection. It has been convincingly demonstrated that with thorough washing and aggressive debridement, replacement of the bone flap does not seem to be associated with an increased risk of infection.[3,17–20] This approach also obviates the need for subsequent cranioplasty.

## SINUS INJURY

### Key Concepts

- Temporal depressed fractures are at higher risk of rapidly expanding epidural hematoma, especially if crossing over the groove of the middle meningeal artery.
- Fractures overlying a dural sinus, especially the superior sagittal, can cause thrombosis, which is usually managed medically.

DSFs overlying a dural venous sinus can constitute a complex problem (Fig. 28.2). If elevation of the fracture is attempted, there is the potential for massive intraoperative hemorrhage and subsequent ischemic complications from sinus thrombosis.[21] Given the risk, most depressed fractures overlying a dural venous sinus are treated nonoperatively.[3,6] Indications for operation include mechanical obstruction of the superior sagittal sinus causing persistent intracranial hypertension via outflow obstruction. Endothelial damage can promote thrombus formation, leading to hemorrhagic infarction that may require decompression. Despite these risks, the presence of significant mass effect or deep contamination may warrant surgical intervention. In such cases, one must be prepared for massive bleeding and the need for blood transfusion.[21]

## MAXILLOFACIAL TRAUMA

### Key Concepts

- The cribriform plate is particularly vulnerable to facial trauma and is associated with CSF rhinorrhea and anosmia.
- Anosmia is a frequent and often unrecognized result of traumatic brain injury (TBI) and can have a very significant effect on the quality of life.

The cribriform plate of the ethmoid, the orbital plate of the frontal bone, portions of the temporal bone, the sphenoid bone, and the occipital bone all contribute to the skull base. The frontal, sphenoid, and ethmoid bones are unique in that they become increasingly pneumatized from early childhood and are lined by respiratory epithelium. The frontal sinus is the last to become pneumatized, rising to the glabella in early adolescence. Much like modern automobiles, the face has crumple zones that dissipate and direct energy away from the most vital structures. Therefore fractures of the skull base and facial bones follow somewhat predictable configurations (Fig. 28.3). Fractures of the frontal bone and sinus occur in patterns, dampening forces transmitted to the frontal lobes. The maxillary sinus and the condylar necks of the mandible commonly fracture to protect brain in the middle cranial fossa. The nasal bones and maxillary frontal processes articulate to the thin laminae papyracea of the ethmoid. Upon impact, these bones telescope backward, distributing force through the ethmoid sinuses. Energy is thus directed away from the globes, optic nerves, and cribriform plate.[22]

## ORBITAL TRAUMA

Some fractures to the face and orbit can result in facial or gaze asymmetry and dental malocclusion (Fig. 28.4). Definitive treatment is often delayed until swelling has resolved, allowing for improved soft tissue mobility and assessment of symmetry, thus enabling improved cosmetic results. In contrast, true orbital entrapment of the extraocular muscles is an uncommon emergency given the risk of ischemic necrosis. In orbital floor reconstruction, the orbital contents are surgically reduced (from the maxillary sinus), and the floor of the orbit is restored typically with either bone grafts or alloplastic implants. The conical shape and volume of the orbit must be precisely reconstructed to prevent orbital dystopia and enophthalmos. A postoperative computed tomography (CT) scan is helpful to determine the adequacy of the reduction.

## CEREBROSPINAL FLUID FISTULAE, MENINGITIS, AND CRANIAL NEUROPATHIES

### Key Concepts

- Basal skull fractures are associated with a higher risk of major injuries to the brainstem, cranial nerves, or arteries.
- Most cases of rhinorrhea and otorrhea do resolve spontaneously over a few days without surgical intervention.

Frontobasilar fractures are of specific importance because the dura is torn easily at the skull base. The potential for ascending meningitis via direct communication between the subarachnoid space and the aerated sinuses is high. Nevertheless, most fractures of the skull base are managed without surgery and usually resolve without sequelae. When surgery is indicated, the general goal is a durable separation of these two spaces. Various open and endoscopic techniques have been developed and may have to be individualized for each case depending on its unique anatomy.[1,22,23]

Fractures of the petrous temporal bone sometimes have to be addressed surgically if there is a facial nerve entrapment/disruption or a persistent cerebrospinal fluid (CSF) fistula. Facial nerve decompression and repair are generally approached via a transmastoid supralabyrinthine approach or a middle fossa subtemporal approach. An avulsed nerve may be repaired primarily or with a nerve graft.[24,25] Dural tears and bony defects are repaired with various materials. Fractures of the occipital condyle deemed mechanically unstable are customarily treated with occipital cervical fusion with rigid internal fixation.[26] Whereas occipital condyle fractures are common, fortunately, resultant instability is not.

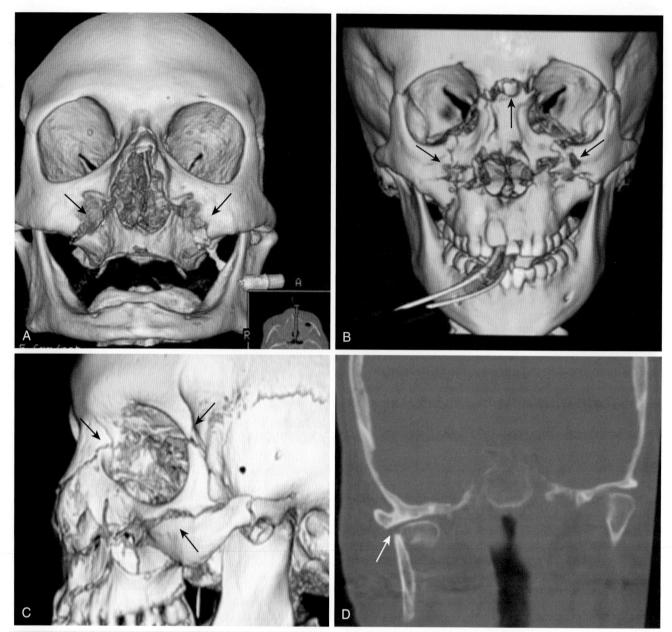

**Fig. 28.3** Le Fort I (**A**), Le Fort II (**B**), and Le Fort IV (**C**) facial fractures. Mandibular condyle fracture with dislocation (**D**).

## Preoperative Considerations

Prehospital care and emergency room care should follow Advanced Trauma Life Support (ATLS) recommendations and special consideration given to unappreciated spinal instability.[4] Glasgow Coma Scale score, pupillary checks, asymmetry in the motor responses, and signs of ICP elevation should be ascertained as part of the ATLS secondary survey. Tetanus immunization should be administered and antithrombotics should be reversed for hemostasis. Urinary toxicology should be checked in case of altered consciousness.

Scalp lacerations may bleed profusely, and direct compression, Raney clips, staples, or sutures should be used to quickly close the wound and gain hemostasis. The threshold for taking a patient to the operating room with uncontrollable bleeding from scalp laceration should be low, given the volume of blood that can be lost. Bruising behind the ear (Battle's sign), in the periorbital area (raccoon eyes), or the

presence of blood behind the tympanic membrane (hemotympanum) is nearly pathognomonic of a basal skull fracture. Insertion of a nasogastric tube or nasopharyngeal airway is best deferred to avoid intracranial penetration.

Fractures of the facial bones are often described in the context of Le Fort's classical descriptions. Facial bone fractures may be evaluated by gentle mobilization of the midface fragments (Fig. 28.3). In the tertiary survey, cranial nerve dysfunction (anosmia, visual acuity, facial paralysis, dysphagia, dysarthria, and deafness) is assessed.[1,27,28] Noncontrast thin-slice CT of the head should be obtained with coronal reformatting. Three-dimensional reconstructions may increase the sensitivity of CT to detection of fractures.

Patients with complex craniofacial fractures should be closely monitored, ideally in a dedicated surgical/trauma intensive care unit (ICU) or neurosurgical ICU where frequent neurological examinations and serial CTs can be

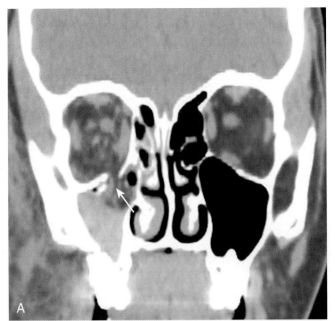

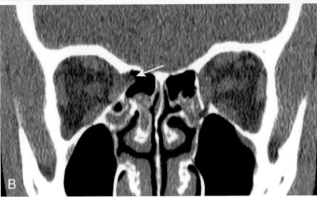

Fig. 28.4 Orbital floor "blow-out" fracture with inferior rectus entrapment **(A)**. Medial orbital wall fracture of ethmoid with medial rectus entrapment **(B)**.

performed to promptly detect any neurological deterioration.[29,30] Brain swelling and evolving hemorrhage may require rapid decompression.

## Clinical Pearls

Facial Fractures

- Nasal bone fractures are the most common facial fractures, and packing may be necessary to control the bleeding.
- The septum should be evaluated for a septal hematoma, which, if untreated, may lead to a saddle-nose deformity and loss of nasal projection.
- Le Fort type I: transverse maxillary fracture separating the lower maxilla from the immobile nasal/forehead segment
- Le Fort type II: pyramid-shaped maxillary fracture up to the nasal bridge responsible for abnormal movement of the entire maxillary and nasal segments
- Le Fort type III: horizontal fracture from the nasal bridge to the lateral wall of the orbit and zygomatic bone responsible for abnormal separation of the entire face from the forehead
- Many facial fractures are combinations of these classical patterns.

# Perioperative Surgical Care

## DEPRESSED SKULL FRACTURES

DSFs are usually evident on the initial CT scan of the head (particularly on the bone windows). Open compound DSFs are sometimes palpable through the laceration as a depression or step-off deformity. However, galeal swelling or hematoma may mimic or conceal this. In our experience, it is quite common for a galeal hematoma to feel like a DSF. DSFs occur in less than 10% of all head injuries, but these patients should command special attention due to the frequency of associated extraaxial hematomas, parenchymal contusions, and cranial nerve injuries.[4,5,9] A DSF alerts the informed clinician to the potential for increased neurological sequelae.[8–11] Fractures in the temporal, parietal, or frontobasal location are associated with more significant neurological deficits,[6,10] seizures,[11] pneumocephalus, central nervous system infection,[18–20,31,32] and intracranial hemorrhage.[5,9,10] Compound DSFs (Figs. 28.1 and 28.2) raise the concern of intracranial contamination. In a large series of open DSFs, infection rates varied between 5% and 11%.[17] When an open DSF is present, cefazolin 1 g tid for 24 h is usually administered empirically at our institution to reduce the risk of subsequent bacterial meningoencephalitis, but there are insufficient data to recommend a particular antibiotic choice or duration.[6,14,31–34]

Current neurosurgical guidelines advocate surgical intervention for compound DSFs, especially in patients with radiological evidence of dural penetration, the presence of a significant intracranial hematoma, greater than 1 cm depression of bone fragments, involvement of the frontal sinus, cosmetic deformity of the skull, or gross contamination of the wound or pneumocephalus.[3,6] With evidence of dural violation, early operation and antibiotics are advocated. Delay may increase the risk of meningitis and cerebritis associated with persistent neurological deficit, epilepsy, and death.[11,17] Open DSFs in patients with no other surgical lesion and without evidence of dural laceration are often managed with local wound washout, closure, and antibiotics alone. There is strong evidence to support the nonoperative management of uncomplicated compound DSFs.[3,6,17] Elevating an uncomplicated closed DSF may lead to better cosmesis, but does not decrease the risk of posttraumatic epilepsy.[11] Reversing neurological deficit by elevating a fracture is not in and of itself a realistic surgical indication. The cortical insult occurs at the time of injury, and surgical intervention may not reverse its effects.[3,6,19,20]

## MANAGEMENT OF VENOUS SINUS THROMBOSIS

Venous thrombosis leading to venous occlusion and hemorrhagic infarction may occur due to skull fractures, especially in the case of compression of the posterior third aspect of the superior sagittal sinus (Fig. 28.2).[35,36] Patients with DSFs overlying a dural sinus should undergo vascular imaging via magnetic resonance venography (MRV) (Fig. 28.5) or CT venography. The possibility of venous sinus thrombosis should be considered throughout the patient's ICU course.[21,36] MRV has significantly facilitated establishment of this diagnosis. Nevertheless, delay

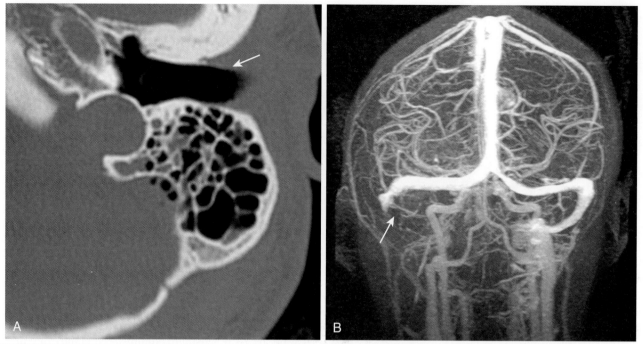

**Fig. 28.5** Subtle fracture of the left mastoid with air in the sigmoid sinus **(A)**. The patient did indeed have a left sigmoid sinus and jugular vein thrombosis and was heparinized **(B)**.

in making the diagnosis is common and may be associated with a poorer outcome.[35] Management generally consists of diligent hydration and in some cases gentle anticoagulation and/or an antiplatelet agent. Some centers have advocated thrombolytic therapy, with promising results.[35] Endovascular interventions are continually being advanced, and these may be valuable in some cases. There is no clear decision-making model to help balance thrombotic and hemorrhagic risks. A decompressive craniectomy may be warranted if there is severe brain swelling with uncontrollable ICP. In the case of mechanical venous outflow obstruction, conservative measures may ultimately fail and surgical intervention may become necessary secondary to high ICP.[21,35,36]

## CEREBROSPINAL FLUID FISTULAE REPAIR

### Key Concepts

- Most cases of rhinorrhea and otorrhea do resolve spontaneously over a few days without surgical intervention (85% within 1 week).
- But after that, the risk of meningitis is related to the duration of CSF leak, and it should be addressed by early closure, rather than by prophylactic antibiosis.

Red-tinged rhinorrhea or otorrhea in a head-injured patient should be inspected for the "halo" sign (aka "target" or "ring" sign), the chromatic dispersion of CSF on the periphery of a bloody stain on gauze that is suspicious for, although not diagnostic of, a CSF leak. Testing samples for glucose is obsolete and results in too many false positives.[37] The presence of beta-2-transferrin in the suspicious fluid is diagnostic but may take several days to obtain a result. A posttraumatic CSF fistula is a strong and

independent predictor of meningitis.[38] Traumatic leaks typically manifest within 2 days of injury, and 95% will present within 3 months. About 85% will resolve spontaneously without surgical intervention within 1 week.[23] Otorrhea is more likely to cease spontaneously than rhinorrhea.

Fractures involving the frontal sinus occur in 2% to 12% of skull fractures. Often, both anterior and posterior walls are fractured, and in 15% to 30% of these cases a CSF leak is present.[38,39] CSF fistulae at other locations along the anterior cranial fossa may not be readily apparent on CT. Rhinorrhea does not necessarily localize the source of the leak to the anterior cranial fossa. The Eustachian tube will drain CSF originating at a temporal bone fracture from the middle ear to the nasopharynx when the tympanic membrane is intact. Often, dedicated temporal bone CT may not clearly localize the leak, but signs such as mastoid air cell opacification, fluid in the middle ear on otoscopic examination and CT, facial nerve weakness, or unilateral hearing loss help localize the leak to the temporal bone.

Regardless of location (rhinorrhea or otorrhea), initial management consists of keeping the head of bed elevated at all times to lower ICP while maintaining a pressure gradient favoring downward flow of CSF; avoidance of noninvasive positive pressure ventilation and incentive spirometry; and avoidance of sneezing, nose blowing, use of straws, or Valsalva maneuvers. If intracranial hematoma necessitates urgent surgical intervention and a CSF leak is also evident, an effort should be made to repair the leak. This may require placement of a pericranial flap over the floor of the frontal fossa along with a biological glue such as fibrin glue.

In the presence of a posttraumatic CSF leak, the risk of meningitis is related to the duration of rhinorrhea, the size of fracture displacement, and the proximity to the midline.

The risk of meningitis is 9% over the first week and doubles to 19% after the second week.[40] Recommendations regarding when to escalate management vary in the literature.[37,41] Many experts believe that prophylactic CSF diversion, preferably via lumbar drainage, should be performed within a week and continue for a period of 7 to 10 days.[23,27] If treated, patients should still be carefully observed for signs of meningitis, overdrainage, and development of pneumocephalus. In the event that air is being drawn through the dural defect, drainage should be promptly discontinued. Whether acute or delayed, successful repair of CSF leaks decreases the 10-year cumulative risk of meningitis from 85% to 7%.[23]

Prophylactic antibiotic administration was at one time the standard of care. In 1997 a metaanalysis of six mostly retrospective case series over 25 years demonstrated a decrease in meningitis from 10% to 2.5% with the use of prophylactic antibiotics.[34] However, a 2011 Cochrane metaanalysis of five randomized controlled clinical trials with 208 patients showed with high significance that antibiotics provided no protection from meningitis.[32] There is also evidence that prophylactic antibiotics could actually increase the incidence and virulence of meningitis by selecting out more pathogenical and antibiotic-resistant bacteria.[32]

## SKULL-BASE FRACTURES

### Key Concepts

- Traumatic carotid-cavernous fistula is a rare but dramatic sequela of a head injury and should be considered when one encounters ocular proptosis or bruit.
- The timing of repair of facial fractures must be weighed against the potential risk of worsening a TBI with long operative procedures and potential for significant blood loss or brain manipulation. Consideration should be given to delaying these definitive repairs to allow for head injury stabilization.

Medial temporal and sphenoid bone fractures extending to the carotid canal should prompt vascular imaging to rule out dissection.[42] The carotid artery is prone to shearing forces within the cavernous sinus that may result in a small tear. In this segment the artery is inside a venous sinus, explaining why skull-base trauma may result in a high-flow connection between the two systems. Carotid-cavernous fistulas occur in up to 4% of patients with basilar skull fracture,[22,42] but this is not a prerequisite for fistula creation. This direct high-flow shunt usually presents acutely with significant venous hypertension within the orbital compartment leading to proptosis, chemosis, orbital bruit, headache, blurry vision, and diplopia. The latter two symptoms represent optic nerve ischemia and cranial nerve compression. When present, the need for intervention becomes more urgent if vision and ocular motility are to be preserved. The diagnosis can be confirmed by CT angiography or conventional cerebral angiography and is best treated by endovascular occlusion of the fistula with coils or liquid embolic agents.[42]

Fractures of the petrous part of the temporal bone are fairly common and can be either longitudinal (70%–90%) or transverse (10%–30%). Facial nerve injury occurs with a frequency of 7% to 10% and is more common in transverse fractures.[24,25] Transverse fractures more commonly disrupt the bony labyrinth leading to sensorineural hearing loss. In temporal bone fractures with facial palsy, surgical decompression is controversial. Generally speaking, patients with any residual function should be managed conservatively with steroids.[27,28] Those with complete palsy are often taken for decompression and repair of the nerve, but it is evident in multiple series that return of function is comparable to non-operated patients.[24,25]

## OCCIPITAL CONDYLAR FRACTURES

Fractures of the occipital condyle imply a significantly serious injury. They are relatively rare and are seen in less than 0.4% of trauma series.[43] There are associated cervical spine fractures in nearly 30% of cases.[5,26] Most fractures of the condyle are stable, but a minority of fractures may be highly unstable secondary to avulsion at the insertion of the alar ligament and tectorial membrane. This disruption is best imaged by magnetic resonance imaging. Significantly displaced condylar fractures, as well as fractures involving the transverse foramen in the cervical spine, may compress and dissect the vertebral artery. Condylar fractures are associated with epidural and subdural hematomas around the foramen magnum in up to 30% of patients, and nearly one third may have hypoglossal nerve palsy.[26] This posterior fossa hematoma may be occult upon presentation and only manifest after several hours with potentially fatal consequences.

## FACIAL FRACTURES

In the trauma patient with significant facial trauma, ensuring a patent airway is the first objective. Swelling and hematoma may progressively distort the airway, so early endotracheal intubation is advisable in order to avoid a rescue cricothyroidotomy. Profuse bleeding and deformity of the face are often challenging. For more superficial bleeding, direct pressure with gauze soaked in lidocaine with epinephrine may be sufficient. Life-threatening hemorrhage can occur from laceration of the internal maxillary artery or its branches in midface fractures. Angiographic embolization may be necessary to stop the bleeding after packing and attempted reduction have failed, and is now the procedure of choice. If angiography is unavailable, the external carotid can be directly ligated or the patient taken directly to the operating room for exploration or for open reduction and fixation.[3,6,22]

Nasal bone fractures are the most common facial fracture. However, Le Fort fractures—zygomatic fractures with trismus and nasal fractures involving the ethmoid bone—all require urgent attention by subspecialist experts from multiple teams.[22] Ophthalmology, otorhinolaryngology, oral and maxillofacial, and/or plastic surgery consultations should be obtained for severe lacerations, facial injuries, impaired vision, impaired extraocular movements or lacrimation, widened intercanthal distance, proptosis, enophthalmos, altered hearing or speaking, or mandibular malocclusion.

Thin-slice CT with coronal reformatting is important to fully evaluate facial and orbital fractures, hematoma, and herniation of orbital contents (Fig. 28.4). Ultrasound of the orbits may also be useful to look for extraocular muscle injury and hematoma, penetrating injury to the globe, lens dislocation, vitreous hemorrhage, and retinal detachment. Pain, proptosis, and decreased visual acuity may suggest a retrobulbar hematoma. Untreated, this may lead to infarction of the optic nerve and permanent blindness. Immediate relief of the pressure may be achieved using a lateral canthotomy, which may be performed at the bedside by an ophthalmologist prior to emergent operating room exploration.

Diplopia (double vision) may result from trauma to the rectus muscles or from entrapment of the periorbita. A forced duction test (manipulation of the sclerae) can be performed to determine whether the rectus muscles are entrapped. Orbital fractures with radiological and clinical entrapment of oculomotor muscles require urgent operative repair. Clinical serial reevaluation can be useful, although guidelines[3,6] remain vague about the optimal schedule.

# Postoperative Complications

## SEIZURES

In patients with depressed skull fracture, it has been demonstrated that approximately 4% to 10% of patients will develop seizures within the first week (early epilepsy), and 7% to 15% thereafter (late epilepsy).[11] In some patients, the risk of late epilepsy may be as high as 60%. Factors that increase this risk include posttraumatic amnesia exceeding 24 hours, presence of dural defects, focal neurological deficit, and early epilepsy.[11] Infection is also significantly associated with persistent neurological deficit, late epilepsy, and death.

Of note, the most cited reviews were published in the 1970s, largely predating the era of continuous electroencephalography (cEEG) to detect nonconvulsive seizures. More recent data suggest a large underestimation in prior cohorts, with up to one in four TBI patients experiencing seizures during the first week.[44,45] Seizures are responsible for varying degrees of metabolic disarray, structural change, and atrophy, which, in the long term, is linked to cognitive impairment mimicking the pathogenicity seen in mesial temporal sclerosis.[45]

The high incidence and cognitive sequelae of traumatic epilepsy have prompted systematic pharmacological prophylaxis and cEEG monitoring in many cases after repair of skull fractures and evacuation of mass lesions. Current guidelines strongly support the use of seizure prophylaxis for 7 days to help prevent posttraumatic seizures after severe TBI.[6] Studies have focused on phenytoin and valproate, although levetiracetam is favored in many neurocritical care centers due to a more favorable side effect profile.[46,47] Duration of prophylaxis varies and depends on the type of injury and electroencephalographic results. If no seizures develop within 1 week, anticonvulsants should be stopped because their value in preventing future seizures is not established.[3,6] Once seizure occurs, treatment is as per therapy detailed in another chapter of this book.

## HEMORRHAGIC AND THROMBOTIC COMPLICATIONS IN THE INTENSIVE CARE UNIT

Cortical venous thrombosis and occlusion of the major venous sinuses are known complications of TBI. These can result in slowing of venous drainage and ICP elevation, sometimes with lethal results. In case of extensive dural venous thrombosis, clinicians may apply IV continuous anticoagulation as recommended by the American Stroke Association for nontraumatic spontaneous cortical venous thrombosis.[48] However, in the presence of recent trauma, the use of anticoagulation is a double-edged sword and often cannot be used.

Reaccumulation of a subdural or epidural hematoma is not uncommon, but with no clearly reported incidence in the literature. Contralateral bleeding may occur by reexpansion of the cerebrum after drainage of a hematoma on the other side.[49] Many small epidural hematomas are venous in etiology and may not require surgical evacuation. However, they need to be carefully monitored with serial CT scans of the head and can be considered to be nonsurgical only after they have remained unchanged over the first few hours. Of course, anticoagulated patients with skull fractures are at very high risk of intracerebral hemorrhage (ICH) and reaccumulation. They should be aggressively reversed and monitored in the acute phase for rebleed, but also in the subacute phase for thrombosis.[50]

Severe TBI significantly raises the odds of deep vein thrombosis.[51] Low-dose heparin or low-molecular-weight heparinoids are useful to prevent this, but the timing for their safe initiation is unclear.[6] Modifications to the Parkland protocol[52] can be tailored to our readers' institutional practice patterns in an effort to avoid excessively early initiation leading to more returns to the operating room, as well as excessively late initiation leading to increased venous thromboembolism rates.[53] Please refer to the American College of Chest Physicians guidelines for the surgical patient[54] and the Brain Trauma Foundation guidelines[6] for more on this topic.

## ADRENAL INSUFFICIENCY

Adrenal insufficiency is seen in 25% of TBI patients, with a predilection for basal skull or facial fractures.[55,56] Direct contusion with edema or hemorrhage along the hypothalamic-pituitary axis or injury to the pituitary stalk is the presumed cause. When the clinical syndrome is present, hormonal repletion is warranted. Three months after TBI, it is judicious to test every symptomatic TBI patient for endocrine dysfunction.[56]

## DELAYED RETURN TO OPERATING ROOM

When obstruction of the nasofrontal duct persists in unrepaired frontal sinus fractures, or during the initial surgery, removal of mucosa was inadequate, a mucocele may develop. This will slowly erode bone, causing progressive deformity characterized by bulging in the area of the glabella and orbit that may become infected. Missed or incompletely repaired fractures of bones comprising the orbit can lead to deformity such as telecanthus, enophthalmos, and vertical dystopia, to name a few. A nasal septal hematoma could lead to a saddle-nose deformity and loss of nasal projection.[22]

Midface Le Fort fractures (Fig. 28.3) when improperly reduced and fixed can lead to malocclusion (poor alignment of the bite) and loss of midface height and projection. An anterior open bite occurs when the early posterior teeth impaction leads to inability of the front teeth to close effectively. A cross bite occurs when the reduction is not properly achieved in a transverse dimension. Dislocation of the mandibular condyle from the glenoid fossa may also be the cause for an open bite, and the temporomandibular joint should be palpated while the patient opens and closes the jaw and inspected for clicking. Once fractures have healed, sometimes return to the operating room for removal of hardware may be necessary to achieve normal occlusion. Mild occlusal impairments may be treated with orthodontics postoperatively.[22]

## FUNCTIONAL OUTCOME AND MORTALITY

Craniofacial trauma can result in permanent neurological deficits (PNDs) and sometimes in mortality. PNDs unfortunately ensue in up to 10% of DSF patients, with overall fatality of about 2% to 20%.[2,3,6,10]

# Conclusions

Skull fractures and their associated injuries have a wide spectrum of complexity and severity. Careful clinical and radiographic evaluation is important in the initial management of the patient. Intracranial hematomas sometimes need to be surgically evacuated, and in other cases, are followed with serial examinations and CT studies for the first few hours or days postinjury. DSFs sometimes need surgical correction, but may be managed conservatively as long as they are not compressing vital structures or are cosmetically unacceptable. Patients with craniofacial injuries often require a multidisciplinary approach for optimal results.

## References

1. Shenaq SM, Dinh T. Maxillofacial and scalp injury in neurotrauma. In: Narayan RK, Wilberger JE, Povlishock JT, eds. Neurotrauma. New York: McGraw-Hill; 1996.
2. Carson HJ. Brain trauma in head injuries presenting with and without concurrent skull fractures. J Forensic Leg Med. 2009;16(3):115–120.
3. Bullock MR, Chesnut R, Ghajar J, et al. Surgical Management of Traumatic Brain Injury Author Group. Surgical management of depressed cranial fractures. Neurosurgery. 2006;58(3 Suppl):S56–S60.
4. Mulligan RP, Mahabir RC. The prevalence of cervical spine injury, head injury, or both with isolated and multiple craniomaxillofacial fractures. Plast Reconstr Surg. 2010;126(5):1647–1651.
5. Macpherson BC, MacPherson P, Jennett B. CT evidence of intracranial contusion and haematoma in relation to the presence, site and type of skull fracture. Clin Radiol. 1990;42(5):321–326.
6. Brain Trauma Foundation. American Association of Neurological Surgeons, Congress of Neurological Surgeons. Guidelines for the management of severe traumatic brain injury. J Neurotrauma. 2007;24(Suppl 1):S1–S106.
7. Meaney DF, Olvey SE, Gennarelli T. Biomechanical basis of traumatic brain injury. In: Winn HR, ed. Youmans Neurological Surgery. 6th ed. Philadelphia: Saunders Elsevier; 2011.
8. Adeolu AA, Shokunbi MT, Malomo AO, et al. Compound elevated skull fracture: a forgotten type of skull fracture. Surg Neurol. 2006;65:503–505.
9. Teasdale GM, Murray G, Anderson E, et al. Risks of acute traumatic intracranial haematoma in children and adults: implications for managing head injuries. Br Med J. 1990;300:363–367.
10. Braakman R. Depressed skull fracture: data, treatment and follow up in 225 consecutive cases. J Neurol Neurosurg Psychiatry. 1972;35(3):395–402.
11. Jennett B, Miller JD, Braakman R. Epilepsy after nonmissile depressed skull fracture. J Neurosurg. 1974;41:208–216.
12. Lam AM. Standards of neuroanesthesia. Acta Neurochir Suppl. 2001;78:93–96.
13. Bohman LE, Heuer GG, Macyszyn L, et al. Medical management of compromised brain oxygen in patients with severe traumatic brain injury. Neurocrit Care. 2011;14(3):361–369.
14. Ratilal B, Sampaio C. Prophylactic antibiotics and anticonvulsants in neurosurgery. Adv Tech Stand Neurosurg. 2011;36:139–185.
15. Williams GW, Cheng YC, Sharma A. Use of ketamine for control of refractory seizures during the intraoperative period. J Neurosurg Anesthesiol. 2014;26(4):412–413.
16. Zeiler FA, Teitelbaum J, West M, et al. The ketamine effect on ICP in traumatic brain injury. Neurocrit Care. 2014;21(1):163–173.
17. Heary RF, Hunt CD, Krieger AJ, et al. Nonsurgical treatment of compound depressed skull fractures. J Trauma. 1993;35(3):441–447.
18. Wylen EL, Willis BK, Nanda A. Infection rate with replacement of bone fragment in compound depressed skull fractures. Surg Neurol. 1999;51:452–457.
19. Al-Haddad S, Kirollos R. A 5 year study of the outcome of surgically treated depressed skull fracture. Ann R Coll Surg Engl. 2002;84:196–200.
20. van den Heever CM, van der Merwe DJ. Management of depressed skull fractures. Selective conservative management of nonmissile injuries. J Neurosurg. 1989;71(2):186–190.
21. LeFeuvre D, Taylor A, Peter JC. Compound depressed skull fractures involving a venous sinus. Surg Neurol. 2004;62(2):121–125.
22. Kellman RM. Maxillofacial trauma. In: Flint PW, Haughey BH, Lund VJ, et al., eds. Cummings Otolaryngology: Head and Neck Surgery. 5th ed. Philadelphia: Mosby; 2010.
23. Boahene K, Dagi TF, Quinones-Hinojosa A. Management of cerebrospinal fluid leaks. In: Quinones-Hinojosa A, ed. Schmidek and Sweet: Operative Neurosurgical Techniques. 6th ed. Philadelphia: Saunders Elsevier; 2012.
24. Brodie HA. ThompsonTC. Management of complications from 820 temporal bone fractures. Am J Otol. 1997;18:188–197.
25. Nash JJ, Friedland DR, Boorsma KJ, Rhee JS. Management and outcomes of facial paralysis from intratemporal blunt trauma: a systematic review. Laryngoscope. 2010;120(7):1397–1404.
26. Hanson JA, Deliganis AV, Baxter AB, et al. Radiological and clinical spectrum of occipital condyle fractures: retrospective review of 107 consecutive fractures in 95 patients. Am J Roentgenol. 2002;178(5):1261–1268.
27. Adegbite AB, Khan MI, Tan L. Predicting recovery of facial nerve function following injury from a basilar skull fracture. J Neurosurg. 1991;75(5):759.
28. Maiman DJ, Cusick JF, Anderson AJ, et al. Nonoperative management of traumatic facial nerve palsy. J Trauma. 1985;25(7):644.
29. Pineda JA, Leonard JR, Mazotas IG, et al. Effect of implementation of a paediatric neurocritical care programme on outcomes after severe traumatic brain injury: a retrospective cohort study. Lancet Neurol. 2013;12(1):45–52.
30. Harrison DA, Prabhu G, Grieve R, et al. Risk Adjustment In Neurocritical care (RAIN)—prospective validation of risk prediction models for adult patients with acute traumatic brain injury to use to evaluate the optimum location and comparative costs of neurocritical care: a cohort study. Health Technol Assess. 2013;17(23):vii–viii. 1–350.
31. Ali B, Ghosh A. Antibiotics in compound depressed skull fractures. Emerg Med J. 2002;19(6):552.
32. Ratilal BO, Costa J, Sampaio C, Pappamikail L. Antibiotic prophylaxis for preventing meningitis in patients with basilar skull fractures. Cochrane Database Syst Rev. 2011;8.
33. Nellis JC, Kesser BW, Park SS. What is the efficacy of prophylactic antibiotics in basilar skull fractures? Laryngoscope. 2014;124(1):8–9.
34. Brodie HA. Prophylactic antibiotics for posttraumatic cerebrospinal fluid fistulae. A meta-analysis. Arch Otolaryngol Head Neck Surg. 1997;123:749–752.

35. Wang WH, Lin JM, Luo F, et al. Early diagnosis and management of cerebral venous flow obstruction secondary to transsinus fracture after traumatic brain injury. *J Clin Neurol.* 2013;9(4):259–268.

36. Fuentes S, Metellus P, Levrier O, Adetchessi T, Dufour H, Grisoli F. Depressed skull fracture overlying the superior sagittal sinus causing benign intracranial hypertension. Description of two cases and review of the literature. *Br J Neurosurg.* 2005;19(5):438–442.

37. Ziu M, Savage JG, Jimenez DF. Diagnosis and treatment of cerebrospinal fluid rhinorrhea following accidental traumatic anterior skull base fractures. *Neurosurg Focus.* 2012;32(6):E3.

38. Sonig A, Thakur JD, Chittiboina P, et al. Is posttraumatic cerebrospinal fluid fistula a predictor of posttraumatic meningitis? A US nationwide inpatient sample database study. *Neurosurg Focus.* 2012;32(6):E4.

39. Yilmazlar S, Arslan E, Kocaeli H, et al. Cerebrospinal fluid leakage complicating skull base fractures: analysis of 81 cases. *Neurosurg Rev.* 2006;29(1):64.

40. Eljamel MS, Foy PM. Acute traumatic CSF fistulae: the risk of intracranial infection. *Br J Neurosurg.* 1990;4(5):381–385.

41. Somasundaram A, Pendleton C, Raza SM, Boahene K, Quinones-Hinojosa A. Harvey Cushing's treatment of skull base infections: the Johns Hopkins experience. *J Neurol Surg B Skull Base.* 2012;73(5):358–362.

42. Ellis J, Goldstein H, Connolly ES, et al. Carotid-cavernous fistulas. *Neurosurg Focus.* 2012;32(5).

43. Maserati MB, Stephens B, Zohny Z, et al. Occipital condyle fractures: clinical decision rule and surgical management. *J Neurosurg Spine.* 2009;11(4):388–395.

44. Vespa PM, Miller C, McArthur D, et al. Nonconvulsive electrographic seizures after traumatic brain injury result in a delayed, prolonged increase in intracranial pressure and metabolic crisis. *Crit Care Med.* 2007;35(12):2830–2836.

45. Vespa PM, McArthur DL, Xu Y, et al. Nonconvulsive seizures after traumatic brain injury are associated with hippocampal atrophy. *Neurology.* 2010;75(9):792–798.

46. Inaba K, Menaker J, Branco BC, et al. A prospective multicenter comparison of levetiracetam versus phenytoin for early posttraumatic seizure prophylaxis. *J Trauma Acute Care Surg.* 2013;74(3):766–771 discussion 771–3.

47. Szaflarski JP, Sangha KS, Lindsell CJ, et al. Prospective, randomized, single-blinded comparative trial of intravenous levetiracetam versus phenytoin for seizure prophylaxis. *Neurocrit Care.* 2010;12(2):165–172.

48. Saposnik G, Barinagarrementeria F, Brown Jr RD, et al. American Heart Association Stroke Council and the Council on Epidemiology and Prevention. Diagnosis and management of cerebral venous thrombosis: a statement for healthcare professionals from the American Heart Association/American Stroke Association. *Stroke.* 2011;42(4):1158–1192.

49. Shen J, Pan JW, Fan ZX, et al. Surgery for contralateral acute epidural hematoma following acute subdural hematoma evacuation: five new cases and a short literature review. *Acta Neurochir (Wien).* 2013;155(2):335–341.

50. Cohen DB, Rinker C, Wilberger JE. Traumatic brain injury in anticoagulated patients. *J Trauma.* 2006;60:553.

51. Knudson MM, Ikossi DG, Khaw L, et al. Thromboembolism after trauma: an analysis of 1602 episodes from the American College of Surgeons National Trauma Data Bank. *Ann Surg.* 2004;240:490–496.

52. Phelan HA. Pharmacologic venous thromboembolism prophylaxis after traumatic brain injury: a critical literature review. *J Neurotrauma.* 2012;29(10):1821–1828.

53. Kapinos G, Ciampa C, Jun P, Narayan RK. Appropriate and effective venous thrombo-embolism (VTE) prophylaxis: Institutional good clinical practice guidelines (GL) for Neurology & Neurosurgery patients. *BMJ Quality & Safety and the European Journal of Hospital Pharmacy.* 2014; supplement.

54. Gould MK, Garcia DA, Wren SM, et al. Prevention of VTE in nonorthopedic surgical patients: Antithrombotic Therapy and Prevention of Thrombosis, 9th ed: American College of Chest Physicians Evidence-Based Clinical Practice Guidelines. *Chest.* 2012;141(2 Suppl):e227S–e277S.

55. Vespa PM. Hormonal dysfunction in neurocritical patients. *Curr Opin Crit Care.* 2013;19(2):107–112.

56. Powner DJ, Boccalandro C. Adrenal insufficiency following traumatic brain injury in adults. *Curr Opin Crit Care.* 2008;14(2):163–166.

# 29 Decompressive Craniectomy for the Treatment of Traumatic Brain Injury

RANDALL M. CHESNUT

The Monro Kellie doctrine holds that intracranial pressure (ICP) is a product of the sum of the volumes of the intracranial contents (i.e., blood, brain, cerebrospinal fluid [CSF], and other).[1] The goal of decompressive craniectomy is to violate the Monro Kellie doctrine, thereby relaxing the physical constraints on compartment volume(s), which manifest as intracranial hypertension.

## Neuroanatomy and Procedure

### Key Concepts

- Choose unilateral decompression for mass effect localized to one hemisphere, producing midline shift.
- Choose bilateral decompression for diffuse swelling or bilateral mass effect.
- Size matters. Decompressions should be as large as possible and include a wide opening of the dura.
- Full decompression of the temporal fossa via craniectomy of the temporal squama is mandatory for all supratentorial decompressions.

The following descriptions apply only to decompressive procedures performed with the specific intent of lowering ICP through provision of space for mass effect. Frequently, the term *decompressive craniectomy (DC)* is applied to procedures aimed at removing intracranial mass lesions (such as subdural hematomas), wherein the bone is not replaced at the end of the case due to intraoperative swelling or the perception that the patient is at risk of such. The initial surgical planning for the latter operations is influenced by the size and location of the mass lesion and its proximity to other structures that may be involved (e.g., air or venous sinuses). If leaving the bone out is considered at the beginning of such operations, however, the following concepts should be included when formulating the approach.

The most frequently quoted description of the DC technique is the bifrontal procedure of Kjellberg and Prieto.[2] Their approach was a radical attempt to minimize the physical constraints on the swollen brain. It involved a large bilateral, bifrontal exposure with removal of all of the bone, including that overlying the sagittal sinus. The dura was opened widely and, uniquely, the falx cerebri was divided just above the floor of the frontal cranial fossa. This involved achieving hemostasis across the usually small but frequently patent anterior sagittal sinus in this region and dissecting back between the hemispheres through the deep margin of the falx cerebri. When this is completed, the frontal lobes generally rise up to some extent, which is felt to represent decompression of the deep structures. Because the Kjellberg procedure is recognized as the classic technique, it is considered by some to be the gold standard. It is, however, possessed of increased morbidity due to the process of removing the bone over the sagittal sinus (often accompanied by bleeding, sometimes significant), sectioning the falx and anterior extent of the sagittal sinus, invasion of the frontal sinuses, and the lack of the physical structure of the frontal bone during care of the patient after surgery, prior to reconstruction. Additionally, the importance of these aspects of this procedure has not been scientifically established. Therefore many variations exist.

The variation generally used by us is to maintain a narrow strip of bone over the sagittal sinus by performing two separate large lateral craniectomies through an ear-to-ear (Sutar) incision, which is curvilinear in nature in order to maximize the ability to retract the skin flap down over the brow (Fig. 29.1). By making the incision posteriorly and maximizing the posterior scalp retraction, the posterior aspect of the craniotomy can be almost as extensive as a single unilateral approach, which is particularly important when a bifrontal craniotomy is used to treat a situation with primarily unilateral swelling. Advantages of this approach are the maintenance of some frontal structure postoperatively, which facilitates nursing care and the wearing of a protective helmet, as well as the ability to leave a "Harborview Peninsula" of bone jutting out from this sagittal bone strip slightly over the hemisphere through which intracranial monitoring devices can be placed and anchored for postoperative care (outlined in red in Fig. 29.1).

When only unilateral decompression is needed, the head will be positioned laterally and a "question mark" incision made, originating at the root of the zygoma, coursing posteriorly over the ear, to eventually join the midline from whence it is continued forward to the hairline or approximately 6 cm anterior to the coronal suture when there is no anterior hair border (Fig. 29.2). The craniotomy closely approximates the scalp incision, with the exception that it will be kept slightly lateral to the sagittal sinus. This can be accomplished by visualizing the sagittal suture and running the craniotomy approximately 2 cm laterally.

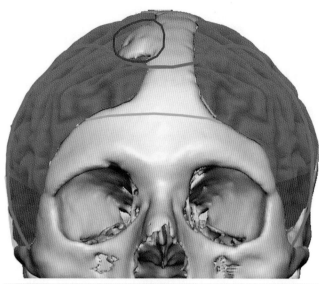

**Fig. 29.1** Modified bifrontal decompressive craniectomy, wherein a strip of bone is left in the midline. The bifrontal (Sutar) incision (*blue line*) allows skull exposure from the brow through the parietal bosses. Large bilateral skull flaps are then removed in a fashion similar to unilateral craniectomies. The temporal (middle cranial) fossae are then decompressed laterally with rongeurs (*red shaded area*). If postoperative intracranial monitoring is planned, one option is to leave a small peninsula of bone over the chosen hemisphere for use to anchor monitoring devices (*red circle*). If a Kjellberg-type procedure is chosen, the craniotomy is carried across the midline (*green line*) and the midline bone strip is removed. The superior sagittal sinus is then ligated as anteriorly as possible and the falx cerebri divided.

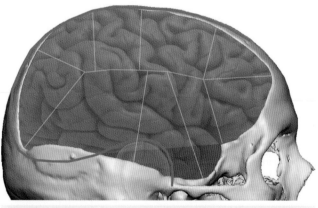

**Fig. 29.2** Unilateral decompressive craniectomy. A "question mark" incision is made from the root of the zygoma and carried back over the ear to meet the midline in the occipital-parietal area after which it is carried forward in the midline (*blue line*). The bone flap is fashioned to be as large as possible, coming to within 1 to 2 cm of the midline. The lateral wall of the temporal (middle cranial) fossa is then decompressed laterally with rongeurs (*red shaded area*). The dura is opened widely, generally in a cruciate fashion (*yellow line*).

If attention has been paid to the size of the ipsilateral frontal air sinus on the preoperative computed tomograph (CT), the frontal limb of the craniotomy can be fashioned to avoid violating this potentially contaminating compartment.

In all cases, the dura is opened widely, generally in a cruciate fashion, in order to afford decompression all the way to the craniotomy margin. When the dura is managed at the close of the procedure, the flaps may be pointed toward their original orientation by one or more very, very loose sutures, but the dura must not be closed tightly. Many surgeons place an autologous or artificial barrier over the exposed brain, again avoiding re-creating a restrictive structure.

Anatomical considerations unique to such decompressions include the determinants of the craniotomy geometry, the physical goals of the operation, and the compartments that require decompression.

Constraints to the size of the craniotomy flap include the limits of soft tissue exposure, the skull base (floors of the middle and frontal cranial fossae), and the midline sagittal sinus and associated draining veins that connect the cortical venous system to the sinus. The closer to the midline, the more risk there is of entering the sagittal sinus or injuring the draining veins. However, it is desirable to open the dura as widely as possible in order to maximize the area through which the brain can swell. Too small a durotomy can result in *fungus cerebri*, with compromise of the venous structures at the dural margin, resulting in infarction of the decompressed tissue.

The middle cranial fossa is particularly important to decompress, as this is a tightly constrained compartment, which forces swelling of the temporal lobe medially toward the third cranial nerve and the brainstem. Therefore the craniectomy needs to include the lateral wall of the temporal fossa, which is the inferior portion of the temporal bone. Due to constraints from the overlying temporalis muscle, this bone is usually not removed as part of the flap, but, rather, taken down piecemeal using rongeurs (areas shaded red in Figs. 29.1 and 29.2). This process involves skeletonizing the lateral portion of the sphenoid ridge wherein lies the middle meningeal artery. Because bleeding from this artery can produce a hematoma at arterial pressure, it is critical that hemostasis be obtained. Once this craniotomy is finished, the dura is opened in the same region to allow the temporal lobe to swell laterally.

There is no clinically established method of estimating how much extra volume is necessary to reverse a given instance of intracranial hypertension. Therefore the goal of decompressive craniotomy is to maximize the volume afforded to the various intracranial compartments, and the optimal procedure involves as large a craniotomy flap as possible, as well as generous durotomy. Closure of the dura, if attempted, should be very loose and nonrestrictive. Techniques have been suggested of bony removal accompanied by fenestration or linear slitting of the dura to avoid brain herniation through the decompression site. Because such a technique markedly decreases the ability of the brain to swell, it should be considered only in cases where minimal volume expansion is expected to be required. As noted earlier, the most important technique for avoiding complications of the brain swelling through the dural defect is to maximize the size of the opening so that the swelling is distributed over a larger area.

Although the elasticity of the scalp is preferable to the rigidity of the skull, part of the benefit of the compressive craniotomy is removal of the volume of the explanted craniotomy bone. For a $10 \times 12$ cm flap, this can be as much as 60 mL of volume. Techniques that "float" the craniotomy flap, maintaining it unsecured but in situ, while potentially avoiding the necessity for cranioplasty, do so at the expense of sacrificing the increased intracranial volume afforded by removal of the bone.

Other than the decision to perform surgical decompression, the major question is unilateral versus bilateral decompression. In general, when there is hemispheric volume asymmetry manifest by midline shift, unilateral decompression is chosen. When the swelling is diffuse with obscuration of the basal cisterns in the absence of significant midline mass effect, bifrontal decompression is usually the choice. In cases where there is significant lateralizing mass effect but also concerning injury to the contralateral hemisphere, an expanded bifrontal technique may be chosen if it is felt that a sufficiently generous decompression of the hemisphere producing the shift can be accomplished.

## Perioperative Considerations

### Key Concepts

- The precise indications for this procedure are unclear, but recent randomized controlled trial evidence suggests that it should not be considered for intracranial hypertension that is not firmly established to be refractory to other first-tier medical interventions.
- Questions of patient salvageability should be addressed prior to proceeding with decompressive craniectomy, and the procedure should be limited to patients without evidence of severe brainstem involvement or signs of persistent herniation.
- Secondary insults must be avoided during transport to and from the operating theater as well as during the procedure. In particular, blood pressure and cerebral perfusion pressure must be maintained.

Decompressive craniotomy has a checkered history. The initial case series of 35 patients reported surprisingly good results.[3] A subsequent report from the same group that included 50 more patients and more detailed follow-up, however, found that increased survivorship was at the expense of a high frequency of vegetative survival.[4] As such, the general teaching was that this operation was not useful. In the 1980s, however, the compressive craniotomy was resurrected after the vast advancements in the acute care of posttraumatic intracranial hypertension. Patients felt to be salvageable but who were expected to die due to uncontrollable intracranial hypertension were reconsidered as candidates for surgical decompression. A large number of case series followed, suggestive of the efficacy of decompressive craniotomy in controlling intracranial hypertension and improving outcome. The frequency of this operation therefore blossomed. Optimal candidates for surgical decompression are those where the primary process felt to threaten the patient was secondary insults due to refractory intracranial hypertension and not widespread, severe primary brain injury. Generally considered contraindications include advanced age, signs of brainstem compression, severe electroencephalogram abnormalities, signs of herniation such as motor posturing or dilated pupils, or protracted episodes of secondary insult such as periods of severe intracranial hypertension or hypoperfusion.[5–8] In some cases, decompressive craniotomy has been considered a prophylactic procedure in patients whose initial ICP was very high or in whom early control was at the expense of markedly escalating or initially elevated therapeutic efforts.

The profound resurgence of decompressive craniotomy prompted randomized controlled investigation. The Decompressive Craniectomy in Patients with Severe Traumatic Brain Injury (DECRA) trial was designed to investigate early, aggressive decompressive craniotomy prompted by *forme fruste* refractory intracranial hypertension (ICP >20 mm Hg for ≥15 min over 1 hour) and was focused on the value of such operation when performed before the occurrence of numerous secondary insults related to intracranial hypertension.[9] The RescueICP trial was concomitantly initiated to study the influence of decompressive craniotomy on intracranial hypertension that was more firmly established as highly refractory (ICP >25 mm Hg for 1–12 hours).[10] The results of the DECRA trial suggested that decompressive craniotomy, although effective in terms of degree of lowering of postrandomization ICP, was not associated with improved outcome. Indeed, some analyses suggested that it produced a worse outcome. Although this was overall a very high-quality trial, issues surrounding patient recruitment, statistical analysis, surgical technique, and experimental design remain. Critiques include that the indications used in this study did not select for sufficiently severe or refractory intracranial hypertension, because the mean postrandomization ICP in both the surgical and nonsurgical groups was acceptably controlled. The value of this study is to demonstrate that determining the proper selection criteria for decompression is critical. In contrast, the RescueICP trial evaluated the effects of salvage, late tier decompressive craniotomy on ICP control and functional outcome as determined by the extended Glasgow Outcome Scale (GOS-E). The results of this randomized controlled trial found a 25% reduction in mortality in the surgical treatment arm, and more importantly, an increase in the percentage of patients with upper severe and moderate disability. These results demonstrate that DC does not simply increase the likelihood of a vegetative state, but that it confers a survival advantage to those with lesser levels of disability, e.g. those who are able to live independently.[11]

Because the purpose of DC is to reverse or minimize the secondary insults related to intracranial hypertension, it is critical not to compound such insults during transport to and from the operating theater or during surgery. In particular, blood pressure, ICP, and cerebral perfusion pressure must be monitored and meticulously managed to every extent possible at all stages. It is well documented that transportation is one of the most risky epochs in severe traumatic brain injury (sTBI) care.[12] Those patients considered for DC are in *extremis*, or at the point of death, and are at exceptional risk of having the potential benefit of the operation nullified by secondary insults related to discontinuous monitoring or oversight.

# Postoperative Complications

## Key Concepts

- Neurological deterioration or the development of a tense scalp flap (or unexplained intracranial hypertension if monitored) early after surgery should prompt rapid CT imaging for postoperative subgaleal hematoma, intraparenchymal hemorrhage, or appearance or expansion of contralateral pathology.
- Monitoring ICP after decompressive craniectomy should be considered in order to assess the influence of the procedure, act as an early warning of untoward effects of decompression (*vide supra*), optimizing cerebral perfusion pressure (CPP), and assessing autoregulation. Such information may be useful for prognosis as well as in guiding therapy.
- Hydrocephalus is a common sequela of decompressive craniectomy, which may manifest as neurological decline or lack of progression of recovery.
- The syndrome of the trephined may present similarly to hydrocephalus, but is associated with a sunken scalp flap and is best treated by cranioplasty.
- Paradoxical herniation is a neurological emergency, presenting as pupillary abnormalities, decreased level of consciousness, focal deficits, or autonomic instability, which may be misdiagnosed as intracranial hypertension, but responds to lowering the head of the bed, stopping ICP treatments, and discontinuing CSF diversion.

## IMMEDIATE POSTOPERATIVE PERIOD

Complications arising in the immediate postoperative period (Box 29.1) may evolve from craniotomy site bleeding, evolution of intracranial mass lesions such as contusions, expansion of contralateral pathology, or diffuse or focal brain swelling as a consequence of the decompression itself (hyperemia, reperfusion injury, etc.). Such complications will generally manifest as a decrease in the level of consciousness, alterations in the pupils, deterioration in the motor examination, or increasing tension in the scalp flap overlying the decompression and are related to

---

### Box 29.1    Postoperative Complications

- Intracranial hypertension
  - Inadequate decompression
  - Increased edema
  - Expansion of contusions/hemorrhages
  - Expansion of contralateral lesion
  - Hyperemia/loss of autoregulation
  - Subgaleal hematoma
- Infection
  - Wound
  - Cerebritis
  - Abscess
- Hydrocephalus
  - Ventricular
  - External (fifth ventricle)
- Syndrome of the trephined
- Paradoxical herniation
- Seizures
- External trauma to the unprotected brain

---

elevated ICP. Under such conditions, evidence of neurological worsening should prompt immediate intervention and CT imaging. Etiologies such as surgical site bleeding or the expansion of a contralateral mass lesion should prompt consideration of return to the operating theater. Other etiologies, such as increased cerebral edema, may indicate failure of the compression to achieve resolution of intracranial hypertension and prompt reconsideration of salvage ability. Indeed, because decompressive craniotomy for intracranial hypertension is frequently a last-ditch intervention, any consideration of return to theater should be accompanied by reassessment of salvageability. One instance where return to theater may be particularly indicated is when the initial craniotomy wasn't sufficient, either due to small size or being unilateral when bilateral decompression is indicated. Such occurrences, however, should be minimized by proper preoperative analysis and decompressive technique.

## Postcraniectomy Intracranial Hypertension

The question of whether to monitor ICP after decompressive craniectomy is controversial. Proponents of not monitoring argue that this procedure is definitive and that further treatment is not required. Recent metaanalysis of the influence of DC on ICP-related parameters in pooled data supported significant acute and sustained reduction of mean ICP and improvement in CPP after surgery.[13] However, complete resolution of intracranial hypertension is not universal. Individual case series have reported failure to reverse intracranial hypertension in up to 20% of cases, wherein it is associated with poor outcome.[6,14–17] Lack of CPP response to decompression has also been reported.[18,19] Rigorous analysis of this problem is hampered by lack of standardization of definitions of intracranial hypertension, inclusion/exclusion criteria, or decompression techniques and the lack of clinical outcome data correlated with ICP control after DC. A primary problem is that there are no data on whether successful management of postdecompressive craniectomy intracranial hypertension independently influences outcome. Therefore the choice to monitor after decompression remains unsettled.

One reason to consider postdecompression monitoring is to avoid iatrogenic exacerbation of cerebral edema consequent to altered intracranial dynamics such as increased postoperative CPP and impairment of cerebrovascular pressure reactivity.[6,19–21] Modulating cerebral blood flow (CBF) toward avoiding hyperemia without inducing ischemia can potentially reduce the risk of driving increased edema[22,23] but requires multimodality monitoring (including ICP) and has not been studied in terms of affecting outcome.

Unfortunately, interpretation of such multimodality monitoring is not straightforward. Parameters such as the cerebrovascular compensatory reserve (RAP), the cerebrovascular pressure-reactivity index (PRx) cerebral blood flow, and cerebral metabolism also vary in their response to decompressive craniectomy in a fashion that appears correlated with outcome. These parameters, however, most likely primarily represent severity of the disease. Whether or not they can be beneficially manipulated as a form of treatment is unclear. It is therefore entirely possible that postdecompression ICP monitoring is primarily useful in prognostication rather than guiding treatment.

In cases where DC is done as a permissive maneuver for the purpose of facilitating treatment of a systemic insult that collides with cerebral management (e.g., acute respiratory distress syndrome), monitoring should be interpreted toward individualizing the ICP and CPP thresholds in the face of confounding extracranial influences. Permissive intracranial hypertension and a CPP adjusted toward 50 mm Hg may be tolerated without ischemia or herniation when the intracranial hypertension is driven entirely by outside influences (e.g., elevated mean intrathoracic pressure). Postoperative monitoring toward facilitating such decisions can be useful in choosing and guiding treatments such as proning, positive end-expiratory pressure elevation, and permissive hypercapnia.

## LATER COMPLICATIONS

When studied prospectively, medical or surgical complications that may arise in the intensive care unit (ICU) after DC occur frequently; 37% of postdecompressive craniectomy patients had one or more such events in the DECRA trial.[9] These complications include those related to surgical ramifications of the procedure (infection, hydrocephalus, paradoxical herniation, and the syndrome of the trephined) as well as medical complications of patients with this severity of TBI (pneumonia, sepsis, pulmonary embolism, acute renal failure).

Infection is a risk at any time and may be difficult to diagnose in patients with multiple candidate sources for fever. Unless there is obvious evidence of local infection, other sources of fever should be ruled out first. Wound breakdown or discharge is obvious but is an uncommon early sign. Frank inflammation, tenderness, or increased local temperature may also not be apparent. Because there are frequently small subgaleal collections below craniectomy closures, plain CT imaging is often not helpful, although new evidence of parenchymal edema or mass effect may suggest cerebritis or abscess. The finding of enhancement on imaging with contrast is suspicious, although false negatives can occur. If there is significant suspicion of an infected subgaleal collection, bedside aspiration of a small fluid sample by neurosurgery can be definitive. Such a procedure must, of course, be performed with strict attention to sterility, and caution is required to avoid damage to the underlying brain.

Subgaleal infections and intracerebral abscesses require drainage. Stereotaxic aspiration/drainage can be considered for abscesses; open débridement and drainage are required for extraaxial collections and still comprise the more common approach to deep infections. Unless the patient is toxic, it is useful to delay antibiotics pending obtaining a definitive bacterial sample via an expeditiously performed access procedure. If preprocedural antibiotics are started, a sample should be sent for polymerase chain reaction identification of the infectious organism(s).

There are no data on which to base recommendations on prophylactic postoperative antibiotics specific to DC. We do not continue perioperative antibiotics beyond 24 hours after surgery.

Hydrocephalus was the most common complication of DC in the DECRA trial, occurring in 10% of decompressed patients versus 1% of those managed nonoperatively. External evidence will include a full flap (which may have been previously sunken) and neurological deterioration or plateauing of recovery. Hydrocephalus may manifest classically, with ventricular enlargement, or as external hydrocephalus with a fifth ventricle consisting of unilateral or bilateral subgaleal hygromas, sometimes with small, compressed lateral ventricles (Fig. 29.3).

The difficulty with managing hydrocephalus in the patient with a surgical decompression is preventing overdrainage, which can precipitate the syndrome of the trephined[24,25] or even paradoxical herniation,[26,27] as well as make it difficult to prevent the development of refractory extraaxial hygromas after eventual cranioplasty. For this reason, we routinely attempt to replace the skull flap at the time of shunting (shuntoplasty) using an adjustable shunt valve, which is initially set high and dialed down subsequently, based on imaging and the neurological examination. In those cases where such extraaxial collections are resistant to prevention and become sizeable, they may be separately shunted to the pleural or peritoneal space (Fig. 29.4).

The syndrome of the trephined was initially described by Grant and Norcross in 1939 as a clinical condition, often occurring after a period of recovery, consisting of seizures, weakness or paralysis, headache, sensory changes, altered mentation, visual disturbances, or speech disturbances.[24] It has become much more common with the resurgence of DC for intracranial hypertension[25,28] and now includes the possibility of brainstem findings as well.[29] The treatment is cranioplasty.

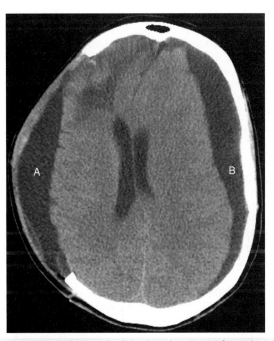

**Fig. 29.3** Subgaleal **(A)** and subdural **(B)** hygromas after right-sided decompressive craniectomy.

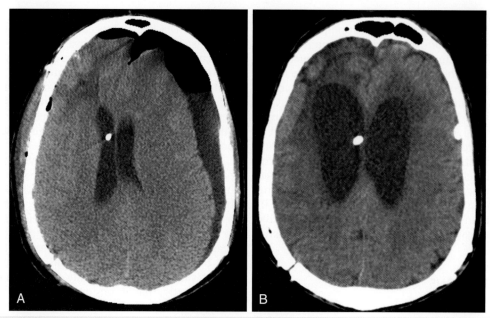

**Fig. 29.4** Left-sided subdural hygroma after a right-sided cranioplasty accompanied by ventriculoperitoneal shunting **(A)**. Persistence of this collection and its associated mass effect prompted internal drainage via a subdural-pleural shunt, which obliterated the extraaxial collection and revealed the general etiology of posttraumatic/postcraniectomy hydrocephalus, which was eventually managed by adjusting the drainage pressure setting of the ventriculoperitoneal shunt.

A much less common but potentially catastrophic complication of DC is that of paradoxical herniation.[26,27] This may occur at any time in decompressed patients, including long after the procedure. Decompressive craniectomy renders the supratentorial space sensitive to atmospheric pressure, which must be buffered across potential herniation sites (e.g., foramen magnum or tentorial incisura) by CSF pressure. When that buffer is compromised, such as by spontaneous, traumatic, or iatrogenic subaxial CSF leaks, paradoxical herniation can occur. This may manifest as decreased level of consciousness, pupillary changes (anisocoria, bilateral dilation, or loss of reactivity), focal neurological deficits, or autonomic instability—signs that are more frequently attributed to elevated ICP, which may lead to incorrect diagnosis and treatment. Efforts to lower ICP will not be effective in paradoxical herniation and may worsen the situation. The proper approach will be to lower the head of the bed (even beyond horizontal), cease any CSF diversionary measures (especially lumbar drainage), hydrate the patient, and discontinue ICP-based interventions such as hyperosmotic agents. If an implanted ventricular drainage system is in place, it should be externalized and clamped. If there is a known site at risk for lumbar CSF leakage such as a lumbar puncture site or recently removed lumbar drain, a blood patch may be performed in the short term, although cranioplasty is the primary consideration after the acute crisis has been managed.

Seizures can occur at any time after TBI or DC and were part of the initial description of the syndrome of the trephined. Of note, seizures were not reported as a complication in either group of the DECRA study, related to either the index procedure or subsequent cranioplasty.[9] There are no data to drive recommendations for altering antiepileptic drug administration practice patterns specifically for DC patients.

The unprotected brain is at risk of external trauma. A prominent notice should be placed at the ICU bedside describing the presence and location of the craniectomy for visitors and practitioners. Patient positioning must avoid lying on the craniectomy site. A protective helmet should be customized as soon as one is feasible to be fitted and worn. One helmet-related caveat is to avoid pressure on the craniotomy incision, because this may precipitate wound breakdown.

There is a growing body of anecdotal evidence (case reports, case series) that cranioplasty may be followed by neurological improvement in patients without obvious signs of the syndrome of the trephined, even when they have apparently plateaued in their recovery.[29–31] There is no evidence to support predicting such a response in individual patients.

The proper timing for cranioplasty is unclear. Traditionally, with little solid evidentiary foundation, such surgery was delayed 3 months. Recent uncontrolled anecdotal evidence has suggested no increased risk of infection, neurological complications, or hydrocephalus associated with shorter delays.[32,33] We routinely consider reimplantation of DC flaps (or a custom orthosis) in uncomplicated cases soon after cerebral mass effect has resolved and there is complete lack of evidence of any local or systemic infection.

## Conclusions

Decompressive craniectomy is a surgical treatment for diffuse brain edema or focal hematomas causing intracranial hypertension that is refractory to medical management.

The putative utility of DC is to decrease ICP and risk of herniation and also to mitigate secondary injury by improving brain tissue oxygenation, cerebral perfusion and cerebral metabolism. However, use of DC as an early stage treatment may result in poor outcomes, possibly due to persistence or intracranial hypertension (despite decompression) or to significant complications of the procedure. Therefore, careful selection of patients for this potentially life-saving therapy is critical.

## References

1. Monro A. *Observations on the Structure and Function of the Nervous System.* Edinburgh: Creech and Johnson; 1783.
2. Kjellberg RN, Prieto Jr A. Bifrontal decompressive craniotomy for massive cerebral edema. *J Neurosurg.* 1971;34(4):488–493. PubMed PMID: 5554353. Epub 1971/04/01. eng.
3. Ransohoff J, Benjamin MV, Gage Jr EL, Epstein F. Hemicraniectomy in the management of acute subdural hematoma. *J Neurosurg.* 1971;34(1):70–76. PubMed PMID: 5539647. Epub 1971/01/01. eng.
4. Cooper PR, Rovit RL, Ransohoff J. Hemicraniectomy in the treatment of acute subdural hematoma: a re-appraisal. *Surg Neurol.* 1976;5(1):25–28.
5. Gaab MR, Rittierodt M, Lorenz M, Heissler HE. Traumatic brain swelling and operative decompression: a prospective investigation. *Acta Neurochir Supp.* 1990;51:326–328.
6. Aarabi B, Hesdorffer DC, Ahn ES, Aresco C, Scalea TM, Eisenberg HM. Outcome following decompressive craniectomy for malignant swelling due to severe head injury. *J Neurosurg.* 2006;104(4):469–479. PubMed PMID: 16619648. Epub 2006/04/20. eng.
7. Whitfield PC, Patel H, Hutchinson PJ, et al. Bifrontal decompressive craniectomy in the management of posttraumatic intracranial hypertension. *Br J Neurosurg.* 2001;15(6):500–507. PubMed PMID: 11814002. Epub 2002/01/30. eng.
8. Sahuquillo J, Arikan F. Decompressive craniectomy for the treatment of refractory high intracranial pressure in traumatic brain injury. *Cochrane Database Systematic Rev (Online).* 2006;1:CD003983. PubMed PMID: 16437469. Epub 2006/01/27. eng.
9. Cooper DJ, Rosenfeld JV, Murray L, et al. Decompressive craniectomy in diffuse traumatic brain injury. *New Eng J Med.* 2011;364(16):1493–1502. PubMed PMID: 21434843. Epub 2011/03/26. eng.
10. Hutchinson PJ, Corteen E, Czosnyka M, et al. Decompressive craniectomy in traumatic brain injury: the randomized multicenter RESCUEicp study (http://www.RESCUEicp.com). *Acta Neurochir Supp.* 2006;96:17–20. PubMed PMID: 16671415. Epub 2006/05/05. eng.
11. Hutchinson PJ, Kolias AG, Timofeev IS, et al. RESCUEicp trial collaborators. Trial of decompressive craniectomy for traumatic intracranial hypertension. *N Engl J Med.* 2016; Sep 22;375(12):1119–1130.
12. Jones PA, Andrews PJ, Midgley S, et al. Measuring the burden of secondary insults in head-injured patients during intensive care. *J Neurosurg Anesthesiol.* 1994;6(1):4–14.
13. Bor-Seng-Shu E, Figueiredo EG, Amorim RL, et al. Decompressive craniectomy: a meta-analysis of influences on intracranial pressure and cerebral perfusion pressure in the treatment of traumatic brain injury. *J Neurosurg.* 2012;117(3):589–596. PubMed PMID: 22794321. Epub 2012/07/17. eng.
14. Jagannathan J, Okonkwo DO, Dumont AS, et al. Outcome following decompressive craniectomy in children with severe traumatic brain injury: a 10-year single-center experience with long-term follow up. *J Neurosurg.* 2007;106(4 Suppl):268–275. PubMed PMID: 17465359. Epub 2007/05/01. eng.
15. Taylor A, Butt W, Rosenfeld J, et al. A randomized trial of very early decompressive craniectomy in children with traumatic brain injury and sustained intracranial hypertension. *Childs Nerv Sys.* 2001;17(3):154–162. PubMed PMID: 11305769. Epub 2001/04/18. eng.
16. Williams RF, Magnotti LJ, Croce MA, et al. Impact of decompressive craniectomy on functional outcome after severe traumatic brain injury. *J Trauma.* 2009;66(6):1570–1574. discussion 4–6. PubMed PMID: 19509616. Epub 2009/06/11. eng.
17. Yoo DS, Kim DS, Cho KS, Huh PW, Park CK, Kang JK. Ventricular pressure monitoring during bilateral decompression with dural expansion. *J Neurosurg.* 1999;91(6):953–959. PubMed PMID: 10584840. Epub 1999/12/10. eng.
18. Münch E, Horn P, Schurer L, Piepgras A, Paul T, Schmiedek P. Management of severe traumatic brain injury by decompressive craniectomy. *Neurosurgery.* 2000;47(2):315–322. discussion 22–3. PubMed PMID: 10942004. Epub 2000/08/15. eng.
19. Timofeev I, Czosnyka M, Nortje J, et al. Effect of decompressive craniectomy on intracranial pressure and cerebrospinal compensation following traumatic brain injury. *J Neurosurg.* 2008;108(1):66–73. PubMed PMID: 18173312. Epub 2008/01/05. eng.
20. Cooper PR, Hagler H, Clark WK, Barnett P. Enhancement of experimental cerebral edema after decompressive craniectomy: implications for the management of severe head injuries. *Neurosurgery.* 1979;4(4):296–300. PubMed PMID: 450227. Epub 1979/04/01. eng.
21. Wang EC, Ang BT, Wong J, Lim J, Ng I. Characterization of cerebrovascular reactivity after craniectomy for acute brain injury. *Br J Neurosurg.* 2006;20(1):24–30. PubMed PMID: 16698605. Epub 2006/05/16. eng.
22. Bor-Seng-Shu E, Hirsch R, Teixeira MJ, De Andrade AF, Marino Jr R. Cerebral hemodynamic changes gauged by transcranial Doppler ultrasonography in patients with posttraumatic brain swelling treated by surgical decompression. *J Neurosurg.* 2006;104(1):93–100. PubMed PMID: 16509152. Epub 2006/03/03. eng.
23. Olivecrona M, Rodling-Wahlstrom M, Naredi S, Koskinen LO. Effective ICP reduction by decompressive craniectomy in patients with severe traumatic brain injury treated by an ICP-targeted therapy. *J Neurotrauma.* 2007;24(6):927–935. PubMed PMID: 17600510. Epub 2007/06/30. eng.
24. Grant FC, Norcross NC. Repair of Cranial Defects by Cranioplasty. *Ann Surg.* 1939;110(4):488–512. PubMed PMID: 17857467. PubMed Central PMCID: PMC1391431. Epub 1939/10/01. eng.
25. Joseph V, Reilly P. Syndrome of the trephined. *J Neurosurg.* 2009;111(4):650–652. PubMed PMID: 19361266. Epub 2009/04/14. eng.
26. Fields JD, Lansberg MG, Skirboll SL, Kurien PA, Wijman CA. "Paradoxical" transtentorial herniation due to CSF drainage in the presence of a hemicraniectomy. *Neurology.* 2006;67(8):1513–1514. PubMed PMID: 17060591. Epub 2006/10/25. eng.
27. Oyelese AA, Steinberg GK, Huhn SL, Wijman CA. Paradoxical cerebral herniation secondary to lumbar puncture after decompressive craniectomy for a large space-occupying hemispheric stroke: case report. *Neurosurgery.* 2005;57(3):E594. discussion E. PubMed PMID: 16145506. Epub 2005/09/08. eng.
28. Honeybul S, Ho KM. Long-term complications of decompressive craniectomy for head injury. *J Neurotrauma.* 2011;28(6):929–935. PubMed PMID: 21091342. Epub 2010/11/26. eng.
29. Gottlob I, Simonsz-Toth B, Heilbronner R. Midbrain syndrome with eye movement disorder: dramatic improvement after cranioplasty. *Strabismus.* 2002;10(4):271–277. PubMed PMID: 12660851. Epub 2003/03/28. eng.
30. Dujovny M, Aviles A, Agner C, Fernandez P, Charbel FT. Cranioplasty: cosmetic or therapeutic? *Surg Neurol.* 1997;47(3):238–241. PubMed PMID: 9068693. Epub 1997/03/01. eng.
31. Honeybul S, Janzen C, Kruger K, Ho KM. The impact of cranioplasty on neurological function. *Br J Neurosurg.* 2013;27(5):636–641. PubMed PMID: 23883370. Epub 2013/07/26. eng.
32. Beauchamp KM, Kashuk J, Moore EE, et al. Cranioplasty after postinjury decompressive craniectomy: is timing of the essence? *J Trauma.* 2010;69(2):270–274. PubMed PMID: 20699735.
33. Bender A, Heulin S, Rohrer S, et al. Early cranioplasty may improve outcome in neurological patients with decompressive craniectomy. *Brain Inj.* 2013;27(9):1073–1079. PubMed PMID: 23662672.

SECTION **3**

# Spinal Surgery

**SECTION OUTLINE**

# 30 Spine Trauma and Spinal Cord Injury

JAMES M. SCHUSTER and PETER SYRE

## Introduction

Spinal trauma, with and without neurological injury, is very common at major trauma centers. Spinal trauma often occurs in the setting of polytrauma, intensifying the complexity of these injuries. The effective management of these patients requires a basic understanding of the pathophysiology of spinal injury, a fundamental knowledge of the principles of treatment, and the ability to identify and appropriately handle potential complications. These basic principles include appropriate triage and resuscitation within the Advanced Trauma Life Support paradigm, appropriate immobilization and protection of the unstable spine, recognition and classification of the spinal injury, formulation and execution of a treatment plan that includes early decompression of neural elements and reestablishing structural integrity and stability, physiological stabilization to minimize secondary injury, and early mobilization to avoid secondary complications and enhance rehabilitation potential. The following sections are organized around key management sections, with the key concepts based on the highest level of available evidence.

## Pathophysiology and Classification

### Key Concepts

- A basic understanding of the common spinal injury patterns facilitates comprehensive management and complication recognition/avoidance.
- Precise documentation and classification of the neurological examination are paramount because this has management and prognostic implications.

### Clinical Pearls

- Bradycardia and hypotension in a trauma patient are concerning for a cervical spinal cord injury until proven otherwise.
- The neurological examination in a spinal cord injured patient can fluctuate for the same examiner and between examiners, so close clinical follow-up is key.

Anatomically and pathophysiologically the spine is regionally subclassified to account for spinal injuries with a predilection for certain regions: occipital cervical junction (occiput to C2) subaxial cervical spine (C3–T1), thoracic (T2–T10), thoracolumbar junction (T11– L2), lower lumbar (L4–S1), and sacrum. An exhaustive description of spinal trauma is beyond the scope of this book, but the next section will provide the basic anatomical and pathophysiological highlights most relevant to neurocritical care.

Occipital condyle fractures generally arise from an axial loading–type injury with either an extension of a skull fracture to the condyle (Anderson Montesano type 2)[1] or a crush type injury between the skull and C1 lateral mass (type 1) (Fig. 30.1A). These axial loading–type injuries are rarely unstable. The third type (type 3)[2] often represents an avulsion type injury of the alar ligament pulling a fragment of bone from the condyle. This often happens in the context of a significant distractive injury and should raise a suspicion of atlantooccipital dissociation (AOD).

AOD is a severe distractive injury resulting in disruption of the major stabilizers of the craniocervical junction, including the tectorial membrane, alar ligaments, apical ligament, O–C1 joints, and often C1–C2 capsular ligaments (Fig. 30.1B). It is most commonly seen in high-speed motor vehicle accident/motorcycle accident and car versus pedestrian accidents. This is a dynamic and highly unstable injury. These patients can have fluctuating neurological examinations. Even with modern imaging the injury can be missed, and the first indication of an issue is a new neurological deficit. Other radiographic findings include subarachnoid hemorrhage/ epidural hematoma at the foramen magnum, vertebral artery injury, and magnetic resonance signal change in the spinal cord. This injury generally requires surgical stabilization (occipital-cervical fusion).[3,4]

The classic C1 fracture injury is the Jefferson fracture, which is an axial loading–type injury with generally two opposing fractures in the ring (Fig. 30.1C). The crucial determination in this injury is the integrity of the transverse ligament. If the transverse ligament is disrupted, manifested by significant lateral displacement of the lateral masses on imaging, surgical stabilization may be indicated.[5,6]

Other C2 fractures include hangman's fractures or traumatic fractures of the C2 pars interarticularis/pedicles (Fig. 30.1D). Although the injury resembles the fracture pattern seen with judicial hangings, the mechanism is more often an axial loading/flexion type injury versus the distraction/extension injury seen with hangings. The need

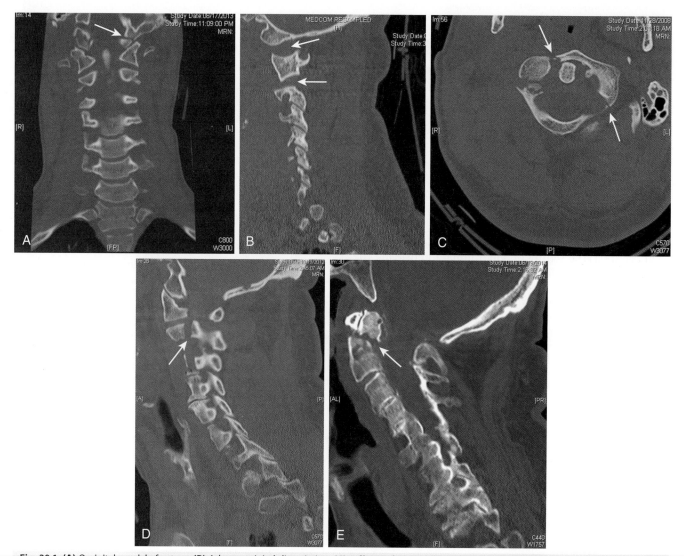

**Fig. 30.1  (A)** Occipital condyle fracture. **(B)** Atlantooccipital dissociation. **(C)** Jefferson fracture. **(D)** Hangman's fracture. **(E)** Type 2 odontoid fracture.

for surgical stabilization depends generally on the amount of resultant angulation and displacement. Other C2 fractures include body fractures and lateral mass fractures, which in isolation generally have a benign course and are treated with an external brace.[7]

The most common types of C2 fractures are odontoid fractures, of which there are three varieties. Type 1 is rare and again often associated with distractive type injuries. Type 2, generally with fracture across the base of the dens, is the most common type, especially in the elderly (Fig. 30.1E). Type 3, with fracture extension into the C1–C2 joints bilaterally, has more fractured bone surface area and is more likely to heal with an external brace (collar or halo). The younger the patient and the less displaced, the more likely a type 2 fracture will heal with a brace. Unfortunately, in general elderly patients do not tolerate halos well, commonly resulting in respiratory and sometimes psychiatric disturbances. This often creates a dilemma because surgical risks related to fixation to avoid a halo are higher in the elderly population.[7] Odontoid fractures as well as other fragility falls from standing such as hip and arm fractures are often a surrogate marker for declining function overall. Surgery for odontoid fractures most commonly

involves posterior C1–C2 fusions with occasional incorporation of the occiput. A smaller percentage is stabilized using an odontoid screw from an anterior approach.

The subaxial cervical spine (C3–T1) is quite mobile, and resultant injury patterns are generally the result of composite forces. Pure axial loading injuries in the mildest form can give benign compression fractures. More significant axial loading can give burst fractures with retropulsion of bone or traumatic discs that can cause spinal cord compression. These forces, in combination with flexion and/or rotation, can cause disruption in the posterior ligamentous complexes, including the interspinous, interlaminar, joint capsules, and disc capsules. This may result in facet fractures or dislocation with significant subluxation and resultant spinal cord injury (SCI). The classic diving injury occurs through axial loading and hyperflexion, resulting in bilateral facet dislocation and SCI (Figs. 30.2A and 30.2B).[8]

The thoracic spine is generally well stabilized by the rib cage, and as a result significant injury generally requires severe disruptive forces. Again, the most common injuries occur along a spectrum from simple compression, to burst fractures, flexion distraction injuries with compressive forces on the vertebral body and posterior ligamentous

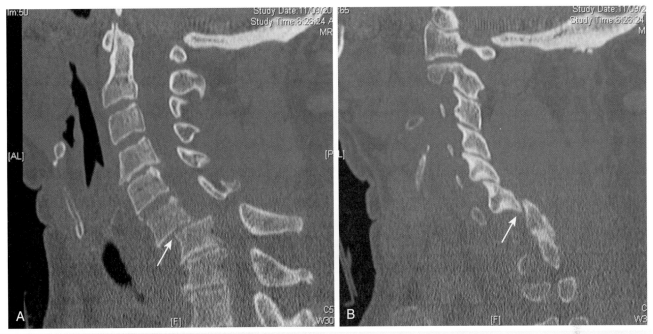

Fig. 30.2 **(A)** Midline view of bilateral jumped facets. **(B)** Right jumped facet.

disruption, to fracture dislocations. The thoracolumbar junction is a common site for more significant injuries because of the transition from rigid thoracic to mobile lumbar spine (Fig. 30.3).

The lower lumbar spine at L3–L5 is inherently stable, and so operative injuries are less common. The sacrum is commonly involved in major pelvic trauma and can sometimes result in lumbopelvic instability and neurological compromise.

**Injury Classification and Surgical Decision Making:** An exhaustive description of the classification of spinal trauma is beyond the scope of this book. The best classification systems are simple, convey meaningful information

with good interobserver reliability, and perhaps give some guidance with regard to management decisions concerning surgical versus nonsurgical options. In the past classification systems have been criticized for not adequately representing the significance of neurological compromise. Two of the newer classification systems place particular emphasis on injury mechanism/description, integrity of the posterior ligamentous complex, and neurological injury: Subaxial Cervical Spine Injury Classification System (SCLICS)[9] and Thoracolumbar Injury Classification and Severity Scale (TLICS)[10] (Table 30.1). The injury is scored and the total score can be used to make management decisions based on published validation studies. The mechanism description

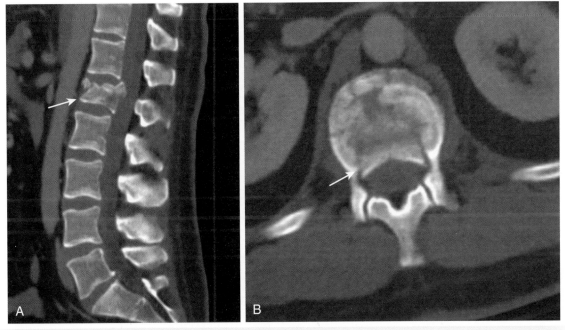

Fig. 30.3 **(A)** Sagittal view of L1 burst fracture. **(B)** Axial view of L1 burst fracture.

**Table 30.1** The Thoracolumbar Injury Classification and Severity Scale (TLICS)

| Points | |
|---|---|
| **Morphology** | |
| No abnormality | 0 |
| Compression | 1 |
| Burst | +1 = 2 |
| Distraction (e.g., facet perch, hyperextension) | 3 |
| Rotation/translation (e.g., facet dislocation, unstable teardrop or advanced staged flexion compression injury) | 4 |
| **Discoligamentous complex (DLC)** | |
| Intact | 0 |
| Indeterminate | 2 |
| Disrupted | 3 |
| **Neurological status** | |
| Intact | 0 |
| Root injury | 2 |
| Complete cord injury | 2 |
| Incomplete cord injury | 3 |

0–3 Nonoperative treatment; 4 Surgeon's choice; ≥5 Operative treatment.

category puts much more weight on distractive and/or subluxation/rotation forces. In the neurological injury category, there is more weight given to an incomplete versus complete cord injury, and a distinction is made between nerve root and cord lesions. These systems are less applicable to the O–C injuries described previously, which have their own classification schemes to help guide management.

## Neurological Status

A detailed and accurate documentation of a patient's neurological status after spinal injury is paramount. We generally recommend the American Spinal Injury Association/International Standards for Neurological Classifications of Spinal Cord Injury (ASIA/ISNCSCI) documentation system. It is comprehensive and allows the ability to detect significant neurological changes and allows transmission of useful information from practitioner to practitioner and institution to institution (Fig. 30.4).[11] A proper neurological examination always includes a detailed rectal examination because sacral sparing has prognostic significance in the spinal cord–injured patient.[12]

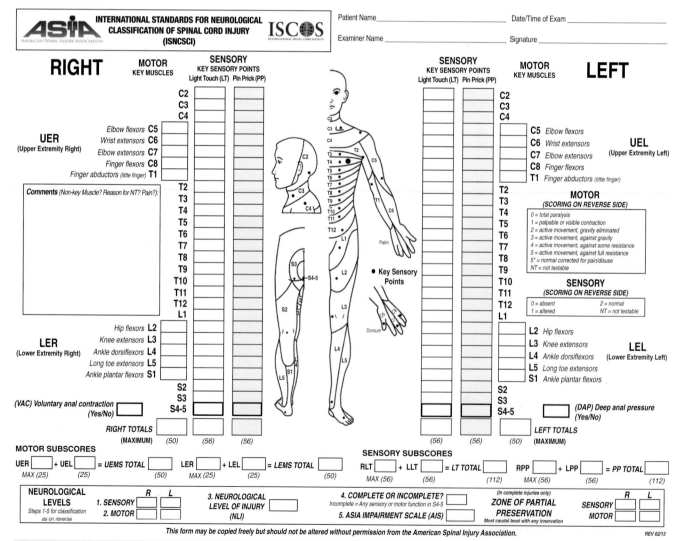

**Fig. 30.4** ASIA scoring chart.

# Management

## Key Concepts

- Early decompression and stabilization of spinal fractures (less than 24 hours) can be carried out safely and may improve outcome, especially in incomplete neurological injuries.
- Early stabilization allows early mobilization that has been associated with reduced pulmonary complications.

## Clinical Pearls

- Although early stabilization is ideal, adequate resuscitation (often indicated by serum lactate levels) and attention to other potentially life-threatening injuries must take precedence.
- Coordination between services, including distinct procedures under the same anesthesia (i.e., lower extremity external fixation and spinal stabilization) to avoid repetitive trips to the operating room, is beneficial to the patient.

Key principles in the management of spinal injury include timely decompression of neural elements, if indicated, and stabilization of the mechanically unstable spine. Spinal instability is somewhat of a nebulous concept but essentially can be described as the loss of structural integrity so that there is a risk of neurological decline, progressive deformity, or persistent pain under normal physiological loads and range of motion. Some fractures can be treated effectively with external brace immobilization (generally with more bony than ligamentous disruption). Other injuries that have significant bone and ligamentous disruption, especially with subluxation, will require internal stabilization. The prevailing trend is early decompression and stabilization of spinal injuries with neurological deficits, especially with incomplete injuries.[13] Even with complete injuries, early surgery allows early mobilizations, which is correlated with decreased risk of significant pulmonary issues.[14] Specific surgical approaches are covered in other portions of this book.

# Cervical Traction

## Key Concept

Cervical traction can be used to rapidly reduce spinal fractures, but should only be carried out by someone with extensive experience with this technique.

## Clinical Pearls

- Cervical traction tong tension pins and pin sites should be checked daily, as should a cross-table x-ray to avoid overdistraction.
- MRI-compatible traction tongs allow MRI imaging with tongs in place.

Decompression of the neural elements can be accomplished indirectly, such as with cervical traction, or with direct surgical decompression. The diving injury with flexion/axial loading injury classically results in bilateral facet dislocation (bilateral jumped facets) with a high incidence of neurological injury (Figs. 30.2A and 30.2B). Rapid decompression of the spinal cord can be achieved with application of cervical traction using Gardner Wells (GW) tongs and progressive weight suspended from the head (Fig. 30.5).[15] Generally this requires an awake and cooperative patient to allow close neurological monitoring. The patients are generally administered analgesics and anxiolytics to facilitate the process. Weight is sequentially added, and with each increment the patient is reexamined and the dislocation is visualized with a lateral x-ray. The process is continued until a reduction is obtained, two thirds of the patient's body weight is reached, the patient has neurological changes, or there is excessive distraction by x-ray (Figs. 30.6A, 30.6B, and 30.6C). This procedure should only be attempted by someone with substantial experience with this process. After reduction, alignment can generally be maintained with substantially less weight than what was needed for reduction. The patient is generally kept in traction until he or she undergoes surgical stabilization. The security of the GW tongs should be checked daily, as should a cross-table x-ray. Because these patients remain supine, a rotating bed is advisable with reverse Trendelenburg to aid nutrition and airway protection. In addition, because they continue to require pain medication and anxiolytics, nasogastric suction for avoidance of aspiration should be considered.

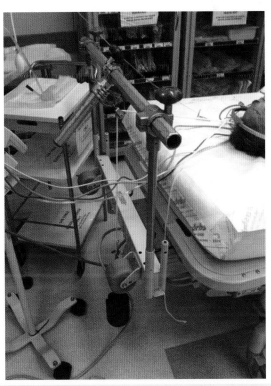

**Fig. 30.5** Gardner-Wells tongs placement and weight application.

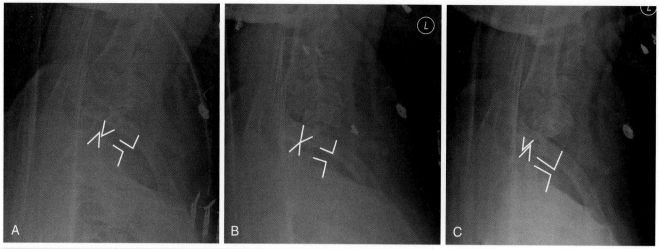

**Fig. 30.6** Sequence of cervical traction reduction of bilateral jumped facets. **(A)** 25 lb, slight distraction but still subluxed. **(B)** 50 lb, facets perched. **(C)** Postreduction.

## Blood Pressure Management

### Key Concepts

- SCI can produce hypotension and in so doing make for a worse SCI.
- Class 3 data suggest a goal mean arterial pressure (MAP) of 85 to 90 for 7 days. However, this must be balanced against the benefit of early mobilization after stabilization and the potential adverse effect of vasopressor treatment.

### Clinical Pearl

Blood pressure augmentation should not be a substitute for early decompression, stabilization, and mobilization.

Cervical and high thoracic injuries block the normal sympathetic response, resulting in bradycardia and hypotension. Hypotension is especially troublesome because the injured spinal cord is at risk for secondary injury from hypoperfusion. SCI management guidelines recommend maintenance of MAP between 85 and 90 for 7 days.[16] This is based on class 3 data. Unfortunately, the pressure parameters and length of treatment were chosen arbitrarily with no consideration of other parameters or lengths of treatment. The risks and benefits have to be determined for each individual patient, especially after having been surgically stabilized, because prolonged immobility and the use of vasopressors can have deleterious effects. Maintaining MAP is generally done with judicious fluid management and vasopressors as needed. Numerous vasopressor agents have been utilized, including dopamine, phenylephrine, epinephrine, norepinephrine, and vasopressin. The choice of vasopressor is addressed in the Consortium for Spinal Cord Medicine guidelines.[17] They suggest that cervical and upper thoracic injuries through T6 warrant a vasopressor with inotropic, chronotropic, and vasoconstrictive properties. They suggest either dopamine or norepinephrine as first choices. A recent study concluded that vasopressor use for MAP goals in spinal cord–injured patients results in a concerning complication rate requiring multiple vasopressor changes.[18] Dopamine has significantly higher complication rates than other vasopressors and a concerning rate of serious arrhythmias and ischemia. Older patients and those with more severe injuries are especially at risk. Phenylephrine, a pure vasoconstrictor, had a higher incidence of bradycardia, which is problematic in a population already at risk for bradycardia.

## Autonomic Derangements

### Key Concept

SCI patients are susceptible to orthostatic hypotension. Various methods are available to help mitigate, including pharmacological, mechanical, and electrical strategies.

### Clinical Pearl

Orthostatic hypotension should be aggressively managed because it impedes mobilization, rehabilitation, and recovery.

As discussed previously, cervicothoracic SCI can result in dysregulated autonomic function. After the initial efforts to maintain adequate spinal cord perfusion with blood pressure augmentation, patients with SCI are especially susceptible to postural hypotension with mobilization. Whether the patient is symptomatic or not, this often delays or limits mobilization, which is key to rehabilitation. Numerous pharmacological and mechanical therapies have been utilized to help with this common problem. The therapeutic goal for management of postural hypotension is not to normalize the blood pressure values but to improve symptoms while avoiding side effects. The strongest data would suggest enterally administered midodrine may be useful for SCI-induced postural hypotension.[19] Ephedrine is also commonly used for this purpose. Abdominal binders and lower extremity compression stockings or wraps are commonly used; however, there is no strong evidence to support this practice. Others modalities, including functional electrical stimulation of the leg muscles, may also be useful to combat orthostatic hypotension.[19]

## Pulmonary/Airway Issues

### Key Concepts

- Cervical spine injury can make securing an airway extremely difficult and requires advanced planning and experience.
- Early tracheostomy is safe after anterior cervical surgery.
- Early mobilization in spinal fractures prevents pulmonary complications.

### Clinical Pearls

- Early intubation in a controlled setting is far better than emergent intubation in an unstable patient with an unstable spinal injury.
- Early tracheostomy is a good option in spinal cord injury patients because of limited functional reserve, risk of repetitive ventilator weaning failure, and difficult airways. Use of a talking tracheostomy device can help with mood and early rehabilitation efforts.

Pulmonary and airway issues are very common in cervical spinal cord injuries. Cervical cord injuries generally result in loss of accessory respiratory muscle function with abdominal breathing, reduced tidal volumes, and poor pulmonary toilet. Injuries above C5 with phrenic nerve involvement will impair diaphragm function to further degrade respiratory function. This puts patients at risk for respiratory failure and difficulty weaning from the ventilator. Intubation requiring maintenance of spinal alignment and the presence of other injuries, including facial injuries, can provide difficult airway management. This requires experienced personnel and perhaps adjuncts such as a fiberoptic scopes. Generally, tracheostomy can be placed safely relatively early after anterior surgical procedures without increased risk of infection.[20] Finally, in patients with polytrauma and thoracolumbar injuries, early stabilization and mobilization are associated with a reduced development of adult respiratory distress syndrome.[14]

## Prevention of Venous Thromboembolism

### Key Concepts

- Early implementation of deep venous thrombosis (DVT) chemoprophylaxis is recommended in spinal cord injury.
- Generally, DVT prophylaxis can be restarted within 24 hours of surgery, but should be individualized for each patient.
- Most venous thromboembolism (VTE) events occur within 3 months of injury, and consideration can be given to discontinuation after that time.

### Clinical Pearl

Because spinal cord injury patients have an extremely high risk of DVT and pulmonary embolism, an aggressive approach to prevention and treatment is reasonable.

Significant SCI and resultant immobility put patients at risk for thromboembolic events. Decisions about short- and long-term prophylaxis have to be weighed against perioperative risk of bleeding and other injuries. Prophylactic treatment of VTE in patients with severe motor deficits due to SCI is recommended (class 1).[21] Early administration of VTE prophylaxis (within 72 hours) after SCI is highly recommended (class II), and holding chemical prophylaxis 1 day prior to and 1 day after surgical intervention is suggested as a reasonable perioperative strategy.[22] Class II medical evidence indicates that the majority of thromboembolic events occur in the first 3 months after acute SCI, and for this reason, it suggested that prophylactic therapy can be discontinued after 3 months unless the patient is at high risk for further VTE events (previous thromboembolic events, obesity, advanced age). It is also reasonable to stop therapy earlier in patients who regained lower extremity motor function because the incidence of VTE events in these patients is substantially lower than those patients with complete motor injuries.[21]

Low-dose heparin in combination with pneumatic compression stockings or electrical stimulation is recommended as a prophylactic treatment strategy, but not low-dose heparin alone. The use of low-molecular-weight heparins, rotating beds, or a combination of modalities is recommended as a prophylactic treatment strategy. Oral anticoagulation alone is not recommended as a prophylactic treatment strategy.[21]

Inferior vena cava filters are not recommended as a routine prophylactic measure in SCI patients but have a role in patients who have suffered thromboembolic events despite anticoagulation and for SCI patients with contraindications to anticoagulation and/or the use of pneumatic compression devices (class III).[21]

Duplex ultrasound can be utilized to screen patients with a clinical suspicion for extremity DVT, and generally a chest computed tomography angiogram (CTA) can be utilized to confirm the presence of a pulmonary embolism. There is significant institutional variability regarding routine surveillance for DVT without clinical suspicion. Currently, there are no strong studies to show routine surveillance improves outcome in SCI patients.[21]

# Vertebral Artery Injury

## Key Concepts

- Patients meeting appropriate criteria should be screened for arterial injury generally by CTA.
- Aspirin is a reasonable treatment for vertebral artery injury.
- The role of endovascular treatment is not well defined.

## Clinical Pearl

Screening for vertebral artery injury is often done for surgical planning because if the vertebral artery is injured on one side, it may determine whether it is prudent to place surgical hardware close to the intact vertebral artery on the other side.

Cervical spinal fractures can put the vertebral arteries at risk for injury. The incidence of vertebral artery injury (VAI) may be as high as 11% after nonpenetrating cervical spinal trauma in patients meeting specific clinical and physical examination criteria. The modified Denver Screening Criteria are used to assist in screening trauma patients for neurovascular imaging (Box 30.1).[23]

C1–C2 fractures through the foramen transversarium, subluxation type injuries, and SCI introduce more concern for vascular injury. CTA is a highly accurate alternative to digital subtraction angiography for screening for VAI in blunt injury trauma patients.[23] The majority of patients with VAI are asymptomatic, even among patients with incidental cerebellar and posterior circulation strokes found on imaging studies at the time of diagnosis or in follow-up. Although no conclusive medical evidence

## Box 30.1   Modified Denver Criteria for Screening for Vascular Injury

Lateralizing neurological deficit (not explained by CT head)

- Infarct on CT head scan
- Cervical hematoma (nonexpanding)
- Massive epistaxis
- Anisocoria/Homer's syndrome
- Glasgow Coma Scale score <8 without significant findings
- Cervical spine fracture
- Severe facial fracture (LeForte II or III only)
- Cervical bruit or thrill

*CT*, computed tomography.

supports a specific treatment for VAI, treatment of symptomatic VAI with either anticoagulation or antiplatelet therapy is suggested. Because of an increased risk of hemorrhagic complications from anticoagulation in polytrauma patients, systemic anticoagulation is not ideal therapy for symptomatic or asymptomatic VAI, especially given no proven treatment superiority. Antiplatelet therapy (aspirin most commonly) appears to be a safe and comparable option for symptomatic patients with VAI after blunt trauma. No treatment or antiplatelet therapy appears to be a reasonable option for the treatment of asymptomatic patients with VAI. The choice of therapy for patients with VAI should be individualized based on the patient's specific VAI, associated traumatic injuries, and the relative risk of bleeding.

Endovascular intervention has been suggested for pseudoaneurysms, dissections, and fistula associated with VAI. However, the need for dual antiplatelet therapy after endovascular procedures is a relative contraindication in multiple-injury trauma patients with VAI. The utility of endovascular treatments, including stenting of dissections or occlusion for persistent embolization in someone who cannot be anticoagulated, is less clearly defined.[23]

# Steroids

## Key Concepts

- Currently there are no convincing data that the administration of steroids for spinal cord injury provides a therapeutic benefit.
- The administration of high-dose steroids does carry a significant risk of complications.

## Clinical Pearl

If a clinician chooses to use steroids for spinal cord injury, it is recommended that he or she strictly adhere to the recommended indications and administration (i.e., not for penetrating injury).

There continues to be significant individual and institutional variability with regard to the use of corticosteroids in the management of acute SCI. Currently the position statement of the Joint Section of Neurological Surgery based on class 1 data states "Administration of methylprednisolone (MP) for the treatment of acute spinal cord injury (SCI) is not recommended. Clinicians considering MP therapy should bear in mind that the drug is not Food and Drug Administration (FDA) approved for this application." There is no class I or class II medical evidence supporting the clinical benefit of MP in the treatment of acute SCI. Scattered reports of class III evidence claim inconsistent effects likely related to random chance or selection bias. However, class I, II, and III evidence exists that high-dose steroids are associated with harmful side effects, including death.[24] If individual clinicians choose to use MP for the treatment of SCI, it is recommended that they adhere to the currently recommended administration guidelines.

# Traumatic Central Cord Syndrome

## Key Concepts

- Early decompression can be performed safely in patients with central cord syndrome with some evidence that it may improve outcome.
- These patients are generally older with more comorbidities and a higher risk for perioperative hypotension.

## Clinical Pearls

- There should be a high suspicion for neurological injury in an elderly patient with a cervical hyperextension mechanism, even without radiographic bony injury.
- Decompression during the initial hospital stay allows early and uninterrupted rehabilitation, as opposed to sending the patient out and bringing him or her back.

Traumatic central cord syndrome, notable for upper extremity weakness with less or no lower extremity weakness, is a very common injury at a level 1 trauma center. It typically is an acute cervical myelopathy generally caused by a hyperextension mechanism in a patient with underlying degenerative cervical stenosis and/or congenital stenosis. It generally occurs in an older patient population where the prevalence of degenerative stenosis is higher, along with more falls, and is less likely to be associated with a fracture. Often the patients do not give a history of underlying cervical problems. Because of the laminated arrangement of tracts in the spinal cord with cervical pathways more centrally located, these injuries are more centrally located in the spinal cord, and therefore the upper extremities may be more affected than the lower extremities. These patients are especially susceptible to hypotension-induced secondary SCI, and therefore maintaining adequate perfusion pressure is especially important perioperatively. Because this injury occurs generally in older patient populations, normal baseline blood pressures and resultant adequate perfusion pressures may be higher than in the younger SCI populations. In addition, these older patients are at higher risk of complications associated with the use of vasopressor agents to maintain blood pressure parameters.[18]

The timing of surgical intervention has been debated, but recent studies have shown that these operations can be carried out early (less than 24 hours after injury) with excellent safety and a suggestion of improved outcome compared with delayed surgical intervention. The surgeries, whether involving anterior, posterior, or both approaches, often involve multiple levels. The choice of approach is dependent on multiple factors, including number of involved levels, spinal alignment, location of pathology, and surgeon's preference.[13,25,26]

# Contracture Prevention

## Key Concepts

- Early mechanical and manual prevention of contractures is generally recommended.
- The use of botulinum injection to prevent contractures is becoming more prevalent.

## Clinical Pearl

Prevention of extremity contractures should be an early priority after injury to prevent long-term sequelae.

A large amount of health care resources are used for the treatment and prevention of contractures in people with SCI. The most widely used interventions for this purpose are stretch and passive movements. There are various ways these interventions can be administered. For example, stretch can be applied using splints, positioning programs, or braces, and passive movements can be administered using mechanical devices or manually by therapists.[27,28]

The evidence to date indicates that intermittent stretch treatments applied for less than 3 months confer little or no added benefit over and above usual care in people with SCI. There is a small benefit from passive movements compared with usual care when applied for 6 months, but it is unclear whether this benefit is clinically worthwhile.[29] Botulinum toxin provides a window of opportunity to improve the outcomes from physical management of the focal and multifocal problems of spasticity.[30]

# Penetrating Spinal Cord Injury

## Key Concepts

- Penetrating spinal injuries from gunshot wounds (GSWs) have a different pathophysiology than blunt trauma due to concomitant blast effects in addition to mechanical trauma.
- Cauda equina–level injuries tend to have a better prognosis than cord-level injuries.
- Transabdominal trajectory injuries do not require extensive debridement or antibiotic coverage.

## Clinical Pearl

Spinal GSWs with civilian weapons are rarely unstable injuries and rarely require surgical stabilization.

Penetrating SCIs, specifically GSWs, are, unfortunately, common injuries at major urban trauma centers. They are considered separately because the pathophysiology is considerably different from blunt injuries. In addition to the direct penetrating effect of bullets and bullet fragments on neural tissue, there can be a considerable blast component that can cause substantial neural injury beyond the level of direct impact, similar to what happens with GSW to the brain. This in part explains the high incidence of complete injuries even when penetration of the canal is less significant and there are no retained bullet fragments in the canal. Evaluation with magnetic resonance imaging (MRI) can be limited by metallic artifact and is limited at many institutions because of the lack of confirmation of the bullet components. However, with most civilian ordnance, the bullet components are not paramagnetic and do not preclude MRI evaluation. In addition, civilian GSWs are rarely unstable and the need for surgical stabilization and/or external braces is less clearly defined. The role of surgical intervention for GSW to the spine is less clearly defined, especially in motor-complete injuries. In general, cauda equina-level injuries do better than cord-level injuries. In addition, retrieving bullet fragments from the canal confers an added risk of further neurological injury and has a high complication rate with regard to cerebrospinal fluid leak, because it is difficult to obtain a watertight closure in most cases.[30,31] These patients often have multiple GSWs and multiple injuries. This includes trajectories through the abdomen and chest with injuries to the gastrointestinal organs before entering the spinal canal. It has been shown that these patients do not need extended antibiotic courses or debridement because of the concern for increased infection risk.[32]

## Cervical Spine Clearance in the Comatose Patient

### Key Concepts

- Missing a significant injury with a normal high-quality spinal CT is unlikely.
- The role of flexion and extension films in spinal clearance, especially in the unexaminable patient, has come into question.
- MRI may overestimate soft tissue injury in patients with normal CT imaging and may actually prolong the amount of time the patient stays in a collar.

### Clinical Pearls

- In the short term it is safer to keep a patient in a collar who cannot be cleared clinically, especially if he or she has higher-priority injuries that need to be attended to, and also if there is a likelihood that he or she will be examinable in the near future.
- Be especially careful in older patients with significant degenerative disease because fractures can be subtle.

In polytrauma patients, the combination of head injury and potential cervical spine injury is a very common problem. Because of the potential for cervical spine injuries with

these complex traumas, the patients are routinely placed in cervical spine collars. Classically, C-spine clearance requires negative imaging studies and no clinically significant pain with palpation and range of motion in a cooperative patient. Obviously in the trauma patient with altered mental status clinical clearance is not an option. The major issue arises with a question of collar clearance and normal cervical spine CT imaging. Realistically, with modern CT imaging the likelihood of missing a significant injury with normal studies is extremely low.[33] However, if the patient has underlying degenerative changes, the sensitivity is reduced. Options at this point would be long-term collar utilization. However, this can be associated with skin breakdown and other issues.[34] Passive flexion and extension films in a patient with altered mental status who cannot give you feedback also continue to be controversial.[35,36] Others advocate MRI scans for clearance; however, it has been shown that in patients with normal C-spine CT scans, MRI may be overly sensitive and nonspecific. Nonspecific signal changes, especially in the paraspinous musculature without significant disruption of the posterior ligamentous complex or disc, do not necessarily imply instability; however, this interpretation requires significant clinical expertise.[37] Additionally, MRI scans can miss significant injuries, again especially in patients with significant degenerative or ankylosing changes. MRI scans also require transporting critically ill patients and are associated with significant cost.[38] Short-term utilization of collars for less than 2 weeks, especially in patients who will likely regain the ability to be cleared clinically within that period of time, is a safe and cost-effective management paradigm. In patients who are likely to be persistently vegetative or unexaminable for longer periods of time (longer than 2 weeks) with normal CT scans, clearance can be institution and clinician specific. Options again include MRI scans (taking into account the limitations of this study), or simply discontinuing the collar.

## Prognosis

### Key Concepts

- A detailed neurological examination, including rectal examination for sacral sparing, has important prognostic significance.
- Although ASIA grade improvement was demonstrated with early decompression of spinal injuries, the effect was much more robust in the incomplete injury patients.

### Clinical Pearls

- The worse the examination and the longer time from injury without improvement, the less likely the patient will make a meaningful recovery.
- Even in complete injuries, an argument can be made for early decompression and stabilization to maximize potential recovery.

Patients and families have questions about neurological recovery after SCI, specifically about regaining the ability to walk and have normal bowel, bladder, and sexual function. Detailed neurological examination at initial evaluation and again at 72 hours has been shown to be highly predictive of future recovery.[12,39] In general, the worse the ASIA grade, the less likely the patient will have significant recovery. In addition, complete thoracolumbar injuries have a much worse prognosis compared with cervical injuries because of the extreme forces needed to produce these injuries in the thoracolumbar spine. Patients are considered to have a complete lesion (AIS impairment A), according to the ASIA Impairment Scale (AIS), in the absence of sensory or motor function at the lowest sacral segments. Incomplete lesions are defined when sensation and/or motor function are preserved below the neurological level of injury, and in particular in the lowest sacral segments (anal sensation, including deep anal pressure and voluntary external anal sphincter contraction).[13]

Fehlings et al. showed that decompressive surgery prior to 24 hours after SCI was performed safely and was associated with improved neurological outcome defined as at least a two-grade AIS improvement at 6 months follow-up, especially in incomplete injuries. The severity of neurological injury, level of injury, and the presence of a zone of partial preservation were consistent predictors of neurological outcome.[13] The effect was much more robust in the incomplete injury group. Practically speaking in the patients who were initially ASIA A and underwent early surgery, 8 of 44 patients (18%) improved to the point where they could potentially ambulate (ASIA C, D). In the ASIA B group 23 of 31 (74%) were ASIA C or better. In the ASIA C group, 20 of 22 (91%) were ASIA D or E.

# Hypothermia

## Key Concept

Currently, there is no strong evidence to support the utilization of hypothermia in the acute management of SCI.

There continues to be interest in the application of hypothermia in the management of acute SCI. This is based on animal data as well as clinical reports of improved outcome in a small series. This includes the utilization of both systemic hypothermia and regional/local hypothermia at the time of surgical decompression.[40–42] The current guidelines from the American Association of Neurological Surgery/Congress of Neurological Surgery joint Section on Spine provide a grade C (level 4 evidence) for the use of modest systemic hypothermia for SCI.[43] The growing body of literature suggests that larger multicenter, randomized trials would be warranted to further address this potential therapy

## References

1. Anderson PA, Montesano PX. Morphology and treatment of occipital condyle fractures. *Spine.* 1988;13(7):731–736.
2. Theodore N, Aarabi B, Dhall SS, et al. Occipital condyle fractures. *Neurosurgery.* 2013;72:106–113.
3. Bellabarba C, Mirza SK, West GA, et al. Diagnosis and treatment of craniocervical dislocation in a series of 17 consecutive survivors during an 8 year period. *J Neurosurg Spine.* 2006;4:429–440.
4. Theodore N, Aarabi B, Dhall SS, et al. The diagnosis and management of traumatic atlanto-occipital dislocation injuries. *Neurosurgery.* 2013;72:114–126.
5. Kakarla UK, Chang SW, Theodore N, et al. Atlas fractures. *Neurosurgery.* 2010 March;66(3) Supplement:60–67.
6. Ryken TC, Aarabi B, Dhall SS, et al. Management of isolated fractures of the atlas in adults. *Neurosurgery.* 2013;72:127–131.
7. Gelb DE, Hadley MN, Aarabi B, et al. Treatment of subaxial cervical spinal injuries. *Neurosurgery.* 2013;72:187–194.
8. Vaccaro AR, Hulbert RJ, Patel AA, et al. Spine Trauma Study Group. The subaxial cervical spine injury classification system: a novel approach to recognize the importance of morphology, neurology, and integrity of the disco-ligamentous complex. *Spine.* 2007 Oct 1;32(21):2365–2374.
9. Vaccaro AR, Lehman Jr RA, Hurlbert RJ, et al. A new classification of thoracolumbar injuries: the importance of injury morphology, the integrity of the posterior ligamentous complex, and neurologic status. *Spine.* 2005 Oct 15;30(20):2325–2333.
10. American Spinal Injury Association. *International Standards for Neurological Classifications of Spinal Cord Injury (revised).* Chicago, IL: American Spinal Injury Association; 2000.
11. Scivoletto G, Tamburella F, Laurenza L, et al. Who is going to walk? A review of the factors influencing walking recovery after spinal cord injury. *Front Hum Neurosci.* 2014 March;8(141):1–11.
12. Fehlings MG, Vaccaro A, Wilson JR, et al. Early versus delayed decompression for traumatic cervical spinal cord injury: results of the Surgical Timing in Acute Spinal Cord Injury Study (STASCIS). *PLoS One.* 2012 Feb;7(2):1–8.
13. Bellabarba C, Fisher C, Chapman JR, et al. Does early fracture fixation of thoracolumbar spine fractures decrease morbidity or mortality? *Spine.* 2010 Apr 20;35(9 Suppl):S138–S145.
14. Gelb DE, Hadley MN, Aarabi B, et al. Initial closed reduction of cervical spinal fracture-dislocation injuries. *Neurosurgery.* 2013;72:73–83.
15. Ryken TC, Hurlbert RJ, Hadley M, et al. The acute cardiopulmonary management of patients with cervical spinal cord injuries. *Neurosurgery.* 2013;72:84–92.
16. Consortium for Spinal Cord Medicine. Early acute management in adults with spinal cord injury: a clinical practice guideline for health-care professionals. *J Spinal Cord Med.* 2008;31:403–479.
17. Inoue T, Manley GT, Patel N, et al. Medical and surgical management after spinal cord injury: vasopressor usage, early surgeries, and complication. *J Neurotrauma.* 2014 Feb 1;31:284–291.
18. Krassioukov A, Eng JJ, Warburton D, et al. A systematic review of the management of orthostatic hypotension following spinal cord injury. *Arch Phys Med Rehabil.* 2009 May;90(5):876–885.
19. Babu R, Owens TR, Thomas S, et al. Timing of tracheostomy after anterior cervical spine fixation. *J Trauma Acute Care Surg.* 2013 Apr;74(4):961–966.
20. Dhall SS, Hadley MN, Aarabi B, et al. Deep venous thrombosis and thromboembolism in patients with cervical spinal cord injuries. *Neurosurgery.* 2013;72:244–254.
21. Christie S, Thibault-Halman G, Casha S. Acute pharmacological dvt prophylaxis after spinal cord injury. *J Neurotrauma.* 2011 Aug;28:1509–1514.
22. Harrigan MR, Hadley MN, Dhall SS, et al. Management of vertebral artery injuries following non-penetrating cervical trauma. *Neurosurgery.* 2013;72:234–243.
23. Hurlbert RJ, Hadley MN, Walters B, et al. Pharmacological therapy for acute spinal cord injury. *Neurosurgery.* 2013;72:93–105.
24. Aarabi B, Hadley M, Dhall SS, et al. Management of acute traumatic central cord syndrome (ATCCS). *Neurosurgery.* 2013;72:195–204.
25. Fehlings MG, Smith JS, Kopjar B, et al. Perioperative and delayed complications associated with the surgical treatment of cervical spondylotic myelopathy based on 302 patients from the AOSpine North America Cervical Spondylotic Myelopathy Study. *J Neurosurg Spine.* 2012 May;16(5):425–432.
26. Craven C, Hitzif SL, Mittmann N. Impact of impairment and secondary health conditions on health preference among Canadians with chronic spinal cord injury. *J Spinal Cord Med.* 2012;35 (5):361–370.
27. Harvey LA, Glinsky JA, Katalinic OM, et al. Contracture management for people with spinal cord injuries. *Neurorehabilitation.* 2011;28:17–20.

28. Ward AB. Spasticity treatment with botulinum toxins. *J Neural Transm.* 2008;115(4):607–616.

29. Sidhu GS, Ghag A, Prokuski V, et al. Civilian gunshot injuries of the spinal cord: a systematic review of the current literature. *Clin Orthop Relat Res.* 2013 Dec;471(12):3945–3955. http://dx.doi.org/10.1007/s11999-013-2901-2.

30. Klimo Jr P, Ragel BT, Rosner M, Gluf W, McCafferty R. Can surgery improve neurological function in penetrating spinal injury? A review of the military and civilian literature and treatment recommendations for military neurosurgeons. *Neurosurg Focus.* 2010 May;28(5): E4, 1–11.

31. Pasupuleti LV, Sifri ZC, Mohr AM. Is extended antibiotic prophylaxis necessary after penetrating trauma to the thoracolumbar spine with concomitant intraperitoneal injuries? *Surg Infect (Larchmt).* 2014 Feb;15(1):8–13.

32. Chew BG, Swartz C, Quigley MR, et al. Cervical spine clearance in the traumatically injured patient: is multidetector CT scanning sufficient alone? Clinical article. *J Neurosurg Spine.* 2013 Nov;19(5):576–581.

33. Chan M, Al-Buali W, Stewart TC, et al. Cervical spine injuries and collar complications in severely injured paediatric trauma patients. *Spinal Cord.* 2013;51:360–364.

34. Theologis AA, Dionisio R, Mackersie R, et al. Cervical spine clearance protocols in level 1 trauma centers in the United States. *Spine.* 2014;39(5):356–61.

35. Tran B, Saxe JM, Ekeh AP. Are flexion extension films necessary for cervical spine clearance in patients with neck pain after negative cervical CT scan? *J Surg Res.* 2013;184:411–413.

36. Horn EM, Lekovic GP, Feliz-Erfan I, et al. Cervical magnetic resonance imaging abnormalities not predictive of cervical spine instability in traumatically injured patients. *J Neurosurg Spine.* 2004;1:39–42.

37. Halpern CH, Milby AH, Guo W, et al. Clearance of the cervical spine in clinically unevaluable trauma patients. *Spine.* 2010;35(18):1721–1728.

38. Wilson JR, Cadotte DW, Fehlings MG. Clinical predictors of neurological outcome, functional status, and survival after traumatic spinal cord injury: a systematic review. *J Neurosurg Spine (Suppl).* 2012;17:11–26.

39. Hansebout RR, Hansebout CR. Local cooling for traumatic spinal cord injury: outcomes in 20 patients and review of the literature. *J Neurosurg Spine.* 2014 May;20(5):550–561.

40. Dididze M, Green BA, Dalton Dietrich W, Vanni S, Wang MY, Levi AD. Systemic hypothermia in acute cervical spinal cord injury: a case-controlled study. *Spinal Cord.* 2013;51:395–400.

41. Levi AD, Green BA, Wang MY, et al. Clinical application of modest hypothermia after spinal cord injury. *J Neurotrauma.* 2009;26:407–415.

42. Ahmad FU, Wang MY, Levi AD. Hypothermia for acute spinal cord injury—a review. *World Neurosurg.* 2014 Jul–Aug;82(1-2):207–214.

# 31 *Anterior Cervical Spine Surgery Complications*

C. RORY GOODWIN, CHRISTINE BOONE, and DANIEL M. SCIUBBA

## Introduction

Anterior cervical operations are some of the most common spinal operations performed, with continually growing numbers as more spine surgeons gain experience with this approach. In general, anterior cervical operations (discectomy, fusion, corpectomy) have excellent outcomes with low overall morbidity and mortality. The most common neurosurgical indications for the treatment of spinal disorders include decompression of the spinal cord and/or neural elements, mechanical instability, deformity correction, neurosurgical debulking or excision of spinal tumors, and treatment of medically intractable pain. Although the region of the anterior cervical spine has a host of complex and critical structures in its vicinity, an understanding of the relevant anatomy can reduce morbidity and mortality and can predict common complications and/or patient complaints. This chapter will describe the relevant neuroanatomy of the anterior cervical spine and anterior neck and then detail the surgical approach to the anterior cervical spine and associated complications.

### NEUROANATOMY AND DETAILS OF THE ANTERIOR APPROACH

#### Key Concepts

- The structures of the neck are organized into the visceral, bilateral vascular, and vertebral compartments separated by layers of deep cervical fascia.
- The cervical spine consists of seven cervical vertebrae (C1–C7), in which a corresponding cervical nerve exits above the vertebrae, except C8, which exits below the C7 vertebral body. T1 is often considered part of the cervical spine because the T1 nerve root (exiting below the T1 pedicle) is important in hand function.

### Cervical Spine Neuroanatomy

The cervical spine consists of seven cervical vertebrae (C1–C7), in which a corresponding cervical nerve exits above the vertebrae. The eighth cervical nerve exits between C7 and the first thoracic vertebra. T1 is often considered part of the cervical spine because the T1 nerve root (exiting below the T1 pedicle) is important in hand function. Cervical vertebrae have small vertebral bodies, which attach bilaterally to superior and inferior articular processes via a pedicle. Each superior and inferior articulating facet forms a joint with the vertebrae above and below.

From the articulating processes, the laminae meet in the posterior midline to form spinous processes that are commonly bifid at C2. Anterolateral to the pedicles, the transverse foramen (foramina transversarium), located commonly from C6 to C2 bilaterally, contains the vertebral arteries, which branch off the subclavian arteries proximally on their way to the cranium distally. The vertebral arteries are most vulnerable laterally to the uncinate process, which can be palpated as a marker of laterality.[1] The anterior and posterior tubercles of the transverse processes serve as muscle attachment points. Cervical nerves exit the spinal canal through foramina formed by a groove between the transverse foramen and the superior articular process. The dorsal root ganglia are located in this space posterior to the vertebral arteries.

Intervertebral discs between the vertebral bodies consist of the nucleus pulposus surrounded by the annulus fibrosus. The intervertebral discs articulate with hyaline cartilage on the inferior and superior aspects of adjacent vertebral bodies. In surgery, the bony vertebral bodies and interceding symphyses form alternating "valleys" and "peaks" that can be palpated to identify spinal levels.

### Neck Anatomy

The structures of the neck are organized into compartments by layers of deep cervical fascia:

- Visceral compartment formed by the pretracheal fascial layer
- Bilateral vascular compartments formed by the carotid sheath fascial layer
- Vertebral compartment formed by the prevertebral fascial layer

Superficial cervical fascia contains the platysma, cutaneous blood vessels, and nerves. The platysma is a thin sheet of muscle originating in the thorax that attaches to the mandible. Deep to the superficial fascia is the deep investing layer, which encircles all structures of the neck.

The investing layer surrounds the sternocleidomastoids (SCMs) bilaterally, infrahyoid muscles anteriorly, and the bilateral trapezius muscles posteriorly. The infrahyoid muscles include the omohyoids, sternohyoids, thyrohyoids, and sternothyroids. The omohyoid muscle is a digastric muscle that passes across the sternohyoid muscle, common carotid artery, and internal jugular vein. The superior belly of the omohyoid muscle inserts into the hyoid bone superiorly and medially and ends in an intermediate tendon, just deep to the SCMs. From the intermediate tendon the inferior belly inserts into the scapula. The sternohyoid muscle is deep and medial to the omohyoid and just medial to the carotid sheath structures; it attaches to the hyoid and sternum. The thyrohyoid and sternothyroid muscles are the deepest of the infrahyoid muscles.

The other fascial layers create four compartments within the neck. The visceral compartment is in the midline and formed by the pretracheal layer of fascia surrounding the trachea, esophagus, right and left recurrent laryngeal nerves, and thyroid and parathyroid glands. Of note, the superior border of the thyroid cartilage, as well as the bifurcation of the common carotid artery into the internal and external carotid arteries, are commonly located between the C3 and C4 levels. The junctions of both the pharynx and the trachea and the larynx and esophagus occur between the C5 and C6 levels. The right and left recurrent laryngeal nerves arise as branches off the descending right and left vagus nerves, respectively, and climb back into the neck along a groove between the trachea and the esophagus to reach the larynx. The right recurrent laryngeal nerve loops under the right subclavian artery, whereas the left recurrent laryngeal nerve travels further down into the thorax to pass under the aortic arch.

The vascular compartment, which is lateral to the visceral compartment, contains the common carotid artery, internal carotid artery, internal jugular vein, and vagus nerve that are all circumscribed by the carotid sheath. The vagus nerve joins and courses along with the internal carotid artery and internal jugular vein as these vascular structures leave the skull. The external carotid artery gives off several branches, the most relevant of which is the superior thyroid artery that travels medially to the thyroid at the C3 level. The inferior thyroid arteries pass posteriorly to the common carotid arteries to the inferior aspect of the thyroid at the C7 level. The structures within the carotid sheath pass through the neck to the thoracic cavity, posterior and lateral to the medial edge of the SCM.

The vertebral compartment, enclosed by the prevertebral fascial layer, occupies the most posterior aspect of the anterior neck/cervical spine. This compartment contains the cervical spinal column and spinal cord. The prevertebral fascia attaches to the surfaces of the vertebral bodies from C1 to C7 and their corresponding transverse processes. The vertebral compartment also contains the cervical spinal nerves as they exit the spinal cord and the muscles that directly support the cervical spine, including the longus colli muscles, which extend between the anterior tubercles of the transverse processes, the anterior surfaces of the cervical vertebral bodies, and the anterior surfaces of the first three thoracic vertebral bodies.

Each of these fascial layers creates a potential space that can serve as a conduit for infection between the neck and thoracic cavity. The pretracheal space, within the pretracheal fascial layer anterior to the esophagus, is continuous with the anterior mediastinum. The retropharyngeal space lies between the fascia covering the posterior aspect of the pharynx and esophagus and the prevertebral fascia and continues from the skull base to the posterior mediastinum. Within the prevertebral fascia, there is a continuous space, known as the *danger space*, that travels from the skull base down to the diaphragm.

## Details of the Procedure

The patient is positioned supine on the operating table, with slight extension of the head. Extension increases access to more spinal levels; however, overextension increases tension on visceral structures. Some surgeons utilize cervical traction with weights to increase spinal-level access and to provide a few millimeters of distraction on the vertebral bodies to allow for improved graft placement when a discectomy and fusion are performed. When planning the location of the skin incision, lateral fluoroscopy may be used to estimate cervical level. Determining the side of approach remains controversial. Anatomy supports a left-sided approach to avoid damage to the shorter right recurrent laryngeal nerve. An association between a right-sided approach and greater risk of recurrent laryngeal nerve injury is inconsistently observed.[2-5] Surgeon preference, desired cosmesis, and number of spinal levels to be exposed dictate the incision type employed. A horizontal incision along a natural crease at the level of disease generally provides good cosmesis and adequate exposure for the majority of spinal pathologies. Some surgeons prefer an incision along the medial border of the SCM, especially in cases of multilevel disease where exposure of the rostral and caudal elements is paramount.

In the superficial cervical fascia, the platysma is identified and incised along the same direction as the skin incision. The platysma is then dissected off the investing fascia below. Along the entire medial border of the SCM, the investing layer is broached, and blunt dissection proceeds downward in the plane between the carotid sheath, located laterally, and the pretracheal fascia, medially, to the anterior surface of the cervical spine (Fig. 31.1). At this point, blunt retractors are inserted between the longus colli muscles and the surface of the vertebral bodies, posterior to the esophagus. The prevertebral fascia may be opened and used to lift the longus colli muscles off the vertebral bodies to

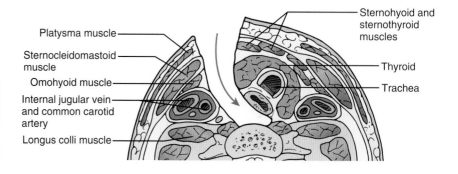

**Fig. 31.1** Schematic representation of anterior approach to cervical spine and structures involved. (Adapted from Wolfla CE and Resnick DK, eds. Neurosurgical Operative Atlas, 2nd ed.: *Spine and Peripheral Nerves.* New York: Thieme; 2007.)

Platysma muscle

Sternocleidomastoid muscle

Omohyoid muscle

Internal jugular vein and common carotid artery

Longus colli muscle

Sternohyoid and sternothyroid muscles

Thyroid

Trachea

insert self-retracting retractors under the muscles. Placing the retractors on the surface of the vertebral bodies reduces risk of recurrent laryngeal nerve injury from placing retractors between the esophagus and trachea. The structures in the visceral compartment, sternohyoid, sternothyroid, and thyrohyoid muscles, medial to the dissection plane, will be retracted medially to the contralateral side of the incision. The lateral structures, SCM, omohyoid muscle, and vascular compartment will be retracted laterally. Blunt or sharp dissection can be used to increase the exposure of the anterior spine. At the C3 and C7 levels, the superior thyroid artery and the inferior thyroid artery may be encountered, respectively, putting them at risk of injury. The superior belly of the omohyoid muscle may be encountered when extending the exposure above the C5 level, but this muscle can be dissected and retracted. Once the appropriate spinal levels are exposed, craniocaudal retractors may be added. Fluoroscopy is employed to confirm that the correct levels have been exposed.

The surgeon is then able to tackle the primary indication for surgery. In cases of diffuse idiopathic skeletal hyperostosis causing dysphagia, drilling the anterior osteophytes can be performed. For cervical neck pain, weakness, or myelopathy, an anterior cervical discectomy and fusion may be performed. For infection, tumors, trauma, or even multilevel spondylosis, a full corpectomy may be indicated. The anterior cervical approach provides adequate exposure to perform a wide array of surgeries utilizing this traditional approach.

## PERIOPERATIVE CONSIDERATIONS

### Key Concepts

- Fiberoptic bronchoscope (FOB)–guided endotracheal intubation (awake or asleep at the discretion of the operative team), direct laryngoscopy with manual in-line stabilization (MILS), or video laryngoscopic intubation should be considered for airway management in patients undergoing cervical spine surgery with a history of symptomatic cervical myelopathy from stenosis, cervical immobility, or concerns for spinal instability.
- Review of preoperative imaging is crucial to determine abnormal anatomy and reduce the risks of surgery.
- The use of cervical collars postoperatively to limit cervical range of motion and promote bone healing is surgeon-dependent; however, it can be associated with skin breakdown, swallowing difficulty, and airway impairment.

### Clinical Pearls

- In patients with previous anterior spinal surgery, the decision to approach from the opposite side warrants preoperative ENT evaluation to rule out silent recurrent laryngeal nerve (RLN) injury because the potential for bilateral injury is devastating.
- Patients with the potential for airway compromise should be kept intubated in the perioperative period until the critical care and neurosurgical staff feel it is safe to extubate. It is often prudent to have anesthesia and/or ENT present for patients with difficult airways.

## Preoperative Considerations

Airway management is another important concern in patients undergoing cervical spine surgery. The goal of this is to reduce manipulation and displacement of the cervical spine. FOB-guided endotracheal intubation, direct laryngoscopy with MILS, and nasal intubation are three commonly used methods.[9] The recent availability of video laryngoscopes may change the approach to airway management in some of these patients. FOB intubation, performed in the awake or anesthetized patient, allows visualization of vocal cords for intubation without excessively manipulating the neck. MILS involves applying countertraction to stabilize the head in place during laryngoscopy and intubation.[10] Nasal intubation, which can be performed blind or with bronchoscopy, involves passing the endotracheal tube through the nares. The patient must be able to take spontaneous breaths, or it is assisted by FOB.

Some measures taken prior to surgery may improve outcomes postoperatively. Postoperative dysphagia can be reduced with tracheal/esophageal traction exercises (TTEs) in the preoperative period. The exercise, performed by medical staff, is thought to increase the compliance of the trachea and esophagus when the thyroid cartilage is pushed back and forth horizontally across the midline twice a day for 3 days before surgery. The exercise is not performed the day before. Increasing the compliance of these structures may decrease pressure on the esophagus from the retractors.[6,7] Although the benefits of the TTE on vocal cord palsy (VCP) have yet to be studied, decreasing the pressure on the wall of the esophagus from retractors and the endotracheal tube (ETT) cuff could reduce likelihood of stretching or pinching the recurrent laryngeal nerves.[8]

### Intraoperative Considerations

Steps to reduce postoperative dysphagia and/or VCP may be taken during the procedure as well. There is moderate evidence to support monitoring and adjusting ETT cuff pressure to reduce the risk of VCP.[11] Maintaining ETT cuff pressure at $\leq 20$ mm Hg during retraction may have mild benefit, but strong evidence is lacking.[12] Once the primary exposure is performed, certain authors have advocated for deflation and reinflation of the cuff after retraction to minimize the pressure on the visceral structures.[13] Another measure to address postoperative VCP and dysphagia is administration of methylprednisolone, which has not been shown to have any significant effect on patients' symptoms of these conditions.[11,12]

Careful analysis of the preoperative imaging should be performed to determine whether the patient has abnormal anatomy that could introduce increased risk to the surgery (Fig. 31.2). For instance, an aberrant, more medially placed vertebral artery that may or may not follow the normal path through the foramina transversarium could result in unforeseen complications during exposure or the surgical procedure itself. In general, vertebral artery injuries may be avoided by observing lateral markers, such as the uncinate process between levels C3 and C6. Drilling should remain in the midline, removing lateral bone or disc should be conservative, and, in the presence of tumor or infection, lateral bone should be inspected for softening.[1] Esophageal perforation is very rare. It may be caused by injury with a

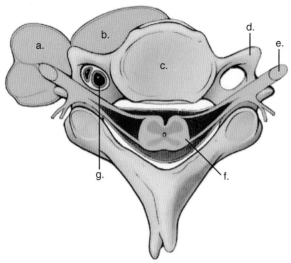

**Fig. 31.2** Anatomical relationships of the cervical spine. Cross-sectional representation of the cervical spine at C5. The anterior scalenus muscle *(a.)*, the longus colli muscle *(b.)*, the vertebral body *(c.)*, and the transverse foramina *(d.)* are noted. The cervical nerve root *(e.)* and the spinal cord *(f.)* are seen relative to the anterior vertebral body *(c.)* and musculature *(a., b.)*. The vertebral artery *(g.)* is noted within the transverse foramina. The vertebral body enters the sixth cervical foramina and extends to the right of C1 posteriorly to become the basilar artery. Injury to the vertebral artery may occur when releasing or dissecting the longus colli muscles. It may also be injured in discectomies that involve dissection in the lateral aspect of the disc near the uncovertebral joint (not shown). (Reprinted from Herkowitz et al. *Rothman-Simeone, The Spine*, 6th ed. Philadelphia, PA: Saunders-Elsevier; 2011: 1728–1776.)

retractor, ETT, fractured bone, overstretching the esophagus, or during the surgical exposure. The earlier this is diagnosed, the better the outcome.[14]

### Clinical Pearl

▪ Injuries to vascular, visceral, and neural tissues can be avoided by developing natural planes of dissection and avoiding the use of excessive sharp dissection or electrocautery. The use of guarded electrocautery tips is advised because unrecognized thermal injury may present in a delayed fashion.

### Postoperative Considerations

Postoperatively, depending on the procedure performed, patients are kept overnight for observation. In cases with expected major anterior swelling and potential for airway compromise, patients can be kept intubated until this period passes. Although the surgical procedure commonly provides stabilization of the spine, in emergency situations when airway management takes priority, manipulation and displacement of the cervical spine, if reintubation is required, could potentially undo some of the work performed during surgery.

Patients may experience temporary esophageal pain or dysphagia immediately after the procedure due to physical manipulation of these structures, but this usually resolves within a week and is minor. Patients can resume their

normal activity upon discharge from the hospital; however, full precautions are not lifted until the first follow-up visit. Routine postoperative radiograph after cervical spine fusion procedures may not be necessary in patients with unremarkable history and postoperative examination.[15] Some surgeons contend that patients wear a cervical collar for the 2 to 3 months after the procedure; however, this is dictated by surgeon preference. Fifty-five percent of patients with single-level anterior cervical discectomy and fusion and 76% of patients with multilevel utilize cervical collars postoperatively.[16] Concerns regarding limiting cervical range of motion with a rigid collar impairing balance, and other negative effects on skin, swallowing, and airway function, have raised questions regarding the necessity of postoperative collars.[17]

## COMPLICATIONS

### Key Concepts

• The most common anterior cervical spine complications are postoperative hematoma, dysphagia, and symptomatic recurrent laryngeal nerve palsy.
• Transient dysphagia occurs secondary to the retraction on the esophagus and trachea and the endotracheal intubation and typically resolves weeks after surgery.
• Rarer complications must be treated on a case-by case basis, beginning with radiographic imaging, depending on the disease process.

The majority of complications can be avoided with adequate analysis of the preoperative imaging and using meticulous and safe technique in the surgical procedure. Common risk factors for increased rate of complications include multilevel surgery because of the extensive dissection and retraction necessary to achieve adequate exposure, revision surgery, aberrant anatomy, excessive coagulation, and/or retraction. The most common complications of an anterior cervical approach include postoperative hematoma, dysphagia, symptomatic recurrent laryngeal nerve palsy, esophageal perforation, Horner syndrome, wound infection, transient dysphagia, vascular injuries, and cerebrospinal fluid (CSF) leaks.

Potential complications can occur, especially in larger exposures or exposures that may require sharp dissection. In cases where there has been previous surgery in this area, scarring may necessitate sharp dissection, increasing the risk of injury. Among the most common complications is VCP caused by recurrent laryngeal nerve injury, which comprises ~17% of all neurological injuries.[18] The incidence in the immediate postoperative period ranges between 2.3% and 24.2%.[4,11,19] VCP is caused by injury to the recurrent laryngeal nerves from pinching or overstretching the nerve, pressure from an ETT cuff, or division of the nerve. Adjustment of the ETT cuff could reduce VCP incidence by 4.8%. There is good evidence for previous surgery in the anterior neck as a risk factor for VCP.[11] Injury to the recurrent laryngeal nerve increases the risk of aspiration and hoarseness of the voice. Referral to an ear/nose/throat (ENT) surgeon for assessment and evaluation of vocal cord function is advised.

Postoperative airway compromise has been reported as high as 6.1% in anterior cervical spine surgery patients.[20] Larger exposures for multilevel disease and longer cases should make the care team especially attentive and cautious about airway issues. In the immediate postoperative period, airway issues are often caused by hematoma[21]; in the first few days after, pharyngeal swelling is a more likely cause.[20] This complication can also be a result of displacement of implants, angioedema, and pseudomeningocele caused by CSF leak. Quickly identifying and closely monitoring airway obstruction are critical to resolving this complication. If there are signs of impending airway compromise (expanding neck mass, tracheal deviation, impaired breathing, stridor, hypoxemia, etc.), then emergent reexploration of the wound should be performed to evacuate the mass and obtain hemostasis. The decision to extubate a patient postoperatively, whether at the end of the case or in a delayed fashion, should be made as a joint discussion between the surgical team, anesthesia, and the critical care team. A clear plan including timing, extubation parameters, and the need for anesthesia or ENT to be present at extubation should be clearly defined and documented. If the patient is classified as a difficult airway, this should also be clearly documented. In general the decision to extubate should be biased toward a more cautious approach, especially after long and complex cases and especially at night or other times when there are fewer critical team members available.[22] One common parameter taken into account when deciding about extubation is a cuff leak with the endotracheal tube. Although the lack of a cuff leak generally would argue against extubation at the time, the presence of an air leak alone does not always indicate that it is safe to extubate.[23,24]

Transient dysphagia is another frequent complication of anterior cervical spine surgery that commonly occurs because of the combination of the retraction on the esophagus and trachea and the endotracheal intubation. Reports estimate that this occurs in roughly 8% of patients[25]; however, some studies demonstrate ranges from 1.7% to 71%.[6,26] The incidence drops the most after 2 months out from surgery.[27] Dysphagia can be caused by recurrent laryngeal nerve injury, esophageal injury, swelling, or scarring. Female patients and elderly patients are more likely to develop dysphagia soon after surgery. High ETT cuff pressure may be related to dysphagia as well.[7,26] Some contend that the incidence of transient dysphagia has risen with the application of anterior cervical plates.

Anterior spinal procedures are often performed for cervical radiculopathy and myelopathy. It is imperative that the team taking care of the patient postoperatively is familiar with the patient's preoperative neurological examination. This background information is required to evaluate for new neurological deficits postoperatively. Neurological deficits can arise from direct injury to the spinal cord and nerve roots intraoperatively, compression from bone grafts or instrumentation, or from hematoma, especially if the posterior longitudinal ligament is removed during the procedure, allowing a connection with the epidural space. If a new deficit is detected, generally imaging with plain x-rays and/or computed tomography (CT) scan is undertaken to rule out a structural problem such as a malpositioned graft or screw. If this is not revealing, a magnetic resonance image (MRI) may be better suited to evaluate for spinal cord compression, hematoma, or other soft tissue abnormalities. If the deficit is progressive, especially if associated with airway issues, immediate reexploration should be considered.[18,28]

Vascular injuries are the most severe complications of the anterior cervical approach, but are also rare. Most vascular injuries can be avoided using blunt dissection. Although uncommon, injury to the carotid artery and/or jugular vein can occur with excessive sharp dissection and/or use of sharp-edged retractors. Similarly, the superior and inferior thyroid arteries, which commonly cross at C3 and C7, respectively, can be injured during the anterior cervical exposure. The incidence of vertebral artery injury is estimated to be 0.3% to 0.5%.[1,9,10] The vertebral arteries are most exposed lateral to the midline between C3 and C7.[1] If a vertebral artery injury is experienced intraoperatively, the incision should be packed to tamponade the bleeding vessel and a cerebral angiogram should be obtained to determine whether there is good collateral flow from the alternative side.[29,30] Depending on the extent of the injury, various modalities can be employed through open or neurointerventional means (Fig. 31.3).

Injuries to the esophagus are rare, but can be life threatening. Given the continuation of the fascial compartments with the mediastinum, esophageal and hypopharynx perforation can lead to potentially lethal infections that may spread via the fascial compartments or spaces.[11] Infections can cause mediastinitis and/or vertebral osteomyelitis secondary to colonization with gut flora. It presents as neck and throat pain, pain and difficulty with swallowing, hoarseness, and aspiration. Esophageal perforation occurs in 0.25% of patients.[14,28,31,32] There are reported cases of

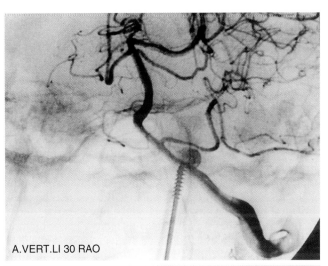

A.VERT.LI 30 RAO

**Fig. 31.3** Angiogram demonstrating a pseudoaneurysm of the left vertebral artery adjacent to the tip of a malpositioned long C2 threaded screw placed for fracture. (Reprinted from Herkowitz et al. *Rothman-Simeone, The Spine*, 6th ed. Philadelphia, PA: Saunders-Elsevier; 2011: 1728–1776.)

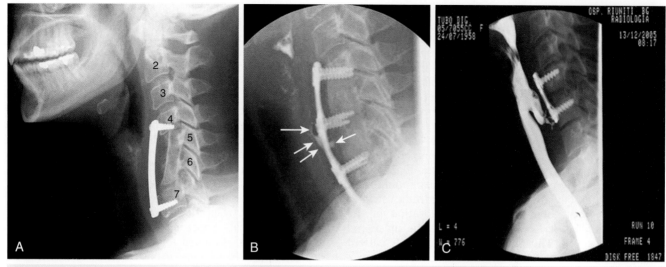

**Fig. 31.4 (A)** Lateral cervical radiograph showing graft dislodgement and subsidence. **(B)** Lateral radiograph demonstrating air (*large arrow*) and dye extravasation (*small arrows*) during Gastrografin swallowing study. **(C)** Barium swallow study showing a pharyngoesophageal diverticulum, which developed after cervical spine surgery. **(A, B** Reprinted from Patel NP et al. Esophageal injury associated with anterior cervical spine surgery. *Surg Neurol.* 2008;69(1): 20–4. **C** Reprinted from Bonavina L. Re: Esophageal injury associated with anteriorcervical spine surgery; 2009;71(6):727–8.)

plate or screw erosion of the esophagus in the literature; however, this is uncommon. If an esophageal perforation is suspected, a swallowing study or upper endoscopy should be obtained to determine the severity of the injury (Fig. 31.4). These patients will likely require broad-spectrum antibiotics to prevent mediastinitis from presumed infection with gut flora and potentially a percutaneous endoscopic gastrostomy tube placement while the perforation heals.

CSF leak is a rare complication that is estimated to occur in 0.2% to 1.0% of cases, although the exact incidence is unknown[22,33,34] (Fig. 31.5). In cases of ossification of the posterior longitudinal ligament, the incidence of CSF leak is greater (4.3%–32%) when an anterior cervical approach is attempted. The majority of dural breaches are seen intraoperatively; however, given the limited view, smaller dural lacerations may not be recognized. In these cases, patients may present postoperatively with neck masses, leakage from the wound, meningitis, dysphagia, or orthopnea. CSF leaks recognized intraoperatively are usually repaired at that time using a combination of treatment strategies, including suture, dural substitutes, and dural sealant; however, the proximity to the spinal cord and limited working corridor make anterior cervical spine durotomies more difficult to repair primarily. After attempted primary repair, there are several different management options that can be employed to reduce the pressure on the repaired dural breach and allow the area to scar in, thus preventing any further morbidity. These include keeping the head of the bed above 30 degrees for a specified number of days postoperatively and/or insertion of a lumbar drain with continuous drainage over a 2- to 3-day period. In refractory cases, a ventriculoperitoneal shunt may be warranted. Regardless of the management algorithm employed, the patient should receive close follow-up to detect any potential return of symptoms.

## Clinical Pearls

- Patients with suspected RLN injury should be kept on nothing by mouth status and have early ENT evaluation because they have aspiration risk. Injection of the affected vocal fold by ENT improves voice quality and may reduce aspiration risk.
- Infections with anterior approaches to the cervical spine are so much less common than posterior approaches that the presence of infection should raise concern for esophageal injury.
- In rare circumstances, for patients who demonstrate recurrent CSF leaks despite primary repair, lumbar drainage, or other measures, a head CT should be obtained to determine whether there is hydrocephalus.

Bicortical screws can iatrogenically injury the spinal cord or result in a durotomy, but these complications are rare, given the widespread use of lateral fluoroscopy and the preference of surgeons to use screws that do not breach the posterior cortex. The graft height can also lead to axial neck pain via increased lordosis, apposition of the facet joints, or narrowing of the neural foramen causing nerve root compression. If the screw backs out it, could potentially perforate the esophagus.

## Conclusion

Anterior cervical procedures are common spinal operations that, in general, have excellent outcomes with low overall morbidity and mortality. The most common complications of an anterior cervical approach include postoperative hematoma, dysphagia, symptomatic recurrent laryngeal

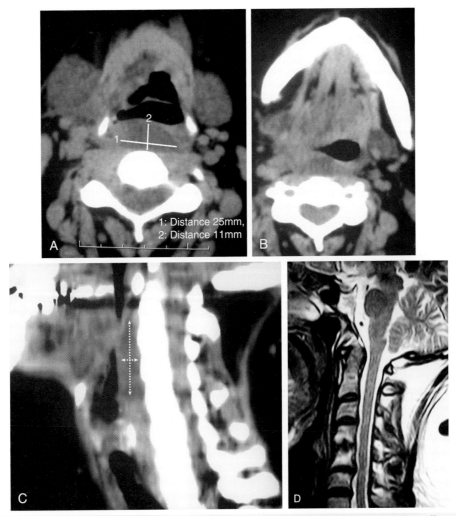

**Fig. 31.5** Postoperative CT scan of the neck demonstrating a low-density retropharyngeal CSF mass **(A)**; exerting mass effect on the right side of the posterior wall of the pharynx **(B)**; and extending in front of C3, C4, and C5 vertebral bodies. Sagittal reconstruction **(C)**. Three months' follow-up of sagittal T2-weighted image MRIs, showing the complete collapse of the collection **(D)**. (Reprinted from Spennato P et al. Retropharyngeal cerebrospinal fluid collection as a cause of postoperative dysphagia after anterior cervical discectomy. *Surg Neurol.* 2007;67(5):499–503.)

nerve palsy, esophageal perforation, Horner syndrome, wound infection, transient dysphagia, vascular injuries, and CSF leaks. However, an understanding of the relevant anatomy, avoidance of excessive dissection or coagulation, and knowledge of potential complications that can be encountered can help to reduce the risks to each individual patient.

## References

1. Russo VM, Graziano F, Peris-Celda M, Russo A, Ulm AJ. The V 2segment of the vertebral artery: anatomical considerations and surgical implications. *J Neurosurg Spine.* 2011 Dec;15(6):610–619.
2. Beutler WJ, Sweeney CA, Connolly PJ. Recurrent laryngeal nerve injury with anterior cervical spine surgery. *Spine.* 2001 Jun;26 (12):1337–1342.
3. Kilburg C, Sullivan HG, Mathiason MA. Effect of approach side during anterior cervical discectomy and fusion on the incidence of recurrent laryngeal nerve injury. *J Neurosurg Spine.* 2007;4 (4):273–277.
4. Jung A, Schramm J, Lehnerdt K, Herberhold C. Recurrent laryngeal nerve palsy during anterior cervical spine surgery: a prospective study. *J Neurosurg Spine J Neurosurg Publishing Group.* 2005;2 (2):123–127.
5. Jung A, Schramm J. How to reduce recurrent laryngeal nerve palsy in anterior cervical spine surgery. *Neurosurgery.* 2010 Jul;67(1):10–15.
6. Chen Z, Wei X, Li F, et al. Tracheal traction exercise reduces the occurrence of postoperative dysphagia after anterior cervical spine surgery. *Spine.* 2012 Jul;37(15):1292–1296.
7. Joaquim AF, Murar J, Savage JW, Patel AA. Dysphagia after anterior cervical spine surgery: a systematic review of potential preventative measures. *Spine J.* 2014 Sep 1;14(9):2246–2260.
8. Mehra S, Heineman TE, Cammisa FP, Girardi FP, Sama AA, Kutler DI. Factors predictive of voice and swallowing outcomes after anterior approaches to the cervical spine. *Otolaryngol Head Neck Surg.* 2014 Feb;150(2):259–265.
9. Manninen PH, Jose GB, Lukitto K, Venkatraghavan L, Beheiry El H. Management of the airway in patients undergoing cervical spine surgery. *J Neurosurg Anesthesiol.* 2007 Jul 1;19(3):190–194.
10. Aziz M. Use of video-assisted intubation devices in the management of patients with trauma. *Anesthesiol Clin.* 2013 Mar 1;31(1):157–166.
11. Tan TP, Govindarajulu AP, Massicotte EM, Venkatraghavan L. Vocal cord palsy after anterior cervical spine surgery: a qualitative systematic review. *Spine J.* 2014 Jul 1;14(7):1332–1342.
12. Riley III LH, Vaccaro AR, Dettori JR, Hashimoto R. Postoperative dysphagia in anterior cervical spine surgery. *Spine.* 2010;35(Supplement):S76–S85.
13. Audu P, Artz G, Scheid S, et al. Recurrent laryngeal nerve palsy after anterior cervical spine surgery. *Anesthesiology.* 2006 Nov;105 (5):898–901.
14. van Berge Henegouwen DP, Roukema JA, de Nie JC. vander Werken C. Esophageal perforation during surgery on the cervical spine. *Neurosurgery.* 1991 Nov;29(5):766–768.

15. Grimm BD, Leas DP, Glaser JA. The utility of routine postoperative radiographs after cervical spine fusion. *Spine J.* 2013 Jul;13 (7):764–769.

16. Bible JE, Biswas D, Whang PG, Simpson AK, Rechtine GR, Grauer JN. Postoperative bracing after spine surgery for degenerative conditions: a questionnaire study. *Spine J.* 2009 Apr;9(4):309–316.

17. Abbott A, Halvorsen M, Dedering A. Is there a need for cervical collar usage post anterior cervical decompression and fusion using interbody cages? A randomized controlled pilot trial. *Physiother Theory Pract.* 2013 May 1;29(4):290–300.

18. Flynn TB. Neurologic complications of anterior cervical interbody fusion. *Spine.* 1982 Nov;7(6):536–539.

19. Zeidman SM, Ducker TB, Raycroft J. Trends and complications in cervical spine surgery. *J Spinal Disord.* 1997 Dec;10(6):523–526.

20. Sagi HC, Beutler W, Carroll E, Connolly PJ. Airway complications associated with surgery on the anterior cervical spine. *Spine.* 2002 May;27(9):949–953.

21. Sethi R, Tandon MS, Ganjoo P. Neck hematoma causing acute airway and hemodynamic compromise after anterior cervical spine surgery. *J Neurosurg Anesthesiol.* 2008 Jan;20(1):69–70.

22. Kwon B, Yoo JU, Furey CG, Rowbottom J, Emery SE. Risk factors for delayed extubation after single-stage, multi-level anterior cervical decompression and posterior fusion. *J Spinal Disord Tech.* 2006 Aug;19(6):389–393.

23. Patel AB, Ani C. Feeney Colin, Cuff leak test and laryngeal survey for predicting post-extubation stridor. *Indian J Anaesth.* 2015 Feb;59 (2):96–102.

24. Zhou T, Zhang HP, Chen WW, Xiong ZY, Wang L, Wang G. Cuff-leak test for predicting postextubation airway complications: a systematic review. *J Evid Based Med.* 2011 Nov;4(4):242–254.

25. Morio Y, Teshima R, Nagashima H, Nawata K, Yamasaki D, Nanjo Y. Correlation between operative outcomes of cervical compression myelopathy and MRI of the spinal cord. *Spine.* 2001 Jun 1;26 (11):1238–1245.

26. Zeng J-H, Zhong Z-M, Chen J-T. Early dysphagia complicating anterior cervical spine surgery: incidence and risk factors. *Arch Orthop Trauma Surg.* 2013 May 21;133(8):1067–1071.

27. Bazaz R, Lee MJ, Yoo JU. Incidence of dysphagia after anterior cervical spine surgery. *Spine.* 2002 Nov;27(22):2453–2458.

28. Seex KA. An anterior cervical retractor utilizing a novel principle. *J Neurosurg Spine.* 2010 Apr 20;12(5):547–551.

29. Park H-K, Jho H-D. The management of vertebral artery injury in anterior cervical spine operation: a systematic review of published cases. *Eur Spine J.* 2012 Jul 12;21(12):2475–2485.

30. Burke JP, Gerszten PC, Welch WC. Iatrogenic vertebral artery injury during anterior cervical spine surgery. *Spine J.* 2005 Sep;5 (5):508–514.

31. Zhong Z-M, Jiang J-M, Qu D-B, et al. Esophageal perforation related to anterior cervical spinal surgery. *J Clin Neurosci.* 2013 Oct;20 (10):1402–1405.

32. Gaudinez RF, English GM, Gebhard JS, Brugman JL, Donaldson DH, Brown CW. Esophageal perforations after anterior cervical surgery. *J Spinal Disord.* 2000 Feb;13(1):77–84.

33. Wang MC, Chan L, Maiman DJ, Kreuter W, Deyo RA. Complications and mortality associated with cervical spine surgery for degenerative disease in the United States. *Spine.* 2007;32 (3):342–347.

34. Syre P, Bohman L-E, Baltuch G, Le Roux P, Welch WC. Cerebrospinal fluid leaks and their management after anterior cervical discectomy and fusion. *Spine.* 2014 Jul;39(16):E936–E943.

# 32 *Posterior Approaches to the Spine*

CRAIG KILBURG, JAMES M. SCHUSTER, SAFDAR ANSARI, and ANDREW DAILEY

## Introduction

Posterior approaches to the spine can be used to treat a wide variety of pathologies, including degenerative conditions, infection, traumatic injuries, vascular lesions, congenital disorders, and neoplasias. Operative planning for these operations involves general surgical details applicable to all posterior approaches, as well as regional considerations specific to the location within the spinal axis where surgery is performed. The goal of this chapter is to highlight how these general principles, such as patient positioning and anesthesia, and regional considerations can help to focus postoperative care and identify potential postoperative complications.

## Neuroanatomy

The skeletal, neurostructural, and vascular anatomy of the spine varies substantially from the occipitocervical junction to the sacrum. There are also substantial regional differences within the cervical spine, which has led to a subclassification of this region into axial (occiput to C2) and subaxial (C3–C7) components. Furthermore, some also consider the cervicothoracic junction (C7–T1) to be a separate entity based on biomechanics and regional anatomy.

The overall alignment of the cervical spine is normally lordotic, and its vertebral segments are relatively more mobile compared with other regions within the spine. This is especially true at the specialized joints from the occiput to C2 where a substantial portion of head rotation and flexion/extension occur. As a result, surgical stabilization across these levels can be quite disabling to patients. The cervical spine is also unique in that the vertebral arteries run along the majority of its length. The arteries generally enter the transverse foramen at C6 (92%)[1,2] and then travel through the foramen transversaria at each level until C1, where they course medially across the top of the C1 ring before going intradurally.

The thoracic spine is normally kyphotic and is incorporated within the bony rib cage, making it relatively stiffer than the remainder of the spine. The region of the thoracic spine also plays a relatively important role in the vascular supply of the spinal cord. The anterior spinal artery originates from the union of an intracranial branch off each vertebral artery and is primarily fed from several segmental vessels throughout the thoracic spine, the most prominent of which is the artery of Adamkiewicz, which is generally found at the thoracolumbar junction.[3,4] Sacrificing this

vessel through a posterior approach could result in an anterior spinal cord infarct. In addition, the midthoracic spine can be a vascular watershed area, and it is susceptible to ischemia. Therefore with more extensive posterior approaches (e.g., lateral extracavitary approaches), care is taken to avoid taking multiple segmental vessels on one side or bilateral segmental vessels.

The spinal cord in an adult generally ends at approximately the T12 to L1 level, and below this are the nerves of the cauda equina, which are generally more tolerant to manipulation than the spinal cord. Advanced degenerative changes in the normally lordotic lumbar spine can lead to loss of alignment and resultant scoliosis. This is treated with deformity correction, which represents some of the most complex spinal procedures with a significant potential for perioperative complications, especially in the older population.[5–9]

## Regional Considerations

### CERVICAL SPINE

#### Key Concepts

- The posterior cervical approach is versatile and allows access for various spinal indications, but it is associated with a higher rate of postoperative hematoma, infection, and postoperative pain than anterior approaches.
- Identification of the correct operative level is imperative and is accomplished using known anatomical landmarks and intraoperative fluoroscopy.
- The vertebral arteries and, to a lesser extent, the internal carotid arteries are at risk for injury during posterior cervical spine surgery, especially during hardware placement.

#### Clinical Pearls

- C5 palsy can occur in a delayed fashion after cervical laminectomy.
- Minimizing lateral dissection and ensuring correct screw trajectory helps to reduce vertebral artery injuries.
- In postoperative patients, increasing neck pain and associated evolving neurological symptoms in the extremities should be considered to indicate a postoperative hematoma until proven otherwise.

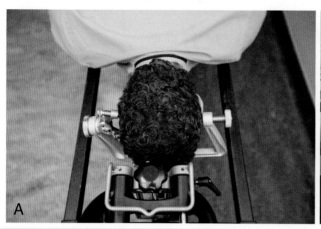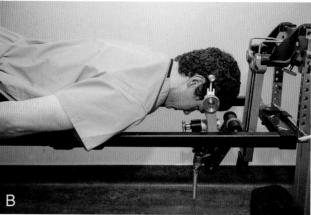

**Fig. 32.1** Anteroposterior and lateral view of Mayfield head holder connected to the Jackson table via the cervical management system. The Mayfield head holder consists of a three-point system pinned to the skull and then attached to the Jackson table via the cervical management system or a standard operating table. It provides rigid immobility at the craniocervical junction for surgeries in this region and prevents pressure on the face and orbits, helping to reduce the incidence of ischemic optic neuropathy. (Courtesy of Mizuho OSI, Union City, CA, USA, http://www.mizuhosi.com/)

Posterior cervical spine surgery allows for the management of pathologies extending from the craniocervical junction through the inferior cervical spine; however, it does have a relatively high rate of postoperative pain, which is related to the extensive paraspinal muscle retraction performed during surgery; infection, especially in obese patients; and hematoma.[10–12] Patients are most commonly positioned prone with the head fixed firmly in a Mayfield head holder (Fig. 32.1). Often, a large incision, extending from the inion (external occipital protuberance), or slightly above, to the C7 spinous process, is used, although more focal surgeries allow a smaller, more localized incision. Midline placement of the incision allows dissection to occur in the relatively avascular midline raphe of the nuchal ligament, significantly reducing blood loss by avoiding dissection through the paraspinal muscles. Dissection is universally carried down to the known landmarks of the spinous processes of the cervical vertebrae before proceeding laterally along the lamina to the lateral masses.

In procedures involving the occipitocervical junction, such as occiput to C2 posterior spinal fusions, C1 to C2 posterior spinal fusions, or Chiari decompressions, exposure of the caudal portion of the cranium, as well as the posterior aspect of the ring of the C1 vertebra and spinous process and bilateral lamina of C2, is required. Care must be taken not to extend the exposure too far laterally to avoid injury to the vertebral arteries (Box 32.1). Injury rates to the vertebral arteries during C1 to C2 posterior spinal fusions as high as 4% have been reported.[13,14] Preoperative planning using a computed tomography angiogram or magnetic resonance imaging (MRI) of the neck can be used to determine the distance from midline at which dissection may be safe; however, a safe benchmark is that the vertebral arteries lie approximately 1.5 cm from midline.[2,15,16] The large venous plexuses that surround the vertebral arteries can also produce rapid, significant bleeding if they are violated.[2] The internal carotid arteries lie in close proximity to the anterior surface of C1 and rarely may be injured during posterior spinal fusions involving screw placement within this vertebra (Box 32.1).[17,18]

---

**Box 32.1   Cervical Spine Complications**

**Regional Complications: Cervical Spine**
Injury to the vertebral or internal carotid arteries
Delayed C5 palsy
Paresthesias/numbness in the dermatomes of the greater occipital nerves

---

The C2 nerve roots, which originate from the second spinal nerve, may be sacrificed or injured during instrumentation placement at C1 to C2. As a result, patients may experience paresthesias or complete sensory loss in the dermatomal distribution of the greater occipital nerves postoperatively.[19] Because there is a relative lack of bony protection in this location, careful dissection is also required around and between the occiput and the C1 vertebra to avoid violation of the dura and cerebrospinal fluid leak or injury to the underlying spinal cord (Box 32.2).

Surgery within the mid- and lower cervical spine also begins via a midline incision and then proceeds with unilateral dissection of the spinous process, lamina, and facet joints in cervical laminoforaminotomies and bilateral dissection in laminectomies, laminoplasties, and posterior cervical fusions. Correct localization of the spinal level to be operated on is imperative in the mid- and lower cervical spine and is frequently achieved with the use of

---

**Box 32.2   Complications Common to All Regions**

**General Complications**
**Deep venous thrombosis/pulmonary embolus**
Injury to spinal cord/nerve roots
Postoperative hematoma
Ischemic optic neuropathy
Cerebrospinal leak
Compression neuropathies/skin necrosis from inadequate padding

intraoperative fluoroscopy prior to the incision and during the procedure prior to any bony decompression.

The extensive lateral dissection needed for exposure of the facet joints may irritate the dorsal rami of the cervical nerve roots, producing minor posterior paresthesias and sensory loss in the associated dermatomes postoperatively.[19] Another well-documented complication of decompressive surgeries involving the midcervical spine is palsy of the C5 nerve root (Box 32.1).[20] The nerve dysfunction will often develop in a delayed fashion and then gradually resolve over a period of time. The deficit is primarily motor and involves the deltoid, but it can also involve the bicep to a variable extent. It can be relatively disabling and concerning to the patient and should be specifically discussed with the patient prior to surgery, because there is a wide range of reported rates of occurrence with a mean incidence of 7.8% in posterior cervical surgeries involving the C4 to C5 level.[20]

Intradural procedures in the cervical spine are most commonly done through a posterior approach. Indications include intramedullary tumors (e.g., astrocytomas, ependymomas), extramedullary tumors (e.g., schwannomas, meningiomas, neurofibromas), and Chiari malformations. To gain access to the spinal canal, the lamina are either removed through laminectomy or replaced at the end of the procedure as a laminoplasty. The dura must also be opened and is then sutured closed at the end of the operation, with or without the application of a dural sealant. Intramedullary tumors require dissection into the spinal cord. This is most often performed in the midline between the posterior columns, and, as a result, patients will often have at least transient dysfunction of the posterior columns postoperatively.

Injury to the vertebral arteries during surgical exposure is rare within the mid- and lower cervical spine because they remain encased within the transverse foramen throughout their course over these levels; however, injury can occur to the arteries and the cervical nerve roots during screw placement for posterior cervical fusions, with rates in the literature reported between 0.1% and 0.5%.[21,22] Care is taken to place lateral mass screws and transpedicular screws with the correct starting trajectory, and these procedures are commonly performed with intraoperative fluoroscopy or with intraoperative computer-assisted navigation to help prevent these injuries or injuries to the dura with resultant cerebrospinal fluid leaks.

If vertebral artery injury occurs on one side, placement of screws on the contralateral side is usually aborted to prevent possible bilateral vertebral artery injury.[15] In addition, if injury to the vertebral artery occurs during screw placement, the screw is often left in place to provide a tamponade effect on the artery, preventing further hemorrhage.[15,16,22] After surgery, the patient is taken for angiography, and the artery may be occluded to prevent embolization from an intimal tear, provided there is adequate flow into the posterior circulation from the contralateral vertebral artery.

Postoperatively, patients should have serial complete neurological examinations, including examinations of the upper and lower extremities, to evaluate for new or worsening neurological deficits. Patients who have had posterior cervical spine surgery should also undergo thorough cranial nerve and cerebellar examinations to evaluate

for possible vertebral artery dissections or occlusions. Although injuries to the vertebral arteries are often quite obvious during surgery, occult injuries can occur.[15] Rapidly increasing neck pain with new neurological deficits should immediately raise the concern for an epidural hematoma, and these patients should undergo emergent magnetic resonance imaging, or immediate return to the operating room if the MRI will be delayed and/or the patient has rapid clinical deterioration.

## THORACIC SPINE

### Key Concepts

- Many pathological conditions traditionally approached through the chest can be approached through extended posterior approaches.
- Extended posterior procedures can result in pulmonary and great vessel injury.
- The thoracic spine is a vascular watershed territory, and the sacrifice of multiple unilateral or bilateral segmental vessels should be avoided to prevent spinal cord ischemia/infarct.
- The sacrifice of thoracic nerve roots is generally well tolerated with the exception of the C8 and T1 nerve roots as a result of their contribution to the brachial plexus.

### Clinical Pearls

- Correct identification of the surgical level is much more difficult in the thoracic spine and may require preoperative placement of a radiopaque marker by interventional radiology.
- Obtaining a chest x-ray 12 to 24 hours after surgery can help to identify occult pneumothoraces not seen on immediate postoperative x-rays.

There are four main posterior approaches to pathologies within the thoracic spine: thoracic laminectomy, the transpedicular approach, costotransversectomy, and the lateral extracavitary approach. The purpose of the lateral extracavitary approach or a costotransversectomy is to allow exposure of the lateral elements of the spine, as well as the anterior vertebral body, providing an alternative surgical route for lesions that previously required an anterior approach through the chest. Localization of the correct operative level is difficult within the thoracic spine; it is often necessary to use intraoperative fluoroscopy for localization as in the cervical spine or preoperative radiopaque markers placed within a pedicle of the operative level by interventional radiology.[23]

The exposures typically begin with a midline or slightly paramedian incision with dissection extended down through the midline raphe, similar to dissection in the cervical spine. The dissection is not as avascular as in the cervical spine because the nuchal ligament does not extend into the thoracic spine, but dissection in the midline affords the least amount of blood loss by minimizing dissection through muscle.

The extent of exposure varies depending on the approach. During a thoracic laminectomy, the spinous processes, lamina, and facet joints are exposed. In a transpedicular approach, these elements along with the transverse process are dissected out, and during a costotransversectomy or lateral extracavitary approach, the dissection is extended out along the rib head, with the most dissection along the rib head occurring during the lateral extracavitary approach. Upon completion of rib head disarticulation and excision, the vertebral body can be resected to the extent needed given the specific operative pathology. Disarticulation of the rib head from the vertebral body and resection of the vertebral body itself destabilize the spine, and patients undergoing these procedures often require spinal fusion with posterior pedicle screw fixation over multiple levels and anterior cage/strut placement to replace the resected vertebral body.

During the spinal canal decompression, it is important to avoid injury to the spinal cord and violation of the dura causing cerebrospinal fluid leaks (Box 32.2). Pedicle screw fixation should also be executed with care to maintain the correct trajectory to avoid injury to the spinal cord, dura, and thoracic nerve roots. As with procedures in the cervical spine, these operations are usually performed with intraoperative fluoroscopy or, less commonly, stereotactic navigation to ensure safe screw placement.

Costotransversectomies and lateral extracavitary approaches can put vascular structures, such as the aorta, at risk (Box 32.3).[24–26] The thoracic region contains vascular watershed areas, and sacrificing multiple segmental arteries on one side or bilaterally should be avoided to prevent possible spinal cord ischemia (Box 32.3).[4] Near the thoracolumbar junction, it is important to identify and avoid if possible the artery of Adamkiewicz, the major arterial supply to the anterior spinal artery.[3,4] If a large segmental artery is encountered, an aneurysm clip can be placed across the vessel temporarily and motor evoked potentials monitored before sacrificing the vessel. If the vessel cannot be safely sacrificed or monitoring is not available, approach from the other side should be considered.[3]

These approaches also risk injury to pulmonary structures (Box 32.3). Care must be taken when resecting the rib heads at any of the thoracic levels to avoid violating the parietal pleura and creating a pneumothorax, which would necessitate placement of a chest tube.[24–26] This is a rare complication, as long as the underlying lung is not injured. All patients undergoing a costotransversectomy or a lateral extracavitary approach should have both an immediate postoperative chest x-ray and, if a chest tube was placed during surgery, serial daily chest x-rays to evaluate for pneumothorax.

The thoracic nerve roots and their ventral rami are often encountered in these approaches during the lateral

exposure. Sacrifice of one or more thoracic nerves at T2 or below is generally well tolerated and allows greater exposure of the rib head and vertebral body without significant neurological deficit[25]; however, the C8 and T1 nerve roots contribute to the brachial plexus and should be spared because their resection will have a significant effect on intrinsic motor function of the ipsilateral hand. Patients undergoing posterior approaches to the thoracic spine that involve these levels should have a detailed neurological examination with special focus on hand intrinsic function to evaluate for new or worsening neurological deficits.

## LUMBAR SPINE AND SACRUM

### Key Concepts

- Large multilevel deformity corrections have significant potential morbidity, including substantial blood loss with coagulopathy and need for resuscitation.
- Patients can have transient new or worsening of symptoms and deficits postoperatively as a result of traction on the lumbar nerve roots during surgery.
- Retroperitoneal structures, including the aorta, vena cava, common iliac arteries and veins, descending colon, and ureters, are at risk for injury.
- Ileus is a common postoperative complication, and an aggressive bowel regimen should be started early in the postoperative period.

### Clinical Pearls

- Cerebrospinal fluid leak is one of the most common complications of lumbar surgical procedures.
- Worsening back and lower extremity pain with new or worsening neurological deficits should be considered to indicate a postoperative hematoma until proven otherwise.

Surgical approaches within the lumbar spine and sacrum begin most often with a midline or slightly paramedian incision similar to those in the cervical and thoracic spine. The correct operative level is intraoperatively localized using known anatomical landmarks (such as the iliac crests to identify the L4–5 interspace), preoperative imaging, and intraoperative fluoroscopy prior to the incision and also prior to any bony decompression.

During a lumbar laminectomy, bilateral laminectomies allow for complete exposure of the dorsolateral spinal canal. The canal is then decompressed via resection of the hypertrophied ligamentum flavum and the bony overgrowth of facet hypertrophy. A microdiscectomy is usually performed unilaterally using a partial laminectomy to allow exposure of the lateral thecal sac and nerve root. Gentle traction is often placed on the nerve root to allow complete exposure and removal of the disc herniation. This may result in transient worsening of preoperative symptoms or neurological deficits or entirely new, transient deficits in the postoperative period. The dura surrounding the nerve

### Box 32.3  Thoracic Spine Complications

**Regional Complications: Thoracic Spine**
Pneumothorax/lung injury
Injury to the great vessels
Spinal cord ischemia/infarct

root is often thinned from chronic compression by the disk, so traction on the nerve root can lead to microtears in the friable dura with subsequent cerebrospinal fluid leaks.

Posterior spinal fusion in the lumbar spine is accomplished using posterolateral fusion (bone placed on and between the lateral bony structures), posterior lumbar interbody fusions (PLIFs), and transforaminal lumbar interbody fusions (TLIFs). Transpedicular fusions are usually not used in isolation in the lumbar spine but are often combined with PLIFs or TLIFs, which were developed to provide a method of fusion across the disc space without requiring an anterior approach. Bilateral laminectomies and medial facetectomies are performed during a PLIF, whereas TLIFs utilize a unilateral approach. The intervertebral disc is then excised, and a graft—either bone or a synthetic cage—is placed to promote interbody fusion. Grafts are placed bilaterally in a PLIF and unilaterally during a TLIF. Placement of the graft requires retraction of the thecal sac and nerve roots, with more retraction required during a PLIF than a TLIF, creating the potential for new or transient worsening of symptoms or deficits postoperatively. These approaches are most commonly augmented with pedicle screw fixation.

Lateral extracavitary approaches can also be performed in the lumbar spine. They proceed as in the thoracic spine, but there are no rib heads that need to be disarticulated. Access to the lateral elements of the spinal canal and vertebral body is instead achieved by dissection of the psoas major muscle off the anterior surface of the transverse process and the lateral surface of the vertebral body. Extreme care must be taken to avoid injury to the exiting lumbar nerve roots during this portion of the dissection.[26]

Large deformity operations frequently involve the posterior lumbar spine and often consist of multilevel fusions extending from the thoracic spine to the pelvis. These procedures require long incisions with extensive dissections, increasing blood loss.[5-9] Patients may require blood product transfusions, including not only packed red blood cells but platelets and fresh frozen plasma as well.[5-9] Transfusion needs are not limited to the operating room, and patients should be monitored closely postoperatively for anemia or coagulopathy. Deformity operations also have a high rate of overall perioperative morbidity, especially in elderly patients.[5-9]

Bony dissection and decompression around the spinal canal and lumbar nerve roots in all lumbar spine operations must be performed with care to avoid injury to these structures and to prevent violations of the dura (Box 32.2). In chronic degenerative disease cases, the hypertrophied ligamentum flavum can be rather calcified and adherent to the dura, and slow, careful dissection is needed to separate it off and excise it without causing a cerebrospinal fluid leak. Placement of hardware, including interbody grafts and transpedicular screws, is also a source of injury to these structures. Therefore direct visualization or fluoroscopic or stereotactic guidance is often used during hardware placement in the lumbar spine, as in the other regions of the spine.

Retroperitoneal structures such as the aorta, vena cava, common iliac arteries and veins, descending colon, and ureters are also at risk for injury during the ventral dissection of the lateral extracavitary approach and during removal of the intervertebral disc in microdiscectomies

---

**Box 32.4  Lumbar Spine and Sacrum Complications**

**Regional Complications: Lumbar Spine and Sacrum**
Vascular injury
Bowel/urological injury
Ileus/Ogilvie syndrome

---

and interbody fusions (Box 32.4). Injuries can be avoided in the lateral extracavitary approach by maintaining constant contact with the bony elements of the vertebral column. During disc space preparation, injury to retroperitoneal structures can be avoided by limiting to 2.5 to 3 cm the depth to which instruments enter the disc space.[27]

Injury to the vascular structures only produces obvious back bleeding at the time of surgery in approximately 50% of cases.[27] Other indications of these injuries can be acute or progressive hypotension or bruising of the flanks (Grey Turner's sign) indicating retroperitoneal hemorrhage. Patients with abdominal pain or decreased urine output postoperatively may have an injury to the ureter, and a patient with a tense, painful abdomen and signs of systemic infection may have an intestinal injury. Progressive back pain with new or worsening neurological deficits should raise the concern for an epidural hematoma. All of these cases should be emergently evaluated with radiological imaging or return to the operating room if clinically indicated.

Postoperative constipation is another common complication encountered by patients after lumbar spine surgery, and an aggressive bowel regimen, including stool softeners and laxatives, should be started early in the postoperative period.[28] The cause is thought to be ileus related to the effect of increased narcotic usage and immobility. Rarely patients can develop acute colonic pseudoobstruction, or Ogilvie syndrome, which is an adynamic ileus that results in severe colonic dilatation and possible rupture (Box 32.4).[28,29] Ogilvie syndrome can often be treated conservatively but may require treatment with neostigmine or colonoscopic decompression.[29]

## General Perioperative and Postoperative Considerations

### Key Concepts

- Maintenance of adequate perfusion pressure is critical in patients with myelopathy or spinal cord injury at any level within the spine.
- Correct patient positioning and padding are important to prevent ocular injury, compression neuropathies, and pressure sores, and patients should be examined for these conditions postoperatively.
- Deep vein thrombosis prevention begins in the operating room with the application of sequential compression devices and compression stockings and should be continued in the postoperative period with the addition of chemoprophylaxis within 12 to 24 hours of surgery.

- Cerebrospinal fluid leaks are common after posterior spine surgery, and treatment may require specific positioning parameters or further procedures, including lumbar drain placement or reoperation.
- Posterior spine operations are often associated with significant blood loss requiring extensive resuscitation both intraoperatively and postoperatively and close monitoring of hemodynamic parameters and laboratory values postoperatively.

## Clinical Pearls

- Antispasmodics are often required in addition to narcotic pain medication for adequate pain control.
- Patients undergoing long and potentially bloody prone spine procedures should be counseled about ischemic optic neuropathy.
- The use of total intravenous anesthesia for monitoring purposes during long operations may delay the patient's emergence from anesthesia and impede the postoperative neurological examination for extended periods after surgery.

## Perioperative Considerations

Perioperative considerations play a prominent role in posterior spine surgery, and they begin with patient positioning. Patients are significantly more susceptible to pressure-related injuries in the operating room than they are in other settings within the hospital because general anesthesia prevents them from protecting themselves. This vulnerability is magnified when patients are positioned prone, as they must be for posterior approaches to the spine, because the prone position is not as natural a position for the human body as the supine position.

It is imperative that pressure points are properly padded (Box 32.2). Particular attention needs to be paid to the axilla to prevent brachial plexus injuries, and all patients undergoing a posterior spinal approach should have a thorough brachial plexus examination postoperatively to ensure there is no evidence of injury.[30] Appropriate padding and positioning of the breasts and nipples in females and the genitalia in males are important to prevent necrosis during extended surgeries. The anterior superior iliac spines and knees should also be carefully padded to prevent skin breakdown (Fig. 32.2), and judicious padding of the elbows and posterior popliteal fossa will prevent ulnar and peroneal nerve compression neuropathies, respectively.[30] Finally, it is imperative that there is no pressure on the eyes, and this should be reevaluated throughout the course of a prone surgical case (Figs. 32.3 and 32.4).[30]

Ischemic optic neuropathy is a rare but devastating complication of prone spine surgery (Box 32.2). It was once thought to be caused by direct pressure to the globes, but it continued to occur even when patients were positioned in Mayfield head holders to ensure there was no pressure on the globes (Fig 32.1). Ischemic optic neuropathy was seen most often in multilevel instrumented cases of the thoracic and lumbar spine that took more than 6 hours and

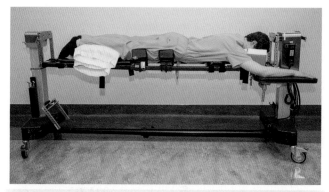

**Fig. 32.2** Jackson table with the foam pillow. The open midline design of this operative table places the lumbar spine in a lordotic position, which is ideal for fusion operations. The design also reduces abdominal compression, helping to improve cardiac function and ventilation and decrease blood loss. (Courtesy of Mizuho OSI, Union City, CA, USA, http://www.mizuhosi.com/)

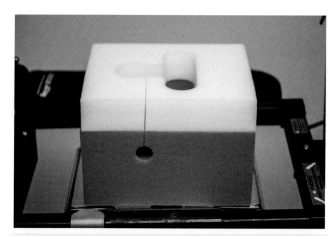

**Fig. 32.3** Foam pillow. Head holder used in short- to medium-length thoracic and lumbar operations. Soft padding helps to reduce pressure on the face and orbits (Courtesy of Mizuho OSI, Union City, CA, USA, http://www.mizuhosi.com/)

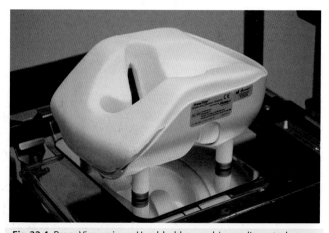

**Fig 32.4** ProneView mirror. Head holder used in medium- to longer-length thoracic and lumbar operations. Foam padding helps to reduce pressure on the face and orbits. The floor of the holder is a mirror that allows the anesthesia team to monitor the airway and check for sites of increased pressure. (Courtesy of Mizuho OSI, Union City, CA, USA, http://www.mizuhosi.com/)

involved an estimated blood loss of 1 liter or more.[30–33] The data regarding the exact cause of ischemic optic neuropathy are unclear, but there is some thought now that it may be related to venous hypertension.[3–33]

The need for precautions to prevent deep venous thrombosis during surgery is also important. Unfortunately, it is often not safe to use prophylactic dosing of heparin or enoxaparin during surgery, especially during operations involving the central nervous system.[34] Instead, deep venous thrombosis prevention relies on the use of compression stockings and sequential compression devices, which are essential during surgery.[35–37] Any significant, acute changes to the patient's hemodynamic status during the operation or in the postoperative period may suggest a pulmonary embolism, and further evaluation should be undertaken.

Neuromonitoring is an important tool to ensure patient safety during posterior approaches to the spine.[38–40] In situations where the spine is unstable, monitoring is initiated while the patient is in the supine position prior to transferring to the prone position so that baseline motor evoked potentials and somatosensory evoked potentials can be obtained. Testing is then repeated shortly after repositioning and periodically throughout the procedure. If there are changes in the signal, the operation is paused, and an informed decision is made regarding the current status of the operation and whether to continue with the procedure or alter technique.[38–40] The use of neuromonitoring and specifically motor evoked potentials generally does not allow the use of volatile anesthetic agents because these agents interfere with the neuromonitoring signals.[38–40] Intravenous anesthetic agents must be used instead, which usually results in prolonged recovery and reemergence from anesthesia, especially with longer cases, which delays reliable neurological evaluation postoperatively.

The prone position creates a unique set of anesthetic considerations as well, with the most important considerations related to cardiac function and ventilation. The prone position, especially on the Wilson frame or gel rolls (Fig. 32.5), which restrict space along the midline, increases intraabdominal and intrathoracic pressures, consequently increasing peak and plateau ventilation pressures, decreasing tidal volumes, and increasing ventilation/perfusion mismatch, making it challenging to adequately ventilate patients.[41,42] These positioning devices also decrease venous return and therefore stroke volume and cardiac output, potentially necessitating increased volume and vasopressor support[43] The cardiopulmonary problems associated with the prone position are magnified in patients who are overweight or obese, who suffer from obesity-hypoventilation syndrome at baseline, who are pregnant, or who have preexisting cardiopulmonary conditions. Occasionally, patients will require paralytic agents to allow adequate ventilation; however, this comes at the cost of not being able to monitor motor evoked potentials during surgery, increasing the risk of inadvertent injury to the nervous system. The use of the Jackson table, with its open midline design that allows the patient's abdomen to hang free, reduces, but does not eliminate, these problems (Fig 32.2)[41–43]

Prone positioning also hinders cardiopulmonary resuscitation efforts in the event they are necessary.[44] Patients are in a suboptimal position to allow the emergent placement of additional peripheral access and are in a position that completely prohibits the safe placement of central venous access. Anterior cardiac compressions are impossible in the prone position, and compressions must be performed posteriorly.[44] Adequate airway management is also severely hindered.[44] As a result, these patients may present to an intensive care unit in an emergent fashion critically underresuscitated or in the process of resuscitation and without adequate venous access. Proper preoperative setup by the anesthesia team can prevent many of these problems.

Patients with compressive myelopathy and traumatic spinal cord injury are at risk for secondary cord injury from inadequate spinal cord perfusion secondary to hypotension.[45,46] This is especially true of elderly patients. Systemic hypotension with systolic blood pressures less than 90 mm Hg should be avoided, and mean arterial pressures should be kept greater than 85 mm Hg.[45,46] This often requires patients to be given intravenous vasopressor therapy, necessitating intensive cardiopulmonary monitoring in an intensive care unit setting.[45,46] Notably, if low blood pressure produces cord ischemia, consequent cord dysfunction can itself further contribute to hypotension as a positive feedback cycle.

## Postoperative Considerations/Complications

The extensive muscular dissection associated with posterior approaches to the spinal column creates a significant burden of pain postoperatively. Patients not only suffer from incision pain, but they also endure a large component of muscle spasm and nearly universally require the addition of antispasmodic medications to their pain control regimens. The judicious use of heat and/or ice therapy is also helpful for control of muscle spasm, as is a program of early neck mobilization for patients undergoing cervical spine procedures and overall mobilization with physical therapy and occupational therapy for all patients. Continuous local or regional anesthesia systems that are placed within the paraspinal musculature at the time of surgery to provide local anesthetic over a set number of days have recently been added to the pain control armamentarium.[47] Patients undergoing spine surgery often have a history of chronic

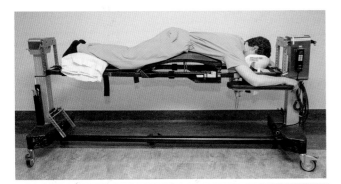

**Fig 32.5** Wilson frame with the ProneView mirror. The arched design of this frame helps to widen the intervertebral spaces of the lumbar spine for decompression operations and microdiscectomies. The frame can be placed on the Jackson table or any standard operative table. (Courtesy of Mizuho OSI, Union City, CA, USA, http://www.mizuhosi.com/)

pain and preoperative, long-term, high-dose narcotic pain medication usage that can make pain control in the postoperative setting difficult and predispose them to withdrawal syndromes if narcotic pain medications are tapered postoperatively[48] or problems with overdose if pain medication is ramped up too aggressively. The use of patient-controlled analgesic systems or the early involvement of acute pain services is often required to achieve adequate pain control. A multimodal approach may be needed.

Patients should be monitored closely in the postoperative period for worsening neurological deficits (Box 32.2). Accurate monitoring requires a thorough knowledge of the patient's presenting symptoms and neurological examination findings. Clues to potential new or worsened deficits are often provided by changes that were observed with the neuromonitoring intraoperatively, but spontaneous deficits can also occur. Deficits and pain that progressively worsen in the postoperative period may be indications of conditions requiring further surgical intervention, such as abdominal injury or developing epidural hematomas (Box 32.2).

The measures to prevent deep venous thrombosis that were initiated in the operating room should be continued in the postoperative period. Patients who undergo extensive spine procedures are often slow to mobilize, which creates a greater risk of venous stasis and deep venous thrombosis formation (Box 32.2). All patients should be fitted with compression stockings and/or sequential compression devices in the postoperative period.[35–37] In addition, chemoprophylaxis with subcutaneous heparin or enoxaparin should be initiated 12 to 24 hours after surgery.[35–37] A program of early mobilization with physical therapy and occupational therapy should also be instituted.

Postoperatively, aggressive and early respiratory therapy, including incentive spirometry or ventilator-assisted recruitment maneuvers, is important for the prevention of atelectasis and pulmonary complications. Patients undergoing lengthy prone procedures can develop facial and laryngeal edema, which may delay safe extubation, hinder postoperative swallowing or reintubation efforts, and increase the risk of delayed extubation failure.

Posterior spine surgeries can involve significant blood loss related to the extensive subcutaneous tissue and muscular dissection necessary for adequate surgical exposure. The extensive epidural venous plexus throughout the spinal axis can also produce rapid and considerable blood loss over a short period of time. Patients are also at risk for postoperative hemorrhages and should be monitored closely for flank hematomas or ecchymoses, which may be indicative of significant subcutaneous or retroperitoneal hemorrhage. Tachycardia in the postoperative period should not be reflexively attributed to pain; instead, it should prompt an evaluation for a possible source of hemorrhage because it may be a sign of early hypovolemic shock.

Patients undergoing posterior approaches to the spine often require extensive resuscitation with crystalloids and occasionally colloids. This can have a significant impact on the hemodynamic functioning of patients with cardiopulmonary comorbidities, and careful observation of these patients postoperatively is necessary to prevent hypervolemic or underresuscitated states. Hemoglobin and hematocrit levels should be monitored daily for several days postoperatively and blood product transfusions judiciously provided to prevent significant acute blood loss anemia. Patients undergoing significant resuscitation should also be monitored closely for the possible development of transfusion-related lung injury.[49]

Cerebrospinal fluid leaks are possible during all of the posterior approaches to the spine (Box 32.2). Leaks are often apparent at the time of surgery and an attempt made to primarily repair the tear in the dura.[50] Occasionally, if the injury to the dura is extensive and an adequate primary repair cannot be accomplished, cerebrospinal fluid diversion techniques, including lumbar drain placement, may be used and continued for several days postoperatively.[50] In addition, specific patient-positioning parameters may be instituted, such as strict maintenance of the head of the bed at 30 to 45 degrees for cerebrospinal fluid leaks within the cervical spine, or flat for leaks within the lumbar spine.[50]

## References

1. Eskander MS, Drew JM, Aubin ME, et al. Vertebral artery anatomy: a review of two hundred fifty magnetic resonance imaging scans. *Spine*. 2010;35(23):2035–2040.
2. Heary RF, Albert TJ, Ludwig SC, et al. Surgical anatomy of the vertebral arteries. *Spine*. 1996;21(18):2074–2080. [Comparative Study].
3. Charles YP, Barbe B, Beaujeux R, Boujan F, Steib JP. Relevance of the anatomical location of the Adamkiewicz artery in spine surgery. *Surg Radiol Anat*. 2011;33(1):3–9.
4. Murakami H, Kawahara N, Tomita K, Demura S, Kato S, Yoshioka K. Does interruption of the artery of Adamkiewicz during total en bloc spondylectomy affect neurologic function? *Spine*. 2010;35(22): E1187–E1192. [Case Reports Research Support, Non-U.S. Gov't].
5. Bridwell KH, Lewis SJ, Edwards C. Complications and outcomes of pedicle subtraction osteotomies for fixed sagittal imbalance. *Spine*. 2003;28(18):2093–2101. [Evaluation Studies Research Support, Non-U.S. Gov't].
6. Cassinelli EH, Eubanks J, Vogt M, Furey C, Yoo J, Bohlman HH. Risk factors for the development of perioperative complications in elderly patients undergoing lumbar decompression and arthrodesis for spinal stenosis: an analysis of 166 patients. *Spine*. 2007;32(2):230–235.
7. Cho KJ, Suk SI, Park SR, et al. Complications in posterior fusion and instrumentation for degenerative lumbar scoliosis. *Spine*. 2007;32 (20):2232–2237. [Multicenter Study].
8. Daubs MD, Lenke LG, Cheh G, Stobbs G, Bridwell KH. Adult spinal deformity surgery: complications and outcomes in patients over age 60. *Spine*. 2007;32(20):2238–2244. [Evaluation Studies].
9. Deyo RA, Cherkin DC, Loeser JD, Bigos SJ, Ciol MA. Morbidity and mortality in association with operations on the lumbar spine. The influence of age, diagnosis, and procedure. *J Bone Joint Surg Am*. 1992;74(4):536–543. [Research Support, U.S. Gov't, Non-P.H.S. Research Support, U.S. Gov't, P.H.S.].
10. Goldstein CL, Bains I, Hurlbert RJ. Symptomatic spinal epidural hematoma after posterior cervical surgery: incidence and risk factors. *Spine J*. 2015 Jun 1;15(6):1179–1187.
11. Lubelski D, Healy AT, Silverstein MP, et al. Reoperation rates after anterior cervical discectomy and fusion versus posterior cervical foraminotomy: a propensity matched analysis. *Spine J*. 2015 Jun 1;15 (6):1277–1283.
12. Pahys JM, Pahys JR, Cho SK, et al. Methods to decrease postoperative infections following posterior cervical spine surgery. *J Bone Joint Surg Am*. 2013;95(6):549–554. [Evaluation Studies].
13. Neo M, Fujibayashi S, Miyata M, Takemoto M, Nakamura T. Vertebral artery injury during cervical spine surgery: a survey of more than 5600 operations. *Spine*. 2008;33(7):779–785. [Multicenter Study].
14. Wright NM, Lauryssen C. Vertebral artery injury in C1-2 transarticular screw fixation: results of a survey of the AANS/CNS section on disorders of the spine and peripheral nerves. American Association of Neurological Surgeons/Congress of Neurological Surgeons. *J Neurosurg [Review]*. 1998;88(4):634–640.
15. Gluf WM, Schmidt MH, Apfelbaum RI. Atlantoaxial transarticular screw fixation: a review of surgical indications, fusion rate,

complications, and lessons learned in 191 adult patients. *J Neurosurg Spine*. 2005;2(2):155–163.

16. Peng CW, Chou BT, Bendo JA, Spivak JM. Vertebral artery injury in cervical spine surgery: anatomical considerations, management, and preventive measures. *Spine*. 2009;9(1):70–76. [Review].

17. Currier BL, Maus TP, Eck JC, Larson DR, Yaszemski MJ. Relationship of the internal carotid artery to the anterior aspect of the C1 vertebra: implications for C1-C2 transarticular and C1 lateral mass fixation. *Spine*. 2008;33(6):635–639. [Comparative Study].

18. Hoh DJ, Maya M, Jung A, Ponrartana S, Lauryssen CL. Anatomical relationship of the internal carotid artery to C-1: clinical implications for screw fixation of the atlas. *J Neurosurg Spine*. 2008;8(4):335–340.

19. Yeom JS, Buchowski JM, Kim HJ, Chang BS, Lee CK, Riew KD. Postoperative occipital neuralgia with and without C2 nerve root transection during atlantoaxial screw fixation: a post-hoc comparative outcome study of prospectively collected data. *Spine J*. 2013;13(7):786–795. [Comparative Study].

20. Guzman JZ, Baird EO, Fields AC, et al. C5 nerve root palsy following decompression of the cervical spine: a systematic evaluation of the literature. *Bone Joint J*. 2014 Jul;96-B(7):950–955.

21. Abumi K, Shono Y, Ito M, Taneichi H, Kotani Y, Kaneda K. Complications of pedicle screw fixation in reconstructive surgery of the cervical spine. *Spine*. 2000;25(8):962–969. [Comparative Study].

22. Lunardini DJ, Eskander MS, Even JL, et al. Vertebral artery injuries in cervical spine surgery. *Spine J*. 2014;14(8):1520–1525. [Research Support, Non-U.S. Gov't].

23. Binning MJ, Schmidt MH. Percutaneous placement of radiopaque markers at the pedicle of interest for preoperative localization of thoracic spine level. *Spine*. 2010;35(19):1821–1825.

24. Lubelski D, Abdullah KG, Mroz TE, et al. Lateral extracavitary vs. costotransversectomy approaches to the thoracic spine: reflections on lessons learned. *Neurosurgery*. 2012;71(6):1096–1102.

25. Lubelski D, Abdullah KG, Steinmetz MP, et al. Lateral extracavitary, costotransversectomy, and transthoracic thoracotomy approaches to the thoracic spine: review of techniques and complications. *J Spinal Disord Tech*. 2013;26(4):222–232. [Meta-Analysis Review].

26. Resnick DK, Benzel EC. Lateral extracavitary approach for thoracic and thoracolumbar spine trauma: operative complications. *Neurosurgery*. 1998;43(4):796–802. discussion 803. [Review].

27. Desaussure RL. Vascular injury coincident to disc surgery. *J Neurosurg*. 1959;16(2):222–228.

28. Fineberg SJ, Nandyala SV, Kurd MF, et al. Incidence and risk factors for postoperative ileus following anterior, posterior, and circumferential lumbar fusion. *Spine J*. 2014;14(8):1680–1685.

29. Ponec RJ, Saunders MD, Kimmey MB. Neostigmine for the treatment of acute colonic pseudo-obstruction. *N Engl J Med*. 1999;34(3):137–141. [Clinical Trial Randomized Controlled Trial Research Support, Non-U.S. Gov't].

30. Kamel I, Barnette R. Positioning patients for spine surgery: avoiding uncommon position-related complications. *World J Orthop*. 2014;5(4):425–443. [Review].

31. Risk factors associated with ischemic optic neuropathy after spinal fusion surgery. *Anesthesiology*. 2012;116(1):15–24. [Multicenter Study Randomized Controlled Trial Research Support, Non-U.S. Gov't].

32. Lee LA. Perioperative visual loss and anesthetic management. *Curr Opin Anaesthesiol*. 2013;26(3):375–381. [Review].

33. Lee LA, Roth S, Posner KL, et al. The American Society of Anesthesiologists Postoperative Visual Loss Registry: analysis of 93 spine surgery cases with postoperative visual loss. *Anesthesiology*. 2006;105(4):652–659. quiz 867–8.

34. Cheng JS, Arnold PM, Anderson PA, Fischer D, Dettori JR. Anticoagulation risk in spine surgery. *Spine*. 2010;35(9 Suppl):S117–S124. [Research Support, Non-U.S. Gov't Review].

35. Agnelli G, Piovella F, Buoncristiani P, et al. Enoxaparin plus compression stockings compared with compression stockings alone in the prevention of venous thromboembolism after elective neurosurgery. *N Engl J Med*. 1998;339(2):80–85. [Clinical Trial Comparative Study Multicenter Study Randomized Controlled Trial Research Support, Non-U.S. Gov't].

36. Gerlach R, Raabe A, Beck J, Woszczyk A, Seifert V. Postoperative nadroparin administration for prophylaxis of thromboembolic events is not associated with an increased risk of hemorrhage after spinal surgery. *Eur Spine J*. 2004;13(1):9–13.

37. Strom RG, Frempong-Boadu AK. Low-molecular-weight heparin prophylaxis 24 to 36 hours after degenerative spine surgery: risk of hemorrhage and venous thromboembolism. *Spine*. 2013;38(23):E1498–E1502.

38. Clark AJ, Ziewacz JE, Safaee M, et al. Intraoperative neuromonitoring with MEPs and prediction of postoperative neurological deficits in patients undergoing surgery for cervical and cervicothoracic myelopathy. *Neurosurg Focus*. 2013;35(1).

39. Epstein NE, Danto J, Nardi D. Evaluation of intraoperative somatosensory-evoked potential monitoring during 100 cervical operations. *Spine*. 1993;18(6):737–747. [Comparative Study].

40. Garcia RM, Qureshi SA, Cassinelli EH, Biro CL, Furey CG, Bohlman HH. Detection of postoperative neurologic deficits using somatosensory-evoked potentials alone during posterior cervical laminoplasty. *Spine J*. 2010;10(10):890–895.

41. Nam Y, Yoon AM, Kim YH, Yoon SH. The effect on respiratory mechanics when using a Jackson surgical table in the prone position during spinal surgery. *Korean J Anesthesiol*. 2010;59(5):323–328.

42. Palmon SC, Kirsch JR, Depper JA, Toung TJ. The effect of the prone position on pulmonary mechanics is frame-dependent. *Anesth Analg*. 1998;87(5):1175–1180. [Clinical Trial Research Support, Non-U.S. Gov't].

43. Dharmavaram S, Jellish WS, Nockels RP, et al. Effect of prone positioning systems on hemodynamic and cardiac function during lumbar spine surgery: an echocardiographic study. *Spine*. 2006;31(12):1388–1393. discussion 1394. [Randomized Controlled Trial].

44. Brown J, Rogers J, Soar J. Cardiac arrest during surgery and ventilation in the prone position: a case report and systematic review. *Resuscitation*. 2001;50(2):233–238. [Case Reports Review].

45. Ryken TC, Hurlbert RJ, Hadley MN, et al. The acute cardiopulmonary management of patients with cervical spinal cord injuries. *Neurosurgery*. 2013;72(Suppl 2):84–92. [Review].

46. Vale FL, Burns J, Jackson AB, Hadley MN. Combined medical and surgical treatment after acute spinal cord injury: results of a prospective pilot study to assess the merits of aggressive medical resuscitation and blood pressure management. *J Neurosurg*. 1997;87(2):239–246.

47. Ross PA, Smith BM, Tolo VT, Khemani RG. Continuous infusion of bupivacaine reduces postoperative morphine use in adolescent idiopathic scoliosis after posterior spine fusion. *Spine*. 2011;36(18):1478–1483.

48. Armaghani SJ, Lee DS, Bible JE, et al. Increased preoperative narcotic use and its association with postoperative complications and length of hospital stay in patients undergoing spine surgery. *Clin Spine Surg*. 2016 Mar;29(2):E93–E98.

49. Clifford L, Jia Q, Subramanian A, et al. Characterizing the epidemiology of postoperative transfusion-related acute lung injury. *Anesthesiology*. 2015;122(1):12–20. [Research Support, Non-U.S. Gov't].

50. Boahene K, Dagi T, Quinones-Hinojosa A. Management of cerebrospinal fluid leaks. In: Quinone-Hinojosa A, ed. *Schmidek & Sweet Operative Neurosurgical Techniques: Indications, Methods, and Results*. 6th ed. Philadelphia: Elsevier Saunders; 2012:1579–1595.

# 33 Transthoracic and Transabdominal Approaches to the Spine

MARK E. OPPENLANDER, CHRISTOPHER M. MAULUCCI, MICHAEL S. WEINSTEIN, and JAMES S. HARROP

## Introduction

The transthoracic and transabdominal approaches to the spine have become standard for a wide array of spinal disorders. What makes these approaches unique is their multidisciplinary nature, where an approach surgeon with general surgery training often works along with the spinal surgeon. This strategy optimizes patient safety during exposures of the viscera within the thorax and abdomen. However, some spine surgeons do perform their own approaches to these procedures.

In addition, patients undergoing transthoracic or transabdominal spinal surgery require vigilant perioperative care, usually in the intensive care unit. Working postoperatively with neurocritical care specialists, further multidisciplinary strategies for patient care are obtained. This chapter outlines the indications, approaches, postoperative care nuances, and complication management for patients undergoing transthoracic or transabdominal approaches to the spine.

## Neuroanatomy and Procedure

### Key Concepts

- The indications for transthoracic and transabdominal approaches to the spine are wide, and the approach should be tailored to the patient and pathology.
- Complete knowledge of thoracic and abdominal anatomy allow for avoidance of intraoperative complications.
- An understanding of transthoracic and transabdominal procedure nuances will theoretically lead to better postoperative care among multidisciplinary clinicians.

### TRANSTHORACIC APPROACHES

#### General Considerations and Indications

The transthoracic approach is utilized for access to the ventral thoracic spine. In general, a classic thoracotomy allows access to T4 to T10 levels. Upper thoracic lesions may be accessed via thoracotomy, a transsternal approach,[1,2] or a posterolateral extracavitary approach.[3] The ventral thoracolumbar region (T10–L2) can be accessed via posterolateral approaches,[4,5] or via a combined transthoracic-retroperitoneal approach,[6] with elevation of the diaphragm. Finally, the thoracoscopic technique is an alternative to thoracotomy for certain pathologies.[7,8]

Indications for the transthoracic approach include tumor, deformity, trauma, infection, and degenerative diseases. Most neoplasms affecting the spinal column are malignant and include metastases[9,10] or primary vertebral tumors such as chordoma.[11] Operative intervention is appropriate for tissue diagnosis, neural decompression, and spinal stabilization.

Coronal or sagittal deformities may be addressed from a transthoracic approach.[12–14] The deformity may be a result of idiopathic or neuromuscular scoliosis, old fracture or infection, or adult degenerative disease. In deformity surgery, the side of the curve's apex is generally chosen as the side of the approach.

Thoracolumbar fractures have undergone multiple permutations of classification systems,[15,16] and the optimal surgical approach for an individual fracture type remains controversial. According to Denis,[17] disruption of two of the three vertebral columns results in an unstable injury requiring internal fixation. The Thoracolumbar Injury Classification and Severity Score system attempts to quantify the severity of biomechanical disruption with the patient's neurological status in order to standardize indications for surgery.[16,18] A ventral approach to the thoracic spine for neural decompression and internal fixation may be indicated for select fracture morphologies.

By far the majority of spinal degenerative disease occurs in the cervical and lumbar regions, but degenerative disease in the thoracic spine becomes clinically relevant in the form of herniated discs. Thoracic disc herniations are less common, yet may cause debilitating thoracic myelopathy or radiculopathy.[19–21] In general, if a herniated thoracic disc is large, centrally located in the spinal canal, and calcified, then a transthoracic approach is preferred for operative decompression.[22]

#### Neuroanatomy

The thoracic spine consists of 12 vertebral segments. The vertebral bodies lie anteriorly, with the spinal canal being bordered posteriorly by the pedicles, laminae, and spinous processes. The transverse processes extend laterally and articulate with the rib head at each level.

The thoracic spinal cord lies within the spinal canal, and the nerve roots exit from vertebral foramen bilaterally at each level. A specific nerve root level exits below the pedicle of its corresponding vertebral level (e.g., the T6 nerve root exits caudal to the T6 pedicle through the T6–7 foramen).

Blood supply to the thoracic spinal cord is derived from the segmental aortic branches, which travel approximately midway along each vertebral body in the craniocaudal dimension (Fig. 33.1). A limited number of radicular arteries actually supply the spinal cord, the largest being the artery of Adamkiewicz, which is the main arterial supply to the cord below the T8 level. This artery is located on the left in approximately 80% of patients and originates between the T9 and L2 levels in nearly 85% of patients.[23] This vascular anatomy is important to remember when approaching the thoracic spine because ligation of multiple segmental vessels may increase the likelihood of postoperative cord ischemia.[24] If in doubt about an artery's importance to the thoracic cord, the artery can be clamped prior to permanent ligation in order to evaluate for changes in neuromonitoring signals.

## Procedure

An initial step in the thoracotomy procedure is determining from which side to approach the pathology, left versus right. Often the pathology dictates the side, as with a herniated disc that is eccentrically located to one side of the spinal canal, or a tumor that has lateral extension from the vertebral body. If the pathology is equivocal in laterality,

then preference in approach relates to several factors. A right-sided approach will avoid the aorta, whereas the left-sided approach avoids the inferior vena cava and the liver. Should a combined thoracoabdominal approach be required for access to the lower thoracic and lumbar spine, then the left side is preferred in order to avoid the liver and venous structures.

Lung isolation is performed with a double lumen endotracheal intubation, or via placement of a bronchial blocker. We generally use lung isolation for approaches above the T9 level. Below that level, retraction alone of the lung usually suffices.

The patient is positioned in the lateral decubitus position with padding applied to all pressure points. An incision is planned over the pathology, along the length of a target rib. The rib articulating with a given spinal level will overlie the level of a vertebral body two levels caudally so that the T6 rib overlies the vertebral body of T8. The pathology can be localized and the incision planned using radiography before starting the procedure (Fig. 33.2).

The length of the incision is dictated by the number of levels that need to be exposed and by the body habitus of the patient. A classic thoracotomy incision generally extends from the lateral margin of the paraspinous muscles to the sternocostal junction of the rib to be resected. In our experience smaller incisions generally suffice. The subcutaneous tissue is dissected with monocautery. The latissimus

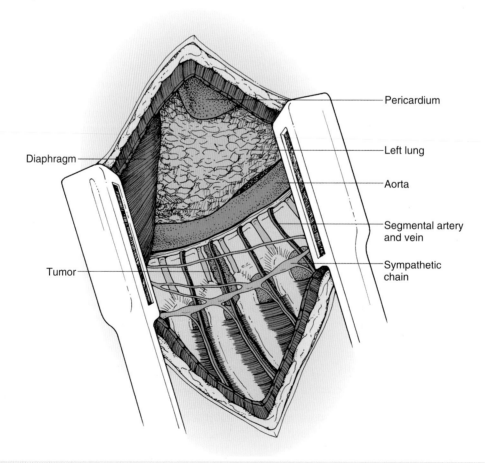

**Fig. 33.1** Surgical anatomy of a left-sided thoracotomy approach. (Reprinted from Benzel EC (Ed.). *Spine Surgery: Techniques, Complication Avoidance, and Management,* 3rd ed. Philadelphia, PA: Elsevier Saunders; 2012: 479, Fig. 50.3.)

Labels on figure: Pericardium, Left lung, Aorta, Segmental artery and vein, Sympathetic chain, Diaphragm, Tumor

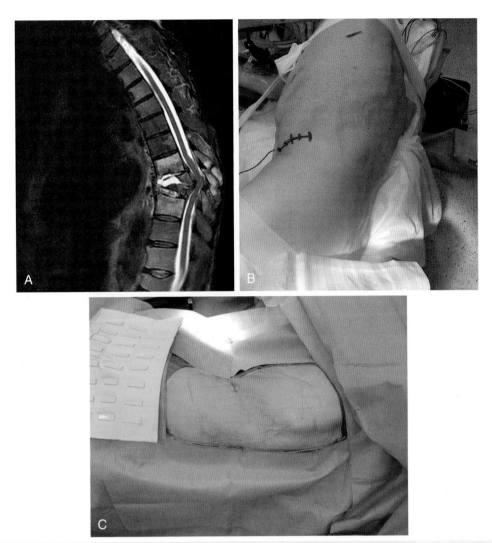

**Fig. 33.2** A 61-year-old man had back pain and was found to have T8–9 vertebral body collapse in the setting of osteodiscitis **(A)**. He underwent a left thoracotomy for decompression and fusion. The patient is positioned in the right-lateral decubitus position **(B)**, then pictured after preparation and draping **(C)**.

dorsi and serratus anterior muscles are split along the course of the underlying rib. Alternatively, the muscles are mobilized and retracted. The rib is freed with blunt dissection, keeping in mind the neurovascular bundle running along the inferior aspect of the rib. If wide access is required, the rib is then cut as far anteriorly and posteriorly as possible with the rib cutter and is set aside for possible use as graft material later in the procedure.

The pleura is then opened. The lung may be isolated as described earlier, ventilating only the dependent lung. The lung and diaphragm are retracted with a covered malleable retractor. A rib spreader maximizes exposure, and the spinal column comes into view. The parietal pleura is elevated off the spine, and the segmental vessels are identified. These may be sacrificed depending on the procedure's exposure requirements. In general, the rib head of the appropriate level is identified first, and this leads to the pedicle of the involved vertebral level.

Once the spinal portion of the procedure is completed, a chest drainage tube is placed and wound closure begins. The ribs are reapproximated with suture; then the

anesthesiologist reinflates the lung. The remainder of the wound is closed in layers.

## TRANSABDOMINAL APPROACH: ANTERIOR APPROACHES

### General Considerations and Indications

The lumbar spine can be approached through an anterior transabdominal approach for a variety of pathologies, including degenerative, tumor, infection, and deformity. One of the most common indications is for anterior lumbar interbody fusion (ALIF). An ALIF reconstructs the anterior column of the lumbar spine. It has the ability to increase lordosis via insertion of a large interbody graft. It therefore helps to provide significant anterior column support when needed. Further, a large, easily accessible surface area for arthrodesis can be obtained, promoting fusion and helping to decrease the risk of pseudarthrosis. However, the neural elements cannot be accessed easily via this approach. Rather, via distraction, the nerve roots are indirectly decompressed.[25]

Careful patient selection is crucial before performing ALIF. Surgical indications for ALIF include lumbar degenerative disc disease without significant stenosis, kyphotic lumbar deformity, anterior column support in long constructs, and patients at high risk for pseudarthrosis. Additional indications for a transabdominal approach to the lumbar spine include tumor biopsy and resection,[26] debridement of infection,[27] and decompression and stabilization after trauma.[28]

Given that the usual approach for ALIF necessitates traversing the retroperitoneal space, many other factors must be considered. The only true contraindication is severe osteoporosis that results in subsidence of a graft into the vertebral bodies. Otherwise, most other contraindications are relative and depend on the experience of the surgical team. Neural compression, as discussed earlier, is a relative contraindication. The indirect decompression achieved via ALIF may be sufficient to provide relief of radicular symptoms. A history of prior retroperitoneal surgery, severe peripheral vascular disease, infrarenal aortic aneurysm, and an anomalous genitourinary system with a solitary ureter are other relative contraindications. Patients who have hypercoagulable disease or take medications that create a hypercoagulable state should be carefully considered before ALIF.

## Neuroanatomy

The typical exposure for ALIF gives the surgeon access to the anterior aspect of the lumbar vertebral body. The anterior longitudinal ligament and the annulus fibrosis are readily recognized overlying the osseous structures. Little to no visualization of the dura and its contents, the cauda equina, is possible through a relatively narrow channel created by the discectomy. If, however, an L1 to L2 discectomy is being performed, one must be cognizant that the conus medullaris may lie at this relatively low level. Important neural structures also lie adjacent to the spine.

The bilateral psoas muscles are pierced by the nerves of the lumbar plexus, which supply sensory and motor function to the proximal lower extremities. The superior hypogastric plexus is located near the abdominal aorta between the origin of the inferior mesenteric artery and the bifurcation of the abdominal aorta into the two common iliac arteries. These nerves control vasomotor, pilomotor, and secretory functions to the skin of the perineum and lower limbs. Notably, this plexus also controls ejaculation in males.

## Procedure

For lumbar levels at and below L2, the patient is positioned supine on a radiolucent table with the lumbar spine in lordosis. A midline or paramedian incision is utilized. For the approach to L1, the patient is placed in the lateral position. An oblique flank incision is utilized in these cases. The retroperitoneum is approached from the left side because it is generally safer to retract the muscular aorta rather than the relatively thin-walled inferior vena cava. Before incision, the lower extremity peripheral pulses should be detected, either via palpation or Doppler probe. This allows a baseline for intraoperative and perioperative monitoring. A pulse oximeter can also be placed on the lower extremity as a means of identifying vascular insufficiency intraoperatively.

As the dissection proceeds the peritoneum is identified. The peritoneal contents are bluntly swept aside from left to right revealing the retroperitoneal space (Fig. 33.3). If a peritoneal rent is created, it is closed with a running Vicryl suture. The ureter must be identified and retracted with the peritoneal sac. The prevertebral space is entered with blunt dissection without the use of monopolar cautery. This helps to reduce the risk of injury to the superior hypogastric plexus in the aortic bifurcation. Proper vessel ligation must be performed during dissection. The left iliolumbar vein, which crosses the L5 body, is best ligated and divided to allow full mobilization of the left common iliac vein.

The intraperitoneal contents are retracted with self-retaining retractors. Major vascular structures are best retracted by an assistant with a handheld retractor. This

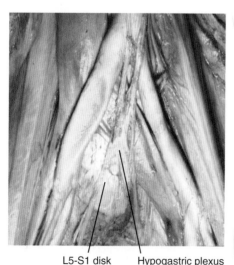 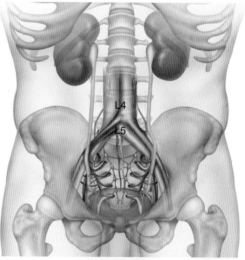

L5-S1 disk    Hypogastric plexus

**Fig. 33.3** Surgical anatomy of a left-sided retroperitoneal approach for anterior lumbar interbody fusion. (Reprinted from Quinones-Hinojosa A (Ed.). *Schmidek and Sweet: Operative Neurosurgical Techniques*, 6th ed. Philadelphia, PA: Elsevier Saunders; 2012: 1959, Fig. 171.6.)

allows for frequent release of retraction to prevent thrombosis, as well as constant visualization of the vessels. The discectomy is then performed and a graft, with or without hardware, is inserted after radiographic localization of the target level. The wound is irrigated and closed in a layered fashion.

## TRANSABDOMINAL APPROACH: LATERAL APPROACH

The lumbar and thoracolumbar spine can also be approached with the patient in the lateral position. This again can be used for a variety of indications, including degenerative, tumor, infection, and deformity. These approaches generally require less mobilization of the vasculature, especially in the upper lumbar and thoracolumbar spine. It sometimes requires mobilization of the diaphragm at the thoracolumbar junction, requiring careful repair at the end of the case. One of the approaches that has gained popularity within the past decade is the lateral lumbar interbody fusion (LLIF). This approach accomplishes similar goals to that of ALIF regarding the ability to insert a large interbody graft, providing excellent anterior column stabilization and a large surface area for arthrodesis. Like ALIF, LLIF provides indirect neural decompression through distraction of the vertebral body. The LLIF can also be considered a powerful tool for correcting a coronal deformity, for example, scoliosis.[29,30] The concavity or convexity of a spinal curve can be reached for reconstruction of the anterior spine. Oftentimes, LLIF must be performed in conjunction with posterior supplemental instrumentation for spinal stability (Fig. 33.4). This can be done in a staged fashion if necessary.

Careful patient selection is crucial before performing LLIF. Indications for LLIF include lumbar degenerative disc disease without significant stenosis, coronal lumbar deformity, anterior column support in long constructs, and patients at high risk for pseudarthrosis.

### Neuroanatomy

The lateral aspect of the vertebral body and the ventral aspect of the transverse process are the osseous structures visible during LLIF. The annulus fibrosis and disc space can be identified between the vertebral bodies. The dura lies dorsal to the body.

The psoas muscle runs obliquely from medial to lateral in the coronal plane and from posterior to anterior in the sagittal plane. Its deep fibers originate from the lumbar transverse processes; the deep fibers originate from the lateral surfaces of the lowest thoracic vertebra, lumbar vertebral bodies, and intervertebral discs. The psoas joins the iliacus, forms the iliopsoas muscle, and inserts on the lesser trochanter of the femur. The lumbar plexus lies between the two layers of the psoas. The plexus runs from posterior to anterior along the lateral aspect of the lumbar vertebrae. It lies at the posterior aspect of the body at the L1 to L2 level and can be as far anterior as the midportion of the body at L4 to L5.

### Procedure

An initial step in the LLIF procedure is determining from which side to approach the pathology. A scoliotic deformity is usually best approached from the side of the concavity

because multiple discs can be reached from a single approach due to the curvature.[29]

The patient is positioned in the lateral decubitus position with padding applied to all pressure points. An incision is planned using intraoperative radiographic guidance, marking the anterior and posterior extents of the disc space in a lateral projection. The skin is incised and dissection carried out identifying the external oblique muscle, internal oblique muscle, transversus abdominis muscle, and fascia. The retroperitoneal adipose tissue is then identified (Fig. 33.5). A self-retaining retractor is placed with the assistance of intraoperative electromyography to ensure that the femoral nerve is not injured.[31,32] Depending on the target level and anatomy, the psoas muscle may or may not have to be traversed in order to reach the disc space. The annulus fibrosis is incised, a discectomy completed, and an interbody graft inserted with radiographic guidance. The wound is closed in layers.

# Perioperative Considerations

## Key Concepts

- Perioperative patient management is generally considered in the context of the specific surgical approach to the spine.
- Patients who undergo thoracotomy will generally require management of a chest tube, whereas transabdominal approaches may have no drainage catheters.
- For all patients undergoing major spine surgery, pain control is pursued aggressively and early mobilization is employed if possible.

After transthoracic or transabdominal approaches to the spine, the patient is usually transferred to an intermediate care or intensive care unit for close observation. Clear communication between the surgical and medical personnel caring for the patient must take place in order to discuss the proceedings of surgery. If there is concern over an intraoperative complication, this must be communicated.

Patients who have undergone major spine surgery should have their pain controlled aggressively.[33] The diet is advanced postoperatively as tolerated. These patients are mobilized as soon as possible in order to decrease risk of deep venous thrombosis and to prevent deconditioning. An external orthosis is applied at the discretion of the surgeon.

### Transthoracic Approaches

## Clinical Pearls

- Chest tubes are quite painful for patients, and every effort should be made for expeditious removal, because this delays mobilization.
- Atelectasis is a common problem related to decreased vital capacity and splinting after thoracotomy.

After a transthoracic approach to the spine, chest tube drainage is monitored and serial chest x-rays are obtained

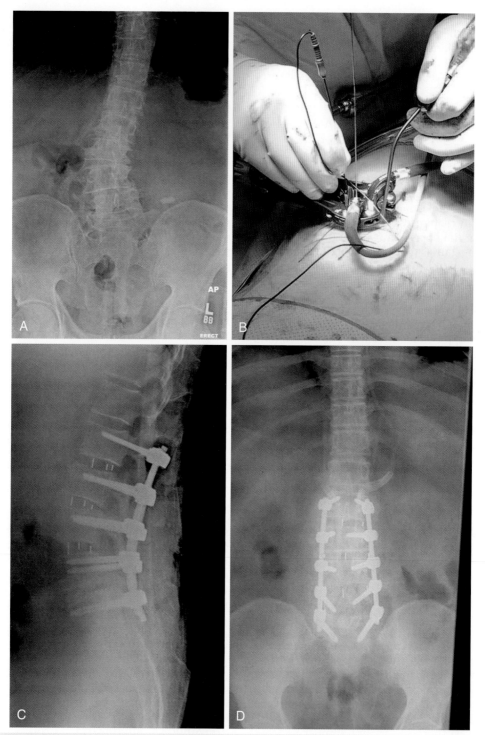

**Fig. 33.4** Case of a 70-year-old man who presented with progressive back pain and right leg weakness. He was found to have degenerative lumbar scoliosis **(A)** and underwent a lateral approach for decompression and interbody fusion. A retroperitoneal approach is undertaken **(B),** and interbody grafts are inserted. The patient underwent a second-stage posterior decompression and fusion with pedicle screws. Postoperative lateral **(C)** and anteroposterior (AP) **(D)** x-rays show correction of deformity.

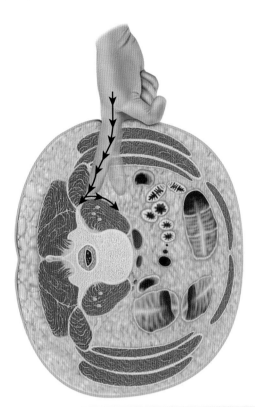

**Fig. 33.5** Retroperitoneal approach for lateral lumbar interbody fusion. (Reprinted from Quinones-Hinojosa A (Ed.). *Schmidek and Sweet: Operative Neurosurgical Techniques*, 6th ed. Philadelphia, PA: Elsevier Saunders; 2012, p. 1967, Fig. 172.5.)

in concern for developing hemothorax, pneumothorax, lung consolidation, atelectasis, or other approach-related complication. The chest tube(s) are removed after output has decreased and chest x-rays are stable, generally after 24 to 48 hours if there is no air leak.

### Anterior Lumbar Interbody Fusion

## Clinical Pearls

■ The postoperative ileus rate appears to be higher from a transperitoneal versus a retroperitoneal approach.
■ Drains that communicate with the peritoneal space can have substantial sustained output. This does not necessarily imply pathology but may just reflect physiological peritoneal fluid.

Urinary retention occurs postoperatively in up to 27% of ALIF cases, but is usually temporary. It most often is due to the use of perioperative narcotics.[34] If, however, this symptom does not resolve within the first few days after surgery, ureteral injury or cauda equina syndromes must be ruled out.

Postoperative ileus is also common after ALIF. It usually resolves within a week after surgery. If nausea or radiographic enlargement of bowel loops is evident, then placement of a nasogastric tube may be necessary.

### Lateral Lumbar Interbody Fusion

Approximately 10% to 20% of postoperative LLIF patients experience a transient numbness, especially in the anterior thigh region.[35] During surgery, the sensory nerves cannot be monitored and therefore are more susceptible to injury than the motor nerves. Most patients experience a near-complete recovery of this deficit by 1 year after surgery. For those patients in whom the psoas muscle was entered, a transient mild hip flexion weakness may exist because the muscle has been damaged. However, this is not considered a complication unless it is accompanied by knee extension weakness, which is indicative of a femoral nerve injury.[32,36]

## POSTOPERATIVE COMPLICATIONS

### Key Concepts

• Patients who undergo thoracotomy will generally require serial chest x-ray while chest drainage tubes are in place, and specific complications are addressed accordingly.
• Most complications after ALIF are related to the surgical approach.
• Most complications after LLIF are typically neurological in nature.
• Any surgery to the chest or superior abdomen risks problems with atelectasis related to decreased vital capacity.

### Clinical Pearls

■ Ventral cerebrospinal fluid (CSF) leaks are notoriously difficult to repair, and so symptoms of CSF hypotension must be monitored for in cases of intraoperative dural lacerations, especially with a chest tube in place.
■ Prolonged lateral positioning can be associated with significant dependent skin breakdown, nerve palsies, and dependent lung edema.

### Transthoracic Approaches

Many complications from a thoracotomy are decreased by appropriate preoperative workup for comorbidities, such as cardiac or pulmonary disease. Smoking cessation should be strongly encouraged.[37] In addition, the assistance from a thoracic surgeon or a general surgeon may decrease approach-related morbidity. Regardless, the possibility of certain complications must be considered in the perioperative period[38,39] (Table 33.1).

A lung laceration may occur during dissection of pleural adhesions or from direct trauma with an instrument, thereby increasing risk for postoperative pneumothorax. A lung laceration may be repaired primarily, using suture or staplers. If using stapling devices, seam guards can decrease the risk of air leak. Fibrin glue may be placed over the laceration to prevent air leak. After repair, a chest tube is placed near the location of potential air leak, biased anteriorly in the chest to account for anterior migration of air within the thoracic cavity.

**Table 33.1** Major Postoperative Complications of Transthoracic and Transabdominal Approaches*

| 1.1 Procedure | 1.2 Complication |
| --- | --- |
| Thoracotomy | Tension pneumothorax |
| | Hemothorax |
| | Pneumothorax |
| | Chylothorax |
| | Atelectasis/lung edema |
| | Infection (pleural abscess) |
| ALIF | Bowel injury |
| | Ureteral injury |
| | Thrombosis (venous or arterial) |
| | Retroperitoneal hematoma |
| | Retrograde ejaculation (men) |
| LLIF | Femoral nerve injury |
| | Abdominal muscle denervation |
| | Anterior thigh numbness |

*ALIF, anterior lumbar interbody fusion; LLIF, lateral lumbar interbody fusion.

In the case of a postoperative pneumothorax, an anteriorly placed chest tube should remain in place until the pneumothorax resolves. An additional chest tube insertion may be required. Pneumothorax recurrences are treated by numerous methods, including observation, replacement of chest tube, or repeat thoracotomy with placement of chest tube.[40] Tension pneumothorax is an emergent complication. Signs of tension pneumothorax include respiratory distress, hypoxemia, decreased unilateral lung sounds, tracheal deviation, distended neck veins, hypotension, and tachycardia.

Lacerations of thoracic vessels are managed by either ligation of the vessel or with primary repair, but still increase the risk for postoperative complications. The azygos vein and segmental vessels can often be ligated in the case of laceration. If laceration of the inferior vena cava occurs, primary repair is attempted, but ligation remains an acceptable damage control technique.[41] The aorta and pulmonary artery require direct suturing, and assistance from an experienced thoracic surgeon is recommended. Superior vena cava ligation can produce acute superior vena cava syndrome and jeopardize vision.

Clinicians should be alert to detect retained hemothorax after thoracotomy. If bleeding is expected in the postoperative period, the chest tube should be placed in the anticipated location of blood accumulation (often oriented posteriorly in the paraspinous region). The chest tube should remain in place until bloody output decreases. If high output continues or increases, then consideration for repeat thoracotomy and direct hemostasis should be given.

Likewise, injury to the thoracic duct requires vigilant postoperative care. The thoracic duct is often not visualized intraoperatively, but a suspected thoracic duct injury can

be oversewn or, alternatively, the thoracic duct can be ligated primarily. Chylothorax is identified by postoperative chest x-ray, combined with a milky fluid emission from the chest tube. Treatment may involve parenteral nutrition with continued chest tube drainage. Thoracentesis or repeat thoracotomy for further repair remain options for continued chyle output.[42,43]

Postoperative infection may result in pleural abscess. If early in development, chest tube drainage with intravenous antibiotics may successfully treat the process. Late-stage pleural abscess may require thoracotomy for decortication and evacuation.[44]

## Anterior Lumbar Interbody Fusion

### Clinical Pearl

The most common major complications from anterior abdominal approaches are vascular and generally involve the venous structures. This can result in significant intraoperative blood loss requiring aggressive intraop and postoperative resuscitation. Even with primary intraoperative repair the deep venous thrombosis (DVT) rate is significant.

Intraoperative or postoperative complications of ALIF mostly relate to the operative approach (Table 33.1). If the peritoneum is violated and not repaired at the time of surgery, a hernia, and possibly bowel obstruction or infarction, can occur. Injury to the bowel is a rare complication requiring immediate detection and treatment.[45] The operative field must be aggressively irrigated and the bowel repair performed by a general surgeon. Prophylactic broad-spectrum antibiotics should be administered and the ALIF aborted. Preoperative bowel prep and intraoperative nasogastric tube insertion can decrease the risk of the complication by decompressing loops of bowel. Should the ureter be damaged during ALIF, a urological surgeon must be contacted immediately. Primary repair of the ureter, with or without stenting, is required.[46,47]

Injury to a major vascular structure occurs in 2% to 4% of ALIF surgeries.[48] Direct repair of the vessel by a vascular surgeon is necessary. Appropriate vascular access and readily available blood products should be present in preparation for this potential complication. If it arises, postoperative issues related to massive transfusion and ongoing hemorrhage may arise.

Thrombosis of either venous or arterial structures is another potential complication of ALIF. Venous thrombosis has been reported in 1% to 11% of ALIF procedures.[49] Arterial thrombosis is quite rare. If thrombosis is suspected, then immediate angiogram should be performed. Treatment consists of open surgical thrombectomy.[45,49]

Intraoperative durotomy during ALIF can be readily recognized. However, it is very difficult to control because access to the thecal sac is limited. Free muscle or fascia grafts should be harvested and may be combined with a fibrin glue to promote healing. A lumbar subarachnoid drain should be inserted to divert cerebrospinal fluid in the immediate postoperative course.

Radiculopathy or symptoms consistent with cauda equina syndrome should be immediately worked up with neuroimaging. If hematoma, retropulsed disc material, or malpositioned hardware is causing compression, dorsal decompression and exploration is the most efficacious treatment strategy.

Injury to the genitofemoral or ilioinguinal nerves may occur after ALIF. This is more common at the upper lumbar levels. Symptoms manifest as numbness in the groin and/or medial thigh. These nerve palsies typically resolve spontaneously within the first 6 months after surgery.[34,50]

Damage to sympathetic nerves on the side of the approach may also occur. This complication may result in ipsilateral vasodilatation in the lower extremity vessels. The patient will usually complain, though, of a cold sensation in the contralateral foot. These symptoms usually resolve in 3 to 6 months. Damage to the sympathetic plexus in males may result in retrograde ejaculation. This complication occurs in 0.5% to 2% of all ALIF procedures.[51] The internal bladder sphincter relaxes during ejaculation, resulting in retrograde flow into the bladder. There is no surgical management strategy for this complication, but 25% to 33% of patients recover normal function by 2 years.[51,52]

A postoperative infection in the form of osteomyelitis or discitis occurs in approximately 1% of all ALIF procedures.[34] Radiographic evidence coupled with increased white cell count, C-reactive protein, or sedimentation rate will increase suspicion of this complication. If there is an epidural component causing compression of the neural elements, ventral or dorsal exploration and debridement is recommended. Otherwise, prolonged antibiotic use with an external orthosis may be attempted with radiographic and clinical surveillance.

## Lateral Lumbar Interbody Fusion

Unlike ALIF, LLIF complications are typically neurological[53,54] (Table 33.1). LLIF carries with it a 3% to 23% incidence of femoral nerve injury resulting in hip flexion and knee extension weakness.[54] Patients with motor weakness regain 50% recovery at 90 days and 90% recovery at 1 year. This complication can be avoided with vigilant neuromonitoring and stimulating the region exposed within the retractor blades in search of motor nerve branches. If no "safe zone" can be located, the procedure should be aborted.

During LLIF exposure, the nerves supplying the musculature to the abdominal flank may be significantly injured resulting in a flank bulge. This complication has been reported in approximately 4% of cases.[30,35] A hernia must be ruled out. Usually this complication is purely esthetic, but can be very troubling to patients.

# Conclusion

Through multidisciplinary care from the spinal surgeon and the neurocritical care specialist, patients undergoing transthoracic or transabdominal spinal surgery can achieve optimal outcomes. Specifically, vigilant postoperative care, often in the intensive care unit, is necessary for the identification and management of potential complications. Because the transthoracic and transabdominal exposures involve viscera outside of the spinal surgeon's specialty, the necessity for this multidisciplinary approach in perioperative patient management becomes even more apparent.

## References

1. Zengming X, Maolin H, Xinli Z, Qianfen C. Anterior transsternal approach for a lesion in the upper thoracic vertebral body. *J Neurosurg Spine*. 2010;13(4):461–468.
2. Jiang H, Xiao Z-M, Zhan X-L, He M-L. Anterior transsternal approach for treatment of upper thoracic vertebral tuberculosis. *Orthop Surg*. 2010;2(4):305–309.
3. Lubelski D, Abdullah KG, Steinmetz MP, et al. Lateral extracavitary, costotransversectomy, and transthoracic thoracotomy approaches to the thoracic spine: review of techniques and complications. *J Spinal Disord Tech*. 2013;26(4):222–232.
4. Le Roux PD, Haglund MM, Harris AB. Thoracic disc disease: experience with the transpedicular approach in twenty consecutive patients. *Neurosurgery*. 1993;33(1):58–66.
5. Simpson JM, Silveri CP, Simeone FA, Balderston RA, An HS. Thoracic disc herniation. Re-evaluation of the posterior approach using a modified costotransversectomy. *Spine*. 1993;18(13):1872–1877.
6. Burrington JD, Brown C, Wayne ER, Odom J. Anterior approach to the thoracolumbar spine: technical considerations. *Arch Surg*. 1976;111(4):456–463.
7. Rosenthal D, Dickman CA. Thoracoscopic microsurgical excision of herniated thoracic discs. *J Neurosurg*. 1998;89(2):224–235.
8. Han PP, Kenny K, Dickman CA. Thoracoscopic approaches to the thoracic spine: experience with 241 surgical procedures. *Neurosurgery*. 2002;51(5 Suppl):S88–S95.
9. Loblaw DA, Perry J, Chambers A, Laperriere NJ. Systematic review of the diagnosis and management of malignant extradural spinal cord compression: the Cancer Care Ontario Practice Guidelines Initiative's Neuro-Oncology Disease Site Group. *J Clin Oncol*. 2005;23(9):2028–2037.
10. Prasad D, Schiff D. Malignant spinal-cord compression. *Lancet Oncol*. 2005;6(1):15–24.
11. Boriani S, Bandiera S, Biagini R, et al. Chordoma of the mobile spine: fifty years of experience. *Spine*. 2006;31(4):493–503.
12. Richardson JD, Campbell DL, Grover FL, et al. Transthoracic approach for Pott's disease. *Ann Thorac Surg*. 1976;21(6):552–556.
13. Lowe TG, Alongi PR, Smith DAB, O'Brien MF, Mitchell SL, Pinteric RJ. Anterior single rod instrumentation for thoracolumbar adolescent idiopathic scoliosis with and without the use of structural interbody support. *Spine*. 2003;28(19):2232–2241. discussion 2241–2.
14. Tis JE, O'Brien MF, Newton PO, et al. Adolescent idiopathic scoliosis treated with open instrumented anterior spinal fusion: five-year follow-up. *Spine*. 2010;35(1):64–70.
15. Magerl F, Aebi M, Gertzbein SD, Harms J, Nazarian S. A comprehensive classification of thoracic and lumbar injuries. *Eur Spine J*. 1994;3(4):184–201.
16. Vaccaro AR, Lehman RA, Hurlbert RJ, et al. A new classification of thoracolumbar injuries: the importance of injury morphology, the integrity of the posterior ligamentous complex, and neurologic status. *Spine*. 2005;30(20):2325–2333.
17. Denis F. The three column spine and its significance in the classification of acute thoracolumbar spinal injuries. *Spine*. 1983;8(8):817–831.
18. Patel AA, Dailey A, Brodke DS, et al. Thoracolumbar spine trauma classification: the Thoracolumbar Injury Classification and Severity Score system and case examples. *J Neurosurg Spine*. 2009;10(3):201–206.
19. Hott JS, Feiz-Erfan I, Kenny K, Dickman CA. Surgical management of giant herniated thoracic discs: analysis of 20 cases. *J Neurosurg Spine*. 2005;3(3):191–197.
20. Arce CA, Dohrmann GJ. Herniated thoracic disks. *Neurol Clin*. 1985 May;3(2):383–392.
21. Currier BL, Eismont FJ, Green BA. Transthoracic disc excision and fusion for herniated thoracic discs. *Spine*. 1994;19(3):323–328.
22. Oppenlander ME, Clark JC, Kalyvas J, Dickman CA. Surgical management and clinical outcomes of multiple-level symptomatic herniated thoracic discs. *J Neurosurg Spine*. 2013 Dec;19(6):774–783.
23. Martirosyan NL, Feuerstein JS, Theodore N, Cavalcanti DD, Spetzler RF, Preul MC. Blood supply and vascular reactivity of the spinal cord under normal and pathological conditions. *J Neurosurg Spine*. 2011;15(3):238–251.

24. Leung YL, Grevitt M, Henderson L, Smith J. Cord monitoring changes and segmental vessel ligation in the "at risk" cord during anterior spinal deformity surgery. *Spine*. 2005;30(16):1870–1874.

25. Mummaneni PV, Haid RW, Rodts GE. Lumbar interbody fusion: state-of-the-art technical advances. Invited submission from the Joint Section Meeting on Disorders of the Spine and Peripheral Nerves, March 2004. *J Neurosurg Spine*. 2004;1(1):24–30.

26. Sundaresan N, Steinberger AA, Moore F, et al. Indications and results of combined anterior-posterior approaches for spine tumor surgery. *J Neurosurg*. 1996;85(3):438–446.

27. Dimar JR, Carreon LY, Glassman SD, Campbell MJ, Hartman MJ, Johnson JR. Treatment of pyogenic vertebral osteomyelitis with anterior debridement and fusion followed by delayed posterior spinal fusion. *Spine*. 2004;29(3):326–332. discussion 332.

28. Vaccaro AR, Lim MR, Hurlbert RJ, et al. Surgical decision making for unstable thoracolumbar spine injuries: results of a consensus panel review by the Spine Trauma Study Group. *J Spinal Disord Tech*. 2006;19(1):1–10.

29. Acosta FL, Liu J, Slimack N, Moller D, Fessler R, Koski T. Changes in coronal and sagittal plane alignment following minimally invasive direct lateral interbody fusion for the treatment of degenerative lumbar disease in adults: a radiographic study. *J Neurosurg Spine*. 2011;15 (1):92–96.

30. Dakwar E, Cardona RF, Smith DA, Uribe JS. Early outcomes and safety of the minimally invasive, lateral retroperitoneal transpsoas approach for adult degenerative scoliosis. *Neurosurg Focus*. 2010;28(3).

31. Tohmeh AG, Rodgers WB, Peterson MD. Dynamically evoked, discrete-threshold electromyography in the extreme lateral interbody fusion approach. *J Neurosurg Spine*. 2011;14(1):31–37.

32. Berjano P, Lamartina C. Minimally invasive lateral transpsoas approach with advanced neurophysiologic monitoring for lumbar interbody fusion. *Eur Spine J*. 2011.

33. Boysen PG. Perioperative management of the thoracotomy patient. *Clin Chest Med*. 1993;14(2):321–333.

34. Loguidice VA, Johnson RG, Guyer RD, et al. Anterior lumbar interbody fusion. *Spine*. 1988;13(3):366–369.

35. Benglis DM, Vanni S, Levi AD. An anatomical study of the lumbosacral plexus as related to the minimally invasive transpsoas approach to the lumbar spine. *J Neurosurg Spine*. 2009;10 (2):139–144.

36. Rodgers WB, Gerber EJ, Patterson J. Intraoperative and early postoperative complications in extreme lateral interbody fusion: an analysis of 600 cases. *Spine*. 2011;36(1):26–32.

37. Barrera R, Shi W, Amar D, et al. Smoking and timing of cessation: impact on pulmonary complications after thoracotomy. *Chest*. 2005;127(6):1977–1983.

38. Baron EM, Albert TJ. Medical complications of surgical treatment of adult spinal deformity and how to avoid them. *Spine*. 2006;31(19 Suppl):S106–S118.

39. De Giacomo T, Francioni F, Diso D, et al. Anterior approach to the thoracic spine. *Interact Cardiovasc Thorac Surg*. 2011;12(5):692–695.

40. Baumann MH, Strange C. The clinician's perspective on pneumothorax management. *Chest*. 1997;112(3):822–828.

41. Sullivan PS, Dente CJ, Patel S, et al. Outcome of ligation of the inferior vena cava in the modern era. *Am J Surg*. 2010;199(4):500–506.

42. Marts BC, Naunheim KS, Fiore AC, Pennington DG. Conservative versus surgical management of chylothorax. *Am J Surg*. 1992;164 (5):532–534. discussion 534–5.

43. Shimizu K, Yoshida J, Nishimura M, Takamochi K, Nakahara R, Nagai K. Treatment strategy for chylothorax after pulmonary resection and lymph node dissection for lung cancer. *J Thorac Cardiovasc Surg*. 2002;124(3):499–502.

44. Renner H, Gabor S, Pinter H, Maier A, Friehs G, Smolle-Juettner FM. Is aggressive surgery in pleural empyema justified? *Eur J Cardiothorac Surg*. 1998;14(2):117–122.

45. Rajaraman V, Vingan R, Roth P, Heary RF, Conklin L, Jacobs GB. Visceral and vascular complications resulting from anterior lumbar interbody fusion. *J Neurosurg Spine*. 1999;91(1):60–64.

46. Gumbs AA, Hanan S, Yue JJ, Shah RV, Sumpio B. Revision open anterior approaches for spine procedures. *Spine J*. 2007;7(3):280–285.

47. Rauzzino MJ, Shaffrey CI, Nockels RP, Wiggins GC, Rock J, Wagner J. Anterior lumbar fusion with titanium threaded and mesh interbody cages. *Neurosurg Focus*. 1999;7(6).

48. Baker JK, Reardon PR, Reardon MJ, Heggeness MH. Vascular injury in anterior lumbar surgery. *Spine*. 1993;18(15):2227–2230.

49. Wood KB, Devine J, Fischer D, Dettori JR, Janssen M. Vascular injury in elective anterior lumbosacral surgery. *Spine*. 2010;35(9 Suppl):S66–S75.

50. Saraph V, Lerch C, Walochnik N, Bach CM, Krismer M, Wimmer C. Comparison of conventional versus minimally invasive extraperitoneal approach for anterior lumbar interbody fusion. *Eur Spine J*. 2004;13(5):425–431.

51. Flynn JC, Price CT. Sexual complications of anterior fusion of the lumbar spine. *Spine*. 1984;9(5):489–492.

52. Carragee EJ, Mitsunaga KA, Hurwitz EL, Scuderi GJ. Retrograde ejaculation after anterior lumbar interbody fusion using rhBMP-2: a cohort controlled study. *Spine J*. 2011 Jun;11(6):511–516.

53. Pumberger M, Hughes AP, Huang RR, Sama AA, Cammisa FP, Girardi FP. Neurologic deficit following lateral lumbar interbody fusion. *Eur Spine J*. 2012;21(6):1192–1199.

54. Cahill KS, Martinez JL, Wang MY, Vanni S, Levi AD. Motor nerve injuries following the minimally invasive lateral transpsoas approach. *J Neurosurg Spine*. 2012;17(3):227–231.

# Endovascular Neurosurgery

# 34  *Carotid and Intracranial Stent Placement*

BRYAN MOORE, ROBERT TAYLOR, CUONG NGUYEN, and MICHELLE J. SMITH

## Neuroanatomy and Procedure

### Key Concepts

- Balloon angioplasty and stenting are commonly performed to treat patients with cervical internal carotid artery stenosis.
- Stent placement for intracranial arterial stenosis has declined in use since the Stenting versus Aggressive Medical Therapy for Intracranial Arterial Stenosis (SAMMPRIS) trial and is indicated only for symptomatic, medically refractory cases.
- Stent-assisted coiling is routinely used to electively treat wide-necked intracranial aneurysms.
- Flow-diversion devices are utilized for large and giant wide-necked intracranial aneurysms.

### CERVICAL CAROTID ARTERY STENT PLACEMENT

The critical care management of patients undergoing carotid stent placement begins with an understanding of the indications for the procedure. The latest American Heart Association/American Stroke Association (AHA/ ASA) guidelines make a statement about the carotid artery stent (CAS) as a reasonable alternative to carotid endarterectomy (CEA) in normal-surgical-risk patients largely based on the results of the Carotid Revascularization Endarterectomy Versus Stenting Trial (CREST) trial:[1,2]

*CAS is indicated as an alternative to CEA for symptomatic patients at average or low risk of complications associated with endovascular intervention when the diameter of the lumen of the internal carotid artery is reduced by more than 70% as documented by noninvasive imaging or more than 50% as documented by catheter angiography and the anticipated rate of periprocedural stroke or mortality is less than 6% (Class IIb, Level of Evidence: B).*

However, CAS tends to be preferentially performed over CEA in patients at high risk for endarterectomy. The AHA/ ASA guidelines' statement about this approach to patient management is as follows:[2]

*Among patients with symptomatic severe stenosis (>70%) in whom anatomical or medical conditions are present that greatly increase the risk for surgery, or when other specific circumstances exist, such as radiation-induced stenosis or restenosis after CEA, CAS is reasonable (Class IIa; Level of Evidence B) (Secondary stroke prevention).*

Therefore it is best to understand the patient's high-risk medical or anatomical factors.[3] These are summarized in Box 34.1.

The next important aspect of managing patients undergoing CAS is having a basic understanding of the procedure. CAS is routinely performed under monitored anesthesia care, as opposed to general endotracheal anesthesia, in order to obtain serial neurological assessments and avoid large fluctuations in heart rate and blood pressure. Typically, a large sheath is placed in the femoral artery. Through this sheath, catheters are navigated under fluoroscopic guidance beyond the aortic arch into the distal common carotid artery (Fig. 34.1A–B). Next, a distal embolic protection (DEP) device is navigated past the area of stenosis into the distal cervical internal carotid artery (Fig. 34.1C). After the DEP device has been deployed, a noncompliant balloon is navigated over the guidewire and is temporarily inflated within the area of stenosis. At this point, communication with the anesthesia team is critical because balloon inflation often induces transient bradycardia, necessitating treatment with an anticholinergic agent such as glycopyrrolate. Once the balloon is deflated and removed, a stent is then guided over the wire and deployed within the area of previous stenosis. Lastly, the DEP device is retrieved and withdrawn. A final angiographic run confirms adequate resolution of the stenosis, no dissection of the artery, and good expansion and placement of the stent (Fig. 34.1D–E).

### INTRACRANIAL STENT PLACEMENT

Contrary to CAS, stent placement for intracranial arterial stenosis has declined in use since the SAMMPRIS trial published in 2011.[4] This trial randomly assigned 451 patients with recent transient ischemic attack (TIA) or stroke attributed to 70% to 99% intracranial arterial stenosis to aggressive medical management alone versus aggressive medical management plus angioplasty with the use of the Wingspan stent system (Stryker, Kalamazoo, MI). The trial was stopped early due to higher 30-day stroke or death rate in the interventional group (14.7%) compared with the medical therapy group (5.8%). The trial reported a high periprocedural complication rate. Of the 32 complications, 9 were hemorrhagic strokes and 23 were ischemic. Of the hemorrhagic strokes, four were due to vessel ruptures likely from microwire perforations and five were thought to be reperfusion hemorrhages. Of the ischemic strokes, most were considered perforator infarcts from the basilar artery.[5]

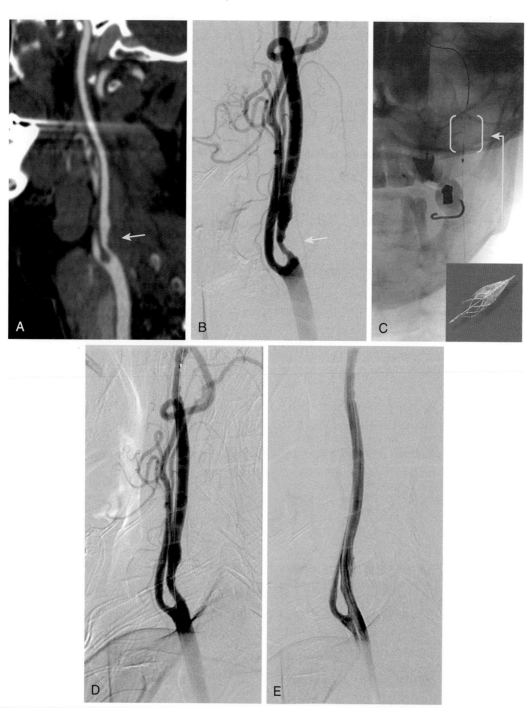

**Fig. 34.1** A 66-year-old female smoker admitted with acute bilateral middle cerebral artery (MCA) watershed infarcts, found to have right internal carotid artery (ICA) occlusion (not shown) and 65% left ICA stenosis as demonstrated on CTA **(A)** and cervical digital subtraction angiography (DSA) **(B)**. The patient underwent CAS with deployment of an Accunet Rx distal embolic protection device **(C)**. Postintervention DSA (**D**: post balloon angioplasty; **E**: post stenting) shows significant reduction in stenosis with approximately 10% residual narrowing after stent placement. (Inset for **(C)** Courtesy of Abbott Vascular. ©2013 Abbott. All Rights Reserved.)

A new postmarket surveillance study of the Wingspan stent system post market surveillance study (WEAVE) is underway to further investigate whether angioplasty and stenting with this system can reach an acceptable stroke or death rate of 6.6% or less. Several considerations for periprocedure risk are being taken into account. Only patients who have a recurrent stroke (not TIA) despite medical therapy are currently being considered for the trial. Patients are being treated after 7 days from the last stroke because patients treated within 7 days had higher complication rates in the SAMMPRIS trial.[4]

When intracranial arterial angioplasty and stenting is utilized for very specific, medically refractory cases, the procedure is performed under general endotracheal anesthesia. Typically a 6 French sheath is placed in the femoral artery and, under fluoroscopic guidance, a guide catheter is navigated into the cervical internal carotid or vertebral artery. At this time, heparin is administered intravenously to achieve an activated clotting time of >250. Next, a noncompliant balloon microcatheter is navigated over a microwire across the area of stenosis. Under fluoroscopic guidance, the balloon is inflated to a nominal pressure to expand the area of stenosis. Care is taken not to overinflate

the balloon in order to avoid vessel rupture. Next, after the balloon microcatheter is withdrawn, a separate microcatheter is navigated beyond the area of stenosis. The stent is then threaded through this microcatheter. As the microcatheter is withdrawn, the stent is "unsheathed" across the area of previous stenosis. Postintervention catheter angiography is then performed, demonstrating appropriate placement of the stent and normal filling of all parent and branch vessels (Fig. 34.2 A–E).

Contrary to its use for stenosis, intracranial stent placement for assistance in elective treatment of brain aneurysms is very common. Prior to detaching coils in wide-necked aneurysms, self-expanding intracranial stents, such as the Neuroform EZ (Stryker, Kalamazoo, MI) and Enterprise (Cordis, Miami, FL), can be deployed and prevent coil loops from herniating into the parent vessel (Fig. 34.3 A–D). This stent-assisted coil technique has been shown to achieve a high rate of long-term aneurysm occlusion with a very acceptable risk profile in patients undergoing elective treatment for aneurysms.[6,7]

Finally, a flow-diversion device, namely the Pipeline Embolization Device (PED) (EV3 Neurovascular, Irvine, CA),

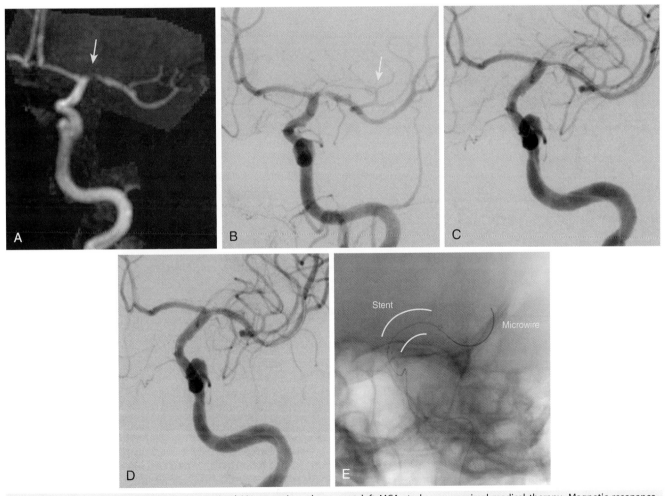

**Fig. 34.2** A 62-year-old man with severe proximal M1 stenosis and recurrent left MCA strokes on maximal medical therapy. Magnetic resonance angiogram (MRA) **(A)** and subsequent cerebral DSA **(B)** showed severe stenosis (>90%) of the proximal M1 MCA. The patient underwent angioplasty and stenting. Postintervention DSA (**C**: post balloon angioplasty; **D**: post stenting) shows significant reduction in stenosis with no significant residual narrowing after stent placement. Unsubtracted image **(E)** shows Wingspan stent in place, extending from the left supraclinoid ICA to mid left M1 MCA.

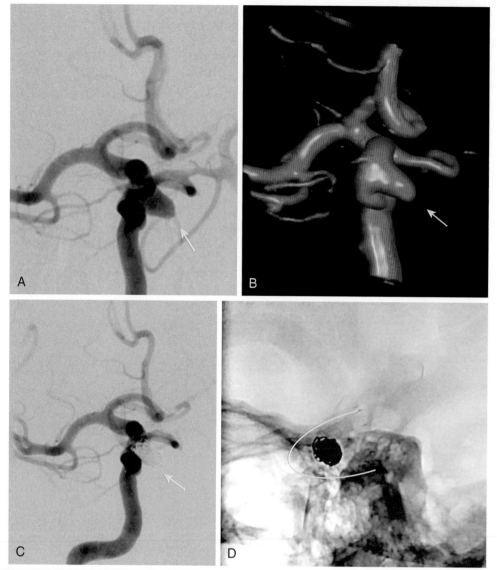

**Fig. 34.3** A 67-year-old woman nonsmoker with history of hypertension and incidental unruptured wide-necked 5.5 × 4.0 × 5.0 mm (dome × diameter × neck) right superior hypophyseal artery aneurysm as demonstrated on cerebral DSA **(A)** and 3D volume-rendered image of a rotational angiogram **(B)**. Angiogram post stent-assisted coil embolization shows exclusion of the aneurysm with minimal filing at the aneurysm base. Unsubstracted image **(D)** shows an Enterprise stent (*curved line*) across the aneurysm neck, extending from the supraclinoid to cavernous segment of the right ICA.

has been approved for use in large and giant wide-necked aneurysms of the internal carotid artery from the petrous to the superior hypophyseal artery segments. This is a sten-tlike device constructed of a fine network of cobalt and chromium mesh resulting in 30% to 35% metal surface area coverage. After microcatheter delivery and deployment of this device, stagnation of blood flow occurs in the aneurysm, leading to chronic occlusion and neoendothelialization of the vessel wall (Fig. 34.4A–F). Early studies have demonstrated a 70% to 90% occlusion rate at 180 days.[8,9] The Flow Re-Direction Endoluminal Device (Microvention-Terumo, Tustin, CA), a similar flow-diversion technology, is currently in phase II and III trials for Food and Drug Administration approval.

Although these devices provide a welcome treatment option for extremely challenging aneurysms with a poor natural history and paucity of other safe and effective treatments,

the risk of adverse event may be higher than with traditional endovascular techniques for simpler aneurysms.[10] Additionally, the PED is being utilized more frequently for off-label purposes, and long-term outcome studies are needed.

The technique for deployment of these devices is similar to those for intracranial arterial angioplasty and stenting; however, no balloon angioplasty is performed. Additionally, for specific cases, two microcatheters are placed within the guide catheter simultaneously in order to performing a "jailing" technique. This includes navigating the first microcatheter into the aneurysm neck, where it will remain while the stent is deployed through the second microcatheter. This enables the first microcatheter to already be in optimal position for coiling as opposed to subsequently navigating that catheter through the stent tines into the aneurysm neck. These procedures are also routinely performed with the patient fully anticoagulated with heparin.

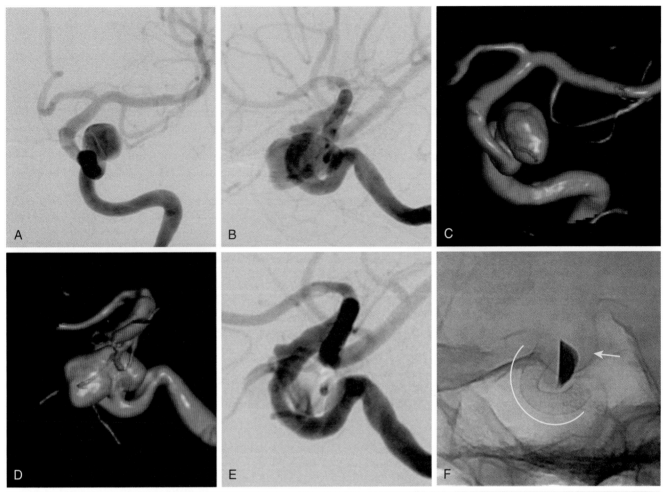

**Fig. 34.4** A 67-year-old woman smoker with incidental unruptured $15 \times 9 \times 5$ mm (dome $\times$ diameter $\times$ neck) left supraclinoid ICA aneurysm as seen on cerebral DSA (**A**: AP projection; **B**: lateral projection) and 3D volume-rendered images of a rotational angiogram (**C** and **D**). Angiogram postdeployment of Pipeline embolization device shows reduction in filling of the aneurysm (**E**) with expected stagnation within aneurysm as seen on unsubtracted image (**F**; Pipeline device outlined by curved line).

## Perioperative Considerations

### Key Concepts

- Maintaining hemodynamic stability while stenting is important and may require anticholinergic agents or pressors.
- Cervical and intracranial stents are thrombogenic.
- Dual antiplatelet therapy for stenting is the current standard of care.
- Individual patients may be resistant to certain antiplatelet medications.
- Platelet function testing with the VerifyNow method is common, although controversial, and generates a P2Y12 reaction unit (PRU) value.
- Increasing the dose of clopidogrel and use of prasugrel or ticagrelor have been proposed as mechanisms to reduce the incidence of thromboembolic events for patients resistant to clopidogrel.

### CERVICAL CAROTID ARTERY STENT PLACEMENT

There are several perioperative considerations when performing balloon angioplasty and stent placement for cervical carotid stenosis. The first is regarding prevention of thromboembolic complications by utilizing adequate antiplatelet medications. Cervical carotid stents are inherently thrombogenic, and the standard regimen includes starting acetylsalicylic acid (ASA) 325 mg and clopidogrel 75 mg daily. The exact regimens used are heterogeneous and often based on regional practice patterns[11]; however, at our institution elective stent patients are routinely premedicated with ASA 325 mg and clopidogrel 75 mg daily for 5 days prior to the procedure and for 3 months afterward. Patients requiring emergency stenting receive a loading dose of ASA 325 mg and clopidogrel 600 mg 1 day prior to the procedure and then continue standard-dose ASA 325 mg and clopidogrel 75 mg daily for 3 months. At that point, clopidogrel is discontinued and ASA 81 mg is continued for life.

Another perioperative consideration regarding CAS includes maintaining adequate control of blood pressure and heart rate. Patients with severe stenosis, especially with contralateral carotid occlusions or tandem stenoses, may be dependent on systemic blood pressure to maintain cerebral perfusion. For this reason, hypotension should be avoided to prevent perioperative ischemia or stroke.

Additionally, balloon angioplasty and catheter manipulation within the carotid bulb can trigger a baroreceptor reflex inducing significant bradycardia or hypotension. Bradycardic episodes are often controlled with anticholinergic agents such as glycopyrrolate or atropine, and hypotension refractory to fluid boluses may be treated with vasopressor agents.

## INTRACRANIAL STENT PLACEMENT

Similar to carotid stents, intracranial stents are also thrombogenic and require adequate dual antiplatelet therapy. Practice patterns regarding these medications are also extremely heterogeneous. At our institution, prior to placement of the Wingspan (Stryker, Kalamazoo, MI), Enterprise (Cordis, Miami, FL), or Neuroform (Stryker, Kalamazoo, MI) stent, a protocol identical to cervical carotid stents is followed. However, the antiplatelet regimen for placement of a flow-diversion device is more involved given the potentially higher rate of thromboembolic and hemorrhagic complications associated with this device. First, a patient is placed on daily ASA 325 mg and clopidogrel 75 mg for a minimum of 5 days. Next, a point-of-care testing (VerifyNow, Accumetrics, Sparta, NJ) is performed to assess for resistance to clopidogrel. If resistance is suspected, clopidogrel is stopped and an alternative antiplatelet agent such as prasugrel (10 mg daily) is initiated. Additionally, if point-of-care testing demonstrates that a patient is a "hyperresponder" to clopidogrel, he or she may be switched to 75 mg every other day. Finally, after PED placement, dual antiplatelet therapy is continued until follow-up imaging demonstrates complete thrombosis of the aneurysm. Practice patterns regarding antiplatelet therapy surrounding flow-diversion devices and point-of-care testing remains controversial.[11]

## CONSIDERATIONS FOR ANTIPLATELET MEDICATION TREATMENT

Controversy surrounding antiplatelet medication regimens and testing exists for several reasons. First, most data regarding these factors are extrapolated from the cardiac literature, given the paucity of studies directly addressing neurovascular patients. Cardiologists have conducted numerous studies looking at the efficacy of dual antiplatelet therapy with aspirin and clopidogrel in the prevention of in-stent thrombosis after coronary artery interventions. Their results have been applied to both carotid and intracranial artery stenting.[12–15] There is significant heterogeneity in the response that patients will have to standard doses of antiplatelet agents. Every measure must be made to administer an adequate antiplatelet regimen in the perioperative period. Preoperative testing of platelet function can serve as a guide to ensure patient response to antiplatelet therapy.

Although most patients benefit from dual therapy with aspirin and clopidogrel after stenting, approximately one-third of the studied population has high residual platelet activity while on clopidogrel and therefore qualifies as "clopidogrel resistant."[16] Numerous laboratory studies can quantify the level of antiplatelet activity that aspirin or clopidogrel achieves in an individual patient. The gold-standard is light transmission aggregometry, a laboratory-based method that is labor intensive and lacks a high level of interlaboratory standardization. Another laboratory-based method is the vasodilator-stimulated phosphoprotein assay, which is somewhat insensitive for low P2Y12 receptor blockade.[17] Common point-of-care testing methods include multiple electrode platelet aggregometry, thrombelastography, Platelet Function Assay 100, and the VerifyNow System. The VerifyNow System (Accumetrics, CA) warrants explanation due to its common use in clinical practice. The test uses citrated whole blood under light transmission–based optical detection to measure adenosine diphosphate–induced platelet aggregation in a cartridge containing fibrinogen-coated beads.[18] The assay generates PRUs that are a metric of resistance to clopidogrel, with higher PRU values indicating more resistance to clopidogrel. A PRU value of 235 to 240 is generally accepted as the cutoff for "clopidogrel resistance."[19]

The CYP2C19 hepatic isoenzyme plays a major role in the bioactivation of the prodrug form of clopidogrel. Variant forms of CYP2C19 may lead to either hypo-activation or hyperactivation of clopidogrel, leading to a low percent inhibition with a high PRU value or a high percent inhibition with a low PRU value, respectively (Table 34.1).

In patients who are clopidogrel resistant and on maintenance therapy, doubling the dose of clopidogrel increases platelet inhibition.[20] A recent multicenter randomized trial studied increased clopidogrel maintenance dosing based on the results of platelet function tests. In patients with high residual platelet reactivity, the Gauging Responsiveness with A VerifyNow Assay–Impact on Thrombosis And Safety trial showed neither benefit nor harm in the high-dose clopidogrel group compared with standard dosing.

Another proposed option to reduce the likelihood of in-stent thrombosis is to place patients with clopidogrel resistance on a different inhibitor of the platelet adenosine diphosphate receptor. Prasugrel and ticagrelor have both been found to have more predictable and homogeneous antiplatelet effects compared with clopidogrel. Both have a faster onset of action than clopidogrel and also have less interpatient variability in their metabolism. However, the Assessment by a Double Randomization of a Conventional Antiplatelet Strategy versus a Monitoring-guided Strategy for Drug-Eluting Stent Implantation and of Treatment Interruption versus Continuation One Year after Stenting

**Table 34.1**  CYP2C19 Isoforms and Clopidogrel Response

| Isoform | Bioactivation of prodrug | Percent Inhibition | PRUs | Clinical result |
|---|---|---|---|---|
| CYP2C19*2 | Decreased | Decreased | Increased | Increased risk of thrombosis |
| CYP2C19*17 | Increased | Increased | Decreased | Increased risk of bleeding |

*PRU*, P2Y12 reaction unit.

trial failed to show a significant reduction in all-cause death, myocardial infarction, stroke, or TIA in the conventional group versus the monitored group.[21]

Personalized antiplatelet therapy continues to be studied, but no randomized controlled trial has shown a benefit in the clinical setting thus far.

# Complications (Table 34.2)

## Key Concepts

- Stroke has been reported in 4.1% of CAS cases and is associated with worse overall functional outcome.
- Stretch applied to carotid baroreceptors during balloon angioplasty can cause significant hypotension and bradycardia, referred to as *CAS dysautonomia*.
- Cerebral hyperperfusion syndrome (CHS) occurs after carotid or intracranial angioplasty due to loss of vessel autoregulation distal to the site of stenosis.
- Periprocedural myocardial infarction (PMI) leads to increased morbidity and mortality after endovascular procedures.
- Access site complication rates can be extrapolated from the coronary intervention literature and are reported between 0.6% and 6.0%.

## ACUTE STROKE AFTER CAROTID STENTING

Perhaps the most feared complication after CAS is stroke. According to results of the CREST trial, 4.1% of 1262 CAS patients experienced perioperative stroke within the first 30 days.[1] Furthermore, stroke was significantly associated with worse functional outcome at 1 year according to the Medical Outcomes Study 36-Item Short-Form Health Survey (SF-36) and mental component scale.[1] Regarding intracranial angioplasty and stenting for intracranial stenosis, the SAMMPRIS trial was a prospective randomized controlled trial studying intervention versus medical management. This study reported periprocedural, nonfatal stroke in 12.5% and fatal stroke in 2.2% of patients receiving intracranial angioplasty and stent placement.[4,22] The study was stopped early because the primary endpoint of stroke or death was reached in a significantly higher percentage of patients undergoing intervention.

Etiology of ischemic stroke after cervical and intracranial stenting is varied but can include embolic events, hypoperfusion, and in-stent thrombosis. The source of embolic material may be air emboli introduced at the time of the procedure, thrombotic emboli from the catheters or stent, and/or atherosclerotic plaque material at the time of balloon angioplasty if distal embolic protection is not possible or fails. Given the technical challenges of CAS, several

**Table 34.2** Complications of Cervical and Intracranial Stent Placement

| Complication | Etiology | Management |
|---|---|---|
| Stroke | | |
| Ischemic | Hypotension<br>Thromboembolic (air, plaque, clot)<br>In-stent thrombosis | Hydration<br>Pressors<br>Anticholinergics<br>Tissue plasminogen activator<br>Glycoprotein IIb/IIIa Inhibitor<br>Angioplasty<br>Mechanical thrombectomy |
| Hemorrhagic | Hyperperfusion<br>Thromboembolic<br>Aneurysm rupture | Anticoagulant reversal<br>Consideration of antiplatelet reversal<br>Aneurysm retreatment<br>Neurosurgical intervention |
| Autonomic dysfunction | Baroreceptor reflex | Hydration<br>Anticholinergics<br>Pressors |
| Cerebral hyperperfusion syndrome | Impaired cerebral autoregulation | Lower blood pressure<br>Antiepileptics |
| Acute coronary syndrome, MI | Ruptured coronary plaque<br>Myocardial demand ischemia | Continue ASA<br>Decrease myocardial demand<br>Cardiac intervention |
| Access site complications | | |
| Hematoma<br>-Superficial<br>-Retroperitoneal | Insufficient compression<br>Puncture above inguinal ligament | Manual compression<br>Ultrasound-guided compression resuscitation<br>Anticoagulant reversal |
| Pseudoaneurysm | Insufficient compression<br>dissection | Manual compression<br>Ultrasound-guided compression<br>Thrombin injection |
| Thromboembolism | Dissection<br>Use of closure device | Anticoagulation<br>Vascular surgery |

*MI*, myocardial infarction; *ASA*, acetylsalicylic acid.

studies have demonstrated an inverse relationship between operator experience and rate of these complications.[23]

Although acute in-stent thrombosis is a rare event reported between 0.5% and 2.0% of CAS procedures, its occurrence can be catastrophic.[24] Early reports of this complication appeared to be related to insufficient anticoagulation and antiplatelet therapy prior to and during the procedure.[25] If a patient experiences stroke symptoms in the acute perioperative period, a stat noncontrast head computed tomogram (CT) followed by a computed tomography angiogram (CTA) of the neck and head should be obtained to rule out hemorrhage and to assess for small- or large-vessel occlusion. If thrombosis is present, the patient may return to the interventional suite for treatment with an intraarterial glycoprotein IIb/IIIa receptor antagonist such as abciximab or tissue plasminogen activator.[24] Occasionally, mechanical intervention with repeat balloon angioplasty or mechanical embolectomy can be performed. Similar to the concept of treatment for acute ischemic stroke, rapid intervention is essential to salvage ischemic brain tissue.

Hemorrhagic stroke occurs less frequently than acute ischemic stroke after CAS. A study evaluating incidence of intracerebral hemorrhage (ICH) after CAS utilizing the Nationwide Inpatient Sample database found a rate of 0.15% in a sample of 13,093 patients.[26] Excluding direct vessel perforation at the time of procedure, hemorrhagic stroke in the perioperative period is often due to cerebral hyperperfusion to previously deprived brain tissue (27). A rapid noncontrast head CT can be used to detect ICH. Treatment should include reversal of heparin with protamine, consideration of reversal of antiplatelet agents, and strict control of blood pressure. A large ICH causing significant mass effect and herniation may require surgical evacuation. All of these interventions must be done in close collaboration with both the interventionalist and neurosurgeon, because treatment decisions will be based on nuances of the preceding CAS procedure.

## AUTONOMIC DYSFUNCTION

### Background

Autonomic dysfunction after carotid revascularization with CAS or CEA has been labeled *hemodynamic instability, hemodynamic depression,* and "*CAS-related dysautonomia* (CAS-D) in the literature.[28–30] The syndrome consists of hypotension with systolic blood pressure less than 90 mm Hg and/or bradycardia with heart rate less than 60 beats per minute that occurs during balloon dilation of the carotid artery prior to stent placement. The hypotension and/or bradycardia may continue in the postprocedural period. The response can be profound enough to induce asystole or complete cessation of postganglionic sympathetic nerve activity.[31] Studies have shown that the incidence of CAS-D is 1.7% to 84%.[30,32] Difference in the incidence between studies is largely attributable to a lack of a standard definition for the syndrome.[33] The risk of CAS-D is higher than the risk of periprocedural stroke and myocardial infarction combined.[28]

### Pathophysiology

Baroreceptors in the carotid sinuses and aortic arch are a part of the vascular system's autoregulation in the setting of hemodynamic changes. Carotid sinus baroreceptors are free-nerve-ending mechanoreceptors that stretch in response to increased arterial blood pressure. Activation of baroreceptors results in increased firing of action potentials with the rapidity proportional to the degree of mechanical stretch.[28] Carotid baroreceptor response during CAS is most prominent during balloon inflation when the arterial wall sustains the greatest degree of acute radial force.[28] When the carotid sinus mechanoreceptors are activated by an increase in pressure, they transmit signals through afferent pathways in the glossopharyngeal nerve (CN IX) and the vagus nerve (CN X). These inputs synapse in the nucleus solitarius. The nucleus solitarius then projects to the caudal ventrolateral medulla, where the incoming excitatory signal from carotid baroreceptor afferent nerves produces inhibitory effects on sympathetic activity. The caudal ventrolateral medulla inhibits the rostral ventrolateral medulla via GABAergic interneurons. The rostral ventrolateral medulla is the origin of efferent sympathetic nerve activity.[28]

### Predictors of Dysautonomia after Carotid Artery Stenting

Studies looking at risk factors and demographic data to predict which patients will develop CAS-D have yielded mixed results. One case series of patients found that the degree of stenosis in the carotid artery prior to stenting was the only variable with significant correlation with occurrence of CAS-D.[33] No other risk factor or demographic data showed significant correlation with CAS-D. Another multicenter study by Qureshi et al. found that a history of myocardial infarction was predictive of CAS-D.[34] The largest study looking at risk factors for CAS-D analyzed 500 consecutive CAS procedures performed over a 5-year period.[29] Atherosclerotic lesions at the carotid bulb or the presence of a calcified plaque independently predicted CAS-D. Baroreceptors are exposed to dampened pressure waves when they are encased in calcium. They then receive an extraordinary stimulation by radial force due to balloon dilation. Calcified plaques may require more aggressive balloon inflation that triggers an amplified baroreflex response.[28] Prior ipsilateral CEA, history of diabetes, and use of a beta-blocker were associated with reduced risk of CAS-D.[29] Patients with prior ipsilateral endarterectomy may have sustained damage to their baroreceptors during surgery, which may explain why they have a lower incidence of CAS-D.[28] Sympathetic output may be impaired in diabetic patients due to underlying autonomic neuropathy. Smoking also provided protection from CAS-D. Smoking is known to increase sympathetic tone through the release of epinephrine and norepinephrine, thereby raising blood pressure and heart rate.[35] Mylonas et al. performed a metaanalysis of 27 studies with 4204 patients that showed that the only statistically significant associations for CAS-D were patient age, less than or equal to 10 mm distance between the carotid bifurcation and the site of minimum lumen diameter, and prior ipsilateral CEA.[36]

### Outcomes

In a case series of 461 patients, Gupta et al. found that persistent hemodynamic depression was associated with an increased risk of periprocedural major adverse clinical events and stroke.[29] Persistent CAS-D was defined as a requirement for continuous pressor infusion. Major adverse events were defined as myocardial infarction, stroke, or death. Howell et al. found a linear correlation between the magnitude of periprocedural systolic blood pressure change and the incidence of adverse neurological events.[37] Conversely, in a series of 471 patients Mlekusch et al. found no differences in the rates of neurological complications between the groups of patients with and without CAS-D. The Mylonas et al. study similarly showed no difference in the rates of death, stroke, TIA, or major adverse events between the groups of patients with and without CAS-D. Based on the results of a prospective study following 223 patients, Cieri et al. concluded that even in severe CAS-D there was no increased risk of adverse cerebrovascular or cardiac events.[38]

## Management

At present there is no standardized approach to the treatment of CAS-D. A frequent strategy includes periprocedural hydration and prophylactic use of anticholinergic agents. Cayne et al. evaluated the use of prophylactic atropine administration before balloon inflation during CAS. They found a decreased incidence of intraoperative bradycardia and a decrease in perioperative cardiac morbidity in patients who received prophylactic atropine compared with patients who did not receive prophylactic atropine.[32] In addition, they noted a lower incidence of perioperative hypotension and vasopressor requirement to maintain goal heart rate or blood pressure in the group that received atropine versus the control group.[32] Nandalur et al. used a retrospective analysis to examine the effect of vasopressor choice on the outcomes in patients treated for CAS-D.[39] The study showed that phenylephrine might be preferable to treat CAS-D. Patients in the phenylephrine treatment group had a lower mean vasopressor infusion time, reduced intensive care unit (ICU) length of stay, and a reduced rate of major adverse events compared with the dopamine treatment group.

The most comprehensive treatment algorithm available was developed by a team of physicians at Yale New Haven Hospital.[28] In this algorithm, all patients are advised to discontinue any atrioventricular nodal blocking agent at least 24 hours prior to planned CAS. The majority of patients are also asked to hold their morning dose of antihypertensive medication. All patients with a pulse less than 60 receive prophylactic atropine prior to dilation of the carotid lesion. All patients receive atropine after dilation and prior to stent placement. If asymptomatic bradycardia persists, then no further intervention is performed. First-line treatment for isolated periprocedural hypotension is an intravenous bolus of 0.9% saline, followed by boluses of phenylephrine, followed by a phenylephrine infusion titrated to a mean arterial pressure greater than 65 mm Hg and/or systolic blood pressure >90 mm Hg. In the case of persistent hypotension lasting longer than 12 hours, midodrine 10 mg PO tid is started.

Other common aspects of care include continuous telemetry for cardiac monitoring and continuous blood pressure monitoring via an arterial line. It is standard to admit patients from the angiography suite to an ICU, where atropine and cardiac pacing devices are immediately available. If home antihypertensives or atrioventricular nodal blocking agents were continued periprocedurally and the patient developed CAS-D, then the medications should be immediately discontinued. In rare instances patients will need placement of a transvenous pacemaker. Prophylactic transvenous pacing is not currently recommended due to the risk of inducing ventricular arrhythmias and of atrial or ventricular perforation.

## CEREBRAL HYPERPERFUSION SYNDROME

CHS is a life-threatening complication that occurs in approximately 3% of all patients after carotid angioplasty with stenting.[40] CHS is defined by a 100% or greater increase in cerebral blood flow over a patient's baseline after angioplasty and stent placement. The pathophysiologic mechanisms involved in increased cerebral blood flow are alterations of cerebrovascular autoregulation and increased postangioplasty systolic arterial blood pressure.[41] The chronic low-flow state caused by severe carotid or intracranial arterial disease results in a compensatory dilation of cerebral vessels distal to the stenosis as part of the normal autoregulatory response to maintain cerebral blood flow. The vessels distal to the region of stenosis lose their ability to autoregulate resistance in response to changes in blood pressure. This results in increased cerebral blood flow after recanalization because autoregulation has been lost and systolic blood pressure and cerebral blood flow have a more linear relationship than if autoregulation was intact.

Risk factors for CHS include postangioplasty hypertension, increased severity of pretreatment stenosis, and the presence of contralateral carotid artery stenosis or occlusion.[42] If measures are not taken to reduce the cerebral blood flow to the at-risk brain parenchyma, then significant edema can develop, as well as intraparenchymal or subarachnoid hemorrhage. Diseased arterioles may not be able to constrict to reduce hydrostatic pressure, contributing to development of edema.[43]

Numerous imaging modalities can play a role in investigating suspected CHS, including transcranial Doppler (TCD) ultrasonography, single-photon emission computed tomography (SPECT), computed tomography with or without perfusion imaging (CT or CT-P), and magnetic resonance imaging (MRI) with diffusion and perfusion imaging. TCD can be used to assess a patient's baseline vasomotor reactivity in the preoperative period. Patients who have exhausted their cerebrovascular reactivity are at increased risk for CHS, which can be confirmed with postoperative TCD showing an increase in flow velocities of more than 100%. Noncontrast CT scan of a patient with CHS may be normal or show patchy edema in the parenchyma distal to the angioplasty site. CT-P and magnetic resonance perfusion can both show an increase in cerebral blood flow over baseline to the vascular territory distal to angioplasty, with MRI possibly showing local edema, infarct, or hemorrhage. SPECT scan can also demonstrate hyperperfusion, although cost limits its use in clinical practice.

## ACUTE CORONARY SYNDROME AND MYOCARDIAL INFARCTION

It is known that PMI leads to increased morbidity and mortality after vascular surgery or endovascular procedures.[44] PMI may be the consequence of rupture of an unstable coronary atherosclerotic plaque. More commonly PMI is due to severe but stable coronary artery disease and occurs within 48 hours of the endovascular procedure.[45] There are six subtypes of myocardial infarction, but only two of the subtypes commonly occur as PMI: type 1 PMI and type 2 PMI. Type 1 PMI involves thrombotic occlusion of a coronary artery. Type 2 PMI is due to a mismatch between myocardial supply and demand in the setting of stable but obstructive coronary atherosclerotic burden and physiological stress induced by a procedure. This is frequently referred to as *demand ischemia* by clinical providers. PMI in the noncardiac perisurgical period is most commonly type 2.[46]

PMI is diagnosed by the combination of elevated cardiac biomarkers, ischemic symptoms, and ischemic changes in a patient's electrocardiogram. In early PMI, any one of these features may be seen in isolation or they may be seen together,[47] and the World Health Organization defines PMI as any biomarker release alone.[48] Biomarker elevation has been associated with long-term morbidity and mortality after noncardiac surgery. The perioperative ischemic evaluation (POISE) trial looked at more than 8000 patients after noncardiac surgery, 40% of which were vascular surgeries other than CEA. POISE found that the incidence of PMI was 5% and that the 30-day mortality was 2.2% in patients without PMI and 11.5% in patients with PMI.

Analysis of outcomes from the CREST trial found an incidence of PMI of 2% in the CAS arm versus 3.4% in the CEA arm. All PMI in CREST imposed a significant increase in mortality risk, including biomarker-only PMI.[49] The percentage of biomarker-only PMI was similar between the CAS and the CEA arms of the CREST trial. Non-ST-elevation myocardial infarction was associated with worse long-term outcomes than ST-elevation myocardial infarction, possibly due to the lack of indication for emergent percutaneous coronary intervention.

## ACCESS SITE COMPLICATIONS

Access site complication rates can be extrapolated from the coronary intervention literature and are reported to range from 0.6% to 6.0%.[50] There are multiple factors associated with increased risk of this complication and include larger sheath size; repeated femoral artery access; thrombolytic, anticoagulant, and antiplatelet use; thrombocytopenia; postprocedural anticoagulation; increased duration of sheath placement; older age; and peripheral vascular disease.[50-52] Similar to coronary interventions, CAS is usually performed through relatively large catheters, namely a 6 French sheath or an 8 French guide catheter. Some centers utilize even larger diameter proximal embolic protection devices.[53]

The first of these access-related complications is hematoma. Superficial hematomas occur due to ineffective manual compression to close the femoral artery access site. They are usually recognized as a firm mass or raised area, deep to the skin, in the femoral region.[54] Small hematomas often only result in ecchymosis and are self-limited. Larger hematomas, especially when remaining in communication with femoral artery lumen, can cause pseudoaneurysm formation.[55-57] Pseudoaneurysms are diagnosed with palpation of a tender, pulsatile groin mass and are confirmed by duplex ultrasonography or CTA. Although usually benign, pseudoaneurysms do have a risk of rupture and are most often treated with ultrasound-guided compression or thrombin injection. Rarely, they require open surgical repair.[54]

A more serious type of hematoma, or bleeding complication, is a retroperitoneal hematoma. If arterial puncture occurs above the ilioinguinal ligament, hematoma may develop in the retroperitoneal space. This event leads to flank pain and hypotension. A CT of the abdomen and pelvis is utilized to confirm the diagnosis. A patient suspected of having a retroperitoneal hematoma must be monitored vigilantly. Treatment is often conservative and includes bed rest, blood transfusion and following serial hemoglobin levels. Anticoagulation may need to be reversed. If bleeding persists, surgical intervention may be required.[54]

Access complications also include thromboembolism at the femoral artery puncture site. Dissection or injury to the femoral artery may occur at the time of sheath placement and is also associated with use of access closure devices.[58] If arterial wall injury is severe, it may lead to complete thrombosis of the artery or thromboembolism to distal peripheral vasculature. Weakened or absent peripheral pulses along with a cool, pale, and painful lower extremity should prompt rapid evaluation with ultrasound or CTA. In cases of vascular compromise, surgery may be needed to extract the thrombus and repair the vessel wall.

## References

1. Mantese VA, Timaran CH, Chiu D, Begg RJ, Brott TG. The Carotid Revascularization Endarterectomy versus Stenting Trial (CREST): stenting versus carotid endarterectomy for carotid disease. *Stroke.* 2010;41(10 Suppl):S31–S34.
2. Furie KL, Kasner SE, Adams RJ, et al. Guidelines for the prevention of stroke in patients with stroke or transient ischemic attack: a guideline for healthcare professionals from the american heart association/american stroke association. *Stroke.* 2011;42 (1):227–276.
3. Roffi M, Mukherjee D, Clair DG. Carotid artery stenting vs. endarterectomy. *Eur Heart J.* 2009;30(22):2693–2704.
4. Chimowitz MI, Lynn MJ, Derdeyn CP, et al. Stenting versus aggressive medical therapy for intracranial arterial stenosis. *N Engl J Med.* 2011;365(11):993–1003.
5. Derdeyn CP, Fiorella D, Lynn MJ, et al. Intracranial stenting: SAMMPRIS. *Stroke.* 2013;44(6 Suppl 1):S41–S44.
6. Hetts SW, Turk A, English JD, et al. Stent-assisted coiling versus coiling alone in unruptured intracranial aneurysms in the matrix and platinum science trial: safety, efficacy, and mid-term outcomes. *Am J Neuroradiol.* 2014;35(4):698–705.
7. Mine B, Aljishi A, D'Harcour JB, Brisbois D, Collignon L, Lubicz B. Stent-assisted coiling of unruptured intracranial aneurysms: long-term follow-up in 164 patients with 183 aneurysms. *J Neuroradiol.* 2014;41(5):322–328.
8. Becske T, Kallmes DF, Saatci I, et al. Pipeline for uncoilable or failed aneurysms: results from a multicenter clinical trial. *Radiology.* 2013;267(3):858–868.
9. Nelson PK, Lylyk P, Szikora I, Wetzel SG, Wanke I, Fiorella D. The pipeline embolization device for the intracranial treatment of aneurysms trial. *Am J Neuroradiol.* 2011;32(1):34–40.
10. Phillips TJ, Wenderoth JD, Phatouros CC, et al. Safety of the pipeline embolization device in treatment of posterior circulation aneurysms. *Am J Neuroradiol.* 2012;33(7):1225–1231.
11. Faught RWF, Satti SR, Hurst RW, Pukenas BA, Smith MJ. Heterogeneous practice patterns regarding antiplatelet medications for neuroendovascular stenting in the USA: a multicenter survey. *J Neurointerv Surg.* 2014;10:774–779.

12. Bhatt DL, Topol EJ. Clopidogrel for High Atherothrombotic Risk and Ischemic Stabilization Management, and Avoidance Executive C. Clopidogrel added to aspirin versus aspirin alone in secondary prevention and high-risk primary prevention: rationale and design of the Clopidogrel for High Atherothrombotic Risk and Ischemic Stabilization, Management, and Avoidance (CHARISMA) trial. *Am Heart J.* 2004;148(2):263–268.

13. Spertus JA, Peterson E, Rumsfeld JS, et al. The Prospective Registry Evaluating Myocardial Infarction: Events and Recovery (PREMIER)—evaluating the impact of myocardial infarction on patient outcomes. *Am Heart J.* 2006;151(3):589–597.

14. Steinhubl SR, Berger PB, Mann 3rd JT, et al. Early and sustained dual oral antiplatelet therapy following percutaneous coronary intervention: a randomized controlled trial. *JAMA.* 2002;288(19):2411–2420.

15. Wallentin L. Dual antiplatelet therapy in the drug-eluting stent era. *Eur Heart J Supp.* 2008;10(D):D38–D44.

16. Siller-Matula J, Schror K, Wojta J, Huber K. Thienopyridines in cardiovascular disease: focus on clopidogrel resistance. *Thromb Haemost.* 2007;97(3):385–393.

17. Judge H, Buckland R, Sugidachi A, Jakubowski J, Storey R. Relationship between degree of P2Y12 receptor blockade and inhibition of P2Y12 mediated platelet function. *Thromb Haemos.* 2010;103(6):1210–1217.

18. Yamaguchi Y, Abe T, Sato Y, Matsubara Y, Moriki T, Murata M. Effects of VerifyNow P2Y12 test and CYP2C19*2 testing on clinical outcomes of patients with cardiovascular disease: a systematic review and meta-analysis. *Platelets.* 2013;24(5):352–361.

19. Bonello L, Tantry US, Marcucci R, et al. Consensus and future directions on the definition of high on-treatment platelet reactivity to adenosine diphosphate. *J Am Coll Cardiol.* 2010;56(12):919–933.

20. Angiolillo DJ, Bernardo E, Palazuelos J, et al. Functional impact of high clopidogrel maintenance dosing in patients undergoing elective percutaneous coronary interventions. Results of a randomized study. *Thromb Haemost.* 2008;99(1):161–168.

21. Collet JP, Cuisset T, Range G, et al. Bedside monitoring to adjust antiplatelet therapy for coronary stenting. *N Engl J Med.* 2012;367 (22):2100–2109.

22. Derdeyn CP, Chimowitz MI, Lynn MJ, et al. Aggressive medical treatment with or without stenting in high-risk patients with intracranial artery stenosis (SAMMPRIS): the final results of a randomised trial. *Lancet.* 2014;383(9914):333–341.

23. Khan M, Qureshi AI. Factors associated with increased rates of postprocedural stroke or death following carotid artery stent placement: a systematic review. *J Vasc Interv Neurol.* 2014;7(1):11–20.

24. Tong FC, Cloft HJ, Joseph GJ, Samuels OB, Dion JE. Abciximab rescue in acute carotid stent thrombosis. *Am J Neuroradiol.* 2000;21(9): 1750–1752.

25. Chaturvedi S, Sohrab S, Tselis A. Carotid stent thrombosis: report of 2 fatal cases. *Stroke.* 2001;32(11):2700–2702.

26. Timaran CH, Veith FJ, Rosero EB, Modrall JG, Valentine RJ, Clagett GP. Intracranial hemorrhage after carotid endarterectomy and carotid stenting in the United States in 2005. *J Vasc Surg.* 2009;49 (3):623–628. discussion 8–9.

27. Lieb M, Shah U, Hines GL. Cerebral hyperperfusion syndrome after carotid intervention: a review. *Cardiol Rev.* 2012;20(2):84–89.

28. Bujak M, Stilp E, Meller SM, et al. Dysautonomic responses during percutaneous carotid intervention: principles of physiology and management. *Catheter Cardiovasc Interv.* 2015;85(2):282–291.

29. Gupta R, Abou-Chebl A, Bajzer CT, Schumacher HC, Yadav JS. Rate, predictors, and consequences of hemodynamic depression after carotid artery stenting. *J Am Coll Cardiol.* 2006;47(8):1538–1543.

30. Ullery BW, Nathan DP, Shang EK, et al. Incidence, predictors, and outcomes of hemodynamic instability following carotid angioplasty and stenting. *J Vasc Surg.* 2011;58(4):917–925.

31. Acampa M, Guideri F, Marotta G, et al. Autonomic activity and baroreflex sensitivity in patients submitted to carotid stenting. *Neurosci Lett.* 2011;491(3):221–226.

32. Cayne NS, Faries PL, Trocciola SM, et al. Carotid angioplasty and stent-induced bradycardia and hypotension: impact of prophylactic atropine administration and prior carotid endarterectomy. *J Vasc Surg.* 2005;41(6):956–961.

33. Kojuri J, Ostovan MA, Zamiri N, Farshchizarabi S, Varavipoor B. Hemodynamic instability following carotid artery stenting. *Neurosurg Focus.* 2011;30(6).

34. Qureshi AI, Luft AR, Sharma M, et al. Frequency and determinants of postprocedural hemodynamic instability after carotid angioplasty and stenting. *Stroke.* 1999;30(10):2086–2093.

35. Grassi G, Seravalle G, Calhoun DA, et al. Mechanisms responsible for sympathetic activation by cigarette smoking in humans. *Circulation.* 1994;90(1):248–253.

36. Mylonas SN, Moulakakis KG, Antonopoulos CN, et al. Carotid artery stenting-induced hemodynamic instability. *J Endovasc Ther.* 2013;20(1):48–60.

37. Howell M, Krajcer Z, Dougherty K, et al. Correlation of periprocedural systolic blood pressure changes with neurological events in high-risk carotid stent patients. *J Endovasc Ther.* 2002;9(6): 810–816.

38. Cieri E, De Rango P, Maccaroni MR, et al. Is haemodynamic depression during carotid artery stenting a predictor of peri-procedural complications? *Eur J Vasc Endovasc Surg.* 2008;35:399–404.

39. Nandalur MR, Cooper H, Satler LF, et al. Vasopressor use in the critical care unit for treatment of persistent post-carotid artery stent induced hypotension. *Neurocrit Care.* 2007;7(3):232–237.

40. Pennekamp CW, Moll FL, De Borst GJ. Role of transcranial Doppler in cerebral hyperperfusion syndrome. *J Cardiovasc Surg.* 2012;53 (6):765–771.

41. Ballesteros-Pomar M, Alonso-Argueso G, Tejada-Garcia J, Vaquero-Morillo F. Cerebral hyperperfusion syndrome in carotid revascularisation surgery. *Rev Neurol.* 2012;55(8):490–498.

42. Abou-Chebl A, Yadav J, Reginelli J, Bajzer C, Bhatt D, Krieger D. Intracranial hemorrhage and hyperperfusion syndrome following carotid artery stenting: risk factors, prevention, and treatment. *J Am Coll Cardiol.* 2004;43(9):1596–1601.

43. Lieb M, Shah U, Hines GL. Cerebral hyperperfusion syndrome after carotid intervention: a review. *Cardiol Rev.* 2012;20(2):84–89.

44. Landesberg G, Shatz V, Akopnik I, et al. Association of cardiac troponin, CK-MB, and postoperative myocardial ischemia with long-term survival after major vascular surgery. *J Am Coll Cardiol.* 2004;42(9):1547–1554.

45. Landesberg G, Mosseri M, Shatz V, et al. Cardiac troponin after major vascular surgery: the role of perioperative ischemia, preoperative thallium scanning, and coronary revascularization. *J Am Coll Cardiol.* 2004;44(3):569–575.

46. Cohen MC, Aretz TH. Histological analysis of coronary artery lesions in fatal postoperative myocardial infarction. *Cardiovasc Pathol.* 1999;8 (3):133–139.

47. Thygesen K, Alpert JS, Jaffe AS, et al. Third universal definition of myocardial infarction. *J Am Coll Cardiol.* 2012;60(16):1581–1598.

48. Cutlip DE, Windecker S, Mehran R, et al. Clinical end points in coronary stent trials: a case for standardized definitions. *Circulation.* 2007;115(17):2344–2351.

49. Stilp E, Baird C, Gray WA, et al. An evidence-based review of the impact of periprocedural myocardial infarction in carotid revascularization. *Catheter Cardiovasc Interv.* 2013;82(5):709–714.

50. Muller DW, Shamir KJ, Ellis SG, Topol EJ. Peripheral vascular complications after conventional and complex percutaneous coronary interventional procedures. *Am J Cardiol.* 1992;69(1):63–68.

51. Popma JJ, Satler LF, Pichard AD, et al. Vascular complications after balloon and new device angioplasty. *Circulation.* 1993;88(4 Pt 1):1569–1578.

52. Blankenship JC, Hellkamp AS, Aguirre FV, Demko SL, Topol EJ, Califf RM. Vascular access site complications after percutaneous coronary intervention with abciximab in the evaluation of c7E3 for the prevention of ischemic complications (EPIC) trial. *Am J Cardiol.* 1998;81(1):36–40.

53. Patel RA. State of the art in carotid artery stenting: trial data, technical aspects, and limitations. *J Cardiovasc Transl Res.* 2014;7(4):446–457.

54. Carrozza J. Complications of diagnostic cardiac catheterization, In: *UpToDate*, Cutlip D (Ed), Waltham, MA. Accessed on 09.03.15.

55. Krueger K, Zaehringer M, Strohe D, Stuetzer H, Boecker J, Lackner K. Postcatheterization pseudoaneurysm: results of US-guided percutaneous thrombin injection in 240 patients. *Radiology.* 2005;236(3): 1104–1110.

56. Katzenschlager R, Ugurluoglu A, Ahmadi A, et al. Incidence of pseudoaneurysm after diagnostic and therapeutic angiography. *Radiology.* 1995;195(2):463–466.

57. Webber GW, Jang J, Gustavson S, Olin JW. Contemporary management of postcatheterization pseudoaneurysms. *Circulation.* 2007;115(20):2666–2674.

58. Koreny M, Riedmuller E, Nikfardjam M, Siostrzonek P, Mullner M. Arterial puncture closing devices compared with standard manual compression after cardiac catheterization: systematic review and meta-analysis. *JAMA.* 2004;291(3):350–357.

# 35 Endovascular Management of Intracranial Aneurysms

ROHAN CHITALE, DAVID KUNG, STAVROPOULA TJOUMAKARIS, PASCAL JABBOUR, and ROBERT H. ROSENWASSER

## Neuroanatomy and Procedure

### Key Concepts

- Aneurysms are treated in order to reduce the risk of initial or repeated subarachnoid hemorrhage.
- Advances in techniques allow most aneurysms to be treated endovascularly.

### Clinical Pearls

- A variety of endovascular techniques may be used to treat aneurysms.
- Small aneurysms pose a higher risk of intraoperative rupture.
- Giant aneurysms have a higher recurrence rate with coil embolization, but lower procedural risk than with clip ligation.

The primary goal of cerebral aneurysm coil embolization is to reduce the risk of initial or repeated subarachnoid hemorrhage. Intracranial aneurysms typically occur at branching sites of intracranial arteries in the subarachnoid space.[1] Due to rapid advances in endovascular techniques, most intracranial aneurysms may be treated endovascularly. Aneurysms in locations such as the basilar tip, cavernous internal carotid artery, or ophthalmic artery are easier to treat with coil embolization than with open microsurgery. However, distal middle cerebral artery aneurysms are more easily treated with surgical clip ligation.[2,3] Very small aneurysms (<3 mm) pose a higher risk of intraoperative rupture.[4] Giant aneurysms have a higher recurrence rate when treated with coiling, which must be weighed against higher initial morbidity when treated with microsurgical clip ligation.

### ANESTHETIC CONSIDERATIONS/PROCEDURAL CONSIDERATIONS

The patient is brought to the endovascular suite after discussion with the patient and family regarding the risks and benefits of the procedure, of alternative treatments, and of no treatment. Although practices may vary, general endotracheal anesthesia is typically performed for aneurysm embolization. This allows for reliable immobilization of the patient for better imaging quality, better patient comfort, and better control of respiratory and cardiovascular variables.[5] The disadvantages of general anesthesia are the loss of neurological examination and the difficulties in controlling blood pressure and intracranial pressure during extubation.[5] An indwelling urinary catheter is placed and an arterial line is used to monitor blood pressure. A 7 Fr sheath is typically placed in the femoral artery contralateral to the site of the pathology. If an unruptured aneurysm is to be coiled, then heparin boluses are administered to maintain activated clotting time (ACT) between two and three times baseline. Neurophysiological monitoring, namely, electroencephalogram and somatosensory-evoked potentials, may be used during the procedure.

### TECHNIQUE OPTIONS

A variety of tools are available for the treatment of aneurysms. Saccular aneurysms with a favorable fundus:neck ratio (>2:1) are ideal for coil embolization. Coils made of soft platinum alloys are available with varying degrees of softness, size, and shapes. Intracranial stents may be deployed to facilitate coiling of wide-necked or complex aneurysms, because they provide an endoluminal scaffold that retains coils within the aneurysm while preserving flow through the parent vessel. Patients who undergo stent placement require long-term antiplatelet therapy. Alternatively, balloon-assisted embolization may be used to treat wide-neck aneurysms and obviates the need for long-term platelet administration. In this method, coils are placed into the aneurysm while the parent vessel is protected by a balloon that is inflated across the aneurysm neck. A liquid embolic agent, Onyx HD 500 (eV3), may also be used to obliterate the lumen of the aneurysm with balloon assistance. Flow diversion is a new technique in which a low-porosity alloy stent is placed across the neck of the aneurysm in order to reconstruct the parent vessel and reduce blood flow into the aneurysm. This technique also requires long-term antiplatelet therapy. On occasion, a deconstructive approach may be used in which the parent vessel of the aneurysm, as well as afferent vessels, are embolized, typically after a temporary balloon occlusion demonstrates safety of the deconstruction.

# Perioperative Considerations

## Key Concepts

- A thorough preoperative evaluation and informed consent are necessary.
- Knowledge of drugs commonly used in endovascular treatment of intracranial aneurysms, such as antiplatelet agents, contrast media, and anticoagulant medications, is important.

## Clinical Pearls

- Peripheral vascular disease may limit treatment options and must be evaluated preoperatively.
- Renal function must be monitored carefully.
- Heparin-induced thrombocytopenia may occur in a delayed fashion and result in significant morbidity.

A thorough preoperative evaluation is essential to the success of any surgical procedure. For endovascular aneurysm embolization, several factors require special attention.

## PERIPHERAL VASCULAR DISEASE

There is significant overlap between the risk factors for cerebral aneurysms and those for atherosclerosis and peripheral vascular disease (e.g., cigarette smoking, hypertension); therefore, these conditions frequently co-occur. Traversing arteries in patients with advanced atherosclerosis is associated with an increased risk of thromboembolism and vessel dissection. For patients undergoing endovascular procedures, preoperative evaluation of pedal pulses and ankle-brachial indices are useful. Computed tomography (CT) angiography of the aorta and lower extremities may help to predefine vascular anatomy and disease, and to determine whether an alternative route of vascular access, such as the brachial, radial, or carotid artery, might be necessary. During the procedure, if distal limb ischemia develops, then prompt anticoagulation or surgical revascularization is often indicated.

## RENAL DISEASE

Contrast-induced nephropathy (CIN) is a potential complication of endovascular embolization. Risks factors include chronic renal insufficiency, diabetes mellitus, dehydration, old age, use of angiotensin-converting enzyme (ACE) inhibitors and hypertension.[6] Serum creatinine should be checked prior to the procedure. Adequate hydration with IV fluid is the most important factor in the prevention of CIN. Nonionic, low osmolar contrast should be used in patients with creatinine $>1$,[7] and the minimum amount of contrast necessary should be used to achieve procedural goals. Administration of acetylcysteine and bicarbonate has been suggested to decrease the risk of developing CIN.[8] However, more recent studies have demonstrated that volume supplementation with sodium chloride is more effective than sodium bicarbonate, with or without acetylcysteine, in the prevention of CIN.[9,10] For patients with end-stage renal disease, there is

**Table 35.1** Medication-Related Complication Rate

| | Complication Rate |
|---|---|
| Contrast allergy | 3% — mild reaction<br>0.04% — severe reaction<br>2–6 per million cases — fatal reaction |
| Heparin-induced thrombocytopenia | 1–5% |

little evidence of significant further renal impairment with contrast administration. There is also no evidence of systemic or organ-specific toxicity from contrast, suggesting that there is no need for urgent dialysis in those patients who are dialysis dependent.[11] Patients taking metformin (Glucophage) for diabetes mellitus should discontinue its use 24 hours prior to and for 48 hours after angiography to avoid lactic acidosis due to reduced renal tubule excretion of the medication from contrast exposure.

## CONTRAST ALLERGY

Mild reactions to nonionic contrast media, such as tachycardia, nausea, or vomiting, occur in approximately 3%. Severe reactions, such as bronchospasm and hypotension, occur in about 0.04%, and fatal reactions in 2–6 per million cases. The incidence of allergic reaction is six times higher for patients with previous contrast allergy.[12–14] It is generally believed that intraarterial injection of contrast media is associated with a lower incidence of allergic reactions than intravenous injection. Patients with history of an allergic reaction to contrast media should be pretreated with antihistamines (diphenhydramine 50 mg) and prednisolone (40 mg 12 hours and 2 hours before the procedure). Mild reactions can usually be treated with antihistamines and IV fluids. Severe reaction should be treated with steroids, epinephrine, and ventilation support (see Table 35.1).

## HEPARIN-INDUCED THROMBOCYTOPENIA

Patients with a history of heparin-induced thrombocytopenia (HIT) must be identified preoperatively to avoid devastating consequences of reexposure to heparin during endovascular procedures. A thorough history must be gathered to prevent this complication, and direct thrombin inhibitors may be used in lieu of heparin during endovascular procedures for patients who have or who are at high risk for HIT (see Table 35.1).

# Intraoperative and Postoperative Complications

## Key Concepts

- The main complications of endovascular treatment of intracranial aneurysm are thromboembolic.
- Intraoperative hemorrhagic events can be devastating, whereas delayed hemorrhagic complications are relatively rare.
- The rate of postsubarachnoid hemorrhage complications such as vasospasm and hydrocephalus are similar between endovascular treatment and traditional microsurgery.

## Clinical Pearls

- Stent placement requires antiplatelet therapy.
- Early placement of ventriculostomy is essential if considering using antiplatelet medications in a patient with subarachnoid hemorrhage.
- Intraprocedural thrombus is thought to be the result of platelet aggregation and is treated with intraarterial glycoprotein IIB/IIIA inhibitors.
- Blood pressure control is paramount.
- Protamine sulfate must be used immediately when hemorrhagic complications occur.

Patients are typically observed in an intensive care unit after aneurysm embolization procedures. Continuous cardiovascular monitoring is performed along with hourly neurological examinations for at least the first 24 hours. The femoral arterial sheath may be removed once the patient's neurological examination has stabilized and ACT values have returned to baseline. Often the femoral arterial sheath is not removed immediately upon completion of the procedure so that vascular access is preserved in case emergent angiography or retreatment is required during the acute postoperative period.

The key complications of cerebral aneurysm embolization include thromboembolic events and hemorrhagic events, including intraoperative aneurysm rupture.

## THROMBOEMBOLIC EVENTS

An inherent risk of endovascular treatment of aneurysms is the potential for ischemic stroke due to disruption and embolization of material from atherosclerotic plaque, or from a clot that forms on the catheter, coils, stents, or balloons (see Table 35.2).

Symptomatic thromboembolism is documented in 2% to 8% of coil embolization cases.[15–20] In the majority, neurological deficits are transient.[17,21]

In balloon-assisted coil embolization, thromboembolic complications are thought to arise from the use of two microcatheters and the hemodynamic stasis caused by balloon inflation.[18,22–24] Sluzewski et al. reported that balloon-assisted techniques resulted in higher thromboembolic complications than coil embolization (14.1% vs. 3%) in 757 consecutively treated patients.[24] However, a more recent series by Cekirge et al. reported a 1.7% rate of thromboembolic events causing morbidity or mortality in 1.3% of cases.[25] In a recent metaanalysis comparing 867 unassisted coiled aneurysms to 273 balloon-assisted coil

embolizations, Shapiro et al. found no statistically significant difference in rates of thromboembolism.[26] A case series of 76 balloon-assisted coiling procedures between 2009 and 2011 from our institution demonstrated a 6% rate of thromboembolism that caused transient morbidity in 5.2% of cases and no permanent morbidity.[22] In the same institution, for patients undergoing endovascular procedures to treat ruptured aneurysms, thromboembolic complications occurred in 7.5%.[27]

With stent-assisted coil embolization for unruptured aneurysms, pretreatment with dual antiplatelet agents is standard of care to minimize the risk of platelet aggregation and thromboembolic events.[28] Typically acetylsalicylic acid 325 mg and clopidogrel 75 mg once a day is given for 7 days prior to placement of a stent, or a loading dose of acetylsalicylic acid 650 mg and clopidogrel 600 mg is given. The antiplatelet effect of acetylsalicylic acid is observed 1 hour after loading and persists for the life span of platelets (7–10 days). Controversy exists regarding "acetylsalicylic acid resistance" because of lack of consensus about its definition, uncertainty about its clinical relevance, and how best to measure it. Currently, data do not support routinely monitoring the antiplatelet effect of acetylsalicylic acid to guide individual treatment.

Clopidogrel is a thienopyridine agent that requires metabolism by hepatic cytochrome P450 enzymes into an active form that irreversibly blocks the platelet adenosine diphosphate (ADP) receptor P2Y12. A 600-mg loading dose is optimal and reaches its effect in 2 to 4 hours.[29–31] Variability in patient response to clopidogrel has been reported.[32] The issue of clopidogrel resistance is also somewhat controversial; in patients who seem to have a suboptimal response to clopidogrel, consideration may be given to the use of newer ADP receptor antagonists, such as prasugrel, which has been shown to cause a more consistent platelet inhibition.[33]

Stent-assisted embolization in the setting of subarachnoid hemorrhage requires weighing the thromboembolic risk against the hemorrhagic risk associated with administration of antiplatelet medications.

The incidence of perioperative in-stent thrombosis varies from 4% to 18.8%.[34–38] In a retrospective series of 65 patients with subarachnoid hemorrhage treated with stent-assisted coiling, 7.7% of patients developed intraoperative in-stent thrombosis.[39] Among several small series, there is no consensus on optimal timing of initiation of antiplatelet therapy to minimize thromboembolic or hemorrhagic complications.[34–36,38] In patients with acute aneurysmal subarachnoid hemorrhage and hydrocephalus, placement of a ventriculostomy prior to the endovascular procedure is preferable, because if stents are used during the procedure, administration of antiplatelet agents becomes necessary and the risk of bleeding from ventriculostomy insertion might increase.[39]

The overall incidence of perioperative thromboembolic complications after flow diversion with the pipeline embolization device (PED) ranges between 0% and 14%.[40] Level of platelet inhibition as measured by P2Y12 reaction units (PRUs) >240 may correlate with higher perioperative thromboembolic risk.[40]

Intraprocedural heparin is used to mitigate thromboembolic risk, along with antiplatelet regimens when stents or

**Table 35.2** Thromboembolic Complication Risk

|  | Thromboembolic Risk |
|---|---|
| Coil embolization | 2%–8% |
| Balloon-assisted coiling | 1.7%–14.1% |
| Stent-assisted coiling | 4%–18.8% |
| Flow diversion | 0%–14% |

flow diverters are used. Intraoperatively, posttreatment angiograms are compared with pretreatment images in order to identify all branching vessels and to assess for thromboembolism or dissection. If a patient has neurological deterioration after the procedure, or neurophysiological monitoring demonstrates intraprocedural changes, then the cause is immediately sought. If the postprocedure head CT demonstrates no hemorrhage, then emergent angiography may be warranted to identify any thromboembolic phenomena, coil herniation, or stent migration/thrombosis. Periprocedural thrombosis is often the result of platelet aggregation or fibrin formation. Consequently, immediate treatment with intraarterial glycoprotein IIB-IIIa inhibitors such as abciximab (ReoPro) may be used at a dosage of 4 to 10 mg over 10 to 20 minutes.[41] Intravenous abciximab is also suggested as a first-line treatment (ReoPro, 0.25 mg/kg IV rapid bolus followed by 125 mcg/kg/min infusion for 12 hours).[42] Intraarterial tissue plasminogen activator and heparin may be used. In the postoperative setting, intravenous abciximab and heparin may also be used for 24 hours. In the case of large-vessel occlusion, placement of stents or the use of embolectomy devices may be warranted. In the intensive care unit, aggressive blood pressure management is essential. Blood pressure should be titrated to minimize the risks both of exacerbating ischemia and of hemorrhagic conversion of infarction.

## HEMORRHAGIC EVENTS

Intracranial hemorrhage (ICH) may occur as a result of intraoperative aneurysm rupture, vessel avulsion, parent artery injury, or hemorrhagic conversion of an infarct. In the intensive care unit, care must particularly be taken to avoid transient spikes in blood pressure during extubation of patients. If the patient suffers from acute neurological change after intervention, a CT scan of the head should be obtained to evaluate for hemorrhage. If the scan is consistent with acute hemorrhage, then heparin is reversed with protamine sulfate (1 mg for every 100 IU heparin, up to 50 mg). If the bleeding is massive or obstructs cerebrospinal fluid (CSF) outflow, then placement of a ventriculostomy or surgical decompression may be considered. Protamine can cause nonimmunogenic histamine release that can result in systemic peripheral vasodilation and mild to moderate hypotension.[43] The reported incidence of anaphylactic reactions to protamine ranges from 0.06% to 10.6%.[44]

Use of antiplatelet medications is a risk factor for ICH, increased ICH volume, and increased mortality.[45] Therefore patients who undergo stent embolization in which both aspirin and clopidogrel are administered are at risk for cerebral hemorrhagic complications. In patients with primary ICH, information obtained from platelet inhibition assays for aspirin (VerifyNow) and clopidogrel (P2Y12, Accumetrics, Inc.) has been shown to correlate with increased ICH volume growth, increased chance of death at 14 days, and poor outcome at 3 months.[45–48] Whether platelet transfusion reduces this risk, and if so, whether the complications of platelet transfusion are outweighed by its benefits are unknown, and transfusion practices vary. Administration of 10 units of platelets after a 300-mg clopidogrel load

or 12.5 units after a 600-mg loading has been shown to normalize platelet function.[49] Some recommend administration of platelets continuously for 4 or 5 days after the last dose of clopidogrel due to persistence of an active metabolite.[50] Other studies question the benefit of antiplatelet reversal. In a retrospective study of patients with ICH who had been taking antiplatelet medications, Ducruet et al. showed no difference in hematoma growth or clinical outcome between those who were treated with platelet transfusions ($n = 35$) and those who were not ($n = 31$).[51] In a literature review, Campbell et al. found no benefit of platelet transfusion and suggested that further study is necessary to definitively determine the impact of transfusion therapy on outcomes.[52]

ICH in patients who have undergone stent-assisted embolization procedures poses a clinical challenge. Discontinuation of antiplatelet agents may minimize morbidity from the hemorrhage, but increases the odds of morbidity from a thromboembolic complication (in-stent stenosis or thrombosis). Reversal of antiplatelet effects in patients with flow-diverting stents may be even more dangerous because these stents have a lower porosity and higher metal surface coverage, which result in a higher risk of thrombosis. The optimal management of these patients is unclear and should be determined on a case-by-case basis. At our institution, when performing flow diversion, a P2Y12 assay is obtained prior to initiation of clopidogrel and immediately preprocedure in order to calculate a percent platelet inhibition. Values between 30% and 70% are thought optimal to balance thrombotic and hemorrhagic risks. In a recent study, preprocedure PRU values <60 and >240 were shown to be the strongest predictor of perioperative hemorrhagic and thromboembolic complications after placement.[40] Although no data exist about how to manage this risk after hemorrhage in a patient with a PED, we administer platelet transfusions as guided by the P2Y12 in theory to maintain an intermediate level of antiplatelet therapy while reducing the risk of hemorrhage expansion. Serial head CTs and clinical examinations are used to monitor progression of bleeding and the patient's clinical course.

Delayed intraparenchymal hematomas have also been described after placement of flow-diverting stents and are theorized to result from hemorrhagic conversion of ischemic lesions, embolized foreign material, and loss of autoregulation in the distal arteries, all in the setting of dual antiplatelet therapy.[53,54] Delayed stent migration is another complication that occurs as a result of a mismatch in arterial diameter between inflow and outflow of the parent vessel and can result in both thromboembolic events and aneurysmal rupture.[55] Finally, delayed aneurysm rupture is a phenomenon that is thought to occur due to hemodynamic changes related to flow diversion and biological changes related to thrombus formation.[56]

One of the most dreaded complications during aneurysm coil embolization is intraoperative aneurysm rupture. The incidence of intraoperative rupture is between 1% and 4% and may occur spontaneously or iatrogenically from microwire, microcatheter, or coil placement into the aneurysm.[57–59] A rapid rise in intracranial pressure occurs and results in acute systemic hypertension. If present, a ventriculostomy may be used to divert CSF and lower intracranial pressure. Osmotic agents, such as mannitol and hypertonic saline, may also be used to treat intracranial hypertension. Blood pressure should be stabilized and cautiously reduced to minimize the risk of aneurysmal rebleeding. Although many operators use anesthetics, such as propofol or barbiturates, to lower cerebral metabolic rate as a neuroprotective strategy, evidence to support this practice is lacking, and use of this strategy in other disease states, such as traumatic brain injury and acute ischemic stroke, has been associated with harm.

When intraprocedural aneurysm rupture occurs, heparin should be reversed with protamine immediately, and platelet transfusion should be considered for patients on antiplatelet medications. Foremost, the aneurysm must be secured quickly. If the microcatheter is within the subarachnoid space, then the catheter should not be pulled backward, but rather coiling should continue from the subarachnoid space back into the aneurysm. If readily available, a balloon may also be used to occlude the parent vessel for proximal control. As a last resort, liquid embolic agents and coils may be used to sacrifice the parent vessel.

## HEPARIN-INDUCED THROMBOCYTOPENIA

Patients are exposed to heparin during endovascular procedures. Flushing lines in sheaths and catheters typically contain unfractionated heparin, and intraoperative systemic anticoagulation with heparin is routine. HIT is a prothrombotic antibody-mediated, potentially life-threatening condition characterized by thrombocytopenia and platelet activation. The incidence is approximately 1% but has been reported as high as 5%.[60] Thrombocytopenia usually develops 5 to 10 days after initial exposure, although it may occur early, within 1 day of reexposure, or late, several weeks after exposure. Sequelae of HIT include both venous and arterial thrombosis (4:1 ratio).[61] These include deep vein thrombosis, pulmonary embolism, stroke, myocardial infarction, and peripheral arterial thromboses that may be limb threatening. Less commonly, necrotizing skin lesions at heparin injection sites or disseminated intravascular coagulation may occur. The mortality associated with HIT is 5% to 10% and is usually due to thrombotic complications[62] (see Table 35.1).

Treatment of HIT begins with immediate discontinuation of all heparins and initiation of an immediate-acting nonheparin anticoagulant that interrupts the coagulation cascade at the level of thrombin or factor X. Parenteral direct thrombin inhibitors are commonly used. Argatroban (Novastan, Abbott, North Chicago, IL), a synthetic direct thrombin inhibitor, is approved by the Food and Drug Administration (FDA) for the treatment of HIT and is currently the anticoagulant of choice in this population. Its onset is immediate, its half-life is 40 to 50 minutes, and it undergoes hepatobiliary clearance. Postprocedure, it should be dosed as an intravenous infusion of 2 ug/kg/min or at 0.5 to 1.2 ug/kg/min in patients with liver disease or critical illness. The infusion rate should be titrated to maintain activated partial thromboplastin time between 1.5 and 3 times baseline values and to no greater than 10 ug/kg/min. There is no antidote. Bivalirudin, a hirudin analog, is a direct thrombin inhibitor that is FDA approved for percutaneous coronary interventions in patients who have or who are at

risk for HIT. It has a half-life of 25 minutes and is cleared renally and by enzymatic degradation. The treatment dose for HIT has not been established. Lepirudin and desirudin are recombinant hirudins. The former is no longer manufactured, and data regarding the latter for HIT are limited. Other nonheparin anticoagulants that do not directly inhibit thrombin include danaparoid and fondaparinux. Danaparoid is no longer available in the United States but is available in Canada, Japan, Europe, and Australia for treatment of HIT. Fondaparinux is administered as a subcutaneous injection and is dosed daily due to its long half-life. It is therefore not ideal for use in the intensive care unit and data for treatment of HIT are limited. Guidelines for the treatment of HIT have been published by the American College of Chest Physicians and by the Hemostasis and Thrombosis Task Force of the British Committee for Standards in Haematology.[63,64]

# Vascular Access Complications

## Key Concepts

- Although endovascular techniques are less invasive than open surgery, they are associated with a unique set of complications.
- Comprehensive preprocedure evaluation can help limit risk of complications.
- Close monitoring after the procedure is critical in order to identify complications early.

## Clinical Pearls

- Ideal femoral puncture site is 2 to 3 centimeters below the inguinal ligament to reduce chances of intraperitoneal or retroperitoneal hemorrhage.
- Pulse oximeter monitoring of the ipsilateral foot can help to identify early limb ischemia.

Endovascular procedures require arterial access. Common femoral artery access is obtained using a single wall puncture technique and placement of a sheath by the Seldinger technique. A femoral arteriogram is performed at the beginning and at the end of each intervention to identify vessel stenosis, occlusion, dissection, and pseudoaneurysm. We routinely access the groin contralateral to the side of the aneurysm for the rare possibility of concurrent cerebral and groin complications. With this strategy, a hemispheric insult will result in hemiparesis of the same leg that might be affected by a femoral artery insult. Choosing to access the contralateral groin helps avoid deficit to bilateral lower extremities of the patient in the uncommon instance of simultaneous cerebral and femoral injuries.

The ideal femoral puncture site is 2 to 3 centimeters below the inguinal ligament. The femoral artery is usually found coursing over the medial third of the femoral head, lateral to the femoral vein. A high entry site poses higher risk of retroperitoneal hemorrhage, and a lower entry site may result in an occlusive sheath. Postoperatively, cardiovascular monitoring helps to identify hypotension and tachycardia. These clinical signs along with back, abdomen, and groin pain or swelling may indicate failure of closure of the femoral artery and resultant retroperitoneal hemorrhage or groin hematoma. Abdominal compartment syndrome and hemorrhagic shock might develop if the diagnosis is delayed. Ecchymosis of the flank (Grey Turner sign) or periumbilical area (Cullen sign) is a late finding and should not be relied upon to make the diagnosis of acute retroperitoneal hematoma. If suspected clinically, the diagnosis of retroperitoneal hematoma should be made with a CT scan of the abdomen and pelvis. Fluid resuscitation, blood transfusion, and reversal of anticoagulation might be adequate in a stable patient. Active extravasation of contrast might require open surgical repair. Alternatively, endovascular treatment with a covered stent across the arteriotomy might be an option.

Dissection and pseudoaneurysm can result from intramural contrast injections or the wire/catheter pushing into a subintimal plane. This complication can occur anywhere between the access site and the target vessel. Fortunately dissection resulting in vessel occlusion is rare.[65] Treatment typically includes observation, antiplatelet agents, or anticoagulation. In the case of a flow-limiting dissection, stent placement may be indicated.[66]

The femoral artery puncture site is closed either with a closure device or by manual compression. A pulse oximeter should be placed on the toe that is ipsilateral to the femoral artery that is used for access. Oxygen saturation may be monitored both perioperatively and postoperatively to identify quickly limb ischemia. Dorsalis pedis and posterior tibial pulses must also be checked before sheath removal and hourly thereafter. Evidence of limb ischemia should prompt urgent evaluation by a vascular surgeon to determine whether thrombectomy or endovascular repair is warranted and feasible. Failure to identify vascular insufficiency may result in loss of the limb.

## References

1. Rhoton Jr AL. Aneurysms. *Neurosurgery.* 2002;51(4 Suppl): S121–S158.
2. Regli L, Uske A, de Tribolet N. Endovascular coil placement compared with surgical clipping for the treatment of unruptured middle cerebral artery aneurysms: a consecutive series. *J Neurosurg.* 1999;90 (6):1025–1030.
3. Johnston SC, Wilson CB, Halbach VV, et al. Endovascular and surgical treatment of unruptured cerebral aneurysms: comparison of risks. *Ann Neurol.* 2000;48(1):11–19.
4. Raymond J, Roy D. Safety and efficacy of endovascular treatment of acutely ruptured aneurysms. *Neurosurgery.* 1997;41(6):1235–1245. discussion 45–6.
5. Varma MK, Price K, Jayakrishnan V, Manickam B, Kessell G. Anaesthetic considerations for interventional neuroradiology. *Br J Anaesth.* 2007;99(1):75–85.
6. Parfrey PS, Griffiths SM, Barrett BJ, et al. Contrast material-induced renal failure in patients with diabetes mellitus, renal insufficiency, or both. A prospective controlled study. *New Eng J Med.* 1989;320 (3):143–149.
7. Porter GA. Radiocontrast-induced nephropathy. *Nephrol Dial Transplant.* 1994;9(Suppl 4):146–156.
8. Schmidt P, Pang D, Nykamp D, Knowlton G, Jia H. N-acetylcysteine and sodium bicarbonate versus N-acetylcysteine and standard hydration for the prevention of radiocontrast-induced nephropathy following coronary angiography. *Ann Pharmacother.* 2007;41(1):46–50.
9. Shavit L, Korenfeld R, Lifschitz M, Butnaru A, Slotki I. Sodium bicarbonate versus sodium chloride and oral N-acetylcysteine for the prevention of contrast-induced nephropathy in advanced chronic kidney disease. *J Intervent Cardiol.* 2009;22(6):556–563.
10. Klima T, Christ A, Marana I, et al. Sodium chloride vs. sodium bicarbonate for the prevention of contrast medium-induced nephropathy: a randomized controlled trial. *Eur Heart J.* Aug;33(16):2071–9.
11. Dawson P. Contrast agents in patients on dialysis. *Sem Dial.* 2002;15 (4):232–236.
12. Lasser EC, Lyon SG, Berry CC. Reports on contrast media reactions: analysis of data from reports to the U.S. Food and Drug Administration. *Radiology.* 1997;203(3):605–610.
13. Katayama H, Yamaguchi K, Kozuka T, Takashima T, Seez P, Matsuura K. Adverse reactions to ionic and nonionic contrast media. A report from the Japanese Committee on the Safety of Contrast Media. *Radiology.* 1990;175(3):621–628.
14. Wolf GL, Mishkin MM, Roux SG, et al. Comparison of the rates of adverse drug reactions. Ionic contrast agents, ionic agents combined with steroids, and nonionic agents. *Invest Radiol.* 1991;26 (5):404–410.
15. Qureshi AI, Luft AR, Sharma M, Guterman LR, Hopkins LN. Prevention and treatment of thromboembolic and ischemic complications associated with endovascular procedures: Part II—Clinical aspects and recommendations. *Neurosurgery.* 2000;46(6):1360–1375. discussion 75–6.
16. Vinuela F, Duckwiler G, Mawad M. Guglielmi detachable coil embolization of acute intracranial aneurysms: perioperative anatomical and clinical outcome in 403 patients. *J Neurosurg.* 1997;86(3):475–482.
17. Pelz DM, Lownie SP, Fox AJ. Thromboembolic events associated with the treatment of cerebral aneurysms with Guglielmi detachable coils. *AJNR.* 1998;19(8):1541–1547.
18. Derdeyn CP, Cross 3rd DT, Moran CJ, et al. Postprocedure ischemic events after treatment of intracranial aneurysms with Guglielmi detachable coils. *J Neurosurg.* 2002;96(5):837–843.
19. Friedman JA, Nichols DA, Meyer FB, et al. Guglielmi detachable coil treatment of ruptured saccular cerebral aneurysms: retrospective review of a 10-year single-center experience. *AJNR.* 2003;24 (3):526–533.
20. Ross IB, Dhillon GS. Complications of endovascular treatment of cerebral aneurysms. *Surg Neurol.* 2005;64(1):12–18. discussion 8–9.
21. Soeda A, Sakai N, Sakai H, et al. Thromboembolic events associated with Guglielmi detachable coil embolization of asymptomatic cerebral aneurysms: evaluation of 66 consecutive cases with use of diffusion-weighted MR imaging. *AJNR.* 2003;24(1):127–132.
22. Chalouhi N, Jabbour P, Tjoumakaris S, Dumont AS, Chitale R, Rosenwasser RH, Gonzalez LF. Single-center experience with balloon-assisted coil embolization of intracranial aneurysms: safety, efficacy and indications. *Clin Neurol Neurosurg.* May;115(5):607–13.
23. Ross IB, Dhillon GS. Balloon assistance as a routine adjunct to the endovascular treatment of cerebral aneurysms. *Surg Neurol.* 2006;66(6):593–601. discussion 602.
24. Sluzewski M, van Rooij WJ, Beute GN, Nijssen PC. Balloon-assisted coil embolization of intracranial aneurysms: incidence, complications, and angiography results. *J Neurosurg.* 2006;105(3):396–399.
25. Cekirge HS, Yavuz K, Geyik S, Saatci I. HyperForm balloon remodeling in the endovascular treatment of anterior cerebral, middle cerebral, and anterior communicating artery aneurysms: clinical and angiographic follow-up results in 800 consecutive patients. *J Neurosurg.* Apr;114(4):944–53.
26. Shapiro M, Babb J, Becske T, Nelson PK. Safety and efficacy of adjunctive balloon remodeling during endovascular treatment of intracranial aneurysms: a literature review. *AJNR.* 2008;29(9):1777–1781.
27. Chitale R, Chalouhi N, Theofanis T, et al. Treatment of ruptured intracranial aneurysms: comparison of stenting and balloon remodeling. *Neurosurgery.* Jun;72(6):953–9.
28. Mocco J, Snyder KV, Albuquerque FC, et al. Treatment of intracranial aneurysms with the Enterprise stent: a multicenter registry. *J Neurosurg.* 2009;110(1):35–39.
29. Hochholzer W, Trenk D, Frundi D, et al. Time dependence of platelet inhibition after a 600-mg loading dose of clopidogrel in a large, unselected cohort of candidates for percutaneous coronary intervention. *Circulation.* 2005;111(20):2560–2564.
30. Muller I, Seyfarth M, Rudiger S, et al. Effect of a high loading dose of clopidogrel on platelet function in patients undergoing coronary stent placement. *Heart (British Cardiac Society).* 2001;85(1):92–93.

31. von Beckerath N, Taubert D, Pogatsa-Murray G, Schomig E, Kastrati A, Schomig A. Absorption, metabolization, and antiplatelet effects of 300-, 600-, and 900-mg loading doses of clopidogrel: results of the ISAR-CHOICE (Intracoronary Stenting and Antithrombotic Regimen: choose Between 3 High Oral Doses for Immediate Clopidogrel Effect) Trial. *Circulation.* 2005;112(19):2946–2950.

32. Serebruany VL, Steinhubl SR, Berger PB, Malinin AI, Bhatt DL, Topol EJ. Variability in platelet responsiveness to clopidogrel among 544 individuals. *J Am Coll Cardiol.* 2005;45(2):246–251.

33. Brandt JT, Payne CD, Wiviott SD, et al. A comparison of prasugrel and clopidogrel loading doses on platelet function: magnitude of platelet inhibition is related to active metabolite formation. *Am Heart J.* 2007;153(1):66 e9–66 e16.

34. Tahtinen OI, Vanninen RL, Manninen HI, et al. Wide-necked intracranial aneurysms: treatment with stent-assisted coil embolization during acute (<72 hours) subarachnoid hemorrhage—experience in 61 consecutive patients. *Radiology.* 2009;253(1):199–208.

35. Meckel S, Singh TP, Undren P, et al. Endovascular treatment using predominantly stent-assisted coil embolization and antiplatelet and anticoagulation management of ruptured blood blister-like aneurysms. *AJNR.* Apr;32(4):764–71.

36. Katsaridis V, Papagiannaki C, Violaris C. Embolization of acutely ruptured and unruptured wide-necked cerebral aneurysms using the Neuroform2 stent without pretreatment with antiplatelets: a single center experience. *AJNR.* 2006;27(5):1123–1128.

37. Benitez RP, Silva MT, Klem J, Veznedaroglu E, Rosenwasser RH. Endovascular occlusion of wide-necked aneurysms with a new intracranial microstent (Neuroform) and detachable coils. *Neurosurgery.* 2004;54(6):1359–1367. discussion 68.

38. Akpek S, Arat A, Morsi H, Klucznick RP, Strother CM, Mawad ME. Self-expandable stent-assisted coiling of wide-necked intracranial aneurysms: a single-center experience. *AJNR.* 2005;26(5):1223–1231.

39. Amenta PS, Dalyai RT, Kung D, et al. Stent-assisted coiling of wide-necked aneurysms in the setting of acute subarachnoid hemorrhage: experience in 65 patients. *Neurosurgery.* Jun;70(6):1415–29; discussion 29.

40. Delgado Almandoz JE, Crandall BM, Scholz JM, et al. Pre-procedure P2Y12 reaction units value predicts perioperative thromboembolic and hemorrhagic complications in patients with cerebral aneurysms treated with the Pipeline Embolization Device. *J Neurointervent Surg.* Nov;5 Suppl 3:iii3–10.

41. Kwon OK, Lee KJ, Han MH, Oh CW, Han DH, Koh YC. Intraarterially administered abciximab as an adjuvant thrombolytic therapy: report of three cases. *AJNR.* 2002;23(3):447–451.

42. Mounayer C, Piotin M, Baldi S, Spelle L, Moret J. Intraarterial administration of Abciximab for thromboembolic events occurring during aneurysm coil placement. *AJNR.* 2003;24(10):2039–2043.

43. Hobbhahn J, Habazettl H, Conzen P, Peter K. Complications caused by protamine. 1: pharmacology and pathophysiology. *Anaesthesist.* 1991;40(7):365–374.

44. Weiler JM, Gellhaus MA, Carter JG, et al. A prospective study of the risk of an immediate adverse reaction to protamine sulfate during cardiopulmonary bypass surgery. *J Allergy Clin Immunol.* 1990;85(4):713–719.

45. James RF, Palys V, Lomboy JR, Lamm JR, Jr., Simon SD. The role of anticoagulants, antiplatelet agents, and their reversal strategies in the management of intracerebral hemorrhage. *Neurosurg Focus.* May;34(5):E6.

46. Naidech AM, Bendok BR, Garg RK, et al. Reduced platelet activity is associated with more intraventricular hemorrhage. *Neurosurgery.* 2009;65(4):684–688. discussion 8.

47. Naidech AM, Bernstein RA, Levasseur K, et al. Platelet activity and outcome after intracerebral hemorrhage. *Ann Neurol.* 2009;65(3):352–356.

48. Naidech AM, Jovanovic B, Liebling S, et al. Reduced platelet activity is associated with early clot growth and worse 3-month outcome after intracerebral hemorrhage. *Stroke.* 2009;40(7):2398–2401.

49. Vilahur G, Choi BG, Zafar MU, et al. Normalization of platelet reactivity in clopidogrel-treated subjects. *J Thromb Haemost.* 2007;5(1):82–90.

50. Herman J, Benson K. Platelet transfusion therapy. In: PD M, ed. *Transfusion Therapy: Clinical Principles and Practice.* 2nd ed. Bethesda, MD: AABB Press; 2004:335–353.

51. Ducruet AF, Hickman ZL, Zacharia BE. et al. Impact of platelet transfusion on hematoma expansion in patients receiving antiplatelet agents before intracerebral hemorrhage. *Neurolog Res.* 2010;32(7):706–710.

52. Campbell PG, Sen A, Yadla S, Jabbour P, Jallo J. Emergency reversal of antiplatelet agents in patients presenting with an intracranial hemorrhage: a clinical review. *World Neurosurg.* 2010;74(2-3):279–285.

53. Chitale R, Gonzalez LF, Randazzo C. et al. Single center experience with pipeline stent: feasibility, technique, and complications. *Neurosurgery.* 2012;3:679–691 discussion 91.

54. Velat GJ, Fargen KM, Lawson MF, Hoh BL, Fiorella D, Mocco J. Delayed intraparenchymal hemorrhage following pipeline embolization device treatment for a giant recanalized ophthalmic aneurysm. *J Neurointervent Surg.* 2012;4(5):e24.

55. Chalouhi N, Satti SR, Tjoumakaris S, et al. Delayed migration of a pipeline embolization device. *Neurosurgery.* 2013;72(2 Suppl Operative):229–234; discussion 34.

56. Kulcsar Z, Houdart E, Bonafe A, et al. Intra-aneurysmal thrombosis as a possible cause of delayed aneurysm rupture after flow-diversion treatment. *AJNR.* 2011;32(1):20–25.

57. Brisman JL, Niimi Y, Song JK, Berenstein A. Aneurysmal rupture during coiling: low incidence and good outcomes at a single large volume center. *Neurosurgery.* 2008;62(6 Suppl 3):1538–1551.

58. Levy E, Koebbe CJ, Horowitz MB, et al. Rupture of intracranial aneurysms during endovascular coiling: management and outcomes. *Neurosurgery.* 2001;49(4):807–811. discussion 11–3.

59. Doerfler A, Wanke I, Egelhof T, et al. Aneurysmal rupture during embolization with Guglielmi detachable coils: causes, management, and outcome. *AJNR.* 2001;22(10):1825–1832.

60. Arepally GM, Ortel TL. Clinical practice. Heparin-induced thrombocytopenia. *New Engl J Med.* 2006;355(8):809–817.

61. Warkentin TE, Kelton JG. A 14-year study of heparin-induced thrombocytopenia. *Am J Med.* 1996;101(5):502–507.

62. Warkentin TE, Kelton JG. Temporal aspects of heparin-induced thrombocytopenia. *New Eng J Med.* 2001;344(17):1286–1292.

63. Linkins LA, Dans AL, Moores LK, et al. Treatment and prevention of heparin-induced thrombocytopenia: Antithrombotic Therapy and Prevention of Thrombosis, 9th ed: American College of Chest Physicians Evidence-Based Clinical Practice Guidelines. *Chest.* Feb;141(2 Suppl):e495S–530S.

64. Keeling D, Davidson S, Watson H. The management of heparin-induced thrombocytopenia. *Br J Haematol.* 2006;133(3):259–269.

65. Fifi JT, Meyers PM, Lavine SD, et al. Complications of modern diagnostic cerebral angiography in an academic medical center. *J Vasc Interv Radiol.* 2009;20(4):442–447.

66. Fusco MR, Harrigan MR. Cerebrovascular dissections: a review. Part II: blunt cerebrovascular injury. *Neurosurgery.* Feb;68(2):517–30; discussion 30.

# 36 *Arteriovenous Malformation and Dural Arteriovenous Fistula Embolization*

DOROTHEA ALTSCHUL, SEAN D. LAVINE, and RAUL G. NOGUEIRA

## Neuroanatomy and Procedure

### Key Concepts

- Arteriovenous malformation (AVM) patients present most commonly in young adulthood with an intracranial hemorrhage.
- Focal neurological signs without hemorrhage are distinctively rare.
- Most dural arteriovenous fistula (DAVF) patients present in their fifth and sixth decades with symptoms related to lesion location and venous drainage patterns.

### CEREBRAL ARTERIOVENOUS MALFORMATIONS

AVMs of the brain are vascular lesions in which an abnormal network of tangled vessels (nidus) permits pathological shunting of blood flow from the arterial to the venous tree without an intervening capillary bed. Although AVMs are uncommon, they can exist anywhere in the neural axis. Therefore any intracranial artery or extracranial collateral artery can supply these lesions.

Since the advent of contemporary brain imaging techniques, brain AVMs are incidental findings in approximately 0.05% of the population.[1] Although AVMs often present in young adulthood (mean age, 35 years),[2] they are thought to form during embryonic development. Some AVMs can be genetic and hereditary, but the majority is not and is likely a result of spontaneous mutation or other environmental factors such as embryonic intracranial venous thrombosis.[3]

Roughly half of patients with brain AVMs present with intracranial hemorrhage (ICH), resulting in a first-ever hemorrhage rate of 0.55 per 100 000 person-years.[2] Hemorrhage location is dependent on the location of the lesion and is usually intraparenchymal and/or intraventricular. These types of ICH are a result of either rupture of an intranidal aneurysm or a sudden change in the angioarchitecture of the nidus, as in a change in the venous outflow. Compared with other causes of ICH, the morbidity associated with AVM rupture is less, although it still can be fatal, particularly if it occurs in the deep midline structures, posterior fossa, or brainstem. The reported long-term annual mortality rates are 1% to 1.5%.[4] Overall, it is estimated that 10% to 30% of survivors have long-term disability. The risk of subsequent hemorrhage is increased when the brain AVM presents with hemorrhage,[5,6] exclusive deep venous drainage,[5,7] presence of a single draining vein,[8] or the presence of intranidal aneurysms.[9,10]

Subarachnoid hemorrhage can also be a presentation of AVM. This is usually a result of prenidal, high-flow-related aneurysms (Fig. 36.1). These aneurysms arise on normal arterial vessels at branch points or bifurcations, similar to spontaneous berry aneurysms. No histological or imaging features have been found to distinguish flow-related aneurysms occurring in association with AVMs from those aneurysms occurring in absence of AVMs. Interestingly many flow-related aneurysms will regress spontaneously after treatment of AVMs. Although rare, AVMs may also present with subdural hematoma.

The next most common presentation is seizure, which occurs in about one third of cases, often alerting the physician to the presence of an AVM.[11] Inconsistent data preclude accurate determination of the relationship between seizures and subsequent risk of ICH. Several types of attacks labeled as seizures occur, and the type of seizure is often unreported in studies. Seizures result from the gliotic parenchyma that surrounds the nidus.

Headache is the presenting symptom in about 15% of AVM patients. Because headaches are a common complaint in the population at large, it has been difficult to determine whether the headaches associated with AVMs are unique to the condition. In contrast to early assumptions, very little evidence supports the claim that recurrent unilateral headaches should arouse suspicion of an ipsilateral AVM. Migraine headaches with and without aura have been documented in patients with AVMs.[12] The postoperative disappearance of migraine is not unusual and may occur after any type of treatment.

Few patients present with slowly progressing neurological deficits (4%–8%).[13,14] Shunting through a low-resistance AVM results in hypoperfusion of the surrounding normal brain tissue, a phenomenon known as *vascular steal*; however, evidence for a causal link with ischemic symptoms is lacking. Venous hypertension and mass effect of the nidus are alternative explanations for slowly progressing focal neurological deficits.

A commonly used grading scale for brain AVMs is the Spetzler-Martin Grade (SMG) scale (Table 36.1), which is a composite score of nidus size, "eloquence" of adjacent brain, and presence of deep venous drainage.[15] If any or all of the venous drainage occurs through deep veins (internal cerebral, basal veins, precentral cerebellar vein), it is

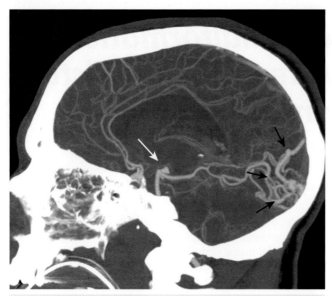

Fig. 36.1 A 51-year-old man was found unconscious in the setting of a subarachnoid hemorrhage. A flow-related left posterior cerebral artery aneurysm (*white arrow*) and left occipital arteriovenous malformation (*black arrows*) were demonstrated on CT angiography.

**Table 36.1** Classification of Arteriovenous Malformations (AVMs) proposed by Spetzler and Martin.[15] A Separate Grade of 6 Is Reserved for Inoperable Lesions

| AVM Characteristics | Grading |
| --- | --- |
| Size of the AVM | |
| Small (<3 cm) | 1 point |
| Medium (3–6 cm) | 2 points |
| Large (>6 cm) | 3 points |
| Localization of the AVM | |
| Noneloquent | 0 points |
| Eloquent | 1 point |
| Venous drainage | |
| Only superficial | 0 point |
| Deep | 1 point |

categorized as deep. An AVM is considered adjacent to eloquent brain parenchyma if it is next to the sensorimotor cortex, language areas, visual cortex, hypothalamus, thalamus, internal capsule, brainstem, cerebellar peduncles, or deep cerebellar nuclei. SMG ranges from 1 to 5, summing the points for each category.

The SMG system was originally developed to predict the perioperative and postsurgical outcomes and reliably correlates with surgical outcome. It has also been evaluated in the combined management of AVMs, including embolization followed by surgical resection, embolization alone, or radiosurgery.[15] Deterioration due to treatment is seen in 19% of patients with SMG I or II lesions, 35% of patients with SMG III lesions, and 42% of patients with SMG IV or V lesions. The scale does not include hemorrhagic risk characteristics such as associated aneurysms, venous stasis, or venous aneurysms. There are no reliable data correlating such features with treatment risk.

The annual hemorrhage risk may be as low as 0.9% in patients with unruptured, superficially located brain

AVMs with superficial drainage and may be as high as 34% in patients with previously ruptured, deeply seated AVMs with deep venous drainage.[16] The treatment paradigm for unruptured, high-grade AVMs (particularly SMG III-V) remains controversial; treatment may be warranted on when anatomical and angiographic findings suggest a relatively high risk of hemorrhage.[17] Given the low morbidity associated with surgical obliteration of SMG I-II AVMs, treatment is recommended for most. Grade III-V AVMs must be dealt with on a case-by-case basis.

Because ruptured brain AVMs have a higher hemorrhage risk (4.5%–34%) than previously unruptured ones (0.9%–8%),[5,16] treatment of ruptured brain AVMs is advisable,[18] despite the absence of evidence from randomized controlled trials that the benefits outweigh the risks.

The ultimate goal of AVM therapy is the complete obliteration of the lesion because partial treatment may actually increase the chances of bleeding.[19]

The available options for treatment include endovascular embolization, microsurgical resection, stereotactic radiosurgery, or a combination of these modalities. (Please see Chapter 10 for a detailed description of microsurgery for AVMs/AVFs and Chapter 25 for stereotactic radiosurgery [SRS].) Therapeutic management of AVMs requires a careful multidisciplinary approach to estimate a risk-to-benefit ratio for the individual patient (Box 36.1).

SRS can often be curative for AVMs. Although this modality can be used for ruptured AVMs, it is important to note that cure is not achieved with radiosurgery until several months to years after treatment. The success of radiotherapy is inversely related to the size of the AVM nidus. AVMs with a volume of less than 10 mL (diameter of less than 3 cm) are frequently suitable for radiosurgery, with estimated rates of cure at 2 years of around 80% to 88%.[20] The major disadvantage of radiation therapy is a persistent risk of intracranial hemorrhage (ICH), which may be as high as 10%, until the lesion disappears. This risk may persist even after obliteration of the AVM.[21] Because of this risk, SRS is often reserved for treatment of unruptured lesions. In certain ruptured cases where other treatment modalities are deemed too risky, it may still be used, acknowledging the continued risk of rupture. Endovascular embolization may be used to shrink the nidus to a smaller single target (Fig. 36.2), often for future radiosurgery. Other goals include the treatment of nidal aneurysms that represent a risk for hemorrhage until the radiosurgically induced

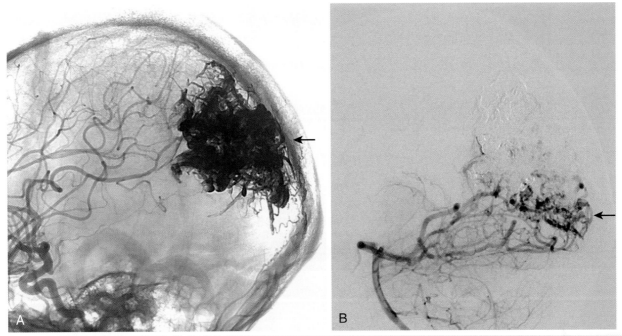

**Fig. 36.2** Final angiographic appearance after five embolization sessions using the "stacking method." **(A)** The anterior circulation component of the AVM was nearly completely obliterated (*black arrow*) with **(B)** persistence of only a small posterior circulation component, which was centered at the visual cortex area (*black arrow*). The patient subsequently underwent radiosurgery.

obliteration occurs and also to attempt to obliterate large arteriovenous fistulae that are typically more refractory to the effects of radiosurgery. For larger, deep nidal lesions, some have advocated staged SRS with multiple treatments. This is usually used in the setting of larger inoperable lesions. There are new reports that flow reduction alone without evidence of reduction of AVM volume may not provide benefit before SRS, and in fact, it may lead to an impaired understanding of the angioarchitecture, thereby causing incorrect mapping and treatment planning.[8]

AVM embolization is most commonly performed as a precursor to surgical resection, particularly for those in central and eloquent locations and for those with deep feeders.[18] Prospective controlled studies comparing surgery with and without embolization do not exist; nevertheless, a number of case series have demonstrated that preoperative embolization results in improved treatment outcomes.[18–25] Advantages include diminished blood loss and shorter surgical times by decreasing the size of the nidus and the amount of blood flow through the AVM. Embolized vessels are also more readily identified during surgery and can provide a road map for the resection of the arterial feeders and nidus while preserving en passage arteries to nearby eloquent parenchyma. Finally, staged embolization resulting in reduced nidal blood flow can decrease the incidence of potentially catastrophic hemorrhage.[26]

AVMs may be cured completely using embolization alone (Fig. 36.3). Published embolization cure rates vary, depending on selection criteria, technique, and nidal size. The chance of a cure appears to be inversely proportional to the AVM volume and the number of feeding pedicles, with complete obliteration rates of 71% for AVMs smaller than 4 mL and only 15% for AVMs ranging from 4 to 8 mL.[27] Others have found that AVM volume does not significantly predict the potential for endovascular cure.[28]

Rather, a 74% rate of curative embolization (overall cure rate of 40%) has been reported in a subgroup of patients with favorable angiographic features, such as one or a few dominant feeding arteries, no perinidal angiogenesis, and a fistulous nidus.[28] With improved techniques and growing experience, the proportion of AVMs that are successfully obliterated with embolizations is increasing.[29]

Palliative embolization does not appear to improve upon conservative medical management of patients with incurable AVMs and may worsen the subsequent clinical course.[30] There is, however, a role for palliative embolization in select circumstances because it may alleviate symptoms due to arterial steal or venous hypertension. Nonetheless, this effect is often only temporary, and symptoms may recur due to rapid development of collateral flow. Palliative embolization may also be undertaken in patients presenting with seizures resistant to medical management. It is believed that partial embolization reduces the severity of arterial shunting and thereby improves perfusion to the surrounding brain parenchyma.

## INTRACRANIAL DURAL ARTERIOVENOUS FISTULAS

Intracranial DAVFs are pathological shunts between dural arteries and dural venous sinuses, meningeal veins, or cortical veins.[31] DAVFs account for 10% to 15% of intracranial AVMs. The term *dural AVM* should be reserved for pediatric dural arteriovenous (AV) shunts because malformation implies a developmental origin, and adult dural AV shunts are acquired lesions. DAVFs are distinguished from parenchymal or pial AVMs by the presence of a dural arterial supply and the absence of a parenchymal nidus.[31] Most DAVFs are located in the transverse, sigmoid, and cavernous sinuses.[32] DAVFs are predominantly idiopathic,

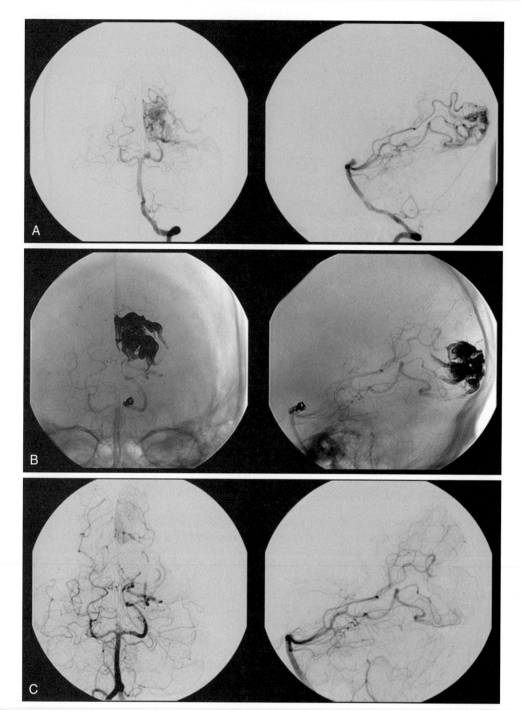

**Fig. 36.3 A-C** Two-staged curative Onyx embolization treatment. Anteroposterior and lateral views **(A)** pretreatment, **(B)** demonstrating Onyx cast, and **(C)** after two-staged ONYX treatment without any evidence of residual arteriovenous shunting.

though a small percentage of patients have a history of previous craniotomy, trauma, or dural sinus thrombosis.[33,34]

### Clinical Pearl

Pulsatile tinnitus is a symptom that results from increased blood flow through the dural venous sinuses, particularly in relation to transverse and sigmoid sinus lesions. Cavernous sinus DAVFs can present with ophthalmoplegia, proptosis, chemosis, retroorbital pain, or decreased visual acuity (Fig. 36.4).

The DAVF venous drainage pattern determines the severity of symptoms and provides the foundation for the classification schemes of Borden et al.[35] and Cognard et al.[36]

The Borden classification stratifies lesions based on the site of venous drainage and the presence or absence of cortical venous drainage (CVD) (Table 36.2). The Cognard classification[36] is based on the direction of dural sinus drainage, the presence or absence of CVD, and venous outflow architecture (nonectatic cortical veins, ectatic cortical veins, or spinal perimedullary veins). Type I lesions drain into the dural sinus, have an antegrade flow direction, and lack CVD. Type II lesions are subdivided into three

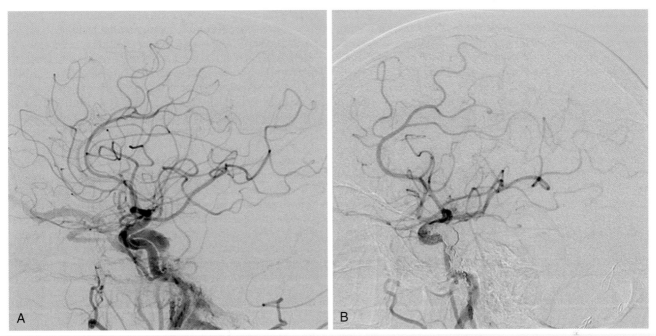

**Fig. 36.4** Lateral view on catheter angiography of a clival dural arteriovenous fistula before **(A)** and after **(B)** transvenous Onyx embolization demonstrating complete obliteration of arteriovenous shunting. Cavernous sinus, dilated superior ophthalmic vein.

**Table 36.2** Borden Classification of DAVFs

| Type | Venous Drainage Site | Cortical Venous Drainage |
|---|---|---|
| Benign | | |
| I | Dural Sinus | No |
| Aggressive | | |
| II | Dural Sinus | Yes |
| III | Cortical Vein | Yes |

categories: type IIa lesions drain retrograde into a dural sinus without CVD, type IIb lesions drain anterograde into a dural sinus with CVD, and type IIa + b lesions drain retrograde into a dural sinus with CVD. Types III to V lesions all have CVD, absent dural venous drainage, and varying cortical venous outflow architecture (III with CVD only, IV with CVD and venous ectasia, and V with CVD and spinal perimedullary drainage). Lack of CVD is a favorable feature and is associated with a benign natural history. DAVF patients typically present incidentally or with symptoms of increased venous pressure, such as seizures, parkinsonism, cerebellar symptoms, cognitive decline, dementia, and cranial nerve abnormalities, including rare cases of trigeminal neuralgia.

The risk of ICH from Borden type I (Cognard types I and IIa) lesions is extremely low.[37] The presence of CVD (Borden type II and III, Cognard types IIb–V) places DAVFs in a higher risk category for hemorrhagic presentations. In these lesions, an annual mortality rate of 10.4%, an annual risk of ICH of 8.1%, and annual risk of neurological deficits of 6.9% have been reported.[38] Subdividing lesions with CVD (Borden types II and III, Cognard types IIb–V) into symptomatic and asymptomatic types may further

improve the accuracy of risk stratification.[39] There is a significant difference in the risk of annual hemorrhage between symptomatic and asymptomatic types: 7.4% versus 1.5%, respectively.[39] Although classifying DAVFs is helpful for risk stratification, these lesions have a dynamic nature. Type I lesions can develop CVD over time due to the development of venous stenosis, venous thrombosis, or increased arterial flow.[40] The risk of conversion is low, having only been reported in 2% of low-grade lesions.[40] Cases of spontaneous thrombosis/resolution of DAVFs have also been reported.[41] Any change in a patient's symptoms can reflect exacerbations of the venous drainage pattern and should prompt further evaluation with neurovascular imaging.

## IMAGING AND ANGIOGRAPHIC ASPECTS

Intracranial AVMs and DAVFs may be diagnosed with a variety of diagnostic noninvasive imaging studies, including computed tomography (CT) and CT angiography (CTA). Magnetic resonance (MR) imaging techniques are more helpful because they can demonstrate dilated vessels, venous pouches, vascular enhancement, and signs of venous hypertension in high-grade DAVF lesions (e.g., white matter hyperintensity, ICH, or venous infarction). However, noninvasive imaging may be completely normal in many cases of DAVF or small AVMs, and unexplained subarachnoid or parenchymal hemorrhages should prompt consideration of catheter angiography, which remains the gold standard for defining the arterial and venous anatomy and plays a crucial role in planning therapy.

Angiographic images should be evaluated carefully for the presence of aneurysms. Because of their propensity to hemorrhage, aneurysms should generally be addressed before the remainder of the lesion. Aneurysms may be located on vessels that are remote from the nidus, on feeding vessels ("flow-related" aneurysms), or within the nidus itself ("intranidal" aneurysms) (Fig. 36.2). These lesions can represent true aneurysms located in the most distal arterial branches adjacent to the AVM nidus, dilated venous pouches, or pseudoaneurysms arising as residua of prior hemorrhages.[7]

The venous phase images represent another critical component of the angiographic evaluation. The presence of any preexisting venous outflow stenoses should be noted because inadvertent occlusion of venous efflux during embolization is dangerous.

Rapid AV shunting may result in superimposition on angiographic imaging of arterial feeders, the nidus, and draining veins, resulting in obscuration of important features, such as small arterial feeders, distal feeding pedicles, nidal aneurysms, direct AV fistulas, and small accessory draining veins. Superselective angiography, using microcatheters advanced into distal aspects of the arterial feeders, is often needed to ascertain the finer details of the lesion.[28]

# Perioperative Considerations

## Key Concepts

- AVM management involves a multidisciplinary team and often a multimodal approach.
- N-butyl-cyanoacrylate (NBCA) glue and Onyx are the most commonly used embolic agents.
- The goal of embolization is to form a solid intranidal cast.

Vascular access for the embolization procedure is achieved through a 5 or 6 French sheath in the femoral artery. Anticoagulation decisions for AVMs are made on a case-by-case basis. Some centers prefer to use heparin to keep the activated clotting time (ACT) at least 2 to 2.5 times the baseline value; other centers do not use heparin.

Direct transduction of arterial pressure is indicated for intracranial embolizations, especially with manipulation of systemic pressure with vasoactive agents, as well as for postprocedure blood pressure management. Hypotension, or even temporary asystole (with adenosine), may be induced to slow flow through the AV shunt and provide more control over deposition of embolic material.[42]

Most centers perform embolizations under general anesthesia, and some use neuroelectrophysiological monitoring (somatosensory evoked potentials and electroencephalography) to monitor neurological function during the procedure. Others use monitored anesthesia care with deep intravenous sedation. There is no evidence that either general endotracheal anesthesia or monitored anesthesia care is associated with a lower rate of complications.[43] Both methods have advantages and disadvantages. Arguments for embolization under general anesthesia include improved visualization of structures with the absence of patient movement, especially with temporary apnea or when the ventilation is timed with digital subtraction angiography contrast injection.

Monitored anesthesia care trades off the potential for patient movement against the increased ability to examine and assess functional anatomy of a given patient. This approach requires deep intravenous sedation to render the patient comfortable during catheter placement and while keeping the patient appropriately responsive for selective neurological testing. In this setting, superselective injection of amobarbital, with or without lidocaine into the feeder vessel, is performed prior to the AVM embolization.[44] Focused neurological examination is then immediately performed. The evoked deficits resolve with dissipation of the injected agent within several minutes.

Embolic agents currently available include liquid embolysates, such as NBCA, ethylene-vinyl alcohol copolymer with dimethyl sulfoxide (Onyx), and undiluted absolute ethyl alcohol (ETOH); particles such as polyvinyl alcohol particles; and solid occlusive devices, such as coils, silk, threads, and balloons. Liquid embolysates are the most widely used.

Liquid adhesive polymer agents offer several important advantages: (1) the potential for penetration deep into the AVM nidus; (2) permanent embolization with durable obliteration of the vessel or pedicle; (3) the ability to be delivered through small, flexible, flow-directed catheters that can be manipulated safely and atraumatically into the most distal locations within the vasculature; and (4) the ability to be delivered into the pedicle quickly. Polyvinyl alcohol (PVA) particles were commonly employed for brain embolization before liquid embolic agents became more widely used. Embolization of brain AVMs with ETOH has been advocated on the basis of its success to eradicate peripheral vascular malformations. These agents are not regularly used because they are less effective than NBCA and Onyx and are potentially associated with higher risks.

NBCA (Trufill NBCA Liquid Embolic, Codman Neurovascular, Raynham, Massachusetts, USA) was approved by the Food and Drug Administration (FDA) for presurgical embolization of cerebral vascular malformations in 2000. NBCA is a liquid monomer, commonly referred to as "glue," that undergoes a rapid exothermic polymerization catalyzed by nucleophiles found in blood and on the vascular endothelium to form a solid adhesive. The rate of polymerization can be adjusted by mixing ethiodized oil into the mixture, which, unlike NBCA, is radio-opaque. Higher concentrations of ethiodized oil decrease the polymerization rate and increase the viscosity of the embolic material. Ratios used in the prospective randomized clinical study of the NBCA liquid embolic system varied from 10% to 70% NBCA and 30% to 80% ethiodized oil by volume. Typically, a 1:1 to 1:3 (NBCA:oil) mixture is used. This translates into a 2- to 7-second polymerization time. Modifications can be made based on the individual's angioarchitecture and hemodynamics. Glacial acetic acid may be added in low concentrations to delay polymerization and lead to increased penetration. This technique is, however, a deviation from the FDA-approved indications for use of the commercially available NBCA. Tantalum powder may be mixed with the NBCA:oil mixture to provide greater radio-opacity. The goal of the embolization is to form a solid intranidal NBCA cast, avoiding early polymerization in the arterial feeder or later polymerization in the venous outflow. Pure NBCA polymerizes almost instantaneously at the catheter tip.

The vessel is permanently occluded when the polymer completely fills the lumen. NBCA provokes an inflammatory response in the wall of the vessel and surrounding tissue leading to thrombosis, vessel necrosis, and fibrous ingrowth. Vessel recanalization is uncommon.

Onyx is a nonadhesive liquid embolic agent with a lava-like flow pattern. It is premixed with ethylene-vinyl alcohol copolymer (EVOH), dimethyl sulfoxide (DMSO), and micronized tantalum powder for radio-opacity.[45] Before injection, the Onyx solution must be vigorously shaken for 20 minutes to fully suspend the micronized tantalum powder. The copolymer coheres as it is injected but it does not adhere to the endothelium or to the microcatheter tip. When the mixture contacts blood, DMSO rapidly diffuses away from the mixture, causing in situ precipitation and solidification of the polymer, with formation of a spongy embolus. The precipitation progresses from the outer surface inward, forming a skin with a liquid center that continues to flow as the solidification continues. The rate of precipitation of the copolymer is proportional to the concentration of EVOH. Complete solidification of both formulations occurs within 5 minutes, which is more slowly than that of NBCA. Because ONYX is nonadherent to the vascular endothelium and the microcatheter, prolonged injection times are possible with better penetration of the vascular bed.

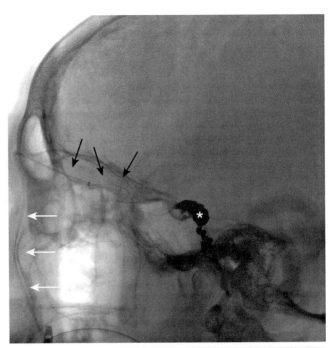

**Fig. 36.5** Onyx transvenous embolization via facial vein (*white arrows*) to superior ophthalmic vein (*black arrows*) and into the cavernous sinus (*white star*). An Onyx cast lies at the expected location of the cavernous sinus (*white star*) extending into the inferior petrosal sinus.

## Clinical Pearl

Onyx has some advantages over NBCA. The operator has the option of stopping the injection if Onyx begins to track toward another arterial pedicle, venous outflow vessel, or suspected dangerous anastomoses. Another advantage is the possibility of obtaining control angiograms during embolization. This allows for assessment of the remaining flow and changing hemodynamic pattern of a complex lesion. However, fluoroscopy times can be longer, and radiation-induced injury has been reported.

DMSO can induce vasospasm, angionecrosis, arterial thrombosis, and vascular rupture.[46] These undesirable consequences are related to the volume of DMSO infused and the endothelial contact time. Severe angiotoxic effects do not occur when the DMSO infusion rate does not exceed 0.25 mL/90 seconds. Only specifically approved microcatheters (Ultraflow, Marathon, Echelon) can be used with Onyx because DMSO dissolves incompatible catheters. Patients may notice a garliclike taste for several hours, and their skin and breath may have a characteristic odor due to the DMSO for 1 to 2 days after an embolization with Onyx.

For DAVFs, endovascular treatment with transarterial, transvenous, or, occasionally, combined-approach embolization, has become a first-line approach. Treatment is aimed at complete elimination of the arteriovenous shunt—incomplete treatment allows recruitment of collateral vessels and persistent risk of hemorrhage. When complete occlusion of the shunt is not feasible or considered too risky, selective disconnection of CVD should be considered. This approach can have an efficacy comparable with DAVF obliteration in preventing neurological morbidity with lower levels of procedural risk. The optimal method of endovascular treatment is controversial. The rates of complete

angiographic obliteration by transvenous embolization have been reported at 71% to 87.5%[47] (Figs. 36.4 and 36.5). Long-term cure rates in the 90% range have been reported with transarterial Onyx embolization.[48]

## Postoperative Complications

### Key Concepts

- Microcatheter retention occurs in less than 3% of embolizations.
- Catheter-induced thromboemboli are the most common cause of cerebral ischemia during embolization.
- Intensive neurological monitoring is recommended for at least 24 hours after embolization.

Complications during endovascular navigation of the cerebral vasculature can be rapid and dramatic and require interdisciplinary collaboration. Embolization of brain lesions can be performed with a high degree of technical success and a relatively low rate of permanent neurological complications. The reported incidence of overall complications from brain AVM embolization varies between 3% and 25%.[49] Mortality rates associated with embolization have been reported to be 2% or less, and permanent neurological deficits 2% to 8.9% with the use of new-generation microcatheters.[27,49] Permanent complications of transvenous embolization have been reported in 4% to 7% of cases.[47]

A serious complication is adherence of the liquid agents to the catheter, making catheter withdrawal traumatic or impossible. Retention of the microcatheter tip in the nidus occurs in less than 3% of all embolizations. Retained catheters can be removed with surgical resection soon after the embolization, or even few weeks after if there is no adhesion to the vessel wall. Straight microcatheters within the vessel lumen do not appear to cause thrombosis. However, some neurointerventionalists prefer a 3- to 6-month course of anticoagulation to prevent thrombosis if deemed safe for the patient. Microcatheter fracture/retention may be more frequent in Onyx embolizations compared with NBCA. However, the advent of DMSO-compatible microcatheters with detachable tips has dramatically reduced microcatheter retention.[50] This technology is currently only available in Europe.

Catheter-induced thromboemboli, embolization of the wrong vessel, and reflux of embolic material into normal cerebral vessels are the most common causes of cerebral ischemia during embolization. Thromboembolism can be prevented with systemic anticoagulation and/or flushing of all catheters with heparinized saline. Reflux of embolic material into normal parenchymal branches during embolization can be prevented with high-quality biplanar imaging systems, general anesthesia, optimal positioning of the microcatheter, and appropriate dilution of the liquid embolic agent to allow for desired polymerization times. In the setting of inadvertent vascular occlusions, blood pressure augmentation, with or without direct thrombolysis, may be used to increase distal perfusion.[42] Given the best available evidence, deliberately induced hypertension in the face of symptomatic cerebral ischemia from vascular occlusion during embolization should not be avoided because of fear of rupturing the malformation.

ICH, during or after embolization, is one of the most feared complications of embolization treatment. In the setting of an intraprocedural hemorrhage, immediate protamine reversal of heparin (if heparin was used during the procedure) should be done as rapidly as possible.[42] Hemorrhagic complication rates associated with AVM embolization range from 2% to 4.7%. The possible etiologies are diverse but most frequently include (1) vessel perforation during microcatheter navigation (the use of flow-directed catheters has significantly reduced the incidence of vessel perforations because they do not require metal guidewires beyond the tip to navigate into the AVM feeders); (2) venous outflow obstruction related to either venous occlusion by the embolic material or late venous thrombosis due to abrupt venous flow reduction; and (3) normal perfusion pressure breakthrough (NPPB) hemorrhage.

NPPB is thought to be due to the sudden increase in perfusion pressure in the surrounding normal brain parenchyma, which theoretically suffers from chronically impaired autoregulation, after AVM embolization or resection. NPPB tends to occur in patients with large high-flow AVMs and multiple large feeding vessels. Reduction of the patient's mean arterial pressure 15% to 20% below the baseline during the first 24 hours after embolization and limiting embolization (staging embolizations) to 30% of the AVM nidus per session are strategies to reduce the risk of ICH due to NPPB.

Hydrocephalus may result from numerous causes after AVM embolization. These include intraventricular hemorrhage and compression of the aqueduct of Sylvius by large draining veins.[18] Choroidal AVMs may be associated with overproduction of cerebrospinal fluid and hydrocephalus.

Typically, hydrocephalus is treated by insertion of a ventricular drainage catheter.

Cranial nerve injuries and transient ophthalmoplegia have been reported in 14% of transvenous cavernous sinus embolizations, but patients typically have a full recovery.[47] The risk of cranial nerve damage from coil mass effect or direct coil injury can be avoided through the use of liquid embolic agents. DMSO-induced angiotoxicity or vasospasm can sometimes be prevented by slow Onyx injection.[51] Avoiding injecting vessels that supply the lower cranial nerves (petrosal branch of the middle meningeal artery, stylomastoid branch of the posterior auricular and occipital arteries, and jugular branch of the ascending pharyngeal artery) helps to avoid cranial nerve injury. A short course of steroids after cranial injury may be considered.[52]

Usually obliteration of AVM/DAVF leads to a decrease in seizure incidence,[53] although this has been best shown after surgical resection. Seizure frequency may increase postoperatively. In a small series, seizures after Onyx embolization occurred in 45% of cases, of which 10% had no other identifiable cause other than a recent Onyx embolization (median days to seizure was 7 days).[54]

Postprocedurally, neurological intensive care monitoring is recommended. Patients are preferably extubated after the procedure to allow for neurological examinations to monitor the patient's condition, although practices vary, and some neurointerventionalists maintain patients intubated to allow for better blood pressure control. The arterial sheath is usually removed after the procedure, but an arterial line may be maintained for blood pressure monitoring. Knowledge of vascular access site complications and management is important in providing quality postoperative care[55] (Table 36.3).

Systemic anticoagulation with heparin after the procedure should be considered for patients with sluggish venous outflow or compromise of an important component of the venous outflow system. Sluggish flow in the veins can lead to venous thrombosis with subsequent hemorrhage from the remaining nidus. In general, a low systolic blood pressure (80–120 mm Hg) is maintained after embolization procedures to avoid the possibility of NPPB hemorrhage. Antihypertensive medications that do not have venodilator properties may be preferred to reduce the likelihood of hemorrhage.

A new neurological deficit after embolization is usually investigated with a noncontrast CT scan to rule out a new ICH or hydrocephalus. Magnetic resonance (MR) imaging scanning with diffusion-weighted imaging may be appropriate if an ischemic infarct is suspected or in cases where a large Onyx cast may prevent adequate CT evaluation. Gadolinium-enhanced spoiled gradient (SPGR) MR sequence and/or time-resolved MR angiogram/CTA may allow for noninvasive evaluation of the venous outflow patency.[56]

## Conclusion

Brain AVMs and DAVFs are vascular lesions, which may be clinically silent or cause devastating ICH. Ruptured lesions require urgent treatment; however, treatment for unruptured lesions is less clear. Treatment options include endovascular embolization, microsurgical resection, stereotactic

**Table 36.3**  Vascular Access Site Complications and Management

| Complication | Description | Clinical findings | Management |
|---|---|---|---|
| Hematoma (most common) Incidence: 5%–23% | Collection of blood in the soft tissue Occurs because of blood loss at the arterial and/or venous access site or perforation of an artery or vein May occur if the arterial puncture is below the femoral bifurcation so the femoral head is not available to assist with compression | Swelling surrounding the puncture (visible) Area of hardening surrounding the puncture site (palpable) Varies in size Often associated with pain in the groin area that can occur at rest or with leg movement Can result in decrease of hemoglobin and blood pressure and increase in heart rate, depending on severity | Apply pressure to site Mark the area to evaluate for any change in size Provide hydration Monitor serial complete blood cell counts Maintain/prolong bed rest Interrupt anticoagulant and antiplatelet medications if necessary Many hematomas resolve within a few weeks as the blood dissipates and is absorbed into the tissue |
| Retroperitoneal hemorrhage Incidence: 0.15 %–0.44% | Bleeding that occurs behind the serous membrane lining the walls of the abdomen/pelvis May occur if the arterial wall puncture is made above the inguinal ligament, resulting in perforation of a suprainguinal artery or penetration of the posterior wall Can be fatal if not recognized early | Back pain/flank pain or abdominal pain Abdominal distention Often not associated with obvious swelling Ecchymosis and decrease in hemoglobin and hematocrit are late signs Hypotension and tachycardia Diagnosed by computed tomography | Provide hydration Perform serial blood cell counts Maintain/prolong bed rest Interrupt anticoagulation and antiplatelet medications if necessary Blood transfusion, if indicated If severe, may require surgical evacuation |
| Pseudoaneurysm Incidence: 0.5%–9% | Communicating tract between a weaker femoral artery wall and surrounding tissue Possible causes include difficulty with cannulation, inadequate compression after sheath removal, and impaired hemostasis | Swelling at insertion site Large, painful hematoma Ecchymosis Pulsatile mass Bruit and/or thrill in the groin Pseudoaneurysms can rupture causing abrupt swelling and severe pain Suspect nerve compression when pain is out of proportion to size of hematoma Nerve compression can result in limb weakness that takes weeks or months to resolve Diagnosed by ultrasound | Maintain/prolong bed rest Small femoral pseudoaneurysms should be monitored; they commonly close spontaneously after cessation of anticoagulant therapy Large femoral pseudoaneurysms can be treated by ultrasound-guided compression, ultrasound-guided thrombin injection, or surgical intervention |
| Arteriovenous fistula Incidence: 0.2%–2.1% | Direct communication between an artery and a vein that occurs when the artery and vein are punctured The communication occurs once the sheath is removed Risk factors: multiple access attempts, punctures above or below proper site level, impaired clotting | Can be asymptomatic Bruit and/or thrill at access site Swollen, tender extremity Distal arterial insufficiency and/or deep venous thrombosis can result in limb ischemia Congestive heart failure Confirmed by ultrasound | Some arteriovenous fistulas resolve spontaneously without intervention Some arteriovenous fistulas require ultrasound-guided compression or surgical repair |
| Arterial occlusion Incidence: <0.8% | Occlusion of an artery by a thromboembolus Most common sources: atherosclerotic plaque, vascular aneurysm, cardiac Thromboemboli can develop at sheath site or catheter tip Embolization can occur during sheath removal Prevention/reduction with anticoagulation, vasodilators, physician/nursing vigilance | Classic symptoms include pain, paralysis, paresthesias, pulselessness, pallor Doppler studies help localize the area Angiogram is required to identify the exact location of occlusion site | Treatment depends on size/type of embolus, location, and patient's ability to tolerate ischemia in affected area Small thromboemboli in well-perfused areas may undergo spontaneous lysis Larger thromboemboli may require thromboembolectomy and/or thrombolytic agents, surgery Distal embolic protections devices (i.e., filters) may be placed in venous occlusions |
| Femoral neuropathy Incidence: 0.21% | Nerve damage caused by injury of the femoral nerve or lateral cutaneous branch during access and/or compression of nerves by hematoma | Local or radiating Pain/tingling/numbness Leg weakness Difficulty moving affected leg Decreased patellar tendon reflex | Identification and treatment of the source and symptoms Most resolve spontaneously Physical therapy |
| Infection Incidence: <0.1% | Colonization by pathogen Causes: compromised technique, poor hygiene, prolonged indwelling sheath time Femoral access closure device (have been linked with increased occurrence of infection) | Pain, erythema, swelling, discharge at access site Fever Increased white blood cell count | Treatment of symptoms (e.g., pain) Antibiotics |

radiosurgery, or a combination of these modalities. Endovascular embolization is most commonly performed as a precursor to microsurgery or radiotherapy. Knowledge of the different embolic agents is paramount. Complications during and after embolization can be rapid and dramatic and require optimal interdisciplinary communication and collaboration. Although embolization of brain lesions can be performed with a high degree of technical success and a relatively low rate of permanent neurological complications, significant morbidity and mortality do occur.

## References

1. Morris Z, Whiteley WN, Longstreth Jr WT, et al. Incidental findings on brain magnetic resonance imaging: systematic review and meta-analysis. *BMJ.* 2009;339:b3016.
2. Stapf C, Mast H, Sciacca RR, et al. The New York Islands AVM Study: design, study progress, and initial results. *Stroke.* 2003;34(5):e29–e33.
3. Kim H, Su H, Weinsheimer S, Pawlikowska L, Young WL. Brain arteriovenous malformation pathogenesis: a response-to-injury paradigm. *Acta Neurochir Suppl.* 2011;111:83–92.
4. Ondra SL, Troupp H, George ED, Schwab K. The natural history of symptomatic arteriovenous malformations of the brain: a 24-year follow-up assessment. *J Neurosurg.* 1990;73(3):387–391.
5. Hernesniemi JA, Dashti R, Juvela S, Vaart K, Niemela M, Laakso A. Natural history of brain arteriovenous malformations: a long-term follow-up study of risk of hemorrhage in 238 patients. *Neurosurgery.* 2008;63(5):823–829. discussion 9–31.
6. Mast H, Young WL, Koennecke HC, et al. Risk of spontaneous haemorrhage after diagnosis of cerebral arteriovenous malformation. *Lancet.* 1997;350(9084):1065–1068.
7. Marks MP, Lane B, Steinberg GK, Snipes GJ. Intranidal aneurysms in cerebral arteriovenous malformations: evaluation and endovascular treatment. *Radiology.* 1992;183(2):355–360.
8. Pollock BE, Flickinger JC, Lunsford LD, Bissonette DJ, Kondziolka D. Factors that predict the bleeding risk of cerebral arteriovenous malformations. *Stroke.* 1996;27(1):1–6.
9. da Costa L, Wallace MC, Ter Brugge KG, O'Kelly C, Willinsky RA, Tymianski M. The natural history and predictive features of hemorrhage from brain arteriovenous malformations. *Stroke.* 2009;40(1):100–105.
10. Redekop G, TerBrugge K, Montanera W, Willinsky R. Arterial aneurysms associated with cerebral arteriovenous malformations: classification, incidence, and risk of hemorrhage. *J Neurosurg.* 1998;89(4):539–546.
11. Brown Jr RD, Wiebers DO, Forbes G, et al. The natural history of unruptured intracranial arteriovenous malformations. *J Neurosurg.* 1988;68(3):352–357.
12. Monteiro JM, Rosas MJ, Correia AP, Vaz AR. Migraine and intracranial vascular malformations. *Headache.* 1993;33(10):563–565.
13. ApSimon HT, Reef H, Phadke RV, Popovic EA. A population-based study of brain arteriovenous malformation: long-term treatment outcomes. *Stroke.* 2002;33(12):2794–2800.
14. Hillman J. Population-based analysis of arteriovenous malformation treatment. *J Neurosurg.* 2001;95(4):633–637.
15. Spetzler RF, Martin NA. A proposed grading system for arteriovenous malformations. *J Neurosurg.* 1986;65(4):476–483.
16. Stapf C, Mast H, Sciacca RR, et al. Predictors of hemorrhage in patients with untreated brain arteriovenous malformation. *Neurology.* 2006;66(9):1350–1355.
17. Mohr JP, Parides MK, Stapf C, et al. Medical management with or without interventional therapy for unruptured brain arteriovenous malformations (ARUBA): a multicentre, non-blinded, randomised trial. *Lancet.* 2014;383(9917):614–621.
18. Ogilvy CS, Stieg PE, Awad I, et al. AHA Scientific Statement: Recommendations for the management of intracranial arteriovenous malformations: a statement for healthcare professionals from a special writing group of the Stroke Council, American Stroke Association. *Stroke.* 2001;32(6):1458–1471.
19. Wikholm G, Lundqvist C, Svendsen P. Embolization of cerebral arteriovenous malformations: part I—Technique, morphology, and complications. *Neurosurgery.* 1996;39(3):448–457. discussion 57–9.
20. Lunsford LD, Kondziolka D, Flickinger JC, et al. Stereotactic radiosurgery for arteriovenous malformations of the brain. *J Neurosurg.* 1991;75(4):512–524.
21. Maruyama K, Kawahara N, Shin M, et al. The risk of hemorrhage after radiosurgery for cerebral arteriovenous malformations. *New Eng J Med.* 2005;352(2):146–153.
22. Deruty R, Pelissou-Guyotat I, Mottolese C, Bascoulergue Y, Amat D. The combined management of cerebral arteriovenous malformations. Experience with 100 cases and review of the literature. *Acta Neurochir (Wien).* 1993;123:101–102.
23. Deruty R, Pelissou-Guyotat I, Amat D, et al. Multidisciplinary treatment of cerebral arteriovenous malformations. *Neurol Res.* 1995;17:169–177.
24. Hartmann A, Mast H, Mohr JP, et al. Determinants of staged endovascular and surgical treatment outcome of brain arteriovenous malformations. *Stroke.* 2005;36:2431–2435.
25. Starke RM, Komotar RJ, Otten ML, et al. Adjuvant embolization with N-butyl cyanoacrylate in the treatment of cerebral arteriovenous malformations: outcomes, complications, and predictors of neurologic deficits. *Stroke.* 2009;40:2783–2790.
26. Jafar JJ, Davis AJ, Berenstein A, Choi IS, Kupersmith MJ. The effect of embolization with N-butyl cyanoacrylate prior to surgical resection of cerebral arteriovenous malformations. *J Neurosurg.* 1993;78(1):60–69.
27. Pierot L, Cognard C, Herbreteau D, et al. Endovascular treatment of brain arteriovenous malformations using a liquid embolic agent: results of a prospective, multicentre study (BRAVO). *Eur Radiol.* 2013;23(10):2838–2845.
28. Valavanis A, Pangalu A, Tanaka M. Endovascular treatment of cerebral arteriovenous malformations with emphasis on the curative role of embolisation. *Intervent Neuroradiol.* 2005;11(Suppl 1):37–43.
29. van Rooij WJ, Jacobs S, Sluzewski M, van der Pol B, Beute GN, Sprengers ME. Curative embolization of brain arteriovenous malformations with onyx: patient selection, embolization technique, and results. *AJNR.* 2012;33(7):1299–1304.
30. Reitz M, Schmidt NO, Vukovic Z, et al. How to deal with incompletely treated AVMs: experience of 67 cases and review of the literature. *Acta Neurochir Suppl.* 2011;112:123–129.
31. Gandhi D, Chen J, Pearl M, Huang J, Gemmete JJ, Kathuria S. Intracranial dural arteriovenous fistulas: classification, imaging findings, and treatment. *AJNR.* 2012;33(6):1007–1013.
32. Kirsch M, Liebig T, Kuhne D, Henkes H. Endovascular management of dural arteriovenous fistulas of the transverse and sigmoid sinus in 150 patients. *Neuroradiology.* 2009;51(7):477–483.
33. Chung SJ, Kim JS, Kim JC, et al. Intracranial dural arteriovenous fistulas: analysis of 60 patients. *Cerebrovasc Dis.* 2002;13(2):79–88.
34. Suh DC, Lee JH, Kim SJ, et al. New concept in cavernous sinus dural arteriovenous fistula: correlation with presenting symptom and venous drainage patterns. *Stroke.* 2005;36(6):1134–1139.
35. Borden JA, Wu JK, Shucart WA. A proposed classification for spinal and cranial dural arteriovenous fistulous malformations and implications for treatment. *J Neurosurg.* 1995;82(2):166–179.
36. Cognard C, Gobin YP, Pierot L, et al. Cerebral dural arteriovenous fistulas: clinical and angiographic correlation with a revised classification of venous drainage. *Radiology.* 1995;194(3):671–680.
37. Davies MA, Ter Brugge K, Willinsky R, Wallace MC. The natural history and management of intracranial dural arteriovenous fistulae. Part 2: aggressive lesions. *Intervent Radiol.* 1997;3(4):303–311.
38. van Dijk JM, terBrugge KG, Willinsky RA, Wallace MC. Clinical course of cranial dural arteriovenous fistulas with long-term persistent cortical venous reflux. *Stroke.* 2002;33(5):1233–1236.
39. Zipfel GJ, Shah MN, Refai D, Dacey Jr RG, Derdeyn CP. Cranial dural arteriovenous fistulas: modification of angiographic classification scales based on new natural history data. *Neurosurg Focus.* 2009;26(5).
40. Satomi J, van Dijk JM, Terbrugge KG, Willinsky RA, Wallace MC. Benign cranial dural arteriovenous fistulas: outcome of conservative management based on the natural history of the lesion. *J Neurosurg.* 2002;97(4):767–770.
41. Luciani A, Houdart E, Mounayer C, Saint Maurice JP, Merland JJ. Spontaneous closure of dural arteriovenous fistulas: report of three cases and review of the literature. *AJNR.* 2001;22(5):992–996.
42. Young WL, Pile-Spellman J. Anesthetic considerations for interventional neuroradiology. *Anesthesiology.* 1994;80(2):427–456.

43. Manninen PH, Gignac EM, Gelb AW, Lownie SP. Anesthesia for interventional neuroradiology. *J Clin Anesth.* 1995;7(6):448–452.

44. Moo LR, Murphy KJ, Gailloud P, Tesoro M, Hart J. Tailored cognitive testing with provocative amobarbital injection preceding AVM embolization. *AJNR.* 2002;23(3):416–421.

45. Jahan R, Murayama Y, Gobin YP, Duckwiler GR, Vinters HV, Vinuela F. Embolization of arteriovenous malformations with Onyx: clinicopathological experience in 23 patients. *Neurosurgery.* 2001;48(5):984–995. discussion 95–7.

46. Chaloupka JC, Huddle DC, Alderman J, Fink S, Hammond R, Vinters HV. A reexamination of the angiotoxicity of superselective injection of DMSO in the swine rete embolization model. *AJNR.* 1999;20(3):401–410.

47. Yoshida K, Melake M, Oishi H, Yamamoto M, Arai H. Transvenous embolization of dural carotid cavernous fistulas: a series of 44 consecutive patients. *AJNR.* 2010;31(4):651–655.

48. Chandra RV, Leslie-Mazwi TM, Mehta BP, et al. Transarterial onyx embolization of cranial dural arteriovenous fistulas: long-term follow-up. *AJNR.* 2014;35(9):1793–1797.

49. Jayaraman MV, Marcellus ML, Hamilton S, et al. Neurologic complications of arteriovenous malformation embolization using liquid embolic agents. *AJNR.* 2008;29(2):242–246.

50. Altschul D, Paramasivam S, Ortega-Gutierrez S, Fifi JT, Berenstein A. Safety and efficacy using a detachable tip microcatheter in the embolization of pediatric arteriovenous malformations. *Childs Nerv Syst.* 2014;30(6):1099–1107.

51. Nogueira RG, Dabus G, Rabinov JD, et al. Preliminary experience with onyx embolization for the treatment of intracranial dural arteriovenous fistulas. *AJNR.* 2008;29(1):91–97.

52. Ogilvy CS, Stieg PE. Awad I, et al, Special Writing Group of the Stroke Council, American Stroke Association. AHA Scientific Statement. Recommendations for the management of intracranial arteriovenous malformations: a statement for healthcare professionals from a special writing group of the Stroke Council, American Stroke Association. *Stroke.* 2001;32:1458–1471.

53. Baranoski JF, Grant RA, Hirsch LJ, et al. Seizure control for intracranial arteriovenous malformations is directly related to treatment modality: a meta-analysis. *J Neurointerv Surg.* 2014;6(9):684–690.

54. de Los Reyes K, Patel A, Doshi A, et al. Seizures after Onyx embolization for the treatment of cerebral arteriovenous malformation. *Intervent Radiol.* 2011;17(3):331–338.

55. Nasser TK, Mohler 3rd ER, Wilensky RL, Hathaway DR. Peripheral vascular complications following coronary interventional procedures. *Clin Cardiol.* 1995;18(11):609–614.

56. Nogueira RG, Bayrlee A, Hirsch JA, Yoo AJ, Copen WA. Dynamic contrast-enhanced MRA at 1.5 T for detection of arteriovenous shunting before and after Onyx embolization of cerebral arteriovenous malformations. *J Neuroimaging.* 2013;23(4):514–517.

# 37 *Acute Stroke Management*

CAITLIN LOOMIS, BRYAN A. PUKENAS, and ROBERT W. HURST

## Introduction

Stroke occurs every 40 seconds in the United States and is the leading cause of long-term adult disability. Ischemic stroke constitutes the vast majority of all strokes.[1] Intravenous recombinant tissue plasminogen activator (IV rt-PA) was approved by the Food and Drug Administration (FDA) in 1996 for the treatment of acute ischemic stroke within 3 hours.[2] The treatment window was extended to 4.5 hours in 2009 for specific patients.[3,4] However, only 2% to 5% of ischemic stroke patients across the United States are treated with IV rt-PA,[5,6] largely due to unknown time of symptom onset and presentation to medical care after the therapeutic time window. A large metaanalysis showed a strong correlation between arterial recanalization and good functional outcome at 3 months,[7] suggesting that recanalization is paramount to recovery. IV rt-PA achieves partial to complete recanalization in 6% to 50% of patients, with less favorable results in proximal artery occlusions. Reocclusion rates after IV rt-PA are as high as 34%.[7–15] Patients who do not respond well to IV rt-PA include patients with large vessel occlusions,[14,16,17] large thrombus burden (thrombi >8 mm),[18] and noncardioembolic etiology of stroke.[19]

The significant burden of stroke combined with high reocclusion rates and less favorable results for those with proximal artery occlusion make endovascular therapy an appealing option for select patients. In this chapter, we will discuss the relevant neuroanatomy, considerations, and indications for endovascular treatment of acute ischemic stroke and perioperative complications.

## Neuroanatomy and Procedure

### Key Concepts

- Several anatomical variants of the aortic arch and circle of Willis (COW) exist, which should not be mistaken for arterial occlusion or disease.
- Anatomical features that affect difficulty with catheterization and therefore time to treatment include disease at the origin of the great vessels, aortic arch variants, and tortuosity of the common carotid arteries (CCAs).
- The majority of emboli from the internal carotid artery (ICA) are carried to the middle cerebral artery (MCA).

Clinical evaluation and noninvasive imaging, usually computed tomography (CT) angiography, are utilized to determine the site of vessel occlusion prior to digital subtraction angiography (DSA).

Entry into the arterial system for DSA is usually accomplished by puncturing the right common femoral artery.

For safe postprocedure hemostasis, the puncture site must be below the inguinal ligament. Puncture in this location permits effective hemostasis by compression and minimizes the chance of retroperitoneal hematoma. After arterial puncture and placement of an arterial sheath, the guidewire and catheter are advanced into the aortic arch.

The configuration of the aortic arch varies with respect to anatomical favorability for selective catheterization of branch vessels.[20] The arch may be classified into three types based on the origins of the branch vessels with respect to the superior and inferior margins of the arch (Fig. 37.1). The three types present progressive difficulty in selective branch vessel catheterization, with types II and III increasing the chance of catheter prolapse into the arch with attempts at selective catheterization. Types II and III also are associated with advancing age, as well as a higher risk of emboli, dissection, and thrombus formation.[21]

### Clinical Pearl

Type II and III arches are associated with higher risk of emboli, dissection, and thrombus formation.

The three major aortic arch branches include the innominate, the left common carotid, and left subclavian artery (Fig. 37.1). The innominate is the first and shortest of the three branches, running for several centimeters before dividing into the right subclavian and right CCA. Next is the left CCA, typically followed by the left subclavian artery. The VAs generally originate as the first branch of the respective subclavian arteries, although in approximately 5% of the population, the left vertebral artery originates directly from the aortic arch just distal to the left CCA.

Additional anatomical factors that affect difficulty with selective catheterization and, consequently, time to treatment in acute ischemic stroke, include disease at the origin of the great vessels; aortic arch variants, including a common origin of the innominate and left common carotid artery; and tortuosity of the CCAs.

After selective catheterization, a long sheath (80–90 cm) is placed proximally in the arterial system to be treated (internal carotid or vertebral artery) using a wire exchange. The sheath provides a stable platform through which more distal catheterization is performed. A flexible introducer catheter may be advanced through the sheath to achieve a more distal position in the extracranial portion of the vessel.

The ICA is often divided into four segments (Fig. 37.2): the cervical, petrous, cavernous, and intradural segments. ICA lesions proximal to the ophthalmic artery (OA) are

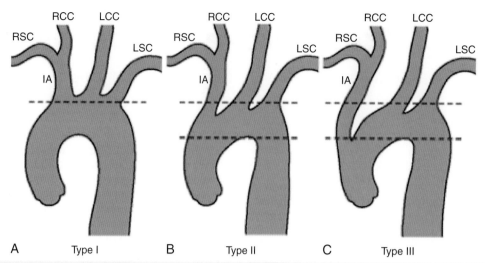

**Fig. 37.1** Aortic arch morphologies. Arch morphology is defined based on the origin of the great vessels. **(A)** Type I arch: all vessels originate at the superior margin of the arch. **(B)** Type II arch: at least one vessel originates between the superior and inferior margins of the aortic arch. **(C)** Type III arch: at least one vessel originates below the inferior margin of the aortic arch. *IA,* innominate artery; *RSC,* right subclavian artery; *RCC,* right common carotid artery; *LCC,* left common carotid artery; *LSC,* left subclavian artery. (Adapted from Rapp, J, et al. Carotid artery stenting. In Morton, J ed. *The Interventional Cardiac Catheterization Handbook,* 3rd ed., pp. 324-339 © 2013, Elsevier, Inc.)

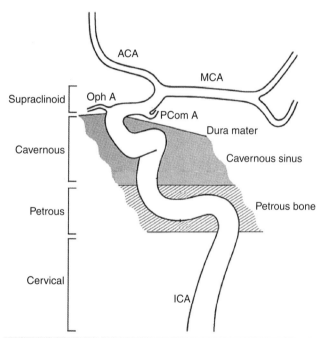

**Fig. 37.2** Segments of the internal carotid artery. The internal carotid artery may be divided into the following four segments: cervical, petrous, cavernous, and supraclinoid. The cervical segment runs from the origin of the ICA until its entry into the carotid canal where the vessel becomes the petrous segment. The cavernous segment runs through the cavernous sinus (CS), surrounded by the venous plexus of the sinus and medial to the cranial nerves of the cavernous sinus (III, IV, V1, V2, and VI). Exiting the cavernous sinus, the supraclinoid ICA penetrates the dura and gives off three major intradural branches. The ophthalmic artery (OA) is the first intradural branch of the ICA and is typically used as a neuroradiologic marker for the site of ICA dural penetration. The posterior communicating artery (PComm), a component of the circle of Willis, is the next intradural branch followed by the anterior choroidal artery (not shown), which originates just proximal to the bifurcation of the ICA into the middle cerebral artery (MCA) and anterior cerebral artery (ACA). (Adapted from Takeuchi S, Karino T. Flow patterns and distributions of fluid velocity and wall shear stress in the human internal carotid and middle cerebral arteries. *World Neurosurg.* 2010 Mar;73(3):174–85.)

extradural in location, whereas those at or distal to the OA origin are located within the subarachnoid space. Ophthalmic collaterals from the external carotid artery may be robust and compensate for occlusion of the ICA, reconstituting the vessel in the supraclinoid portion.

The VAs have also been divided into four segments, designated V1 through V4 (Fig. 37.3). V1, V2, and V3 are extradural, whereas V4 is intradural. V4 gives origin to the only major branch of the VA, the posterior inferior cerebellar artery (PICA). The portion of V4 distal to PICA may be congenitally hypoplastic in 5% to 15% of the population, an anomaly that occurs most commonly on the right and should not be confused with acquired occlusion or atherosclerotic disease. Asymmetry of the VAs is common, with the left VA being as large or larger than the right VA in approximately 80% of the population. Consequently, the relative ease of access and typically larger size dictate selection of the left VA for endovascular treatment of most cases of posterior circulation occlusion.

## Clinical Pearl

Congenitally hypoplastic vertebral artery distal to PICA is present in 5% to 15% of the population and should not be confused with acute occlusion or atherosclerotic disease.

Diagnostic angiography is performed through the sheath or introducer catheter, usually from the CCA, the cervical segment of the ICA, or the V2–V3 segment of the VA. Evaluation of the diagnostic angiogram determines the site of occlusion, as well as the anatomy of the intracranial circulation. Of particular importance is the evaluation of potential collateral routes and the configuration of the COW.

The COW is an important anastomotic arterial structure at the base of the brain that may provide collateral flow from left to right, as well as between the anterior and posterior circulations (Fig. 37.4).

Asymmetry, hypoplasia, or aplasia of one or more portions of the COW is common. Approximately 40% of the population demonstrates angiographic asymmetry of the A1 segments. Importantly, hypoplasia (4%) or aplasia (1%) of one A1, configurations that inhibit left-to-right collateral flow in ICA occlusion, are not rare. In addition, a significant portion of the population has hypoplasia of one (20%) or both (2%) P1s. This configuration results in the posterior cerebral artery distribution receiving major supply from the PComm and is referred to as a *fetal configuration of the PComm*.[22] The variable anatomy of the COW has major implications for the effects of proximal vessel occlusion and emboli in acute ischemic stroke.

### Clinical Pearl

Strokes in the PCA territory may be supplied by the ICA: 20% of the population has hypoplasia of one P1, resulting in anterior circulation supply of the posterior cerebral artery territory via the PComm.

The MCA receives the major outflow from the ICA and, consequently, most emboli from the ICA are carried into the MCA distribution.[23] The M1 portion runs from the MCA origin to the Sylvian fissure and gives origin to the lateral lenticulostriate (LST) arteries. These perforating arteries provide blood flow to deep gray nuclei, including the putamen and globus pallidus. Consequently, occlusion of the M1 can result in blockage of the poorly collateralized LST distribution, as well as ischemia of more distal portions of the MCA. In the Sylvian fissure, the MCA divides into superior and inferior trunks, which course over the insula and around the operculum, giving rise to cortical branches supplying the lateral aspects of the frontal, parietal, and temporal lobes.

The anterior cerebral artery (ACA) also originates at the ICA bifurcation, running medially as the A1 until its junction with the AComm. The more distal portions of the ACA run in the interhemispheric fissure, giving rise to cortical branches supplying the medial frontal and parietal lobes.

The major vessel of the posterior circulation, the basilar artery, originates at the vertebrobasilar junction and runs superiorly along the surface of the pons and midbrain. The basilar artery gives rise to perforating arteries as well as transverse branches supplying brainstem and portions of the cerebellum. The two named cerebellar branches of the basilar artery include the anterior inferior cerebellar artery (AICA) and the superior cerebellar artery (SCA). The AICA originates approximately one third along the length of the basilar artery and runs laterally across the pons to supply pontine perforating arteries. The SCA originates from the distal basilar artery and courses laterally around the midbrain before giving rise to superior hemispheric and vermian branches to the cerebellum.

At its apex, the basilar artery divides into the posterior cerebral arteries (PCAs). The P1 portions give origin to the majority of blood supply to the thalamus via the proximally located thalamoperforating arteries. Hypoplasia of P1 is common (see earlier) and should not be confused with acquired occlusion. The PCA then courses around the

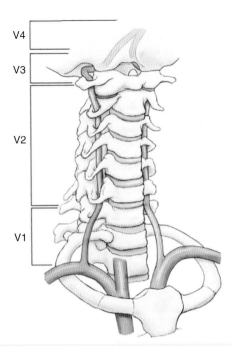

**Fig. 37.3** The four segments of the vertebral artery. The V1 or preforaminal segment includes that portion of the VA from the origin until the vessel enters the transverse foramen of the lower cervical vertebrae, usually at C6. The V2 or foraminal portion runs through the transverse foramina to the C2 level. The V3 or suboccipital portion of the VA runs through the transverse foramina of C2, C1, and along the superior margin of C1 before penetrating the dura, a transition often marked by mild normal narrowing of the vessel. The intradural or V4 portion runs in the subarachnoid space to join the contralateral VA at the vertebrobasilar junction to form the basilar artery. (Adapted from Charbel, FT, et al. Extracranial Vertebral Artery Diseases, In: Winn, HR ed. *Youmans Neurological Surgery* Copyright © 2011, Elsevier Inc.)

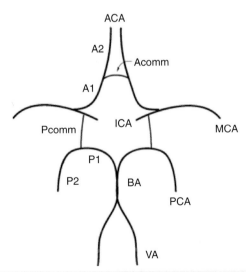

**Fig. 37.4** Arteries comprising a complete circle of Willis. *ICA*, internal carotid artery; *ACA*, anterior carotid artery; *MCA*, middle cerebral artery; *PCA*, posterior cerebral artery; *BA*, basilar artery; *VA*, vertebral artery *AComm*, anterior communicating artery; *PComm*, posterior communicating artery; *A1, A2, P1, P2*, branches of the anterior and posterior communicating arteries. (Adapted from Cucchiara, B, et al. *Medical Hypotheses*. 2008, 70: pp. 860–65.)

midbrain, giving rise to inferior temporal branches. The PCAs then approach the midline and enter the posterior interhemispheric fissure, providing supply to the medial portions of the occipital and parietal lobes.

After identification of the site of occlusion, microcatheters for endovascular treatment are placed through the sheath or introducer catheter and into the intracranial circulation. Current techniques for endovascular therapy of acute ischemic stroke include intraarterial (IA) infusion of thrombolytic medication and/or mechanical techniques for removal of acute clot.

The MERCI retriever, the earliest device approved in the United States, consists of a corkscrewlike device to snare thrombus within the intracranial vessels. The device and thrombus are then withdrawn under suction.[24]

The Penumbra System utilizes an aspiration microcatheter connected to a suction pump to remove the clot. A teardrop-shaped separator is placed through the aspiration microcatheter, then advanced and retracted just distal to the microcatheter to break up the clot, thereby enhancing aspiration.[25] Direct aspiration using only the microcatheter may also be performed.[26] Variable sizes of aspiration microcatheters may allow access to relatively distal branches, including M2–3, A2, and P2.

Stent retrievers, including the Solitaire FR and Trevo devices, are stent devices attached to a wire that are deployed into the occlusive thrombus and left open across the occluded segment for various periods of time to allow integration of the clot into the stent cells. The device with the incorporated clot is then withdrawn while maintaining suction on the introducer catheter or sheath[27] (see Fig. 37.5).

## CONSIDERATIONS AND INDICATIONS FOR ENDOVASCULAR THERAPY

### Key Concepts

- Certain patient populations are eligible for endovascular therapy for acute ischemic stroke, including those with large vessel occlusion who do not respond to IV rt-PA, or patients out of the window for IV rt-PA, but within 6 to 8 hours of time last normal.
- The time window for basilar artery thrombosis is extended to 12 hours, with reports of benefit up to 48 hours, given the poor prognosis that the diagnosis carries.
- Mechanical thrombectomy is generally favored over IA rt-PA by most interventionalists.

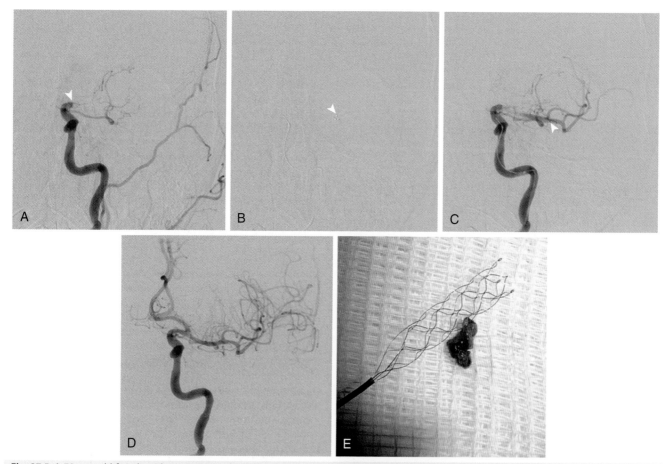

**Fig. 37.5** A 78-year-old female with acute onset of right hemiparesis and aphasia. **(A)** AP view of left internal carotid (LICA) injection demonstrating occlusion at ICA bifurcation (*arrowhead*). **(B)** AP view, preinjection, with Solitaire deployed (*arrowhead demonstrates distal tines of Solitaire device*). **(C)** AP view during injection with Solitaire deployed (*arrowhead demonstrates distal tines of Solitaire device*). Solitaire opens distal ICA and MCA with distal filling. **(D)** AP view post Solitaire removal with complete reopening of MCA and ACA. **(E)** Solitaire device after removal with adherent clot.

A number of studies have been published comparing the effectiveness of the available devices. The newer devices, particularly the Penumbra System and stent retrievers, have been found to have higher rates of reopening and improved clinical outcome than that of earlier devices or IA thrombolytic treatment alone.[28–31] Importantly, very few of these devices were utilized in early randomized trials comparing IV thrombolysis to endovascular treatment in acute ischemic stroke.

The Middle Cerebral Artery Embolism Local Fibrinolytic Intervention Trial (MELT) and the Prolyse in Acute Cerebral Thromboembolism (PROACT) II trials evaluated the safety and efficacy of IA urokinase in MCA occlusion, comparing IA urokinase to standard of care. PROACT II showed improved recanalization, with more patients achieving slight or no disability. MELT was stopped early due to IV rt-PA approval in Japan; although its primary endpoint of modified Rankin Scale (mRS) of $\leq 2$ was not significantly different among the two groups, it did show a higher rate of recovery to normal or near normal (mRS $\leq 1$) in the treatment group. Of note, PROACT II had significantly higher rates of intracerebral hemorrhage (ICH).[32,33] The Mechanical Embolus Removal in Cerebral Ischemia (MERCI), Multi-MERCI, and PENUMBRA trials evaluated mechanical thrombectomy in acute ischemic stroke. Although they achieved improved recanalization rate and showed a trend toward improved outcomes, they did not unequivocally prove benefit.[24,25,34]

In 2013 the results of the Interventional Management of Stroke (IMS) III, SYNTHESIS (Synthesis Expansion: A Randomized Controlled Trial on Intra-Arterial Versus Intravenous Thrombolysis in Acute Ischemic Stroke), and the Mechanical Retrieval and Recanalization of Stroke Clots Using Embolectomy (MR RESCUE) trials were published, comparing various reperfusion strategies, including IV rt-PA, IA rt-PA, mechanical thrombectomy, and a combination of these. IMS III was stopped prematurely due to futility, although it did show higher rates of reperfusion in the IA-rtPA + interventional techniques group and an increased proportion of patients with mRS $\leq 2$ at 90 days with greater reperfusion. SYNTHESIS did not show a benefit to patients receiving endovascular treatment compared with IV rt-PA, although on average patients receiving endovascular therapy were treated 1 hour after patients receiving IV rt-PA. In MR RESCUE, embolectomy was not proven to be better than standard of care, although only the MERCI and PENUMBRA devices were used.[35–37]

In 2015 five randomized prospective trials evaluating the effect of endovascular therapy for acute ischemic stroke were published.[38–42] Each trial demonstrated that endovascular treatment was highly beneficial compared with IV t-PA alone in patients with occlusions of the intracranial ICA or MCA who were treated within specific durations, usually within 6 hours, after symptom onset. In these trials, endovascular treatment was typically used in addition to IV-tPA; however, some trials included patients who were ineligible for IV-tPA.

These trials resulted in major changes in recommended management for acute ischemic stroke. Important lessons from the trials include the fact that endovascular thrombectomy is a potently effective treatment for patients with severe neurological deficit and proven occlusion of the distal internal carotid or proximal MCA in the face of a relatively normal head CT. In addition, there are benefits of receiving IV-tPA prior to endovascular therapy, and IV-tPA should not be withheld in patients who meet criteria for its administration. Importantly, the benefits were demonstrated when endovascular treatment was performed in an endovascular stroke center by a coordinated multidisciplinary system that minimizes time to recanalization using current thrombectomy devices.[43]

Based on these trials, an American Heart Association/American Stroke Association Focused Update of the 2013 Guidelines for the Early Management of Patients With Acute Ischemic Stroke Regarding Endovascular Treatment was published in 2015.[44] Important recommendations for management of acute ischemic stroke contained in the guidelines include:

Eligible patients with acute ischemic stroke and significant neurological deficit presenting within 4.5 hours of symptom onset should receive IV-tPA.

If endovascular therapy is contemplated, noninvasive vascular imaging (CT angiogram) is recommended to detect large proximal arterial occlusions (intracranial ICA and MCA).

Endovascular treatment with stent retrievers is recommended for patients with large proximal arterial occlusions (Class I; Level of Evidence A); however, other devices may be reasonable in some circumstances.

Endovascular treatment should be initiated within 6 hours of symptom onset.

The guidelines emphasize system-based management of acute ischemic stroke patients. It is recommended that patients be transported rapidly to the closest available certified primary stroke center or comprehensive stroke center (Class I; Level of Evidence A). The guidelines further note that in some instances, this may involve air medical transport and bypass of the nearest hospital.

A metaanalysis of eight recent stroke trials found that compared with standard medical therapy, acute endovascular stroke therapy was associated with greater functional independence and higher rates of angiographic revascularization, but no difference in symptomatic ICH or all-cause mortality at 90 days.[45]

Exceptions to the standard therapeutic time window are typically made for basilar artery occlusion and thrombosis, as it carries an 80% to 90% mortality rate without thrombolysis. Mortality decreases to 42% to 70% with endovascular therapy, with patients faring better with earlier treatment.[46–48] Given this prognosis, interventionalists have considered revascularization over 12 hours after symptom onset,[49] with reports of improvement occurring up to 48 hours from onset[50] (see Table 37.1 and Fig. 37.6).

IA thrombolytic infusion has theoretical advantages over IV administration, including delivery of medication directly into the occluding clot, thereby allowing lower doses with a potentially decreased risk of ICH IV rt-PA.[51] In addition, immediate angiographic confirmation of reopening is possible. Compared with mechanical thrombectomy, IA rt-PA has fewer complications related to guidewires and catheters, including arterial dissection, perforation, and vessel rupture.[52,53] Furthermore, IA rt-PA is able to travel distally and reach occluded vessels that could not otherwise be reached by devices.

**Table 37.1**   Possible Selection Criteria for Acute Ischemic Stroke Endovascular Revascularization Therapy (ERT)

| | |
|---|---|
| Inclusion criteria for ERT | Neurological deficit attributable to a medium to large vessel occlusion<br>Procedure initiated within 6–8 hours from time last normal for anterior circulation, 12 hours for posterior circulation<br>Treatment beyond 6–8 hours guided by advanced imaging<br>Potentially disabling neurological deficit<br>Persistent or worsening deficits after IV rt-PA |
| Exclusion criteria for ERT | Arterial stenosis precluding safe access<br>Suspicion of aortic dissection<br>Uncontrolled HTN (SBP > 185 mm Hg or SBP > 110 mm Hg) that cannot be treated with medication<br>Platelet count <30,000<br>INR >3.0<br>Known bleeding diathesis<br>Deficits attributable to glucose <50 mg/dL<br>Seizure at onset, if deficits are attributable to postictal state<br>Imaging findings: significant mass effect with midline shift, intracranial hemorrhage, subacute infarct that occupies >1/3 MCA territory or >100 cc brain tissue, CNS lesion with high likelihood of bleeding (brain tumor, abscess, vascular malformation, aneurysm, contusion) |
| Relative contraindications for ERT | Intracranial or spinal surgery, head trauma, or stroke in different vascular territory within 3 months<br>History of intracerebral hemorrhage (ICH)<br>Terminal illness with short life expectancy or comorbid illness<br>Pregnancy: perform risk versus benefit analysis, ability to shield patient<br>Known subacute bacterial endocarditis with or without mycotic aneurysm and stroke<br>Special consideration to patients on novel anticoagulants |
| Relative contraindications for adjunctive ERT following IV rt-PA | Glucose >400 mg/dL, based on increased ICH risk<br>Ongoing hemodialysis or peritoneal dialysis, due to possibly increased ICH risk |

*HTN*, hypertension; *SBP*, systolic blood pressure; *INR*, international normalization ratio; *MCA*, middle cerebral artery; *CNS*, central nervous system.
Adapted from Lazzaro MA, Novakovic RL, Alexandrov AV, et al. Developing practice recommendations for endovascular revascularization for acute ischemic stroke. *Neurology.* 2012;79(13 Suppl 1):S243–55.

rtPA is currently the thrombolytic medication of choice for IA thrombolysis. Typical doses do not exceed 22 mg IA, but IA rt-PA may be administered in addition to previously administered full-dose IV rt-PA. In addition, various amounts of heparin are often administered during the procedure to minimize clot formation on endovascular devices. Although these doses typically do not exceed a bolus of 2000 units and an infusion of 500 units/hr, consultation with personnel performing the procedure is important to evaluate risk of postprocedural hemorrhage.[49]

Current mechanical techniques have the advantage of avoiding administration of thrombolytic medications. These techniques utilize a number of devices, including the MERCI retriever, Penumbra System, and stent retrievers, as described earlier. Mechanical thrombectomy is available to patients who are otherwise ineligible for IA

rt-PA, including those with known bleeding complications, coagulopathy, or who are recently postoperative.[51]

Despite the known complications of mechanical thrombectomy, most interventionalists prefer it to IA rt-PA, reserving IA rt-PA for those patients in whom mechanical devices have failed or are unable to be used safely.[54]

## PERIOPERATIVE CONSIDERATIONS

### Key Concepts

- Attempts to increase cerebral blood flow should be made, including permissive hypertension, adequate hydration, and maintaining the head of bed flat. There are currently insufficient data to recommend augmentation of blood pressure with vasopressors for endovascular therapy.
- General anesthesia has been shown in small studies to be potentially harmful, although it must be used in certain situations. Particular attention to blood pressure is warranted, especially during induction and emergence from anesthesia.
- Neuroimaging should be obtained after an endovascular procedure to assess for ICH.
- Pyrexia and hyperglycemia should be avoided in all patients.

### Blood Pressure Management

Antihypertensive medications should be held prior to endovascular therapy, as is standard of care in patients with acute ischemic stroke. Increasing systemic blood pressure may augment cerebral blood flow, increase perfusion to the area of ischemia, and facilitate opening of collateral vessels.[55] Guidelines for blood pressure parameters are adapted from recommendations for patients with acute ischemic stroke with and without IV rt-PA: blood pressure should be maintained less than 180/105 mm Hg in those receiving thrombolytics and <220/110 mm Hg in those not receiving thrombolytics.[56]

Augmentation of blood pressure with vasopressors has been studied as a means of improving cerebral blood flow and perfusion to penumbral tissue. Several small studies have been conducted in patients with acute ischemic stroke. A small pilot study showed that the National Institutes of Health Stroke Scale (NIHSS) improved and volume of hypoperfused tissue decreased with augmentation of blood pressure.[57] A larger retrospective review of patients who received vasopressors for acute stroke demonstrated that the practice was not associated with increased risk of hemorrhage or mortality, but that the benefit of blood pressure augmentation decreased within 24 to 48 hours after onset.[58,59] What remains unclear is how these data pertain to patients undergoing endovascular therapy. For now, blood pressure augmentation is reasonable in the setting of frank arterial hypotension, but is not otherwise recommended outside the scope of clinical trials.[56]

### Hydration

Adequate hydration is essential, particularly to minimize the risk of contrast nephropathy.[55] Isotonic fluids should be used, so as to avoid aggravation of cerebral edema, and fluid should contain no dextrose, except in the case of frank hypoglycemia.[55,56] Total intake and output should

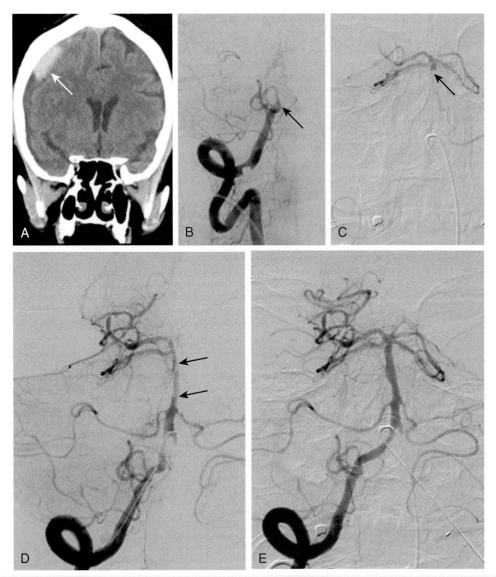

**Fig. 37.6** A 74-year-old woman with right subdural hematoma and acute onset right-sided weakness. **(A)** Coronal CT scan shows right hemispheric subdural hematoma. **(B)** AP view right vertebral artery injection, occlusion at vertebrobasilar junction (*arrow*). **(C)** Microcatheter injection at basilar tip shows filling of bilateral PCA and SCCAs (*arrow*). **(D)** Repeat AP angiogram of right vertebral artery post angioplasty and Penumbra. Reopening of basilar artery with residual irregular intraluminal thrombus (*arrows*). **(E).** Postthrombolysis angiogram after use of a Solitare device.

be recorded before and during the procedure in order to adjust fluid requirements and maintain euvolemia postprocedure. Patients with a known history of congestive heart failure or a low ejection fraction should be monitored carefully; presence of neurocritical care or anesthesia expertise may be helpful to guide management.[55]

## Head of Bed

Lowering the head of bed has been shown in small studies to increase MCA mean flow velocity, suggesting increased cerebral perfusion in those patients.[60,61] The benefit of lowering the head of bed must be weighed against the risk of aspiration and airway maintenance.

## Antithrombotic Therapy Prior to Endovascular Therapy

Antithrombotic therapy should be avoided in patients who have received IV rt-PA in the past 24 hours, according to the National Institute of Neurological Disorders and Stroke (NINDS) study protocol.[2] Special consideration should be given to patients with planned intracranial stenting in order to avoid in-stent thrombosis. However, there are little data to guide the antithrombotic management of these patients. In general, patients should receive loading doses of two antiplatelet medications prior to and after the procedure. In the first FDA-approved trial of intracranial stenting for acute ischemic stroke, patients received clopidogrel 600 mg and aspirin 650 mg prior to the procedure.[62]

## Anesthesia

Whether general anesthesia or conscious sedation is preferable remains an area of controversy. Benefits to general anesthesia include maintenance of a secure airway—of paramount importance in patients with bulbar dysfunction or airway compromise[63]; lack of patient movement during the procedure, which might decrease the risk of arterial perforation; and ability to optimize analgesia, as mechanical force applied to cerebral vessels may result in pain.[64] Disadvantages to general anesthesia include hypotension on induction, which may exacerbate ischemic injury, delay in therapy due to intubation, and loss of neurological examination.[55]

Conscious sedation similarly has many advantages and disadvantages. Advantages include decreased time to reperfusion and relative hemodynamic stability. Disadvantages include risk of patient movement during the procedure and lack of fasting in most patients prior to the procedure, with subsequent concern for aspiration. Conscious sedation may be particularly risky for patients with aphasia or neglect, who may be less cooperative during the procedure.[49]

> ### Clinical Pearl
>
> Patients with severe aphasia or neglect may be less cooperative during the procedure and therefore may benefit from general anesthesia.

Several studies have looked at general anesthesia versus conscious sedation for acute ischemic patients undergoing endovascular therapy. A large retrospective multicenter trial demonstrated no difference in ICH rates between the two groups; however, patients who received general anesthesia had nearly twice the risk of worse neurological outcomes at 90 days.[65] A small retrospective study also demonstrated better clinical outcomes, smaller final infarct volume, and decreased in-hospital mortality in patients who were not intubated during the procedure.[66] A subset of the IMS II trial evaluated general anesthesia versus conscious sedation and found that patients who received conscious sedation had higher rates of recanalization and fewer complications, with patients undergoing general anesthesia experiencing higher rates of infection.[67] Therefore although no publication has shown that general anesthesia is better than conscious sedation, three publications have demonstrated that general anesthesia may, in fact, be harmful, possibly due to delay in treatment and complications from intubation and sedation.[65,68]

If general anesthesia must be used, blood pressure should be strictly controlled, particularly at induction, to prevent transient hypotension and worsening neurological status. When contemplating general anesthesia, the patient's baseline blood pressure, stroke syndrome, and general medical condition should be considered.[63] Target blood pressure should be within 10% to 20% of admission blood pressure, unless the patient has received IV rt-PA, in which case blood pressure should be maintained <180/105 mm Hg.[55]

> ### Clinical Pearl
>
> During general anesthesia, providers must be vigilant about monitoring blood pressure to avoid hypoperfusion and extension of the infarct.

## Antithrombotic Management: Intraprocedure

There are no clear guidelines regarding the optimal use of intraoperative antithrombotic and anticoagulant medications. Limited data, however, exist on the safety of heparin administered during the procedure. Variable protocols have been reported for thromboprophylaxis, including an unfractionated heparin bolus during the procedure, followed by a continuous infusion for the remainder of the procedure.[33,35,69] Risk of hemorrhage attributable to heparin administration is unclear, given that those patients also received IA rt-PA. A subgroup analysis of the MERCI trial looked at 51 patients, 47% of whom received periprocedural heparin, and found no association with risk of hemorrhage or 90-day mortality.[70] The role of glycoprotein IIb/IIIa inhibitors in acute ischemic stroke patients undergoing endovascular therapy is unclear, and administration is not recommended outside of clinical trials.[71] After endovascular intervention, there is no clear indication to continue either unfractionated heparin or glycoprotein IIb/IIIa inhibitors.[64]

## Neuroimaging and Monitoring

Neuroimaging is often performed immediately postprocedure and should be obtained within 16 to 32 hours after endovascular intervention, with either a noncontrast head CT or magnetic resonance imaging (MRI) of the brain with susceptibility-weighted sequences. In the setting of clinical deterioration, a noncontrast head CT should be obtained immediately to rule out hemorrhage.[49] All patients should be admitted to the neurology intensive care unit (ICU) postprocedure to ensure frequent neurological and peripheral vascular examinations.

## Blood Pressure: Postprocedure

Careful monitoring of blood pressure is essential after endovascular intervention to avoid excessive hypertension and reperfusion hemorrhage. Although it is clear that systolic blood pressures below 120 mm Hg should be avoided,[72] the optimum blood pressure after intervention has not yet been determined. The degree of recanalization and patient's neurological status should be taken into consideration; if complete recanalization with improvement in neurological function has been achieved, a reasonable goal systolic blood pressure (SBP) is 120 to 140 mm Hg to avoid reperfusion hemorrhage.[55] However, some interventionalists favor higher blood pressure in order to promote collateral blood flow and clear distal emboli from the vasculature.[73] Post-IV-rt-PA blood pressure parameters have also been recommended for those patients who have achieved recanalization but have not received IV rt-PA.[74] It is reasonable to implement post-IV-rt-PA monitoring parameters for endovascular patients, ensuring that both blood pressure and neurological examination are checked frequently.

> ### Clinical Pearl
>
> The degree of recanalization and neurological status should be taken into consideration prior to determining goal blood pressure.

## Antithrombotic Therapy: Postprocedure

Unfractionated heparin has been used in some centers after endovascular procedures and was part of the MERCI trial protocol, to be used at the discretion of the treating physician.[34] Data to support this practice, however, are limited, with concern for hemorrhagic transformation after endovascular intervention. Subcutaneous heparin dosed for deep vein thrombosis prophylaxis, however, has been shown to independently be associated with improved outcomes after acute stroke and should be implemented as soon as neuroimaging confirms the absence of hemorrhage, or after 24 hours after rt-PA administration.[55,75] Pneumatic compression boots can be used immediately.

Antithrombotic medications are typically avoided in all patients who have received IA rt-PA in the first 24 hours after intervention[56]; exceptions include patients who have received a stent. For patients who underwent mechanical thrombectomy only, antithrombotics can be started earlier if neuroimaging confirms the absence of hemorrhage.[55]

## Postoperative Complications

### Key Concepts

- There are many complications of cerebral endovascular therapy that are unrelated to cerebral ischemia/infarction; the majority of these complications are common to all endovascular procedures.
- Five percent to 6% of acute ischemic stroke patients experience ICH related to endovascular intervention, largely due to reperfusion injury.
- Air emboli, although rare, may cause significant neurological deficits and should be treated with 100% oxygen or hyperbaric therapy (see Table 37.2).

Several complications of endovascular treatment of acute ischemic stroke exist, many of which are common to all interventional vascular procedures. These complications include complications of arterial access, medication and contrast media, anesthesia, and systemic complications. Complications specific to catheters and guidewires can also occur, including perforation, embolization, dissection, formation of pseudoaneurysm, and arterial vasospasm. The remainder of this section will focus on complications that occur specifically in the context of the endovascular treatment of acute ischemic stroke (see Box 37.1).

### Intracranial Hemorrhage

ICH is a well-described and feared complication of endovascular therapy for acute ischemic stroke, occurring in approximately 5% to 6% of patients who undergo IA recanalization.[56] ICH in the setting of endovascular therapy is typically due to reperfusion injury after recanalization; other etiologies include direct vessel perforation by a catheter, microwire, or device. The pattern of ICH in the setting of endovascular therapy tends to be more variable than what is seen with post-IV-rt-PA hemorrhage, with a higher

**Table 37.2** List of Common Complications

| | |
|---|---|
| Arterial Access | Hematoma<br>Retroperitoneal hemorrhage<br>Pseudoaneurysm and dissection<br>Arterial venous fistula<br>Groin infection<br>Arterial thrombosis |
| Medication and Contrast Media | Hemorrhage<br>Nausea/vomiting<br>Vasovagal syncope<br>Allergic reaction<br>Hypotension<br>Arrhythmias<br>Acute renal failure<br>Congestive heart failure |
| Systemic Complications | Myocardial infarction<br>Arrhythmias<br>Hypotension<br>Renal insufficiency |
| Anesthesia-Related | Nausea/vomiting<br>Aspiration<br>Hypotension<br>Arrhythmias |
| Device-Related Complications | Perforation<br>Arterial dissection/pseudoaneurysm<br>Thrombus formation<br>Embolization (air/particulate)<br>Subintimal contrast injection<br>Arterial spasm<br>External carotid occlusion<br>Device fracture<br>Cavernous carotid fistula |
| Stent-Related | Stent thrombosis<br>Stent migration<br>Post deployment stent compression<br>Deployment failure |
| Balloon-Related | Balloon rupture<br>Embolization (air/particulate)<br>Vasospasm<br>Perforation |

Adapted from Darkhabani Z, Nguyen T, Lazzaro MA, et al. Complications of endovascular therapy for acute ischemic stroke and proposed management approach. *Neurology.* 2012;79(13 Suppl 1):S192–8.

### Box 37.1 Complications Secondary to Endovascular Intervention of Acute Stroke in Order of Severity

Intracerebral hemorrhage
Emboli to new vascular territories and in situ thrombosis
Air emboli
Arterial dissection
Carotid cavernous fistula

*Note: depending on the severity of the complication, the order of this list may change.*

risk of subarachnoid hemorrhage (SAH).[76] Factors known to increase the risk of developing ICH include higher NIHSS, elevated serum glucose, platelet count <200,000, time to treatment, poor pial collaterals, and tandem occlusions.[77–79] Independent predictors of SAH include procedure-related vessel perforation, rescue angioplasty after thrombectomy, distal MCA occlusion, and hypertension.[53]

Any change in neurological examination, acute rise in blood pressure, nausea, vomiting, or new-onset headache should prompt immediate investigation with noncontrast head CT and serum labs, including complete blood count, prothrombin time/international normalized ratio/partial thromboplastin time, type and screen, and fibrinogen level.[56] It is essential to differentiate between acute hemorrhage and contrast extravasation on neuroimaging; brain MRI with susceptibility-weighted imaging is helpful in this setting.[80] If ICH is found, all antithrombotics and anticoagulants should be reversed; although there are no standard guidelines for reversal agents, cryoprecipitate is typically used in the setting of IV or IA rt-PA to replete fibrinogen levels.[56] Surgical decompression and clot evacuation remain an area of controversy. Although there are no definitive data regarding the role of surgery in the setting of symptomatic ICH, neurosurgical evaluation should be considered in the appropriate clinical setting, taking into account the patient's neurological and medical status.[56] Decompressive surgery for cerebellar hemorrhages, however, has been shown to be effective for spontaneous ICH, and is therefore reasonable to consider for postendovascular hemorrhage.[56,81]

Blood pressure should be tightly controlled after ICH. Although there are no definitive data, it is prudent to maintain SBP between 120 and 160 mm Hg and diastolic blood pressure <90 mm Hg.[82] In the setting of SAH, ICU management should focus on prevention, early recognition, and treatment of vasospasm, and prophylactic antiepileptic medication might be considered.[82]

## Air Emboli

Although uncommon, air emboli accounted for 0.08% of significant neurological deficits in a review of over 4500 patients undergoing neuroangiographic procedures; all air emboli occurred during interventional procedures, and none during conventional angiography.[83] In the SWIFT trial, comparing the MERCI device with the Solitaire device, air emboli occurred in two patients (1.4%), one of which was considered a serious adverse event.[28,29] The cause of air emboli is thought to be flushing of the arterial line or negative pressure suddenly applied to the catheter, enabling air to enter the artery.[82] Careful measures should be taken to avoid air emboli, including gently prepping and flushing all catheters and devices prior to insertion (to remove air bubbles) and minimizing the number of microcatheter runs.[82] If air emboli result in symptomatic neurological deficits, 100% oxygen or hyperbaric chamber should be considered.[84]

## Arterial Dissection

Arterial dissection is an uncommon complication of interventional neuroangiographic procedures. In a large review of over 3000 patients undergoing both diagnostic angiograms and interventional procedures, 0.4% of patients experienced arterial dissection, with 0.7% occurring in the interventional group.[85] The SWIFT trial had a much higher arterial dissection rate of 3.5%.[28,76] In patients who experience arterial dissection, close neurological monitoring is required. For arterial dissections that do not

compromise blood flow or the patient's neurological status, antithrombotic or antiplatelet medications may be considered[82] (see Fig. 37.7).

## Carotid Cavernous Fistula

Carotid cavernous fistulae are a known complication of endovascular procedures and are typically due to direct wire perforation.[82] They have, however, also been reported to occur from angioplasty.[86] Several treatment strategies have been described, including stent placement,[86] stent-assisted coil occlusion of the fistula,[87] and Onyx embolization into the cavernous sinus with direct transorbital[88] or transvenous access.[89] In addition, Onyx embolization can be performed directly through the arterial perforation into the cavernous sinus if the interventionalist is able to maintain access to the perforation.[82]

## Emboli to New Vascular Territories and In Situ Thrombosis

During endovascular intervention, clot can migrate distally to either another single branch or multiple smaller branches, causing ischemic strokes.[82] Emboli to new vascular territories may also occur.[76] In situ thrombosis can also occur, likely due to platelet activation and induction of the coagulation process. Thrombosis can be exacerbated by decreased blood flow in the region of the IA device, which may already be compromised by acute stroke.[82] Thrombosis accounts for a large proportion of neurological deterioration secondary to endovascular interventions. Prevention includes infusion of heparinized normal saline, whereas thrombosis can be treated with heparin boluses. Limited data exist on the role of glycoprotein IIb/IIIa inhibitors. If anticoagulants and antithrombotics fail to achieve recanalization, mechanical thrombectomy can be considered.[82]

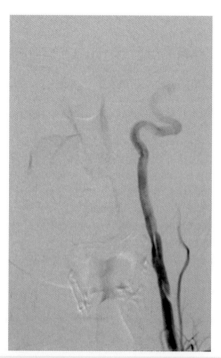

**Fig. 37.7** Frontal projection of left vertebral artery injection demonstrating a nonflow-limiting dissection of the V2 segment.

# Conclusion

Endovascular treatment of acute ischemic stroke is a critical tool in the management of patients who are ineligible for IV rt-tPA or are otherwise not improving despite treatment. Anatomical, radiographic, and clinical considerations are necessary prior to initiation of endovascular therapy. Patients should be monitored closely before, during, and after the procedure to ensure adequate treatment of ischemic stroke and avoidance of any complications.

## References

1. Go AS, Mozaffarian D, Roger VL, et al. Heart disease and stroke statistics—2014 update: a report from the American Heart Association. *Circulation*. 2014;129(3):e28–e292.
2. Tissue plasminogen activator for acute ischemic stroke. The National Institute of Neurological Disorders and Stroke rt-PA Stroke Study Group. *New Engl J Med*. 1995;333(24):1581–7.
3. Hacke W, Kaste M, Bluhmki E, et al. Thrombolysis with alteplase 3 to 4.5 hours after acute ischemic stroke. *New Eng J Med*. 2008;359 (13):1317–1329.
4. Del Zoppo GJ, Saver JL, Jauch EC, Adams Jr HP. American Heart Association Stroke C. Expansion of the time window for treatment of acute ischemic stroke with intravenous tissue plasminogen activator: a science advisory from the American Heart Association/American Stroke Association. *Stroke*. 2009;40(8):2945–2948.
5. Adeoye O, Hornung R, Khatri P, Kleindorfer D. Recombinant tissue-type plasminogen activator use for ischemic stroke in the United States: a doubling of treatment rates over the course of 5 years. *Stroke*. 2011;42(7):1952–1955.
6. Kleindorfer D, Lindsell CJ, Brass L, Koroshetz W, Broderick JP. National US estimates of recombinant tissue plasminogen activator use: ICD-9 codes substantially underestimate. *Stroke*. 2008;39 (3):924–928.
7. Rha JH, Saver JL. The impact of recanalization on ischemic stroke outcome: a meta-analysis. *Stroke*. 2007;38(3):967–973.
8. Alexandrov AV, Molina CA, Grotta JC, et al. Ultrasound-enhanced systemic thrombolysis for acute ischemic stroke. *New Eng J Med*. 2004;351(21):2170–2178.
9. Daffertshofer M, Gass A, Ringleb P, et al. Transcranial low-frequency ultrasound-mediated thrombolysis in brain ischemia: increased risk of hemorrhage with combined ultrasound and tissue plasminogen activator: results of a phase II clinical trial. *Stroke*. 2005;36 (7):1441–1446.
10. Alexandrov AV, Grotta JC. Arterial reocclusion in stroke patients treated with intravenous tissue plasminogen activator. *Neurology*. 2002;59(6):862–867.
11. del Zoppo GJ, Poeck K, Pessin MS, et al. Recombinant tissue plasminogen activator in acute thrombotic and embolic stroke. *Ann Neurol*. 1992;32(1):78–86.
12. Wunderlich MT, Goertler M, Postert T, et al. Recanalization after intravenous thrombolysis: does a recanalization time window exist? *Neurology*. 2007;68(17):1364–1368.
13. Wolpert SM, Bruckmann H, Greenlee R, Wechsler L, Pessin MS, del Zoppo GJ. Neuroradiologic evaluation of patients with acute stroke treated with recombinant tissue plasminogen activator. The rt-PA Acute Stroke Study Group. *AJNR*. 1993;14(1):3–13.
14. Linfante I, Llinas RH, Selim M, et al. Clinical and vascular outcome in internal carotid artery versus middle cerebral artery occlusions after intravenous tissue plasminogen activator. *Stroke*. 2002;33 (8):2066–2071.
15. Lee KY, Han SW, Kim SH, et al. Early recanalization after intravenous administration of recombinant tissue plasminogen activator as assessed by pre- and post-thrombolytic angiography in acute ischemic stroke patients. *Stroke*. 2007;38(1):192–193.
16. Kharitonova T, Ahmed N, Thoren M, et al. Hyperdense middle cerebral artery sign on admission CT scan—prognostic significance for ischaemic stroke patients treated with intravenous thrombolysis in the safe implementation of thrombolysis in Stroke International Stroke Thrombolysis Register. *Cerebrovascular Dis*. 2009;27 (1):51–59.
17. De Silva DA, Brekenfeld C, Ebinger M, et al. The benefits of intravenous thrombolysis relate to the site of baseline arterial occlusion in the Echoplanar Imaging Thrombolytic Evaluation Trial (EPITHET). *Stroke*. 2010;41(2):295–299.
18. Riedel CH, Zimmermann P, Jensen-Kondering U, Stingele R, Deuschl G, Jansen O. The importance of size: successful recanalization by intravenous thrombolysis in acute anterior stroke depends on thrombus length. *Stroke*. 2011;42(6):1775–1777.
19. Molina CA, Montaner J, Arenillas JF, Ribo M, Rubiera M, Alvarez-Sabin J. Differential pattern of tissue plasminogen activator-induced proximal middle cerebral artery recanalization among stroke subtypes. *Stroke*. 2004;35(2):486–490.
20. Naggara O, Touze E, Beyssen B, et al. Anatomical and technical factors associated with stroke or death during carotid angioplasty and stenting: results from the endarterectomy versus angioplasty in patients with symptomatic severe carotid stenosis (EVA-3S) trial and systematic review. *Stroke*. 2011;42(2):380–388.
21. Bajzer CT. Anatomical considerations. In: Bhatt DL, ed. *Guide to Peripheral and Cerebrovascular Interventions*. London: Remedica Publishing; 2004: 1–20.
22. Yaşargil MG. *Microneurosurgery*. New York: Georg Thieme Verlag; Thieme Medical Publishers; 1987.
23. Ng YS, Stein J, Ning M, Black-Schaffer RM. Comparison of clinical characteristics and functional outcomes of ischemic stroke in different vascular territories. *Stroke*. 2007;38(8):2309–2314.
24. Smith WS, Sung G, Saver J, et al. Mechanical thrombectomy for acute ischemic stroke: final results of the Multi MERCI trial. *Stroke*. 2008;39 (4):1205–1212.
25. Penumbra Pivotal Stroke Trial I. The penumbra pivotal stroke trial: safety and effectiveness of a new generation of mechanical devices for clot removal in intracranial large vessel occlusive disease. *Stroke*. 2009;40(8):2761–2768.
26. Turk 3rd AS, Campbell JM, Spiotta A, et al. An investigation of the cost and benefit of mechanical thrombectomy for endovascular treatment of acute ischemic stroke. *J Neurointev Surg*. 2014;6 (1):77–80.
27. Castano C, Dorado L, Guerrero C, et al. Mechanical thrombectomy with the Solitaire AB device in large artery occlusions of the anterior circulation: a pilot study. *Stroke*. 2010;41(8):1836–1840.
28. Saver JL, Jahan R, Levy EI, et al. Solitaire flow restoration device versus the Merci Retriever in patients with acute ischaemic stroke (SWIFT): a randomised, parallel-group, non-inferiority trial. *Lancet*. 2012;380(9849):1241–1249.
29. Leker RR, Eichel R, Gomori JM. Ramirez de Noriega F, Ben-Hur T, Cohen JE. Stent-based thrombectomy versus intravenous tissue plasminogen activator in patients with acute middle cerebral artery occlusion. *Stroke*. 2012;43(12):3389–3391.
30. Beadell NC, Lutsep H. New stent retriever devices. *Curr Atherosclerosis Rep*. 2013;15(6):333.
31. Almekhlafi MA, Menon BK, Freiheit EA, Demchuk AM, Goyal M. A meta-analysis of observational intra-arterial stroke therapy studies using the Merci device, Penumbra system, and retrievable stents. *AJNR*. 2013;34(1):140–145.
32. Ogawa A, Mori E, Minematsu K, et al. Randomized trial of intraarterial infusion of urokinase within 6 hours of middle cerebral artery stroke: the middle cerebral artery embolism local fibrinolytic intervention trial (MELT) Japan. *Stroke*. 2007;38(10):2633–2639.
33. Furlan A, Higashida R, Wechsler L, et al. Intra-arterial prourokinase for acute ischemic stroke. The PROACT II study: a randomized controlled trial. Prolyse in Acute Cerebral Thromboembolism. *JAMA*. 1999;282(21):2003–2011.
34. Smith WS, Sung G, Starkman S, et al. Safety and efficacy of mechanical embolectomy in acute ischemic stroke: results of the MERCI trial. *Stroke*. 2005;36(7):1432–1438.
35. Broderick JP, Palesch YY, Demchuk AM, et al. Endovascular therapy after intravenous t-PA versus t-PA alone for stroke. *New Engl J Med*. 2013;368(10):893–903.
36. Ciccone A, Valvassori L, Nichelatti M, et al. Endovascular treatment for acute ischemic stroke. *New Engl J Med*. 2013;368(10):904–913.
37. Kidwell CS, Jahan R, Gornbein J, et al. A trial of imaging selection and endovascular treatment for ischemic stroke. *New Engl J Med*. 2013;368(10):914–923.
38. Berkhemer OA, Fransen PS, Beumer D, et al. A randomized trial of intraarterial treatment for acute ischemic stroke. *New Engl J Med*. 2015;372:11–20.

39. Campbell BC, Mitchell PJ, Kleinig TJ, et al. Endovascular therapy for ischemic stroke with perfusion-imaging selection. *New Engl J Med.* 2015;372:1009–1018.

40. Goyal M, Demchuk AM, Menon BK, et al. Randomized assessment of rapid endovascular treatment of ischemic stroke. *New Engl J Med.* 2015;372:1019–1030.

41. Jovin TG, Chamorro A, Cobo E, et al. Thrombectomy within 8 hours after symptom onset in ischemic stroke. *New Engl J Med.* 2015;372:2296–2306.

42. Saver JL, Goyal M, Bonafe A, et al. Stent-retriever thrombectomy after intravenous t-PA vs. t-PA alone in stroke. *New Engl J Med.* 2015;372:2285–2295.

43. Grotta JC, Hacke W. Stroke neurologist's perspective on the new endovascular trials. *Stroke.* 2015;46:1447–1452.

44. Powers WJ, Derdeyn CP, Biller J, et al. 2015 American Heart Association/American Stroke Association focused update of the 2013 Guidelines for the Early Management of Patients with Acute Ischemic Stroke Regarding Endovascular Treatment: a guideline for healthcare professionals from the American Heart Association/American Stroke Association. *Stroke.* 2015;46:3020–3035.

45. Badhiwala JH, Nassiri F, Alhazzani W, et al. Endovascular thrombectomy for acute ischemic stroke: a meta-analysis. *JAMA.* 2015;314 (17):1832–43.

46. Lazzaro MA, Novakovic RL, Alexandrov AV, et al. Developing practice recommendations for endovascular revascularization for acute ischemic stroke. *Neurology.* 2012;79(13 Suppl 1):S243–S255.

47. Eckert B, Kucinski T, Pfeiffer G, Groden C, Zeumer H. Endovascular therapy of acute vertebrobasilar occlusion: early treatment onset as the most important factor. *Cerebrovasc Dis.* 2002;14(1):42–50.

48. Schulte-Altedorneburg G, Hamann GF, Mull M, et al. Outcome of acute vertebrobasilar occlusions treated with intra-arterial fibrinolysis in 180 patients. *AJNR.* 2006;27(10):2042–2047.

49. Arnold M, Nedeltchev K, Schroth G, et al. Clinical and radiological predictors of recanalisation and outcome of 40 patients with acute basilar artery occlusion treated with intra-arterial thrombolysis. *J Neurol Neurosurg Psychiatry.* 2004;75(6):857–862.

50. Berg-Dammer E, Felber SR, Henkes H, Nahser HC, Kuhne D. Long-term outcome after local intra-arterial fibrinolysis of basilar artery thrombosis. *Cerebrovasc Dis.* 2000;10(3):183–188.

51. Nguyen TN, Babikian VL, Romero R, et al. Intra-arterial treatment methods in acute stroke therapy. *Frontiers Neurol.* 2011;2:9.

52. Nguyen TN, Lanthier S, Roy D. Iatrogenic arterial perforation during acute stroke interventions. *AJNR.* 2008;29(5):974–975.

53. Shi ZS, Liebeskind DS, Loh Y, et al. Predictors of subarachnoid hemorrhage in acute ischemic stroke with endovascular therapy. *Stroke.* 2010;41(12):2775–2781.

54. Hennerici MG, Kern R, Szabo K. Non-pharmacological strategies for the treatment of acute ischaemic stroke. *Lancet Neurol.* 2013;12 (6):572–584.

55. Tarlov N, Nien YL, Zaidat OO, Nguyen TN. Periprocedural management of acute ischemic stroke intervention. *Neurology.* 2012;79(13 Suppl 1):S182–S191.

56. Jauch EC, Saver JL, Adams Jr HP, et al. Guidelines for the early management of patients with acute ischemic stroke: a guideline for healthcare professionals from the American Heart Association/American Stroke Association. *Stroke.* 2013;44(3):870–947.

57. Hillis AE, Ulatowski JA, Barker PB, et al. A pilot randomized trial of induced blood pressure elevation: effects on function and focal perfusion in acute and subacute stroke. *Cerebrovasc Dis.* 2003;16(3):236–246.

58. Rordorf G, Cramer SC, Efird JT, Schwamm LH, Buonanno F, Koroshetz WJ. Pharmacological elevation of blood pressure in acute stroke. Clinical effects and safety. *Stroke.* 1997;28(11):2133–2138.

59. Rordorf G, Koroshetz WJ, Ezzeddine MA, Segal AZ, Buonanno FS. A pilot study of drug-induced hypertension for treatment of acute stroke. *Neurology.* 2001;56(9):1210–1213.

60. Wojner AW, El-Mitwalli A, Alexandrov AV. Effect of head positioning on intracranial blood flow velocities in acute ischemic stroke: a pilot study. *Crit Care Nurs Q.* 2002;24(4):57–66.

61. Wojner-Alexander AW, Garami Z, Chernyshev OY, Alexandrov AV. Heads down: flat positioning improves blood flow velocity in acute ischemic stroke. *Neurology.* 2005;64(8):1354–1357.

62. Levy EI, Siddiqui AH, Crumlish A, et al. First Food and Drug Administration-approved prospective trial of primary intracranial stenting for acute stroke: SARIS (stent-assisted recanalization in acute ischemic stroke). *Stroke.* 2009;40(11):3552–3556.

63. Froehler MT, Fifi JT, Majid A, Bhatt A, Ouyang M, McDonagh DL. Anesthesia for endovascular treatment of acute ischemic stroke. *Neurology.* 2012;79(13 Suppl 1):S167–S173.

64. Abou-Chebl A. Intra-arterial therapy for acute ischemic stroke. *Neurotherapeutics.* 2011;8(3):400–413.

65. Abou-Chebl A, Lin R, Hussain MS, et al. Conscious sedation versus general anesthesia during endovascular therapy for acute anterior circulation stroke: preliminary results from a retrospective, multicenter study. *Stroke.* 2010;41(6):1175–1179.

66. Jumaa MA, Zhang F, Ruiz-Ares G, et al. Comparison of safety and clinical and radiographic outcomes in endovascular acute stroke therapy for proximal middle cerebral artery occlusion with intubation and general anesthesia versus the nonintubated state. *Stroke.* 2010;41 (6):1180–1184.

67. Nichols C, Carrozzella J, Yeatts S, Tomsick T, Broderick J, Khatri P. Is periprocedural sedation during acute stroke therapy associated with poorer functional outcomes? *J Neurointervent Surg.* 2010;2 (1):67–70.

68. Gupta R. Local is better than general anesthesia during endovascular acute stroke interventions. *Stroke.* 2010;41(11):2718–2719.

69. Investigators IIT. The Interventional Management of Stroke (IMS) II Study. *Stroke.* 2007;38(7):2127–2135.

70. Nahab F, Walker GA, Dion JE, Smith WS. Safety of periprocedural heparin in acute ischemic stroke endovascular therapy: the multi MERCI trial. *J Stroke Cerebrovascr Dis.* 2012;21(8):790–793.

71. Nahab F, Kass-Hout T, Shaltoni HM. Periprocedural antithrombotic strategies in acute ischemic stroke interventional therapy. *Neurology.* 2012;79(13 Suppl 1):S174–S181.

72. Sheth KN, Sims JR. Neurocritical care and periprocedural blood pressure management in acute stroke. *Neurology.* 2012;79(13 Suppl 1): S199–S204.

73. Caplan LR, Hennerici M. Impaired clearance of emboli (washout) is an important link between hypoperfusion, embolism, and ischemic stroke. *Arch Neurol.* 1998;55(11):1475–1482.

74. Leslie-Mazwi TM, Sims JR, Hirsch JA, Nogueira RG. Periprocedural blood pressure management in neurointerventional surgery. *J Neurointervent Surg.* 2011;3(1):66–73.

75. Bravata DM, Wells CK, Lo AC, et al. Processes of care associated with acute stroke outcomes. *Arch Intern Med.* 2010;170 (9):804–810.

76. Akins PT, Amar AP, Pakbaz RS, Fields JD, Investigators S. Complications of endovascular treatment for acute stroke in the SWIFT trial with solitaire and Merci devices. *AJNR.* 2014;35(3):524–528.

77. Kidwell CS, Saver JL, Carneado J, et al. Predictors of hemorrhagic transformation in patients receiving intra-arterial thrombolysis. *Stroke.* 2002;33(3):717–724.

78. Vora NA, Gupta R, Thomas AJ, et al. Factors predicting hemorrhagic complications after multimodal reperfusion therapy for acute ischemic stroke. *AJNR.* 2007;28(7):1391–1394.

79. Christoforidis GA, Karakasis C, Mohammad Y, Caragine LP, Yang M, Slivka AP. Predictors of hemorrhage following intra-arterial thrombolysis for acute ischemic stroke: the role of pial collateral formation. *AJNR.* 2009;30(1):165–170.

80. Greer DM, Koroshetz WJ, Cullen S, Gonzalez RG, Lev MH. Magnetic resonance imaging improves detection of intracerebral hemorrhage over computed tomography after intra-arterial thrombolysis. *Stroke.* 2004;35(2):491–495.

81. Morgenstern LB, Hemphill 3rd JC, Anderson C, et al. Guidelines for the management of spontaneous intracerebral hemorrhage: a guideline for healthcare professionals from the American Heart Association/American Stroke Association. *Stroke.* 2010;41 (9):2108–2129.

82. Darkhabani Z, Nguyen T, Lazzaro MA, et al. Complications of endovascular therapy for acute ischemic stroke and proposed management approach. *Neurology.* 2012;79(13 Suppl 1):S192–S198.

83. Gupta R, Vora N, Thomas A, et al. Symptomatic cerebral air embolism during neuro-angiographic procedures: incidence and problem avoidance. *Neurocrit Care.* 2007;7(3):241–246.

84. Murphy BP, Harford FJ, Cramer FS. Cerebral air embolism resulting from invasive medical procedures. Treatment with hyperbaric oxygen. *Ann Surg.* 1985;201(2):242–245.

85. Cloft HJ, Samuels OB, Tong FC, Dion JE. Use of abciximab for mediation of thromboembolic complications of endovascular therapy. *AJNR.* 2001;22(9):1764–1767.
86. Kim SH, Qureshi AI, Boulos AS, et al. Intracranial stent placement for the treatment of a carotid-cavernous fistula associated with intracranial angioplasty. Case report. *J Neurosurg.* 2003;98 (5):1116–1119.
87. Moron FE, Klucznik RP, Mawad ME, Strother CM. Endovascular treatment of high-flow carotid cavernous fistulas by stent-assisted coil placement. *AJNR.* 2005;26(6):1399–1404.
88. Elhammady MS, Peterson EC, Aziz-Sultan MA. Onyx embolization of a carotid cavernous fistula via direct transorbital puncture. *J Neurosurg.* 2011;114(1):129–132.
89. Bhatia KD, Wang L, Parkinson RJ, Wenderoth JD. Successful treatment of six cases of indirect carotid-cavernous fistula with ethylene vinyl alcohol copolymer (Onyx) transvenous embolization. *J Neuro Ophthalmol.* 2009;29(1):3–8.

# 38 *Tumor Embolization*

HESHAM MASOUD, THANH NGUYEN, and ALEXANDER NORBASH

In this chapter, we review the head and neck tumors most often encountered for embolization, with special attention to tumor appearance on neuroangiography. Neuroanatomical considerations and angioarchitectural features, such as tumor vasculature and anastomoses, are also highlighted. In addition, a description of the procedural and perioperative management, including postoperative complications, are discussed with the goal of providing a comprehensive overview of the issues critical to management of the tumor embolization patient.

## Clinical Pearls

- Patients with hypervascular tumors may benefit from preoperative embolization, reducing surgical morbidity by minimizing blood loss and shortening operative time.
- The ascending pharyngeal artery represents the main blood supply to carotid body tumors.
- Severe bradycardia requiring atropine can occur due to the trigeminocardiac reflex in association with external carotid artery branch manipulation.

## Introduction

Tumor embolization refers to any procedure, either percutaneous via direct puncture of the tumor or endovascular (commonly a transfemoral approach), in which particles, liquid embolic agents, coils, gel foam, or other materials are injected, typically with the goal of reducing tumor vascularity prior to surgical excision.[1]

The proposed goals for preoperative tumor embolization include (1) controlling surgically inaccessible arterial feeders; (2) reducing surgical morbidity by lowering blood loss; (3) shortening operative procedure time; (4) increasing the chances of complete surgical resection; (5) decreasing the risk of damage to adjacent normal tissue; (6) relieving intractable pain; (7) decreasing expected tumor recurrence; and (8) facilitating visualization of the surgical field with decreased surgical complications.

Palliative tumor embolization may be indicated as the sole treatment in patients who are poor candidates for surgery, radiation therapy and chemotherapy to treat intractable pain, hemorrhage, or increasing neurological deficit.[2]

Hypervascular tumors that may benefit from preoperative embolization include paragangliomas, juvenile nasopharyngeal angiofibromas, meningiomas, hemangiomas, hemangioblastomas, hemangiopericytomas, esthesioblastomas, and hypervascular metastases.

## Tumor Vascular Supply

### Key Concepts

- Tumors that frequently require presurgical embolization include juvenile nasal angiofibroma, paragangliomas, and meningiomas.
- Tumor blood supply is derived from the regional vasculature.
- The embolization is performed by placement of a microcatheter in the targeted tumor-feeding vessel and delivery of embolic material into the vascular tumor bed.

The blood supply to tumors of the head and neck is derived from the regional vasculature, including dural or extracranial branches of the external carotid artery (ECA) or pial supply by distal branches of the intracranial circulation. Fig. 38.1 demonstrates the normal ECA anatomy. Depending on tumor location there may also be feeding branches from the vertebral artery, internal carotid artery (ICA), adjacent parenchymal central nervous system (CNS) small branch feeding vessels, thyrocervical, and costocervical trunks.[3] Large tumors may redirect flow from nearby vasculature, and preexisting anastomoses may undergo dramatic enlargement due to increased flow requirement.

## Tumors Frequently Requiring Embolization

### JUVENILE NASAL ANGIOFIBROMA

Juvenile nasal angiofibromas (JNAs) are highly vascular, benign tumors found almost exclusively in adolescent males. Rare in the United States and Europe, JNAs account for 0.5% of all head and neck tumors. Nasal obstruction and epistaxis are common symptoms. JNAs originate near the sphenopalatine foramen and can spread into the nasal cavity, from the pterygopalatine fossa to the palate and the zygomaticomaxillary fissure, orbit, sphenoid sinus, and cavernous sinus.

On conventional angiography a lobulated vascular mass with an intense, prolonged vascular stain is observed. Vascular supply is via an enlarged internal maxillary artery. The ascending pharyngeal and vidian arteries may also supply JNAs (see Fig. 38.2).[4]

### PARAGANGLIOMAS

Paragangliomas, also known as *glomus tumors*, are highly vascular tumors that account for 0.6% of all head and

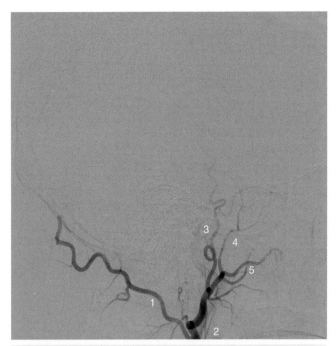

**Fig. 38.1** Angiography of the major external carotid artery branches: 1, occipital artery; 2, ascending pharyngeal artery; 3, superficial temporal artery; 4, middle meningeal artery; and 5, internal maxillary artery are demonstrated.

neck tumors.[5] Hereditary head and neck paragangliomas (HNPs) are frequently caused by mutation of the succinate dehydrogenase subunit genes. Rarely gene mutations causing endocrine neoplasia type 2, von-Hippel-Lindau disease, and neurofibromatosis type 1 can be associated with HNP.[6]

Glomus tumors can present as a slowly growing mass. Later in the course, lower cranial neuropathies (Vernet's syndrome; CN IX–CN XI), additional cranial nerve XII involvement (Collet-Sicard syndrome), and Horner's syndrome (ptosis, miosis, anhidrosis, and enophthalmos) may be observed.[34,36]

Paragangliomas arise from neural crest derivatives of the autonomic nervous system and are named by tumor location. Glomus tympanicum tumors arise from the tympanic nerve (Jacobson's nerve) in the middle ear and may cause hearing loss and pulsatile tinnitus. Glomus jugulare tumors arise from the jugular foramen. If the tumor is large enough to extend into the middle ear, the term *glomus jugulotympanicum* is used. Table 38.1 demonstrates the Fisch jugulotympanic paraganglioma classification. Carotid body tumors occur at the carotid bifurcation and represent one third of HNPs. Table 38.2 shows the commonly used Shamblin carotid body tumor classification. Vagal paragangliomas (glomus vagale and juxtavagale) occur along the course of the vagal nerve and may present with hoarseness and dysphagia.

Up to 3% of paragangliomas have secretory activity associated with elevated catecholamine release inducing tachycardia, hypertension, and diaphoresis.[6] Such metabolically active paragangliomas are also categorized as chromaffin paragangliomas, compared with nonchromaffin paragangliomas that are not metabolically active. Catecholamine assays are necessary to make the diagnosis; a 24-hour urine collection of metanephrine, normetanephrine, and vanillylmandelic acid will almost always exceed the normal range. Recent recommendations for testing include high-performance liquid-phase chromatography measurements of plasma-free metanephrines or 24-hour urine unfractionated metanephrines.[7] Rarely, angiography in these cases may precipitate life-threatening hypertensive crisis.[8] In these patients, angiography and surgical intervention require perioperative alpha adrenergic blockade.[9]

Carotid body tumors characteristically splay apart the ECAs and ICAs. The most common feeding vessel identified is the ascending pharyngeal artery (APA), which in such cases may be challenging to angiographically isolate and enter, because they may overlap the most rapid and densely

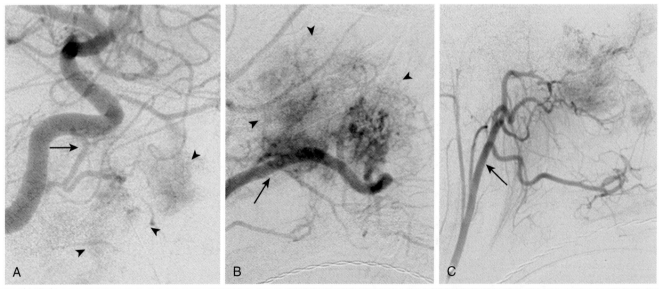

**Fig. 38.2** **(A)** Angiography of the internal carotid artery revealing a nasopharyngeal tumor blush (*arrowheads*) fed by the inferolateral trunk (*black arrow*). **(B)** External carotid artery angiogram demonstrating tumor supply from the internal maxillary artery (*black arrow*) to the juvenile nasopharyngeal angiofibroma (*arrowheads*). **(C)** Tumor supply is also seen from the pharyngeal trunk of the ascending pharyngeal artery (*black arrow*).

**Table 38.1**  Fisch Classification of Jugulotympanic Paragangliomas

| Class | Tumor characteristics |
| --- | --- |
| A | Tumors arise along promontory tympanic plexus; confined to middle ear |
| B | Tumors arise in the tympanic canal and invade the hemotympanum and mastoid |
| C | Tumors originate in the dome of the jugular bulb and invade petrous bone and pyramid; C1–4 subgrouping based on degree of carotid canal erosion from the carotid foramen to the cavernous sinus |
| D | Tumors with posterior fossa intracranial extension; subdivided by depth of invasion<br>De: extradural<br>De1—dura displacement < 2 cm<br>De2—dura displacement > 2 cm<br>Di: intradural<br>Di1—intradural invasion < 2 cm<br>Di2—intradural invasion > 2 cm<br>Di3—inoperable |

Reprinted from Fisch U, Mattox DE. *Microsurgery of the Skull Base*. Stuttgart: Thieme Medical Publishers, Inc.; 1988.

**Table 38.2**  Shamblin Classification of Carotid Body Tumors

| Class | Tumor Characteristics |
| --- | --- |
| I | Splaying of the carotid bifurcation with little attachment to the carotid vessels; complete resection with very little morbidity |
| II | Partial surrounding of internal and external carotid artery; complete resection more challenging |
| III | Complete surrounding of the carotid vessels; complete resection often requires major vessel reconstruction |

Reprinted from Boedeker CC, Ridder GJ, Schipper *J Fam Cancer*. 2005;4(1):55–9.

opacifying portion of the paraganglioma. Larger lesions may recruit supply from nearby ECA branches. Glomus vagale tumors displace the ECA and ICA anteromedially. Arterial supply is similar to carotid body tumors, however, without involvement of carotid bifurcation branches. Arterial supply of glomus jugulare and tympanicum tumors include the inferior tympanic branch of the APA, the stylomastoid branch of the occipital artery (OA), the petrosquamous branch of the middle meningeal artery (MMA), and the anterior tympanic branch of the internal maxillary artery (IMA). Larger tumors invading the skull base may recruit branches from the petrocavernous ICA and/or muscular branches of the vertebral artery (VA). Glomus jugulare tumors often obstruct the jugular vein.

On angiography, paragangliomas appear similar, regardless of tumor location; a well-delineated hypervascular, round or lobulated mass is observed with prolonged dense contrast staining. Vessel encasement and narrowing can also be seen with larger tumors, and arteriovenous shunting may also be present (see Fig. 38.3).

## MENINGIOMAS

Meningiomas are benign intracranial or spinal tumors characterized by dural attachment or "tail," slow growth, and variable although occasionally very high vascularity. Meningiomas are often incidentally found, but patients may present with headache, seizures, or focal neurological deficit due to local mass effect. Most commonly, meningiomas are located on the cerebral convexity, followed by sphenoparietal, parasagittal, and petroclival meningiomas.[10] Patients with neurofibromatosis 2 (NF2) are at an elevated risk for developing meningiomas.

Branches of the ECA are ordinarily involved in extraaxial cranial tumors such as meningiomas. Meningioma blood supply based on location is listed in Table 38.3. The middle and accessory meningeal branches of the IMA supply the meninges over the frontal, parietal, and temporal lobes. Posterior meningeal branches of the vertebral artery can supply posterior fossa meningiomas. Transosseous branches of the occipital arterial branch of the ECA may also be recruited by larger meningiomas.

A well-circumscribed, highly vascular mass with a homogenous, intense vascular stain is characteristically seen on angiography. The stain arrives early in the arterial phase and persists late into the venous phase. Enlarged dural arterial supply to the tumor core may give the appearance of a sunburst or spoke and wheel pattern. Pial supply to the tumor periphery may also be observed.

## HEMANGIOMAS

Hemangiomas represent the most common tumors of infancy and enlarge due to proliferation of endothelial cells. Hemangiomas commonly present as an isolated lesion in the head and neck region. Multifocal lesions with systemic involvement can also be encountered. Superficial lesions have a strawberry-like appearance; bright red and raised, they may be pulsatile with an audible bruit on auscultation. Deeper lesions can appear blue due to overlying dilated draining veins.

Angiography demonstrates dilated feeding arteries, a dense parenchymal blush with multisegmental glandlike angioarchitecture, possibly with rapid venous drainage indicating arteriovenous shunting.[11]

## HEMANGIOBLASTOMAS

Hemangioblastomas are rare vascular tumors, accounting for less than 3% of CNS tumors. Mostly located in the cerebellum, brainstem, and spinal cord, they may include benign, well-circumscribed, highly vascular neoplasm with variable and occasionally conspicuous cystic components. Symptoms occur as a result of local compression of the neural structures and rarely may cause bleeding or paraneoplastic complication (see Fig. 38.4).[12]

## HEMANGIOPERICYTOMAS

Hemangiopericytoma (HPC) is a rare hypervascular tumor sarcoma arising from smooth muscles cells in or around bone. HPC tends to involve the musculoskeletal system. On angiography, HPC is highly vascular, often with observed rapid

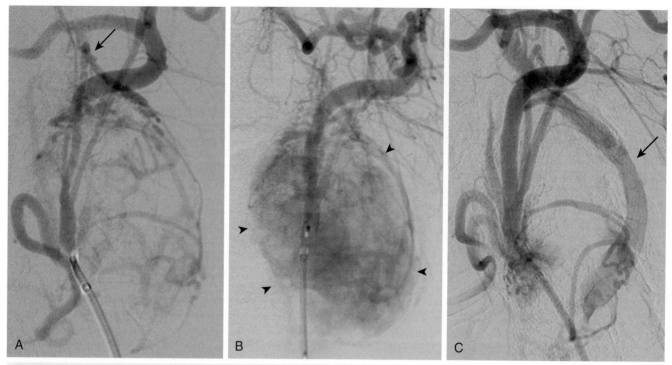

**Fig. 38.3** **(A)** Angiography of the right external carotid artery showing the carotid body tumor predominantly fed by the ascending pharyngeal artery (*black arrow*). **(B)** The intense contrast tumor blush is shown delineating the hypervascular tumor margins (*arrowheads*). **(C)** Postembolization angiography demonstrates significant reduction in hypervascularity. Overflow contrast filling of the internal carotid artery is seen (*black arrow*). The tumor was resected 2 days postembolization and 50 mL of blood loss was reported.

**Table 38.3**  Meningioma Blood Supply Based on Location

| Location | Blood supply |
|---|---|
| Parasagittal/falx | MMA (including contralateral), anterior ethmoidal |
| Olfactory groove | Anterior/posterior ethmoidal |
| Sphenoid wing | Sphenoidal branches of MMA |
| Parasellar | ICA branches, MMA, artery of foramen rotundum |
| Tentorial | Marginal tentorial artery, basal tentorial artery |
| Posterior fossa | MMA, OA, APA |

*MMA*, middle meningeal artery; *OA*, occipital artery; *ICA*, internal carotid artery; *APA*, ascending pharyngeal artery.
Reprinted from Gupta R, Thomas AJ, Horowitz M. *Neurosurgery.* Nov 2006:59 (5); S3–251.

arteriovenous shunting.[13] Innumerable tiny irregular feeding vessels sprouted from a main trunk and an intense fluffy contrast stain with prolonged tumor circulation time are common angiographic findings.[14]

## Details of Procedure

The embolization procedure can be performed in a single session, simultaneously with diagnostic angiography, or alternatively it may need to be staged over multiple sessions depending on the size and target location. The procedure is often performed 24 to 72 hours prior to a planned surgical resection to optimize tumor devascularization at the time of surgery. The procedure is performed under conscious sedation or general endotracheal anesthesia in the neuroangiography suite; the latter may be required depending on the need for temporary neuromuscular blockade to perform the embolization safely. Periprocedurally it is important to ensure that the patient is well hydrated to help protect the kidneys from the iodinated contrast load.

Transfemoral access is secured in the standard fashion, and a 4 F or 5 F multipurpose catheter and 0.035-in hydrophilic guidewire are used to perform the initial diagnostic angiography. Dedicated injections of the ICAs and ECAs, bilateral VAs, and cervical vessels may be necessary, depending on tumor location. Superselective angiography of the arterial feeders to the tumor is performed using a hydrophilic microcatheter and microguidewire. Superselective distal positioning of the microcatheter with consideration of gentle wedging avoids the possibility of reflux embolization into critical or eloquent territories. To protect from embolization of normal structures, the microcatheter is typically positioned as close to the tumor bed as possible.

Embolic material (particles or liquid embolic agents) is injected under fluoroscopy until tumor blush disappears or maximal allowable reflux is encountered. The embolic solution is carefully formulated to permit a reasonable concentration of embolic material that does not have a propensity to overconcentrate and accidentally occlude the microcatheter, and that is sufficiently opacified with contrast material to confidently permit visualization of unwanted reflux during embolization. A slow, steady, pulsatile rate of injection is maintained while watching for subtle reflux that alerts the operator to discontinue the now-successful pedicle embolization. Once the

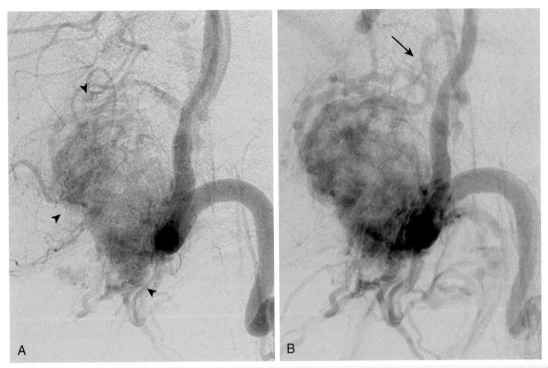

**Fig. 38.4** **(A)** Angiography of the vertebral artery (*black arrow*) demonstrates innumerable feeding branches to the dense tumor blush of a posterior fossa hemangioblastoma (*arrow heads*). **(B)** The late arterial phase more clearly demonstrates tumor supply from the posterior inferior cerebellar artery (*black arrow*).

tumor is adequately embolized, perhaps after single- or multiple-branch embolizations as deemed appropriate in a particular case, the proximal feeding vessel can be occluded with Gelfoam (Upjohn Co., Kalamazoo, MI) or platinum coils before targeting any remaining arterial feeders.[15]

To minimize the risk of stroke during embolization of internal carotid or VA branches, a temporary balloon may be inflated across or distal to the origin of the target vessel depending on the location of vessels to be protected. Under these circumstances anticoagulation is typically also required.[16] Frequently, certain vascular territories are not amenable to embolization due to shared eloquent territorial supply, such as pial leptomeningeal supply to a meningeal-based tumor, or ethmoidal supply (via the ophthalmic artery) to an olfactory groove meningioma, where such directly embolized anastomoses could endanger the CNS or globe.

However, in the event that balloon protection is chosen in such cases, this requires additional instrumentation and careful aspiration at the guide catheter prior to balloon deflation to prevent any reflux of particle embolization intracranially. Recently balloon-augmented tumor embolization using a dual-lumen balloon catheter (Scepter C, MicroVention, Inc., Tustin, CA) has been reported with proposed advantages over older devices, including improved catheter navigation and reduction of procedural time.[17]

Bradycardia from the trigeminocardiac reflex can occur in association with external carotid artery branch manipulation. Atropine should be on hand during the procedure in case of severe bradycardia.

Direct percutaneous puncture and tumor embolization under fluoroscopy, ultrasound, or computed tomography can be performed in cases unsuitable for transarterial embolization such as inaccessible vascular tortuosity,

hazardous atherosclerotic disease, diminutive size of arterial feeders, or involvement of vascular anastomoses to the ICA or VA. An 18- or 20-gauge needle may be used to puncture the target lesion under imaging guidance after completion of initial traditional angiography delineating the tumor vasculature. Lesions at the skull base can be directly punctured using an infrazygomatic, transnasal, transpalatal, or transoral approach.[18]

## Perioperative Considerations

### Key Concepts

- Depending on tumor location, vessel sacrifice during surgical resection may be necessary. If so, a preoperative balloon test occlusion of the vessel may be requested to assess feasibility.
- Tumor embolization is typically performed 24 to 72 hours before planned surgical resection.
- Knowledge of cranial nerve vascular supply and external-internal carotid artery anastomosis is critical to the safety of the procedure.

### Clinical Pearls

- Smaller-sized embolic agents optimize tumor necrosis but are associated with increased risk of unintended embolization.
- Dangerous ECA-ICA anastomoses may appear due to changes in flow during the embolization procedure.
- Embolic material sized less than 150 microns may devascularize vasa nervosum causing cranial neuropathy.

## CHOOSING EMBOLIC MATERIAL

Ideally an embolic agent is chosen that will maximally penetrate the tumor vascular bed while sparing normal adjacent tissue.[2] Current embolic agents include particles such as polyvinyl alcohol (PVA), gelatin sponge (Gelfoam; Upjohn, Kalamazoo, MI), Embospheres (BioSphere Medical, Rockland, MA), liquid embolic agents (alcohol, glue [n-butyl cyanoacrylate (NBCA)], ethylvinyl alcohol copolymer [EVOH], or Onyx [eV3, Irvine, CA]), and coils.[19]

### Polyvinyl alcohol

PVA embolic agents are fragmented sterilized foam particles with a wide range of sizes. Smaller particles (45–150 microns) infiltrate the tumor capillary vascular bed, aiding in devascularization and are associated with higher rates of postembolization tumor necrosis.[20] Larger particles (150–250 microns) embolize arterioles in the tumor bed. Smaller particles will allow for more distal penetration, however, with the caveat of an increased potential for unintended systemic embolization. Adequate anterograde flow in the target vessels is required to deliver particles to the tumor bed. Flow arrest due to catheter-related vasospasm may cause reflux of the PVA particles, increasing the risk of nontarget embolization. One technique is to target distal vessels with smaller particles, gradually increasing the particle size for subsequent injections.[21] Delayed recanalization occurs with particle embolization, thus diminishing the chance of durable long-term devascularization, in addition to minimizing the risk of long-term sequelae from inadvertent nontarget tissue embolization.[22]

### Gelfoam

Gelfoam can be found in sponge and powder form for use in tumor embolization. It is a water-insoluble, porous agent that resorbs completely in 4 to 6 weeks. Gelfoam strips can be advanced through the microcatheter to the target vessel using a technique similar to particle embolization.[21]

### Embospheres

Trisacryl gelatin microspheres are nonabsorbable, round embolic agents with precise size. Available in sizes ranging from 40 to 1300 microns, they are uniform in size and shape. The hydrophilic coating may reduce aggregation, facilitating injection through the delivery microcatheter.

### N-butyl cyanoacrylate

NBCA, also known as *super glue*, is a liquid embolic agent that undergoes rapid polymerization on exposure to ionic solutions such as blood or saline. NBCA and ethiodol are combined in a customized manner that alters the speed of polymerization, and radioopaque tantalum powder (Trufill; Codman Neurovascular, Inc., Raynham, MA) may be added to further improve fluoroscopic visualization. Polymerization time can be managed by adjusting the volumetric concentration of ethiodol relative to the NBCA. Successful delivery of glue requires extensive familiarity with the material and procedural technique with careful control of polymerization time, microcatheter manipulation, and speed of injection. To avoid the risk of microcatheter retention with glue, injections must be performed quickly and relatively continuously and, in doing so, precise control may be sacrificed. In addition, the microcatheter must be replaced for each vessel embolized.

### Alcohol

For tumors with small feeders arising from larger vessels supplying normal brain, a liquid embolization technique using alcohol has been described.[15,23] Flow control techniques using a balloon catheter are employed to direct flow of alcohol preferentially to the target feeding branches and away from normal brain supply. This technique is considered controversial due to the risk of residual floating particles embolizing distally when the balloon is deflated.

### Onyx (ethylene vinyl alcohol)

Onyx is a nonadhesive and cohesive liquid embolic agent dissolved in dimethyl sulfoxide (DMSO). Once the polymer solution is injected into a vessel, the DMSO is absorbed transmurally, leaving the unsuspended polymer within the vessel to gradually solidify as an intravascular polymeric plug conforming to the configuration of the containing vessels. Tantalum powder is added for fluoroscopic visualization. Onyx is mechanically occlusive without being adherent to the vessel wall, allowing for a slow single injection of the embolic agent over a prolonged period, often measuring in the tens of minutes for injection duration. Onyx is supplied as a formulaic suspension in DMSO and is available in 6% (Onyx 18) and 8% (Onyx 34) EVOH concentrations. Selection of concentration is based on flow velocity within the tumor. Embolization of each feeding pedicle is performed until vessel stasis is achieved and maximal allowable reflux is encountered. If unfavorable filling of normal vasculature occurs, the injection can be paused for 30 seconds to 2 minutes, to allow for solidification of the embolized portion of tumor. When resuming injection, Onyx will take the path of least resistance to fill another portion of the tumor. Due to the deliberate and gradual nature of Onyx injections, Onyx typically advances in a single column, reducing the risk of involuntary venous migration. To prevent reflux during embolization, an initial plug is allowed to form at the microcatheter tip. The risk of catheter retention is less than with NBCA due to the nonadhesive properties of Onyx. At the end of the procedure, the microcatheter is withdrawn to further minimize risk of catheter retention.[24] Microcatheters used must be DMSO compatible and replaced after each vessel embolization. Microcatheters and syringes that are not DMSO compatible may dissolve or deform rather quickly when exposed to DMSO, permitting inadvertent, accidental, and dangerous leakage of embolic material.

## DANGEROUS ANASTOMOSES

Anastomotic pathways exist between the ECA, ICA, VA, ophthalmic artery, ascending cervical artery, deep cervical artery, and spinal arteries.[3] It is important to note that these anastomoses may not be apparent on initial angiography, but can reveal themselves with changes in regional blood flow during the embolization procedure as the embolization proceeds and the flow of blood and angiographic contrast material find formerly unopacified vascular channels. As such, multiple interval hand injections are necessary to evaluate for intraprocedurally manifesting anastomoses before targeting previously discovered feeding branches for intraprocedural embolization.

Functional vascular anatomical knowledge of the ECA branches and mindfulness of certain intraextracranial anastomotic routes is critical to avoid unintended embolic stroke or cranial nerve palsies. Cranial nerve palsies can result from ischemia of the vasa nervosum investing and supplying the cranial nerves with their own vascular supply. The three geographical regions that serve as major anastomotic pathways are the orbital, petrocavernous, and upper cervical regions, summarized in Table 38.4.

A summary of the cranial nerve supply is presented in Table 38.5. The most important ECA cranial nerve supply is to CN VII and the lower CNs (IX–XII). In general, the size of the nonvisualized anastomotic arteries ranges from 50 to 80 microns. Therefore particles sized larger than 150 microns will be unable to penetrate the anastomoses, avoiding potential embolic complications. When embolizing the arterial supply of cranial nerves such as the stylomastoid branch of the OA or the neuromeningeal trunk of the ascending pharyngeal artery, increasing particle size to 300 to 500 microns is recommended. Several techniques can be used to prevent embolic material from entering collaterals if particles are to be infused proximal to the tumor branches: mechanical obstruction of the proximal collateral branch with large particles or coils, or flow control or flow reversal techniques using a proximal balloon catheter to occlude the collateral ECA vessel, leading to redirection of flow from the ICA to the ECA region. This technique may still lead to complications as residual particles floating in the ICA may embolize distally causing stroke.[15,25] Provocative testing for suspected cranial nerve supply can be performed with local injection of lidocaine to observe neurological deficit. If neurological signs are elicited, then the microcatheter may be repositioned.

## BALLOON TEST OCCLUSION

When a large number of feeding branches arise from the ICA and/or the tumor encases the ICA, surgical consideration may be given to the possibility of sacrificing the ICA, and a balloon test occlusion (BTO) is often requested. The BTO is performed under conscious sedation and systemic anticoagulation. A guiding catheter is used to advance the balloon catheter into the cervical ICA segment. A catheter may be placed in the contralateral carotid artery to verify adequate collateral inflow to the occluded territory from adjoining circulations during BTO. After systemic anticoagulation with heparin (activated clotting time of 250–350 seconds), the balloon is slowly inflated to occlude

**Table 38.4** Summary of the Major Extracranial and Intracranial Anastomoses

| Extracranial | | | Intracranial | |
|---|---|---|---|---|
| Major artery | Location | Branch | Branch | Artery |
| Internal maxillary artery | Proximal | MMA | Orbital branches, anterior branch (anterior falcine artery) | Ophthalmic artery |
| | | | Cavernous branches | ILT |
| | | | Petrous branch | CN VII supply |
| | Proximal | AMA | Artery of foramen ovale | ILT |
| | Distal | Vidian artery | | Petrous ICA |
| | Distal | Artery of foramen rotundum | | ILT |
| | Distal | Anterior deep temporal artery | | Ophthalmic artery |
| Superficial temporal artery | Frontal branch | | Supraorbital branch | Ophthalmic artery |
| Ascending pharyngeal artery | Pharyngeal trunk | Superior pharyngeal artery | Carotid branch (foramen lacerum) | Lateral clival artery |
| | Neuromeningeal trunk | Odontoid arch | | Vertebral artery (C1) |
| | | Hypoglossal and jugular branch | | Meningohypophyseal trunk of ICA |
| Posterior auricular-occipital artery | Stylomastoid branch | | | CN VII supply |
| Occipital artery | Muscular branches | | | Vertebral artery (C1-C2) |
| Ascending and deep cervical arteries | | | | Vertebral artery (C3-C7) |

*ILT*, inferolateral trunk; *ICA*, internal carotid artery; *CN*, cranial nerve; *MMA*, middle meningeal artery; *AMA*, accessory meningeal artery.
Reprinted from Geibprasert S, Pongpech S, Armstrong D et al. *AJNR*. 2009;30(8):1459–68.

**Table 38.5**  Summary of Cranial Nerve Supply

| Cranial Nerve | Location | Arterial Supply | |
|---|---|---|---|
| III, IV | Cisternal | Mesencephalic perforators (common trunk for CN III) | Vertebrobasilar system |
| | Cavernous sinus | CN III: ILT only; CN IV; marginal artery of the tentorium cerebelli (meningohypophyseal trunk)+ILT | |
| | Superior orbital fissure | Anteromedial branch of ILT | |
| VI | Cisternal | | Vertebrobasilar system |
| | Dorsum sella | Jugular branch of APA, medial branch of lateral clival artery, meningohypophyseal trunk | |
| | Cavernous sinus | ILT | |
| | Superior orbital fissure | Anteromedial branch of ILT | |
| V | Cisternal | Basilar vestige of trigeminal artery (between SCA and AICA) | |
| | Meckel cave | Lateral artery of trigeminal ganglion, cavernous branch of MMA, carotid branch of APA, ILT | |
| V2 | Foramen rotundum | Artery of foramen rotundum | ILT, distal IMA |
| V3 | Foramen ovale | Posteromedial branch | ILT, AMA |
| VII, VIII | Cisternal+IAC | Internal auditory artery | AICA |
| | Geniculate ganglion | Petrosal branch of MMA, stylomastoid artery of posterior auricular artery/occipital artery | |
| IX, X | Cisternal, jugular foramen | Jugular branch of neuromeningeal trunk | VA, APA |
| XI | Spinal root | C3 segmental branch | Cervical arteries, musculospinal branch of APA |
| | Cranial root | Jugular branch of neuromeningeal trunk | APA |
| XII | Cisternal hypoglossal canal | Hypoglossal branch of neuromeningeal trunk | VA, APA |

*APA*, ascending pharyngeal artery; *ILT*, inferolateral trunk; *SCA*, superior cerebellar artery; *AICA*, anterior inferior cerebellar artery; *MMA*, middle meningeal artery; *IMA*, internal maxillary artery; *AMA*, accessory meningeal artery; *IAC*, internal auditory canal.
Reprinted from Geibprasert S, Pongpech S, Armstrong D et al. *AJNR.* 2009;30(8):1459–68.

the vessel of interest (typically the ICA). The patient is then examined over a period of 30 minutes to see whether ICA sacrifice can be tolerated. To further evaluate adequacy of collaterals, the blood pressure is pharmacologically lowered (20 mm Hg below baseline) for an additional 15 minutes, and the patient is reassessed for neurological deficit. To further increase the sensitivity of the BTO, a stump pressure measurement may be performed; a microcatheter is placed beyond the inflated occlusive balloon catheter to record the mean stump pressure distal to the occluded ICA. A stump pressure ratio greater than 60% (calculated by comparing mean stump pressure to the radial systemic mean arterial pressure during the ICA occlusion time) in an asymptomatic patient suggests that ICA sacrifice, if necessary, is safe.[26] The venous phase technique is performed by contrast injection from the contralateral ICA. A delay of longer than 2 seconds between opacification of the bihemispheric cortical veins suggests that ICA sacrifice is not safe (a failed test). Transcranial Doppler monitoring of ipsilateral middle cerebral artery blood flow velocities during BTO may also be used to assess tolerance. A 30% drop in velocity while the balloon is inflated indicates borderline collateralization, and a 40% decrease suggests inadequate collaterals to support cerebral perfusion.[27,28] Cerebral single-photon

emission computed tomography imaging may assist in evaluation on perfusion during BTO. Risks of BTO include stroke and local blood vessel injury in addition to the overall risks related to cerebral angiography.

## TIMING OF PRESURGICAL EMBOLIZATION

Ideally, embolization is performed 24 to 72 hours prior to surgical resection to permit maximal thrombosis of the occluded vessels and prevent recanalization of the occluded arteries or development of collateral arterial channels.[19] If large pedicles are embolized, delay in tumor resection can lead to neoangiogenesis and revascularization of the tumor bed. The use of permanent liquid embolic agents (glue and Onyx) when combined with a greater delay of surgery may permit maximal tissue necrosis and softening. In such instances the optimal gap between embolization and surgical resection may increase to between 7 and 9 days. Such intentional necrotizing embolization may also be achieved with very small-particle embolization, although as described earlier in this chapter, small-particle embolization is also accompanied with a greater risk of inadvertent occlusion of anastomotic arcades and cranial nerve vasa arteriosum. Embolization of large tumors carries risk of tumor necrosis and associated swelling, which may produce symptoms and force earlier surgery (within 12–24 hours). A recent review reported an average time to surgery postembolization of 6.3 days, ranging between 0 and 30 days.[10]

## Postoperative Complications

### Key Concepts

- Reported complication rates related to tumor embolization range from 2.8% to 12.6%.
- Major complications include thromboembolism, cranial neuropathy, and postembolization increased tumor mass effect.
- Mild risks of cerebral angiography include groin hematoma, blood vessel injury, and contrast nephropathy.
- Postprocedure care includes standard postcatheterization groin protocol, IV hydration, and close monitoring for delayed swelling in the case of large tumors. If the tumor is small and/or the resection is delayed, the patient may return home after 24 hours of observation.

### Clinical Pearls

- Severe bradycardia can occur in association with ECA manipulation and may require atropine.
- Cranial nerve palsy and blindness may occur due to unintended embolization to normal structures or the ophthalmic artery.
- Rapid tumor necrosis with malignant edema may occur after embolization of large tumors, forcing early surgical resection.
- Three percent of paragangliomas may have secretory activity with elevated catecholamine release. Hypertensive crises can occur if beta-blockers are administered without prior to alpha adrenergic blockade.

A review of 459 patients reported a complication rate of 4.6% directly related to embolization.[10] Other studies have reported complication rates ranging from 2.8% to 12.6%[29–32] (mean of 6.8% for 749 tumors embolized).

Proposed guidelines for tumor embolization have been published,[1] and the suggested complication thresholds are listed in Table 38.6. The most common transient complications are fever and localized pain. A noninfectious fever is associated with necrosis of larger lesions and can persist for 2 to 3 weeks; however, cultures should be obtained in all febrile patients to rule out a treatable infectious etiology.

Puncture site complications, such as groin hematoma, are usually clinically inconsequential unless very large in size or if bleeding is retroperitoneal. Additional risks of catheter angiography include blood vessel injury from arterial catheterization and contrast nephropathy. Iatrogenic arterial perforation may cause epidural, subdural, or subarachnoid hemorrhage, depending on location, and may require emergent neurosurgical intervention (e.g., craniotomy, hematoma evacuation, extraventricular drain placement, etc.).

Serious complications directly related to embolization include nerve and tissue damage, blindness from

**Table 38.6** Proposed Complication Thresholds that Should Prompt Review If Exceeded

| Indicator | Threshold (%) |
| --- | --- |
| Nerve Palsy | |
| Transient | >2 |
| Permanent | >1 |
| Neurological deficit | |
| Major permanent | >1 |
| Minor permanent | >2 |
| Death | >0 |
| Unintended vascular occlusion | >5 |
| Total complications | >5 |

Reprinted from American Society of Interventional and Therapeutic Neuroradiology. *AJNR.* 2001;22:S14–S15.

ophthalmic artery occlusion, and stroke. Lower cranial nerve palsy with subsequent difficulty swallowing increases aspiration risk and may necessitate percutaneous endoscopic gastrostomy and/or tracheostomy. For these patients, intensive swallowing therapy with a speech therapist is required. Potential airway compromise should be anticipated if there is suspicion of cranial neuropathy, signaling extra caution during extubation postprocedure. If arteriovenous shunting is present within the tumor, smaller particles may travel through the lesion and embolize to the lungs. Skin necrosis can occur if cutaneous branches of the ECA are embolized and may necessitate topical antiseptics or antibiotics.

Intratumor hemorrhage has been associated with embolization of meningiomas.[20] The presumed pathophysiology of hemorrhage includes distal occlusion of abnormal, friable microvasculature, or continued pulsation within the proximal vessels resulting in rupture of small occluded vessels.[33] Postprocedure edema may be reduced by treating the patient with steroids before embolization,[37] and its use is recommended for large tumors and meningiomas, especially if resection is delayed.[1] However, rapid tumor necrosis and associated symptomatic tissue swelling may still occur after tumor embolization, precipitating earlier surgical resection (within 12–24 hours). Patients with posterior fossa meningiomas should be monitored closely due to increased risk of brainstem herniation. Any signs of brainstem compression should be managed aggressively, and urgent posterior fossa craniotomy may be indicated.

As previously described, rarely, paragangliomas may have secretory activity. Secretion of excess catecholamines causes symptoms similar to those encountered in patients with pheochromocytoma. Hypertensive crises can be precipitated if beta-adrenergic antagonists are administered before alpha-adrenergic antagonists due to unopposed alpha-adrenergic activity. Phenoxybenzamine, an irreversible alpha-adrenergic blocking agent, is preferred in dose and timing to produce adequate alpha-adrenergic blockade. Beta blockade can then be then initiated cautiously with a low-dose beta-blocker (e.g., propranolol) initially, followed by a single long-acting dose to achieve a goal heart rate between 60 and 80 beats per minute. If blood pressure control is inadequate, a calcium channel blocker (e.g., nicardipine, verapamil) may be added and is also recommended for use in patients with supraventricular tachycardia or contraindication to beta blockers.[35] Neuropeptide secretion may also be present, and high circulating levels of cholecystokinin have been associated with prolonged postoperative ileus.[38]

It is our practice that patients who undergo embolization of large tumors are admitted to the intensive care unit where they are closely monitored for changes in neurological examination or airway compromise due to tumor swelling. In some cases, patients may be monitored overnight and subsequently discharged to home the next day if clinically stable and surgical resection is to be delayed. We emphasize the importance of adequate pain control and a regimen tailored to the individual patient's degree of discomfort.

## Summary

Preoperative tumor embolization may result in decreased surgical morbidity and mortality through the provision of greater hemostasis, consequential decreased procedural time, and decreased need for blood replacement. Such procedures have a relatively low risk but demand attention to potentially dangerous anatomical vascular considerations and specific technical variables. They require expertise related to angiographic methods, tools, and approaches utilized to successfully accomplish their goals.

### References

1. Duffis JE, Gandhi CD, Prestigiacomo CJ, et al. Head, neck, and brain tumor embolization guidelines. *J NeuroIntervent Surg.* 2012;4(4):251–255.
2. American Society of Interventional and Therapeutic Neuroradiology. *AJNR.* 2001;22:S14–S15.
3. Gemmete JJ, Ansari SA, McHugh J, et al. Embolization of vascular tumors of the head and neck. *Neuroimag Clin N Am.* 2009;19(2):181–198.
4. Osborn AG. *Diagnostic Cerebral Angiography.* 2nd ed. Philadelphia: Lippincott Williams & Wilkins; 1999.
5. Sykes JM, Ossoff RH. Paragangliomas of the head and neck. *Otolaryngol Clin North Am.* 1986;19(4):755–767.
6. Offergeld C, Brase C, Yaremchuk S, et al. Head and neck paragangliomas: clinical and molecular genetic classification. *Clinics (Sao Paulo).* 2012;67(Suppl 1):19–28.
7. Colen TY, Mihm FG, Mason TP, et al. Catecholamine-secreting paragangliomas: recent progress in diagnosis and perioperative management. *Skull Base.* 2009;19(6):377–385.
8. Hu WY, TerBrugge KG. The role of angiography in the evaluation of vascular and neoplastic disease in the external carotid artery circulation. *Neuroimag Clin N Am.* 1996;6(3):625–644.
9. Hahn S, Palmer JN, Adappa ND. A catecholamine-secreting skull base sinonasal paraganglioma presenting with labile hypertension in a patient with previously undiagnosed genetic mutation. *J Neurol Surg Rep.* 2012;73(1):19–24.
10. Shah AH, Patel N, Raper DM, et al. The role of preoperative embolization for intracranial meningiomas. *J Neurosurg.* 2013;119(2):364–372.
11. Song JK, Niimi Y, Berenstein A. Endovascular treatment of hemangiomas. *Neuroimag Clin N Am.* 2007;17(2):165–173.
12. Bamps S, Calenbergh FV, Vleeschouwer SD, et al. What the neurosurgeon should know about hemangioblastoma, both sporadic and in Von Hippel-Lindau disease: A literature review. *Surg Neurol Int.* 2013;4:145 eCollection 2013.
13. Santillan A, Zink W, Lavi E, et al. Endovascular embolization of cervical hemangiopericytoma with Onyx-18: case report and review of the literature. *J NeuroIntervent Surg.* 2011;3(3):304–307.
14. Marc JA, Takei Y, Schecter MM, et al. Intracranial hemangiopericytomas. Angiography, pathology and differential diagnosis. *Am J Roentgenol Radium Ther Nucl Med.* 1975;125(4):823–832.

15. Gupta R, Thomas AJ, Horowitz M. Intracranial head and neck tumors: endovascular considerations, present and future. *Neurosurgery.* 2006;59(5 Suppl 3):S251–S260.
16. Tymianski M, Willinsky RA, Tator CH, et al. Embolization with temporary balloon occlusion of the internal carotid artery and in vivo proton spectroscopy improves radical removal of petrous-tentorial meningioma. *Neurosurgery.* 1994;35(5):974–977.
17. Spiotta AM, Miranpuri A, Vargas J, et al. Balloon augmented Onyx embolization utilizing a dual lumen balloon catheter: utility in the treatment of a variety of head and neck lesions. *J Neurointervent Surg.* 2014;6(7):547–555.
18. Gemmete JJ, Chaudhary N, Pandey A, et al. Vinyl Alcohol Copolymer in Conjunction with Standard Endovascular Embolization Techniques for Preoperative Devascularization of Hypervascular Head and Neck Tumors: Technique, Initial Experience, and Correlation with Surgical Observations. *AJNR.* 2010;31(5):961–966.
19. Gandhi D, Gemmette JJ, Ansari SA, et al. Interventional neuroradiology of the head and neck. *AJNR.* 2008;29(10):1806–1815.
20. Wakhloo AK, Juengling FD, Van Velthoven V, et al. Extended preoperative polyvinyl alcohol microembolization of intracranial meningiomas: assessment of two embolization techniques. *AJNR.* 1993;14(3):571–582.
21. Lazzaro MA, Badruddin A, Zaidat OO, et al. Endovascular embolization of head and neck tumors. *Frontiers Neurol.* 2011;2:64.
22. Sorimachi T, Koike T, Takeuchi S, et al. Embolization of cerebral arteriovenous malformations achieved with polyvinyl alcohol particles: angiographic reappearance and complications. *AJNR.* 1999;20(7):1323–1328.
23. Horowitz M, Whisnant RE, Jungreis C, et al. Temporary balloon occlusion and ethanol injection for preoperative embolization of carotid-body tumor. *Ear Nose Throat J.* 2002;81(8):536–538, 540, 542.
24. Gemmete JJ, Pandey AS, Kasten SJ, et al. Endovascular methods for the treatment of vascular anomalies. *Neuroimag Clin N Am.* 2013;23(4):703–728.
25. Geibprasert S, Pongpech S, Armstrong D, et al. Dangerous extracranial-intracranial anastomoses and supply to the cranial nerves: vessels the neurointerventionalist needs to know. *AJNR.* 2009;30(8):1459–1468.
26. Mazza A, Armigliato M, Marzola MC, et al. Anti-hypertensive treatment in pheochromocytoma and paraganglioma: current management and therapeutic features. *Endocrine.* 2014;45(3):469–478.
27. Sekhar LN, Biswas A, Hallam D, et al. Neuroendovascular management of tumors and vascular malformations of the head and neck. *Neurosurg Clin N Am.* 2009;20(4):453–485.
28. Kofke WA, Brauer P, Policare R, et al. Middle cerebral artery blood flow velocity and stable xenon computed tomographic blood flow during balloon test occlusion of the internal carotid artery. *Stroke.* 1995;26(9):1603–1606.
29. Waldron JS, Sughrue ME, Hetts SW, et al. Embolization of skull base meningiomas and feeding vessels arising from the internal carotid circulation. *Neurosurgery.* 2011;68(1):162–169.
30. Bendszus M, Monoranu CM, Schutz A, et al. Neurologic complications after particle embolization of intracranial meningiomas. *AJNR.* 2005;26(6):1413–1419.
31. Carli DF, Sluzewski M, Beute GN, et al. Complications of particle embolization of meningiomas: frequency, risk factors, and outcome. *AJNR.* 2010;31(1):152–154.
32. Rosen CL, Ammerman JM, Sekhar LN, et al. Outcome analysis of preoperative embolization in cranial base surgery. *Acta Neurochir (Wein).* 2002;144(11):1157–1164.
33. Kallmes DF, Evans AJ, Kaptain GJ, et al. Hemorrhagic complications in embolization of a meningioma: case report and review of the literature. *Neuroradiology.* 1997;39(12):877–880.
34. Krings T, Geibprasert S, ter Brugge KG. *Case-Based Interventional Neuroradiology.* New York, NY: Thieme Medical Publishers, Inc.; 2011.
35. Fisch U, Mattox DE. *Microsurgery of the Skull Base.* Stuttgart: Thieme Medical Publishers, Inc.; 1988.
36. Boedeker CC, Ridder GJ, Schipper J. Paragangliomas of the head and neck: diagnosis and treatment. *Fam Cancer.* 2005;4(1):55–59.
37. Wang AY, Chen CC, Lai HY, et al. Balloon Test Occlusion of the Internal Carotid Artery with Stump Pressure Ratio and Venous Phase Delay Technique. *J Stroke Cerebrovasc Dis.* 2013;22(8):e533–e540.
38. Jackson CG, Gulya AJ, Knox GW, et al. A paraneoplastic syndrome associated with glomus tumors of the skull base? Early observations. *Otolaryngol Head Neck Surg.* 1989;100(6):583–587.

# 39 *Spinal Vascular Lesions*

SANTIAGO ORTEGA GUTIERREZ, IAN KAMINSKY, NEENA I. MARUPUDI, and SANDRA NARAYANAN

## Neuroanatomy and Procedure

### Key Concepts

- Vascularization of the spinal axis consists of somatotopically organized, transversely oriented, paired segmental arteries connected by several longitudinal channels.
- Most segmental arteries are limited to supply nerve roots, dura, vertebrae, and epidural soft tissue. Only a few segmental arteries give rise to radiculomedullary feeders that will anastomose with the spinal cord arteries.
- Variability of segmental and longitudinal connections is common. The anterior and posterior spinal arteries comprise the primary spinal cord supply.
- Venous drainage occurs from longitudinal intraspinal veins through medullary veins into the longitudinal epidural and paraspinal plexus.

### Embryology

Vascularization of the spinal axis is determined during the first few weeks of intrauterine development. Each of 31 somites receives one pair of segmental arteries from the dorsal aorta to supply each developing metamere. As the spinal cord enlarges, longitudinal connections form between transverse arteries. These connections merge in the midline, giving rise to the future spinal artery. Concomitantly, the distalmost portions of the segmental arteries (future radicular arteries) gradually regress; these will primarily supply vertebral bodies, paraspinal muscles, dura, and nerve roots. Few dominant segmental arteries remain (future radiculomedullary arteries) to supply the spinal cord (Fig. 39.1).[1]

### Spinal Vascular Unit

The spinal axis vasculature consists of two segmental arteries arising from the dorsal aorta. The vessels traverse posteriorly around the vertebral body, send small perforating branches to supply the anterolateral aspect of the vertebral body, and divide into dorsal and ventral branches.[2] The spinal branch of the dorsal intercostal artery enters the vertebral canal through the intervertebral foramen and divides into (1) an anterior arcade beneath the longitudinal ligament that vascularizes the posterior vertebral body; (2) a posterior branch traveling in the posterior epidural space to supply the anterior lamina and part of the spinous process; and (3) a radicular artery, which supplies the dura and nerve root at every segmental level. At some levels, radicular arteries maintain their embryonic anastomoses with the anterior spinal arteries (ASAs) and posterior spinal arteries (PSAs) and also supply a large segment of the spinal cord. Radicular arteries that anastomose with the ASAs are called *anterior*

*radiculomedullary arteries* (average of six anastomoses). Those that anastomose posteriorly with the PSAs are known as *radiculopial* or *posterior medullary arteries* (average of 11–16). They may originate separately or as common trunks and follow the nerve root, supplying collaterals to it and the surrounding dura (radiculomeningeal branches). The main trunk of the dorsal branch of the segmental artery traverses posteriorly beneath the ipsilateral transverse process along the outer surface of the lamina, forming an arterial plexus close to the spinal process and providing middle and lateral muscular branches to the dorsal muscular group (Fig. 39.2).[3]

### Anatomical Variations of the Spinal Segments

In the cervical, upper thoracic, and sacral regions, segmental vessels arise from vessels other than the aorta. In the cervical region, the development and persistence of consecutive intersegmental anastomotic channels established three dominant craniocaudal vascular systems: the ascending cervical artery, the vertebral artery (VA), and the deep cervical artery. The upper thoracic region is supplied by the supreme intercostal arteries, costocervical trunks, or directly from the subclavian artery. The sacral arteries and iliolumbar artery (supplying the L5 level) derived from each internal iliac artery are the main supply to the caudal spine. The median sacral artery arising from the aortic bifurcation may produce several segmental sacral vessels.[1]

### Spinal Anastomosis

Important anastomoses occur between successive vertebral levels along longitudinal and transverse (across the midline) connections. Longitudinal anastomoses between extraspinal segments of consecutive segmental arteries are highly developed in the cervical regions. The intraspinal extradural system has mainly transverse anastomoses, although longitudinal interconnections are also present. Transverse anastomoses occur dorsal and ventral to the dural sheath, forming an extradural ring with branches supplying adjacent osseous and dural structures. Vessels entering the anterior epidural space have a characteristic hexagonal branching pattern comprising the retrocorporeal collateral network (Fig. 39.3).[4]

### Extrinsic and Intrinsic Supply of the Spinal Cord

The spinal cord is mainly perfused by the ASA, located in the anterior median sulcus and supplying the majority of the gray matter through sulcal branches. Pial branches on the anterior and lateral surface of the cord supply the ventral two thirds of the vasocorona.[5] Various radiculomedullary arteries from the vertebral; ascending; and deep cervical, intercostal, and lumbar arteries contribute to the ASA. The largest radiculomedullary artery, the artery

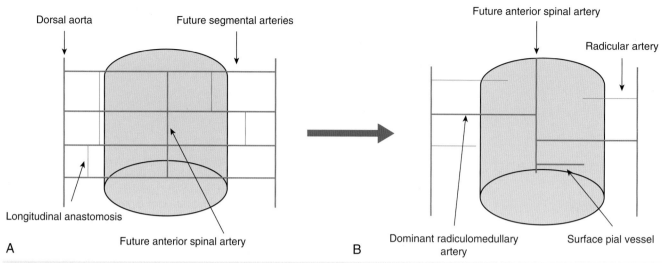

**Fig 39.1** Scheme of embryological development of the spinal cord vasculature.

of Adamkiewicz, or artery of the lumbar enlargement, arises >70% of the time from a left-sided intercostal artery between T9 and T12. The posterior spinal arteries supply the dorsal one third of the vasocorona and posterior horn and marginal part of the central gray matter (Fig. 39.4).[6]

## Spinal Venous System

Knowledge of the venous system is vital for a full understanding of the breadth of spinal vascular pathology. Venous drainage of the spinal cord is divided into intrinsic and extrinsic venous networks and the extradural venous plexus. The intramedullary veins, which drain the spinal cord parenchyma, empty into surface veins, including dorsal, sulcal, and ventral spinal cord veins. Two longitudinally oriented veins, the posterior spinal and anterior medial spinal veins, are valveless and drain through the radicular veins into the extradural venous plexus. Upon dural penetration, functional valves are formed at the level of the radicular veins, preventing retrograde flow from the epidural vertebral veins into the intradural extrinsic system. These radicular veins have no secondary dural support network, making them vulnerable sites for thrombosis and secondary venous hypertension in patients with spinal dural arteriovenous fistulas (DAVFs). The internal vertebral veins consist of two interconnecting longitudinal channels situated anteriorly and posteriorly within the spinal epidural space and drain into paravertebral veins through the intervertebral foramen (Fig. 39.5).

## Classification of Vascular Spinal Lesions

### Key Concepts

- Spinal vascular lesions are rare but are associated with significant morbidity.
- Magnetic resonance imaging (MRI) should be the initial diagnostic test; however, spinal angiogram remains the gold standard to better define the disease and select appropriate therapies.
- Classifications emphasizing vascular anatomy and pathology are most clinically relevant.

Spinal vascular lesions are rare, underdiagnosed, and poorly understood entities that, if not treated promptly and adequately, could cause progressive spinal cord injury and myelopathy. Depending on the lesion type, symptoms vary between acute intramedullary/subarachnoid hemorrhage and subacute venous hypertension. Diagnosis is usually made by identifying abnormal flow-voids on MRI (Table 39.1); however, a more complete understanding of the disease process and appropriate therapeutic planning is best achieved through spinal angiography (Box 39.1).

Multiple classifications considering biological features, location, and genetic predisposition have been proposed.[7,8] For practical reasons, we present a recent modified classification that distinguishes vascular lesions based on anatomy and pathological factors to aid in optimal treatment selection[8-10]:

*Extradural Arteriovenous Fistulae (AVF, aka Epidural Fistulae)* represents an abnormal communication between a ventral epidural arcade branch and the adjacent ventral epidural venous plexus. Although it might be primarily asymptomatic, enlargement of the veins could cause mass effect on the adjacent nerve roots and spinal cord. These rare fistulas are primarily treated by endovascular techniques that aim to close the fistula.

*Intradural Dorsal AVFs (aka Type 1 DAVF)* are by far the most common spinal vascular malformations in patients 40 to 60 years of age. They are composed of a radicular feeding artery communicating with the dorsal coronal venous plexus at the spinal cord. The fistula point is typically in the nerve root dural sleeve and primarily obstructs venous outflow of the cord, leading to venous hypertension and myelopathy. These lesions can be treated by endovascular or surgical means. Key to the procedure is identification and preservation of the arterial feeders and radiculomedullary arteries, especially artery of Adamkiewicz (Fig. 39.6A).

*Intramedullary arteriovenous malformation (AVMs, aka Glomus or Type II AVM)* are lesions entirely within the spinal cord parenchyma receiving single or multiple feeders from the ASA and PSA. Histologically, they are composed of subpial shunts and may be compact or diffuse, based on the angioarchitecture of the nidus. They often present with

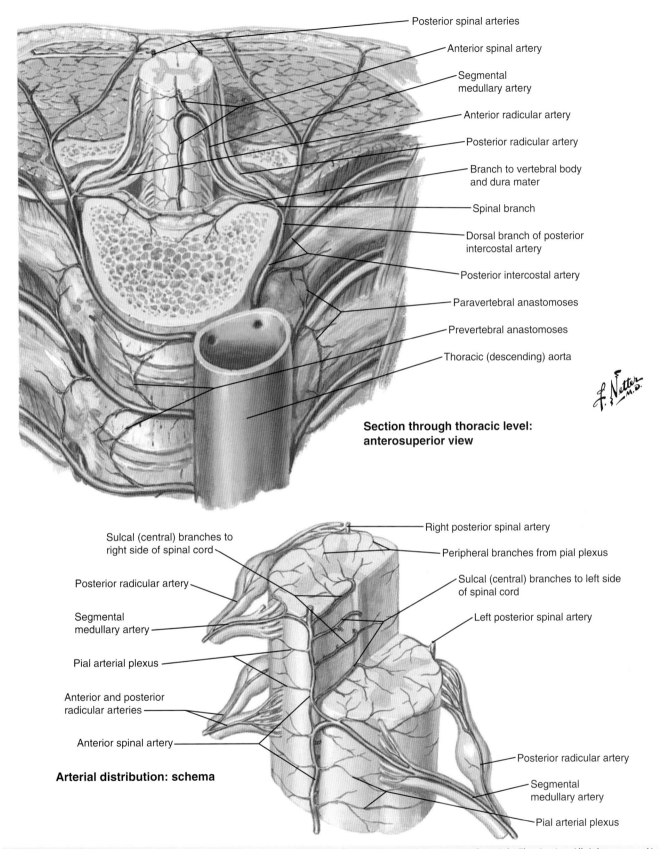

Posterior spinal arteries

Anterior spinal artery

Segmental
medullary artery

Anterior radicular artery

Posterior radicular artery

Branch to vertebral body
and dura mater

Spinal branch

Dorsal branch of posterior
intercostal artery

Posterior intercostal artery

Paravertebral anastomoses

Prevertebral anastomoses

Thoracic (descending) aorta

**Section through thoracic level:
anterosuperior view**

Sulcal (central) branches to
right side of spinal cord

Posterior radicular artery

Segmental
medullary artery

Pial arterial plexus

Anterior and posterior
radicular arteries

Anterior spinal artery

**Arterial distribution: schema**

Right posterior spinal artery

Peripheral branches from pial plexus

Sulcal (central) branches to left side
of spinal cord

Left posterior spinal artery

Posterior radicular artery

Segmental
medullary artery

Pial arterial plexus

**Fig. 39.2** Arteries of the spinal cord: intrinsic distribution. (Netter illustration from www.netterimages.com.  Copyright Elsevier, Inc. All rights reserved.)

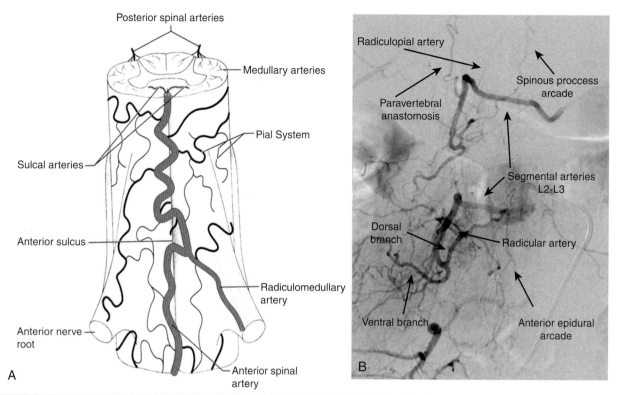

Fig 39.3 (A) Illustration of the anterior view of the spinal cord with visualization of longitudinal anastomosis. (B) Selective left L3 DSA posteroanterior view. Several levels are seen due to the existence of longitudinal anastomoses.

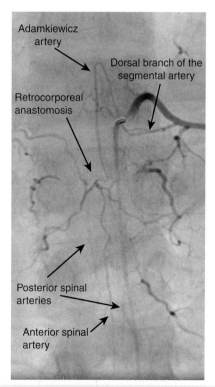

Fig. 39.4 Selective digital subtraction angiography (DSA) injection of left L1 level with visualization of the anterior and posterior spinal arteries.

fulminant neurological deficit, usually due to subarachnoid or intramedullary hemorrhage, before 20 years of age. Both endovascular and surgical treatments may be useful, although resection carries the advantage of removing mass effect. In diffuse multipediculated lesions, preoperative embolization is recommended to reduce blood loss during surgery (Fig. 39.6B).

*Extradural-Intradural AVMs (aka Juvenile or Metameric or Type III AVMs)* are extensive lesions affecting tissues from layers of a discrete somite level. In addition to the spinal cord and nerve roots, the bone, paraspinal muscles, and skin of a given metamere are also affected, although symptoms are mostly due to the intramedullary component. AVM involvement of the entire somite is known as *Cobb's syndrome*. Multiple palliative endovascular treatments are the norm for this complex condition, which is mostly diagnosed in young adults.

*Intradural Ventral AVFs (aka Type IV pial fistula)* are located in the ventral, midline subarachnoid space with the fistulous point between any artery supplying the spinal cord (predominantly the ASA) and an enlarged venous network. Depending on size, they can be divided into type A (single small feeder), type B (several feeders at the level of the fistula), and type C (giant multipediculated lesion with massive dilated venous channels). The latter can cause a substantial steal phenomenon with ischemic cord symptoms. Anterior/anterolateral surgical approaches are preferred for type A lesions, given the risk of catheterizing and embolizing the anterior spinal artery. Type B and C lesions, however, are better suited to endovascular

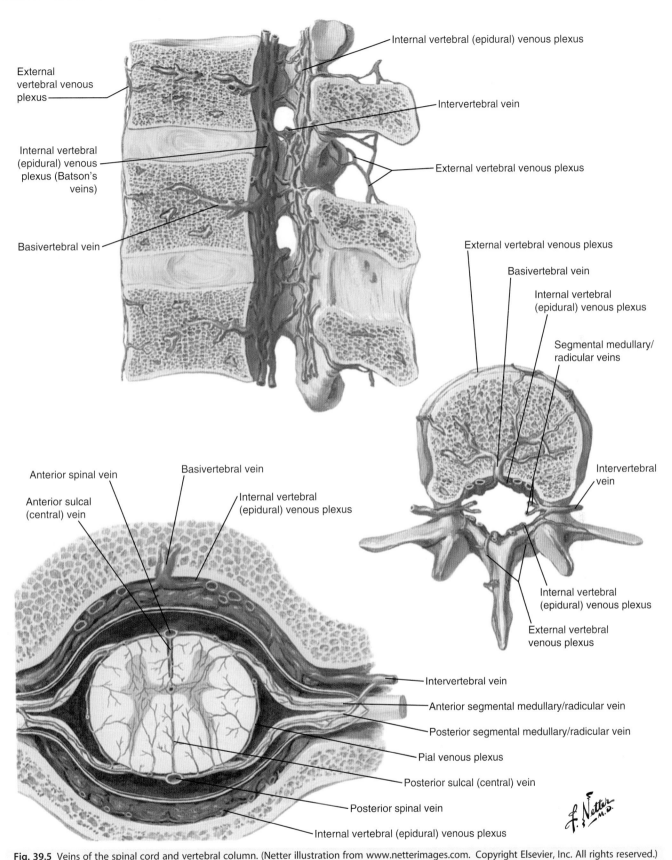

External vertebral venous plexus

Internal vertebral (epidural) venous plexus (Batson's veins)

Basivertebral vein

Internal vertebral (epidural) venous plexus

Intervertebral vein

External vertebral venous plexus

External vertebral venous plexus

Basivertebral vein

Internal vertebral (epidural) venous plexus

Segmental medullary/ radicular veins

Intervertebral vein

Internal vertebral (epidural) venous plexus

External vertebral venous plexus

Anterior spinal vein

Anterior sulcal (central) vein

Basivertebral vein

Internal vertebral (epidural) venous plexus

Intervertebral vein

Anterior segmental medullary/radicular vein

Posterior segmental medullary/radicular vein

Pial venous plexus

Posterior sulcal (central) vein

Posterior spinal vein

Internal vertebral (epidural) venous plexus

**Fig. 39.5** Veins of the spinal cord and vertebral column. (Netter illustration from www.netterimages.com. Copyright Elsevier, Inc. All rights reserved.)

**Table 39.1**    Routine Magnetic Resonance Sequences and Findings on the Evaluation of Spinal Vascular Malformations

| Sequence | Orientation | What to look for | How it looks |
|---|---|---|---|
| T2-weighted | Sagittal | Congestive edema/myelopathy<br>Dilated perimedullary vessels<br>Dilated intramedullary vessels | Hyperintensity and expansion of cord<br>Hypointense ectatic tubular structures (flow-voids) anterior/posterior to cord<br>Tangle of flow-voids within cord |
| T1-weighted | Sagittal | Intramedullary hemoglobin | Mixed hypointense/hyperintense vascular structures |
| FLAIR | Axial | Extramedullary hemorrhage (SAH) | Hyperintense areas within subarachnoid space |
| Gradient Echo | Sagittal | Intramedullary hemosiderin | Variably hypointense regions within cord |
| T1 TSE postgadolinium | Sagittal | Intramedullary/perimedullary contrast enhancement | Enhancement of abnormal vessels |

## Box 39.1   Fundamental Information to Be Obtained from the Diagnostic Spinal Angiogram

1. Differentiation among AVFs, intradural shunts, and fistulous AVMs with identification of the exact vertebral level and fistula point.
2. Identify arterial feeders and their relationship with radiculomedullary (particularly artery of Adamkiewicz) and radiculopial arteries that are not feeding the fistula.
3. Identify the presence of aneurysms and venous varices and their relationship with the symptoms.

treatment due to their complex structure and multiple arterial feeder involvement.

*Conus medullaris AVMs* are characterized by multiple direct shunts from ASA and PSA feeders into dilated veins, leading to venous hypertension and mass effect in the conus medullaris. This unique location produces upper and lower motor neuron deficits. Transarterial embolization combined with surgical decompression of the cauda equina can result in a good outcome.

Other *spinal vascular masses* include benign tumors (hemangioma, hemangioblastoma, aneurysmal bone cyst, osteoid osteoma, osteoblastoma), malignant tumors (multiple myeloma, plasmacytoma, hemangiopericytoma, giant cell tumor, chondrosarcoma, osteogenic sarcoma), certain metastatic tumors (renal cell and thyroid carcinoma), and cavernous malformations.[11] Surgical resection is the best treatment, particularly as some lesions (e.g., cavernous malformations) are angiographically occult.[12]

*Isolated spinal artery aneurysms* are rare in the absence of other spinal vascular lesions and are occasionally associated

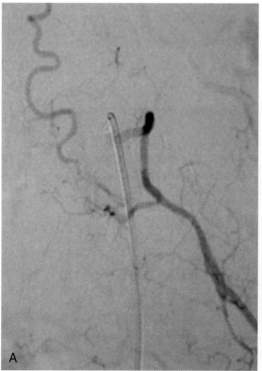 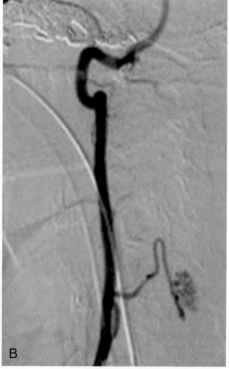

**Fig. 39.6** **(A)** Selective angiographic injection showing an intradural dorsal AVF with feeders from the left T12 radicular artery and early shunting into dilated tortuous perimedullary veins. **(B)** Intramedullary AVM receiving feeders from the anterior spinal artery at the right cervical region. (Courtesy of Dr. Mario Martinez-Galdámez, Director, Interventional Neuroradiology Unit, Department of Radiology, University Clinic Hospital of Valladolid, Spain.)

with dysplastic conditions, such as aortic coarctation, or represent infectious sequelae (mycotic aneurysm). They usually occur in the ASA at the hairpin junction between the radiculomedullary artery and ASA and present with subarachnoid hemorrhage or mass effect.[12]

## Perioperative Considerations: Endovascular Treatment

### Key Concepts

- Use of intraoperative monitoring may help prevent nontarget embolization.
- Therapeutic endovascular interventions are performed using embolizate (NBCA, Onyx) or coiling or both, depending on lesion anatomy and flow.
- Spinal DAVF eradication requires embolization of the proximal draining vein. Spinal AVM treatment requires embolic penetration of the nidus and ideally, preservation of all draining veins to prevent nidal rerupture or venous thrombosis. A multidisciplinary-approach team is essential to appropriately manage spinal vascular lesions.

A repetitive systematic approach is critical in performing the spinal angiogram. A radiolucent ruler with radiopaque markings should be placed below the table pad (Fig. 39.7). Number markings are positioned slightly

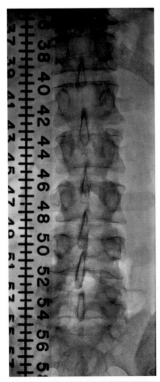

**Fig. 39.7** AP fluoroscopic image with appropriate positioning of the marking ruler just to the right of the spine. When initially counting levels throughout the spine, the level of interest must be centered in the image to avoid parallax and incorrect numbering.

lateral to the right lateral vertebral body margin on anteroposterior (AP) view with the spinous processes centered equidistant from the pedicles, enabling a well-collimated image without obscuring potential pathology due to subtraction artifact. An assistant documents the vertebral levels with their corresponding ruler number. Knowing the exact level of the catheter ensures interrogation of every level, reducing radiation dose from recounting and undercollimating. Many cases are referred for an obvious vascular malformation on MRI but a "negative" spinal angiogram. When reviewing these images, it is often apparent that the same level was injected more than once and labeled differently. Such oversight can delay diagnosis and treatment with devastating consequences.

All means to achieve a crisp image (and thereby avoid missing a critical finding due to a preventable artifact) should be utilized. These include secure positioning of the catheter in the vessel ostium to prevent catheter displacement, suboptimal injection, or unnecessary contrast reflux into the aorta; use of a micro or small (0.3–0.6 mm) focal spot[11] for precise microvascular imaging; application of filters to sharpen the image periphery when filming over less dense tissues, such as the lungs; adequate sedation to maximize patient cooperation/minimize movement; use of apnea to minimize diaphragmatic motion when filming intercostal vessels; and administration of Glucagon to decrease peristalsis. Glucagon 1 to 2 mg IV or IM is indicated in abdominal digital vascular imaging to relax smooth muscles in the gastrointestinal tract and improve image quality.[13] Due to its very short half-life, additional boluses are needed at 10- to 20-minute intervals to maintain the antiperistaltic effect. Minor motion artifact can be corrected by "pixel shifting" of acquired images.

During selective injections of segmental arteries, 4 to 5 mL of nonionic contrast diluted 50% in heparinized saline is injected at a rate of ~2 mL/second. Catheterization of bilateral vertebral arteries and thyrocervical and costocervical trunks might be needed to fully understand the anatomy of cervical spine lesions.

### Clinical Pearl

Delayed venous drainage after anterior spinal artery injection is highly suggestive of venous hypertension and the presence of a shunting lesion at another level.

Delayed filming to properly understand the venous drainage is essential. The pattern of drainage, the presence or absence of normal veins, and the presence of venous ectasia or thrombosis should be noted.[1] Anticoagulation decisions for AVMs are made on a case-by-case basis. Some centers heparinize to an activated clotting time of 2 to 2.5 times baseline or 250 to 300 seconds; others do not use heparin.

Most centers perform embolization under general anesthesia, and some use neuroelectrophysiological monitoring (somatosensory evoked potentials and electroencephalography) to monitor intraprocedural neurological function with appropriate adjustments in anesthetic technique to permit acquisition of satisfactory signals. Superselective injection of amytal sodium with or without lidocaine into the feeder (in an awake patient) may be performed to avoid embolization of normal anatomy.[14] Embolization is achieved primarily by Trufill N-butyl-cyanoacrylate (NBCA or "glue"), ethylene vinyl alcohol copolymer (Onyx), coils, or a combination thereof. Other agents such as polyvinyl alcohol particles are temporarily occlusive and as such, are rarely used. For detailed descriptions of these embolic agents, please refer to Chapters 36 and 38.

There are two main conceptual differences in endovascular therapy, depending on the pathology. In spinal DAVFs or AVMs with fistulous feeders, the treatment goal is to close the fistula by delivering embolic agent into the draining vein and prevent subsequent recanalization via intradural collaterals. Success rate of endovascular therapy in this regard is 25% to 75%.[15,16] In contrast, complete fistula occlusion is achieved >90% of the time with open surgery.[17] The therapeutic goal for spinal AVMs with distinct nidus is to obliterate the nidus with liquid embolic agent (Onyx may be superior to NBCA for nidal penetration and controlled backfilling of other feeders). Premature venous penetration with embolizate prior to nidal occlusion can facilitate a rapid increase in intranidal pressure and hemorrhage.

---

**Clinical Pearl**

Permanent occlusion of a DAVF via endovascular means is best achieved with penetration of a liquid embolic agent into the distal arterial feeder/nidus and the foot of the draining vein. Parent vessel occlusion alone with failure to occlude the proximal draining vein is associated with high DAVF recurrence rates.

---

Radiation dose and contrast volume are variables easily controlled by the operator to help prevent radiation injury and contrast-induced nephropathy. A low-dose protocol is the first step. Three pulses per second are more than adequate for catheter manipulation in most situations,[18] but many fluoroscopy machines are preset at pulse rates of 7.5 to 15/second. Variable frame rate digital subtraction angiography acquisition further reduces the radiation dose. Utilizing the ruler, vessels should be selected with tight collimation, with the level of interest in the center of the image and including approximately half of the vertebral body above and below. With these precautions, radiation injury should not occur, except in patients with increased radiosensitivity. An entire spinal angiogram can be performed with minimal contrast injection to find each lumbar or intercostal branch. Watching the deflection of a posteriorly directed catheter tip is often enough to select the vessel in the hands of a well-trained angiographer, further reducing the total contrast load.

## Postoperative Complications

Complications of spinal angiography and intervention can typically be avoided if appropriate safety measures are in place and if a systematic approach is used by a thoroughly trained operator. This should be performed with a team approach because multiple observers and participants can assist in preventing complications.

Procedural complications can arise during each aspect of the procedure: vascular access, use of contrast media, catheter manipulation, vessel selection, radiation exposure, and embolization/intervention. Spinal angiography complications can also be divided into neurological and nonneurological. The main neurological complication is spinal cord infarction from nontarget embolization. The most common nonneurological complication is, by far, access site hematoma (Box 39.2).

Spinal angiography and intervention is almost exclusively performed via the transfemoral approach. Complication rates are mostly quoted from cerebral angiography series. Significant groin hematomas have been reported at a rate of up to 10.7%.[19,20] This seemingly high rate was seen in patients with larger size sheaths and those with higher levels of heparinization and other anticoagulant use. Another factor affecting the rate of hematoma formation is patient age. A majority of patients who developed a groin hematoma were >60 years old.[20,21] The largest single-center retrospective review revealed a groin hematoma risk of 1% after spinal angiography, all of which were managed conservatively.[22]

---

**Clinical Pearl**

Nearly all spinal angiograms, including interventions, can be performed via a 5 F sheath, which is well tolerated by most adult femoral arteries.

---

Other access site complications include femoral artery pseudoaneurysm and arterial dissection. Published pseudoaneurysm rates after femoral artery access are only 0.05% to 0.55%[23] but may be somewhat higher in the current age of multiantiplatelet therapies and aggressive intraprocedural and postprocedural heparinization. Arterial dissections are also rare (0.4%) and typically occur during initial sheath placement or catheter/guidewire manipulation.[24] Because femoral artery access is retrograde, a dissection here is not typically flow limiting. The dissection can become flow limiting if an overzealous sheath injection is performed or if there is aggressive wire and catheter advancement into the false lumen.

---

**Box 39.2 Complications of Spinal Vascular Lesion Embolization**

- Ischemic or hemorrhagic infarction of spinal cord
- Nontarget embolization
- Spinal venous thrombosis
- Arterial rupture
- Microcatheter implantation
- Arterial dissection
- Allergy to contrast media
- Contrast-induced nephropathy
- Access site or retroperitoneal hematoma
- Femoral artery pseudoaneurysm

With the prevalent use of nonionic iodinated contrast, allergic reactions to contrast media are generally mild. The overall reaction rate has been reported as high as 3.13%, with severe and very severe reactions occurring at rates of 0.04% and 0.004%, respectively.[25] Patients with prior anaphylactic reaction to contrast have a 17% to 35% risk of repeat anaphylaxis during their next exposure.[26–28] The rate of repeat anaphylaxis can be reduced to 0.3% when using a pretreatment regimen of prednisone 50 mg PO at 13, 7, and 1 hour(s) before the angiogram, in addition to diphenhydramine 50 mg at 1 hour prior.[29,30]

Contrast-induced nephropathy, defined as a rise in serum creatinine of >25% above baseline or a rise of 0.5 mg/dL within 48 hours of contrast administration, primarily affects elderly patients or those with preexisting renal insufficiency, diabetes, and congestive heart failure and is exacerbated by insufficient preprocedural, intraprocedural, and postprocedural IV hydration while NPO. Otherwise healthy patients can also suffer this renal injury due to the sometimes excessive contrast volumes utilized during spinal angiography.

Vascular injury during a diagnostic spinal angiogram is unlikely with proper technique and modern catheter technology. Small-vessel perforation is also unlikely but can occur with aggressive microguidewire/microcatheter manipulation that irreversibly damages a delicate vascular feeder. This not only creates intimal injury, but also may eliminate endovascular access to the underlying lesion. Additionally, vessel avulsion can occur during microcatheter removal at the completion of a long liquid embolic injection or when there is excessive tension or embolizate pinning the distal microcatheter in place (Fig. 39.8).

In addition to vascular injury, the risk of thromboembolic complications increases as more complex catheter systems are introduced. Each lumen, from the femoral artery sheath to the distal microcatheter, must remain under continuous heparinized saline flush to prevent thrombus formation. The associated flush lines should be actively checked by multiple team members to ensure that all of the lines remain freely flowing, bags are adequately pressurized, and that the saline bags have adequate volume to make use of the applied pressure.

One of the most important preventable complications of spinal intervention relates to inadvertent embolization of a radiculomedullary branch by a liquid embolic agent and subsequent spinal cord infarction. Extensive interrogation of the vascular levels surrounding the vessel of interest is of paramount importance. If a spinal artery arises at any of the levels supplying a lesion, whether tumor or vascular malformation, then nontarget embolization may result when using a liquid embolic agent. Shunting may occur within the lesion, and in some cases of high-flow arteriovenous shunts or highly vascular tumors, an adjacent spinal artery may not be recognized due to preembolization steal phenomena. This is identified too late when slowing of flow diverts embolic agent into a newly apparent spinal artery. In the case of preoperative embolization to decrease blood loss for a subsequent spinal tumor resection, coils can be used instead of a liquid if a spinal artery arises from one of the feeding vessels. When evaluating vascular malformations, many can be treated surgically if the endovascular route is not deemed safe.

A specific complication that may arise when treating a spinal vascular malformation is spinal venous thrombosis. If the fistula and most proximal aspect of the draining vein are successfully penetrated with a liquid embolic agent, then the lesion is likely obliterated and flow within the chronically enlarged, previously arterialized draining vein

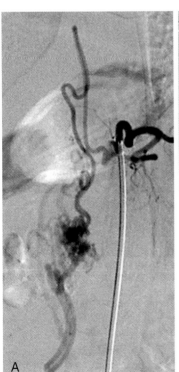 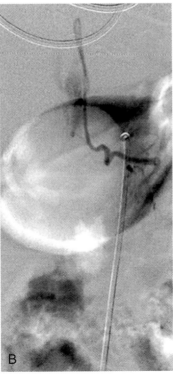

**Fig. 39.8 (A)** AP preembolization view: a perimedullary AVF is supplied by a spinal branch arising on the left at T11. **(B)** AP view after glue embolization and sudden hemodynamic change demonstrates active extravasation of contrast from the anterior spinal artery at T11. Arterial avulsion after rapid microcatheter removal is the presumed etiology.

will be drastically reduced. Flow stagnation, especially in larger vessels, is a major risk for thrombosis. Some have recommended short-term prophylactic anticoagulation after occlusion of the vascular malformation to prevent this complication.[15,31]

When performing preoperative embolization of a tumor, the possibility of tumoral edema must be considered. Cessation of flow to a tumor, in combination with inflammatory properties of certain liquid embolic agents, can result in tumor swelling, which may worsen mass effect upon the spinal cord or nerve roots. If swelling is anticipated, then dexamethasone 10 mg IV may be administered at the beginning of the procedure, followed by 4 mg IV every 6 hours for a 24-hour period. When pharmacological measures are insufficient, surgery and spinal decompression may need to be expedited. The goal of preoperative embolization is to decrease blood loss during resection. This must be performed with the lowest possible risk to ensure that an endovascular complication does not exceed the total risk of the surgery or, at the very least, does not compromise the future resection and patient outcome.

In general, the risks of significant complications during spinal angiography and interventions are quite low in the hands of an experienced neurointerventionalist. Adequate training of the angiographer should be emphasized as one of the most important aspects of complication prevention. In addition to gaining experience in a standardized approach, adequate training bolsters understanding of displayed anatomy and pathology. Neurointerventional procedures require a high level of diagnostic expertise, not only of the angiogram but also of complementary imaging modalities. A well-trained angiographer will have reviewed any pertinent imaging prior to the procedure to aid in the search for a diagnosis and prevent or minimize complications related to the patient's unique anatomy or disease.

Although newer, more minimally invasive techniques have lent themselves to treatment of spinal vascular malformations via endovascular obliteration, microsurgical treatment of spinal vascular malformations remains an integral part of a neurosurgeon's armamentarium. Surgery should be performed early in the disease course to prevent the development of neurological deficits. The patient's preoperative neurological status may be predictive of the overall postoperative outcome.

## Clinical Pearl

The patient's preoperative neurological status may be predictive of the overall postoperative outcome.

Surgical treatment typically involves a broad laminectomy and dural opening while keeping the arachnoid intact, using microsurgical technique. Once the extent of the lesion is determined via inspection through the arachnoid layer, the arachnoid is opened to begin resection of the malformation. In cases of laterally or ventrally positioned malformations, releasing the dentate ligaments between the ventral and dorsal nerve roots can allow for gentle rotation of the spinal cord. In many cases, the entire malformation need not be removed; interruption of the fistula between the major

arterial supply and the arterialized venous system typically treats the lesion and its associated symptoms (Fig. 39.9).

General surgical risks of treating spinal vascular malformations include superficial skin infections, bleeding, chronic pain syndromes, thrombosis of intraepidural or epidural veins resulting in progressive neurological deficits, recurrence of fistula, and spinal cord infarction. Postoperative complications after open neurosurgical treatment of spinal vascular lesions, possibly requiring reoperation, include cerebrospinal fluid (CSF) leak, meningitis, and epidural or subdural hematoma. Other complications include ischemic or hemorrhagic infarctions of the spinal cord and mechanical injury to the spinal cord, nerve roots, or dorsal root ganglia (Box 39.3). Patients must be monitored frequently in the immediate postoperative period. Early identification of neurological decline is essential for implementing therapy and maintaining a good patient outcome. The usual presentation of spinal epidural hematoma is intense, focal pain with radicular symptoms preceding the development of symmetrical motor and sensory weakness by a few hours.[32] Rapid surgical treatment of epidural hematomas correlates with better outcomes, with greater neurological recovery occurring when the interval from symptom onset to surgery is <12 hours.[33]

Due to the need for a wide and lengthy laminectomy and dural opening in most surgeries for spinal vascular malformations, a few technical complications are particularly important to consider. An important but uncommon microsurgical complication after laminectomy is spinal instability. Spinal instability after exposure of a dural AVF or intramedullary AVM can be avoided by limiting the facet removal to <50%.[17] Instrumented or bony fusion should be performed when stability or future development of deformity is a concern. Another possible complication after multilevel spinal exposure is development of pseudomeningocele, a CSF collection adjacent to a dural defect. Meticulous closure of the dura, muscle approximation, and skin closure minimize this complication. Pseudomeningoceles are often initially treated with CSF diversion via lumbar drain, but may eventually require primary closure of the dural defect.

Bipolar coagulation near the spinal cord can result in thermal injury to adjacent neural tissue, nerve roots, and ganglia. Alternatively, aneurysm clips can be used to interrupt a spinal AVF to minimize bipolar coagulation near the spinal cord. Spinal AVM feeders tend to be vestigial in character and thin walled; therefore, clips must be applied very tightly to prevent continued intraoperative and postoperative bleeding.[34] Patients in whom fistulas were clipped and excised had statistically better outcomes than those in whom only a clip was placed.[35] Identifying the point of fistulization can be difficult in complex spinal dural AVF. One useful method to localize the fistula is endovascular placement of a coil in a distal arterial feeder close to the fistula. Intraoperative fluoroscopy can then be used to target the fistula in surgery.

### Surgical Complications Specific to Spinal DAVFs

Elimination of spinal cord venous congestion is a primary treatment goal for spinal DAVFs. The current mode of treatment involves the obliteration of the nidus and interruption of venous drainage. If an ectatic, arterialized coronal

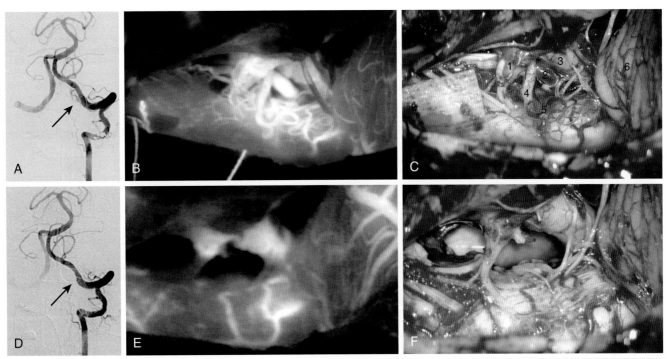

**Fig. 39.9** Preresection **(A–C)** and postresection **(D–F)** resection images of a Cognard V DAVF at the cervicomedullary junction. **(A)** Preoperative angiogram demonstrating an 11 × 5.9 × 5.1-mm triangular nidus *(arrow)* at the left cervicomedullary junction with early venous drainage into a left medullary vein inferior to the left V4 segment. **(B)** Indocyanine green (ICG) injection for intraoperative angiography prior to resection of DAVF. **(C)** Intraoperative view of DAVF with triangular nidus, supplied by a small left V3–4 muscular branch. *1,* C1 ganglion; *2,* medullary vein/draining vein; *3,* left vertebral artery; *4,* V3-4 muscular branch; *5,* DAVF nidus; *6,* cerebellum. Not shown here is the drainage into the anterior spinal, anterior pontomedullary, and right petrosal veins. **(D)** Postoperative angiogram with no residual DAVF or early draining veins. **(E)** Intraoperative ICG injection after resection of DAVF. **(F)** Postresection intraoperative view. The nidus was coagulated and resected fully, and the draining vein was coagulated and cut. (Intraoperative images courtesy of Dr. Sandeep Mittal, Department of Neurosurgery, Wayne State University)

## Box 39.3  Complications of Spinal Vascular Lesion Surgery

- Ischemic or hemorrhagic infarction of spinal cord
- Epidural, subdural, or intramedullary spinal cord hematoma
- Mechanical injury to the spinal cord, nerve roots, or dorsal root ganglia
- Spinal instability
- CSF leak, pseudomeningocele formation
- Chronic pain syndromes
- Superficial skin infections

venous plexus is mistaken as the nidus and resected, venous congestion can be exacerbated. These veins are typically normal intradural extramedullary veins that are transformed in appearance and sometimes become nonfunctional due to chronically elevated pressure and flow. Worsening myelopathy or neurological deficits in the postoperative period may suggest spinal venous congestion and thrombosis.

Rarely, patients may have postoperative persistence of a spinal dural AVF after surgical interruption of the draining vein. This may be due to more than one medullary vein draining the dural AVF or due to having both extradural and intradural drainage of the fistula. Failure to interrupt all proximal draining veins can be avoided or minimized by careful study of preoperative angiography.[36]

Surgical approaches for type IV spinal DAVFs are more challenging due to the typical anterior location of the fistula with respect to the spinal cord and close association with the ASA. If the fistula occurs at the conus medullaris or filum terminale, then it can be safely managed via a posterior approach. Anterior lesions above or high on the conus may require an anterior or anterolateral approach. Approaching a fistula located at the superior conus may require more manipulation, possibly resulting in postoperative neurological deficits.[37]

### Surgical Complications Specific to Spinal Intramedullary AVMs

High-flow spinal AVMs typically contain neural tissue in the interstitial space between AVM vessels. These lesions have a higher risk of intramedullary hemorrhage, which manifests as acute onset of severe back and radicular pain, followed immediately by loss of muscle tone below the lesion and sphincter dysfunction. Ascending and descending tracts are displaced and compressed, but immediate surgical evacuation may preserve the more lateral spinothalamic tracts.[38] Because juvenile-type intramedullary spinal AVMs derive their torrential supply from multiple medullary arteries that also supply the spinal cord and other metameric segments, open surgical intervention is more complicated and poses a higher risk of hemorrhagic, arterial, or venous infarction.

Intramedullary AVMs in the thoracic and lumbar regions have higher operative risk of spinal stroke and postoperative neurological deficits. There is higher risk of AVM persistence due to more tenuous collateral supply in comparison to intramedullary AVMs in the cervical region).[39-41] Very limited long-term data exist regarding the incidence of persistent AVMs, and no long-term data exist on the incidence of clinical relapse or progression from incomplete surgical obliteration.

## References

1. Nelson PK, Setton A, Berenstein A. Vertebrospinal angiography in the evaluation of vertebral and spinal cord disease. *Neuroimaging Clin N Am.* 1996;6(3):589–605.
2. Chiras J, Morvan G, Merland JJ. The angiographic appearances of the normal intercostal and lumbar arteries. Analysis and the anatomic correlation of the lateral branches. *J Neuroradiol.* 1979;6(3):169–196.
3. Fazio C, Agnoli A. The vascularisation of the spinal cord—anatomical and pathophysiological aspects. *Vasc Surg.* 1970;4(4):245–257.
4. Grunwald I, Thron A, Reith W. Spinal angiography: vascular anatomy, technique and indications. *Radiologe.* 2001;41(11):961–967.
5. Lazorthes G, Gouaze A, Zadeh JO, et al. Arterial vascularization of the spinal cord. Recent studies of the anastomotic substitution pathways. *J Neurosurg.* 1971;35(3):253–262.
6. Lazorthes G, Gouaze A. Supply routes of arterial vascularization of the spinal cord. Applications to the study of vascular myelopathies. *Bull Acad Natl Med.* 1970;154(1):34–41.
7. Rodesch G, Hurth M, Alvarez H, et al. Spinal cord intradural arteriovenous fistulae: anatomic, clinical, and therapeutic considerations in a series of 32 consecutive patients seen between 1981 and 2000 with emphasis on endovascular therapy. *Neurosurgery.* 2005;57(5): 973–983.
8. Krings T, Mull M, Reinges MH, et al. Double spinal dural arteriovenous fistulas: case report and review of the literature. *Neuroradiology.* 2004;46(3):238–242.
9. Kim LJ, Spetzler RF. Classification and surgical management of spinal arteriovenous lesions: arteriovenous fistulae and arteriovenous malformations. *Neurosurgery.* 2006;59(5 Suppl 3):S195–S201. discussion S3–13.
10. Krings T, Thron AK, Geibprasert S, et al. Endovascular management of spinal vascular malformations. *Neurosurg Rev.* 2010;33(1):1–9.
11. Narayanan S, Hurst RW, Abruzzo TA, et al. Standard of practice: embolization of spinal arteriovenous fistulae, spinal arteriovenous malformations, and tumors of the spinal axis. *J Neurointerv Surg.* 2013;5(1):3–5.
12. Spetzler RF, Detwiler PW, Riina HA, et al. Modified classification of spinal cord vascular lesions. *J Neurosurg.* 2002;96(2 Suppl):145–156.
13. Chernish SM, Maglinte DD. Glucagon: common untoward reactions—review and recommendations. *Radiology.* 1990;177(1):145–146.
14. Niimi Y, Sala F, Deletis V, et al. Neurophysiologic monitoring and pharmacologic provocative testing for embolization of spinal cord arteriovenous malformations. *AJNR.* 2004;25(7):1131–1138.
15. Niimi Y, Berenstein A, Setton A, Neophytides A. Embolization of spinal dural arteriovenous fistulae: results and follow-up. *Neurosurgery.* 1997;40(4):675–682. discussion 82–3.
16. Van Dijk JM, TerBrugge KG, Willinsky RA, et al. Multidisciplinary management of spinal dural arteriovenous fistulas: clinical presentation and long-term follow-up in 49 patients. *Stroke.* 2002;33(6): 1578–1583.
17. Steinmetz MP, Chow MM, Krishnaney AA, et al. Outcome after the treatment of spinal dural arteriovenous fistulae: a contemporary single-institution series and meta-analysis. *Neurosurgery.* 2004;55(1): 77–87. discussion 88.
18. Pearl MS, Torok C, Wang J, et al. Practical techniques for reducing radiation exposure during cerebral angiography procedures. *J Neurointerv Surg.* 2015;7(2):141–145. http://dx.doi.org/10.1136/neurintsurg-2013-010982.
19. Olivecrona H. Complications of cerebral angiography. *Neuroradiology.* 1977;14(4):175–181.
20. Dion JE, Gates PC, Fox AJ, et al. Clinical events following neuroangiography: a prospective study. *Stroke.* 1987;18(6):997–1004.
21. Thomson KR, Thomson SM. Complications of cerebral angiography in a teaching hospital. *Australas Radiol.* 1986;30(3):206–208.
22. Chen J, Gailloud P. Safety of spinal angiography: complication rate analysis in 302 diagnostic angiograms. *Neurology.* 2011;77 (13):1235–1240.
23. Coley BD, Roberts AC, Fellmeth BD, et al. Postangiographic femoral artery pseudoaneurysms: further experience with US-guided compression repair. *Radiology.* 1995;194(2):307–311.
24. Cox N. Managing the femoral artery in coronary angiography. *Heart Lung Circ.* 2008;17(4 Suppl):S65–S69.
25. Katayama H, Yamaguchi K, Kozuka T, et al. Adverse reactions to ionic and nonionic contrast media. A report from the Japanese Committee on the Safety of Contrast Media. *Radiology.* 1990;175(3):621–628.
26. Witten DM, Hirsch FD, Hartman GW. Acute reactions to urographic contrast medium: incidence, clinical characteristics and relationship to history of hypersensitivity states. *Am J Roentgenol Radium Ther Nucl Med.* 1973;119(4):832–840.
27. Shehadi WH. Adverse reactions to intravascularly administered contrast media. A comprehensive study based on a prospective survey. *Am J Roentgenol Radium Ther Nucl Med.* 1975;124(1):145–152.
28. Fischer HW, Doust VL. An evaluation of pretesting in the problem of serious and fatal reactions to excretory urography. *Radiology.* 1972;103(3):497–501.
29. Greenberger PA, Patterson R, Simon R, et al. Pretreatment of high-risk patients requiring radiographic contrast media studies. *J Allergy Clin Immunol.* 1981;67(3):185–187.
30. Greenberger P, Patterson R, Kelly J, et al. Administration of radiographic contrast media in high-risk patients. *Invest Radiol.* 1980; 15(6 Suppl):S40–S43.
31. Knopman J, Zink W, Patsalides A, et al. Secondary clinical deterioration after successful embolization of a spinal dural arteriovenous fistula: a plea for prophylactic anticoagulation. *Interv Neuroradiol.* 2010;16(2):199–203.
32. Mattle H, Sieb JP, Rohner M, et al. Nontraumatic spinal epidural and subdural hematomas. *Neurology.* 1987;37(8):1351–1356.
33. Lawton MT, Porter RW, Heiserman JE, et al. Surgical management of spinal epidural hematoma: relationship between surgical timing and neurological outcome. *J Neurosurg.* 1995;83(1):1–7.
34. Krayenbühl H, Yaşargil MG, McClintock HG. Treatment of spinal cord vascular malformations by surgical excision. *J Neurosurg.* 1969; 30(4):427–435.
35. Tacconi L, Lopez Izquierdo BC, Symon L. Outcome and prognostic factors in the surgical treatment of spinal dural arteriovenous fistulas. A long-term study. *Br J Neurosurg.* 1997;11(4):298–305.
36. Malis LI. Microsurgery for spinal cord arteriovenous malformations. *Clin Neurosurg.* 1979;26:543–555.
37. Barrow DL, Colohan AR, Dawson R. Intradural perimedullary arteriovenous fistulas (type IV spinal cord arteriovenous malformations). *J Neurosurg.* 1994;81(2):221–229.
38. Pullarkat VA, Kalapura T, Pincus M, et al. Intraspinal hemorrhage complicating oral anticoagulant therapy: an unusual case of cervical hematomyelia and a review of the literature. *Arch Int Med.* 2000;160 (2):237–240.
39. Connolly Jr ES, Zubay GP, McCormick PC, et al. The posterior approach to a series of glomus (Type II) intramedullary spinal cord arteriovenous malformations. *Neurosurgery.* 1998;42(4):774–785.
40. Rosenblum B, Oldfield EH, Doppman JL, et al. Spinal arteriovenous malformations: a comparison of dural arteriovenous fistulas and intradural AVMs in 81 patients. *J Neurosurg.* 1987;67(6):795–802.
41. Yaşargil MG, Symon L, Teddy PJ. Arteriovenous malformations of the spinal cord. *Adv Tech Stand Neurosurg.* 1984;11:61–102.

# Intracranial Monitors and Special Procedures

# 40 Shunt Placement and Management

JASON J. CHANG and ANTHONY M. AVELLINO

## Introduction

Hydrocephalus is a clinical diagnosis characterized by symptoms of elevated intracranial pressure (ICP) secondary to an imbalance in the production or absorption of cerebrospinal fluid (CSF). CSF diversion and management of associated complication remains fundamental tenets of neurocritical care transcending pediatric and adult populations. This chapter will review issues pertaining to CSF diversion in the acute setting with placement of external ventricular drains (EVDs) as well as ventriculoperitoneal, atrial, or pleural shunts in the chronic setting. Shunt failures can be situations requiring critical care observations and timely surgical intervention.

## Neuroanatomy and Procedure

### Key Concepts

- The cerebral aqueduct is the CSF channel that connects the third to the fourth ventricle.
- An upward gaze paresis is diagnostic for a pineal or tectal region mass contributing to a noncommunicating hydrocephalus.
- Seven percent to 10% of patients with aneurysmal subarachnoid hemorrhage will require a shunt.
- The three general categories of valves are fixed pressure, flow regulating, and programmable pressure.

### VENTRICULAR SYSTEM ANATOMY

The ventricular system is characterized by four large fluid-filled spaces interconnected by openings between the supratentorial and infratentorial compartments (Fig. 40.1). The lateral ventricles are bilateral C-shaped structures that span the entire cerebrum. These spaces merge into the anterior aspect of the third ventricle via the foramen of Monro. At the posterior extent, the cerebral aqueduct serves as the connection to the fourth ventricle and is prone to obstruction by pineal region masses (Fig. 40.2, Box 40.1). CSF is able to exit the ventricular system via the foramen of Magendie and foramina of Luschka located along the medial and lateral walls of the fourth ventricle.

### DIAGNOSIS

Intracranial hypertension amenable to CSF diversion may initially present as nonspecific symptoms followed by rapidly progressive neurological deterioration. Regardless of patient age, the initial neurological examination should assess cranial nerves (e.g., examination of pupillary size and reactivity to light), as well as motor, sensory, reflex, and cerebellar functions. Signs of increased ICP include headache, nausea, vomiting, lethargy, decreased level of consciousness, papilledema, double vision secondary to compression of the abducens cranial nerve, and difficulty concentrating. Cushing's triad of bradycardia, hypertension, and an irregular breathing pattern represents the autonomic dysfunction secondary to brainstem compression signifying increased ICP.

If increased ICP is severe, herniation of portions of brain from their normal location into other compartments over the dural membranes may occur compressing adjacent brain structures. Uncal, central transtentorial, and downward herniations are three important brain herniation syndromes. Uncal or unilateral transtentorial herniation results when the uncus is compressed into the tentorial notch, and the midbrain compression leads to an ipsilateral dilated and fixed pupil, decreased consciousness, respiratory and cardiac irregularities, and generally contralateral motor abnormalities. Central or bilateral transtentorial herniation results when both cerebral hemispheres compress the diencephalon and midbrain into the tentorial notch leading to pupillary constriction and then dilation, decreased consciousness, respiratory irregularities, and decerebrate or decorticate rigidity. Downward cerebellar herniation results when the cerebellum is compressed into the foramen magnum. Brainstem compression leads to neck stiffness or head tilt, impaired upward gaze, decreased consciousness, and lower cranial nerve palsies.[1] A lumbar puncture should be carefully considered in any patient suspected of having increased ICP because it may increase the chance of brain herniation.

In neonates and infants younger than 6 months of age, it is difficult to measure ICP invasively. Palpation of open cranial fontanel fullness and sutures splaying provide a rough estimate of the degree of ICP elevation. Other surrogates for increased ICP in neonates and infants include increased occipitofrontal circumference (OFC), decreased level of consciousness, irritability, poor feeding, inappropriate sleepiness, and limited upgaze or forced downgaze (i.e., sun-setting sign) (Fig. 40.2). Papilledema is rare in infants and has low diagnostic sensitivity for detecting elevated ICPs in children.[2] Once increased ICP is diagnosed, urgent neuroimaging studies (i.e., head computed tomography [CT], ultrasound, or magnetic resonance imaging) are critical to facilitate proper treatment.

### SURGICAL APPROACH FOR PLACEMENT OF VENTRICULAR CATHETER

Placement of an EVD can be done at bedside in the intensive care unit or in the operating room. Anatomical reference

**Left lateral phantom view**

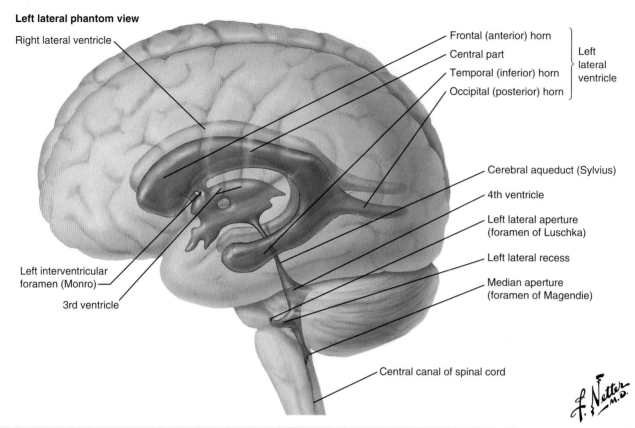

**Fig. 40.1** Normal ventricular anatomy and CSF composition. (Reprinted with permission from Felten DL. Ventricles and the Cerebrospinal fluid. In: *Netter's Atlas of Neuroscience*. Saunders, Elsevier; 2010:67–73.)

points on the skull serve as landmarks to approximate a perpendicular trajectory to the frontal horn of the lateral ventricle. Kocher's point is the most common approach for both acute and long-term ventricular catheter placement and requires a drilled hole through the frontal bone of the skull.[3] The point is approximated 3 cm off midline (i.e., midpupillary line) to avoid damage to bridging veins draining into the sagittal sinus. This point should be 1 to 2 cm anterior to the coronal suture and thus well in front of the motor strip. Once the dura is opened with an 18-gauge needle or scalpel, a ventricular catheter is passed perpendicularly to approximately 6 cm from the inner table of the skull. This technique is safe and accurate for urgent drainage of CSF.

Frazier's point (3 cm lateral and 6 cm above the inion) and Keen's point (3 cm posterior and 3 cm superior to the pinna) are alternative access points at the posterior parietal position to the ventricle used primarily for long-term CSF diversion via an internalized shunt system. Image guidance assists in the accuracy of this approach to place the tip of the ventricular catheter in the lateral ventricle that terminates in the frontal horn (Fig. 40.3).[4] These three access points target the frontal horn of the lateral ventricle to avoid invasive choroid plexus overgrowth, with time occluding the small fenestrations at the catheter tip. Intraoperative ventricular access via Paine's point is occasionally required for brain relaxation. Hyun and Park have modified Paine's point to a more cranial (Park) and caudal (Hyun) position to minimize the risk of injuring eloquent brain.[5–7]

## INDICATIONS FOR EXTERNAL VENTRICULAR DRAINAGE

Increasing ventricular size on neuroimaging with accompanying clinical deterioration should alert the care team to consider EVD placement. Common signs of elevated ICPs likely to respond to ventriculostomy include presence of dilated temporal horns, lateral ventricles, and effacement of the cerebral aqueduct with ventriculomegaly, excluding the fourth ventricle. In most circumstances an EVD is used to accomplish this; however, alternative options, including lumbar punctures or a lumbar drain, may be possible in the absence of a posterior fossa mass lesion or aqueductal stenosis.

## Clinical Pearls

Neurosurgical ventriculostomy access points

| | |
|---|---|
| **Kocher** | 10 cm posterior from nasion and 3 cm lateral in the midpupillary line |
| **Frazier** | 3 cm lateral and 6 cm above the inion |
| **Keen** | 3 cm posterior and 3 cm superior to the pinna |
| **Paine** | 2.5 cm superior to the lateral orbital roof and 4.5 cm anterior to the sylvian fissure. |

**Hydrocephalus**

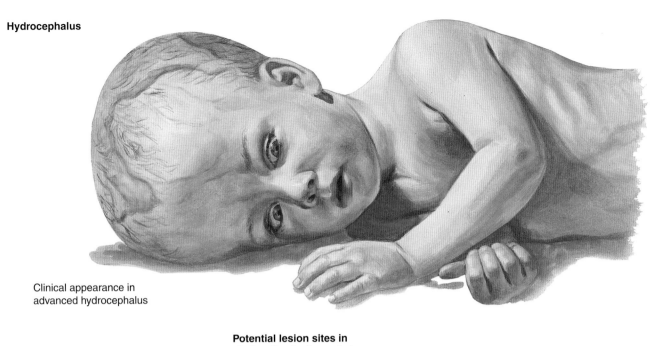

Clinical appearance in
advanced hydrocephalus

**Potential lesion sites in
obstructive hydrocephalus**

1. Interventricular foramina (of Monro)
2. Cerebral aqueduct (of Sylvius)
3. Lateral apertures (of Luschka)
4. Median aperture (of Magendie)

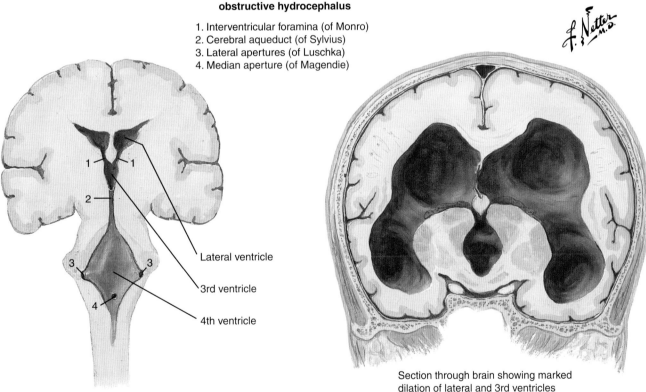

Lateral ventricle

3rd ventricle

4th ventricle

Section through brain showing marked
dilation of lateral and 3rd ventricles

**Fig. 40.2** A child with commons signs of hydrocephalus: bulging fontanel and sun-setting sign. Common intraventricular sites of CSF flow obstruction. (Reprinted with permission from Felten DL. Ventricles and the Cerebrospinal fluid. In: *Netter's Atlas of Neuroscience*. Saunders, Elsevier; 2010:67–73.)

## TREATMENT

The treatment of hydrocephalus can be divided into non-surgical approaches and surgical approaches, which in turn can be divided into nonshunting or shunting procedures. The goals of any successful management of hydrocephalus are (1) optimal neurological outcome and (2) preservation of cosmesis.[8] The radiographic finding of normal-sized ventricles should not be considered the goal of any therapeutic modality.

### Nonsurgical Options

No effective medical treatment exists to definitively treat hydrocephalus. Even if CSF production were to be reduced by 33%, ICP would modestly decrease by only 1.5 cm $H_2O$ pressure. Acetazolamide and furosemide have been

## Box 40.1   Causes of Hydrocephalus Based on Site of Obstruction

Lateral Ventricle
  Choroid plexus tumor
  Intraventricular region glioma
Foramen of Monro
  Congenital atresia
  Iatrogenic functional stenosis
  Stenotic gliosis secondary to intraventricular hemorrhage or ventriculitis
Third Ventricle
  Colloid cyst
  Ependymal cyst
  Arachnoid cyst
  Neoplasms such as craniopharyngioma, chiasmal-hypothalamic astrocytoma, or glioma
Cerebral Aqueduct
  Congenital aqueduct malformation
  Arteriovenous malformation
  Congenital aqueduct stenosis
  Neoplasms such as pineal region germinoma or periaqueductal glioma
Fourth Ventricle
  Dandy-Walker cyst
  Neoplasms such as medulloblastoma, ependymoma, astrocytoma, or brainstem glioma
  Basal foramina occlusion secondary to subarachnoid hemorrhage or meningitis
  Chiari malformations

Reprinted with permission from Singer HS, Kossoff EH, Hartman AL, et al. (eds). *Treatment of Pediatric Neurologic Disorders*. Boca Raton, FL: Taylor and Francis; 2005.

historically used to treat hydrocephalus. Both agents can decrease CSF production for a few days, but do not significantly reduce ventriculomegaly.[8] Acetazolamide is a carbonic anhydrase inhibitor historically used to treat premature infants with posthemorrhagic hydrocephalus. Contemporary studies have shown it to be ineffective in avoiding ventricular shunt placement and associated with increased neurological morbidity. High doses (25 mg/kg/day divided into three daily doses) are required, and side effects include lethargy, poor feeding, tachypnea, diarrhea, nephrocalcinosis, and electrolyte imbalances (e.g., hyperchloremic metabolic acidosis). Acetazolamide is contraindicated in patients with sulfa allergies).

### Surgical: Nonshunting Options

Obstructive lesions causing hydrocephalus should be surgically removed when possible. Resection of tumors in the vicinity of the third and fourth ventricles oftentimes effectively addresses the secondary hydrocephalus without the need for CSF diversion. Unfortunately, most congenital forms of hydrocephalus will not have a surgical mass. Adults with persistent hydrocephalus after trauma, infection, or subarachnoid hemorrhage will require a shunt.

For CSF obstruction at or distal to the aqueduct (e.g., tectal plate tumors, acquired aqueductal stenosis, or posterior fossa tumors), a potential surgical treatment is the endoscopic third ventriculostomy. By surgically creating an opening at the floor of the third ventricle, CSF can be diverted without placing a permanent ventricular shunt. Recent studies report a high success rate for endoscopic

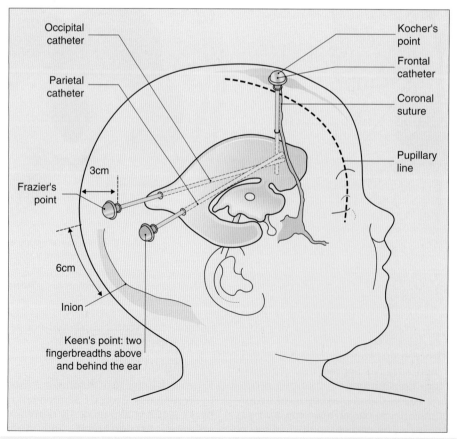

**Fig. 40.3** Common cranial access points for ventricular catheter. (Reprinted with permission from Rengachary SS, Ellenbogen RG, eds. *Principles of Neurosurgery*. 2nd ed. St Louis, MO: Elsevier Mosby; 2005:117–33.)

third ventriculostomies among specific pediatric patients. Age <1 year, hydrocephalus associated with aqueductal stenosis and myelomeningoceles appear to respond favorably to an endoscopic third ventriculostomy.[9] In comparison, communicating hydrocephalus is generally not an indication for a third ventriculostomy.

### Surgical: CSF Shunts

#### Components

There are three components to a shunt: a proximal (ventricular) catheter (as described earlier), a valve, and a distal catheter. The tubing is made of silicone rubber that can be impregnated with antibiotics or barium and may become brittle over time. The system diverts CSF out of the ventricular system to an alternative location (i.e. peritoneal, atrium, or pleural space) where it can be physiologically absorbed (Fig. 40.4).

The distal catheter is typically tunneled beneath the scalp from the ventricular access point and externalized at an abdominal incision to confirm functional patency prior to peritoneal placement (Fig. 40.4). An intermediate release incision may be made posterior to the pinna to facilitate tunneling of the distal catheter. Peritoneal shunts are placed with direct visualization of the peritoneal space. The minilaparotomy is a common approach consisting of a paramedian incision allowing direct inspection of motile abdominal viscera and omentum. Peritoneal access can be challenging in obese patients and those with significant scarring from multiple abdominal surgeries. In those patients, laparoscopic assistance is desired and is the best approach. Some surgeons routinely use laparoscopy for peritoneal access.

---

#### Clinical Pearls

**Peritoneal access**

- A mini-laparotomy incision at least 3 cm off of midline allows better visualization of the layers of the rectus sheath.
- Laproscopic access can be very useful especially in patients with difficult access

---

Alternative locations for distal shunt drainage span the atrial/venous system, pleural cavity, or gallbladder. Atrial/venous shunts are prone to cause thrombosis around the tip in approximately 40% of patients.[10] A one-way valve prevents the backflow of blood into the ventricular catheter and any potential valve obstruction. Atrial/venous shunts can be associated with pulmonary emboli or complicated cardiovascular changes such as cor pulmonale, cardiac tamponade, and arrhythmias.[11] Pleural shunts are placed via a small incision over the lateral and superior rib through where a catheter is introduced into the pleural space while positive pressure is maintained. A pneumothorax is of concern, and thus a postoperative chest x-ray is recommended to verify the placement as well.

When long-term drainage of CSF is needed in the setting of small ventricles such as pseudotumor cerebri, lumboperitoneal shunts may be more desirable given a lower risk of

cerebral complications and decreased likelihood of proximal catheter tip occlusion.[12,13] An intrathecal catheter threaded through a Tuohy needle can access the lumbar intrathecal space at the L4–5 level. Intraoperative fluoroscopy is used to ensure desired placement of the intrathecal portion of the shunt.

At present time, three general valve categories are recognized to treat hydrocephalus: fixed pressure, flow regulated, and programmable pressure (Table 40.1). The earliest valves used were fixed pressure and plagued by continuous CSF drainage that could vary with head position. Symptoms of overdrainage resulted in patients requiring operations to change the valve pressure threshold. Flow-regulating valves were subsequently developed to keep flow constant in the face of changing pressure differentials and patient position. The antisiphon component in these valves is accomplished by ball and spring mechanisms that are activated by specific positions and pressures, thus decreasing the likelihood for overdrainage. More recent designs have implemented a programmable pressure valve allowing incremental outflow adjustments without subjecting patients to repeat operations.

## Perioperative Considerations

---

#### Key Concepts

- Intravenous anesthetics tend to have a favorable effect on ICP, cerebral blood flow (CBF), and cerebral metabolism.
- The Monro-Kellie doctrine requires the skull to be nonexpandable with a constant total volume of the brain, blood, and CSF.
- Compliance describes the exponential relationship between changes in CSF volume and ICP.
- The Pressure Volume Index (PVI) is a mathematical derivative of compliance. It quantifies the amount of fluid associated with a tenfold change in ICP.

---

### ANESTHETIC CONSIDERATIONS

Drug selection is often tailored to the patient and care team needs. Attention to the etiology of the hydrocephalus and need for a complete neurological examination must be considered (see Neuroanesthesia and Perioperative Care). In a patient with progressive deterioration secondary to hydrocephalus, slight changes in intracranial volume can have a dramatic effect depending on reserve compliance. Intravenous anesthetics tend to have a favorable profile on ICP, CBF, and metabolism, whereas some inhalational anesthetics can exacerbate the hydrocephalus (Tables 40.2 and 40.3). Nitrous oxide is generally avoided in situations when CSF diversion is required because it is an inhalational anesthetic that can increase both the cerebral blood flow and ICP. After shunt insertion, rapid declines in ICP on occasion may result in cardiac dysrhythmias.

### INTRACRANIAL PRESSURE AND CEREBROSPINAL FLUID DYNAMICS

ICP has been best conceptualized by the Monro-Kellie doctrine. It holds the intracranial contents constant and

**Shunt Procedure for Hydrocephalus**

Cannula inserted into anterior horn of lateral ventricle through trephine hole in skull

Reservoir at end of cannula implanted beneath galea permits transcutaneous needle puncture for withdrawal of CSF or introduction of antibiotic medication or dye to test patency of shunt

One-way, pressure-regulated valve placed subcutaneously to prevent reflux of blood or peritoneal fluid and control CSF pressure

Drainage tube may be introduced into internal jugular vein and thence into right atrium via neck incision, or may be continued subcutaneously to abdomen

Drainage tube is most often introduced into peritoneal cavity, with extra length to allow for growth of child

Head measurement is of value in diagnosis, especially in early cases, and serial measurements will indicate progression or arrest of hydrocephalus

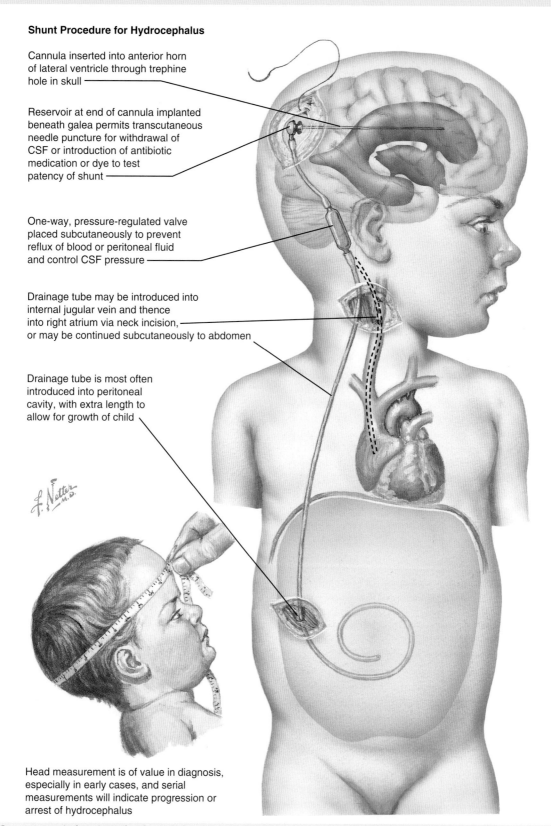

**Fig. 40.4**  Common ventriculoperitoneal and ventriculoatrial shunt placement. (Reprinted with permission from Felten DL. Ventricles and the Cerebrospinal fluid. In: *Netter's Atlas of Neuroscience*. Saunders, Elsevier; 2010:67–73.)

**Table 40.1** Shunt Valves

| Fixed pressure | Flow regulated | Programmable pressure |
|---|---|---|
| Hakim<br>Microprecision<br>(Codman – a Johnson and Johnson company)<br>▪ 0–5 cm H$_2$O outflow resistance<br>▪ Siphonguard (ball and cone) can prevent overdrainage | Orbit-Sigma<br>OSV II<br>(Integra)<br>▪ First flow-regulated valve<br>▪ Three-stage variable resistance mechanism<br>▪ Magnet neutral/MRI safe | Strata<br>(Medtronic)<br>▪ Ball/spring mechanism with magnet<br>▪ Programmable/noninvasive<br>   Incorporated Delta chamber |
| PS Medical<br>(Medtronic)<br>▪ Injectable reservoir<br>▪ Nonmetabolic<br>▪ Low-low, low, medium, and high-pressure outflow available | Delta<br>(Medtronic)<br>▪ Elsatomer diaphragm mechanism<br>▪ 0.5, 1.0, 1.5, 2.0, 2.5 levels available | Codman Hakim<br>(Codman – a Johnson and Johnson company)<br>▪ Noninvasive programs among 18 preset levels<br>▪ Ball/spring mechanism |
| | | Sophy<br>(Sophysa)<br>▪ First adjustable valve<br>▪ Silicone-coated polycarbonate chamber<br>▪ Ball-cone mechanisms with variable pressure spring |
| | | Polaris<br>(Sophysa)<br>▪ MRI compatible variable valve<br>▪ Self-locking magnetic system |
| | | proGAV<br>(Aesculap)<br>▪ MRI-compatible variable valve<br>▪ Self-locking magnetic system<br>▪ Ball/spring mechanism<br>▪ Gravity dependent addition to minimize overdrainage |

*MRI*, magnetic resonance imaging.

Adapted with permission from Blount JP. Effects of Anesthetic Agents and Other Drugs on Cerebral Blood Flow, Metabolism, and Intracranial Pressure. In: *Youmans Neurological Surgery*. 6th ed. Philadelphia, PA: Saunders; 2011:78-94.

**Table 40.2** Summary of Effects of Inhalational Anesthetics on CBF, CMR, and ICP

| | CBF | CMR | ICP |
|---|---|---|---|
| N$_2$O | ↑↑ | ↑ or → | ↑↑ |
| Xenon | ↓(gray) ↑ (white) | ↓ | ↑ or → |
| Isoflurane | ↑ or → | ↓↓ | → or ↗ or ↑ |
| Sevoflurane | ↓ or→or ↗ | ↓ or ↓↓ | → or ↗ or ↑ |
| Desflurane | ↓ or ↑ | ↓↓ | ↑ or → |

*CBF*, cerebral blood flow; *CMR*, cerebral metabolic rate; *ICP*, intracranial pressure.

Arrows indicate semiquantitative changes.

↗:slight increase, ↑:increase, ↑↑:marked increase, →:unchanged ↓:decrease, ↓↓:marked decrease

Reprinted with permission from Sakabe T. Effects of Anesthetic Agents and Other Drugs on Cerebral Blood Flow, Metabolism, and Intracranial Pressure, In: *Cottrell and Young's Neuroanesthesia*. Philadelphia, PA: Mosby, Inc; 2010:78–94.

**Table 40.3** Summary of Effects of Intravenous Anesthetics on CBF, CMR, and ICP

| | CBF | CMR | ICP |
|---|---|---|---|
| Barbiturate | ↓↓ | ↓↓ | ↓↓ |
| Etomidate | ↓↓ | ↓↓ | ↓↓ |
| Ketamine | ↓↓ | ↓↓ | ↓↓ |
| Benzodiazepines | ↓ | ↓ | ↑ or → |
| Synthetic opioids | → or ↗ ↘ | → or ↓ | → or ↗ |
| Dexmedetomidine | ↓ | → or ↓ | → |

*CBF*, cerebral blood flow; *CMR*, cerebral metabolic rate; *ICP*, intracranial pressure.

Reprinted with permission from Sakabe T. Effects of Anesthetic Agents and Other Drugs on Cerebral Blood Flow, Metabolism, and Intracranial Pressure, In: *Cottrell and Young's Neuroanesthesia*. Philadelphia, PA: Mosby, Inc.; 2010:78–94.

composed of brain (80%), CSF (10%), and blood (10%) volumes. The doctrine requires the brain to be in a nonexpandable case of bone, thus limiting the application of the doctrine to patients with open fontanels.[14] Given the constant nature of the intracranial vault and the incompressibility of the brain, changes in CSF volume can be initially partially compensated by compression of venous sinuses thus slightly decreasing cerebral blood volume, however this has a minimal and transient effect.

CSF is normally secreted from the choroid plexus by active transport, and its rate decreases only when CBF begins to decline.[15] Its absorption occurs passively by a hydrostatic gradient through the arachnoid granulations into the venous circulation. This rate is linearly related to ICP.[16] Therefore either an increase in CSF formation or a resistance to absorption will lead to an increased ICP. The normal rate of CSF production and total CSF volume during childhood varies as the child matures

(Table 40.4). It is estimated that the average total CSF volume in a neonate is 40 to 50 mL.[17] In contrast, the average total CSF volume in an adult is 150 mL, with a secretion rate of about 20 mL/hr (0.34 mL/min.[15]

A change in CSF volume is the primary method to treat elevated ICP secondary to hydrocephalus. The majority of CSF is found in subarachnoid spaces, and only 10% in the intracranial ventricular system. The change in volume of CSF to compensate for changes in pressure is expressed as the compliance ($\Delta V/\Delta P$) or PVI.[18,19] The PVI is the volume of fluid injected or withdrawn that would result in a tenfold change in ICP and is calculated as $PVI = \Delta V / Log\ P_f / P_o$, where $\Delta V$ = volume of fluid injected or withdrawn, $P_f$ = final ICP, and $P_o$ = initial ICP. The PVI varies in proportion to the estimated neural axis volume. The PVI is 8 mL in an infant and 25 mL in a 14-year-old. Therefore a 10-mL volume added to the neural axis of a 14-year-old may produce a modest elevation in ICP, whereas the same volume would be lethal in an infant (Fig. 40.5).

## PATHOPHYSIOLOGY AND NEED FOR CSF DIVERSION

An imbalance of CSF dynamics arises in various pathological states of hydrocephalus. It is estimated that at least 7% to 10% of patients with hydrocephalus after ruptured aneurysmal subarachnoid hemorrhage will require a shunt.[20-22] Posttraumatic hydrocephalus (PTH) is commonly seen after severe head injury. This typically develops within the first 3 months after injury but may be confounded by cortical atrophy that develops gradually over at least 6 months or more postinjury. Risk factors predisposing patients to PTH have included age, duration of coma, presence of a decompressive craniectomy, and cortical atrophy attributed to axonal injury and hypoxia.[23-26] Only approximately 10% of patients with severe PTH will develop radiographic and clinical deterioration potentially responsive to shunt placement.

### Clinical Pearls

**Prevalence of hydrocephalus requiring shunting**

- Although 70% of patients with hydrocephalus associated with aneurysmal subarachnoid hemorrhage will improve with acute CSF diversion, only 10% will require shunting.[22]
- Posttraumatic hydrocephalus requiring shunting is more likely to develop after extensive craniectomies abutting the sinus.

**Table 40.4**  Normal Intracranial Pressure by Age

| Age | Normal ICP range (mm Hg) |
| --- | --- |
| Young Child | 3–7 |
| Adults and Older Children | <15 |

*ICP*, intracranial pressure.
Reprinted with permission from Greenberg M. *Handbook of Neurosurgery.* 7th ed. New York, NY: Thieme Publishers, Inc; 2010.

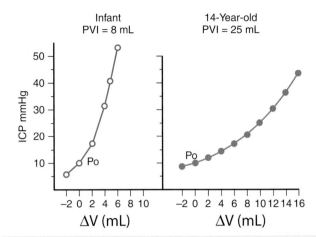

**Fig. 40.5** Compliance differences between an infant and a 14-year-old patient. The pressure volume index (PVI) is the volume of fluid injected or withdrawn that would result in a tenfold change in ICP and is calculated as $PVI = \Delta V / Log\ P_f / P_o$, where $\Delta V$ = volume of fluid injected or withdrawn, $P_f$ = final ICP, and $P_o$ = initial ICP. (Adapted from Cheek WR, et al., eds. *Pediatric Neurosurgery: Surgery of the Developing Nervous System.* 3rd ed. Philadelphia, PA: W.B. Saunders; 1994:307–19.)

## Postoperative Complications

### Key Concepts

- The three types of shunt complications are infections, inadequate flow regulation, and mechanical failures.
- *Staphylococcus epidermidis* causes approximately 60% of shunt infections; *Staphylococcus aureus* is responsible for 30%; and coliform bacteria, propionibacteria, streptococci, or *Haemophilus influenzae* cause the remainder.

### SHUNT COMPLICATIONS

Shunt complications and failure remain a significant problem in treating hydrocephalus. Only 30% to 37% of shunts will remain revision free in the first 10 years after placement.[27,28] In adults undergoing a shunt placement for the first time, up to half will require a revision in the first 6 months.

### Clinical Pearls

**Shunt complications**

- Forty percent of all shunts fail within the first year of placement.[41,48,52]
- Infection can affect up to 10% of shunts.[41,53]
- Only a third of shunts will remain revision free by 10 years of placement.
- Hemorrhage associated with ventriculostomies is more likely to occur in infants and is associated with shorter time to shunt revision.

Immediate complications after implantation relate to intracranial hemorrhage, valve occlusion, and trauma from distal catheter placement. At least 7% of ventriculostomies are associated with hemorrhages, but only 0.8% are clinically significant hemorrhages.[29,30] Intraventricular hemorrhage is a potential complication seen in up to 31% of shunts placed in children.[30] Although not as common, iatrogenic hemorrhagic complications can be associated with approximately 3% of EVD placements and can influence plans for internalization. In situations where an immediate postoperative shunt placement failure is suspected, requisite imaging can confirm disconnections, and a shunt reservoir tap can definitively demonstrate the patency of the system.

Shunt complications fall into three major categories: (1) infection of the CSF or the shunt device, (2) functional failure because of too much or too little flow of CSF, and (3) mechanical failure of the device. A list of shunt complications is outlined in Table 40.5. The two most common complications are infection and obstruction.

## SHUNT INFECTION

Multiple methods have been used to decrease infections such as double gloving, antibiotic-impregnated catheters, iodine-embedded drapes, handling hardware with instruments, perioperative antibiotics, and intrathecal antibiotics at the time of surgery.[10,31–36] Yet up to 15% of all shunting procedures are still complicated by infection. It is believed that most bacteria are introduced at the time of surgery. Pediatric patients tend to have more complications and shunt infections within the first 3 months of placement. This rate seems to be constant and according to some sources stratifying premature infants with the greatest risk.[41]

---

### Clinical Pearls

**Most effective interventions to preventing shunt infections**

- Intravenous antibiotics close to the time of incision
- Intrathecal antibiotics
- Minimal handling of shunt components, frequent glove changes, and utilizing antibiotic-impregnated catheters

---

The offending organism is most often a member of the skin flora. S. epidermidis causes approximately 60% of shunt infections; S. aureus is responsible for 30%; and coliform bacteria, propionibacteria, streptococci, or . influenzae cause the remainder.[42,37] In general, gram-positive organisms correlate with a better prognosis than gram-negative organisms. Common symptoms of a shunt infection include irritability and anorexia. Clinical signs include low-grade fever and elevated C-reactive protein. S. aureus infections often present with erythema along the shunt track. Infected ventriculoatrial shunts may present with subacute bacterial endocarditis and shunt nephritis, an immune-complex disorder that resembles acute glomerulonephritis.[8]

Prophylactic use of antibiotics has been studied in numerous prospective, randomized trials demonstrating statistically significant improvement in shunt infection rates when children were treated with systemic oxacillin, systemic trimethoprim-sulfamethoxazole, or intraventricular vancomycin.[31,39] Of these studies, a prospective multicenter-tested comprehensive strategy incorporating intraventricular antibiotics has been the most influential in establishing the use of systemic cefazolin or vancomycin prior to incision followed by intraventricular vancomycin and gentamicin injected into the shunt reservoir.[32] Across the 21 surgeons at four research institutions, the infection rate was decreased from 8.8% to 5.7% (Fig. 40.6).

The diagnosis of a shunt infection is generally made after sampling the CSF. An accepted CSF profile consistent with an infection includes an elevated white blood cell (WBC) count (1000–5000 mcL) with a predominance of neutrophils, high protein concentration (100–500 mg/dL), and decreased glucose concentration <40 mg/dL.[38] The most effective and widely used treatment of a shunt infection is to remove the shunt hardware and to place an EVD for temporary CSF diversion during a period of systemic antibiotics tailored to the sensitivities. When the infection is cleared, a new ventricular shunt system may be implanted and the external ventriculostomy is removed. A generally accepted criteria includes (1) five to seven consecutive daily negative CSF cultures, (2) CSF WBC count <50 mcL, and (3) CSF protein <500 mg/dL. On occasion, in situ treatment of shunt infections is possible but does not uniformly lead to success.

Infections associated with external ventricular drainage are similar to internalized shunt infections.[35] Staphylococcus tends to be commonly associated with nosocomial ventriculitis. In addition to the techniques to minimize internalized shunt infections, tunneling the ventricular drain out from beneath the scalp at a point >3 cm from the cranial access incision has been found to be important in minimizing the risk for nosocomial infections. Most EVD-associated ventriculitis and meningitis occur within the first 12 days after placement, with highest risk for infection between postplacement days 4 and 9.[34] Prolonged

---

**Table 40.5** Shunt Complications

| COMMON COMPLICATIONS | Cranial | UNCOMMON COMPLICATIONS | | |
| --- | --- | --- | --- | --- |
| | | Subcutaneous | Peritoneal | Atrial |
| Infection | Subdural hygroma | Shunt migration | Peritonitis | Endocarditis |
| Obstruction | Subdural hematoma | Shunt disconnection | Pseudocysts | Nephritis |
| Inadequate flow or overdrainage | Hemiparesis | Shunt fracture | Perforation | |
| | Hematoma | | Hernias | |

Reprinted with permission from Wang PP. Hydrocephalus in Adults, In: Rengachary SS, Ellenbogen RG, eds. *Principles of Neurosurgery*. 2nd ed. St Louis, MO: Elsevier Mosby; 2005:117–33.

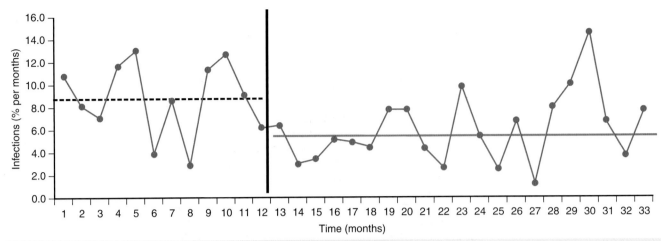

**Fig. 40.6** Graph comparing mean monthly shunt infection rate before and after a standardized protocol implementing the administration of intravenous cefazolin or vancomycin prior to incision and injection of gentamicin and vancomycin into the shunt reservoir at time of placement. The infection rate before implementation of the protocol (first 12 months) was 8.8% (dashed line); after implementation, it was 5.7% (solid line; chi-square = 8.93, $p = 0.0028$). (Adapted with permission from Kestle JR, Riva-Cambrin J, Wellons JC, et al. A standardized protocol to reduce cerebrospinal fluid shunt infection: The Hydrocephalus Clinical Research Network Quality Improvement Initiative. *J Neurosurg Pediatr.* 2011;8(1):22–9.)

periods of drainage did not increase the likelihood of acquiring an associated ventriculitis.[40]

## SHUNT OBSTRUCTION

Shunt obstruction is a common complication that can present with many nonspecific symptoms. Mechanical failures or obstructions can occur at any time within any of the three components. The most common proximal obstruction takes place when the choroid plexus or debris occludes the ventricular catheter tip.[41,42] In growing patients with a shunt placed at infancy, it is common to encounter a distal malfunction once the catheter tip dislodges from the peritoneal cavity. The surgical assessment is a combination of clinical findings interpreted on the backdrop of objective measures. Clinical findings consist of headache, CN VI palsies, upward gaze paresis, irritability, lethargy, nausea, and/or vomiting. Infants with a shunt malfunction may display irritability, poor feeding, increased OFC, and/or inappropriate sleepiness. It is important to inquire if the presenting signs and symptoms are the same as when the shunt malfunctioned in the past.

When a shunt malfunction is suspected, imaging studies consisting of a head CT as well as anteroposterior and lateral x-rays of the skull, chest, and abdomen should be performed (Fig. 40.7).[43] Proper imaging can detect changes in ventricular size, catheter disconnections, and fractures. Confirmation of the programmable valve setting with a skull x-ray film perpendicular to the valve is important in shunt-dependent patients and serves as a reference for symptoms with equivocal objective changes.

Noninvasive methods to demonstrate an obstruction include an evaluation of the scalp for a subcutaneous fluid collection. More invasive methods consist of a percutaneous puncture and aspiration of the valve reservoir by a 23-gauge or smaller needle. This can rapidly diagnose a proximal catheter obstruction based on the ease of fluid egress.[44] It can be a temporizing measure for intracranial hypertensive emergencies if immediate operative intervention is not feasible and allows the collection of CSF for analysis. A nuclear medicine shuntogram can be obtained by injecting radioactive tracer into the valve reservoir to determine the patency of the shunt system. Patients who are diagnosed with a shunt malfunction must be taken urgently to the operating room for a shunt revision.

In less urgent situations and indeterminate clinical data, a dilated fundoscopic examination may be of some use to monitor changes over time. The presence of papilledema is specific, but not sensitive, for detecting elevated ICPs. Age, duration of hydrocephalus, optic atrophy, and intrinsic properties of the brain all contribute to the variable presence of funduscopic clues of malignant ICP.[2,45]

The majority of patients with a shunt malfunction present with increased ventricular size on neuroimaging studies. Patients with stiff ventricles, slit ventricle syndrome, or overdrainage symptoms present challenges in diagnosing a shunt malfunction. In poorly responsive patients with diminished brain compliance, a sterile shunt tap to test the proximal and distal shunt flow is warranted.

### Clinical Pearls

Critical shunt-related terms

- **Slit ventricle syndrome:** Intermittent headaches unrelated to posture often accompanied by nausea, vomiting, drowsiness, irritability, and impaired cognition
- **Overdrainage:** Headaches associated with position affecting activities of daily living
- **Stiff ventricle:** Ventricles that do not change in size due to diminished brain compliance

These symptoms are oftentimes confusing and may overlap with the slit ventricle syndrome in up to 22% of children with headaches and radiology characterized by collapsed ventricles.[46,47] Incontinence, worsening focal neurological deficits, seizures, and lethargy in patients with slit ventricle syndrome may represent a sudden increase in ICP. In

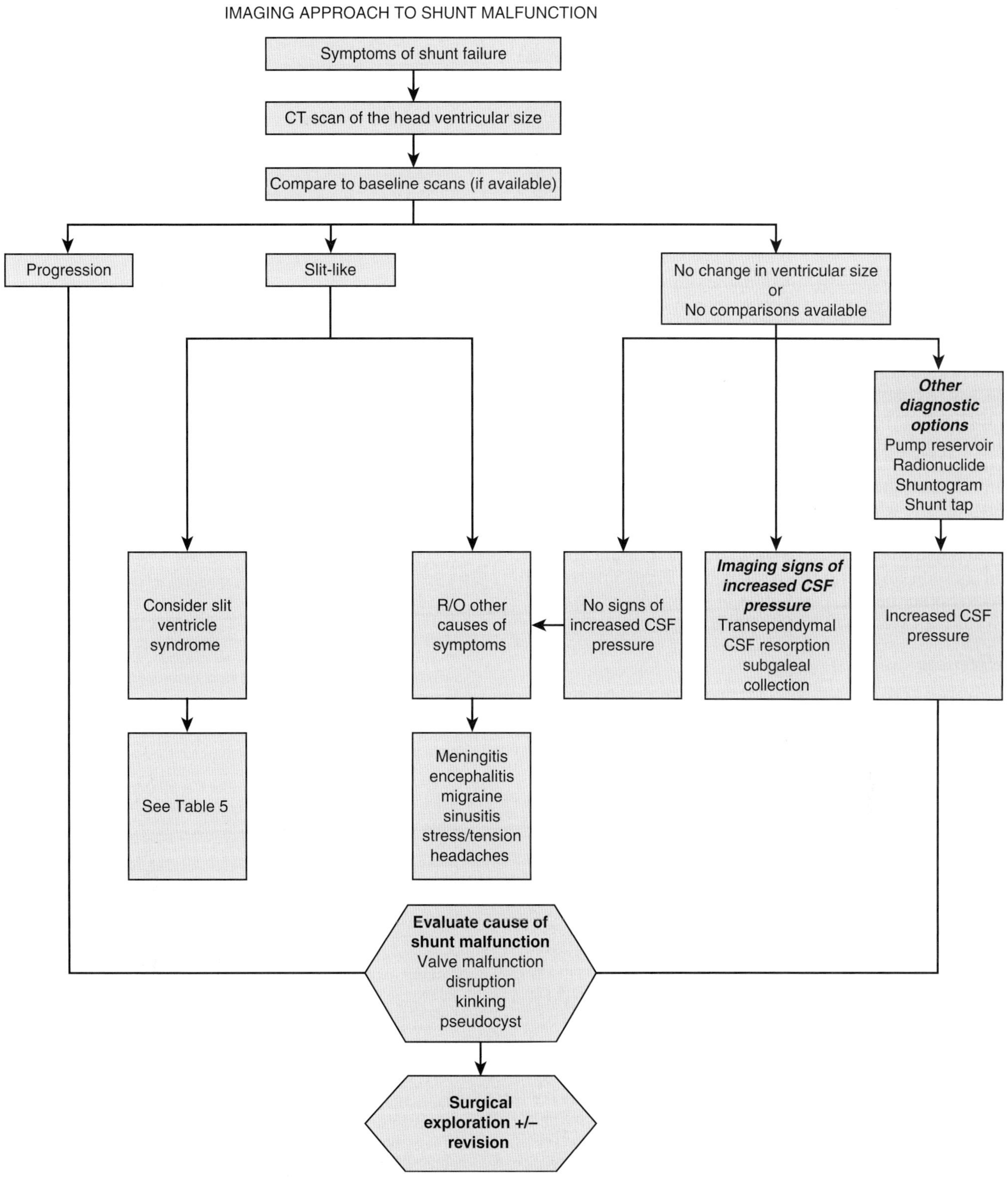

IMAGING APPROACH TO SHUNT MALFUNCTION

Fig. 40.7 An algorithm to guide radiographic and clinical assessments of a potential shunt malfunction. (Adapted with permission from Sivaganesan A, Krishnamurthy R, Sahni D, et al. Neuroimaging of ventriculoperitoneal shunt complications in children. *Pediatr Radiol.* 2012;42(9):1029–46.)

adults, the most common reasons for shunt revisions relate to suboptimal drainage of CSF. With prolonged overdrainage, about 10% of patients may develop subdural hematomas, stenosis/ occlusion of the cerebral aqueduct, slit ventricle syndrome, intracranial hypotension, or premature closure of the skull sutures.[47,48]

Complications that affect distal drainage locations range from inadequate placement to obstructions. In the setting of shunt-dependent hydrocephalus, abdominal discomfort preceding symptoms of inadequate CSF drainage and the presence of an abdominal mass are highly suggestive of a pseudocyst. An abdominal CT or ultrasound can confirm the presence of the fluid collection. Although the etiology for a delayed CSF malabsorption is unclear, an inflammatory reaction resulting in thickened peritoneum is observed.[49,50] Current theories suggest an infectious source, CSF protein moiety, or autoimmune allergic response. The cysts may be percutaneously aspirated, and the fluid cultured. If a potential infection is suspected, a shunt tap and/or period of externalized drainage may be necessary until an infection has effectively been ruled out.

## UNCOMMON SHUNT COMPLICATIONS

Table 40.5 lists several uncommon shunt complications. Subdural hygromas and hematomas may develop after the insertion of a ventricular shunt into a child with very large ventricles and a thin cerebral cortical mantle. Treatment of symptomatic subdural hygromas and hematomas consists of changing the shunt valve to a higher pressure setting and/or by introducing a catheter into the subdural effusion and connecting it to the distal shunt system.[51] Ventricular catheter migration out of the ventricular system occurs if the shunt has not been properly fixed at the burr hole site where it exits the skull. Complications affecting the distal aspect of the shunt include hernias that can develop within 3 months of shunt insertion at the abdominal incision accessing the peritoneum. These are treated like any other hernia. Perforation of intraperitoneal organs is a rare but well-recognized complication.

## References

1. Avellino AM, Carson BS. Increased intracranial pressure. In: Maria BL, ed. *Current Management in Child Neurology*. 2nd ed. Hamilton, Ontario: B.C. Decker; 2002:481–486.
2. Nazir S, O'Brien M, Qureshi NH, Slape L, Green TJ, Phillips PH. Sensitivity of papilledema as a sign of shunt failure in children. *J AAPOS*. 2009;13(1):63–66.
3. Schultke E. Theodor Kocher's craniometer. *Neurosurgery*. 2009;64(5):1001–1004. discussion 4–5.
4. Levitt MR, O'Neill BR, Ishak GE, et al. Image-guided cerebrospinal fluid shunting in children: catheter accuracy and shunt survival. *J Neurosurg Pediatr*. 2012;10(2):112–117.
5. Hyun SJ, Suk JS, Kwon JT, Kim YB. Novel entry point for intraoperative ventricular puncture during the transsylvian approach. *Acta Neurochir*. 2007;149(10):1049–1051. discussion 51.
6. Park J, Hamm IS. Revision of Paine's technique for intraoperative ventricular puncture. *Surg Neurol*. 2008;70(5):503–508. discussion 8.
7. Mortazavi MM, Adeeb N, Griessenauer CJ, et al. The ventricular system of the brain: a comprehensive review of its history, anatomy, histology, embryology, and surgical considerations. *Childs Nerv Syst*. 2014;30(1):19–35.
8. Avellino AM. Hydrocephalus. In: Singer HS, Kossoff ES, Hartman AL, Crawford TO, eds. *Treatment of Pediatric Neurologic Disorders*. Boca Raton, FL: Taylor and Francis; 2005:25–35.
9. Teo C, Jones R. Management of hydrocephalus by endoscopic third ventriculostomy in patients with myelomeningocele. *Pediatr Neurosurg*. 1996;25(2):57–63.
10. Li V. Methods and complications in surgical cerebrospinal fluid shunting. *Neurosurg Clin North Am*. 2001;12(4):685–693. viii.
11. Vernet O, Rilliet B. Late complications of ventriculoatrial or ventriculoperitoneal shunts. *Lancet*. 2001;358(9293):1569–1570.
12. Aoki N. Lumboperitoneal shunt: clinical applications, complications, and comparison with ventriculoperitoneal shunt. *Neurosurgery*. 1990;26(6):998–1003. discussion 1004.
13. Wang VY, Barbaro NM, Lawton MT, et al. Complications of lumboperitoneal shunts. *Neurosurgery*. 2007;60(6):1045–1048. discussion 9.
14. Mokri B. The Monro-Kellie hypothesis: applications in CSF volume depletion. *Neurology*. 2001;56(12):1746–1748.
15. Bruce D. Concepts of intracranial volume and pressure. In: James H, Anas N, Perkin R, eds. *Brain Insults in Infants and Children: Pathophysiology and Management*. Orlando, FL: Grune & Stratton; 1985:19–23.
16. McComb J, Zlokovic B. Cerebrospinal fluid and the blood-brain interface. In: Cheek WR, Marlin AE, McLone DG, eds. *Pediatric Neurosurgery: Surgery of the Developing Nervous System*. Philadelphia, PA: W B Saunders Co; 1994.
17. Hazinski MF, van Stralen D. Physiologic and anatomic differences between children and adults. In: Levin DL, Morriss FC, eds. *Essentials of Pediatric Intensive Care*. St. Louis, MO: Quality Medical Publishing; 1990:5–17.
18. Shapiro K, Morris WJ, Teo C. Intracranial hypertension: mechanisms and management. In: Cheek WR, Marlin AE, McLone DG, eds. *Pediatric Neurosurgery: Surgery of the Developing Nervous System*. 3rd ed. Philadelphia, PA: W.B. Saunders; 1994:307–319.
19. Shapiro K, Marmarou A, Shulman K. Abnormal brain biomechanics in the hydrocephalic child. In: Neurosurgery ASoP, ed. *Concepts in Pediatric Neurosurgery*. 2nd ed. Basel, Switzerland: Karger; 1993:76–88.
20. Germanwala AV, Huang J, Tamargo RJ. Hydrocephalus after aneurysmal subarachnoid hemorrhage. *Neurosurg Clin North Am*. 2010;21(2):263–270.
21. Vassilouthis J, Richardson AE. Ventricular dilatation and communicating hydrocephalus following spontaneous subarachnoid hemorrhage. *J Neurosurg*. 1979;51(3):341–351.
22. Milhorat TH. Acute hydrocephalus after aneurysmal subarachnoid hemorrhage. *Neurosurgery*. 1987;20(1):15–20.
23. Wilson JT, Wiedmann KD, Hadley DM, Condon B, Teasdale G, Brooks DN. Early and late magnetic resonance imaging and neuropsychological outcome after head injury. *J Neurol Neurosurg Psychiatry*. 1988;51(3):391–396.
24. Takeuchi S, Nawashiro H, Otani N, Shima K. Post-traumatic hydrocephalus following decompressive craniectomy. *J Neurotrauma*. 2012;29(5):1028.
25. Mazzini L, Campini R, Angelino E, Rognone F, Pastore I, Oliveri G. Posttraumatic hydrocephalus: a clinical, neuroradiologic, and neuropsychologic assessment of long-term outcome. *Arch Phys Med Rehabil*. 2003;84(11):1637–1641.
26. De Bonis P, Pompucci A, Mangiola A, Rigante L, Anile C. Post-traumatic hydrocephalus after decompressive craniectomy: an underestimated risk factor. *J Neurotrauma*. 2010;27(11):1965–1970.
27. Kulkarni AV, Riva-Cambrin J, Butler J, et al. Outcomes of CSF shunting in children: comparison of Hydrocephalus Clinical Research Network cohort with historical controls: clinical article. *J Neurosurg Pediatr*. 2013;12(4):334–338.
28. Drake JM, Kestle JR, Tuli S. CSF shunts 50 years on—past, present and future. *Childs Nerv Syst*. 2000;16(10–11):800–804.
29. Bauer DF, Razdan SN, Bartolucci AA, Markert JM. Meta-analysis of hemorrhagic complications from ventriculostomy placement by neurosurgeons. *Neurosurgery*. 2011;69(2):255–260.
30. Brownlee RD, Dold ON, Myles ST. Intraventricular hemorrhage complicating ventricular catheter revision: incidence and effect on shunt survival. *Pediatr Neurosurg*. 1995;22(6):315–320.
31. Ragel BT, Browd SR, Schmidt RH. Surgical shunt infection: significant reduction when using intraventricular and systemic antibiotic agents. *J Neurosurg*. 2006;105(2):242–247.
32. Kestle JR, Riva-Cambrin J, Wellons 3rd JC, et al. A standardized protocol to reduce cerebrospinal fluid shunt infection: the Hydrocephalus Clinical Research Network Quality Improvement Initiative. *J Neurosurg Pediatr*. 2011;8(1):22–29.
33. Flint AC, Rao VA, Renda NC, Faigeles BS, Lasman TE, Sheridan W. A simple protocol to prevent external ventricular drain infections. *Neurosurgery*. 2013;72(6):993–999. discussion 9.
34. Zabramski JM, Whiting D, Darouiche RO, et al. Efficacy of antimicrobial-impregnated external ventricular drain catheters: a prospective, randomized, controlled trial. *J Neurosurg*. 2003;98(4):725–730.
35. Thomas R, Lee S, Patole S, Rao S. Antibiotic-impregnated catheters for the prevention of CSF shunt infections: a systematic review and meta-analysis. *Br J Neurosurg*. 2012;26(2):175–184.
36. Choudhury AR. Avoidable factors that contribute to the complications of ventriculoperitoneal shunt in childhood hydrocephalus. *Childs Nerv Syst*. 1990;6(6):346–349.

37. Kulkarni AV, Drake JM, Lamberti-Pasculli M. Cerebrospinal fluid shunt infection: a prospective study of risk factors. *J Neurosurg.* 2001;94(2):195–201.

38. Wells DL, Allen JM. Ventriculoperitoneal shunt infections in adult patients. *AACN.* 2013;24(1):6–12. quiz 3–4.

39. Al-Jeraisy M, Phelps SJ, Christensen ML, Einhaus S. Intraventricular vancomycin in pediatric patients with cerebrospinal fluid shunt infections. *JPPT.* 2004;9(1):36–42.

40. Scheithauer S, Burgel U, Bickenbach J, et al. External ventricular and lumbar drainage-associated meningoventriculitis: prospective analysis of time-dependent infection rates and risk factor analysis. *Infection.* 2010;38(3):205–209.

41. Browd SR, Ragel BT, Gottfried ON, Kestle JR. Failure of cerebrospinal fluid shunts: part I: obstruction and mechanical failure. *Pediatr Neurol.* 2006;34(2):83–92.

42. Dickerman RD, McConathy WJ, Morgan J, et al. Failure rate of frontal versus parietal approaches for proximal catheter placement in ventriculoperitoneal shunts: revisited. *J Clin Neurosci.* 2005;12(7):781–783.

43. Sivaganesan A, Krishnamurthy R, Sahni D, Viswanathan C. Neuroimaging of ventriculoperitoneal shunt complications in children. *Pediatr Radiol.* 2012;42(9):1029–1046.

44. Noetzel MJ, Baker RP. Shunt fluid examination: risks and benefits in the evaluation of shunt malfunction and infection. *J Neurosurg.* 1984;61(2):328–332.

45. Salgarello T, Falsini B, Tedesco S, Galan ME, Colotto A, Scullica L. Correlation of optic nerve head tomography with visual field sensitivity in papilledema. *Invest Ophthalmol Vis Sci.* 2001;42(7):1487–1494.

46. Rekate HL. The slit ventricle syndrome: advances based on technology and understanding. *Pediatr Neurosurg.* 2004;40(6):259–263.

47. Pudenz RH, Foltz EL. Hydrocephalus: overdrainage by ventricular shunts. A review and recommendations. *Surg Neurol.* 1991;35(3):200–212.

48. Browd SR, Gottfried ON, Ragel BT, Kestle JR. Failure of cerebrospinal fluid shunts: part II: overdrainage, loculation, and abdominal complications. *Pediatr Neurol.* 2006;34(3):171–176.

49. Popa F, Grigorean VT, Onose G, Popescu M, Strambu V, Sandu AM. Laparoscopic treatment of abdominal complications *following* ventriculoperitoneal shunt. *J Med Life.* 2009;2(4):426–436.

50. Anderson CM, Sorrells DL, Kerby JD. Intra-abdominal pseudocysts as a complication of ventriculoperitoneal shunts: a case report and review of the literature. *Curr Surg.* 2003;60(3):338–340.

51. Yamamura K, Kodama O, Kajikawa H, et al. Rare intra-abdominal complications of a ventriculoperitoneal shunt: report of three cases. *No Shinkei Geka.* 1998;26(11):1007–1011.

52. Bergsneider M, Stiner E. Shunting. In: *Youmans Neurological Surgery [Internet].* Philadelphia, PA: Elsevier SaundersManagment of Adult Hydrocephalus; 2011:515–524.

53. Al-Tamimi YZ, Sinha P, Chumas PD, et al. Ventriculoperitoneal shunt 30-day failure rate: a retrospective international cohort study. *Neurosurgery.* 2014;74(1):29–34.

# 41 Placement and Complications of Intracranial Monitors and Lumbar Drains

WILLIAM ARES, RAMESH GRANDHI, BRADLEY J. MOLYNEAUX, and DAVID OKONKWO

There is a frequent need for invasive central nervous system monitoring in neurosurgical patients in the neurocritical care setting. Indications for close monitoring are widely varied and include patients with both intracranial and spinal indications for neurosurgical intervention. Although placement of intracranial monitors and lumbar drains are common neurosurgical procedures often performed at the bedside, they are not without their own intraoperative and perioperative risks. We will discuss procedure guidelines, as well as relevant anatomy, common complications from these procedures, and perioperative considerations. (Table 41.1).

## Neuroanatomy and Procedure

### Key Concepts

- The ipsilateral foramen of Monro is the target for the external ventricular drain (EVD) catheter. This target is best approximated by using a burr hole at Kocher's point and aiming along a trajectory that terminates at the intersection of a point that is even with the ipsilateral medical canthus (in the sagittal plane) and 1.5 cm anterior to the tragus (in the coronal plane).
- An intraspinous length of 40 cm is appropriate to facilitate adequate cerebrospinal fluid (CSF) diversion when utilizing a lumbar drain. Care must be taken when removing the insertion stylet as to not fracture the catheter.

### External Ventricular Drain

#### Clinical Pearl

Placement of an EVD in a trauma patient, even without ventricular dilatation, can be a very effective way of managing intracranial pressure. Current guidelines would recommend intracranial pressure monitoring in neurotrauma patients with Glasgow Coma Scale scores of 3–8.[1]

EVD placement is a common neurosurgical procedure performed when measurement of intracranial pressure (ICP) or diversion of (CSF) is indicated. Common indications for placement of an EVD include traumatic brain injury, subarachnoid hemorrhage, posterior fossa mass lesions, and other neurological conditions where the patient is at risk for development of intracranial hypertension or hydrocephalus. EVDs play a crucial role in neurocritical care in guiding therapy, as well as serving as a therapeutic modality by reducing ICP on a sustained basis.[2]

Except in cases where a lesion prevents placement, right-sided EVDs are usually preferred in order to avoid the dominant hemisphere. The patient is maintained in a supine position with his or her head brought to the edge of the bed, with the head of bed elevated to roughly 45 degrees. Hair clippers are used for purposes of widely shaving the head on the same side of the EVD cannulation, and the head is prepared in standard sterile fashion. Two lines are drawn on the scalp in order to establish Kocher's point: one line in the midline from the nasion to a point 10 cm back and another from the previous point to a spot 3 cm lateral to it. This location is where the burr hole placement will occur and should be in the ipsilateral midpupillary line. Finally, two lines are drawn that guide the trajectory of ventricular cannulation—one line is drawn from Kocher's point to the ipsilateral medial canthus of the eye, and a second line is drawn from Kocher's point to a point roughly 1.5 cm anterior to the ipsilateral tragus. After administration of a local anesthetic containing epinephrine, a small linear skin incision is made down to bone and the periosteum is scraped

**Table 41.1** Potential Complications of Implanted Devices

| Device | Complication |
|---|---|
| EVD | Hemorrhage |
| | Brain injury |
| | Infection |
| | Overdrainage/SDH |
| Intracranial monitor | Hemorrhage |
| | Brain injury |
| | Infection |
| Lumbar drain | Overdrainage/herniation/hemorrhage |
| | Nerve root/cord injury |
| | Retained catheter |
| | Infection |

*EVD*, external ventricular drain; *SDH*, subdural hematoma.

off. A twist drill is used to open the cranium, bone fragments and dust are removed, and the dura and pia mater are pierced with a scalpel or sharp object (Fig. 41.1).

Using the demarcated lines as a guide, the trajectory at which the drill is used to create the burr hole is the same trajectory used for passing the ventricular catheter: aiming in the coronal plane toward the medial canthus of the ipsilateral eye and in the anteroposterior plane toward a point 1.5 cm anterior to the ipsilateral tragus. This trajectory is exceedingly important because it delineates the trajectory of the ventricular cannulation; if the burr hole is not created in an appropriate trajectory, the EVD cannot be optimally positioned due to being limited by its bony opening, especially if the cranium is thick. The ventricular catheter is passed to a depth of approximately 6.25 cm using the previously described trajectory. Entrance into the ventricle can often be detected tactilely as a slight change in resistance.

One may alternatively pass the ventriculostomy catheter using Dandy's principle, which states that employing a trajectory directly perpendicular to the skull will allow for ventricular cannulation. Regardless, the ventricular catheter is never passed to a depth greater than 7 cm, due to the risk of damaging the brainstem. Once the EVD is in place, it is tunneled through the skin away from the incision through a separate stab incision and is secured in place. A postprocedural head computed tomography (CT) is then obtained.

There are cases where ventricular cannulation can challenge even the most experienced of neurosurgeons. Our experience is to use the same landmarks and trajectory as outlined earlier, regardless of whether a mass lesion or significant shift is present. Most often, errant EVD passes are due to a lateral trajectory, and one must pay particular attention to avoiding an injury to the ipsilateral internal capsule. In cases in which the ventricle is believed to be cannulated with no egress of CSF, one may consider attaching a small, plungerless syringe filled with sterile saline to the ventriculostomy catheter. If the ventricle is indeed cannulated, saline should flow from the syringe, through the catheter, and into the ventricle. Of note, if one does not obtain CSF flow through the ventriculostomy after three passes, the EVD should be left in place and a head CT scan obtained to determine its position. Alternatively, image guidance or ultrasound guidance techniques may be employed (see later).

## Intracranial Pressure Monitor

Other ICP monitoring devices are used, sometimes as an adjunctive means of monitoring ICP when they are placed in tandem with an EVD, and, at other times, when slitlike ventricles preclude EVD placement. The scalp incision is made in the same location as for a ventriculostomy with a smaller drill bit and small stylet used to puncture the dura. When using microtip strain gauge or fiberoptic parenchymal monitors, the probe is advanced between 1 and 2 cm into the subcortical white matter. The microtip strain gauge probe requires being tunneled through the skin via a separate stab incision and then secured in place. The fiberoptic monitor, on the other hand, can be held in place by a fixation bolt screwed into the skull. The reduced accuracy, reliability, increased propensity for malfunction, and high cost in comparison to EVD placement are factors that must be considered prior to using these alternative ICP monitors.

## Lumbar Drain

Although cannulation of the ventricular system with an EVD is optimal in many cases, lumbar drain (LD) placement is an alternative option for a variety of pathologies. Common indications for LD placement include craniofacial trauma with CSF leak, iatrogenic CSF leak after spinal surgery, assessment for shunt responsiveness in normal-pressure hydrocephalus, and intraoperative CSF diversion for brain relaxation during operative skull-base approaches. Lumbar drainage can also be used as an adjunct in abdominal aortic aneurysm repair procedures where CSF drainage is thought to help facilitate perfusion of the spinal cord.[3]

LD placement is often undertaken at the bedside or in the operating room without fluoroscopic assistance. The patient is placed on a cardiac monitor, administered adequate sedation and analgesia, and placed in the lateral recumbent position. The L4–5 interspace is approximated by palpating the iliac crest, similar to assessment prior to lumbar puncture. After appropriate preparation of the field, a 14-gauge Tuohy needle is inserted in a midline fashion with the bevel oriented parallel to the intraspinous ligament. Once CSF has been encountered, the needle is rotated to a position where the curved end is directed cranially to allow for the insertion of the LD catheter in a cranial direction. After removal of the stylet and free egress of CSF is noted from the Tuohy needle, an 85-cm, barium-impregnated catheter is placed through the needle to a length of 40 cm. Subsequently,

**Fig. 41.1** Axial, coronal, and sagittal views of the internal and external landmarks of the skull for EVD placement are shown. The pathway of the ventricular catheter to the foramen of Monro is approximated by lines from Kocher's point to the ipsilateral medial canthus in the coronal plane and 1.5 cm anterior to the tragus in the sagittal plane. (Reprinted from *The Mont Reid Surgical Handbook*, 6th ed., Wolfgang Stehr pp. 73, 815–18. Copyright © 2008 by Saunders, an imprint of Elsevier, Inc.)

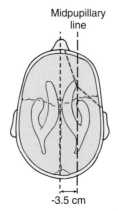
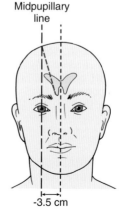
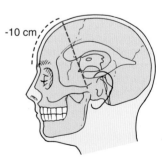

the Tuohy needle is carefully removed so as to not fracture or lacerate the catheter. Redundant catheter is secured to the lumbar skin in a circular fashion to avoid catheter displacement and reduce the risk of infection. Postprocedural imaging is not required after LD placement.

# Postoperative Complications of External Ventricular Drains and Intracranial Pressure Monitors

## Key Concepts

- Central nervous system (CNS) infection is the most common risk associated with EVD placement. Duration of drainage may play a role in incidence of infection. Institution of a standardized evidence-based protocol for EVD placement has been shown to decrease the risk of CNS infection associated with EVD use.
- Although some measure of catheter-associated hemorrhage may affect 6% to 7% of EVD placements, clinically significant hemorrhage only affects approximately 1% of patients requiring EVDs.
- Freehand placement of EVDs utilizing external landmarks results in appropriate CSF diversion approximately 90% of the time. Neurotrauma and midline shift have been shown to be predictors of catheter misplacement.

EVD and/or ICP monitor placement is one of the most commonly performed bedside procedures in the neurology intensive care unit. There are myriad indications for intracranial monitoring via EVD or intracranial pressure monitor (IPM); however, intracranial monitoring is a fundamental component in the management of primary or secondary hydrocephalus and in patients with severe traumatic brain injury. Although generally considered to be a safe bedside procedure, placement of EVDs and IPMs do carry a risk of complication, most notably, infections, hemorrhage, and misplacement.

## Infection

The most common complication associated with EVD placement is infection. In a 2006 study by Lozier et al., infection rates were found to range from 0% to 22%, with the average across 23 large studies to be 8.8%.[4] The disparate rate of infections seen among the individual studies is likely multifactorial; however, lack of a standardized definition of what constitutes a catheter-associated infection may provide a significant contribution to this confusion. The most readily accepted definition of catheter-related infection in published literature most closely resembles that advocated by Mayhall et al. and requires a positive CSF culture drawn from the ventriculostomy.[5] In contrast, Sundbärg et al. advocated for a more stringent definition of catheter-associated infection by requiring not only a positive CSF culture but also CSF pleocytosis, as well as clinical signs of fever or peripheral leukocytosis.[6] Although there are less data pertaining to the infectious complications associated with IPMs, there is a suggestion that the overall rate of infection may be lower than that of EVD, as evidenced by Guyot et al. finding a 0%

infection rate in IPMs placed in 229 neurotrauma patients.[7] Of note, when IPMs are placed in conjunction with an EVD, the combination appears to approach or exceed the infection rate of ventriculostomies alone.[8]

Gram-positive skin flora tend to be the predominant isolate from CSF cultures in patients with catheter-associated infections because they are responsible for greater than 80% of the catheter-related infections.[6] A 2005 study of both EVDs and LDs by Schade et al. supported these findings, as the group reported that gram-positive cocci were the pathogen in nearly 70% of infections in their series.[9] Antibiotic administration represents a key confounding factor; however, a 1998 study by Poon et al. found gram-positive cocci to be responsible in 26% of infections.[10] There were significantly higher proportions of resistant bacterial isolates, presumably due to continuous antibiotic use in the study population.

A number of studies have been undertaken to determine risk factors associated with CSF infection in patients undergoing ventricular catheter placement. In their review of EVD-related infections, Lozier and colleagues noted the most common and most likely factors to be associated with EVD infection (Box 41.1).[4] Of the risk factors listed as positive predictors, all but duration of catheterization were found to be highly supported in the literature. Duration of catheterization as a risk factor for CSF infection appears to be a matter of clinical equipoise: in the Lozier metaanalysis, the authors found 10 studies, totaling 2046 catheters in 1698 patients, that found a correlation between catheterization duration and CSF infection, and 7 studies,

---

**Box 41.1   Risk Factors for CSF Infection in Patients Undergoing External Ventricular Drain Placement**

**Risk factors for cerebrospinal fluid infection in patients who underwent ventriculostomy[a]**
Factors associated with CSF infection

Intraventricular hemorrhage
Subarachnoid hemorrhage
Operative depressed cranial fracture
Basilar cranial fracture with CSF leak
Neurosurgical operation
Ventriculostomy irrigation
Systemic infection
Duration of catheterization

Factors not associated with CSF infection

Venue of ventriculostomy insertion
Corticosteroids
CSF pleocytosis
Catheter manipulations and leaks

Multiple catheters
Concomitant ICP monitors
CSF drainage
Closed head trauma
Tumor
Intracerebral hemorrhage

[a]CSF, cerebrospinal fluid; ICP, intracranial pressure.
Reprinted from Lozier AP, et al. Ventriculostomy-related infections: a critical review of the literature. *Neurosurgery.* 2002;51(1): 170–82.

consisting of 2199 catheterizations in 2113 patients, that did not report a correlation between duration and catheterization. In a retrospective analysis of 584 patients undergoing EVD placement, Holloway et al. found that there was a steadily increasing daily rate of infection until day 10, after which the infection rate reached a plateau.[11] Notably, the group also found that the prophylactic replacement of catheters prior to day 5 did not decrease the infection rate in this population. Winfield et al., however, found that the daily rate of infection across the duration of catheterization was unchanged and independent of duration of catheter placement.[12] Similarly, Park et al. found that after a plateau at day 4, daily infection rates appear to stay stable in a 1% to 2% range until day 14.[13]

There is evidence to support a reduction in EVD-related infections by instituting a bundled evidence-based protocol for drain insertion and management. van Hall et al. found a greater than 300% reduction in EVD-related infections (37%–11.2%) at their institution after initiating a standardized protocol involving hygienic training of those involved with bedside catheter management (disinfection of Luer lock connections when sampling CSF and sterile glove use) and changes in catheter insertion and maintenance practices (use of single-dose prophylactic antibiotics, total hair removal with clippers, and a whole head dressing).[14] Dasic and colleagues also found a significant reduction in EVD-related infections (27%–12%) at their institution following a protocol that mandated EVD placement in the operating room, requiring the use of prophylactic antibiotics on catheter placement, and subcutaneous tunneling of the catheter at least 10 cm.[15]

## Hemorrhage

The reported rate of EVD-related hemorrhage in the literature ranges widely. Recent metaanalyses by both Binz and Bauer have found the cumulative hemorrhage rate associated with EVD placement to be 6% to 7%, with an incidence of a clinically significant hemorrhage of less than 1%.[16,17] The definition of clinically significant hemorrhage in both of these metaanalyses was hemorrhage that (1) caused a change in neurological examination, (2) required surgical evacuation, or (3) led to patient death. The routine use of postoperative CT scanning does appear to influence the rate of discovering both significant and nonsignificant hemorrhages. Both Maniker and Gardner reported greater than 30% rates of catheter associated hemorrhage at centers where routine post procedural CT scan is the accepted practice.[18,19] Interestingly, most of these hemorrhages appear to be nonsignificant, because the rate of neurological changes or need for surgical intervention across both studies (2.5 and 0.6%, respectively) was not significantly different than that seen in larger meta analyses (Fig. 41.2, Table 41.2).

Risk factors associated with EVD-related hemorrhage have not been systematically investigated in the existing literature; however, a number of single-center studies have demonstrated interesting correlations. Maniker et al. found that patients with preexisting cerebrovascular disease were more likely to have hemorrhagic complications, but did not mention use of antiplatelet or anticoagulant medications as a possible confounding factor. Huh and colleagues also confirmed the findings of the former study and showed a trend toward significance ($p = 0.056$) between incidence of hemorrhagic complications and premorbid antiplatelet or anticoagulant therapy use.[20] The authors also found increased age and bilateral catheter placement to be independent risk factors for hemorrhagic complications.

Formal recommendations regarding venous thromboembolism prophylaxis for patients with or requiring external ventricular drainage do not exist; however, there does not appear to be an increased risk in catheter-related hemorrhage in patients who begin chemical prophylaxis 24 hours after placement.[21] Equally limited data exist for

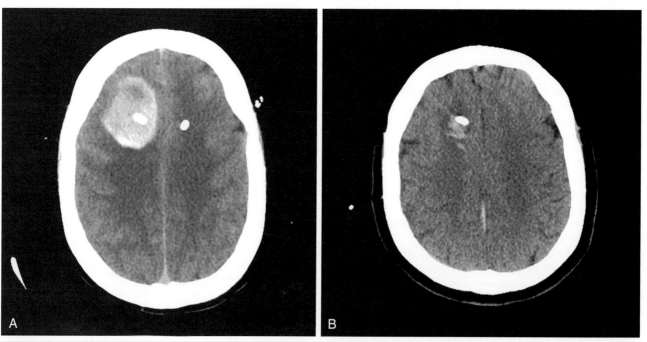

**Fig. 41.2** Noncontrast CT scans demonstrating significant EVD-related hemorrhage (**A,** patient required placement of a contralateral EVD for management) and incidentally found EVD-related hemorrhage (**B,** patient was observed with serial scans).

**Table 41.2** Hemorrhage Rates Associated with External Ventricular Drain Placement.

STUDIES WITH ROUTINE POSTPROCEDURE CT SCANS

| Studies | Hemorrhages | Significant | EVDs |
|---|---|---|---|
| Ehtisham et al. [8] | 6 | 0 | 29 |
| Maniker et al. [1] | 52 | 4 | 160 |
| Paramore and Turner [4] | 2 | 2 | 253 |
| Rhodes et al. [6] | 6 | 0 | 66 |
| Anderson et al. [7] | 12 | 1 | 68 |
| Wiesmann and Mayer [13] | 6 | 0 | 92 |
| Naryan et al. [12] | 4 | 1 | 207 |
| Total | 88 | 8 | 875 |

Hemorrhage rate (10.06%); significant rate (0.91%)

STUDIES WITHOUT ROUTINE POSTPROCEDURE CT SCANS

| Studies | Hemorrhages | Significant | EVDs |
|---|---|---|---|
| Guyot et al. [3] | 9 | 2 | 274 |
| North and Reilly [5] | 2 | 1 | 199 |
| Roitberg et al. [10] | 1 | 0 | 103 |
| Leung et al. [2] | 1 | 0 | 133 |
| Friedman and Vries [11] | 1 | 0 | 100 |
| Khanna et al. [9] | 0 | 0 | 106 |
| Total | 14 | 3 | 915 |

Hemorrhage rate (1.53%); significant rate (0.33%).
CT, computed tomography; EVDs, external ventricular drains
Reprinted from Binz DD, Toussaint III LG, Friedman JA. Hemorrhagic complications of ventriculostomy placement: a meta-analysis. Neurocrit Care 2009;10(2): 253–56.

anticoagulant management during the process of EVD removal. At our institution, a single dose of low-molecular-weight heparin or subcutaneous heparin is held prior to the removal of the hardware, after which the medication is allowed to continue on its regular dosing schedule.

Whereas the infectious risk of IPMs appears to be lower than that of EVDs, the risk for hemorrhage appears to be similar, and in some cases (generally due to indication for monitoring) greater than its counterpart. In a large single-center study of 1000 patients undergoing placement of the Camino IPM (Integra, Inc., Plainsboro, NJ), Gelabert-Gonzalez et al. found that 8.7% of patients with preexisting coagulopathy (abnormality in at least one coagulation parameter) and 1.2% of patients without experienced a hemorrhage associated with IPM placement.[22] Six of these patients (0.6% of the study population) required surgical evacuation of the associated hematoma. Interestingly, among the six patients who underwent surgery, none were coagulopathic prior to IPM placement.

Due to its association with intracranial hypertension, ICP monitoring has become commonplace in patients with fulminant hepatic failure. Given the baseline coagulopathy as a result of their condition, this cohort represents a key subsegment of the population, and putatively, one especially predisposed to hemorrhagic complications after IPM placement. A 1993 study by Blei and colleagues demonstrated

that 1% of epidural monitor placements and 4% to 5% of intraparenchymal or subdural monitor placements in patients with fulminant hepatic failure were complicated by fatal hemorrhage.[23] One decade later, apparently due to a trend toward decreased intraparenchymal and subdural monitor use, Vaquero and colleagues reported an improved 10.8% risk of procedure-related hemorrhage with only two fatalities (both of which were associated with subdural placement of epidural monitors).[24]

## Misplacement

Given that EVD placement is generally done freehand, one of the potentially expected complications of placement is malpositioning of the catheter. Analysis of freehand catheter placement at a single high-volume neurosurgical center was undertaken by Kakarla et al. in 2008 and demonstrated 87% functional accuracy (functional placement in either the ipsilateral frontal horn [77%] or functional placement in the contralateral frontal horn or noneloquent cortex [10%]).[25] Traumatic injury as an indication for catheter placement and presence of midline shift were both associated with catheter misplacement; however, operator experience was not. Similarly, both Patil and Saladino found that nearly 90% of catheters were placed in an appropriate location.[26,27] Patil et al. went on to describe that traumatic indication was the only factor associated with misplacement and that despite the fact that a Ghajar guide was used in 15% of the study population, its use was not associated with an increase in the accuracy of catheter placement (Fig. 41.3).

# Postoperative Complications of Lumbar Drains

## Key Concepts

- Intracranial hemorrhage, intracranial hypotension, and infection have all been rare but reported complications of LD placement.
- Postural and overdrainage headaches are common in patients undergoing lumbar drainage and will resolve with a decrease in drainage rate and analgesia.

## Clinical Pearl

Unintended rapid drainage from a lumbar drain after cranial surgery (i.e., drain placed for skull-base case with potential CSF leak) can cause central herniation and rapid deterioration.

Though relatively noninvasive by its nature, lumbar CSF diversion can carry with it significant consequences, namely intracranial hemorrhage, intracranial hypotension, and infection.

### Intracranial Hemorrhage

In a 2008 study assessing the use of lumbar drainage for normal-pressure hydrocephalus in 233 patients, Governale

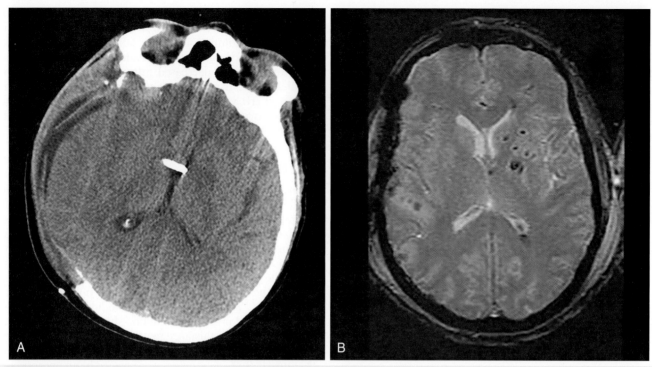

**Fig. 41.3** A noncontrast CT scan of the head demonstrating catheter crossing the septum and terminating in the contralateral caudate **(A)**. Axial SWAN MRI demonstrating a number of punctate areas of cortical injury from misplaced catheters **(B)**.

et al. found a 1.7% frequency of symptomatic intracranial hemorrhage associated with lumbar drainage.[28] Only one of the three patients with lumbar drainage–associated subdural hematomas in the study required surgical drainage. Similarly, in a series of 486 patients treated with lumbar drainage for abdominal aortic aneurysm repair, Wynn et al. found a 3.5% rate of intracranial hemorrhage with two patients requiring subdural hematoma evacuation, and three patients (including the two operative subdural hematomas) died secondary to intracranial processes.[29] Higher volume of spinal fluid drainage during abdominal aortic aneurysm surgery was found to be a significant risk factor in developing intracranial hemorrhage after the procedure.

### Intracranial Hypotension

Intracranial hypotension leading to transtentorial herniation or an acquired Chiari malformation has been reported in the literature as possible side effects of lumbar drainage. Although not described in large trials, a number of case reports have documented neurological dysfunction with radiographic evidence of intracranial hypotension (tonsillar herniation, diffuse meningeal enhancement, obliteration of basal cisterns) that have largely been reversible, if detected early, with cessation of lumbar drainage or administration of an epidural blood patch to a persistent leak from an LD catheter.[30–32]

### Infection

Rates of CNS infection associated with lumbar drainage appear to be less than that of external ventricular drainage. Rates observed in the reviewed studies ranged from 0.8% to 7%.[9,28,33] In the one study that reported bacteriology, contaminants were largely skin flora and not dissimilar to infectious profiles of EVDs.

### Minor Side Effects

Temporary nerve root irritation and transient headache are the two most common minor complications discussed in the literature. Shapiro et al. reported a 24% rate of temporary radiculopathy that resolved upon removal of the indwelling catheter. Three of the six patients in the Governale et al. normal-pressure hydrocephalus trial who complained of radiculopathy required premature removal of the catheter and discontinuation of the trial. Transient "low pressure" headaches can be seen in upwards of 60% of patients undergoing lumbar spinal drainage and typically resolve with a reduction in drainage rate and analgesia.[33,34]

## Perioperative Considerations of Intracranial Monitoring and Lumbar Drainage

### Key Concepts

- Antimicrobial catheters and percutaneous tunneling of catheters have been shown to reduce the incidence of ventriculostomy-related infections in patients requiring EVDs.
- Routine prophylactic antibiotics, catheter exchange, and daily CSF sampling are not supported in the literature as factors that reduce ventriculostomy-associated infections.

### Clinical Pearl

Slow wean (over 96 hours with progressive increase in height draining apparatus) of ventriculostomies may not have any benefit over rapid wean (immediate closure) in preventing long-term shunt dependence.[35]

## Adjunct Technologies for Catheter Placement

As described earlier, the freehand, external landmark-assisted placement of EVDs can occasionally lead to misplaced and nonfunctional catheters. Some have advocated the use of noninvasive instrumentation, such as the Ghajar guide (Neurodynamics, New York, NY), a rigid tripod device through which the catheter is placed to ensure a perpendicular trajectory from the burr hole location to the ventricular space. In a prospective comparison between Ghajar guide use and freehand placement, O'Leary et al. found that the Ghajar guide did allow for more accurate placement of the catheter tip in/near the foramen of Monro but did not lead to an increased rate of ventricular cannulation.[36] With regard to noninvasive imaging techniques, bedside ultrasound utilizing a "burr hole" probe has also been used in pediatric and adult populations with good results, especially in patients with challenging anatomy or mass lesions.[37,38] Noninvasive image guidance techniques comparable to intraoperative neuronavigation have been described in the literature and may increase catheter accuracy, but will require further analysis prior to widespread acceptance.[39,40]

## Catheter Selection

A number of antimicrobial-impregnated catheters are available and have been utilized with good results. Zabramski et al. published one of the first randomized controlled trials comparing standard silicone catheter use to rifampin- and minocycline-impregnated catheters, finding that the use of antibiotic-impregnated catheters led to a sevenfold decrement in the rate of positive CSF cultures and a twofold reduction in catheter colonization.[41] Outside of the study group, the only variables that were noted to correlate with positive CSF cultures were the location in which the catheter placement occurred (emergency room) and presence of another infection. This result was echoed in a study by Abla et al., who demonstrated that the use of rifampin/minocycline- and rifampin/clindamycin-impregnated catheters resulted in no documented CSF infections across 129 study patients over an 18-month period.[42] Silver-impregnated catheters have been studied with similar results to antibiotic-impregnated catheters, reducing infections by one half compared with plain catheters.[43] Both silver-impregnated and standard catheters demonstrated an infectious peak on the fifth day after catheter placement, but only the standard catheters demonstrated a second, larger peak on the tenth day after placement. Interestingly, the authors also noted that the silver-impregnated catheter group had a significantly lower shunt conversion rate, hypothesizing that the silver impregnation not only had an effect on late infections while the catheter was in place, but also after its removal. Conversely, Kaufman et al. noted that hydrophilic-coated catheters did not provide a reduction in infection rates compared with standard silastic catheters.[44]

## Percutaneous Tunneling

Since the 1980 report by Friedman et al. regarding infectious control associated with the percutaneous tunneling of external ventricular catheters, the standard protocol for EVD placement has involved tunneling of the catheter to a separate exit corridor approximately 5 cm from the placement of the burr hole.[45] In 1995 Khanna et al. expanded upon this concept, developing the long tunnel ventriculostomy as a form of infection control for patients who require CSF diversion for an extended period.[46] The procedure is largely similar to that involved with standard ventriculostomy placement, with the exception of involving percutaneous tunneling of the catheter to the upper chest area. Although the authors of the original study did not encounter any CNS infections in the first 16 days of drainage and only 4% infection rate overall, a follow-up study by Leung et al. demonstrated both early infections and a total infectious rate similar to their standard counterparts.[47]

## Prophylactic Antibiotics

The use of continuous prophylactic antibiotics in patients with EVDs is not supported by current evidence.[48-52] A 1999 survey by Prabhu et al. found that 72% of responding university programs used some form of prophylactic antibiotic in patients receiving EVDs; however, greater than 60% of the group reported significant intrainstitutional variances in application of antibiotics, suggesting a nonstandardized practice.[49] In a recent metaanalysis, Sonabend et al. suggested that prophylactic antibiotics may lead to decreased incidence of CSF infection in patients with EVDs, but noted that studies that would support this conclusion were widely heterogeneous in their design and tended to have been performed prior to the advent of antibiotic-impregnated catheters.[50] In fact, only two randomized controlled trials investigating the use of prophylactic antibiotics were cited in the metaanalysis: one demonstrated no benefit with prophylactic antibiotic administration. Furthermore, as mentioned earlier, use of broad-spectrum antibiotics may select for resistant bacterial strains, lead to increased incidence of antibiotic-related complications (allergies, *Clostridium difficile* colitis), and a significant increase in costs. In a study of 308 patients over 2 years, Alleyne et al. demonstrated that prophylactic antibiotics did not reduce the rate of ventriculitis in patients with EVDs and suggested that discontinuation of the use of prophylactic antibiotics would significantly decrease the institutional direct drug costs for this patient population.[51] Additionally, May et al. observed that in a cohort of 279 trauma patients who underwent ICP monitor placement (ventriculostomies, intraparenchymal pressure monitors, or subarachnoid bolts) that broad-spectrum antibiotics did not reduce the risk of CNS infection and only stood to increase the shift to resistant organisms in subsequent infectious complications.[52]

## Catheter Exchange

Regular catheter exchange at 5-day intervals has been postulated in the past to be an effective way of reducing catheter-related CSF infections. The results of randomized controlled trials by Wong and Holloway demonstrate that this practice does not achieve the desired results; rather, Wong et al. demonstrated a nonsignificant increase in infection rates (7.8% vs. 3.8%) in the patient population that underwent regular catheter exchange.[11,53] Additionally, Lo et al. found that among patients who underwent routine catheter exchange, the second and third catheters placed had a significantly higher risk of infection than the first, theorizing that infection may be introduced into the CNS on placement of the drain, not due to retrograde colonization.[54]

## Routine Cerebrospinal Fluid Analysis

In planning frequency of CSF sampling for a patient with an indwelling ventricular catheter and closed CSF collection system, published data would not support daily sampling as a method for predicting CNS infection. Hader et al. analyzed seven catheter-related CNS infections from a sample of 160 catheters over 13 years and found that routine daily CSF cell count and culture analysis did not predict infections before clinical signs and symptoms (peripheral leukocytosis and fever) appeared.[55] Similarly, in a series of 230 patients, Schade et al. discovered that among the 22 patients who developed catheter-related bacterial meningitis, there was no difference in CSF parameters (leukocyte count, protein concentration, glucose concentration, and CSF/blood glucose ratio) in the 3 days preceding diagnosis of meningitis, compared with controls.[56] The authors also suggested that the low specificity of CSF Gram stain makes it a less reliable diagnostic tool when screening for catheter-related infection. Conversely, Pfisterer et al. found that leukocytosis on CSF cell count was associated with catheter infection; however, this was only correlated on the same day as the positive CSF culture.[57]

## References

1. Brain Trauma Foundation, American Association of Neurological Surgeons, Congress of Neurological Surgeons, Joint Section on Neurotrauma and Critical Care, AANS/CNS, Bratton SL, Chestnut RM, et al. Guidelines for the management of severe traumatic brain injury. VIII. Intracranial pressure thresholds. *J Neurotrauma.* 2007;(24 suppl 1):S55–S58.
2. Timofeev I, Dahyot-Fizelier C, Keong N, et al. Ventriculostomy for control of raised ICP in acute traumatic brain injury. *Acta Neurochir Supp.* 2009;99–104. [Internet]. Springer Vienna [cited 2014 Mar 24]. Available from: http://link.springer.com/chapter/10.1007/978-3-211-85578-2_20.
3. Acher CW, Wynn MM, Hoch JR, Popic P, Archibald J, Turnipseed WD. Combined use of cerebral spinal fluid drainage and naloxone reduces the risk of paraplegia in thoracoabdominal aneurysm repair. *J Vasc Surg.* 1994;19(2):236–249.
4. Lozier AP, Sciacca RR, Romagnoli MF, Connolly Jr ES. Ventriculostomy-related infections: a critical review of the literature. *Neurosurgery.* 2002;51(1):170–182.
5. Mayhall CG, Archer NH, Lamb VA, et al. Ventriculostomy-related infections. *N Engl J Med.* 1984;310(9):553–559.
6. Sundbärg G, Nordström C-H, Söderström S. Complications due to prolonged ventricular fluid pressure recording. *Br J Neurosurg.* 1988;2(4):485–495.
7. Guyot LL, Dowling C, Diaz FG, Michael DB. Cerebral monitoring devices: analysis of complications. In: *Intracranial Pressure and Neuromonitoring in Brain Injury:* (71):1998:47–49.
8. Bekar A, Gören S, Korfali E, Aksoy K, Boyaci S. Complications of brain tissue pressure monitoring with a fiberoptic device. *Neurosurg Rev.* 1998;21(4):254–259.
9. Schade RP, Schinkel J, Visser LG, Van Dijk JMC, Voormolen JH, Kuijper EJ. Bacterial meningitis caused by the use of ventricular or lumbar cerebrospinal fluid catheters. *J Neurosurg.* 2005;102(2):229–234.
10. Poon WS, Ng S, Wai S. CSF antibiotic prophylaxis for neurosurgical patients with ventriculostomy: a randomised study. In: *Intracranial Pressure and Neuromonitoring in Brain Injury [Internet]:* 1998: 146–148. [cited 2014 Mar 24]. Available from: http://link.springer.com/chapter/10.1007/978-3-7091-6475-4_43.
11. Holloway KL, Barnes T, Choi S, et al. Ventriculostomy infections: the effect of monitoring duration and catheter exchange in 584 patients. *J Neurosurg.* 1996;85(3):419–424.

12. Winfield JA, Rosenthal P, Kanter RK, Casella G. Duration of intracranial pressure monitoring does not predict daily risk of infectious complications. *Neurosurgery.* 1993;33(3):424–431.
13. Park P, Garton HJ, Kocan MJ, Thompson BG. Risk of infection with prolonged ventricular catheterization. *Neurosurgery.* 2004;55(3):594–601.
14. Leverstein-van Hall MA, Hopmans TE, van der Sprenkel JWB, et al. A bundle approach to reduce the incidence of external ventricular and lumbar drain-related infections: clinical article. *J Neurosurg.* 2010;112(2):345–353.
15. Dasic D, Hanna SJ, Bojanic S, Kerr RC. External ventricular drain infection: the effect of a strict protocol on infection rates and a review of the literature. *Br J Neurosurg.* 2006;20(5):296–300.
16. Binz DD, Toussaint III LG, Friedman JA. Hemorrhagic complications of ventriculostomy placement: a meta-analysis. *Neurocrit Care.* 2009;10(2):253–256.
17. Bauer DF, Razdan SN, Bartolucci AA, Markert JM. Meta-analysis of hemorrhagic complications from ventriculostomy placement by neurosurgeons. *Neurosurgery.* 2011;69(2):255–260.
18. Maniker AH, Vaynman AY, Karimi RJ, Sabit AO, Holland B. Hemorrhagic complications of external ventricular drainage. *Neurosurgery.* 2006;59(4):ONS419–ONS424.
19. Gardner PA, Engh J, Atteberry D, Moossy JJ. Hemorrhage rates after external ventricular drain placement: clinical article. *J Neurosurg.* 2009;110(5):1021–1025.
20. Huh J, Joo WI, Chough CK, Park HK, Lee KJ, Rha HK. Hemorrhagic complications induced by external ventricular draining catheters. *Korean J Cerebrovasc Surg.* 2011;13:256–262.
21. Tanweer O, Boah A, Huang PP. Risks for hemorrhagic complications after placement of external ventricular drains with early chemical prophylaxis against venous thromboembolisms. *J Neurosurg.* 2013;119(5):1309–1313.
22. Gelabert-Gonzalez M, Ginesta-Galan V, Sernamito-Garcia R, Allut AG, Bandin-Diéguez J, Rumbo RM. The Camino intracranial pressure device in clinical practice. Assessment in a 1000 cases. *Acta Neurochir (Wien).* 2006;148(4):435–441.
23. Blei AT, Olafsson S, Webster S, Levy R. Complications of intracranial pressure monitoring in fulminant hepatic failure. *Lancet.* 1993;341(8838):157–158.
24. Vaquero J, Fontana RJ, Larson AM, et al. Complications and use of intracranial pressure monitoring in patients with acute liver failure and severe encephalopathy. *Liver Transpl.* 2005;11(12):1581–1589.
25. Kakarla UK, Chang SW, Theodore N, Spetzler RF, Kim LJ. Safety and accuracy of bedside external ventricular drain placement. *Neurosurgery.* 2008;63(1):ONS162–ONS167.
26. Patil V, Lacson R, Vosburgh KG, et al. Factors associated with external ventricular drain placement accuracy: data from an electronic health record repository. *Acta Neurochir (Wien).* 2013;155(9):1773–1779.
27. Saladino A, White JB, Wijdicks EFM, Lanzino G. Malplacement of ventricular catheters by neurosurgeons: a single institution experience. *Neurocrit Care.* 2009;10(2):248–252.
28. Governale LS, Fein N, Logsdon J, Black PM. Techniques and complications of external lumbar drainage for normal pressure hydrocephalus. *Neurosurgery.* 2008;63(4):379–384.
29. Wynn MM, Mell MW, Tefera G, Hoch JR, Acher CW. Complications of spinal fluid drainage in thoracoabdominal aortic aneurysm repair: a report of 486 patients treated from 1987 to 2008. *J Vasc Surg.* 2009;49(1):29–35.
30. Snow RB, Kuhel W, Martin SB. Prolonged lumbar spinal drainage after the resection of tumors of the skull base: a cautionary note. *Neurosurgery.* 1991;28(6):880–883.
31. Guido LJ, Patterson Jr RH. Focal neurological deficits secondary to intraoperative CSF drainage: successful resolution with an epidural blood patch: Report of two cases. *J Neurosurg.* 1976;45(3):348–351.
32. Samadani U, Huang JH, Baranov D, Zager EL, Grady MS. Intracranial hypotension after intraoperative lumbar cerebrospinal fluid drainage. *Neurosurgery.* 2003;52(1):148–152.
33. Shapiro SA, Scully T. Closed continuous drainage of cerebrospinal fluid via a lumbar subarachnoid catheter for treatment or prevention of cranial/spinal cerebrospinal fluid fistula. *Neurosurgery.* 1992;30(2):241–246.
34. Kitchel SH, Eismont FJ, Green BA. Closed subarachnoid drainage for management of cerebrospinal fluid leakage after an operation on the spine. *J Bone Jt Surg.* 1989;71(7):984–987.

35. Klopfenstein JD, Kim LJ, Feiz-Erfan I, et al. Comparison of rapid and gradual weaning from external ventricular drainage in patients with aneurysmal subarachnoid hemorrhage: a prospective randomized trial. *J Neurosurg.* 2004;100(2):225–229.
36. O'Leary ST, Kole MK, Hoover DA, Hysell SE, Thomas A, Shaffrey CI. Efficacy of the Ghajar Guide revisited: a prospective study. *J Neurosurg.* 2000;92(5):801–803.
37. Phillips SB, Gates M, Krishnamurthy S. Strategic placement of bedside ventriculostomies using ultrasound image guidance: report of three cases. *Neurocrit Care.* 2012;17(2):255–259.
38. Whitehead WE, Jea A, Vachhrajani S, Kulkarni AV, Drake JM. Accurate placement of cerebrospinal fluid shunt ventricular catheters with real-time ultrasound guidance in older children without patent fontanelles. *J Neurosurg.* 2007 Nov;107(5 suppl):406–410.
39. Mahan M, Spetzler RF, Nakaji P. Electromagnetic stereotactic navigation for external ventricular drain placement in the intensive care unit. *J Clin Neurosci.* 2013;20(12):1718–1722.
40. Gautschi O, Smoll N, Kotowski M. Non-assisted versus neuro-navigated and XperCT-guided external ventricular catheter placement: a comparative cadaver study. *Acta Neurochir (Wien).* 156(4):777–785.
41. Zabramski JM, Whiting D, Darouiche RO, et al. Efficacy of antimicrobial-impregnated external ventricular drain catheters: a prospective, randomized, controlled trial. *J Neurosurg.* 2003;98(4):725–730.
42. Abla AA, Zabramski JM, Jahnke HK, Fusco D, Nakaji P. Comparison of two antibiotic-impregnated ventricular catheters: a prospective sequential series trial. *Neurosurgery.* 2011;68(2):437–442.
43. Keong NCH, Bulters DO, Richards HK, et al. The SILVER (silver impregnated line versus EVD randomized trial): a double-blind, prospective, randomized, controlled trial of an intervention to reduce the rate of external ventricular drain infection. *Neurosurgery.* 2012;71(2):394–404.
44. Kaufmann AM, Lye T, Brevner A, et al. Infection rates in standard vs. hydrogel coated ventricular catheters. *Can J Neurol Sci.* 2004;31(4):506–510.
45. Friedman WA, Vries JK. Percutaneous tunnel ventriculostomy: summary of 100 procedures. *J Neurosurg.* 1980;53(5):662–665.
46. Khanna RK, Rosenblum ML, Rock JP, Malik GM. Prolonged external ventricular drainage with percutaneous long-tunnel ventriculostomies. *J Neurosurg.* 1995;83(5):791–794.
47. Leung GKK, Ng KB, Taw BBT, Fan YW. Extended subcutaneous tunnelling technique for external ventricular drainage. *Br J Neurosurg.* 2007;21(4):359–364.
48. Wyler AR, Kelly WA. Use of antibiotics with external ventriculostomies. *J Neurosurg.* 1972;37(2):185–187.
49. Prabhu VC, Kaufman HH, Voelker JL, et al. Prophylactic antibiotics with intracranial pressure monitors and external ventricular drains: a review of the evidence. *Surg Neurol.* 1999;52(3):226–237.
50. Sonabend AM, Korenfeld Y, Crisman C, Badjatia N, Mayer SA, Connolly Jr ES. Prevention of ventriculostomy-related infections with prophylactic antibiotics and antibiotic-coated external ventricular drains: a systematic review. *Neurosurgery.* 2011;68(4):996–1005.
51. Alleyne Jr CH, Hassan M, Zabramski JM. The efficacy and cost of prophylactic and periprocedural antibiotics in patients with external ventricular drains. *Neurosurgery.* 2000;47(5):1124–1129.
52. May AK, Fleming SB, Carpenter RO, et al. Influence of broad-spectrum antibiotic prophylaxis on intracranial pressure monitor infections and subsequent infectious complications in head-injured patients. *Surg Infect.* 2006;7(5):409–417.
53. Wong GKC, Poon WS, Wai S, Yu LM, Lyon D, Lam JMK. Failure of regular external ventricular drain exchange to reduce cerebrospinal fluid infection: result of a randomised controlled trial. *J Neurol Neurosurg Psychiatry.* 2002;73(6):759–761.
54. Lo CH, Spelman D, Bailey M, Cooper DJ, Rosenfeld JV, Brecknell JE. External ventricular drain infections are independent of drain duration: an argument against elective revision. *J Neurosurg.* 2007;106(3):378–383.
55. Hader WJ, Steinbok P. The value of routine cultures of the cerebrospinal fluid in patients with external ventricular drains. *Neurosurgery.* 2000;46(5):1149–1155.
56. Schade RP, Schinkel J, Roelandse FW, et al. Lack of value of routine analysis of cerebrospinal fluid for prediction and diagnosis of external drainage-related bacterial meningitis. *J Neurosurg.* 2006;104(1):101–108.
57. Pfisterer W, Mühlbauer M, Czech T, Reinprecht A. Early diagnosis of external ventricular drainage infection: results of a prospective study. *J Neurol Neurosurg Psychiatry.* 2003;74(7):929–932.

# 42 *Management of Flaps*

ANTHONY J. WILSON, CATHERINE S. CHANG, and SUHAIL KANCHWALA

## Introduction

### Key Concepts

- Free flap reconstruction is the most complex form of reconstruction.
- Multiple types of free flaps exist based on their composition.
- Commonly used free flaps are the anterolateral thigh (ALT) flap, free latissimus, and the transversus abdominus myocutaneous (TRAM) flap.

Reconstructive surgery aims to safely provide lasting wound coverage while simultaneously restoring form and function with minimal donor site morbidity. Plastic surgeons are often consulted for closure of complex defects. To determine optimal closure methods with minimal morbidity, the reconstructive ladder is utilized. The ladder starts with the simplest and ends with the most complex reconstructive option: autologous free tissue transfer. This chapter will focus specifically on free tissue transfer for coverage of common neurosurgical defects. Principles of flap selection, perioperative care, and potential complications are discussed.

Free flap reconstruction in neurosurgical patients is indicated when there is significant local tissue loss and/or lack of periosteum, making either local flap or skin graft nonviable options. Free tissue transfer may also be the preferred means of reconstruction in the setting of radiated wound or prior to local reconstruction when the likelihood of delayed healing and development of a chronic wound is highest (Fig. 42.1).[1–4] Ultimately, the decision to pursue free flap reconstruction is dependent on extensive conversation and consultation between the plastic surgeon and neurosurgical colleagues. Given the donor site morbidity and potential for repeated surgical procedures, thorough patient counseling is also a necessity.

Autologous free tissue transfer, or "free flap," reconstruction is a microsurgical procedure based on elevating an anatomically defined segment of donor tissue and directly transferring this donor tissue to a recipient bed via microanastomosis of artery and vein(s). A flap is characterized by its own distinct blood supply. Flap selection is based upon its anatomy, application, and composition. Flaps are often classified based upon anatomical components. There are eight different types: (1) fascial, (2) fasciocutaneous, (3) muscle, (4) musculocutaneous, (5) musculomucosal, (6) enteric, (7) omentum, and (8) osseus. With respect to neurosurgical wounds, the most commonly used free flaps are muscle with a separate skin graft and musculocutaneous flaps.

The major vascular supply of a free flap is referred to as its *pedicle*. Pedicles are composed of an artery, vein, and usually the motor nerve(s) to the muscle. A dominant pedicle is sufficient to independently sustain the entire muscle and flap. A minor pedicle, in contrast, will supply a certain portion of the muscle but is not sufficient to sustain the entire muscle. Many muscles have multiple discrete sources of blood supply that individually supply a segment of the muscle; as a result, they are termed *segmental pedicles*. In the case of a myocutaneous flap or cutaneous flap, the pedicle or segmental pedicle further divides into branches termed *perforators*. These perforators are essential for perfusion of any skin and subcutaneous tissue transferred with the flap. A lack of sufficient perforators may result in partial or total flap loss (i.e., fat necrosis) or skin sloughing.[5]

The most commonly used flaps to reconstruct wounds after neurosurgical procedures include the ALT, latissimus dorsi flap, and TRAM.[1,6] In the following sections the principle anatomy and surgical technique are described for each of these commonly seen free flaps. Awareness of the intraoperative sequence will provide an important foundation for perioperative and postoperative management of patients with free flap reconstructions.

## ANTERIOR LATERAL THIGH FLAP (FIG. 42.2)

### Anatomy

This is a fasciocutaneous flap located over the middle third of the lateral thigh between the rectus femoris and vastus lateralis. The dominant pedicle is the septocutaneous branch of the descending branch of the lateral femoral circumflex artery and its venae comitantes. Along with the pedicle runs the nerve to the vastus lateralis. This flap can be harvested with both muscle and a skin island. Skin graft is not necessary.

### Flap Elevation

A line is drawn from the anterosuperior iliac spine to the lateral patella. This marks the septum between the rectus femoris and vastus lateralis. Individual perforators are found along this line. An incision is made medially in a vertical fashion and incised through the deep fascia until the rectus femoris muscle is identified. The septum between the rectus femoris and vastus lateralis is dissected to locate the pedicle, which is then followed proximally to its connection with the descending branch of the lateral femoral circumflex artery. There are usually two veins accompanying the artery. Sometimes there is a lack of septocutaneous perforators. In these cases the dissection is continued deep to the medial border of the vastus lateralis. If no appropriately sized perforators from the descending lateral femoral circumflex to the vastus lateralis are identified, dissection

439

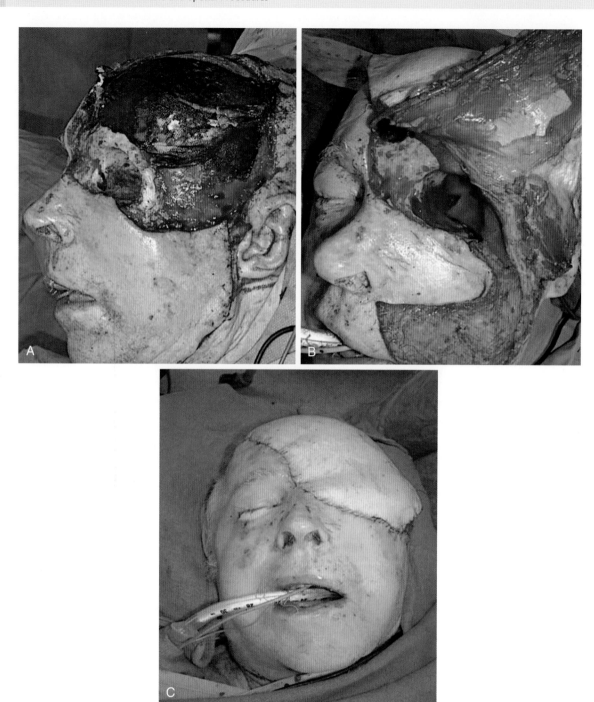

**Fig. 42.1 (A)** This patient has a large defect secondary to invasive squamous cell carcinoma without local reconstructive options. **(B)** Free ALT (musculofasciocutaneous) was used for reconstruction. The pedicle was anastomosed to the facial arteries. **(C)** The flap with its skin paddle is now inset, providing good coverage.

proceeds proximally to locate the transverse branch of the lateral femoral circumflex artery.

After suitable perforators have been identified, the inferior and lateral borders of the flap are determined. Flap elevation then is completed in the subfascial plane. The pedicle is then traced as proximally as the profunda femoris artery and vein, depending on the length needed.

The flap donor site is usually closed primarily. However, if the donor site is wider than 8 centimeters, a skin graft from the contralateral thigh may be harvested.

## LATISSIMUS DORSI FLAP (FIG. 42.3)

### Anatomy

This is a muscle/musculocutaneous flap. The muscle originates at the spinous processes of vertebrae T7–L5, thoracolumbar fascia, iliac crest, inferior third or fourth rib, and inferior angle of the scapula and inserts onto the floor of the humerus. The dominant pedicle is the thoracodorsal artery and venae comitantes. The pedicle is usually located in the deep surface of the muscle in the posterior axilla,

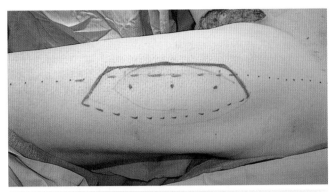

**Fig. 42.2** Anterolateral thigh flap (ALT). Here the flap is marked out with the three main perforators marked by the asterisks.

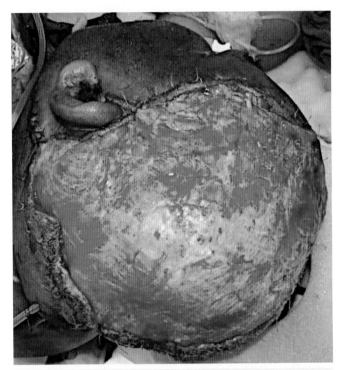

**Fig. 42.3** Free latissimus muscle. Unlike the ALT, this flap is not usually transferred with a skin paddle for neurosurgical reconstruction. At this stage a split-thickness skin graft has not yet been applied. Prior to return to the ICU, a graft will be placed.

10 cm inferior to the latissimus insertion into the humerus. The secondary segmental pedicles consist of the lateral row perforating arterial branches and venae comitantes from the posterior intercostal artery and vein and the medial row perforators from the lumbar artery and vein. The thoracodorsal nerve (C6–8) is the motor branch and enters the latissimus adjacent to the dominant pedicle. The sensory nerves are typically divided during flap elevation.

## Flap Elevation

The patient is placed in the lateral decubitus or prone position with the ipsilateral arm prepped, which allows for shoulder abduction during the dissection. The superomedial origin of the latissimus is divided from the scapula, and the dissection is continued distally to the vertebral

column at the point of origin. Dissection is continued toward the axilla. After the thoracodorsal vessels have been identified, the muscle can be divided from the humerus.

The pedicle is traced proximally until adequate pedicle length is achieved or until it joins with axillary and vein. During the pedicle dissection branches to the teres major and circumflex scapula artery and venae comitantes are sacrificed. For scalp reconstruction this flap is typically harvested without a skin paddle. Split-thickness skin graft is placed superficial to the muscle. The donor site is closed primarily over several drains.

## TRANSVERSE RECTUS ABDOMINUS FLAP (FIG. 42.4)

### Anatomy

The paired rectus muscles extend from the pubic symphysis and pubic crest and insert between the fifth and seventh costal cartilages. The dominant pedicles are the superior and inferior epigastric artery and vein from the internal mammary artery and vein and the external iliac artery and vein, respectively. The motor nerves to the rectus muscles are branches of the seventh through twelfth intercostal nerves and the lateral cutaneous nerves from the seventh to the twelfth intercostal nerve provide sensation to skin overlying the rectus.

### Flap Elevation

The rectus muscle is located between the costal margins and the pubic ramus. A flap is designed correlating to the defect and centered over the rectus muscle. The anterior sheath of the rectus is incised, and the muscle separated from the anterior sheath. Flap elevation is continued from both the medial and lateral aspects of the rectus sheath. The muscle is separated from the posterior sheath with care not to enter the abdominal cavity. This flap is harvested with a large skin island.

The donor site usually requires closure of the anterior sheath with mesh.

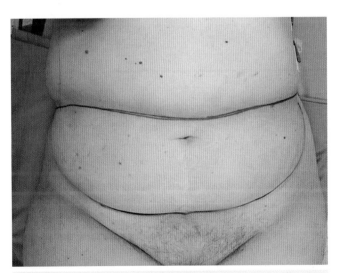

**Fig. 42.4** Markings for the free TRAM site.

# Perioperative Care

## Key Concepts

- Postoperatively patients must be monitored in a dedicated unit.
- Careful attention must be paid to patient hemodynamics, temperature, and volume status.
- Ultimately, the goal of perioperative care is to maintain patent anastomoses and flap perfusion.

Understanding how and why a flap may fail is essential for proper flap monitoring and postoperative patient care. Successful free flap–based reconstruction depends on equal inflow and outflow of flap blood supply. Flap failure results from a deviation from this equal flow state. Common causes for flap failure include arterial and venous thrombosis, mechanical kinking of vessels, vasospasm of the vascular pedicle, and external pressure on the flap from positioning or hematoma.[7] This section is dedicated to preventing and identifying flap compromise. Trained staffing, appropriate patient positioning, and optimization of hemodynamics are all critical variables in flap care and must be addressed to ensure flap success (Table 42.1).

**Table 42.1** Important Parameters for Postoperative Flap Care

| | Intervention | Potential Consequence |
|---|---|---|
| Nursing | ICU or dedicated flap monitoring unit with potential for hourly flap checks (physical examination and Doppler) for first 48–72 hours postoperatively by trained professional. | Delay in recognition of vascular compromise results in decreased potential of flap salvage. Majority of microvascular events occur in the first 48 hours after initial procedure. |
| Positioning | Identification of flap pedicle location. No pressure on flap or pedicle (including eyeglasses, nasal cannula, etc.). Care during all transfers. | Pressure on pedicle can result in mechanical kinking, avulsion, and potential thrombosis of pedicle requiring operative take-back and possible flap loss. |
| Temperature | Euthermia necessary. Patients may require warming blanket in the initial postoperative period. | Hypothermia results in increased vasoconstriction and possible vasoconstriction of the flap pedicle, resulting in both decreased sensitivity of monitoring and possible flap loss. |
| Hemodynamics | Adequate volume resuscitation with goal-directed urine output parameters (30–60 cc/hr). Avoidance of all vasopressors. | Underresuscitation results in decreased perfusion of the free flap. Vasopressors can potentially cause vasospasm of the flap pedicle. |

Early detection of a compromised flap is essential and best achieved with intensive care unit (ICU) monitoring or a nursing unit with flap-specific capabilities, regardless of flap location, type, and overall patient health.[8] The incidence of vascular compromise in a flap is highest within the first 48 hours after initial anastomosis. Any delay from initial event to operative take-back results in an increased likelihood of overall failure. Patients should have the flap assessed with both physical examination and Doppler flow checks every hour for the first 48 hours. These checks should be performed by one or two trained individuals, either a nurse or physician, who are aware of the initial appearance and details of the flap. Handoffs should be limited in number and frequency. Given the potential of a return trip to the operating room during these initial 48 hours, all patients should remain NPO or, at most, on a clear diet until the greatest potential for flap compromise has passed.

> ### Clinical Pearl
>
> The highest likelihood of thrombotic complications after free flap reconstruction occurs during the first 48 hours after the initial procedure. Patients should be in an ICU or dedicated flap-monitoring unit during this period.

Optimization of patient hemodynamics can prevent flap complications. Adequate volume resuscitation provides essential profusion to the free flap, although excessive resuscitation can lead to both patient and flap morbidity.[9,10] In patients with normal renal and cardiac function, urine output is followed closely, and a goal of 30 to 60 cc per hour is ideal to ensure appropriate fluid balance and flap perfusion. Vasopressors should be avoided in all flap patients. Vasopressors may have a direct impact on the flap pedicle, resulting in decreased flap perfusion and potential thrombosis. In any patient with hemodynamic instability, vasopressor use in the ICU should be discussed with the plastic surgeon prior to initiation. Volume resuscitation is preferred whenever feasible and safe for the patient.

Hypothermia is detrimental to flap perfusion and should be avoided. Any hypothermia results in increased adrenergic tone and an increase in systemic vascular resistance. Such physiological response can, in turn, cause vasospasm of the flap pedicle, resulting in reduced monitoring sensitivity and potential flap failure. Postoperatively all patients should be warmed with external warming devices (i.e., forced air warming) until euthermia is achieved.

> ### Clinical Pearl
>
> The ICU team should make all attempts to limit peripheral vasoconstriction in patients with free flap reconstructions.

Close attention must be applied to patient positioning. Any pressure on the flap pedicle can result not only in a transient decrease in blood flow, but also a prothrombotic state and potential frank anastomotic thrombosis.[11] Although practices and patient needs may dictate

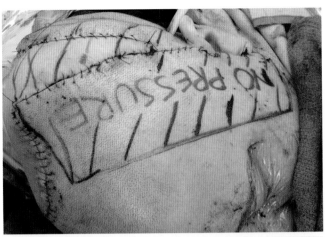

**Fig. 42.5** Key markings demonstrating where the pedicle and anastomosis are located. To prevent mechanical kinking, no pressure should be placed at this site.

**Table 42.2** Essentials of the Free Flap Physical Examination and Monitoring Parameters

| | Normal | Arterial Insufficiency | Venous Insufficiency |
|---|---|---|---|
| Color | Normal skin tone, color of donor site | Pale | Blue or purple |
| Temperature | 1–3 C of core body temperature | Cool to touch | Variable |
| Capillary Refill | 2–3 seconds | >3 seconds | <2 seconds |
| Pinprick | Presence of oxygenated blood | Lack of any bleeding | Excessive bleeding, dark color |
| Doppler | Biphasic arterial | Loss of signal | Changing signal biphasic to monophasic |

otherwise, typically anastomoses in the neurosurgical patient are at the superficial temporal or facial vessels located at or near the temporal fossa and mandible, respectively. Patients should not have any pressure at these sites. Additionally, extreme care must be observed during any transfers or position changes to prevent sheer or avulsing stress on the pedicle. It is the responsibility of the plastic surgeon to denote the location of the pedicle and anastomosis. In case there is any doubt where the pedicle or anastomosis is located, the ICU team should clarify with the plastic surgeon (Fig. 42.5). There are reports of flap compromise and failure from events as small as pressure from eyeglasses and nasal cannulas. Both the patient and unit staff must be provided specific instructions to prevent any pressure- and position-related complications.

Anticoagulation for the prevention of both anastomotic thrombosis and venous thromboembolism remains variable among plastic surgeons and is constantly debated in the literature.[12,13] In most centers, the decision of whether or not to pursue anticoagulation and what agent to use for anticoagulation is surgeon dependent. Often, patients without any contraindication will receive either subcutaneous low-molecular-weight heparin or 325 mg of acetylsalicylic acid daily. Although less common, some practices use IV heparin at low infusion rates (typically 300–500 units per hour) for prophylaxis of anastomotic thrombosis. Dosing specifics and duration, regardless of selected regimen, should be clarified with the surgeon of record.

## Flap Monitoring

### Key Concepts

- Physical examination remains the most important and reliable method of flap monitoring.
- It is essential to identify a compromised flap in a timely fashion.
- Trained staff should monitor a flap, paying attention to temperature, color, and turgor.
- Doppler monitoring is an important adjunct in flap monitoring.

Despite constant technological advancements and novel monitoring techniques, physical examination remains the standard of flap monitoring.[14,15] Changes in the physical examination represent underlying changes in the flow state of the flap. Nurses and physicians in the neurosurgical ICU must have basic training in identifying these changes. Special attention must be paid to the color, turgor, and temperature of a flap because significant changes can indicate a failure of vascular flow (Table 42.2). A flap with normal inflow and outflow should be pink, soft but full, and have a temperature between 1 and 3 degrees Celsius of the core body temperature. Flaps with compromised inflow will often be pale or white, with diminished turgor (excessively soft or wrinkled), and cool to the touch. Flaps with venous congestion will have a bluish or purple color and be firm to the touch. Temperature will be variable depending on the length of time and degree of congestion. Care must be taken to compare the color of the flap with its donor site. Given differing degrees of sun exposure, the color and texture of a flap may vary from the recipient site.

### Clinical Pearl

Monitor flap color, turgor, and temperature hourly during the first 48 hours. Confirm physical examination findings with presence of audible Doppler signal

In the setting of changes in the basic physical examination, further maneuvers such as evaluating the capillary refill and pinpoint bleeding of the flap can help determine adequate flow state. Capillary refill in a normal flap should be approximately 2 to 3 seconds. Capillary refill can be assessed on any clean and dry flap with an instrument or a finger. In a flap with compromised arterial inflow, capillary refill will be either delayed or longer than 3 seconds. Flaps with venous insufficiency but continued arterial inflow will have brisk capillary refill—less than 2 seconds. Physicians can also perform a pinprick test. For this test a 22-gauge needle is inserted into the flap and removed. Brisk, dark bleeding after this maneuver is associated with venous congestion. Little or no bleeding is associated with arterial insufficiency.

Doppler monitoring of free flaps remains an essential adjunct to the physical examination.[16] Doppler monitors can be external handheld probes or internal wires placed intraoperatively around pedicle vessels. Use of external versus internal monitoring is based on surgeon preference and presence of an externally detectable signal. Both internal and external Doppler probes can assess for arterial and venous flow.[17] Typically arterial signals alone are monitored; however, when there is concern for flap compromise, venous signals may provide insight into the overall flow state of the flap. Normal arterial signals are biphasic in nature. Arterial thrombosis and loss of arterial inflow are associated with softer or even absent signal. Venous thrombosis or insufficiency will result in a loss of venous signal and a change in the arterial signal. Typically, the arterial signal changes from biphasic to monophasic, which is described as a "water hammer" sound.

As discussed earlier, not all flaps employed for reconstruction will have an associated skin paddle. The latissimus dorsi muscle flap will often be a muscle-only flap with a separate skin graft. The basic principles of flap physical examination remain largely unchanged in this situation. Like flaps with skin paddles, muscle-only flaps will exhibit changes associated with either venous or arterial insufficiency. A flap with venous insufficiency will swell and have dark, brisk blood flow when pricked. The opposite will occur in the setting of arterial insufficiency. The Doppler can be used just as in the case of a flap with an intact skin paddle.

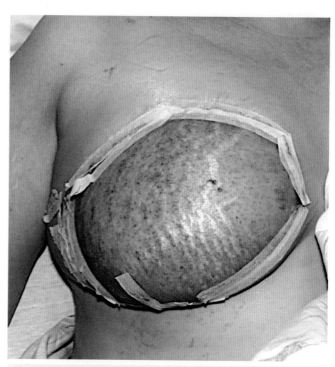

**Fig. 42.6** Postoperative congestion. This figure illustrates the physical examination findings of a flap with venous insufficiency either from thrombosis of the pedicle vein, mechanical kinking of the pedicle, or lack of sufficient intrinsic venous flow despite normal and patent pedicle. The flap is firm and capillary refill is <2 seconds. This flap requires exploration to rule out venous thrombosis.

### Clinical Pearl

Flap monitoring of a muscle-only flap with a skin graft is more challenging than is the case in a flap with a skin island. Temperature, turgor, and pinprick bleeding remain reliable examination findings. Doppler monitors can be used both externally and internally.

Fig. 42.6 and Fig. 42.7 illustrate venous and arterial insufficiency, respectively. Fig. 42.6 demonstrates the appearance of a flap with venous compromise. It is important to recognize a change in color and fullness, which will likely precede any change in Doppler signal. Here the flap is clearly purple and mottled relative to the surrounding tissues. In contrast, the flap in Fig. 42.7 shows classic signs of arterial insufficiency. The arterially insufficient flap is pale and without any capillary refill. Further examination demonstrates it to be cool and excessively soft relative to the surrounding tissues. Both of these flaps require operative intervention urgently.

## Postoperative Complications

### Key Concepts

- Complications include dehiscence, infection, seroma/hematoma, partial flap loss, venous insufficiency, arterial insufficiency, and complete flap loss.
- Early identification of flap complication is critical to flap salvage.

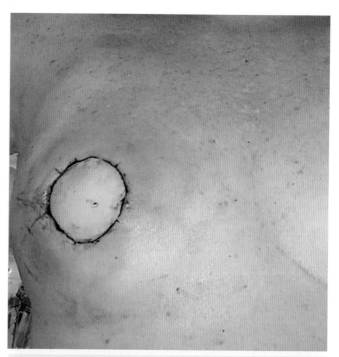

**Fig. 42.7** Postoperative arterial insufficiency. This figure illustrates the examination findings of arterial insufficiency either secondary to arterial thrombosis or mechanical kinking of the pedicle. The flap is soft, cool to the touch, and has no capillary refill. When pricked, it does not bleed. Like venous insufficiency, this flap requires urgent operative evaluation.

**Table 42.3** Postoperative Complications

| | Presentation | Management | Potential Consequences |
|---|---|---|---|
| Hematoma/seroma | Palpable fluid collection | Radiological or surgical drainage | Mechanical pressure on pedicle |
| Venous Thrombosis/ insufficiency | Hyperemic flap with brisk capillary refill | Operative evaluation possible additional venous anastomosis | Eventual arterial thrombosis, flap loss |
| Arterial thrombosis | Pale, cold flap without Doppler signal | Operative evaluation with reanastomosis | Flap kiss |
| Partial flap loss | Skin paddle sloughing, fat necrosis | Conservative vs. operative debridement | Potential operative debridement |

Postoperative complications after free flap reconstruction include dehiscence, local infection, seroma, hematoma, partial flap loss (skin paddle and fat necrosis), venous thrombosis, arterial thrombosis, flap congestion, and potential total flap loss.[17] In cases where a split-thickness skin graft is also used, partial or total loss of skin graft is another possibility (Table 42.3). Complications must be handled in a timely manner to prevent the potentially devastating total loss of the flap.

Flap compromise, whether secondary to overt arterial or venous thrombosis or unclear etiology, occurs in up to 5% to 10% of all flaps.[18] Total flap failure can occur either immediately (i.e., within the first 48 hours of the procedure) or in a delayed fashion.[19] The majority of devastating vascular events occur within the first 48 hours, and salvage rate is dependent on both underlying cause and time to operative assessment and correction. All attempts should be made at getting the patient into the operating room within 1 hour of initial diagnosis.

ICU staff should have a basic understanding of intraoperative events after an unexpected take-back. Flap exploration will involve potential evaluation of both venous and arterial anastomotic sites. Prior anastomoses may be resected, whereas new anastomoses may be performed with or without the need for vein grafting. Vein grafts will require a new donor site, most often the greater saphenous vein overlying the medial malleolus. Patients may therefore return with a new wound requiring modification in care. It is not uncommon for a patient to return more than once for intervention on a compromised flap. However, subsequent returns are associated with decreased likelihood of flap salvage.[13,20,21]

In the case of a thrombotic event, either arterial or venous, the surgeon may elect to use systemic heparin or flap-directed pharmacological thrombolysis with tissue plasminogen activator, urokinase, or streptokinase.[19,22,23] Often a patient postoperative from flap exploration will return to the ICU with a heparin infusion. Goal partial thromboplastin time (PTT) is dependent on surgeon preference and patient comorbidities.

### Clinical Pearl

During flap take-back, original anastomoses are often resected and replaced with new anastomoses. Patients will likely be therapeutically anticoagulated after flap take-back, resulting in an increased risk of hematoma formation and subsequent further surgical intervention. Recently revised flaps should be treated as new flaps, and hourly surveillance should be restarted and continued for an additional 48 hours, or even longer, depending on surgeon preference.

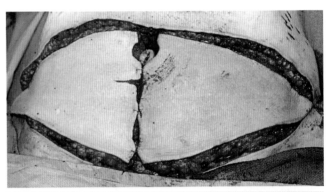

**Fig. 42.8** This illustrates intrinsic venous thrombosis in a TRAM flap. The flap on the patient's left is blue to purple in color with brisk capillary refill. This flap has not been harvested and therefore has normal pedicle anatomy and flow; however, loss of perforators has limited the flap's intrinsic outflow and congestion has resulted.

Venous insufficiency without anastomotic thrombosis is a potential concern after free flap reconstruction (Fig. 42.8).[5] In this situation an audible venous signal may be appreciated in the setting of congested appearance, that is, full, firm, and hyperemic flap. The absence of a clot should be confirmed intraoperatively under direct visualization of the pedicle. Venous insufficiency alone without thrombosis may require treatment with a second anastomosis, referred to as *supercharging*. If no vessels are available for a second anastomosis, leech (*Hirudo medicinalis*) therapy may be indicated. This form of therapy is not without its own complications and is often met without success.[24] All patients treated with leeches under the direction of a plastic surgeon will require an active blood bank specimen for potential transfusion, as well as prophylactic antibiotics (typically fluoroquinolone or cephalosporin) for potential infection with *Aeromonas spp.*[25]

Partial flap loss is a potential complication of any free flap reconstruction. Partial flap loss can be secondary to a salvaged flap where a portion of the flap was not reperfused within a sufficient window, or it can be secondary to an overall deficient intrinsic blood supply of the flap despite patent pedicle vasculature. The latter occurs when the size and volume of harvested tissue exceed the perfusion ability of the pedicle and perforators. Depending on the type of flap (cutaneous, myocutaneous, fasciocutaneous), the presentation of partial flap loss can vary. Loss of skin edges and fat necrosis are typically seen. The majority of cases of partial flap loss are managed conservatively. In cases of excess slough or contamination, operative debridement may be required.

Fluid collections, either seroma or hematoma, are often managed with surgical or radiologically guided percutaneous drainage. Any fluid collection has a potential to cause a mechanical stress and pressure on the vascular pedicle to the flap. The majority of free flap recipient and donor sites will have surgical drains (either Jackson-Pratt or Blake) to prevent seroma and hematoma. ICU nurses and staff must ensure that drains are properly stripped, emptied, and functioning. Any palpable collection should prompt the notification of the plastic surgeon. Notably, minor dehiscence should not be overlooked. Dehiscence can be an early indicator of flap congestion or partial flap loss. Evidence of dehiscence should prompt early evaluation by a plastic surgeon and continued hourly monitoring.

> ### Clinical Pearl
>
> Complications sometimes considered minor in other surgical procedures can be devastating in free flap reconstruction. Hematoma, seroma, and dehiscence must be addressed immediately because they may either lead to or cause further complications, including flap failure.

Contour irregularities and other esthetic concerns, although not complications, deserve mention here. The initial appearance of any free flap reconstruction will change over time as tissue settles and atrophies to a steady state. It is possible to return to the site of a free flap to elevate the flap, thin the flap, and adjust the contour. This is particularly important in patients who may need revision cranioplasty after removal of an infected bone flap or cranioplast. Flap elevation for further procedures should be performed with the assistance of a plastic surgeon.

# Conclusion

Autogenous free tissue transfer, the free flap, serves an important and often utilized means of reconstruction in neurosurgical patients. Physicians and staff caring for patients with free flap reconstructions should recognize the type of flap performed, location of donor site, and possible presence of skin graft. A basic knowledge of potential complications, their presentation, and management is essential. All patients should be initially resuscitated in an ICU or dedicated nursing unit for 48-72 hours with hourly flap checks entailing assessment of color, turgor, temperature, and Doppler signal. Attention to patient position should not be overlooked, and vasopressors should be avoided. Complications of flap surgery require prompt assessment and intervention; any delay can result in suboptimal outcome or even total flap loss. Ultimately free tissue reconstruction is multidisciplinary, and care providers should communicate openly with plastic surgery colleagues for optimal results and successful reconstruction.

## References

1. Oh SJ, Lee J, Cha J, Jeon MK, Koh SH, Chung CH. Free-flap reconstruction of the scalp: donor selection and outcome. *J Craniofac Surg.* 2011;22(3):974–977.
2. Yuen JC, Hochberg J. Free flap coverage of scalp defects following radiation. *J Ark Med Soc.* 2003;100(6):194–195.
3. Chang KP, Lai CH, Chang CH, Lin CL, Lai CS, Lin SD. Free flap options for reconstruction of complicated scalp and calvarial defects: report of a series of cases and literature review. *Microsurgery.* 2010;30(1):13–18.
4. Han DH, Park MC, Park DH, Song H, Lee IJ. Role of muscle free flap in the salvage of complicated scalp wounds and infected prosthetic dura. *Arch Plast Surg.* 2013;40(6):735–741.
5. Blondeel PN, Arnstein M, Verstraete K, et al. Venous congestion and blood flow in free transverse rectus abdominis myocutaneous and deep inferior epigastric perforator flaps. *Plast Reconstr Surg.* 2000;106(6):1295–1299.
6. Hierner R, van Loon J, Goffin J, van Calenbergh F. Free latissimus dorsi flap transfer for subtotal scalp and cranium defect reconstruction: report of 7 cases. *Microsurgery.* 2007;27(5):425–428.
7. Giunta R, Geisweid A, Feller AM. Clinical classification of free-flap perfusion complications. *J Reconstr Microsurg.* 2001;17(5):341–345.
8. Cornejo A, Ivatury S, Crane CN, Myers JG, Wang HT. Analysis of free flap complications and utilization of intensive care unit monitoring. *J Reconstr Microsurg.* 2013;29(7):473–479.
9. Booi DI. Perioperative fluid overload increases anastomosis thrombosis in the free TRAM flap used for breast reconstruction. *Eur J Plast Surg.* 2011;34(2):81–86.
10. Fischer JP, Nelson JA, Mirzabeigi MN, Serletti JM, Kanchwala S. Perioperative hemodynamics in free flap breast reconstruction: incidence, predictors, and management of tachycardia. *Ann Plast Surg.* 2012;69(4):356–360.
11. Garg S, Deschler D. Saving a free flap with close clinical postoperative monitoring. *JAAPA.* 2013;26(1):47–49.
12. Ashjian P, Chen CM, Pusic A, Disa JJ, Cordeiro PG, Mehrara BJ. The effect of postoperative anticoagulation on microvascular thrombosis. *Ann Plast Surg.* 2007;59(1):36–39. discussion 9–40.
13. Fosnot J, Jandali S, Low DW, Kovach 3rd SJ, Wu LC, Serletti JM. Closer to an understanding of fate: the role of vascular complications in free flap breast reconstruction. *Plast Reconstr Surg.* 2011;128(4):835–843.
14. Chao AH, Lamp S. Current approaches to free flap monitoring. *Plast Surg Nurs.* 2014;34(2):52–56.
15. Lohman RF, Langevin CJ, Bozkurt M, Kundu N, Djohan R. A prospective analysis of free flap monitoring techniques: physical examination, external Doppler, implantable Doppler, and tissue oximetry. *J Reconstr Microsurg.* 2013;29(1):51–56.
16. Salgado CJ, Moran SL, Mardini S. Flap monitoring and patient management. *Plast Reconstr Surg.* 2009;124(6 suppl):e295–e302.
17. Williams JG, French RJ, Lalonde DH. Why do free flap vessels thrombose? Lessons learned from implantable Doppler monitoring. *Can J Plast Surg.* 2004;12(1):23–26.
18. Selber JC, Angel Soto-Miranda M, Liu J, Robb G. The survival curve: factors impacting the outcome of free flap take-backs. *Plast Reconstr Surg.* 2012;130(1):105–113.
19. Agostini T, Lazzeri D, Agostini V, Spinelli G, Shokrollahi K. Delayed free flap salvage after venous thrombosis. *J Craniofac Surg.* 2012;23(3):e260–e261.
20. Chang EI, Carlsen BT, Festekjian JH, Da Lio AL, Crisera CA. Salvage rates of compromised free flap breast reconstruction after recurrent thrombosis. *Ann Plast Surg.* 2013;71(1):68–71.
21. Mirzabeigi MN, Wang T, Kovach SJ, Taylor JA, Serletti JM, Wu LC. Free flap take-back following postoperative microvascular compromise: predicting salvage versus failure. *Plast Reconstr Surg.* 2012;130(3):579–589.
22. D'Arpa S, Cordova A, Moschella F. Pharmacological thrombolysis: one more weapon for free-flap salvage. *Microsurgery.* 2005;25(6):477–480.
23. Panchapakesan V, Addison P, Beausang E, Lipa JE, Gilbert RW, Neligan PC. Role of thrombolysis in free-flap salvage. *J Reconstr Microsurg.* 2003;19(8):523–530.
24. Pannucci CJ, Nelson JA, Chung CU, et al. Medicinal leeches for surgically uncorrectable venous congestion after free flap breast reconstruction. *Microsurgery.* 2014 Oct;34(7):522–526.
25. Kalbermatten DF, Rieger UM, Uike K, et al. Infection with *Aeromonas hydrophila* after use of leeches (*Hirudo medicinalis*) in a free microvascular osteo-(myo-)cutaneous flap—suggestions for successful management. *Handchir Mikrochir Plast Chir.* 2007;39(2):108–111.

# 43 Combined and Specialty Surgery: Otolaryngology, Plastics

LORI A. SHUTTER, CARL H. SNYDERMAN, and PAUL A. GARDNER

## Neuroanatomy and Procedures

### Key Concepts

- Head and neck surgery may affect critical structures at the cranial base.
- Craniofacial procedures may produce dural defects.
- Skull-base surgery must consider key neural and vascular structures.
- Collaborative planning between otolaryngology and neurosurgery is crucial to these procedures.
- Reconstruction of defects and healing can be significantly affected by postoperative care.

Anatomical knowledge is the foundation for a patient history, physical diagnosis, and surgical management. Many head and neck surgeries involve the upper airway from the nasal passages to the pharynx. The paranasal sinuses are juxtaposed to the skull base and bounded by critical structures such as the internal carotid arteries, orbits, and cranial nerves. Neurocritical structures that traverse the cranial base have relevance for both specialties during surgery and in the postoperative period.

Sinonasal tumors, both benign and malignant, can involve the base of the cranium. The classic surgical approach for a sinonasal malignancy such as an esthesioneuroblastoma (olfactory neuroblastoma) is a craniofacial resection (Fig. 43.1). This consists of a bifrontal craniotomy and a transfacial approach to achieve an en bloc resection of the tumor-involved cranial base. The dural defect is reconstructed with a sutured graft and a pericranial scalp flap, and the frontal bone flap is replaced. The same surgical goals can be achieved using a completely endoscopic endonasal approach; reconstruction is achieved with fascial grafts, vascularized nasoseptal flap, or extracranial pericranial flap. The medial walls of the orbit (lamina papyracea) are often resected on one or both sides. The cranial base defect extends from the frontal sinus anteriorly to the planum sphenoidale posteriorly. Posteriorly, the resection is limited by the optic nerves and chiasm. Laterally, it is bounded by the orbital tissues and the ethmoidal arteries (branches of the ophthalmic artery). With a transcranial approach, the frontal sinus is usually cranialized (removal of posterior table and mucosa) to remove all remnants of the frontal sinus. With an endonasal approach, the frontal sinus is preserved with a drainage pathway into the nasal cavity.

Surgery through the sphenoid sinus is performed for the treatment of pituitary tumors and other skull-base pathology (craniopharyngiomas, meningiomas) and is discussed in other chapters. Primary sphenoid pathologies include sinonasal malignancy and inflammatory disease (chronic bacterial sphenoid sinusitis, invasive and noninvasive fungal sinusitis, and mucocele). The sphenoid sinus is surrounded by key neural and vascular structures such as the optic nerves, pituitary gland, internal carotid artery (ICA), and cavernous sinus (Fig. 43.2). The clivus (ventral aspect of the occipital bone that abuts the posterior and inferior surface of the sphenoid bone) is roughly divided into thirds. The upper clivus extends from the posterior clinoids to the floor of the sella and is associated intracranially with the oculomotor nerves and the apex of the basilar artery. The middle clivus extends from the floor of the sella to the floor of the sphenoid sinus and is associated intracranially with the abducens nerves and the trunk of the basilar artery. The remainder of the lower clivus extends to the foramen magnum and is associated intracranially with the vertebral arteries and hypoglossal nerves. Tumors that involve the clivus include chordomas and benign meningiomas. Clival defects are reconstructed in a similar manner with fascial grafts, adipose tissue, and a vascularized nasoseptal flap.

The petrous apex is accessible through the sphenoid sinus. Expansile lesions of the petrous apex such as cholesterol granulomas are preferentially drained endoscopically into the sphenoid sinus because access is usually superior and the potential morbidity of transtemporal and middle cranial fossa approaches is avoided (Fig. 43.3). Other indications for petrous apex surgery include tumors and petrous apicitis. The petrous apex is situated posterior to the paraclival segment of the ICA at the level of the clival recess (sphenoid sinus depression below the sella). The bone of the midclivus is drilled to access the petrous apex; it is bounded by the dura of the posterior fossa posteriorly and the ICA anteriorly. The abducens nerve runs along an oblique course deep to the midportion of the paraclival ICA to enter Dorello's canal.

The nasopharynx extends from the sphenoid rostrum (attachment of nasal septum to sphenoid bone) to the level of the soft palate. It is bounded laterally by the cartilaginous portions of the Eustachian tubes. Posterior to the Eustachian tube is the fossa of Rosenmüller, a mucosal recess behind the torus tubarius. The parapharyngeal segment of the ICA is situated posterolaterally and may be less than 1 cm in proximity. Nasopharyngectomy consists of resection of the soft tissues of the nasopharynx. The most

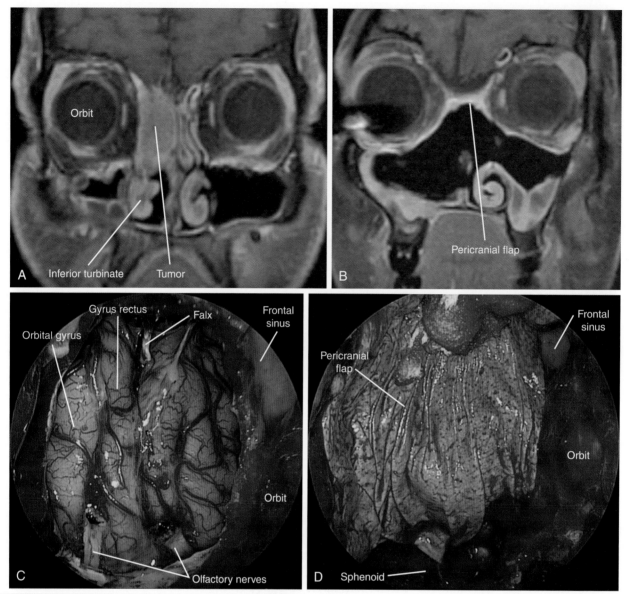

**Fig. 43.1** Preoperative **(A)** and postoperative **(B)** magnetic resonance image (MRI) of an esthesioneuroblastoma. The postoperative MRI demonstrates complete resection of tumor and enhancement of the reconstructive flap. Intraoperative endoscopic view of the dural defect after tumor resection **(C)** and reconstruction with an extracranial pericranial flap **(D)**.

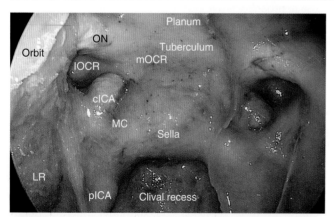

**Fig. 43.2** Anatomical features of the sphenoid sinus include the orbit, optic nerves *(ON)*, lateral optic-carotid recess *(lOCR)*, medial optic-carotid recess *(mOCR)*, cavernous internal carotid artery *(cICA)*, middle clinoid *(MC)*, paraclival internal carotid artery *(pICA)*, lateral recess *(LR)*, planum, tuberculum, sella, and clival recess.

common indications are the treatment of primary malignancy arising from minor salivary glands or residual/recurrent nasopharyngeal cancer. The underlying bone of the clivus may be drilled to achieve clear resection margins. Laterally, the resection is limited by the course of the parapharyngeal ICA. If possible, an exposed ICA is covered with vascularized tissue after the nasopharyngectomy is completed. An exposed ICA is susceptible to delayed rupture, especially in a heavily irradiated tissue bed.

Another collaborative surgery for otolaryngology and neurosurgery is the excision of angiofibromas (Fig. 43.4). These benign tumors arise in adolescent males and can be very large at presentation with erosion of the skull base and intracranial extension. Angiofibromas are hypervascular tumors that often derive part of their blood supply from the ICA when advanced. They arise from the base of pterygoid region and expand the pterygopalatine space (PPS). The PPS is posterior to the maxillary sinus and connects the masticator space with the nasal cavity. Branches of the

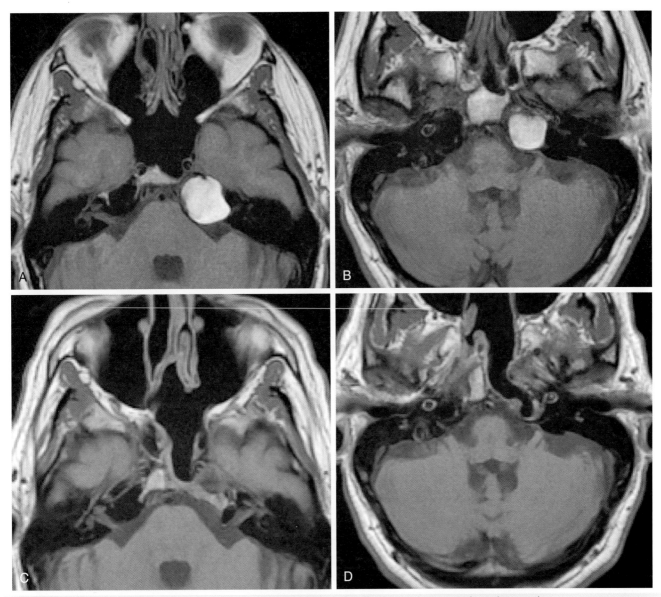

**Fig.43.3** Cholesterol granuloma of the left petrous apex before **(A, B)** and after **(C, D)** an endoscopic endonasal approach.

internal maxillary artery course through the PPS; the sphenopalatine artery is a terminal branch of the internal maxillary artery and exits the PPS at the sphenopalatine foramen. It is the primary blood supply of a nasoseptal flap and inferior turbinate flap. A transpterygoid approach provides access to the lateral recess of the sphenoid sinus and is a starting point for suprapetrous approaches to the middle cranial fossa. After sacrifice of the sphenopalatine artery, the contents of the PPS can be displaced to expose the base of the pterygoid region. The pterygoid canal transmits the vidian nerve and artery and is immediately posterior to the sphenopalatine artery. The vidian nerve is an important landmark for locating the petrous segment of the ICA and crosses superior to the horizontal segment of the artery. Superolateral to the pterygoid canal is the foramen rotundum with the maxillary nerve. A pneumatized lateral recess of the sphenoid sinus extends between these two nerves and is a window to Meckel's cave. The third division of the trigeminal nerve (mandibular nerve) is directly inferior to the

foramen rotundum, posterior to the lateral pterygoid plate. A common route of intracranial extension of angiofibromas is growth from the PPS via the inferior orbital fissure to the superior orbital fissure to the middle cranial fossa (lateral to the cavernous sinus). Both lateral infratemporal and anterior endonasal/transmaxillary approaches are used to remove angiofibromas. With a lateral infratemporal approach, a zygomatic osteotomy and temporalis muscle transposition provide access to the infratemporal skull base and masticator space. A temporal craniotomy may be employed for intracranial extension, but the tumor is almost always extradural. Endoscopic techniques are performed endonasally and via an anterior transmaxillary (Caldwell Luc) approach. Loss of the vidian nerve results in absence of emotional tearing of the ipsilateral eye. Injury to the second and third divisions of the trigeminal nerve results in facial hypesthesia in the affected dermatomes and denervation of the muscles of mastication. Surgery in the masticator space often results in temporary trismus

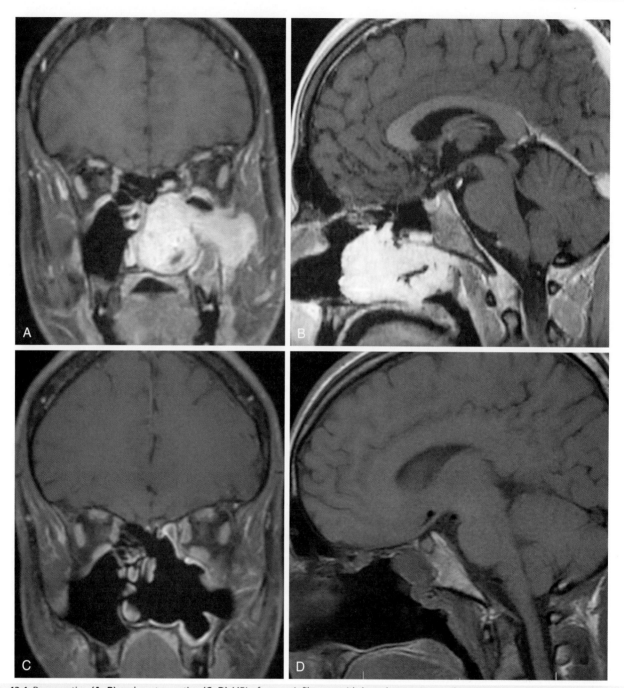

**Fig. 43.4** Preoperative **(A, B)** and postoperative **(C, D)** MRI of an angiofibroma with lateral extension to the masticator space. Endonasal access is provided by a medial maxillectomy.

due to pain and scarring. Angiofibromas are extremely vascular tumors that require preoperative embolization, but may still have significant operative blood loss.

Surgeries of the temporal bone that are relevant to neurosurgery are combined with approaches to the cerebellopontine angle (acoustic neuroma) and are covered elsewhere. Surgery of the parapharyngeal space is performed for neurogenic tumors of the poststyloid parapharyngeal space, as well as paragangliomas (glomus vagale, glomus jugulare). These tumors can extend intracranially through the jugular foramen. The lower cranial nerves are anteromedial to the internal jugular vein at the jugular foramen. A combined approach for transcranial tumors requires a far lateral approach with mastoidectomy and upper cervical

dissection. If necessary, the vertical segment of the facial nerve can be mobilized from the fallopian canal and transposed anteriorly. The lower cranial nerves are dissected superiorly from the neck, and the entire course of the internal jugular vein is visualized.

## Clinical Pearls

- The vidian nerve is a key landmark for intraoperative identification of the petrous ICA.
- The vidian artery from the ICA often contributes significant vascularity to a large angiofibroma.

# Perioperative Considerations

## Key Concepts

- Airway management poses unique challenges in this patient population.
- Nasal instrumentation should not be performed after surgeries that involve the upper airway.
- Special attention and monitoring of cranial nerve function are required.
- Collaborative discussions between otolaryngology, neurosurgery, and neurocritical care are crucial for management of these patients.
- Skull-base surgeries are often long and may involve a moderate amount of blood loss.

After completion of surgery, it is critical that there be good communication among the members of the surgical team, anesthesia, and critical care surrounding the transport of the patient. The primary concern is the stability of the airway and whether the patient should be extubated in the operating room or recovery room, or remain intubated for direct transfer to the intensive care unit. If a patient needs early postoperative imaging, it is preferable to stabilize the patient prior to transport to radiology. The patient's neurological status and level of sedation can be assessed while intubated. The use of checklists or a structured protocol for handoffs is recommended to encourage good communication and minimize risk of errors.

Head and neck procedures often involve the upper airway. Generally, procedures that are above the plane of the hard palate will not cause sufficient upper airway edema to cause airway obstruction. Reconstruction of large palatal defects with a microvascular free flap may cause partial airway obstruction due to the bulk of the flap. Airway options include a prolonged intubation, oral airway, nasal trumpet (nasal tube that extends to the pharynx), or a tracheostomy. After extubation, mask ventilation is usually contraindicated in skull-base procedures due to the risk of forcing air through the dural defect, resulting in pneumocephalus. Air may also be forced into soft tissues if there is a bone defect, resulting in subcutaneous emphysema; the orbital tissues are particularly susceptible.

Obese patients are a special population due to underlying risk factors for obstructive sleep apnea (OSA) and elevated cerebrospinal fluid (CSF) pressures. They may have undiagnosed OSA or be receiving treatment with continuous positive airway pressure (CPAP) at home, which often must be avoided, depending on the presence of a skull-base defect. Although many of these patients can forego CPAP while in the hospital, they should be monitored carefully for sustained periods of hypoxia. Episodes of airway obstruction cause fluctuations in CSF pressures that increase the risk of a postoperative CSF leak.

In surgeries that involve the nasal airway, nasal instrumentation is contraindicated. Signs should be posted in the patient's room to *not* pass any tubes through the nasal cavity. If necessary, passage of a feeding tube transnasally should only be done by the surgical service under direct observation with an endoscope. Blind passage of a tube can disrupt the dural repair and extend intracranially. Transoral passage of tubes should also be performed under direct observation because they can be misdirected into the nasopharynx.

Patients should be cautioned to avoid nose blowing and activities that increase CSF pressure such as straining. A stool softener is routinely prescribed, and the head of the bed is constantly elevated to minimize intracranial venous congestion. Spinal drains are often used to lower CSF pressures in patients undergoing a skull-base dural repair.

In many patients with combined procedures, careful regulation of blood pressure is needed to avoid episodes of hypoperfusion. This is especially important in patients with preoperative visual loss who may have compromised blood flow to the optic chiasm and optic nerves. Avoidance of hypertensive episodes is important to prevent intracranial hemorrhage.

Special attention to the cranial nerves is necessary in these patients. Patients should be closely monitored for worsening of existing cranial nerve deficits or the onset of new deficits. Assessment of visual acuity includes separate assessment of each eye because patients may not be aware of a unilateral visual loss. Pupillary responses to light should be noted; loss of an afferent pupillary reflex implies a compromised unilateral optic nerve. Decreased ability to detect red color is an early indication of visual compromise. Visual field deficits can also be assessed at the bedside. Extraocular motility and the presence of diplopia with lateral or upward gaze are noted. Any change in visual function should prompt a thorough evaluation by an ophthalmologist. Assessment of the corneal reflex can determine the integrity of the first division of the trigeminal nerve. This should be accomplished with drops of normal saline to avoid corneal trauma from testing with cotton or gauze.

Hearing loss may be conductive or sensorineural. A conductive hearing loss results from Eustachian tube dysfunction with pressure changes in the middle ear and fluid collection. This can be ameliorated with a myringotomy or amplification. A sensorineural hearing loss is a consequence of direct injury to the cochlear nerve or inner ear. Unrecognized hearing loss contributes to patient confusion (especially in the elderly) and fosters miscommunication.

Injury to the nerves associated with eating and swallowing (glossopharyngeal, vagus, and hypoglossal nerves) and laryngeal function (vagus nerve) compromises the ability of the patient to protect the airway. Injury to the vagus nerve affects both sensory and motor function of the larynx. Unilateral vocal cord paralysis causes partial airway obstruction, hoarseness, and decreases the effectiveness of coughing. Patients at risk for aspiration should be evaluated by a swallowing therapist prior to resuming an oral diet. A functional endoscopic evaluation of swallowing performed at the bedside is useful in directing swallowing therapy. Temporary feeding with a nasogastric tube may be necessary.

## Clinical Pearls

- Obese patients are at risk for postoperative airway problems as well as CSF leaks.
- Nasal tubes should not be passed blindly after surgery due to the risk of intracranial passage.
- One of the earliest signs of optic nerve compression is a decreased ability to detect red colors.
- Patients who undergo surgical procedures of the nasopharynx should be evaluated for a conductive hearing loss resulting from Eustachian tube dysfunction.

# Postoperative Complications

## Key Concepts

- Early identification of complications is critical.
- Specific complications of concern include airway compromise, hematoma, CSF leaks, pneumocephalus, visual deterioration, and cranial nerve deficits.
- Airway management is a priority, and positive pressure must be avoided.
- Prophylactic antibiotics are not recommended for more than 24 hours postoperatively unless nasal or oral packing is in place.

Early identification of any postoperative complications after cranial base surgery is crucial to management. In addition to the standard assessment for wound infections and postoperative bleeding, care must be taken to assess for airway compromise, dural integrity, and neural injuries. Incidence of these injuries varies greatly based on the surgical approach, procedure, and baseline neurological function. Recent reviews of endoscopic skull-base surgery for parasellar lesions report that the major nonpituitary-related complications seen postoperatively include CSF leakage (7.4%–23.4%), meningitis (5.4%–7.8%), respiratory failure (3.7%), visual deterioration (3.6%), neural (4.1%–11.1%), and vascular injuries (2.7%).[1-4]

## Airway Compromise

Postoperative stridor that is mild may be managed medically (Table 43.1), but there should be a low threshold for airway intervention. In the event of acute airway compromise of any etiology, special awareness is needed regarding intubation techniques for this patient population because there is potential for a difficult airway scenario. A rapid sequence induction may be performed as long as positive pressure mask ventilation is avoided. Rescue airway methods should be available at bedside. An awake fiberoptic intubation, video laryngoscopy, or laryngeal mask airway are options to be considered.

## Vascular Injuries/Bleeding

Epistaxis is a frequent occurrence after upper airway surgery. The significance of the hemorrhage is dependent on the type of surgery and prior therapy. Minor oozing is expected after any nasal/sinus surgery and is not cause for concern. This situation can usually be managed non-surgically with nasal packing, such as an intranasal tampon or balloon catheter. Although effective, they may contribute to development of sinusitis, middle ear effusion, patient discomfort, and hypoxia. Brisk bleeding from the nasal cavity is less common and usually arises from the sphenopalatine artery or, less commonly, the anterior ethmoid artery. In patients with traumatic injuries of the skull base, bleeding is more likely to originate from the ethmoidal arteries. Nasal endoscopy is helpful in identifying the source and placement of nasal packing.

Epistaxis can also be the harbinger of more serious bleeding from an injured ICA or cavernous fistula (Fig. 43.5). A pseudoaneurysm of the ICA or carotid-cavernous fistula can be the consequence of skull-base trauma (fracture of

**Table 43.1**  Medical Management of Airway Edema and Stridor

| Intervention | Comments/Dosage |
|---|---|
| Supplemental oxygen | Nasal cannula, face tent, or mask No positive pressure |
| Head positioning | Upright at 45–90 degrees |
| Nebulized racemic epinephrine | 0.5–0.75 mL of 2.25% racemic epinephrine added to 2.5–3 mL of normal saline Quick and effective |
| Dexamethasone (Decadron) | 4–8 mg IV q8–12 h Delayed effect |
| Inhaled Heliox | 70% helium, 30% oxygen Rapid effect |

sphenoid bone) or iatrogenic injury during sinus or endonasal skull-base surgery. In particular, patients who have had prior irradiation of the nasopharynx for cancer are susceptible to carotid "blow-out" (spontaneous dehiscence) secondary to radiation necrosis. There are tumors that can even require endonasal dissection of the posterior circulation. A high level of suspicion is necessary in such situations, and prompt evaluation with a computed tomography (CT) angiogram or angiography (four vessel) should be performed to identify the source of bleeding. The greatest risk of severe hemorrhage in the upper airway is loss of the airway. Elective intubation or tracheostomy should be considered to protect the airway while the bleeding is addressed. Bleeding from the ICA is temporized with focal packing but will require management using endovascular techniques (vascular stent, coiling, or sacrifice).

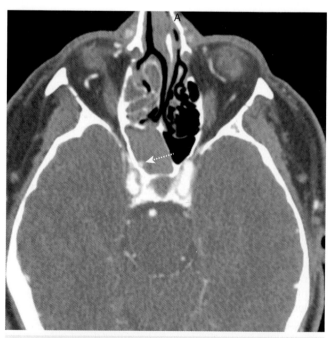

**Fig. 43.5** Pseudoaneurysm (*arrow*) of the cavernous segment of the right internal carotid artery, which resulted from an iatrogenic injury during endoscopic sinus surgery.

## Lower Cranial Nerve Injury

Surgical interventions at the base of the skull require close attention to the cranial nerves perioperatively. In particular, consequences of lower cranial nerve dysfunction may result in airway obstruction and aspiration. Injury to the glossopharyngeal nerves produces a loss of muscle tone of the soft palate resulting in a mechanical upper airway obstruction. Urgent intubation is often necessary, and tracheostomy may be needed. Airway obstruction due to vagal nerve injury is rarely an issue unless both nerves are affected, resulting in bilateral vocal cord paralysis. At rest, the patient may be able to breathe comfortably, but increased respiratory demands or any vocal cord edema may precipitate stridor. Fiberoptic examination of the airway reveals paradoxical movement (medial displacement) with inspiration. Immediate treatment options include medical treatments to decrease airway edema, intubation, and tracheostomy. Options for medical management of airway edema include supplemental oxygen, proper positioning, nebulized racemic epinephrine, dexamethasone, and inhaled Heliox (Table 43.1).

## Cerebrospinal Fluid Leaks

One of the most common complications of cranial base surgery is a CSF leak, occurring in approximately 5% of patients after endoscopic endonasal surgery and 10% of lateral skull-base surgeries.[5] Potential risk factors include diabetes, obesity, prior skull-base surgery, malnutrition, and prior radiation therapy. A root-cause analysis for CSF leak is shown in Table 43.2. CSF rhinorrhea is characterized by clear or xanthochromic watery rhinorrhea that may not become apparent until nasal packing is removed. Posterior drainage into the nasopharynx may induce coughing, which should raise suspicion for a leak. If suspected, a small sample of fluid should be collected and tested for beta-2-transferrin, which has higher sensitivity and specificity than traditional glucose testing.[6] Patients should be cautioned to avoid nose blowing due to the risk of pneumocephalus and bacterial contamination. If a CSF leak is detected in the early postoperative period, head elevation and CSF diversion with a spinal drain may be effective in sealing the leak. The rate of CSF drainage is typically 5 to 15 mL/hr for 5 to 7 days.[7] Overdrainage should be avoided because it may produce meningeal inflammation and low-pressure headaches. These symptoms could mimic the symptoms of meningitis, thus clouding the picture and potentially having a negative impact on medical decisions. Prolonged CSF diversion should also be avoided because it increases the risk of meningitis and development of intracranial abscesses.[8] Prophylactic antibiotics are not recommended because they do not reduce the rate of meningitis and may actually contribute to selection of more virulent organisms.[9] If CSF diversion does not resolve the leak, then surgical exploration and repair may be necessary. Prompt reexploration is preferred over lumbar drainage after endonasal skull-base surgery, given the size of potential defects and lack of intervening tissue.

Spinal drains require attention and aggressive management. CSF samples should be analyzed for infection. Volume of drainage must be monitored closely because overdrainage can occur and produce pneumocephalus, low-pressure headaches, nausea, vomiting, vocal cord paralysis, and even obtundation. In addition, other problems encountered include fracture and retention of drain fragments, chemical meningitis, hemorrhage, occlusion of the posterior cerebral artery, and lumbar radiculopathy.[10,11]

## Pneumocephalus

The incidence of air in the cranial vault, or pneumocephalus, is rare after endoscopic sinus surgery or microscopic skull-base surgery.[12] Perioperative risk factors that may contribute to the development of pneumocephalus are listed in Box 43.1. Symptoms reported with pneumocephalus include mental status changes, new or worsened headache, nausea, vomiting, and seizures. In rare occasions, tension pneumocephalus with flattening of the frontal lobes may develop, producing mass effect and increased intracranial pressure (ICP). The extent of pneumocephalus should be assessed with a CT scan. Some degree of pneumocephalus is to be expected after cranial base surgery that includes opening of the dura; gradual resolution over a week is to be expected. Treatment of pneumocephalus after skull-base surgery should initially be managed with conservative measures such as bed rest, head elevation, supplemental oxygen via a face tent or 100% nonrebreather with absolute avoidance of positive pressure, and pain control.[13] In patients who fail conservative therapy, or with evidence of tension pneumocephalus, surgical exploration of the repair should be considered to address ICP and repair the dural defect. Obese patients with OSA are particularly prone to pneumocephalus. In severe or persistent cases, diversion of the airway with intubation or tracheostomy may be necessary.

## Reconstruction

Failure of reconstruction of the skull base can result in any of the previously mentioned complications. If a patient has a free flap for reconstruction, there are typically very tightly controlled hemodynamic criteria applied. In addition, the type of pressor or antihypertensive agent used should be carefully considered given its potential effects on cerebral or flap arterial supply.

**Table 43.2** Potential Risk Factors for Cerebrospinal Fluid Leak

| Patient Factors | Material | Technique | Perioperative Care |
|---|---|---|---|
| Prior therapy | Allograft | Flap harvest | Lumbar drain |
| High-flow leak | Nonvascularized autograft | Inlay graft | Debridement |
| Recipient bed | Vascularized flap | Flap placement | Patient activity |
| Increased CSF pressure | | Packing | Packing |
| Tumor type | | | |

*CSF*, cerebrospinal fluid.

## Box 43.1   Perioperative Risk Factors for Development of Pneumocephalus

Head position
Duration of surgery
Anesthesia related

- Use of nitrous oxide ($N_2O$) anesthesia
- Spinal anesthesia
- Epidural anesthesia

Hydrocephalus
Intraoperative osmotherapy
Hyperventilation
Barotrauma
Continuous CSF drainage via lumbar drain
Infection (otitis media)
Neoplasms
Skull-base injury
Incomplete reconstruction after skull-base surgeries (fistula)
Positive pressure events in the postoperative period

- Coughing
- Straining
- Vomiting
- Valsalva maneuvers including sneezing, nose blowing

*CSF*, cerebrospinal fluid.

## Visual Deterioration

Endoscopic endonasal and skull-base surgeries can produce visual deficits through injury to the optic nerves, ischemia, or hematoma formation. Complaints of visual changes should prompt an immediate evaluation. Visual loss can occur as a result of complications anywhere along the visual pathways after skull-base surgery. Chiasmal compression from postoperative intracranial hematoma will result in a bitemporal hemianopsia.

Hemorrhage into the orbital tissues can cause a sudden loss of vision and is an ophthalmological emergency. Retraction of an incompletely coagulated, transected ethmoidal artery can cause a retro-orbital hematoma, sudden increase in intraorbital pressure, and an anterior orbital compartment syndrome. Physical examination may demonstrate proptosis, eyelid ecchymosis, chemosis, ophthalmoplegia, afferent pupillary defect, decreased visual fields and acuity, papilledema, and central retinal artery pulsation. Emergency consultation of ophthalmology and otolaryngology should be obtained for bedside evaluation. Measurement of intraocular pressure guides the medical and surgical management. Although radiographic studies may confirm the diagnosis, evaluation and treatment should not be delayed to obtain imaging. If there is acute visual loss, intraocular pressure greater than 40 mm Hg, or proptosis, an emergent lateral canthotomy and cantholysis is recommended to release pressure. Secondary and less sensitive indications for surgical intervention include an afferent pupillary defect, ophthalmoplegia, and severe pain.[14]

## Cranial Nerve Deficits

Risk of cranial neuropathy depends on the pathology, approach, and tumor location within the skull base. Dysfunction of ocular motility can result from direct mechanical, orbital manipulation, or cranial nerve injury and will produce diplopia that can be managed acutely with an eye patch or application of an occlusive lenses to glasses. Persistent symptoms may require the use of Fresnel prisms or surgical intervention. Patients with a sensory deficit of the first division of the trigeminal nerve require eye protection with ocular lubricants, eyelid closure with taping, or an eye patch to avoid corneal injury. The eye patch must not be allowed to contact the cornea because irritation from the patch could contribute to a corneal abrasion. If the patient also has a facial palsy with incomplete eye closure, a temporary tarsorrhaphy may be necessary in addition to the aforementioned precautions.

Hearing loss can potentially be addressed through amplification techniques. Vestibular nerve injury may contribute to orthostatic hypotension, impaired balance, poor spatial memory and navigation, and episodes of vertigo. Rehabilitation and physical therapy can assist with balance and spatial perception. Management of vertigo may require pharmacological interventions.

Although the impact of lower cranial nerve injuries on airway integrity is potentially life threatening, there are other functions of these cranial nerves that can have an impact on long-term recovery. Patients may experience disruptions in taste perception from injury to the facial or glossopharyngeal nerve. This can lead to poor appetite and contribute to malnutrition. Dietary supplements and vitamins may be necessary. Difficulty with swallowing and speech can develop from injury to the glossopharyngeal, vagus, or hypoglossal nerves. Swallowing assessments are required prior to initiation of oral intake to assess for coordination of oral, pharyngeal, and esophageal phases of swallowing and risk for aspiration. Patients at high risk for aspiration require aggressive pulmonary hygiene and may benefit from placement of a feeding tube. Placement of a nasogastric tube should be performed under direct visualization. If long-term nutritional support is necessary, then placement of a percutaneous gastrostomy tube may be warranted.

## Pituitary Dysfunction

The treatment of many anterior cranial base tumors harbors some small but real risk of pituitary compromise. Careful monitoring of morning cortisol levels and fluid and sodium balance are critical when indicated. Urine output over 250 cc/hour for 2 consecutive hours should trigger an evaluation for diabetes insipidus with urine specific gravity (SG) and serum sodium checks. A urine SG <1.005 and serum sodium >145 in this setting should generally be treated with IV or subcutaneous DDAVP. Care should be taken to avoid hyponatremia in the setting of cerebral edema, either from tumor involvement or intraoperative retraction or venous injury. A patient with hyponatremia in this setting has many potential causes, including adrenal insufficiency, syndrome of inappropriate antidiuretic hormone secretion, and cerebral salt wasting. Careful monitoring of fluid balance and urine output is therefore critical.

## Infection

In addition to systemic infections related to prolonged surgery and recovery, the higher rates of CSF leak and fistula should result in a low threshold for spinal fluid sampling. Purely endoscopic endonasal surgery has been shown to have similar rates of meningitis as standard craniotomy[15] but should still be constantly remembered as a potential source of fever in the convalescing skull-base patient. Risk of pneumonia increases with prolonged intubation, but this must be balanced with aspiration risk in patients with lower cranial neuropathies.

## Systemic Complications

The length of combined skull-base procedures and resultant recovery places patients at greatly increased risk of systemic complications. Thromboembolus should be closely monitored with routine screening lower-extremity Dopplers. In addition, early mobilization is key, even in the face of concerns over microvascular flaps, CSF leak, and cranial neuropathy. Patients with sinonasal malignancies or preoperative nutritional compromise are at greater risk for all of the previously mentioned complications and should be carefully monitored for nutritional status.

---

### Clinical Pearls

- Postoperative epistaxis is usually from a branch of the sphenopalatine artery or anterior ethmoid artery.
- Postoperative epistaxis can be an early indication of a pseudoaneurysm of the ICA.
- A sudden change in mental status may be due to pneumocephalus without clinical evidence of a CSF leak.

---

## References

1. Koutourousiou M, Fernandez-Miranda JC, Stefko ST, Wang EW, Snyderman CH, Gardner PA. Endoscopic endonasal surgery for suprasellar meningiomas: experience with 75 patients. *J Neurosurg.* 2014;120(6):1326–1339.
2. Koutourousiou M, Gardner PA, Fernandez-Miranda JC, Paluzzi A, Wang EW, Snyderman CH. Endoscopic endonasal surgery for giant pituitary adenomas: advantages and limitations. *J Neurosurg.* 2013;118(3):621–631.
3. Koutourousiou M, Gardner PA, Fernandez-Miranda JC, Tyler-Kabara EC, Wang EW, Snyderman CH. Endoscopic endonasal surgery for craniopharyngiomas: surgical outcome in 64 patients. *J Neurosurg.* 2013;119(5):1194–1207.
4. Yano S, Hide T, Shinojima N, Hasegawa Y, Kawano T, Kuratsu J. Endoscopic endonasal skull base approach for parasellar lesions: Initial experiences, results, efficacy, and complications. *Surg Neurol Int.* 2014;16(5):51.
5. Zanation AM, Carrau RL, Snyderman CH, et al. Nasoseptal flap reconstruction of high flow intraoperative cerebral spinal fluid leaks during endoscopic skull base surgery. *Am J Rhinol Allergy.* 2009;23(5):518–521.
6. McCudden CR, Senior BA, Hainsworth S, et al. Evaluation of high resolution gel $\beta(2)$-transferrin for detection of cerebrospinal fluid leak. *Clin Chem Lab Med.* 2013;51(2):311–315.
7. Rodrigue T, Selman WR. Postoperative management in the neurosciences critical care unit. In: Suarez JI, ed. *Critical Care Neurology and Neurosurgery.* Totowa: Humana Press; 2004:433–448.
8. Horowitz G, Fliss DM, Margalit N, et al. Association between cerebrospinal fluid leak and meningitis after skull base surgery. *Otolaryngol Head Neck Surg.* 2011;145(4):689–693.
9. Klastersky J, Sadeghi M, Brihaye J. Antimicrobial prophylaxis in patients with rhinorrhea or otorrhea: a double-blind study. *Surg Neurol.* 1976;6(2):111–114.
10. Allen KP, Isaacson B, Purcell P, et al. Lumbar subarachnoid drainage in cerebrospinal fluid leaks after lateral skull base surgery. *Otol Neurotol.* 2011;32(9):1522–1524.
11. Yeo NK, Cho GS, Kim CJ, et al. The effectiveness of lumbar drainage in the conservative and surgical treatment of traumatic cerebrospinal fluid rhinorrhea. *Acta Otolaryngol.* 2013;133(1):82–90.
12. Schirmer CM, Heilman CB, Bhardwaj A. Pneumocephalus: case illustrations and review. *Neurocrit Care.* 2010;13(1):152–158.
13. Delgaudio JM, Ingley AP. Treatment of pneumocephalus after endoscopic sinus and microscopic skull base surgery. *Am J Otolaryngol.* 2010;31(4):226–230.
14. Peak DA, Green TE. Acute orbital compartment syndrome. Medscape. Last updated May 10, 2013.
15. Kono Y, Prevedello DM, Snyderman CH, et al. One thousand endoscopic skull base surgical procedures demystifying the infection potential: incidence and description of postoperative meningitis and brain abscesses. *Infect Control Hosp Epidemiol.* 2011;32(1):77–83.

# 44 *Management of Traumatic Brachial Plexus Injuries*

ZARINA S. ALI, LUKE MACYSZYN, and ERIC L. ZAGER

## Neuroanatomy and Procedure

### Key Concepts

- Traumatic injuries are the most common cause of brachial plexus lesions in children and adults.
- The pathophysiology of nerve injury correlates with the clinical presentation and diagnostic findings and guides treatment options.
- Restoration of motor and sensory function in a timely fashion and alleviation of pain are the goals of surgical management of brachial plexus injuries.
- In cases of nerve root avulsion, nerve transfer procedures are commonly used, whereas in postganglionic injuries, nerve grafting options also exist.
- Priorities for restoration of function include elbow flexion and shoulder stabilization. Functional recovery of the forearm, wrist, and hand is not expected in adults.

The brachial plexus is typically formed by contributions from four cervical roots and one thoracic root, including C5, C6, C7, C8, and T1 (Fig. 44.1). There may be additional contributions from the C4 (prefixed plexus) or T2 levels (postfixed plexus) as well.[1,2] At the level of the spinal nerves, a few branches are formed. Specifically, the dorsal scapular nerve, derived from the C5 spinal nerve, innervates the rhomboid muscles, and the long thoracic nerve—formed by the C5, C6, and C7 nerves—innervates the serratus anterior. The spinal nerves then come together to form the different segments of the brachial plexus. C5 and C6 spinal nerves merge to form the upper trunk. The C7 spinal nerve forms the middle trunk. C8 and T1 spinal nerves join to form the lower trunk.

The upper trunk gives off a nerve to subclavius muscle and also forms the suprascapular nerve, which innervates the supraspinatus and infraspinatus muscles. Each trunk then divides into an anterior and posterior division, which then form cords. The upper trunk gives rise to the lateral cord (from anterior division) and posterior cord (from posterior division). The lateral cord gives rise to the lateral pectoral nerve, which innervates the clavicular head of the pectoralis major. The middle trunk divides into the lateral cord (from anterior division) and posterior cord (from posterior division). Finally, the lower trunk forms the posterior cord (from posterior division) and medial cord (from anterior division). The medial cord forms the medial pectoral nerve, which innervates the sternocostal head of the pectoralis major muscle. Cutaneous branches from this cord include the medial brachial cutaneous nerve, which carries sensation from the lower medial portion of the arm, as well as the medial antebrachial cutaneous, which carries sensation from the ulnar portion of the forearm.

The cords then give rise to the terminal branches of the brachial plexus. Specifically, the lateral cord branches into the musculocutaneous nerve and also contributes to the median nerve. The posterior cord branches into the axillary nerve and then forms the radial nerve. The medial cord branches and contributes to the median nerve and then forms the ulnar nerve. There are varying contributions of motor and sensory fibers from each of the spinal nerves, with C5 and C6 having the greatest motor contribution and C7 having the greatest number of sensory fibers.[3]

Brachial plexus injuries can occur at any of these anatomical locations, resulting in a wide variety of clinical sequelae. The literature reports that 10% to 20% of peripheral nerve injuries are brachial plexus injuries, and 80% to 90% of these traumatic brachial plexus injuries in adults are caused by motorcycle and car accidents.[4] Traumatic brachial plexus injuries are usually a result of stretch or traction injuries or compressive/crush injuries. However, sharp lacerations can also occur. Traction injuries occur when the angle of the head and shoulder is increased supraphysiologically, resulting in an upper trunk injury, involving the C5 or C6 spinal nerves most commonly, also known as *Erb-Duchenne palsy*. The C7 nerve may occasionally be involved, which is also known as *extended Erb-Duchenne palsy*. Alternatively, when the arm is forcefully abducted over the head, traction of the lower elements of the brachial plexus occurs, typically involving C8 and T1, termed *Dejerine-Klumpke palsy*.

It is important to understand the distinction between preganglionic and postganglionic injuries, as this has important clinical implications. Preganglionic injuries occur when the nerve roots are forcefully avulsed from the spinal cord, proximal to the dorsal root ganglion, where the cell bodies of sensory axons reside. These injuries are the most severe type of injury, resulting in motor neuron cell death within the spinal cord and discontinuity of proximal sensory axons from the central nervous system. There is a poor likelihood for any spontaneous recovery in these cases. The C5, C6, and C7 spinal nerves have fibrous attachments between the epineurium and the cervical transverse process that afford some protection from avulsion injury, whereas the absence of these ligaments at C8 and T1 makes them vulnerable to preganglionic injuries. Postganglionic injuries, in contrast, occur distal to the sensory nerve cell bodies and allow for the possibility of nerve regeneration, depending on the extent of injury.

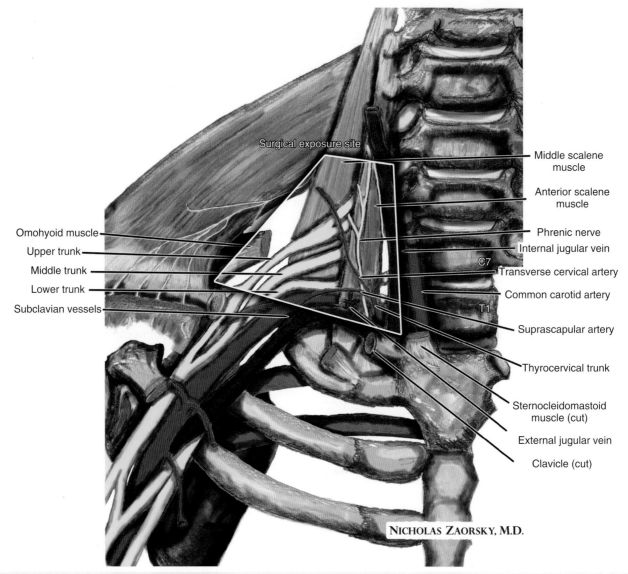

Fig. 44.1 Brachial plexus anatomy. (Illustration courtesy of Nicholas Zaorsky, MD.)

The pathophysiology of nerve injury is also a critical concept to understand when evaluating brachial plexus injuries. Seddon's classification scheme of nerve injury includes categorization of injuries into neurapraxia, axonotmesis, and neurotmesis.[5] Sunderland later introduced a classification scheme based on five grades of micropathology of the nerve injury to categorize the extent of injury and direct subsequent management (Table 44.1).[6] The mildest form of nerve injury, Sunderland type I, involves disruption of the axon's myelin sheath, resulting in a focal conduction block known as *neurapraxia*. Demyelination may occur, but spontaneous recovery is anticipated. Sunderland type II injuries involve more significant nerve injury with accompanying Wallerian degeneration, known as *axonotmesis*. However, the endoneurium remains intact, thereby allowing for spontaneous regeneration. Sunderland type III injuries involve disruption of the endoneurium, reducing the potential for spontaneous regeneration. Sunderland type IV injuries involve injury of the perineurium, with

a high likelihood of no spontaneous recovery. Complete rupture of all elements of the nerve, including the epineurium, a Sunderland type V injury, or Seddon's neurotmesis, portends a poor prognosis for recovery without surgical intervention.

**Table 44.1** Sunderland and Seddon Classifications of Nerve Injuries

| Sunderland Classification | Seddon Classification | Histology |
|---|---|---|
| I | Neurapraxia | Focal conduction block |
| II | Axonotmesis | Endoneurium and perineurium intact |
| III | Axonotmesis | Perineurium intact |
| IV | Axonotmesis | Epineurium intact |
| V | Neurotmesis | All layers disrupted |

**Table 44.2** Five Levels of Brachial Plexus Injuries

| Level of injury | Location |
|---|---|
| Level 1 | Supraclavicular, involving avulsion of the roots |
| Level 2 | Supraclavicular, involving lesions of the anterior branch of the spinal nerves outside the foramina, with or without avulsion, or lesions of the primary trunks |
| Level 3 | Retroclavicular lesions, usually involving the posterior or lateral cord, or both |
| Level 4 | Lesions of the distal part of the cords |
| Level 5 | Lesions of the terminal branches close to the origin at the plexus |

Classically, four levels of brachial plexus injury have been described (Table 44.2).[7] A level 1 injury involves a preganglionic root injury, including spinal cord, rootlets, and root injuries. Level 2 injuries may have a component of avulsion injuries but are also marked by disruption of the spinal nerve distal to the neural foramen, or at the level of the primary trunks of the brachial plexus. Level 3 injuries are retroclavicular and involve the cords, usually sparing the medial cord. Level 4 injuries involve the distal part of the cords. Level 5 injuries affect the terminal branch of the brachial plexus at their origin. An understanding of the level of injury has important surgical treatment implications.

Each type of brachial plexus injury requires a unique reconstructive strategy to allow for functional recovery. Until the 1970s, in cases of brachial plexus avulsion, amputation procedures were routinely performed due to lack of effective treatment options. Other strategies included arthrodesis of the shoulder, elbow, and wrist, depending on the level of the injury. In postganglionic brachial plexus injuries, a conservative "watch-and-wait" strategy was employed to determine whether any spontaneous return of function occurred. Now, with advances in diagnostic imaging and electrophysiology, most surgeons tend to favor early surgery. Many advocate exploratory surgery 3 to 6 months after the injury because delay in surgery is often associated with worse prognosis.[8,9]

A level 1 injury, or preganglionic, nerve root avulsion is the most common type of injury and occurs in about 70% of cases.[7] The only option for recovery of function in these cases relies on the use of nerve transfers, free muscle transplantation, and other palliative approaches. Nerve transfer involves the sacrifice of a physiologically healthy nerve to regenerate within a distal, more functionally important, but degenerating nerve. Thorough internal neurolysis of both the proximal and distal ends of the donor and recipient nerves is critical to allow for direct coaptation without the use of an interposed graft. At the level of the nerve transfer, the donor nerve branch should be cut as far distal (donor distal) as possible to decrease the length of regeneration required for these nerve fibers to reach the target muscle.[10] This process is known as *neurotization*. Several donor nerves exist and can be classified as extraplexal or intraplexal donor nerves.

Extraplexal nerve transfers are aimed at providing motor reinnervation of important muscle groups in the setting of

severe brachial plexus injury involving multiple spinal nerves. Therefore, suitable extraplexal donors include motor neural elements outside of the brachial plexus, including the phrenic nerve, spinal accessory nerve, intercostal nerves, deep motor branches of the cervical plexus, hypoglossal nerve, and the contralateral C7 spinal nerve.[11–13] Extraplexal sensory nerve transfers have also been performed utilizing the supraclavicular sensory nerves, intercostobrachial, and intercostal sensory branches to the median nerve to provide sensation to the paralytic hand.[14] Another option for reconstruction of level 1 injuries is intraplexal nerve transfers. This approach, however, is only possible in a partial plexus avulsion injury, in which fibers from a healthy terminal branch of the brachial plexus are transferred to the distal nerve segments of an avulsed root. This approach is highly dependent on intraoperative findings and availability of donor nerves, along with the patient's clinical status and level of function. Some of the more commonly employed nerve transfers include a posterior approach for spinal accessory nerve transfer to the suprascapular nerve in the setting of an upper trunk avulsion injury,[9] a partial ulnar nerve transfer to the biceps branch of the musculocutaneous nerve, termed *the Oberlin procedure*,[15] which allows for restoration of elbow function in cases of upper trunk avulsions, medial pectoral nerve to musculocutaneous nerve transfer, and a radial nerve triceps branch to axillary nerve transfer for recovery of deltoid function.[16–18] In the case of global nerve root avulsion, a contralateral C7 transfer to the median nerve using a vascularized ulnar nerve graft is employed to regain some hand function.[19] Intercostal nerve transfers to the musculocutaneous nerve, as well as phrenic nerve transfers to the suprascapular nerve, are used to restore elbow flexion and shoulder abduction, respectively.[20] Preferential use of a motor graft for restoration of critical motor function has also been advocated by some, but is not universally accepted.[21]

Free muscle transfer (FMT) is the transfer of a muscle using microvascular and microneural anastomoses to the denervated motor nerve.[22] A variety of free-functioning muscles can be transferred, including the latissimus dorsi (thoracodorsal nerve), the rectus femoris (femoral nerve), and the gracilis (anterior division of the obturator nerve). The gracilis myocutaneous FMT is the most common donor muscle used in brachial plexus reconstruction due to its long tendon length (which has the potential to restore elbow flexion, wrist extension, or finger flexion).[23–25] The FMT must be innervated by a healthy nerve, and either two intercostal motor nerves or the spinal accessory nerve is typically used to power a gracilis muscle flap. Proximally, the gracilis is secured to the clavicle, and distally, the gracilis tendon is woven into the biceps tendon. At least grade 4 elbow flexion is achieved in 79% of gracilis FMTs.[26] Local muscle transfers have also been used in brachial plexus injury repairs, but the outcome is directly related to the preoperative donor muscle strength, which is often impaired in extensive brachial plexus injuries.[12]

Tendon transfers are also useful, primarily in promoting shoulder stabilization and improving elbow flexion.[27] However, many limitations exist. For example, sensation and certain motor functions cannot be restored with this approach. In addition, surgery involves a large region of

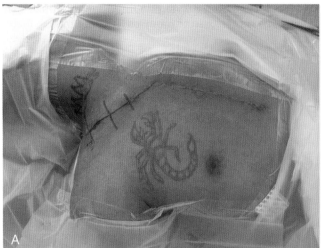
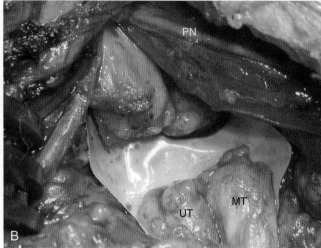

**Fig. 44.2** A 26-year-old patient with a stab wound to the right neck and chest **(A)** who underwent emergent mediastinal exploration for vascular injury, followed by brachial plexus exploration **(B)**, which revealed a laceration of the upper trunk (*UT*) and middle trunk (*MT*). *PN*, Phrenic nerve.

dissection with subsequent significant scarring and adhesions. Complications such as tendon rupture, inadequate tensioning, and stretch are also problematic.[10]

For level 2 to 4 injuries involving primarily postganglionic nerve injuries, the brachial plexus elements are often disrupted with neuroma formation and dense scar tissue. Reconstruction options include neurolysis, nerve repair, nerve grafts, and even nerve transfers, if an associated level 1 injury exists. Neurolysis is employed when the nerve injury is in continuity, implying that some healthy axons are present and capable of undergoing spontaneous recovery. Either an external neurolysis, in which dissection is performed around the epineurium, or internal neurolysis, in which an interfascicular dissection is performed, are options. In brachial plexus lesions, external neurolysis is typically performed, allowing for neural elements to be freed from surrounding, sometimes compressive, connective tissue and muscle scarring. Fascicular transfers, such as the Oberlin procedure, require internal neurolysis.

Direct nerve repair is only possible after clean, sharp penetrating injuries and should be performed acutely to allow for optimal chance of recovery of function. This usually involves direct suture coaptation of severed nerve stumps (Figs. 44.2 and 44.3). In some instances, jagged lacerations of the nerve can be tagged for delayed repair, which allows for appropriate trimming of the injured nerve stumps and grafting, if necessary.

Nerve grafting was introduced by Seddon in 1963[28] and remains the most commonly employed technique in brachial plexus reconstruction surgery. Most commonly, this is performed using a free nerve graft from a donor autologous site, such as the sural nerve graft (Fig. 44.4). The medial cutaneous nerves of the arm and forearm, the radial sensory nerve, and the saphenous nerve from the thigh are sometimes also used. Outcomes after nerve grafting are highly dependent on the length of the graft, the timing of intervention, presence of scar tissue at the wound site, number of grafts used, and the presence of a healthy proximal stump available for grafting.[14] Nerve repair with interposed graft is also employed when direct suture coaptation of ruptured nerve ends cannot be achieved without tension.

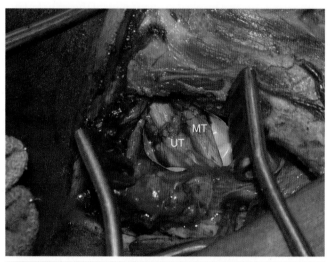

**Fig. 44.3** Coaptation suture and fibrin glue repair of upper trunk (*UT*) and middle trunk (*MT*) laceration injury of patient in Fig. 44.2.

Common examples of interpositional nerve grafting include coaptation of C5 spinal nerve to suprascapular nerve or axillary nerve (for shoulder abduction), C6 to musculocutaneous nerve (for elbow flexion), and C7 to triceps or radial nerve (for elbow extension and wrist extension).[12] Because donor nerve grafts are generally limited, autologous tissue such as vein grafts and manufactured conduits are also used.[29,30] However, outcomes are improved with autologous nerve grafting.[31]

A variety of surgical approaches to the brachial plexus have been described, including the anterior supraclavicular and infraclavicular approaches, as well as the posterior approach. Here, we describe the anterior supraclavicular approach because it is most commonly used by plexus surgeons.[32] General anesthesia is administered with short-acting neuromuscular blockade for induction to allow for subsequent nerve monitoring. The patient is then positioned supine with a standard shoulder roll under the ipsilateral scapula with the head turned toward the contralateral side and can rest on a donut pillow with

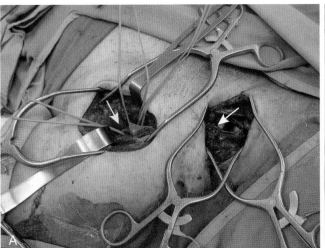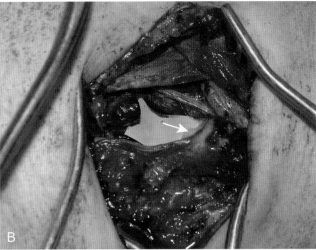

**Fig. 44.4  (A)** Intraoperative view of 20-year-old male involved in a skiing collision who underwent left C5 to musculocutaneous (*yellow arrow*) sural nerve graft (*white arrow*) and left C5 to axillary nerve sural nerve graft. The supraclavicular incision is on the right and infraclavicular incision on the left of the figure. **(B)** High-power view of same patient demonstrating the supraclavicular portion of the left C5 to musculocutaneous sural nerve graft (*white arrow*).

the head of the bed elevated at 15 to 20 degrees. The ipsilateral neck, thorax, upper extremity, and bilateral lower extremities (for possible sural nerve graft in cases of trauma) should be prepped and draped with the upper extremity resting on an arm board table. The surgeon should be able to freely manipulate the arm position during surgery. Needle electromyogram (EMG) electrodes are placed in appropriate muscles of the upper extremity for compound motor action potentials (CMAPs). Somatosensory and motor evoked potentials may also be used. Hook electrodes should be available for nerve action potential (NAP) monitoring.

An incision is made parallel and just superior to the clavicle in a natural skin crease at the base of the posterior cervical triangle (Fig. 44.5). Some surgeons prefer an L-shaped incision with the vertical limb overlying

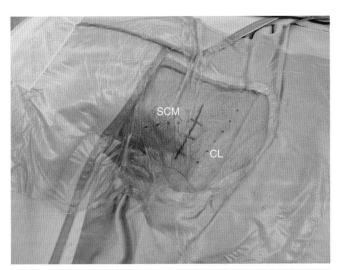

**Fig. 44.5** Right supraclavicular brachial plexus exploration planned skin incision (*solid line*) demonstrating lateral border of sternocleidomastoid (*SCM*) and superior border of clavicle (*CL*) (*dotted lines*) as an approach to the posterior triangle of the neck.

the posterior border of the sternocleidomastoid muscle (SCM). The platysma is immediately encountered and sharply incised. The posterior cervical triangle is then encountered, which is bounded medially by the posterior border of the SCM, laterally by the anterior border of the trapezius muscle, and inferiorly by the clavicle. Dissection proceeds along the posterior border of the SCM, and the lateral aspect of its insertion on the clavicle may be released to enhance exposure. The supraclavicular fat pad is mobilized along its medial and inferior borders and is retracted laterally. The transverse cervical artery and vein are identified at this level and are either retracted or ligated and transected. The posterior belly of the omohyoid muscle is then encountered and also retracted. Lymphatic vessels are either coagulated with the bipolar or ligated. After the SCM is retracted medially and the fat pad laterally, the phrenic nerve is identified at the surface of the anterior scalene muscle (ASM) beneath its thin fascial investment. The phrenic nerve follows a typical course from lateral to medial as it descends over the ASM. In cases of severe trauma, the nerve may not be visible initially and may require electrical stimulation to induce hemidiaphragm contraction. Care should be taken to protect this fragile neural structure and gently retract it to avoid injury. The phrenic nerve serves as an important landmark for identifying the C5 spinal nerve.

The upper trunk is identified lateral to the ASM. The C5 spinal nerve can be identified joining the C6 spinal nerve to form the upper trunk. Exposure of the middle and lower trunks requires C7, C8, and T1 spinal nerve visualization. This can be accomplished by dividing or resecting the ASM. Similarly, the middle scalene muscle may also contain fibrous elements near the attachment to the first rib. These bands must be meticulously divided. The subclavian artery lies deep to the ASM inferiorly, and careful dissection and retraction of this vessel and its branches are required to protect it from injury. Excision of the suprapleural membrane (Sibson's fascia) lying between the lower cervical transverse processes and the parietal pleura allows for access to the C8 and T1 spinal nerves and the lower trunk. Depending on the extent of injury, extensive neurolysis (360-degree dissection) is then performed on all plexus elements. In cases of trauma, the trunks are dissected distally and beneath the clavicle to identify the anterior and posterior divisions and the suprascapular nerve. Infraclavicular brachial plexus exposure through the deltopectoral groove is often necessary in these cases.

CMAPs are recorded to confirm the identity of each neural element and to establish functionality. The surgeon can record NAPs across a traumatic lesion to identify internal fascicular disruption and to determine the extent of axonal regeneration. Lesions with positive NAPs should not be excised after external neurolysis is performed because spontaneous functional recovery occurs in approximately 90% of cases.[33]

At the completion of the procedure, the wound is flooded with saline and the anesthesiologist performs a Valsalva maneuver to check for an air leak, indicating the presence of a pneumothorax. Meticulous hemostasis is achieved using bipolar cautery prior to closure. The surgeon should also recheck for leakage of lymphatic fluid because chylothorax may be a major complication. A drain is optional. The platysma and subcutaneous layers are closed with interrupted 3-0 Vicryl suture followed by 4-0 running subcuticular absorbable suture for the skin. The incision is covered with a dressing for 24 hours. In cases of nerve repair, we maintain the arm in a sling for 3 weeks and then prescribe progressive range-of-motion exercises under supervision of an experienced physical therapist.

## Perioperative Considerations

### Key Concepts

- Imaging studies and electrophysiological studies are used in conjunction with the clinical examination of the patient to determine the best treatment course.
- Intraoperative neurophysiological assessment guides the surgeon with the type and extent of surgical intervention.
- The optimal timing of traumatic brachial plexus exploration and reconstruction is controversial, but early identification of the injury and referral to a neurosurgeon can have dramatic implications for recovery of function.

Planning brachial plexus reconstruction surgery requires thorough preoperative and perioperative evaluation. Often, imaging studies along with electrophysiological studies are used to supplement the clinical examination of the patient. Among the imaging studies, computed tomography myelogram is able to detect nerve root avulsions with a sensitivity of 85% and a specificity of 95%.[34] More advanced magnetic resonance imaging has also been used to identify both evidence of avulsion injury and the precise location of injury along the brachial plexus.[35] Chest x-rays help to reveal rib fractures, which may indicate injury to intercostal nerves and limit their use as potential donors

for nerve transfer. In addition, inspiration and expiration views allow for assessment of diaphragmatic paralysis.

### Clinical Pearls

**Traumatic brachial plexus injuries and management**

- Appropriate patient selection and correct localization of the lesion using detailed history and physical examination remain the most critical aspects of successful peripheral nerve surgery.
- Appropriate diagnostic studies, including EMG and imaging, are essential for determining the proper timing and approach for surgical intervention.
- Complete dissection of all injured brachial plexus elements, along with intraoperative electrophysiological studies, are necessary to identify the optimal surgical management with neurolysis, nerve grafts, and/or nerve transfers.
- The phrenic nerve is particularly vulnerable to retraction injury during exposure of the supraclavicular brachial plexus.

Electrodiagnostic studies can be instrumental in supporting the clinical examination to determine which nerves are injured, the location of the injury, and the presence of regeneration. Baseline EMG and nerve conduction studies are typically performed 3 to 4 weeks after injury. On EMG studies, denervated muscle exhibits positive sharp waves and fibrillations as Wallerian degeneration occurs along the injured motor nerve. EMG can also identify reinnervation potentials (nascent motor units, polyphasic action potentials), which may precede functional recovery. Because these findings imply spontaneous recovery, repeat electrodiagnostic studies are recommended prior to surgical intervention. Preganglionic injuries can also be identified electrophysiologically because an injury proximal to the dorsal root ganglion will spare distal sensory axons. Therefore sensory nerve action potentials (SNAPs) are preserved despite clinical loss of sensation. Similarly, the presence of SNAPs with the absence of voluntary motor unit potentials suggests preganglionic injury.

Intraoperative electrodiagnostic studies are invaluable in brachial plexus reconstruction surgeries. Electrical stimulation of the brachial plexus elements can be performed during surgery to provide the surgeon insight into the relative health or degeneration of particular nerve fibers. In the case of a nerve in continuity with neuroma formation, the NAP becomes critical in the surgeon's decision of whether to perform external neurolysis versus resection of neuroma and nerve grafting. Briefly, the NAP is performed by applying one electrode proximal to the neuroma and one distal to it to enable quantitative assessment of the number of viable nerve fibers.[36,37] More than 90% of patients with a preserved NAP will gain clinically useful recovery.[33] Intraoperative nerve stimulation is also useful in nerve transfer surgery in order to identify donor fascicles that are expendable and confirm nonfunctionality of the recipient nerve fiber.

One of the most critical aspects of brachial plexus reconstruction requires perioperative decision making regarding the goals and timing of surgery. Given that in many of these cases few functioning neural elements exist, prioritization of functional recovery becomes paramount. Many authors advocate for elbow flexion and shoulder stability as fundamental priorities for improved outcome.[12] Secondary priorities include hand sensation and wrist and finger extension and flexion. Hand function, due to its poor potential for recovery, is rarely a priority in adult brachial plexus reconstruction. These priorities are quite different in infants.

With respect to timing of surgery, there has recently been significant interest in performing very early nerve transfers and/or nerve grafting, both in the adult and pediatric populations.[38–44] There is strong evidence that the earlier the nerve repair or transfer surgery is performed, the more effective the target reinnervation, nerve regeneration, and neuromuscular function. This aggressive approach is supported by the natural history of neuronal cell death due to axotomy. It is even more important in preganglionic injuries, in which up to 80% of motoneurons undergo cell death in animal models.[45] Early repair strategies rely on the coordination of trauma surgeons and critical care intensivists to identify patients with a high-velocity mechanism of injury, clinically flail arm with loss of rhomboid and serratus anterior function and evidence of Horner's syndrome, severe neuropathic pain, and associated injuries, such as first rib or clavicular fracture or subclavian vessel injury. These patients require early consultation with a peripheral nerve surgeon in order to determine indications for early brachial plexus exploration or nerve transfer. One of the most common reasons for delayed brachial plexus repair is the presence of other associated major injuries, which may distract from the diagnosis of critical nerve injury. Multidisciplinary care in the intensive care unit (ICU) setting should promote prompt identification of the peripheral nerve injury patient because the timing of intervention can have dramatic implications for recovery of function.

## Postoperative Complications

### Key Concepts

- Most postoperative complications from brachial plexus surgery involve wound healing and infection of the surgical site, as well as the donor nerve site.
- Postoperative chest x-ray is necessary to assess for iatrogenic phrenic nerve injury.
- Patients should be counseled on the risk of failed surgery, which can occur up to 40% of the time.
- Neuropathic pain from brachial plexus injury is best treated by a combination of pharmacological agents and can require the need for pain management referral.

Although most patients do not require postoperative ICU admission, there are several complications that must be avoided and assessed in the postoperative period while the patient is recovering from surgery on the hospital ward (Box 44.1). Most complications in brachial plexus surgery are not dramatically different from those of any other surgery and include delayed wound healing and/or infection, especially of sural nerve harvest incision sites. This is more common in high-risk populations, including diabetic and renal failure patients. Seromas and hematomas in the

**Box 44.1   Complications of Brachial Plexus Reconstruction for Traumatic Brachial Plexus Injuries**

Injury to the subclavian artery or vein
Further injury to the brachial plexus
Phrenic nerve injury
No improvement from surgery/persistent disability
Pneumothorax
Chylothorax
Donor nerve site morbidity
Neuropathic pain, causalgia
Delayed wound healing/infection

operative areas can be minimized by judicious use of drains. An immediate postoperative chest x-ray is necessary to assess for pneumothorax and for evidence of hemidiaphragm elevation, which indicates ipsilateral phrenic nerve injury. In the event of either of these complications, transfer of the patient to the ICU for further respiratory monitoring and/or chest tube placement may be indicated.

Donor site morbidity from nerve harvesting is also a recognized complication of brachial plexus reconstruction surgery. For example, intercostal nerve transfers are associated with pleural tear during nerve elevations, occurring in approximately 9% of cases.[46] Symptomatic pleural effusion, acute respiratory distress syndrome, and seroma formation are much rarer, but potentially more severe sequelae. Additional surgical complications include chylothorax, causalgia, and further injury to the plexus, including total paralysis and complete sensory loss. Other surgical complications that occur relatively infrequently but can pose significant morbidity include injury to the subclavian artery and vein. This intraoperative complication is typically identified and addressed at the time of surgery. Intraoperative vascular surgery consultation may be required in cases of extensive arteriotomy.

Some believe that one of the most significant postoperative complications from brachial plexus reconstruction is failed surgery. The literature reports improved function in only approximately 60% of brachial plexus injury patients, including those treated at experienced centers. Specifically, intercostal to musculocutaneous nerve transfers result in 65% to 72% of patients obtaining M3 or greater biceps function.[47,48] In contrast, spinal accessory nerve transfer to the musculocutaneous nerve produces greater than M3 function in 77% of patients and greater than or equal to M4 function in 29%.[48] The Oberlin procedure has very favorable results, including 85% recovery of M3 or greater biceps strength, with more recent data indicating 94% M4 strength or better.[15] For shoulder abduction and flexion, spinal accessory nerve to suprascapular nerve transfer offers greater than or equal to M3 function at 60 degrees abduction in 80% of patients.[47] This result is enhanced with a second nerve transfer, radial nerve triceps branch to axillary nerve, resulting in an average of 124 degrees of abduction by 28 months.[18] Despite some of these favorable results, many patients remain disabled, with half of those previously employed remaining disabled.

Neuropathic pain is common after brachial plexus injury and can persist until nerve regeneration is complete.[49,50] A combination of sympatholytics, antiinflammatory agents, antiepileptics such as gabapentin and pregabalin, and antidepressants with a narcotic can be used for severe pain. Pain management referrals are usually appropriate for patients with avulsion injuries because they may require high doses of narcotics and possibly procedural intervention (stellate ganglion blocks, peripheral nerve stimulator, and dorsal column stimulator).[50–53] Over time, 80% of these patients have complete recovery from neuropathic pain by 3 years.[54] In severe cases, avulsion pain can be surgically managed by lesioning the dorsal root entry zone of the traumatized spinal cord.[55]

## References

1. Büyükmumcu M, Ziylan T, Uysal II, et al. Brachial plexus variations in human fetuses. *Neurosurgery*. 2003;53(3):676–684. discussion 84. Epub 2003/08/29.
2. Kerr AT. The brachial plexus of nerves in man, the variations in its formation and branches. *Am J Anat*. 1918;23:285–395.
3. Ferrante MA, Wilbourn AJ. The utility of various sensory nerve conduction responses in assessing brachial plexopathies. *Muscle Nerve*. 1995;18(8):879–889. Epub 1995/08/01.
4. Flores LP. Epidemiological study of the traumatic brachial plexus injuries in adults. *Arq Neuropsiquiatr*. 2006;64(1):88–94. Epub 2006/04/20.
5. Seddon HJ. Three types of nerve injury. *Brain*. 1943;66:237–288.
6. Sunderland S. A classification of peripheral nerve injuries producing loss of function. *Brain*. 1951;74(4):491–516. Epub 1951/12/01.
7. Narakas AO. The treatment of brachial plexus injuries. *Int Orthop*. 1985;9(1):29–36. Epub 1985/01/01.
8. Bertelli JA, Ghizoni MF. Results and current approach for Brachial Plexus reconstruction. *J Brachial Plex Peripher Nerve Inj*. 2011;6 (1):2. Epub 2011/06/17.
9. Narakas AO, Hentz VR. Neurotization in brachial plexus injuries. Indication and results. *Clin Orthop Relat Res*. 1988;237:43–56. Epub 1988/12/01.
10. Fox IK, Mackinnon SE. Adult peripheral nerve disorders: nerve entrapment, repair, transfer, and brachial plexus disorders. *Plast Reconstr Surg*. 2011;127(5):105e–118e. Epub 2011/05/03.
11. Gu Y, Xu J, Chen L, et al. Long term outcome of contralateral C7 transfer: a report of 32 cases. *Chin Med J (Engl)*. 2002;115(6):866–868. Epub 2002/07/19.
12. Giuffre JL, Kakar S, Bishop AT, et al. Current concepts of the treatment of adult brachial plexus injuries. *J Hand Surg Am*. 2010;35 (4):678–688. quiz 88. Epub 2010/04/01.
13. Chuang DC. Neurotization procedures for brachial plexus injuries. *Hand Clin*. 1995;11(4):633–645. Epub 1995/11/01.
14. Chuang DC. Brachial plexus injury: nerve reconstruction and functioning muscle transplantation. *Semin Plast Surg*. 2010;24 (1):57–66. Epub 2011/02/03.
15. Oberlin C, Beal D, Leechavengvongs S, et al. Nerve transfer to biceps muscle using a part of ulnar nerve for C5-C6 avulsion of the brachial plexus: anatomical study and report of four cases. *J Hand Surg Am*. 1994;19(2):232–237. Epub 1994/03/01.
16. Leechavengvongs S, Witoonchart K, Uerpairojkit C, et al. Combined nerve transfers for C5 and C6 brachial plexus avulsion injury. *J Hand Surg Am*. 2006;31(2):183–189. Epub 2006/02/14.
17. Witoonchart K, Leechavengvongs S, Uerpairojkit C, et al. Nerve transfer to deltoid muscle using the nerve to the long head of the triceps, part I: an anatomic feasibility study. *J Hand Surg Am*. 2003;28 (4):628–632. Epub 2003/07/25.
18. Leechavengvongs S, Witoonchart K, Uerpairojkit C, et al. Nerve transfer to deltoid muscle using the nerve to the long head of the triceps, part II: a report of 7 cases. *J Hand Surg Am*. 2003;28(4):633–638. Epub 2003/07/25.
19. Gu YD, Zhang GM, Chen DS, et al. Seventh cervical nerve root transfer from the contralateral healthy side for treatment of brachial plexus root avulsion. *J Hand Surg Br*. 1992;17(5):518–521. Epub 1992/10/01.
20. Gu YD, Wu MM, Zhen YL, et al. Phrenic nerve transfer for treatment of root avulsion of the brachial plexus. *Chin Med J (Engl)*. 1990;103 (4):267–270. Epub 1990/04/01.
21. Nichols CM, Brenner MJ, Fox IK, et al. Effects of motor versus sensory nerve grafts on peripheral nerve regeneration. *Exp Neurol*. 2004;190 (2):347–355. Epub 2004/11/09.
22. Tamai S, Komatsu S, Sakamoto H, et al. Free muscle transplants in dogs, with microsurgical neurovascular anastomoses. *Plast Reconstr Surg*. 1970;46(3):219–225. Epub 1970/09/01.
23. Chuang DC. Functioning free muscle transplantation for brachial plexus injury. *Clin Orthop Relat Res*. 1995;314:104–111. Epub 1995/05/01.
24. Doi K. Management of total paralysis of the brachial plexus by the double free-muscle transfer technique. *J Hand Surg Eur Vol*. 2008;33(3):240–251. Epub 2008/06/20.
25. Shin AY, Spinner RJ, Steinmann SP, et al. Adult traumatic brachial plexus injuries. *J Am Acad Orthop Surg*. 2005;13(6):382–396. Epub 2005/10/15.
26. Bishop AT. Functioning free-muscle transfer for brachial plexus injury. *Hand Clin*. 2005;21(1):91–102. Epub 2005/01/26.
27. Chen WS. Restoration of elbow flexion by modified Steindler flexorplasty. *Int Orthop*. 2000;24(1):43–46. Epub 2000/04/25.
28. Seddon HJ. Nerve grafting. *J Bone Joint Surg Br*. 1963;45:447–461. Epub 1963/08/01.
29. Chiu DT. Autogenous venous nerve conduits. A review. *Hand Clin*. 1999;15(4):667–671. ix. Epub 1999/11/24.
30. Chiu DT, Strauch B. A prospective clinical evaluation of autogenous vein grafts used as a nerve conduit for distal sensory nerve defects of 3 cm or less. *Plast Reconstr Surg*. 1990;86(5):928–934. Epub 1990/11/01.
31. Whitlock EL, Tuffaha SH, Luciano JP, et al. Processed allografts and type I collagen conduits for repair of peripheral nerve gaps. *Muscle Nerve*. 2009;39(6):787–799. Epub 2009/03/18.
32. Tender GC, Kline DG. Anterior supraclavicular approach to the brachial plexus. *Neurosurgery*. 2006;58(4 suppl 2) ONS-360–4; discussion ONS-4–5. Epub 2006/04/04.
33. Kline DGHA. *Nerve Injuries: Operative Results for Major Nerve Injuries, Entrapments, and Tumors*. Philadelphia, PA: WB Saunders; 1995.
34. Carvalho GA, Nikkhah G, Matthies C, et al. Diagnosis of root avulsions in traumatic brachial plexus injuries: value of computerized tomography myelography and magnetic resonance imaging. *J Neurosurg*. 1997;86(1):69–76. Epub 1997/01/01.
35. Yoshikawa T, Hayashi N, Yamamoto S, et al. Brachial plexus injury: clinical manifestations, conventional imaging findings, and the latest imaging techniques. *Radiographics*. 2006;26(suppl 1):S133–S143. Epub 2006/10/20.
36. Kline DG, Happel LT. Penfield Lecture. A quarter century's experience with intraoperative nerve action potential recording. *Can J Neurol Sci*. 1993;20(1):3–10. Epub 1993/02/01.
37. Flores LP. The importance of the preoperative clinical parameters and the intraoperative electrophysiological monitoring in brachial plexus surgery. *Arq Neuropsiquiatr*. 2011;69(4):654–659. Epub 2011/08/31.
38. Little KJ, Zlotolow DA, Soldado F, et al. Early functional recovery of elbow flexion and supination following median and/or ulnar nerve fascicle transfer in upper neonatal brachial plexus palsy. *J Bone Joint Surg Am*. 2014;96(3):215–221. Epub 2014/02/07.
39. Mohammad-Reda A. Early post-operative results after repair of traumatic brachial plexus palsy. *Turk Neurosurg*. 2013;23(1):1–9. Epub 2013/01/25.
40. Duclos L, Gilbert A. Obstetrical palsy: early treatment and secondary procedures. *Ann Acad Med Singapore*. 1995;24(6):841–845. Epub 1995/11/01.
41. Kawabata H, Masada K, Tsuyuguchi Y, et al. Early microsurgical reconstruction in birth palsy. *Clin Orthop Relat Res*. 1987;215:233–242. Epub 1987/02/01.
42. Alanen M, Halonen JP, Katevuo K, et al. Early surgical exploration and epineural repair in birth brachial palsy. *Z Kinderchir*. 1986;41 (6):335–337. Epub 1986/12/01.
43. Terzis JK, Vekris MD, Soucacos PN. Outcomes of brachial plexus reconstruction in 204 patients with devastating paralysis. *Plast Reconstr Surg*. 1999;104(5):1221–1240. Epub 1999/10/08.
44. Jivan S, Kumar N, Wiberg M, et al. The influence of pre-surgical delay on functional outcome after reconstruction of brachial plexus injuries. *J Plast Reconstr Aesthet Surg*. 2009;62(4):472–479. Epub 2008/05/20.

45. Koliatsos VE, Price WL, Pardo CA, et al. Ventral root avulsion: an experimental model of death of adult motor neurons. *J Comp Neurol.* 1994;342(1):35–44. Epub 1994/04/01.

46. Kovachevich R, Kircher MF, Wood CM, et al. Complications of intercostal nerve transfer for brachial plexus reconstruction. *J Hand Surg Am.* 2010;35(12):1995–2000. Epub 2010/11/26.

47. Songcharoen P, Wongtrakul S, Spinner RJ. Brachial plexus injuries in the adult. nerve transfers: the Siriraj Hospital experience. *Hand Clin.* 2005;21(1):83–89. Epub 2005/01/26.

48. Merrell GA, Barrie KA, Katz DL, et al. Results of nerve transfer techniques for restoration of shoulder and elbow function in the context of a meta-analysis of the English literature. *J Hand Surg Am.* 2001;26 (2):303–314. Epub 2001/04/03.

49. Schwartzman RJ, Maleki J. Postinjury neuropathic pain syndromes. *Med Clin North Am.* 1999;83(3):597–626. Epub 1999/07/01.

50. Merritt WH. The challenge to manage reflex sympathetic dystrophy/ complex regional pain syndrome. *Clin Plast Surg.* 2005;32 (4):575–604. vii–viii. Epub 2005/09/06.

51. Bittar RG, Teddy PJ. Peripheral neuromodulation for pain. *J Clin Neurosci.* 2009;16(10):1259–1261. Epub 2009/07/01.

52. Novak CB, Mackinnon SE. Outcome following implantation of a peripheral nerve stimulator in patients with chronic nerve pain. *Plast Reconstr Surg.* 2000;105(6):1967–1972. Epub 2000/ 06/06.

53. North R, Shipley J, Prager J, et al. Practice parameters for the use of spinal cord stimulation in the treatment of chronic neuropathic pain. *Pain Med.* 2007;8(suppl 4):S200–S275. Epub 2007/11/13.

54. Zorub DS, Nashold Jr BS, Cook Jr WA. Avulsion of the brachial plexus. I. A review with implications on the therapy of intractable pain. *Surg Neurol.* 1974;2(5):347–353. Epub 1974/09/01.

55. Friedman AH, Nashold Jr BS, Bronec PR. Dorsal root entry zone lesions for the treatment of brachial plexus avulsion injuries: a follow-up study. *Neurosurgery.* 1988;22(2):369–373. Epub 1988/02/01.

# Specific Intensive Care Unit Complications

# 45 Delayed Emergence after Neurosurgery

ANURAG TEWARI, RAFI AVITSIAN, and EDWARD M. MANNO

## Introduction

The quote "It ain't over till it's over" may be a good opening statement for this topic. Similar to a flight, which needs a successful landing, anesthesia needs a well-planned and managed emergence. Although the common understanding of an anesthesiologist is the doctor who "can put me to sleep," we should also not forget about her or his role in "waking me up"!

Emergence is a gradual return to the mental and physical capabilities that existed prior to induction of anesthesia. Emergence is an active process whereby the first three of the four components of anesthesia, namely amnesia, hypnosis, and muscle relaxation, are reversed while ensuring adequate analgesia (the fourth component). An important part of the previous definition is the term *gradual*. Nevertheless a timely emergence after neurosurgical procedures is important to demonstrate the success and safety of the surgical procedure. The goal is to have a medically stable patient who is awake and alert, spontaneously ventilating, and maintaining an adequate airway. Thus delayed emergence, defined as a longer-than-expected emergence, may alert the anesthesiologist to an early diagnosis of intracranial complications.

After stopping sedation the patient should rapidly become awake and alert. Delayed emergence is usually described as failure to regain consciousness 20 to 30 minutes after a neurosurgical procedure. Although one of the most feared complications after craniotomy, intracranial hemorrhage, may manifest as delayed emergence, there are other etiologies that need rapid diagnosis and treatment. For purposes of this chapter, when discussing delayed emergence, we will refer to cases in which the emergence from general anesthesia and extubation is not deliberately postponed. This chapter will first review the anesthetic goals and considerations for determining the best time of emergence and extubation after neurosurgical procedures; the main focus, however, will be on a systematic approach to diagnosis and treatment of patients with noninduced delayed emergence after a neurosurgical procedure.

## Emergence from Neurosurgical Procedures

### Key Concepts

- A controlled emergence from neurosurgery is important to the success of the surgery.
- Too rapid an emergence can lead to secondary complications.
- Delayed emergence and extubation may be required in certain circumstances.

Emergence after a neurosurgical procedure should be rapid and well controlled. These features may seem incompatible, but recent advances in pharmacology have given us newer adjuncts in anesthesia to emerge a patient from anesthesia for an early neurological examination in a smooth manner with minimal hemodynamic changes. A particular problem postoperatively is coughing. Coughing induced by the endotracheal tube can result in a series of hemodynamic changes that lead to a rapid increase in intracranial pressure (ICP), venous pressure, and arterial blood pressure. In patients with disturbed cerebral autoregulation due to residual anesthetics, hypertension (HTN) can result in cerebral hyperemia and potentially breakthrough bleeding in the postoperative brain. Thus stable hemodynamics is an important goal during emergence.

During the early stages of emergence oxygenation and ventilation may also be suboptimal. Hypoventilation may lead to respiratory acidosis with subsequent intracranial hyperemia and increased ICP. This process may be exacerbated in situations of prolonged hyperventilation during surgery.

Delayed emergence from anesthesia may be needed under conditions where a neurosurgical complication is suspected. In these circumstances, delayed emergence is needed to allow better control of hemodynamic and ventilatory physiology. In one large prospective study at least one complication was observed in 54.5% of patients after a neurosurgical procedure. Nausea or vomiting (38%) was found to be the most common complication, followed by cardiovascular (6.7%), neurological (5.7%), and respiratory (2.8%) complications.[1] Other retrospective studies have reported the incidence of major complications to be between 13% and 27.5%.[2-4]

Hasty uncontrolled emergence and extubation may cause a higher incidence of complications than a slow and controlled emergence. In a prospective study, Magni et al.[5] reported complications in 92 of 162 patients (57%), with respiratory impairment (28%) as the most frequent adverse event. They confirmed that the recovery period after neurosurgical procedures remains a time of great danger to patients, given the high incidence of postoperative adverse events. These events appear to be independent of the anesthetic strategy. In a retrospective analysis of common complications of neurosurgery, Li et al.[6] found a higher incidence (52.7%) of complications during the first 2 hours of surgery. In a prospective review of general pediatric neurosurgery, Lindert et al.[7] reported a complication rate of 20.2%, with 2.7% occurring during surgery and 17.5% in the postoperative period.

Due to the frequency of complications associated with early emergence, a period of longer postoperative sedation

**Table 45.1**　Systemic and Cerebral Conditions Contributing to Delayed Emergence

| Systemic | Cerebral |
|---|---|
| Hypothermia <35°C | Preoperative altered consciousness |
| Hypertension SBP >150 mm Hg | Cerebral swelling, herniation, midline shift |
| Hypotension-hypovolemia | Brain ischemic, infarction, bleeding |
| Hematocrit <25% | Surgical duration (>6 h) |
| Hypoxia or hypercapnia | Posterior fossa surgery, injury to cranial nerves (IX, X, XII) |
| Ineffective spontaneous ventilation | Seizures |
| Hypoosmolality (<280 mOsmol/kg) | |
| Residual neuromuscular blockade | |
| Underlying metabolic disorders | |

*SBP*, systolic blood pressure.

and mechanical ventilation has become common in some neurosurgical centers after intracranial procedures. In one neuroanesthesiology practice in Germany, 39% of patients with brain tumors were managed with prolonged postoperative ventilation.[8]

Delayed extubation may be required in cases of longer surgery (>6 hours), large tumor resections, injury to the cranial nerves (especially IX, X, and XII), complications during surgery, hypothermia, or when there are severe respiratory or cardiovascular complications during emergence[9] (Table 45.1). Manninen et al. in a prospective study noted that 11% of patients remained intubated for more than 4 hours after the end of surgery.[1] Cai et al. in a prospective study reported delayed extubation in almost one-half of their patients. They concluded that brainstem procedures and lower cranial nerve dysfunction were the main factors delaying extubation.[10]

# Approach to Delayed Emergence

## Key Concepts

- The approach to the neurosurgical patient who is slow to emerge from anesthesia should occur in a systemic fashion.
- Causes for delayed emergence can be categorized as due to preoperative, intraoperative, or postoperative causes.
- Previous medical conditions, medications, or habitual use of drugs or over-the-counter supplements can complicate emergence from neurosurgical procedures.
- Prolonged pharmacological effects of medications may contribute to delayed emergence.
- Early postoperative diagnosis of neurological complications is an important step in limiting cerebral complications and improving outcome.

An effective way to approach delayed emergence is to identify all possible causes leading to a slower-than-expected return of consciousness and preoperative ventilatory and hemodynamic status. The etiologies of delayed emergence can be categorized into preoperative, intraoperative, and immediate postoperative causes.

## PREOPERATIVE CAUSES

The preoperative mental status and cognitive function of patients undergoing neurosurgical procedures is probably the most important predictor of postoperative mental acuity. Preoperative neurological and mental status evaluation and documentation is an important part in determining an anesthetic plan. During this evaluation, baseline conditions should be identified that may affect the speed of postoperative anesthetic recovery.

The anesthetic dose must also be corrected for age; failure to do so may lead to excess administration of anesthetics and a slower recovery. Elderly patients are also more prone to postoperative delirium.[11] Age also affects the pharmacokinetics of any medications used in the perioperative period.[12]

Another important determinant of anesthetic depth and emergence is the perioperative use of alcohol and recreational drugs. Chronic alcoholism increases the volatile anesthetic needs of a patient defined as the minimal alveolar concentration (MAC) of volatile anesthetic that inhibits movement from a painful stimulus in 50% of patients. Conversely, acute alcohol intoxication decreases the MAC. Chronic use of opioids can also change receptor sensitivity to narcotics and cause an increased need for these medications.

Use of over-the-counter medications as well as some herbal supplements can also affect emergence (Table 45.2).[13] Kava-kava can potentiate the effect of barbiturates and benzodiazepines and cause excessive sedation. Saw palmetto can alter the pharmacokinetics of benzodiazepines (e.g., alprazolam) or dextromethorphan. Ephedra can potentially interact with volatile general anesthetic agents (e.g., halothane, isoflurane, desflurane) and cardiac glycosides (e.g., digitalis) and may cause cardiac dysrhythmias. Patients taking ephedra for prolonged periods can deplete peripheral catecholamine stores. Thus under general anesthesia, these patients may have profound intraoperative hypotension, which must be controlled with a direct vasoconstrictor (e.g., phenylephrine) instead of ephedrine (an indirect sympathomimetic). Use of ephedra with phenelzine or other monoamine oxidase inhibitors may result in insomnia, headache, and tremulousness. Concomitant use with oxytocin has been shown to cause HTN. Ginger enhances barbiturate effects and, as a result of its inotropic effect, can interfere with cardiac medications. Large quantities of ginger may also cause cardiac arrhythmias and central nervous system (CNS) depression.

Patients who have a history of diabetes should have periodic monitoring of their blood sugar, especially during prolonged procedures. Special attention should be given to the diabetic treatment modality because preoperative fasting can elicit hypoglycemia with some diabetic medications if dosing is not adjusted. Mental status changes in these patients could be a result of hypoglycemia or hyperglycemia.

In patients with a history of Parkinson's disease, special attention should be directed at the frequency and dosing

**Table 45.2** Popular Herbal Products and Possible Concerns for Anesthesiologists

| | |
|---|---|
| Black Cohosh | Hypotension; predisposes to bleeding |
| Echinacea | Potentiates barbiturate toxicity, immune suppression; nephrotoxic; inflammation of the liver; antagonizes the immunosuppressive actions of corticosteroids and cyclosporine; inhibits hepatic microsomal enzymes |
| Ephedra | Sympathomimetic, interacts with volatile general anesthetic agents, profound intraoperative hypotension |
| Feverfew | Migraine, insomnia, anxiety, and joint stiffness; inhibits platelet activity |
| Garlic | β-adrenergic antagonist action modulated by garlic dialysate; augments the effects of anticoagulants |
| Ginger | Sedative effects; increases risk of bleeding if patient on anticoagulants; enhances barbiturate effects |
| Ginkgo Biloba | Inhibits hepatic microsomal enzymes; may increase bleeding, immune-stimulating effects |
| Ginseng | Hypertension, insomnia, and irritability; risk of cardiac effects; avoid in patients on anticoagulants; use cautiously in diabetic patients |
| Hoodia | Fluctuations in blood sugar levels; probable arrhythmia |
| Kava | Possible liver toxicity; sedative effects; risk of potentiating effect to medications |
| Saw Palmetto | Can interact with benzodiazepines or medications such as dextromethorphan |
| St. John's Wort | Induces the cytochrome P450 system (CYP 3A4), not recommended with monoamine oxidase inhibitors, β-sympathomimetic amines, or selective serotonin reuptake inhibitors; may prolong anesthesia, delayed emergence |
| Valerian | Increases sedative effects |

of their medications. Delayed administration of anti-Parkinson's medications, which often happens during prolonged surgical procedures, can contribute to delayed emergence. Other neuromuscular disorders such as amyotrophic lateral sclerosis or myasthenia gravis can increase susceptibility to neuromuscular blocking agents. This may lead to a prolonged need for continued tracheal intubation postoperatively. Thus a careful review of the patient's medical and habitual history, as well as careful evaluation of current medications, is essential in evaluating a patient with delayed emergence.

## INTRAOPERATIVE CAUSES

### Anesthetic/Medication-Related Causes

To diagnose an intraoperative cause of delayed emergence, it is essential to review the anesthetic record for both physiological changes and medication administration. The best starting point in an algorithmic approach to delayed emergence is confirmation of adequate perioperative oxygenation and ventilation with stable hemodynamics. Verifying discontinuation and/or reversal of anesthetic agents and muscle relaxants is the next step. Although at lower levels

of exhaled volatile anesthetic concentrations some patients may become responsive to verbal stimulation, it is when the exhaled concentration (as a biomarker for brain concentration) is zero and there is still no response that one becomes concerned about delayed emergence.[14]

Prolonged pharmacological effects of medications may contribute to delayed emergence. Ideal dosages of medications may vary among patients. Benzodiazepines are sedatives with minimal systemic side effects; however, when combined with high-dose opioids, they may cause profound respiratory depression, producing hypoxia and hypercapnia.[15] For preoperative sedation in neurosurgical patients, the use of benzodiazepines should be limited because they can induce respiratory depression mainly in patients with craniotomy or with chronic obstructive pulmonary disease.[16] If benzodiazepines are to be used, then midazolam may be the preferred agent due to its shorter duration of action.[17]

### Clinical Pearl

Age is probably the most important factor in the metabolism of medications. Older patients take longer to emerge from anesthesia. Delayed emergence in a young patient should raise particular concern.

If intravenous anesthetics or opioids are used as an infusion, then the half-life of these agents should be reviewed to estimate the time of emergence after discontinuation. For intravenous anesthetic agents, early recovery depends on redistribution from blood and brain into muscle and fat. Propofol is rapidly metabolized by the liver and other extrahepatic sites. It generally does not accumulate, leading to a faster recovery. The initial drug effect of thiopentone is terminated by redistribution within 5–15 minutes. Elimination is by oxidative metabolism in the liver occurring at the rate of 15% per hour, and as much as 30% of the dose may remain in the body at 24 hours. Cumulative effects may therefore become apparent when more than one dose is given, delaying recovery. Opioids have variable analgesic, sedative, and respiratory depressive effects. Dose response is affected by coadministered anesthetics and other patient factors. Opioids reduce brainstem chemoreceptor sensitivity to carbon dioxide, resulting in hypoventilation with subsequent decreased clearance of volatile agents. The direct opioid receptor effect varies with drug potency, half-life, metabolism, and patient sensitivity. Active metabolites of morphine and meperidine prolong the duration of action, especially in the presence of renal failure.[15] If delayed emergence is thought to be a result of opioids, small doses of naloxone may be used cautiously to reverse the opioid effect. It is important to note that naloxone may have adverse reactions, including significant pain, pulmonary complications, and allergic reactions. Another important consideration is that the half-life of naloxone will be shorter than the opioid used during surgery, and thus sedation and hypoventilation may recur. Therefore if residual opioid is identified as the cause of slow emergence, then it may be prudent to delay emergence and extubation until the opioids are metabolized and excreted.

**Table 45.3**   Factors That May Prolong Neuromuscular Blockade

| | |
|---|---|
| Pharmacological Agents | Antibiotics |
| | Anticholinesterases |
| | Beta-blockers |
| | Calcium channel blockers |
| | Dantrolene |
| | Furosemide |
| | Local anesthetics |
| | MAOIs |
| | Lithium/magnesium (inhibit acetylcholine release) |
| | Local anesthetics (decrease propagation action potentials) |
| | Volatile anesthetics |
| Physiological Conditions | Pseudocholinesterase deficiency |
| | Liver disease |
| | Hypothermia |
| | Hypothyroidism |
| Electrolyte Abnormalities | Metabolic acidosis |
| | Hyponatremia |
| | Hypocalcemia |
| | Hypokalemia |
| Neurological Conditions | Amyotrophic lateral sclerosis |
| | Malignant hyperthermia |
| | Muscular dystrophy |
| | Familial periodic paralysis |
| | Hereditary hepatic porphyria |
| | Myasthenia gravis/Eaton-Lambert syndrome |

*MAOI,* monoamine oxidase inhibitor.

Residual neuromuscular blockade may occur with increased dosing or incomplete reversal of nondepolarizing muscle relaxants (Table 45.3). A nerve stimulator can assist in making the diagnosis, and the train-of-four muscle twitch monitor is a useful device in determining residual muscle relaxation. A fade in the train of four or absence of twitches may indicate residual muscle relaxation or weakness. Correct positioning of the monitor is essential to the interpretation of the result. Clinically, the inability to maintain head lift for 5 seconds in a patient who could normally comply indicates residual block of greater than 30% of receptors. Prolonged apnea after succinylcholine is due to genetically abnormal or absent plasma cholinesterase enzyme. In liver disease, levels of this enzyme also tend to be lower, and prolonged muscle relaxation may be observed. Repeated doses of succinylcholine (>6-8 mg/kg total dose) may produce a phase 2 block (similar to that seen with nondepolarizing agents), which is prolonged and slow to recover. Renal failure reduces elimination of nondepolarizing muscle relaxants such as pancuronium and vecuronium. Large doses of aminoglycoside antibiotics and acidosis can also prolong muscle relaxant duration of action.[14] If continued neuromuscular blockade is the cause of delayed emergence, a dysphoric hyperadrenergic state may develop in a paralyzed but awake patient.

Other pharmacological agents used in the course of the operation should also be reviewed. Antiseizure medications may cause sedation and prolong emergence. Nitrous oxide, due to poor solubility, can increase the size of any air pocket inside the cranium after closure; pneumocephalus can be a reason for slow emergence.

## Metabolic Causes

The use of intraoperative hyperventilation to decrease ICP and improve surgical exposure raises cerebrospinal fluid pH. Rapid normalization of the $Paco_2$ at the time of emergence may cause a relative acidosis in the CNS. An arterial blood gas evaluation can provide important information and guide in diagnosing oxygenation, ventilation, and pH abnormalities.

## Hemodynamic Causes

Cerebral hypoxia or ischemia may occur during neurosurgery due to inadequate cerebral perfusion secondary to low mean arterial pressure. Various cranial vascular surgeries and operations in a sitting position pose a potential threat to cerebral perfusion and is one reason for leveling the arterial transducer at the midbrain level in such procedures. Furthermore intracranial hemorrhage (ICH), thrombosis, or infarction can occur due to changes in intraoperative hemodynamics, arrhythmias, or in patients with abnormal cerebral vasculature. The postoperative outcome of such intraoperative ischemic events varies from minor functional deficits to hemiparesis and coma.[15]

## POSTOPERATIVE CAUSES

Confirmation of adequate oxygenation and ventilation is the first step in investigating delayed emergence. Postoperative respiratory failure can cause hypoxemia, hypercapnia, or both. The causes of respiratory failure may be neurological, pulmonary, and muscular. Central respiratory drive may be lost due to drug overdose, intracranial pathology, chronic obstructive pulmonary disease, or sleep apnea. Ventilation is impaired by primary muscle problems, metabolic imbalance, obesity, and residual neuromuscular blockade. Hypoxemia results in cerebral hypoxia and depresses cortical functioning. Hypercapnia, sensed by central chemoreceptors, initially stimulates respiration but with progression depresses the regulatory respiratory centers of the brain causing further hypoventilation. Hypercapnia results in cerebral vasodilatation leading to increases in cerebral blood volume, and in a head-injured patient with impaired intracranial compliance yields elevations in ICP, which may result in secondary neuronal injury.[15]

Attention to hemodynamics, especially blood pressure, is also essential during emergence. The pathophysiology of emergence HTN is complex. Systemic HTN is a major problem associated with early emergence, because acute HTN in the neurosurgical patient may lead to cerebral hyperemia and breakthrough bleeding. The incidence of postoperative HTN in neurosurgical patients has been reported as high as 70% to 90%.[18,19] This may be a consequence of increased sympathetic stimulation as demonstrated by an increase in circulating catecholamines.[20] Pain during surgical closure may contribute to sympathetic stimulation leading to emergence HTN.[21]

The relationship between cardiac output or blood pressure and cerebral blood flow during emergence is not clear, but there appears to be a link between emergence sympathetic output and cerebral hyperemia. Bruder et al. found a linear relationship between oxygen consumption and cerebral blood flow velocity (by transcranial Doppler) at extubation.[22]

Emergence HTN (systolic blood pressure >200 mm Hg) may be a risk factor for ICH after intracranial surgery. In a randomized prospective trial of low-dose anesthetics in neurosurgical patients, Bhagat et al. reported emergence HTN in 38% of patients.[21] The same results were observed by Bilotta et al., where the use of remifentanil/sufentanil along with propofol resulted in HTN after craniotomy in 37% of patients.[23] Talke et al. reported hypertensive episodes in 50% of their patients, whereas Magni et al. observed HTN during recovery from intracranial surgery in 29% of their patients.[24,25] In a retrospective case control study, Basali et al.[26] reported that neurosurgical patients were 3.6 times more likely to develop postoperative HTN than their matched controls. They found that 62% patients with ICH had intraoperative HTN, compared with only 34% of controls (P<0.001). Again 62% percent of the ICH group had prehemorrhage HTN in the initial 12 postoperative hours versus 25% of controls (P<0.001, odds ratio 4.6) for postoperative ICH. Hospital stay (median, 24.5 vs. 11.0 days) and mortality (18.2 vs. 1.6%) were significantly greater in the ICH than in the control groups. This is of particular concern for the neurosurgeon, who might achieve hemostasis at a low or normal blood pressure, but encounter bleeding at higher pressures.

Because systemic HTN is common during emergence, prophylactic infusion of esmolol (or other sympatholytic drugs) may be considered. Doses as high as 200 to 300 mg/kg/min have been used to control systemic hypertension.[18] Beta-blockers may blunt cerebral hyperemia during emergence caused by hypertension. Various intravenous antihypertensive agents (labetalol, urapidil, or nicardipine) are available to control the immediate rise in systemic hypertension during emergence. A comparative study of labetalol and nicardipine for the control of emergence hypertension after craniotomy showed that the group treated with nicardipine experienced a higher incidence of hypotension and tachycardia.[27] The combination of diltiazem and nicardipine may be effective, with the advantage of producing less tachycardia than nicardipine alone. The use of low doses of fentanyl during craniotomy closure may also be effective for preventing early postoperative hypertension.[21]

Including the measurement of electrolytes and blood glucose in the blood gas analysis can also help in ruling out metabolic reasons of delayed emergence. A patient with cerebral salt wasting or diabetes insipidus may have acute changes of blood sodium levels leading to mental status changes and even seizures. Mild hyponatremia is usually asymptomatic, but serum sodium concentration <120 mmol/L will cause confusion and irritability. Further decreases to <110 mmol/l can cause seizures and coma. The syndrome of inappropriate antidiuretic hormone secretion causes hyponatremia and can result from brain trauma, subarachnoid hemorrhage, and various drugs (e.g. opioids, haloperidol, and vasopressin). Cerebral salt-wasting syndrome, with similar consequences, may also occur in the brain-injured patient.

Extreme hypernatremia (Na > 160 mmol/l) may rarely occur in the postoperative period. Excess sodium dehydrates brain cells potentially leading to ruptured vessels and ICH. The clinical effects of uremia are varied, but when severe, intracerebral changes may produce drowsiness,

confusion, and coma.[15] Attention to other electrolytes is also important; intravenous magnesium administered intraoperatively to prevent seizures can also cause muscle weakness or potentiate neuromuscular blockade.

Because the brain is totally dependent on glucose as its energy source, neuroglycopenia may cause confusion, abnormal behavior, seizures, and coma. It can occur in small children and in poorly controlled diabetes, starvation, and alcohol consumption.[14] Severe hyperglycemia can also prolong unconsciousness after anesthesia. It causes an osmotic diuresis and dehydration in the untreated patient leading to drowsiness and acidosis. In severe cases, blood hyperosmolality and hyperviscosity predispose to cerebral sinus or venous thrombosis and cerebral edema. Intraoperative vascular occlusion in diabetics with microvascular and macrovascular disease may result in ischemic stroke.[15]

Intravenous anesthetics used to initiate burst suppression and to provide brain protection during temporary arterial clipping can prolong emergence. The timing of emergence will depend on the dose given and the pharmacokinetics of the agent used.

### Clinical Pearl

Depending on the nature of the neurosurgical procedure, the likelihood of postoperative seizures may be high and could be a potential source of delayed emergence. Seizures may be subtle in the emerging patient and may be nonconvulsive or include continued nystagmus, subtle finger and toe movements, or twitching movements in the corner of the mouth.

Another important requirement for timely emergence is normothermia. If induced hypothermia is used during neurosurgery or body temperature drops due to inadequate warming techniques, the temperature will be low at the time of emergence. The effects of hypothermia are multiple and widespread. With decreasing temperature, confusion (<35°C), unconsciousness (<30°C), apnea (<24°C), and absent cerebral activity (<18°C) can occur. With a significant decrease in temperature, cardiac output decreases and arrhythmias can occur. Low cardiac output affects circulation and tissue perfusion, as well as drug pharmacokinetics.[15]

### Clinical Pearl

Hypothermia is common in the neurosurgical patient because hypothalamic structures may be affected during surgery, making thermoregulation more difficult.

Hypothermia-induced shivering on emergence can increase oxygen consumption and lead to acidosis. Hypothermia can cause other complications such as delayed wound healing, myocardial ischemia, and coagulopathy.[28] Shivering will increase cerebral metabolic demands and in some cases can be misinterpreted as seizure activity, particularly in the context of incomplete reversal of neuromuscular blockade. The best way to control postoperative shivering is to maintain normothermia, which can be achieved using forced-air warming during neurosurgery. Oxygen consumption and blood catecholamine increases are less during recovery immediately after surgery in normothermic patients.[20] Pharmacological methods can be used to prevent postoperative shivering, keeping in mind that these pharmacological agents may by themselves cause sedation.[29] It is also important to realize that hyperthermia is undesirable during neurosurgical procedures.[30]

## Surgical Causes

Although there is a long list of anesthetic causes for delayed emergence, one should not delay considering potential surgical complications. An algorithmic approach as mentioned earlier to identify the cause and treatment is the best course of action. Communication between the anesthesiologist and neurosurgeon at the time of emergence should be continuous and timely. If there is any possibility that the delay in emergence is not a result of anesthetic causes, the surgeon should be immediately notified. Intracranial hemorrhage arising postoperatively from a bleeding source caused by inadequate hemostasis may rapidly expand. Although some anesthesia and reversal agents may affect pupillary size and reactivity, unequal pupillary size should raise concern for an ICH. Intraoperative trauma and injury to vital cerebral areas may also delay emergence, hence justifying the use of short-acting agents to enhance rapid neurological examination.

Seizures after neurosurgery may be particularly problematic. Although there is no evidence that seizure prophylaxis with an antiepileptic drug should be used for all intracranial procedures,[31] these medications are routinely used in clinical practice. As mentioned earlier, these agents may cause prolonged emergence from sedation.

The vacuum system connected to the extradural drainage system may be a source of postoperative bleeding. It should be checked closely for greater-than-anticipated bleeding that may lead to severe hypotension if not discovered in time. An often overlooked cause of cerebral hemorrhage is the negative pressure of the drains.[32,33] Transient bradycardia after connecting the vacuum device is a warning sign of this complication.

## Residual Anesthetic Drug Causes

Early postoperative diagnosis of neurological complications is an important step in limiting cerebral complications and improving outcome. Some postoperative anesthetics, however, can mimic focal neurological deficits. Low doses of midazolam or fentanyl can exacerbate or unmask focal neurological deficits in more than 60% of patients with prior compensated neurological dysfunction. Transient reemergence of focal symptoms in patients with remote (chronic) stroke can also occur.[34] This observation may explain some of the reports of dramatic reversal of postoperative neurological deficits with naloxone[35] and the observation of transient neurological deficits during the recovery period after neurosurgery. Using short-acting anesthetics during neurosurgical anesthesia avoids unnecessary cranial computed tomography scans or emergency reopening of the cranium.

Systemic and central causes for delayed emergence are summarized in Table 45.1.

## Conclusion

In the immediate postoperative period, many complications may manifest as delayed in emergence. The goal is to have a mentally alert patient who will enable the anesthesiologist and neurosurgeon to perform a neurological evaluation along with ensuring adequate oxygenation, ventilation, and stable hemodynamics. Early evaluation of delayed emergence is facilitated by awareness of the pathophysiological variations occurring at the time of emergence, as well as the pharmacology of the agents used. Being well prepared to preempt any untoward outcome is essential to ensure neurosurgical patient safety.

## References

1. Manninen P, Raman S, Boyle K, et al. Early postoperative complications following neurosurgical procedures. *Can J Anaesth.* 1999;46(1):7–14.
2. Cabantog AM, Bernstein M. Complications of first craniotomy for intra-axial brain tumour. *Can J Neurol Sci.* 1994;21(3):213–218.
3. Brell M, Ibanez J, Caral L, et al. Factors influencing surgical complications of intra-axial brain tumours. *Acta Neurochir (Wien).* 2000;142(7):739–750.
4. Sawaya R, Hammoud M, Schoppa D, et al. Neurosurgical outcomes in a modern series of 400 craniotomies for treatment of parenchymal tumors. *Neurosurgery.* 1998;42(5):1044–1055.
5. Magni G, La Rosa I, Gimignani S, et al. Early postoperative complications after intracranial surgery: comparison between total intravenous and balanced anesthesia. *J Neurosurg Anesthesiol.* 2007;19(4):229–234.
6. Li X, Wang H, Hou C, et al. Retrospective analysis of common complications in neurosurgical postanesthesia care unit. *Chin J Contemp Neurol Neurosurg.* 2010;10(4):452–455.
7. Lindert EJV, Delye H, Leonardo J. Prospective review of a single center's general pediatric neurosurgical intraoperative and postoperative complication rates. *J Neurosurg Pediatr.* 2014;13(1):107–113.
8. Himmelseher S, Pfenninger E. Anesthetic management of neurosurgical patients. *Curr Opin Anaesthesiol.* 2001;14(5):483–490.
9. Bruder N, Ravussin P. Recovery from anesthesia and postoperative extubation of neurosurgical patients: a review. *J Neurosurg Anesthesiol.* 1999;11(4):282–293.
10. Cai Y, Zeng H, Shi Z, et al. Factors influencing delayed extubation after infratentorial craniotomy for tumour resection: a prospective cohort study of 800 patients in a Chinese neurosurgical centre. *J Int Med Res.* 2013;41(1):208–217.
11. Robinson TN, Eiseman B. Postoperative delirium in the elderly: diagnosis and management. *Clin Interv Aging.* 2008;3(2):351–355.
12. Mangoni AA, Jackson SHD. Age-related changes in pharmacokinetics and pharmacodynamics: basic principles and practical applications. *Br J Clin Pharmacol.* 2004;57(1):6–14.
13. Rudra A, Chatterjee S, Sengupta S, Kumar P. Herbal Medications and their Anaesthetic Implications. *Internet J Anesthesiol.* 2008;19(1).
14. Radhakrishnan J, Jesudasan S, Jacob R. Delayed awakening or emergence from anaesthesia. *Update Anaesth.* 2001;13:4–6.
15. Sinclair RCF, Faleiro RJ. Delayed recovery of consciousness after anaesthesia. *Contin Educ Anaesth Crit Care Pain.* 2006;6(3):114–118.
16. Tassonyi E, Fuchs T, Forster A. Role of benzodiazepines in neuroanesthesia. *Agressologie.* 1991;32(8–9):402–404.
17. Revelly JP, Chiolero R, Ravussin P. Use of benzodiazepines in neurosurgical resuscitation. *Agressologie.* 1991;32(8–9):387–390.
18. Lim SH, Chin NM, Tai HY, et al. Prophylactic esmolol infusion for the control of cardiovascular responses to extubation after intracranial surgery. *Ann Acad Med Singapore.* 2000;29(4):447–451.
19. Todd M, Warner D, Sokoll M, et al. A prospective, comparative trial of three anesthetics for elective supratentorial craniotomy. *Anesthesiology.* 1993;78(6):1005–1020.
20. Bruder N, Stordeur JM, Ravussin P, et al. Metabolic and hemodynamic changes during recovery and tracheal extubation in neurosurgical patients: immediate versus delayed recovery. *Anesth Analg.* 1999;89(3):674–678.

21. Bhagat H, Dash HH, Bithal PK, et al. Planning for early emergence in neurosurgical patients: a randomized prospective trial of low-dose anesthetics. *Anesth Analg.* 2008;107(4):1348–1355.

22. Bruder NJ. Awakening management after neurosurgery for intracranial tumors. *Curr Opin Anaesthesiol.* 2002;15(5):477–482.

23. Bilotta F, Caramia R, Paoloni FP, et al. Early postoperative cognitive recovery after remifentanil-propofol or sufentanil-propofol anaesthesia for supratentorial craniotomy: a randomized trial. *Eur J Anaesthesiol.* 2007;24(2):122–127.

24. Talke P, Caldwell JE, Brown R, et al. A comparison of three anesthetic techniques in patients undergoing craniotomy for supratentorial intracranial surgery. *Anesth Analg.* 2002;95(2):430–435.

25. Magni G, Baisi F, La Rosa I, Imperiale C, et al. No difference in emergence time and early cognitive function between sevoflurane-fentanyl and propofol- remifentanil in patients undergoing craniotomy for supratentorial intracranial surgery. *J Neurosurg Anesthesiol.* 2005;17(3):134–138.

26. Basali A, Mascha E, Kalfas I, et al. Relation between perioperative hypertension and intracranial hemorrhage after craniotomy. *Anesthesiology.* 2000;93(1):48–54.

27. Kross R, Ferri E, Leung D, et al. A comparative study between a calcium channel blocker (nicardipine) and a combined alpha-beta-blocker (labetalol) for the control of emergence hypertension during craniotomy for tumor surgery. *Anesth Analg.* 2000;91(4): 904–909.

28. Reynolds L, Beckmann J, Kurz A. Perioperative complications of hypothermia. *Best Pract Res Clin Anaesthesiol.* 2008;22(4):645–657.

29. Kranke P, Eberhart LH, Roewer N, et al. Pharmacological treatment of postoperative shivering: a quantitative systematic review of randomized controlled trials. *Anesth Analg.* 2002;94(2):453–460.

30. Kilpatrick MM, Lowry DW, Firlik AD, et al. Hyperthermia in the neurosurgical intensive care unit. *Neurosurgery.* 2000;47 (4):850–856.

31. Wu AS, Trinh VT, Suki D, et al. A prospective randomized trial of perioperative seizure prophylaxis in patients with intraparenchymal brain tumors. *J Neurosurg.* 2013;118(4):873–883.

32. Hernandez-Palazon J, Tortosa J, Sanchez-Bautista S, et al. Cardiovascular disturbances caused by extradural negative pressure drainage systems after intracranial surgery. *Br J Anaesth.* 1998;80 (5):599–601.

33. Honegger J, Zentner J, Spreer J, et al. Cerebellar hemorrhage arising postoperatively as a complication of supratentorial surgery: a retrospective study. *J Neurosurg.* 2002;96(2):248–254.

34. Lazar R, Fitzsimmons B, Marshall R, et al. Reemergence of stroke deficits with midazolam challenge. *Stroke.* 2002;33(1):283–285.

35. Hans P, Brichant JF, Longerstay E, et al. Reversal of neurological deficit with naloxone: an additional report. *Intensive Care Med.* 1992;18 (6):362–363.

# 46 *Management of Postoperative Hemorrhage*

RAHUL DAMANI and JOSE I. SUAREZ

## Introduction

Postoperative hemorrhage in the neurocritical care unit could be divided into postoperative intracranial hemorrhage (POICH) and extracranial hemorrhage, with retroperitoneal hemorrhage being the most important.

POICH is one of the most common and serious complications of neurosurgical procedures and is frequently associated with significant morbidity and mortality. Historically, because of the potential for dismal outcomes, the practice of neurosurgery has been described as inherently more sensitive to any defect in hemostasis than other surgical disciplines.[1] It is important to point out that there is no clear and universally accepted definition of what constitutes POICH, as we discuss in more detail later.[2-9]

Similarly retroperitoneal hematoma is most dreaded complication of neuroendovascular therapy. The possibility of retroperitoneal bleeding in patients undergoing preoperative, intraoperative, or postoperative cerebral angiography should always be entertained.[10,11]

In this chapter, we present an overview of the epidemiology, risk factors, clinical presentation, and management of neurosurgical patients experiencing POICH and retroperitoneal hemorrhage based on current literature and our clinical experience.

## Epidemiology

### Key Concepts

- The best definition of significant POICH is one that requires surgical intervention.
- Most POICHs will occur within the first 24 hours after surgical intervention.
- Remote intracranial hemorrhage (ICH) is a rare but significant complication.
- The incidence of systemic bleeding in postoperative neurosurgical patients is currently unknown.

### POSTOPERATIVE INTRACRANIAL HEMORRHAGE

The rates of POICH after intracranial procedures reported in the literature vary greatly due to the lack of a standardized definition. Some studies use clinical deterioration criteria,[2-4] whereas other studies use abnormalities found on brain imaging[5,6] or a combination of the two.[7-9] Therefore incidence figures vary depending on the definition used, with rates of 0.8% to 6.9% reported for postoperative clinical deterioration[2-4] and 10.8% to 50.0% based on routine radiological monitoring.[5,6] Currently, most practitioners agree that the best definition for a significant POICH is one requiring surgical evacuation. The critical time period after neurosurgery during which a significant hematoma may develop is considered to be 6 hours. However, POICH can become evident after 24 to 48 hours[6] and occasionally up to 7 days after neurosurgery.[5] Remote ICH, defined as bleeding that occurs in a location remote from the operative site, is an interesting and relatively rare type of POICH. Remote ICH occurs in 0.6% of all supratentorial craniectomies, in 2.8% of craniotomies for clipping of unruptured aneurysms, in 1.4% of craniotomies for temporal lobectomies,[12] and rarely after spine surgery, thought to be related to dural laceration.[12] Although there are studies reporting on the frequency of POICH, the incidence of systemic hemorrhage after intracranial procedures is currently unknown.

### RETROPERITONEAL HEMATOMA

Retroperitoneal bleeding occurs in 0.2% to 0.6% of all patients undergoing cerebral angiography.

## Risk Factors

### Key Concepts

- The main risk factors associated with POICH include diabetes mellitus, hypertension, and cerebral amyloid angiopathy.
- Blood pressure control during the preoperative, intraoperative, and postoperative period is important to reduce the frequency of POICH.
- The main hematological factors associated with POICH include thrombocytopenia, disseminated intravascular coagulation (DIC), factor XIII deficiency, and platelet function inhibition.
- The most serious hemorrhagic complication in patients undergoing cerebral angiography is retroperitoneal hematoma, especially in patients with the following risk factors: female gender, use of a large sheath, antiplatelet agent administration, and excessive anticoagulation.

### POSTOPERATIVE INTRACRANIAL HEMORRHAGE

Various studies have reported on risk factors for the development of POICH. Currently, there is no evidence linking demographic factors such as age, gender, and race to risk of POICH. However, other factors such as diabetes mellitus, hypertension, and cerebral amyloid angiopathy have been associated with the development of POICH. Diabetes mellitus causes a vasculopathy and impaired wound healing, which increase the risk of POICH. However, the exact increase in the risk of POICH due to diabetes is unknown.[13,14] In elderly patients, cerebral amyloid angiopathy causes replacement of smooth muscle cells with amyloid protein deposits, which may increase the risk of POICH.[15,16] Chronic hypertension is a risk factor for vascular disease and increases the risk of primary ICH, as well as aneurysm formation and rupture. Preoperative, intraoperative, and postoperative hypertension have all been implicated in the development of ICH and POICH.[9,17–19]

---

### Clinical Pearls

- Careful blood pressure control during the preoperative, intraoperative, and postoperative period is paramount to minimize the occurrence of POICH.
- Patients who are most likely to experience POICH are those with a history of diabetes mellitus, hypertension, and cerebral amyloid angiopathy.

---

Other hematological risk factors that could increase the risk of systemic hemorrhage and POICH include thrombocytopenia, DIC, and coagulation factor deficiencies. Any condition that reduces platelet count below 100,000/µL might increase the risk of POICH.[20,21] In addition, POICH has a potential to enlarge if the platelet count drop is acute in onset rather than chronic.[20] DIC and factor XIII deficiency have been identified as risk factors for POICH. A large prospective study[7] suggested that the screening of factor XIII levels in patients undergoing neurosurgery and particularly in those who develop a POICH should be undertaken; however, this is not a common practice.

Preoperative use of antiplatelet agents such as aspirin and clopidogrel and oral anticoagulants increases risk of POICH. It is our general practice to stop antiplatelet agents 7 days before a planned surgery. In addition to cases of emergency surgery, we transfuse and assess platelet function assay before and after the procedure. Furthermore we discontinue warfarin at least 5 days prior to elective neurosurgery; if required, low-molecular or unfractionated heparin might be used as a bridge preoperatively. For emergent reversal of warfarin, intravenous (IV) vitamin K should be administered, along with fresh frozen plasma (FFP) and/or prothrombin complex concentrate (PCC), as discussed later.

### RETROPERITONEAL BLEEDING

The possibility of retroperitoneal bleeding in patients undergoing preoperative, intraoperative, or postoperative cerebral angiography should always be entertained.[10,11] Retroperitoneal bleeding is usually caused by inadvertent puncture of the posterior wall of the femoral or iliac arteries. The main risk factors associated with this complication are female gender, use of a large sheath, low platelet count, and excessive anticoagulation.

# Clinical Presentation

---

### Key Concepts

- Failure to awaken from general anesthesia or neurological deterioration should prompt urgent clinical imaging to detect POICH.
- Persistent postoperative hypertension in absence of obvious cause as described later should prompt immediate head computed tomography (CT) imaging to assess for POICH after routine causes of hypertension have been ruled out (e.g., withdrawal of chronic medications like beta adrenergic blockers or surgical pain/anxiety).
- The presence of hypotension, resting tachycardia, and reduced urine output should prompt clinicians to look for a source of blood loss. However, such systemic signs do not arise from the volume of blood lost in an intracranial hematoma (in adults).
- The signs of retroperitoneal bleeding may be vague; it frequently presents with relative hypotension and resting tachycardia, which respond transiently to IV fluids.

---

### POSTOPERATIVE INTRACRANIAL HEMORRHAGE

The timing of presentation of POICH after intracranial procedures is, despite some debate, highest between 6 and 24 hours,[9,15] but might present up to 7 days after neurosurgery.[5] This evidence has led to the suggestion for close clinical and neurological monitoring of these patients at least for the first 24 hours after the surgical procedure. Failure to awaken from general anesthesia or neurological deterioration should prompt urgent clinical imaging to detect POICH.

Postoperative hypertension has been implicated in the development of intraoperative and postoperative hemorrhage.[9,17–19] Persistent hypertension without other typical and treatable causes in the postoperative period should prompt immediate head CT imaging to rule out POICH. In patients who have a Glasgow Coma Scale (GCS) <8, or those who require sedation after surgery, close monitoring of intracranial pressure (ICP) is vital. A rise in ICP after a neurosurgical procedure should raise the suspicion of cerebral swelling and/or intracranial hematoma, and head imaging studies should be performed expeditiously.

### RETROPERITONEAL HEMATOMA

The presence of signs of shock—for example, hypotension (systolic blood pressure [SBP] <90 mm Hg), resting tachycardia (heart rate >90/minute), and reduction in urine output (<0.5 mL/kg/h)—should prompt evaluation for a source of blood loss. However, it is worth noting that resting tachycardia and hypotension might not be evident in the supine patient and only become more obvious in cases of moderate to severe blood loss. The clinical presentation of patients with retroperitoneal bleeding may vary and is often vague.[10,11] Frequently, these patients may experience relative hypotension and resting tachycardia, which respond transiently to bolus IV fluid administration. However, tachycardia may be absent if patients are receiving beta-blockers. Patients with retroperitoneal bleeding may experience back, lower abdominal, or groin discomfort and swelling, followed by hemodynamic instability and a fall in the hematocrit.

### Clinical Pearl

Changes in the level of consciousness or persistent hypertension in the postoperative period should prompt immediate head CT scanning to assess for POICH.

## Laboratory Evaluation and Imaging

### Key Concepts

- Patients at high risk for POICH should have factor XIII concentration measured prior to surgical procedure.
- Intraoperative head imaging may help in early detection of POICH.
- Monitoring of oxygen transport parameters will help identify patients with significant intravascular volume loss.
- Abdominal and pelvic imaging should be considered in patients who present with signs of decreased intravascular volume or unexplained decrease in hemoglobin after cerebral catheter angiography.

Preoperative assessment, not only of platelet count and platelet function, but also of factor XIII concentration,[7] should be considered. Postoperative and 24-hour laboratory evaluation of platelet count, hemoglobin, and hematocrit is routine. However, hematocrit often does not change in the setting of acute blood loss, and a drop in hematocrit might reflect dilution of red blood cell concentration from intraoperative IV fluid administration. In such cases, monitoring of oxygen transport parameters, such as arterial base deficit, arterial lactate concentration, and mixed venous oxygen saturation ($SvO_2$), helps identify patients with hypovolemic shock from systemic (extracerebral) hemorrhage. In patients with significant blood loss, an elevated base deficit is a marker of global tissue acidosis from impaired tissue oxygenation.[22] The normal range for base deficit is +2 to −2 mmol/L. Abnormal elevations in base deficit are classified as mild (−2 to −5 mmol/L), moderate (−6 to −14 mmol/L), and severe (−15 mmol/L). Clinical studies have shown a direct correlation between the magnitude of the increase in base deficit at presentation and the extent of blood loss.[23] In addition, correction of the base deficit within hours after volume replacement is associated with a favorable outcome,[23] whereas persistent elevations in base deficit are often a harbinger of multiorgan failure. Similarly, lactate concentration is a prognostic factor in circulatory shock.[24] Whole blood or serum lactate concentrations above 2 mEq/L are abnormal. Blood lactate levels show a closer correlation with both the magnitude of blood loss[24] and the risk of death from hemorrhage.[24,25] In patients with a central venous line, $SvO_2$ should be monitored either serially or continuously. $SvO_2$ seems to be a reliable and sensitive parameter to detect hemorrhage.[26] $SvO_2 < 70\%$ suggests tissue dysoxia.

### POSTOPERATIVE INTRACRANIAL HEMORRHAGE

In patients at high risk for POICH, intraoperative computed tomography (iCT) and intraoperative magnetic resonance imaging (iMR) have been used in various neurosurgical procedures and should be utilized whenever available. Both iMR and iCT are useful and rapid tools to identify POICH, particularly in areas that are not visible in the surgical field of view. Most neurointensivists and neurosurgeons also prefer routine postoperative imaging with either CT or MRI at 24 hours, which is the time frame that has been suggested to represent the highest risk for the development of POICH.[9,15]

### RETROPERITONEAL HEMATOMA

In patients who have undergone a cerebral angiography for either diagnostic purposes or coadjuvant endovascular therapies, the presence of any signs of shock or hypovolemia should prompt clinicians to evaluate for retroperitoneal hematoma by either abdominal ultrasound (USG) or preferably abdominal and pelvic CT imaging.

## Management

### Key Concepts

- Serial neurological examinations aid in detecting subtle changes that might prompt recognition and treatment of POICH.
- Blood pressure should be adequately managed with a target blood pressure goal of SBP <140 mm Hg for the first 24 hours. Adequate pain control should be achieved because untreated pain might cause hypertension.
- Prompt replacement of intravascular volume and correction of tissue dysoxia are crucial to successful management of hypovolemic shock.
- If initial fluid resuscitation fails to correct hypotension, then vasopressors should be used.
- After initial resuscitation, management should be focused on identifying and treating hemorrhage.
- Thrombocytopenia and coagulopathy should be promptly corrected.

In this section we present an overview of the management of patients with POICH and systemic bleeding after neurosurgery. We divide management into general postoperative care and management of hemorrhagic complications (Box 46.1).

### GENERAL POSTOPERATIVE CARE

The high-risk nature of neurosurgical and neuroendovascular procedures requires attentive postoperative care. Given the life-threatening nature of complications associated with these procedures, patients should be admitted to a critical care unit, preferably a neurocritical care unit, for the first few postoperative hours. Serial clinical and neurological examinations are the cornerstone of good postoperative care. It is paramount to have certainty of the baseline neurological functioning of the patient prior to

**Box 46.1**   Summary of Management of Hemorrhagic Complications

**General postoperative care**

- Admission to ICU/neurology ICU for first few hours postoperative
- Serial neurological examinations
- Head of the bed > 30 degrees
- Pain management
- Blood pressure control: goal SBP <140 mm Hg
- Management of nausea and vomiting
- Glucose control: maintain serum glucose between 120 and 200 mg/dL
- Avoid fever and correct hypothermia
- Deep venous thrombosis prophylaxis with mechanical devices only for first 24 hours
- Gastrointestinal prophylaxis
- Extubate as soon as feasible; maintain plateau pressure <30 cm $H_2O$

**Management of bleeding complications**

- Resuscitation with crystalloids
- IV vasopressors for ongoing hypotension (SBP <90 mm Hg or MAP <65 mm Hg) despite IV fluid resuscitation
- If $O_2$ extraction <50%, then transfuse packed red blood cells
- Identify source of bleeding
- Correct coagulopathy: platelet transfusion, FFP, cryoprecipitate, or PCC administration
- Consider ICP monitoring and treat intracranial hypertension
- Surgical evacuation in symptomatic patients
- Vascular surgery consultation in patients with suspected retroperitoneal bleeding

*ICU*, intensive care unit; *SBP*, systolic blood pressure; *MAP*, mean arterial pressure; *FFP*, fresh-frozen plasma; *PCC*, prothrombin complex concentrate; *ICP*, intracranial pressure.

undergoing surgical or endovascular procedures. This facilitates appreciation of changes, often subtle, that might prompt recognition and treatment of POICH.

Adequate pain control should be achieved because untreated pain results in hypertension, which is a risk factor for POICH. Fentanyl (25–50 μg IV every 2–4 hours) or morphine sulfate (1–4 mg IV every 2–4 hours) should be used judiciously to achieve adequate analgesia without change in sensorium. Postoperative nausea and vomiting, which are common and could lead to aspiration pneumonia, arterial/venous hypertension, and increased ICP, should be promptly treated with either ondansetron (4–8 mg IV every 4–8 hours) or metoclopramide (5–10 mg IV every 6 hours).

Patients should have their head elevated to greater than 30 degrees to reduce ICP, promote venous drainage, and decrease the risk of aspiration pneumonia. Blood pressure should be adequately managed with a target blood pressure goal of SBP <140 mm Hg for the first 24 hours, ensuring adequate cerebral perfusion pressure (CPP > 60 mm Hg). Postoperative hypertension should promptly be treated with IV infusion of nicardipine (5–15 mg/h) or IV labetalol (5–10 mg every 15 minutes). Fast-onset antihypertensive effect can be achieved by a bolus of nicardipine, 100 to 500 μg.[27] This generally has to be a physician-administered treatment. Persistent hypertension should prompt clinicians to look for complications, including POICH.

Postoperative extubation should occur as soon as is safe. Factors that contribute to safe extubation include correction of stable POICH or systemic bleeding, adequate oxygenation ($Sao_2$ > 92% with $Fio_2$ < 50%), acceptable

minute ventilation, absence of hypotension or shock, rapid shallow breathing index <105, no requirement of continuous IV sedation, adequate level of consciousness (GCS >8), and ability to protect their airway.[28] In patients who cannot be extubated safely, ventilator care should be protocolized with the aim of keeping plateau pressure below 30 cm $H_2O$, minimizing coughing, and performing daily weaning trials.[29,30]

Fever defined as a body temperature of >37.5° Celsius should be avoided, and acetaminophen or ibuprofen and external cooling or warming devices should be used if necessary. Hypothermic coagulopathy may predispose to postoperative hemorrhage.

Insulin should be used to maintain glucose between 120 and 200 mg/dL. Prophylaxis against stress ulcers and venous thromboembolism should be systematically prescribed, initially with mechanical methods, and subsequently with low-molecular-weight or unfractionated heparin once POICH or systemic bleeding has been ruled out or stabilized; however, currently there is no literature to guide clinicians on optimal timing of restarting prophylactic anticoagulants. All patients should be started on appropriate diet, and enteral nutrition should be considered for patients who are mechanically ventilated or unable to swallow for more than 24 hours after surgery.

## MANAGEMENT OF HEMORRHAGIC COMPLICATIONS

### Postoperative Intracranial Hemorrhage

In cases of POICH, patients are often found to be hypertensive. In such situations, it is imperative to control the blood pressure. Even though there is no evidence, most neurointensivists prefer to treat hypertension urgently with a target of SBP <140 mm Hg (data extrapolated from primary ICH trials[31,32]). Simultaneously, clinicians should be aware of the possibility of increased ICP, and an effort should be made to maintain CPP >60 mm Hg. If patients do not have ICP monitor, an external ventricular drain should be placed, which would not only help monitor ICP and CPP, but also help to reduce ICP by draining cerebrospinal fluid. In addition, any evidence of thrombocytopenia should be promptly corrected with platelet transfusion. Platelet dysfunction should be monitored and corrected as necessary. Furthermore, FFP, cryoprecipitate, and PCC transfusion must be instituted in the setting of abnormal international normalized ratio or coagulation factors. Factor XIII should be monitored in the postoperative period.

After initial stabilization patients with POICH should be promptly taken back to the operating room, and ICH should be surgically evacuated, especially in cases of subdural, epidural, superficial intraparenchymal, and infratentorial hematoma.[33,34]

### Extracerebral hemorrhage and retroperitoneal hemorrhage

Extracerebral hemorrhage in the postoperative period may be severe, leading to hypovolemic shock and tissue hypoperfusion. Prompt replacement of intravascular volume and correction of tissue dysoxia are critical for successful management of hypovolemic shock.

Treatment should begin with immediate fluid resuscitation with crystalloids as the preferred IV fluids. Based on the degree of intravascular depletion, the initial requirement for fluid resuscitation can vary from 20 to 30 mL/kg, which should be administered through large-bore IV access. Further fluid resuscitation should be aimed at restoring adequate blood flow (SBP >90 mm Hg and mean arterial pressure [MAP] >65 mm Hg) to prevent tissue hypoperfusion and correct tissue dysoxia as evidenced by monitoring arterial base deficit, arterial lactate concentration, and $SvO_2$.[23-26] Central venous pressure (CVP) and stroke volume variation (SVV) can be used to help clinicians determine the patient's intravascular volume and the need for further IV fluid administration. Conventionally CVP is probably the most used parameter for judging whether fluids should be administered. However, a large number of studies[35-37] show that CVP fails to discriminate responders from nonresponders, and overall, the predictive power of the CVP for fluid responsiveness is poor.[36] Given the lack of accuracy of static indices in predicting fluid responsiveness, there has been great interest in using dynamic indices to predict fluid responsiveness, and with SVV being foremost. SVV is calculated from percentage changes in stroke volume during the ventilatory cycle. Normal SVV values are less than 10% to 15% on controlled mechanical ventilation. SVV has repeatedly been shown to accurately predict fluid responsiveness well in various clinical settings.[38-41] Some of the limitation of SVV is that its use has not been validated in patients who are not on a mechanical ventilator; furthermore in mechanically ventilated patients SVV can be affected by arrhythmias and changes in positive end-expiratory pressure and other ventilator parameters. Despite the theoretical superiority of colloids over crystalloids for increasing plasma volume and promoting cardiac output, crystalloids should be used as the fluid of choice for resuscitation. This preference is due to the lack of documented survival benefit with colloid resuscitation, the lack of universal availability, and cost.[41,42] After correction of volume status, the clinician should focus on correcting the oxygen-carrying capacity of blood. A drop of hemoglobin and hematocrit is generally used to trigger the transfusion of packed red blood cells (PRBCs). However, as mentioned earlier in the chapter, during the initial phase of the resuscitation, hematocrit may not accurately reflect the amount of blood loss, and hence oxygen extraction should be used. Oxygen extraction can be calculated by measuring the oxyhemoglobin saturation in both arterial blood ($Sao_2$) and mixed venous blood ($Sv\,o_2$) ($O_2$ extraction % $= Sao_2 - Sv\,o_2$). Oxygen extraction less than 50% suggests tissue dysoxia and is usually used as a trigger for requirement of PRBC transfusion. If initial fluid resuscitation fails to restore blood flow (SBP >90 mm Hg and MAP >65 mm Hg) vasopressors should be used. Norepinephrine (Levophed) is considered a first-line vasopressor to restore blood flow. Other vasopressors that can be used include vasopressin, phenylephrine, and dopamine.

After the initial resuscitation, the focus of patient management should be on identifying and treating the specific hemorrhage. In those patients who have undergone neuroendovascular procedures, an abdominal USG or CT of the abdomen and pelvis should be considered. In addition, a vascular surgery consultation should be sought in all patients with suspected retroperitoneal bleeding.[10,11]

### Clinical Pearls

- Any hypotensive event, especially if accompanied by resting tachycardia and reduced urine output, after endovascular procedures warrants an abdominal or pelvic CT scanning to evaluate for retroperitoneal bleeding if supported by history of femoral or iliac artery instrumentation.
- Attention should be paid to prompt correction of any thrombocytopenia or coagulopathy in the postoperative period.

## Prognosis

Clinical outcomes have been reported to be markedly worse in patients who develop POICH.[19] It has been estimated that approximately 36% to 55% of these patients are dead, vegetative, or severely disabled at 3 months. The overall mortality can be as high as 32%. Due to these alarming statistics, practitioners should pay careful attention to controlling treatable risk factors and early detection of POICH.

## Summary

POICH is one of the most dreaded and catastrophic complications of neurosurgical and neuroendovascular procedures. Many of the risk factors associated with POICH are treatable and could be prevented by good perioperative care. Any worsening of the patient's neurological status should prompt immediate head imaging to detect and treat POICH. The presence of intravascular volume depletion, especially in those patients undergoing cerebral angiography, should raise the suspicion for systemic bleeding, with retroperitoneal hematoma as the most severe form.

### References

1. Merriman E, Bell W, Long DM. Surgical postoperative bleeding associated with aspirin ingestion. Report of two cases. *J Neurosurg.* 1979;50(5):682–684. PubMed PMID: 430164.
2. Samii M, Matthies C. Management of 1000 vestibular schwannomas (acoustic neuromas): surgical management and results with an emphasis on complications and how to avoid them. *Neurosurgery.* 1997;40(1):11–21. discussion 23. PubMed PMID: 8971819.
3. Taylor WA, Thomas NW, Wellings JA, Bell BA. Timing of postoperative intracranial hematoma development and implications for the best use of neurosurgical intensive care. *J Neurosurg.* 1995;82(1):48–50. PubMed PMID: 7815133.
4. Dickinson LD, Miller LD, Patel CP, Gupta SK. Enoxaparin increases the incidence of postoperative intracranial hemorrhage when initiated preoperatively for deep venous thrombosis prophylaxis in patients with brain tumors. *Neurosurgery.* 1998;43(5):1074–1081. PubMed PMID: 9802851.
5. Fukamachi A, Koizumi H, Nukui H. Postoperative intracerebral hemorrhages: a survey of computed tomographic findings after 1074 intracranial operations. *Surg Neurol.* 1985;23(6):575–580. PubMed PMID: 3992457.

6. Touho H, Hirakawa K, Hino A, Karasawa J, Ohno Y. Relationship between abnormalities of coagulation and fibrinolysis and postoperative intracranial hemorrhage in head injury. *Neurosurgery.* 1986;19 (4):523–531. PubMed PMID: 3785592.

7. Gerlach R, Tolle F, Raabe A, Zimmermann M, Siegemund A, Seifert V. Increased risk for postoperative hemorrhage after intracranial surgery in patients with decreased factor XIII activity: implications of a prospective study. *Stroke.* 2002;33(6):1618–1623. PubMed PMID: 12053001.

8. Bullock R, Hanemann CO, Murray L, Teasdale GM. Recurrent hematomas following craniotomy for traumatic intracranial mass. *J Neurosurg.* 1990;72(1):9–14. PubMed PMID: 2294191.

9. Vassilouthis J, Anagnostaras S, Papandreou A, Dourdounas E. Is postoperative haematoma an avoidable complication of intracranial surgery? *Br J Neurosurg.* 1999;13(2):154–157. PubMed PMID: 10616584.

10. Kasotakis G. Retroperitoneal and rectus sheath hematomas. *Surg Clin North Am.* 2014;94(1):71–76. PubMed PMID: 24267499.

11. Chan YC, Morales JP, Reidy JF, Taylor PR. Management of spontaneous and iatrogenic retroperitoneal haemorrhage: conservative management, endovascular intervention or open surgery? *Int J Clin Pract.* 2008;62(10):1604–1613. PubMed PMID: 17949429.

12. Friedman JA, Piepgras DG, Duke DA, et al. Remote cerebellar hemorrhage after supratentorial surgery. *Neurosurgery.* 2001;49 (6):1327–1340. PubMed PMID: 11846932.

13. Yamamoto H, Hirashima Y, Hamada H, Hayashi N, Origasa H, Endo S. Independent predictors of recurrence of chronic subdural hematoma: results of multivariate analysis performed using a logistic regression model. *J Neurosurg.* 2003;98(6):1217–1221. PubMed PMID: 12816267.

14. Zetterling M, Ronne-Engstrom E. High intraoperative blood loss may be a risk factor for postoperative hematoma. *J Neurosurg Anesthesiol.* 2004;16(2):151–155. PubMed PMID: 15021285.

15. Izumihara A, Ishihara T, Iwamoto N, Yamashita K, Ito H. Postoperative outcome of 37 patients with lobar intracerebral hemorrhage related to cerebral amyloid angiopathy. *Stroke.* 1999;30(1):29–33. PubMed PMID: 9880384.

16. Leblanc R, Carpenter S, Stewart J, Pokrupa R. Subacute enlarging cerebral hematoma from amyloid angiopathy: case report. *Neurosurgery.* 1995;36(2):403–406. PubMed PMID: 7731523.

17. Haines SJ, Maroon JC, Jannetta PJ. Supratentorial intracerebral hemorrhage following posterior fossa surgery. *J Neurosurg.* 1978;49 (6):881–886. PubMed PMID: 731306.

18. Basali A, Mascha EJ, Kalfas I, Schubert A. Relation between perioperative hypertension and intracranial hemorrhage after craniotomy. *Anesthesiology.* 2000;93(1):48–54. PubMed PMID: 10861145.

19. Kalfas IH, Little JR. Postoperative hemorrhage: a survey of 4992 intracranial procedures. *Neurosurgery.* 1988;23(3):343–347. PubMed PMID: 3226512.

20. Chan KH, Mann KS, Chan TK. The significance of thrombocytopenia in the development of postoperative intracranial hematoma. *J Neurosurg.* 1989;71(1):38–41. PubMed PMID: 2738639.

21. Harker LA, Slichter SJ. The bleeding time as a screening test for evaluation of platelet function. *N Engl J Med.* 1972;287(4):155–159. PubMed PMID: 4537519.

22. Kincaid EH, Miller PR, Meredith JW, Rahman N, Chang MC. Elevated arterial base deficit in trauma patients: a marker of impaired oxygen utilization. *J Am Coll Surg.* 1998;187(4):384–392. PubMed PMID: 9783784.

23. Davis JW, Shackford SR, Mackersie RC, Hoyt DB. Base deficit as a guide to volume resuscitation. *J Trauma.* 1988;28(10):1464–1467. PubMed PMID: 3172306.

24. Moomey Jr CB, Melton SM, Croce MA, Fabian TC, Proctor KG. Prognostic value of blood lactate, base deficit, and oxygen-derived variables in an LD50 model of penetrating trauma. *Crit Care Med.* 1999;27(1):154–161. PubMed PMID: 9934910.

25. Husain FA, Martin MJ, Mullenix PS, Steele SR, Elliott DC. Serum lactate and base deficit as predictors of mortality and morbidity. *Am J Surg.* 2003;185(5):485–491. PubMed PMID: 12727572.

26. Scalea TM, Hartnett RW, Duncan AO, et al. Central venous oxygen saturation: a useful clinical tool in trauma patients. *J Trauma.* 1990;30(12):1539–1543. PubMed PMID: 2258969.

27. Cheung AT, Guvakov DV, Weiss SJ, et al. Nicardipine intravenous bolus dosing for acutely decreasing arterial blood pressure during general anesthesia for cardiac operations: pharmacokinetics, pharmacodynamics, and associated effects on left ventricular function. *Anesth Analg.* 1999;89(5):1116–1123. Epub 1999/11/30.

28. Dellinger RP, Levy MM, Rhodes A, et al. Surviving sepsis campaign: international guidelines for management of severe sepsis and septic shock: 2012. *Crit Care Med.* 2013;41(2):580–637. PubMed PMID: 23353941.

29. Esteban A, Alia I, Tobin MJ, et al. Effect of spontaneous breathing trial duration on outcome of attempts to discontinue mechanical ventilation. Spanish Lung Failure Collaborative Group. *Am J Respir Crit Care Med.* 1999;159(2):512–518. Epub 1999/02/02.

30. Esteban A, Frutos F, Tobin MJ, et al. A comparison of four methods of weaning patients from mechanical ventilation. Spanish Lung Failure Collaborative Group. *N Engl J Med.* 1995;332(6):345–350. Epub 1995/02/09.

31. Anderson CS, Heeley E, Huang Y, et al. Rapid blood-pressure lowering in patients with acute intracerebral hemorrhage. *N Engl J Med.* 2013;368(25):2355–2365. PubMed PMID: 23713578.

32. Qureshi AI, Tariq N, Divani AA, et al. Antihypertensive Treatment of Acute Cerebral Hemorrhage i. Antihy-pertensive treatment of acute cerebral hemorrhage. *Crit Care Med.* 2010;38(2):637–648. PubMed PMID: 19770736.

33. Kao FC, Tsai TT, Chen LH, et al. Symptomatic epidural hematoma after lumbar decompression surgery. *Eur Spine J.* 2015;24 (2):348–357. PubMed PMID: 24760464.

34. Koizumi H, Fukamachi A, Nukui H. Postoperative subdural fluid collections in neurosurgery. *Surg Neurol.* 1987;27(2):147–153. PubMed PMID: 3810442.

35. Magder S, Bafaqeeh F. The clinical role of central venous pressure measurements. *J Intensive Care Med.* 2007;22(1):44–51. PubMed PMID: 17259568.

36. Osman D, Ridel C, Ray P, et al. Cardiac filling pressures are not appropriate to predict hemodynamic response to volume challenge. *Crit Care Med.* 2007;35(1):64–68. PubMed PMID: 17080001.

37. Kumar A, Anel R, Bunnell E, et al. Pulmonary artery occlusion pressure and central venous pressure fail to predict ventricular filling volume, cardiac performance, or the response to volume infusion in normal subjects. *Crit Care Med.* 2004;32(3):691–699 .PubMed PMID: 15090949.

38. Hofer CK, Muller SM, Furrer L, Klaghofer R, Genoni M, Zollinger A. Stroke volume and pulse pressure variation for prediction of fluid responsiveness in patients undergoing off-pump coronary artery bypass grafting. *Chest.* 2005;128(2):848–854. PubMed PMID: 16100177.

39. Marx G, Cope T, McCrossan L, et al. Assessing fluid responsiveness by stroke volume variation in mechanically ventilated patients with severe sepsis. *Eur J Anaesthesiol.* 2004;21(2):132–138. PubMed PMID: 14977345.

40. Wiesenack C, Fiegl C, Keyser A, Prasser C, Keyl C. Assessment of fluid responsiveness in mechanically ventilated cardiac surgical patients. *Eur J Anaesthesiol.* 2005;22(9):658–665 PubMed PMID: 16163911.

41. Myburgh JA, Mythen MG. Resuscitation fluids. *N Engl J Med.* 2013;369(13):1243–1251. PubMed PMID: 24066745.

42. Annane D, Siami S, Jaber S, et al. Effects of fluid resuscitation with colloids vs crystalloids on mortality in critically ill patients presenting with hypovolemic shock: the CRISTAL randomized trial. *JAMA.* 2013;310(17):1809–1817. PubMed PMID: 24108515.

# 47 *Management of Postoperative Intracranial Hypertension*

JENNIFER GUTWALD MILLER, CHRISTOPHER MELINOSKY, and NEERAJ BADJATIA

## Introduction

Principles for management of intracranial hypertension largely derive from studies of patients with acute severe traumatic brain injury (TBI). For this population there exists a firmly entrenched, tiered, or stepwise clinical algorithm that is endorsed by formal guidelines.[1] These treatments are appropriate in causes specific in patients with global brain swelling after trauma, but are often applied to patients with intracranial hypertension from other causes as well (e.g., ischemic stroke). However, the causes of intracranial hypertension in patients who have undergone elective neurosurgery surgery may differ both in pathophysiology and incidence from those of patients with acute TBI. It is therefore important to recognize predisposing surgery-related factors and to alter treatment accordingly, so that it, too, is cause specific. In the postoperative neurosurgical patient with intracranial hypertension, a focused, pathology-driven process, rather than a general stepwise approach, may be more appropriate.

### PATHOPHYSIOLOGY OF INTRACRANIAL HYPERTENSION

The principle of intracranial compliance is described by the Monro-Kellie doctrine,[2,3] which states that changes in intracranial pressure (ICP) are dependent on changes in intracranial volume compartments composed of cerebrospinal fluid, blood, and parenchymal tissue (Fig. 47.1). Increases in intracranial volume (e.g., tumor) can initially displace both vascular and cerebrospinal fluid without leading to raised ICP; however, due to the rigid intracranial vault, pressure eventually begins to increase exponentially and can suddenly result in catastrophic intracranial hypertension. Theoretically, this can be quantified by measuring the difference between the arterial (P1 – percussion) wave and the venous (P2 – tidal) wave on the ICP waveform (Fig. 47.2). Normally the P1 waves are higher than P2 waves, and as compliance is lost, so is the gradient between P1 and P2. This occurs before there is a rise in ICP, although timing varies based on the acuity of the injury. At the bedside, intracranial compliance can be assessed in patients with an external ventricular drainage system by dividing the amount of drainage by the difference in intracranial pressure predrainage and postdrainage. Unfortunately, there is no current standard method by which to measure intracranial compliance in patients with fiberoptic monitoring, and the interpretation of compliance at the bedside is greatly dependent on the

quality of the waveform, with a realization of the limitations of such an approach.

A discussion of intracranial compliance and management of raised intracranial pressure is incomplete without understanding the relationship between cerebral perfusion pressure (CPP) and cerebrovascular autoregulation. CPP is calculated by subtracting ICP from mean arterial pressure (MAP), with a normal range >50 mm Hg and <150 mm Hg (Fig. 47.3).[4] Beyond the upper and lower limits of autoregulation, cerebral blood flow (CBF) varies with CPP in a linear fashion; these limits are shifted to the right in patients with chronic hypertension (Fig. 47.2). Acute neurological diseases such as ischemic stroke, severe TBI, and subarachnoid hemorrhage (SAH) may impair cerebrovascular autoregulation in zones of injury so that CBF becomes entirely pressure passive (Fig. 47.3).

When intracranial compliance is reduced as a result of an intracranial mass lesion or brain edema, autoregulation-triggered vasodilation increases cerebral blood volume (CBV) and can therefore raise ICP. Patients with increased ICP are especially vulnerable from decreases in MAP because CPP (by definition) is reduced when ICP is high, and vasodilatory compensation only aggravates the situation. Failure of autoregulation at the extremes of CPP and the relationship between ICP and CBF are shown in Fig. 47.3. Beyond the lower limit of autoregulation, passive vessel collapse occurs and ischemic damage predominates; above the upper limit, autoregulatory breakthrough leads to increased intravascular pressure and volume, hyperperfusion injury, and vasogenic edema.

## Common Clinical Scenarios

### POSTOPERATIVE BLEEDING

Postoperative bleeding into the surgical bed is an important consideration in evaluating the cause of increased intracranial pressure and clinical deterioration, and treatment is specifically aimed at achieving hemostasis.[5] Particular surgeries are commonly associated with this complication, with glioblastoma multiforme tumor resections carrying the greatest risk of postoperative bleeding, likely due to the invasive and vascular nature of these tumors, as well as typically incomplete resections, which leave residual tumor that may bleed.[6] Moreover, vascular malformation surgery, with possible relation to normal perfusion pressure breakthrough, may also have increased susceptibility to postoperative bleeding.

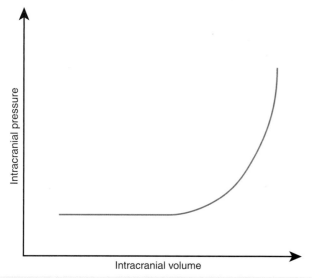

**Fig. 47.1** Relationship between intracranial pressure (ICP) and intracranial volume (ICV). As ICV initially begins to increase, there is a minimal increase in ICP due to compensatory mechanisms (egress of cerebral venous blood and CSF from the cranial vault). However, once these compensatory mechanisms are exhausted, there is a rapid rise in ICP as ICV continues to increase.

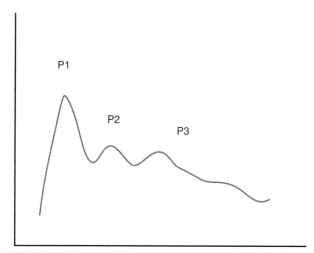

**Fig. 47.2** Intracranial pressure waveform. *P1* is known as the percussion wave and corresponds with the arterial systolic wave. *P2* is known as the tidal wave and is a reflection of venous drainage at the skull base. It is normally less than P1, but can rise when there is an increase in intracranial volume, prior to a change in the mean ICP value. *P3* represents the dicrotic wave and is a reflection of aortic valve closure.

Basali et al.[5] reported an association of postoperative hypertension with intracranial hemorrhage.[7] Intracranial hemorrhage in the postoperative neurosurgical patient may result in elevated intracranial pressure and frequently requires treatment with cerebrospinal fluid (CSF) diversion and osmotic therapy in order to minimize secondary neurological injury. Definitive treatment often requires reoperation to control the bleeding and/or to reduce mass effect from the hematoma. The role of surgical decompression in this population is not well studied, and practice varies. Clinical studies that have evaluated the efficacy of surgical decompression have included patients with spontaneous intracerebral

hemorrhages (ICHs) rather than postoperative ICHs. Potential surgical approaches include open craniotomy, endoscopic aspiration, and stereotactic aspiration. To date, the largest published studies are the Surgical Treatment of Intracerebral Hemorrhage (STICH) trials. In STICH, patients with spontaneous ICH were randomized to early surgery versus conservative management. The patients with early hematoma evacuation had slightly improved outcomes that did not reach statistical significance if craniotomy was the technique employed and if the hematoma was less than 1 cm from the cortical surface.[8] STICH II utilized the subgroup analysis from STICH to determine whether open craniectomy might benefit select patients. It reaffirmed that early surgical intervention and conservative management had similar outcomes.[9] Infratentorial surgical bed rebleeding may cause compression of the brainstem and occlusion of the fourth ventricle (acute hydrocephalus), which can lead to rapid or sudden death. Surgical decompression is indicated for patients with cerebellar hemorrhages who are clinically declining or whose hemorrhages are larger than 3 cm in diameter.[10]

## DURAL VENOUS SINUS THROMBOSIS

Cerebral venous sinus thrombosis (CVT) can occur after neurosurgical instrumentation, particularly after surgeries that are interhemispheric, include sagittal sinus instrumentation, or involve a subtemporal approach.[11] This risk is related to (often intentional) sacrifice of a cortical vein, which can lead to flow disruptions and ultimately thrombosis. CVT can present insidiously with headache that progresses to focal neurological signs when infarction occurs. CVT also may present with clinical signs of acute intracranial hypertension (headache, vomiting, papilledema). It can also present as a nonfocal encephalopathy or with focal neurological deficits. CVT can frequently present as seizures, leading to status epilepticus. The pathogenesis of CVT involves obstruction of the venous structures, which then results in increased venous pressure, decreased capillary perfusion pressure, and increased CBV. The subsequent dilatation of cerebral veins and recruitment of collateral pathways play an important role in the early phases of CVT and may initially compensate for changes in pressure. The increase in venous and capillary pressure causes blood–brain barrier disruption, which leads to vasogenic edema, with leakage of plasma into the interstitial space. As intravenous pressure continues to increase, severe cerebral vasogenic edema and venous hemorrhage can occur due to venous or capillary rupture. The increased intravenous pressure may then lead to an increased intravascular pressure and subsequently a lowering of CPP, resulting in decreased CBF and failure of energy metabolism. In turn, this allows intracellular entry of water from failure of the Na+/K+ ATPase pump and consequent cytotoxic edema added to preceding vasogenic edema. The cytotoxic and vasogenic edema can exacerbate intracranial hypertension, which can itself further interfere with venous drainage.[12] CVT also leads to impaired CSF absorption, which then directly exacerbates increased intracranial pressure.[13] To diagnose CVT, magnetic resonance imaging using gradient echo T2* susceptibility-weighted sequences in combination with magnetic resonance venography has

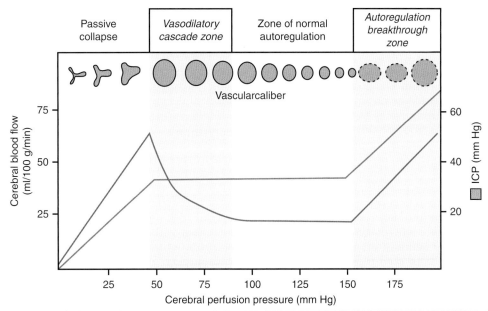

**Fig.47.3** Interaction between cerebral blood flow, cerebral perfusion pressure, and intracranial pressure. The relationship between cerebral blood flow (CBF) and cerebral perfusion pressure (CPP) results in vasoactive changes that directly affect intracranial pressure (ICP). This figure represents a patient with elevated ICP but some autoregulating brain tissue, accounting for the increase in blood volume and increase in ICP at the lower end of the normal autoregulatory range.[4] (Adapted from Rose JC and Mayer SA. *Neurocrit Care.* 1(3):287–99.)

been shown to be the most sensitive imaging method.[14] Computed tomography (CT) should still be the first imaging modality to exclude other causes of increased ICP and sometimes can show abnormalities that raise suspicion for CVT. There are several described findings on CT in CVT: the dense triangle sign, the empty delta sign, and the cord sign. The dense triangle sign is seen as a hyperdensity with a triangular or round shape in the posterior part of the superior sagittal sinus caused by the venous thrombus. The empty delta sign is seen on head CT performed with contrast as a triangular pattern of contrast enhancement surrounding a central region that is lacking contrast enhancement in the posterior part of the superior sagittal sinus. The cord sign can be seen on head CT performed with contrast as a curvilinear or linear hyperdensity over the cerebral cortex, which is caused by a thrombosed cortical vein.[15–17]

## HYDROCEPHALUS

The concern for new-onset hydrocephalus after neurosurgical intervention is usually related to the location of the surgery, with ventricular, infratentorial, and periventricular surgeries being the highest risk. In small case series of skull-base or transsphenoidal surgery, it has been in reported 5% to 8% of cases.[18–20] The most common etiologies are a new hemorrhage into the ventricular system, CSF leak, or focal edema leading to obstructive hydrocephalus. Additionally, risk factors that have been identified include prior craniotomy, prior radiation therapy, and CSF infection.[18]

Patients undergoing foramen magnum decompression for a Chiari I malformation are also at risk for developing new acute hydrocephalus postoperatively. Chiari I malformation is the descent of the cerebellar tonsils below the level of the foramen magnum, which alters the flow of

CSF leading to associated syringomyelia in up to half of cases.[21] Foramen magnum decompression by craniectomy of the posterior fossa and/or C1 arch 5, with or without dural opening and graft to enlarge the cisterna magna, has become the standard of treatment for symptomatic cases. Even after excluding those with hydrocephalus or raised ICP preoperatively, it has been noted that up to 8% of patients develop hydrocephalus or raised ICP as a postoperative consequence of foramen magnum decompression.[21]

The treatment of acute hydrocephalus often necessitates the placement of an external ventricular drain (EVD) as the first line of therapy. Infratentorial lesions may need urgent attention, given the vulnerability of the brainstem. In these cases, a small amount of edema may obstruct the normal drainage pathways of the CSF, leading to hydrocephalus, resulting in mass effect on the brainstem and requiring emergent intervention.

## PNEUMOCEPHALUS

As a result of neurosurgery, air may accumulate in the epidural, subarachnoid, intraventricular, intracerebral, or subdural spaces, with the subdural space most frequent. The most common site is frontal, followed by the occipital and temporal areas.[22]

At least two possible mechanisms for the development of pneumocephalus are described.[23] The first is the so-called *ball-valve effect*, where the air enters from the extracranial space through CSF leakage (e.g., from a dural tear), which allows air to enter but not to exit. A second possibility can be due to the excessive loss of CSF during surgery, which can lead to negative intracranial pressure, resulting in entry of air that replaces CSF as the pressure in the two cavities balance. Although pneumocephalus most commonly results from trauma, it is not unusual after either cranial or spinal surgery and after ear/nose/throat operations, such as paranasal sinus surgery, nasal septum resection, or nasal polypectomy.[22] Pneumocephalus can result in headaches, nausea, vomiting, irritability, dizziness, and seizures. Rarely, pneumocephalus may be under tension, resulting in mass effect (brain compression) and raised ICP. The use of nitrous oxide as an anesthetic has been reported to be a contributing factor to the postoperative development of tension pneumocephalus, because it rapidly can increase the presence of existing pneumocephalus.[24] The mechanism by which this occurs is due to the properties of $N_2O$, which rapidly is dissolved in the blood and enters the closed dural space faster than nitrogen can be removed.[24] Arguably, this chemical property, although enhancing $N_2O$ entry into closed air spaces in the head during surgery, should also promote smaller pneumocephalus postoperatively after $N_2O$ administration is discontinued. However, this notion has not been rigorously evaluated. Clinical symptoms associated with tension pneumocephalus are nonspecific and indistinguishable from other postop complication presentations (such as space-occupying bleeding or increased ICP). These patients can have increased agitation, focal deficits, rapidly decreasing level of arousal, and even cardiac arrest. As with any postop patient with acute neurological deterioration, a rapid CT scan of the head without contrast is indicated. The "Mt. Fuji sign" describes the radiological appearance of acute tension pneumocephalus (Fig. 47.4). This occurs when the presence of subdural free air compresses and separates the frontal lobes.[25]

Pneumocephalus usually gets absorbed without any clinical manifestations, although it may take up to 2

to 3 weeks to fully resolve. Initial management consists of placing the patient in the Fowler position of 30 degrees. Occasionally, hyperbaric oxygen therapy has been utilized to relieve the symptoms referable to pneumocephalus.[26] Tension pneumocephalus in a patient with impaired consciousness is treated with emergent surgical decompression.

## SEIZURES

Seizures are a risk of performing almost any supratentorial neurosurgical procedure. Incidence is estimated to be 15% to 20% in the postoperative population.[27–31] Seizures are most likely to occur in the first month after surgery, and overall risk decreases with time. Risk of seizures is increased with longer duration of surgery; involvement of cortex in the procedure; history of preoperative seizures; and surgery for supratentorial meningioma, low-grade glioma, or aneurysm.[31] Multiple factors contribute to an increased risk of seizures, including tissue irritation, local hypoxia, hemorrhage, and the overall stress of the procedure.[32]

Seizures are a common presenting manifestation of low-grade tumors[33] but can also occur in patients harboring high-grade tumors and may cause acute elevations in ICP. The location of the tumor is also an important consideration because supratentorial tumors are associated with a higher degree of seizure activity, with those tumors located in or adjacent to the perirolandic cortex and temporal lobe being especially prone to epileptogenic activity.[34] In patients undergoing cerebrovascular surgery for aneurysm obliteration or arteriovenous malformation resection, seizures have been reported in 5%[35] and at a rate of 0.16 patients per year,[36] respectively. Unlike tumor surgery, there does not appear to be an anatomical predilection, and in the case of aneurysm clipping or coiling, the majority of the seizures occur within 24 hours of intervention.[35]

Both partial and generalized seizures have been shown to have association with increased ICP, likely due to changes in blood flow.[37] Status epilepticus is rare and may be divided into convulsive or nonconvulsive (NCSE). Convulsive status epilepticus is easily recognized, but NCSE may be difficult to detect, especially in the immediate postoperative period. The hallmarks of NCSE are nonspecific and may include failure to wake when sedation is held, new gaze preference, stereotyped activity, fluctuating level of consciousness, isolated rise in ICP without other cause, or autonomic instability.

If NCSE is suspected, an electroencephalogram (EEG) should be obtained. Empiric administration of a benzodiazepine may result in "paradoxical" improvement in mental status; however, a benzodiazepine trial should not substitute diagnostically for an EEG. A number of studies have investigated the routine use of antiepileptic drugs (AEDs) after craniotomy[30] to prevent seizures or status epilepticus, but none has conclusively shown that the routine prophylactic use of an AED is efficacious. Given the low incidence of status epilepticus, routine use of continuous EEG in all postoperative patients has a low-yield.[38] However, if continuous EEG is already in place, it may provide additional evidence for increased ICP of otherwise unknown etiology.

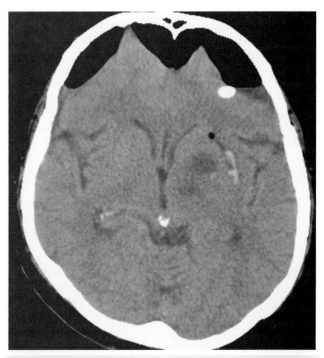

**Fig. 47.4** "Mount Fuji" sign. Axial image on noncontrast CT demonstrates air in the subdural space over the frontal convexities and between the frontal lobes imparting a peaked appearance to the frontal lobes. This suggests tension pneumocephalus.

# General Approach to Raised Intracranial Pressure

## CLINICAL SIGNS AND SYMPTOMS OF INCREASED INTRACRANIAL PRESSURE

The initial neurological evaluation is vital, and both preoperative and postoperative assessments are essential to detect signs and symptoms of raised ICP and neurological deterioration. Papilledema, headaches that are worse in the supine position, nausea and vomiting, abnormal eye movements, pupillary changes, and impaired consciousness are the classic signs of raised ICP. In most cases, a decreasing level of consciousness is the earliest sign of increasing ICP. However, this may be difficult to discern from the side effects of analgesics or sedatives. Therefore it is important to characterize the change in mental status within the context of additional neurological findings to improve diagnostic accuracy. Vomiting is more common in children than in adults and is more often associated with infratentorial lesions that lead to obstructive hydrocephalus. Hemodynamic changes are a late sign, reflecting pressure on the brainstem, and often indicate impending herniation.

Herniation syndromes are important to recognize because irreversible neurological injury may rapidly follow the onset of these signs.[39] Uncal herniation is the most common type of herniation and classically presents with impaired consciousness, a fixed and dilated ipsilateral pupil, and contralateral hemiparesis. The uncus is the anatomical structure located within the mesial temporal lobe that can herniate over the tentorial edge and compress the oculomotor nerve. Further herniation can result in compression of the midbrain and down into the posterior fossa causing impaired consciousness as well as contralateral hemiplegia (by compressing the corticospinal tract). In patients with large temporal lobe tumors and prolonged periods of uncal herniation, the posterior cerebral artery can be compressed between the uncus and the midbrain resulting in an occipital lobe infarct. Subfalcine herniation can occur after a frontal lobe surgery, as a result of local mass on the cingulate gyrus. This is commonly seen in patients with supratentorial metastasis, as well as low- or high-grade gliomas. Branches of the anterior cerebral artery run in close proximity to the free edge of the interhemispheric falx and can be compressed by displacement of the cingulate gyrus, resulting in ischemia or infarction. This would be reflected as changes in tone and strength in the lower extremities. With mass lesions that are superior and cause a downward vector of force (e.g., bilateral subdural hematomas), the entire midbrain may shift downward, causing central (diencephalic) herniation. Patients are usually obtunded, have an altered breathing pattern, pinpoint pupils, and loss of upward gaze. With expansion of the posterior fossa contents, such as in cases of infratentorial tumors, the cerebellum may herniate down through the foramen magnum and compress the caudal medulla. This can lead to cardiorespiratory dysfunction, altered breathing patterns, and impaired consciousness. An abducens nerve palsy in isolation or in combination with other clinical signs is often considered a "false localizing" sign, given that it may be present due to increased ICP on the brainstem or anywhere along the intracranial course of the nerve.[40] Notably, a herniation syndrome may be induced with only mild frontal edema if a lumbar drain had been placed and removed, with a residual dural lumbar CSF leak producing a craniocaudal pressure gradient.[41]

## INTRACRANIAL PRESSURE MONITORING

ICP monitoring may be performed using several different methods with varying degrees of accuracy and with individual complications. The most common method used is an intraventricular catheter (also called an EVD), which involves direct insertion of a catheter into the ventricle. This technique has several advantages; in addition to directly monitoring pressure, the system can be used therapeutically, by allowing for CSF drainage, and diagnostically, by allowing for CSF sampling. This method uses a pressure transducer for monitoring of the ICP waveform while collecting excess fluid in a pressure-dependent fashion. This catheter may be placed in the operating room under direct visualization or at the bedside using anatomical landmarks. The drain is leveled at the tragus or the external auditory meatus, which is an approximation of the level of the foramen of Monro. The pressure is only transduced when the drainage system is closed. There is no standard practice as to whether to maintain the drainage system constantly or intermittently closed. Rather this decision is often made in relation to the acute need for drainage. Newer systems that utilize an air pouch mounted in the tip region of a dual lumen probe allow for simultaneous drainage and pressure monitoring.[42] Given the direct path to the ventricles, ventriculitis may occur in 11% to 20% of catheters. In several small randomized controlled trials, antibiotic- or silver-impregnated probes have generally demonstrated a reduction in ventriculitis rates, although the single most important factor remains the overall duration of drain placement, with an increase in risk for every day beyond 5 days.[43] Additional factors to consider when utilizing EVDs for ICP monitoring are that the catheter may become clogged, there may be tract hemorrhage, or there may be accidental overdrainage. The catheter may entirely stop draining if it becomes displaced. EVD guidelines have been published by the Neurocritical Care Society[44] and by the American Association of Neuroscience Nurses.[45]

Other monitoring methods involve placement of a pressure monitor through the skull into parenchyma, the subarachnoid space, the subdural space, or the epidural space. The most common approach is a parenchymal probe, which rests in white matter, usually in a standard location within either the right or left frontal lobe. These monitors are useful in focal pathologies, but overall are considered less accurate, cannot be recalibrated once placed, are not able to drain fluid, and carry a risk of infection or hemorrhage, albeit lower than with the EVD.

## UNIVERSAL MEASURES

With the first signs of increasing ICP, patient positioning can be vital. The head of the bed should be raised to

30 degrees incline, with the head slightly above the level of the heart. The exception to this approach is with those patients who develop bifrontal edema due to compression from pneumocephalus or occasionally subdural hygroma. The patient's head should be placed in a neutral position without any restrictive device on the neck (such as a collar or tape) in order to prevent jugular compression. Blood pressure should be titrated to optimize CPP; hypotension might raise ICP through reactive vasodilation while decreasing cerebral perfusion. Endotracheal suctioning and other techniques that might suddenly raise intraabdominal or intrathoracic pressure should be avoided if possible during episodes of intracranial hypertension.[46–49] Normothermia should maintained because every 1 C rise in core temperature can increase the cerebral metabolic rate for oxygen by up to 10%, resulting in an increase in CBF, and therefore intracranial blood volume and ICP.[50]

## SEDATION AND ANALGESIA

Adequate sedation and pain control are important first steps in managing raised ICP. Many of the agents utilized are effective in lowering ICP by a coupled reduction in cerebral metabolic rate of oxygen and CBF. However, analgosedatives should not be used as the primary method by which to lower ICP. The goal is to attain adequate sedation and pain control without obscuration of the clinical examination. This is best achieved if sedation and analgesia are titrated to established scales. These scales require clinical assessment of arousability and interaction and do not take into account patients who may be comatose. Nonetheless sedation rating scales can remove the effects of external influences and provide a clearly understood goal for nurses and physicians. The overall effect is a decreased tendency toward oversedation and a reduction in days of mechanical ventilation, need for tracheostomy, and cost.[51,52]

There are both general and neurospecific properties that are important to understand when selecting sedating agents. Foremost, there should be a quick onset and offset with a predictable clearance independent of end organ function. This allows for easier titration to effect, while also permitting continued neurological assessment. Minimal cardiovascular depressant effects are also important, so as not to require additional infusion therapies to maintain goal blood pressures. An ideal agent should reduce ICP by reducing cerebral blood volume by coupling a reduction of both CBF and cerebral metabolic rate for oxygen. This implies that autoregulation not be disturbed, which is not universally observed with all sedatives.

Although there is no ideal agent that fulfills all these criteria, propofol is commonly utilized and is the only agent that has Class I evidence to support its use in lowering ICP.[53] Propofol is a substituted phenol with rapid anesthetic but no analgesic properties. It reduces ICP by a dose-dependent fall in CBF coupled to metabolic rate. Additionally, it has anticonvulsant action via gamma-aminobutyric acid (GABA)–dependent chloride channels, which also contributes to central nervous system depression. Propofol can result in a series of biochemical and cardiac complications, the most severe of which is a constellation of findings characterized as the propofol infusion syndrome. Many of these side effects can be avoided by

limiting the dose and duration of therapy. Dexmedetomidine is a central alpha 1 agonist that has multiple sites of action resulting in an overall decrease in sympathetic activity, shivering, and anxiolytic effects. Unique to this drug is the ability to maintain arousability and sedation, which makes it an attractive agent for neurologically injured patients. This overall lack of significant impact on $CMRO_2$ renders dexmedetomidine a weak ICP-lowering agent. Further, there may be an uncoupling of $CMRO_2$ and CBF, placing patients at risk for cerebral ischemia.[54a] Definitive clinical studies are lacking to indicate whether this concern translates into a quantifiable risk. Benzodiazepines are a commonly used class of sedative drugs that work by acting on the $GABA_A$ receptor causing sedative, hypnotic, and anxiolytic effects. They have a minimal impact on $CMRO_2$ or CBF at sedative doses.[54b] Additionally, they can lead to a reduction in CPP by systemic hypotension, a rise in $Paco_2$ by respiratory depression, and prolonged sedation with long-term use, which make benzodiazepines suboptimal for primary ICP-lowering therapy.

## HYPERVENTILATION

In a mechanically ventilated patient, hyperventilation may be one early technique that can be utilized to rapidly lower ICP by focusing on the blood volume component of the Monro-Kellie doctrine.[3] Decreases in arterial carbon dioxide lead to cerebral vasoconstriction, which decreases intracranial blood volume and in turn decreases ICP. CBF changes 4% for every millimeter mercury change in $Paco_2$.[55] The effects of hyperventilation can be seen in minutes, making it a simple and effective technique to emergently decrease ICP.

However, studies have demonstrated negative consequences of hyperventilation,[56–58] especially early after injury. With hyperventilation, there is an initial compensatory increased oxygen extraction, but this effect does not last. In tissue that is already at risk for ischemia, the added hypoperfusion can increase the risk of infarction. With extended use, there is increased production of mediators of secondary damage such as lactate and glutamate. Therefore hyperventilation is used as a temporary bridging therapy but not as a long-term or prophylactic solution.[56]

## OSMOTIC THERAPY

Hyperosmolar therapy is considered the core medical treatment for elevated ICP.[59–62] Both mannitol and hypertonic saline are commonly used as osmotic agents, most often as bolus treatments.

Mannitol is administered in bolus dosing, with a range of 0.25 to 1.0 g/kg/dose. It acts as an osmotic diuretic, filtered at the glomerulus and reabsorbed. Its peak effects occur 15 to 120 min after administration. To reduce ICP, it increases the osmotic gradient across the blood–brain barrier, because it does not cross it. This favors the movement of water from the brain tissue, thereby decreasing brain water content. Additional favorable side effects include increasing plasma volume and thereby decreasing hematocrit, and viscosity, which thereby improves blood flow in the microvasculature. Mannitol is administered in a 20% solution. Studies have shown a dose-response relationship, with doses below 0.5 g/kg less effective and shorter acting, whereas more effective reduction in ICP occurs with doses between 0.5 and 1.0 g/kg.[60,61] Serum osmolarity or, better yet, the serum osmolar gap, should be measured before and after mannitol administration.

Renal failure is a potential but unusual adverse effect of mannitol therapy—the mechanism proposed involves intrarenal vasoconstriction combined with relative intravascular volume depletion.[46] The incidence in the neurocritical care patient population varies widely due to variations in definitions of renal failure, and data for incidence of clinically significant renal failure are lacking. Mannitol administration can cause hyponatremia, hypochloremia, hyperkalemia, increased osmolar gap, volume overload, and hypotension at rapid infusion rates, that is, total dose given over less than 5 minutes.

Hypertonic saline (HTS) has been shown to decrease intracranial hypertension in patients with TBI, SAH, ischemic and hemorrhagic stroke, liver failure, and mass lesions. It acts by directly increasing serum osmolarity. It is used at various concentrations, including 2% or 3% solutions (150 mL bolus), 7.5% solutions (75 mL bolus), or 23.4% solutions (30 mL bolus). HTS is used in bolus treatment doses for acute management of brain herniation and acute elevations in ICP. In practice, 3% hypertonic saline is also often used as a continuous infusion for prophylactic elevation in serum sodium, titrating to serum sodium levels 145 to 155. Adverse effects of HTS are related to the sustained induction of a hyperosmolar state, where renal failure can result, in addition to the adverse effects of iatrogenic hyperchloremic metabolic acidosis. Hypervolemia may also be problematic in some patients with impaired cardiac reserve. It has been shown that hypernatremia (sodium >160 mEq/l), when induced for osmotic therapy in neurocritical care patients, is an independent predictor of mortality.[63] Central pontine myelinolysis is often discussed as a potential complication of therapy in chronic alcoholics and malnourished patients, but has not been shown to occur in this setting in published studies.

## STEROIDS

Despite the long-standing clinical use of steroids in neurooncology, the exact mechanisms by which their effects are exerted remain unclear. It has been suggested that the effects on edema are due to the reduction in permeability of tumor capillaries.[64,65] Dexamethasone is the most commonly used steroid with a longer half-life, relatively low mineralocorticoid activity, and lower likelihood for prolonged immunosuppression. It has been described that 70% of patients with symptoms related to peritumoral vasogenic edema have symptom improvement with the initiation of steroids.[66] Perioperatively, administration of glucocorticoids has shown to limit the formation of edema during tumor resection.[66] Typically, treatment is started 24 to 48 hours prior to the procedure for best effects. Studies are lacking in describing an optimal dose of dexamethasone, but typically in practice an initial dose of 10 to 20 mg intravenously is given for acute symptoms from mass effect, followed by divided doses for a total 10 to 20 mg daily.[66] Aside from their well-described efficacy in treating peritumoral vasogenic edema, steroids have not

been found to be useful in other causes of intracranial hypertension.[67,68]

## HYPOTHERMIA

There are numerous controlled trials studying the impact of hypothermia on outcome in patients with severe TBI and refractory intracranial hypertension predominantly demonstrating that hypothermia is an effective method for reducing ICP, although the data on outcomes are mostly not favorable.[69] The magnitude of the effect of hypothermia on ICP reduction is estimated to be approximately 10 mm Hg (range 5–23 mm Hg). Across the studies analyzed, the effect on ICP reduction is superior to that achieved with moderate hyperventilation, barbiturates, and mannitol, but less effective than hemicraniectomy and HTS.[70] However, there is no evidence for the use of hypothermia for postoperative ICP reduction. In general, the temperature goal should be the avoidance of fever with the use of antipyretics.

## SURGICAL DECOMPRESSION

Surgical decompression for refractory elevated ICP is considered when standard medical therapies are failing to prevent secondary brain injury. Its indication and timing vary, depending on the etiology of the primary process. In the postop neurosurgical patient, complications including postoperative subdural and epidural hematoma, as well as large space-occupying hemorrhages, would potentially require decompression. Decompression has been studied extensively in TBI, large hemispheric stroke, posterior fossa hemorrhage, and supratentorial ICH, and is indicated in some situations and controversial in others.[71–73]

## References

1. The Brain Trauma Foundation. The American Association of Neurological Surgeons. The Joint Section on Neurotrauma and Critical Care. Intracranial pressure treatment threshold. *J Neurotrauma.* 2000;17:493–495.
2. Marik P, Chen K, Varon J, Fromm Jr R, Sternbach GL. Management of increased intracranial pressure: a review for clinicians. *J Emerg Med.* 1999;17:711–719.
3. Mokri B. The Monro-Kellie hypothesis: applications in CSF volume depletion. *Neurology.* 2001;56:1746–1748.
4. Rose JC, Mayer SA. Optimizing blood pressure in neurological emergencies. *Neurocrit Care.* 2004;1:287–299.
5. Basali A, Mascha EJ, Kalfas I, Schubert A. Relation between perioperative hypertension and intracranial hemorrhage after craniotomy. *Anesthesiology.* 2000;93(1):48–54.
6. Constantini S, Cotev S, Rappaport ZH, Pomeranz S, Shalit MN. Intracranial pressure monitoring after elective intracranial surgery. A retrospective study of 514 consecutive patients. *J Neurosurg.* 1988;69:540–544.
7. Rangel-Castilla L, Spetzler RF, Nakaji P. Normal perfusion pressure breakthrough theory: a reappraisal after 35 years. *Neurosurg Rev.* 2015;38(3):399–404. http://dx.doi.org/10.1007/s10143-014-0600-4. discussion 404–405. Epub 2014 Dec 9.
8. Mendelow AD, Gregson BA, Fernandes HM, et al. Early surgery versus initial conservative treatment in patients with spontaneous supratentorial intracerebral haematomas in the International Surgical Trial in Intracerebral Haemorrhage (STICH): a randomised trial. *Lancet.* 2005;365:387–397.
9. Mendelow AD, Gregson BA, Rowan EN, et al. Early surgery versus initial conservative treatment in patients with spontaneous supratentorial lobar intracerebral haematomas (STICH II): a randomised trial. *Lancet.* 2013;382:397–408.

10. Morgenstern LB, Hemphill 3rd JC, Anderson C, et al. Guidelines for the management of spontaneous intracerebral hemorrhage: a guideline for healthcare professionals from the American Heart Association/American Stroke Association. *Stroke.* 2010;41:2108–2129.

11. Nakase H, Shin Y, Nakagawa I, Kimura R, Sakaki T. Clinical features of postoperative cerebral venous infarction. *Acta Neurochir (Wien).* 2005;147:621–626. discussion 626.

12. Grände PO. The "Lund Concept" for the treatment of severe head trauma—physiological principles and clinical application. *Intensive Care Med.* 2006;32(10):1475–1484. Epub 2006 Aug 2.

13. Gotoh M, Ohmoto T, Kuyama H. Experimental study of venous circulatory disturbance by dural sinus occlusion. *Acta Neurochir (Wien).* 1993;124:120–126.

14. Dormont D, Anxionnat R, Evrard S, Louaille C, Chiras J, Marsault C. MRI in cerebral venous thrombosis. *J Neuroradiol.* 1994;21:81–99.

15. Boukobza M, Crassard I, Bousser MG. When the "dense triangle" in dural sinus thrombosis is round. *Neurology.* 2007;69:808.

16. Lee EJ. The empty delta sign. *Radiology.* 2002;224:788–789.

17. Virapongse C, Cazenave C, Quisling R, Sarwar M, Hunter S. The empty delta sign: frequency and significance in 76 cases of dural sinus thrombosis. *Radiology.* 1987;162:779–785.

18. Sharma M, Ambekar S, Sonig A, Nanda A. Factors predicting the development of new onset post-operative hydrocephalus following trans-sphenoidal surgery for pituitary adenoma. *Clin Neurol Neurosurg.* 2013;115:1951–1954.

19. Duong DH, O'Malley S, Sekhar LN, Wright DG. Postoperative hydrocephalus in cranial base surgery. *Skull Base Surg.* 2000;10:197–200.

20. Burkhardt JK, Zinn PO, Graenicher M, et al. Predicting postoperative hydrocephalus in 227 patients with skull base meningioma. *Neurosurg Focus.* 2011;30:E9.

21. Zakaria R, Kandasamy J, Khan Y, et al. Raised intracranial pressure and hydrocephalus *following* hindbrain decompression for Chiari I malformation: a case series and review of the literature. *Br J Neurosurg.* 2012;26:476–481.

22. Solomiichuk VO, Lebed VO, Drizhdov KI. Posttraumatic delayed subdural tension pneumocephalus. *Surg Neurol Int.* 2013;4:37.

23. Dabdoub CB, Salas G, Silveira Edo N, Dabdoub CF. Review of the management of pneumocephalus. *Surg Neurol Int.* 2015;6:155.

24. Artru AA. Nitrous oxide plays a direct role in the development of tension pneumocephalus intraoperatively. *Anesthesiology.* 1982;57:59–61.

25. Michel SJ. The Mount Fuji sign. *Radiology.* 2004;232:449–450.

26. Paiva WS, de Andrade AF, Figueiredo EG, Amorim RL, Prudente M, Teixeira MJ. Effects of hyperbaric oxygenation therapy on symptomatic pneumocephalus. *Ther Clin Risk Manag.* 2014;10:769–773.

27. Foy PM, Copeland GP, Shaw MD. The incidence of postoperative seizures. *Acta Neurochir (Wien).* 1981;55:253–264.

28. Milligan TA, Hurwitz S, Bromfield EB. Efficacy and tolerability of levetiracetam versus phenytoin after supratentorial neurosurgery. *Neurology.* 2008;71:665–669.

29. North JB, Penhall RK, Hanieh A, Frewin DB, Taylor WB. Phenytoin and postoperative epilepsy. A double-blind study. *J Neurosurg.* 1983;58:672–677.

30. Pulman J, Greenhalgh J, Marson AG. Antiepileptic drugs as prophylaxis for post-craniotomy seizures. *Cochrane Database Syst Rev.* 2013;2. CD007286.

31. Shaw MD, Foy PM. Epilepsy after craniotomy and the place of prophylactic anticonvulsant drugs: discussion paper. *J R Soc Med.* 1991;84:221–223.

32. Kuijlen JM, Teernstra OP, Kessels AG, Herpers MJ, Beuls EA. Effectiveness of antiepileptic prophylaxis used with supratentorial craniotomies: a meta-analysis. *Seizure.* 1996;5:291–298.

33. Chang EF, Potts MB, Keles GE, et al. Seizure characteristics and control following resection in 332 patients with low-grade gliomas. *J Neurosurg.* 2008;108:227–235.

34. Tandon N, Esquenazi Y. Resection strategies in tumoral epilepsy: is a lesionectomy enough? *Epilepsia.* 2013;54(suppl 9):72–78.

35. Lai LT, O'Donnell J, Morgan MK. The risk of seizures during the in-hospital admission for surgical or endovascular treatment of unruptured intracranial aneurysms. *J Clin Neurosci.* 2013;20:1498–1502.

36. Mohr JP, Parides MK, Stapf C, et al. Medical management with or without interventional therapy for unruptured brain arteriovenous malformations (ARUBA): a multicentre, non-blinded, randomised trial. *Lancet.* 2014;383:614–621.

37. Gabor AJ, Brooks AG, Scobey RP, Parsons GH. Intracranial pressure during epileptic seizures. *Electroencephalogr Clin Neurophysiol.* 1984;57:497–506.

38. McNamara B, Ray J, Menon D, Boniface S. Raised intracranial pressure and seizures in the neurological intensive care unit. *Br J Anaesthes.* 2003;90:39–42.

39. Stevens RD, Huff JS, Duckworth J, Papangelou A, Weingart SD, Smith WS. Emergency neurological life support: intracranial hypertension and herniation. *Neurocrit Care.* 2012;17(suppl 1):S60–S65.

40. Larner AJ. False localising signs. *J Neurol Neurosurg Psychiatry.* 2003;74:415–418.

41. Samadani U, Huang JH, Baranov D, Zager EL, Grady MS. Intracranial hypotension after intraoperative lumbar cerebrospinal fluid drainage. *Neurosurgery.* 2003;52(1):148–151. discussion 151–152.

42. Brain Trauma F, American Association of Neurological S, Congress of Neurological S, et al. Guidelines for the management of severe traumatic brain injury. VII. Intracranial pressure monitoring technology. *J Neurotrauma.* 2007;(24 suppl 1):S45–S54.

43. Sonabend AM, Korenfeld Y, Crisman C, Badjatia N, Mayer SA, Connolly Jr ES. Prevention of ventriculostomy-related infections with prophylactic antibiotics and antibiotic-coated external ventricular drains: a systematic review. *Neurosurgery.* 2011;68:996–1005.

44. Fried HI, Nathan BR, Rowe AS, et al. The insertion and management of external ventricular drains: an evidence-based consensus statement: a statement for healthcare professionals from the Neurocritical Care Society. *Neurocrit Care.* 2016;24(1):61–81. http://dx.doi.org/10.1007/s12028-015-0224-8.

45. http://www.aann.org/uploads/AANN11_ICPEVDnew.pdf.

46. Meyer MJ, Megyesi J, Meythaler J, et al. Acute management of acquired brain injury part II: an evidence-based review of pharmacological interventions. *Brain Inj.* 2010;24:706–721.

47. Meyer MJ, Megyesi J, Meythaler J, et al. Acute management of acquired brain injury part I: an evidence-based review of non-pharmacological interventions. *Brain Inj.* 2010;24:694–705.

48. Rosner MJ, Coley IB. Cerebral perfusion pressure, intracranial pressure, and head elevation. *J Neurosurg.* 1986;65:636–641.

49. Wolfe TJ, Torbey MT. Management of intracranial pressure. *Curr Neurol Neurosci Rep.* 2009;9:477–485.

50. Polderman KH. Mechanisms of action, physiological effects, and complications of hypothermia. *Crit Care Med.* 2009;37:S186–S202.

51. Halpern SD, Becker D, Curtis JR, et al. An official American Thoracic Society/American Association of Critical-Care Nurses/American College of Chest Physicians/Society of Critical Care Medicine policy statement: the Choosing Wisely(R) Top 5 list in Critical Care Medicine. *Am J Respir Crit Care Med.* 2014;190:818–826.

52. Riker RR, Fugate JE. Participants in the International Multidisciplinary Consensus Conference on Multimodality M. Clinical monitoring scales in acute brain injury: assessment of coma, pain, agitation, and delirium. *Neurocrit Care.* 2014;(21 suppl 2):S27–S37.

53. Kelly DF, Goodale DB, Williams J, et al. Propofol in the treatment of moderate and severe head injury: a randomized, prospective double-blinded pilot trial. *J Neurosurg.* 1999;90:1042–1052.

54a. Drummond JC, Dao AV, Roth DM, et al. Effect of dexmedetomidine on cerebral blood flow velocity, cerebral metabolic rate, and carbon dioxide response in normal humans. *Anesthesiology.* 2008;108(2):225–232.

54b. Giffin JP, Cottrell JE, Shwiry B, et al. Intracranial pressure, mean arterial pressure, and heart rate following midazolam or thiopental in humans with brain tumors. *Anesthesiology.* 1984;60(5):491–494.

55. Cold GE. Cerebral blood flow in acute head injury. The regulation of cerebral blood flow and metabolism during the acute phase of head injury, and its significance for therapy. *Acta Neurochir Supp.* 1990;49:1–64.

56. Marion DW, Puccio A, Wisniewski SR, et al. Effect of hyperventilation on extracellular concentrations of glutamate, lactate, pyruvate, and local cerebral blood flow in patients with severe traumatic brain injury. *Crit Care Med.* 2002;30:2619–2625.

57. Coles JP, Minhas PS, Fryer TD, et al. Effect of hyperventilation on cerebral blood flow in traumatic head injury: clinical relevance and monitoring correlates. *Crit Care Med.* 2002;30:1950–1959.

58. Muizelaar J, Marmarou A, Ward J, et al. Adverse effects of prolonged hyperventilation in patients with severe head injury: a randomized clinical trial. *J Neurosurg.* 1991;75:731–739.

59. Ropper AH. Hyperosmolar therapy for raised intracranial pressure. *New Engl J Med.* 2012;367:746–752.

60. Marko NF. Hypertonic saline, not mannitol, should be considered gold-standard medical therapy for intracranial hypertension. *Crit Care.* 2012;16:113.

61. Torre-Healy A, Marko NF, Weil RJ. Hyperosmolar therapy for intracranial hypertension. *Neurocrit Care.* 2012;17:117–130.

62. Diringer MN. New trends in hyperosmolar therapy? *Curr Opinion Crit Care.* 2013;19:77–82.

63. Aiyagari V, Deibert E, Diringer MN. Hypernatremia in the neurologic intensive care unit: how high is too high? *J Crit Care.* 2006;21:163–172.

64. Hedley-Whyte ET, Hsu DW. Effect of dexamethasone on blood-brain barrier in the normal mouse. *Ann Neurol.* 1986;19:373–377.

65. Papadopoulos MC, Saadoun S, Binder DK, Manley GT, Krishna S, Verkman AS. Molecular mechanisms of brain tumor edema. *Neuroscience.* 2004;129:1011–1020.

66. Bebawy JF. Perioperative steroids for peritumoral intracranial edema: a review of mechanisms, efficacy, and side effects. *J Neurosurg Anesthesiol.* 2012;24:173–177.

67. Edwards P, Arango M, Balica L, et al. Final results of MRC CRASH, a randomised placebo-controlled trial of intravenous corticosteroid in adults with head injury-outcomes at 6 months. *Lancet.* 2005;365:1957–1959.

68. Poungvarin N, Bhoopat W, Viriyavejakul A, et al. Effects of dexamethasone in primary supratentorial intracerebral hemorrhage. *New Engl J Med.* 1987;316:1229–1233.

69. Polderman KH, Ely EW, Badr AE, Girbes AR. Induced hypothermia in traumatic brain injury: considering the conflicting results of meta-analyses and moving forward. *Intensive Care Med.* 2004;30:1860–1864.

70. Schreckinger M, Marion DW. Contemporary management of traumatic intracranial hypertension: is there a role for therapeutic hypothermia? *Neurocrit Care.* 2009;11:427–436.

71. Taylor B, Lopresti M, Appelboom G, Sander Connolly Jr E. Hemicraniectomy for malignant middle cerebral artery territory infarction: an updated review. *J Neurosurg Sci.* 2015;59:73–78.

72. Barthelemy EJ, Melis M, Gordon E, Ullman JS, Germano I. Decompressive craniectomy for severe traumatic brain injury: a systematic review. *World Neurosurg.* 2016;88:411–420.

73. Takeuchi S, Wada K, Nagatani K, Otani N, Mori K. Decompressive hemicraniectomy for spontaneous intracerebral hemorrhage. *Neurosurg Focus.* 2013;34:E5.

# *Management of Postoperative Stroke*

PEGGY NGUYEN, CHRISTINA HUANG, JAMES M. WRIGHT, and GENE SUNG

## Introduction

### EPIDEMIOLOGY

Guidelines for the acute management of ischemic stroke are established in the American Stroke Association (ASA)/American Heart Association (AHA) guidelines, but the critical care management of postoperative strokes, particularly in the neurosurgical population, is poorly defined.[1] Prior epidemiological studies have established higher rates of stroke with certain surgeries, including cardiac, neurological, and vascular procedures, ranging from 2.2% to 5.2%.[2] Although the exact incidence of postoperative stroke in various neurosurgical procedures has not been fully delineated, the risk of ischemic stroke after carotid endarterectomy has been shown to be 5.5% to 6.1% and the risk of stroke after resection of head and neck tumors has been shown to be 4.8%.[3,4] This chapter will focus on the critical care management of postoperative ischemic strokes after neurosurgical procedures.

### STROKE ETIOLOGIES

In the general surgery population, strokes have been shown to be predominantly embolic; in one study, cardiogenic embolism was the cause of perioperative stroke in 42% of patients in the general surgery population.[4-6] Other common etiologies of stroke include atrial fibrillation at the time of stroke, hypotension during the perioperative or postoperative period, and artery-to-artery embolus in the setting of large-vessel atherosclerotic disease.

During neurosurgical cases, perioperative strokes can be either venous or arterial. Within the neurosurgical population, stroke etiologies vary widely, ranging from embolic strokes, occlusion of perforating vessels due to surgical clipping, clamping of vessels during anastomoses, vascular injury or occlusion secondary to tumor manipulation during resection, or retraction ischemia. In aneurysm clipping studies, reported stroke rates range from 5% to 20%.[7,8] A metaanalysis found no statistically significant difference in the rates of postoperative infarction between patients who had aneurysm clipping (16.1 %) and those who had aneurysm coiling (20.9%).[8]

Tumor resection is also associated with postoperative arterial and venous ischemic events. Data vary significantly in terms of surgeon experience, extent of tumor resection, and patient age and comorbidities. One study of 720 patients found the rate of venous infarctions in meningioma resections to be approximately 2%, with the surgical approach being the most important risk factor in venous ischemic events.[9] Another study of 825 patients undergoing surgical resection of meningiomas found the rate of venous infarction to be 6.8% with large meningiomas (>4 cm) and 1.2% with smaller meningiomas (<4 cm).[10] Tumors invading dural sinuses predispose to venous strokes, particularly meningiomas invading the posterior third of the superior sagittal sinus. An analysis of data on 3812 patients who underwent elective cranial surgery using the American College of Surgeons National Surgical Quality Improvement Program database found the rate of perioperative cerebrovascular accidents to be 1.67%, with patients developing a stroke on average 4 days after surgery.[11]

Sacrifice of draining veins during neurosurgical procedures may result in cerebral venous circulatory disturbances that cause venous infarction. Symptoms may include headache, focal neurological deficits, seizures, diplopia, or encephalopathy. Kageyama et al. reported a rate of 13% in 120 cases, and Saito et al. reported a rate of 2.6% (number of patients). Al-Mefty and Krisht both reported evidence of brain edema in 10% of cases after sacrifice of the superficial Sylvian vein.[12-14] Cerebral veins are valveless, so compensatory circulation and drainage depend on the degree of collateral flow.

## Management

### THROMBOLYTIC AND ANTIPLATELET THERAPY

#### Thrombolytic Drug Therapy

The first goal in acute stroke management is reperfusion; however, reperfusion in the postoperative period has its limitations. Intravenous thrombolysis with tissue plasminogen activator (tPA) leads to a favorable outcome with an Odds Ratio (OR) of 1.9 (95% confidence interval [CI] 1.2–2.9) if given within 3 hours of stroke onset and an OR of 1.28 (95% CI 1.00–1.65) if given within 3.0 to 4.5 hours after stroke onset. Intravenous thrombolysis is one of the few therapies for acute stroke that has proven efficacy, but is contraindicated in the first 2 weeks after surgery.[15] Similarly, although intraarterial thrombolysis (IAT) has been explored as a possible alternative due to lower doses of thrombolytics being used and local delivery, it has a poor safety profile in the neurosurgical population. In one study evaluating the safety of IAT in the postoperative period, investigators concluded that IAT appeared to be a viable therapeutic alternative to IV tPA with the exception of the neurosurgical population, in which IAT after craniotomies had an unacceptable rate of major complications.[16] Therefore IAT is probably contraindicated in the neurosurgical patient.

## Mechanical Thrombectomy

The landmark trial, Multicenter Randomized Clinical Trial of Endovascular Treatment for Acute Ischemic Stroke in the Netherlands (MR CLEAN), was the first large randomized trial demonstrating the benefit of mechanical thrombectomy, which may prove to be the best alternative to IV tPA and IAT.[17] Although no subgroup analyses were done specifically on neurosurgical patients, it is the only acute intervention currently available for the treatment of ischemic stroke in which surgery is not a contraindication. Mechanical thrombectomy should therefore be considered for treatment of patients with postoperative strokes, especially because the most common mechanism of postoperative stroke is embolic, which predominantly affects the large vessels of the anterior circulation. More recently three more randomized trials, Extend-IA, Endovascular treatment for Small Core and Anterior circulation Proximal occlusion with Emphasis on minimizing CT to recanalization times (ESCAPE), and Solitaire with the Intention for Thrombectomy as Primary Endovascular Treatment (SWIFT-PRIME), have corroborated the benefits of embolectomy in large-vessel occlusion.[18–20]

## Antiplatelet Therapy

Low-dose aspirin should be initiated as soon as medically feasible for secondary stroke prevention. There are few evidence-based guidelines for the resumption of aspirin therapy after surgery. In cases of postcraniotomy patients, it may be reasonable to resume low-dose aspirin as soon as 24 hours postoperatively, although in practice, many wait 1–4 weeks before administration of aspirin. In general, patients undergoing spinal surgery may resume aspirin therapy in 3 to 7 days. Treatment with dual antiplatelet agents (e.g., aspirin and clopidogrel) has a high risk of hemorrhagic complications and should therefore be avoided in the postoperative setting.

## HEMODYNAMIC STABILIZATION AND FLUID OPTIMIZATION

Given that blood pressure is a dynamic parameter, it is recommended to monitor blood pressure frequently, especially during the first 24 hours after ischemic stroke.[1] Guidelines for the acute management of ischemic stroke recommend permissive hypertension to a systolic blood pressure of 220 mm Hg over a diastolic blood pressure of 120 mm Hg.[1] The goal of permissive hypertension is to allow cerebral perfusion to the ischemic penumbra. However, allowing hypertension can be problematic in the neurosurgical patient in whom elevated systemic blood pressures after delicate neurovascular surgeries, craniotomies, or spinal surgeries may lead to surgical site hemorrhages. In order to maintain adequate perfusion, it would be reasonable to maintain a systolic blood pressure within 120 mm Hg to 160 mm Hg. In situations where more direct cardiac monitoring is available, mean arterial

pressure (MAP) would also be a reasonable measurement to follow, with a goal MAP of 80 mm Hg or above, translating to a cerebral perfusion pressure of 70.

In the patient with acute ischemic stroke, hypotonic intravenous fluids should be avoided because they may exacerbate ischemic brain edema.[1] Patients requiring fluid resuscitation should therefore be treated with isotonic crystalloid, such as 0.9% saline.

## FEVER

Hyperthermia has been shown to increase mortality in the setting of acute ischemic stroke.[21,22] Although the exact mechanism underlying worsened neurological outcomes after hyperthermia remains unclear, a number of theories have been proposed, including the production of free radicals, increased metabolic demand, and the release of injurious neurotransmitters such as glutamate, $\gamma$-aminobutyric acid, and glycine. In light of these findings, strict measures should be taken to maintain normothermia in the setting of acute ischemic stroke, with a goal body temperature of 38 degrees Celsius.

## GLYCEMIC CONTROL

Hyperglycemia is common in the stroke population, with more than 40% of patients having elevated blood glucose.[1] Several studies have demonstrated the association between hyperglycemia and poorer radiological, as well as clinical, outcomes.[23,24] It is important to note, however, that despite these findings, a recent Cochrane review of several clinical trials has failed to identify a benefit to strict glycemic control with intravenous insulin therapy.[25] Therefore it is recommended to maintain glycemic control as per the current AHA/American Stroke Association guidelines, between 140 and 180 mg/dL, and until further clinical trials demonstrate a consistent safety profile.[1] Intravenous fluids containing dextrose should be avoided.

## INTRACRANIAL PRESSURE CONTROL

Large strokes are often associated with significant cerebral edema and may result in brain herniation. The role of invasive intracranial pressure (ICP) monitoring in these cases is unclear because herniation may occur with focal mass lesions due to local pressure gradients that might not be reflected as an elevation in global ICP. When clinical signs of herniation or ICP are observed, treatments include head-of-bed elevation, maintenance of normocapnia to hypocapnia, use of osmotic agents (e.g., mannitol or hypertonic saline), and temperature control. Many massive strokes result in edema that is refractory to medical management, in which case a craniectomy may prove lifesaving.

## Summary

The management of the ischemic stroke patient in the postoperative neurosurgical patient is complex, especially given the paucity of literature. Published guidelines for management of stroke in the general population must be modified and adapted on a case-by-case basis for the patient with stroke immediately after neurosurgery. Initial management involves a decision about whether reperfusion via intraarterial mechanical embolectomy is warranted. In general, a milder degree of permissive hypertension should be considered, and the timing of aspirin administration must be judged based on the perceived risks and benefits. Routine measures to mitigate secondary injury are employed, including maintenance of euvolemia. Temperature and serum glucose levels should be monitored and controlled.

## References

1. Jauch EC, Saver JL, Adams Jr HP, et al. Guidelines for the early management of patients with acute ischemic stroke: A guideline for healthcare professionals from the American Heart Association/American Stroke Association. *Stroke*. 2013;44:870–947.
2. Wong GY, Warner DO, Schroeder DR, et al. Risk of surgery and anesthesia for ischemic stroke. *Anesthesiology*. 2000;92:425–432.
3. Selim M. Perioperative stroke. *N Engl J Med*. 2007;356:706–713.
4. Nosan DK, Gomez CR, Maves MD. Perioperative stroke in patients undergoing head and neck surgery. *Ann Otol Rhinol Laryngol*. 1993;102:717–723.
5. Limburg M, Wijdicks EF, Li H. Ischemic stroke after surgical procedures: clinical features, neuroimaging, and risk factors. *Neurology*. 1998;50:895–901.
6. Hart R, Hindman B. Mechanisms of perioperative cerebral infarction. *Stroke*. 1982;13:766–773.
7. Suzuki M, Yoneda H, Ishihara H, et al. Adverse events after unruptured cerebral aneurysm treatment: a single center experience with clipping/coil embolization combined units. *J Stroke Cerebrovasc Dis*. 2015;24(1):223–231.
8. Li H, Pan R, Wang H, et al. Clipping versus coiling for ruptured intracranial aneurysms: a systematic review and meta-analysis. *Stroke*. 2013;44(1):29–37.
9. Sughrue M, Rutkowski M, Shangari G, et al. Incidence, risk factors and outcome of venous infarction after meningioma surgery in 705 patients. *J Clin Neurosci*. 2011;18(5):628–632.
10. Jang W, Jung S, Jung T, Moon K, Kim I. Predictive factors related to symptomatic venous infarction after meningioma surgery. *Br J Neurosurg*. 2012;26(5):705–709.
11. Abt N, Bydon M, De la Garza-Ramos R, et al. Concurrent neoadjuvant chemotherapy is an independent risk factor of stroke, all-cause morbidity, and mortality in patients undergoing brain tumor resection. *J Clin Neurosci*. 2014;21(11):1895–1900.
12. Al-Mefty O, Kristh AF. The danger veins. In: Hakuba A, ed. *Surgery of the Intracranial Venous System*. Berlin Heidelberg, New York: Springer; 1996:338–345.
13. Kageyama Y, Watanabe K, Kobayashi S. Postoperative brain damage due to cerebral vein disorders resulting from the pterional approach. In: Hakuba A, ed. *Surgery of the Intracranial Venous System*. Berlin Heidelberg, New York: Springer; 1996:311–315.
14. Saito F, Haraoka J, Ito H, Nishioka H, Inaba I, Yamada Y. Venous complications in pterional approach; About frontotemporal bridging veins. *Surg Cereb Stroke*. 1998;26:237–241.
15. Tissue plasminogen activator for acute ischemic stroke. The national institute of neurological disorders and stroke rt-pa stroke study group. *New Engl J Med*. 1995;333:1581–1587.
16. Chalela JA, Katzan I, Liebeskind DS, et al. Safety of intra-arterial thrombolysis in the postoperative period. *Stroke*. 2001;32:1365–1369.
17. Berkhemer OA, Fransen PS, Beumer D, et al. A randomized trial of intraarterial treatment for acute ischemic stroke. *New Engl J Med*. 2015;372:11–20.
18. Campbell BCV, Mitchell PJ, Kleinig TJ, et al. Endovascular Therapy for Ischemic Stroke with Perfusion-Imaging Selection. *New Engl J Med*. 2015;372:1009–1018.
19. Goyal M, Demchuk AM, Menon BK, et al. Randomized Assessment of Rapid Endovascular Treatment of Ischemic Stroke. *N Engl J Med*. 2015;372:1019–1030.
20. Saver JL, Goyal M, Bonafe A, et al. Solitaire with the Intention for Thrombectomy as Primary Endovascular Treatment. *N Engl J Med*. 2015;372:2285–2295.
21. Hajat C, Hajat S, Sharma P. Effects of poststroke pyrexia on stroke outcome: a meta-analysis of studies in patients. *Stroke*. 2000;31:410–414.
22. Azzimondi G, Bassein L, Nonino F, et al. Fever in acute stroke worsens prognosis. A prospective study. *Stroke*. 1995;26:2040–2043.
23. Baird TA, Parsons MW, Phan T, et al. Persistent poststroke hyperglycemia is independently associated with infarct expansion and worse clinical outcome. *Stroke*. 2003;34:2208–2214.
24. Rosso C, Pires C, Corvol JC, et al. Hyperglycaemia, insulin therapy and critical penumbral regions for prognosis in acute stroke: further insights from the insulinfarct trial. *PLoS One*. 2015;10:e0120230.
25. Bellolio MF, Gilmore RM, Ganti L. Insulin for glycaemic control in acute ischaemic stroke. *Cochrane Database Sys Rev*. 2014;1. Cd005346.

# 49 Management of Postoperative Seizures

BRIAN MAC GRORY, LAWRENCE J. HIRSCH, EMILY GILMORE, and KEVIN N. SHETH

## Introduction

Postoperative seizures are a common phenomenon occurring in approximately a fifth of patients undergoing neurosurgical intervention. Their occurrence in the acute setting is associated with a number of potentially devastating complications, but they also act as a harbinger of a possible long-term diathesis to seizures. Incidence varies based on the type of surgical procedure taking place as well as the reason for surgery. The risk of seizures is associated with the invasiveness of the surgery, underlying pathology, and the number of interventions. Pharmacological management is directed at preventing early seizures, minimizing the risk of late seizures, and protecting the fragile brain. There is a lack of consensus guidelines on which patients warrant prophylactic treatment—if any—and an often-conflicting evidence base for the treatment of postoperative seizures.

In this review, we will discuss the incidence, pathophysiology, and management of postoperative seizures. We will review the occurrence of posttraumatic seizures because they have many similarities to postoperative seizures. Options for specific pharmacological agents will be discussed, as will the acute management of seizures in the neurosurgical intensive care unit (ICU) with particular focus on the postoperative patient and the importance of considering nonconvulsive seizure activity via electroencephalogram (EEG) monitoring.

## Background

### Key Concepts

- Postoperative seizures are associated with worse outcomes in neurosurgical patients and are independently associated with worsening midline shift, increasing hemorrhage size, and increased risk of aspiration.
- Postoperative seizures can be classified into immediate, early, or late.
- The risk of postoperative seizures varies with the type of operation and the underlying disease state. Intracerebral abscesses are associated with a particularly high risk of seizure activity.
- Seizures are common after traumatic brain injury (TBI), but there is no established efficacy for prophylactic treatment for more than 7 days.

Seizures are commonly encountered in postoperative neurosurgical patients. Early postoperative seizures are associated with an increased risk of an ongoing liability to late, recurrent unprovoked seizures, that is, epilepsy.[1,2] Early seizure activity can cause neuronal injury due to increased metabolic demand, increased cerebral edema, elevated glutamate concentrations, and raised intracranial pressure (ICP) superimposed on vulnerable brain tissue.[3] Seizures complicate the clinical examination. Seizures—including nonconvulsive ones—are independently associated with worsening of midline shift[4] and increasing hemorrhage size[5] in nontraumatic intracerebral hemorrhage and increase the risk of aspiration. In patients with TBI, nonconvulsive seizures are associated with increased ICP, elevated lactate/pyruvate ratios, and increased glutamate on cerebral microdialysis (to levels known to be associated with neuronal injury), elevated glycerol (suggesting membrane breakdown), and permanent hippocampal atrophy on the side of the seizures.[3] Seizures account for 8.9% of patients requiring reintubation after craniotomy.[6]

Seizures occur after neurosurgical intervention acutely ("immediate"—defined as within 24 hours—or "early"—defined as those occurring between 24 hours and 1 week postoperatively) or after 1 week postoperatively (late postoperative seizures, strongly associated with risk of epilepsy).[7] Acute symptomatic seizures and late, unprovoked seizures vary in terms of etiology, pathogenesis, prognostic importance, and management (Table 49.1).

### THE PATHOGENESIS OF SEIZURES AFTER CRANIOTOMY

There is a rich body of basic science and clinical research regarding seizures due to craniotomy. In general, early seizures are due to cerebral edema, inflammation at the surgical site, oxidative stress, and disruption of the integrity of the neuronal cell membrane.[8] Increased manipulation of cerebral tissue during procedures increases the risk of postoperative seizures.[9] There is also a positive correlation between the number of interventions and the incidence of postoperative epilepsy.[10] There are three main mechanisms by which neurosurgical intervention causes seizure proclivity:

1. *Free radical generation:* Tissue trauma causes extravascular leakage of blood components. Extravasation of erythrocytes leads to hemolysis and deposition of hemoglobin within neural tissue. Iron released from hemoglobin reacts with hydrogen peroxide in surrounding tissue to generate free radicals, which leads to immediate cortical hyperexcitability as well as epileptogenic focus formation.[11] In experimental models, antioxidant pretreatment has been shown to prevent the formation of iron-induced seizure foci.[12] Free radical production

497

**Table 49.1** The Temporal Definition of Postoperative Seizures

| Seizure type | Time course |
| --- | --- |
| Immediate | <24 hours |
| Early | 24 hours–7 days* |
| Late | ≥7 days |

*Some studies define early as 24 hours to 14 days.

correlates with cell death in an in vitro model of epilepsy.[13] Therefore free radical generation has a reciprocal relationship with the second mechanism of seizure induction.

2. *Disturbance of ion balance across the cell membrane:* Ischemia or hypoxia leads to depletion of adenylpyrophosphatase reserves, which in turn leads to failure of the Na + − K + ATP-ase resulting in disturbance in the ion balance across the cell membrane as the ratio of intracellular to extracellular [K] decreases (and vice versa with [Na]). This manifests as glutamate efflux and neuronal hyperexcitability.[14]

3. *Dysregulation of inhibitory interneurons by anesthetic agents:* Commonly used anesthetic agents can increase the liability to seizure activity. Subanesthetic doses of thiopental have been shown to precipitate both clinical and electrographic seizures in patients after insertion of intracranial electrodes.[15] Opioids produce limbic system hypermetabolism as evidenced by increased temporal lobe glucose utilization[16] and a decreased seizure threshold in response to electroconvulsive therapy in patients anesthetized with remifentanil.[17] In experimental rodent models, alfentanil induces seizures, and this is correlated with hippocampal damage.[18]

## THE INCIDENCE OF POSTCRANIOTOMY SEIZURES

The incidence of postoperative seizures at any point after supratentorial surgery has been reported between 17% and 37% in adults[19,20] and 12% in children.[21] This is highly dependent on the specific lesion and the operation in question. In those with cerebral abscesses the incidence of late, unprovoked postoperative seizures with many years of follow-up is 92%.[22] In the case of infratentorial neurosurgery the incidence ranges from 0% to 5.9% within 2 weeks.[23,24] The incidence of postoperative seizures varies greatly depending on the patient's conditions such as primary disease and the type and location of surgery. In general, the risk of developing seizures decreases with the passage of time after surgery, with the risk of developing new seizure activity falling to less than 10% by 6 months,[25] although patients with surgically treated abscesses have a risk of developing new seizures that persists after 5 years. A study of 877 patients in a neurosurgical center in the United Kingdom in the early 1970s (none with prior history of epilepsy) who underwent supratentorial neurosurgery reported that 17% developed postoperative seizures.[25] In this cohort, the incidence was reported at 92% for those with an abscess and 22% for those undergoing vascular intervention. Of those who had postoperative seizures, 77% occurred within 1 year and 92% occurred within 2 years.[25] Of those who developed postoperative seizures

at any time interval, it was a single seizure in 21% of cases. In children who underwent supratentorial craniotomy for a variety of diagnoses and none of whom had prior epilepsy, 12% had at least one seizures and were on an antiepileptic drug (AED) at 6 months after surgery.[26] In an observational longitudinal study of 100 patients who had supratentorial interventions by craniotomy (33 of whom had had seizures prior to intervention), 13% had at least one early seizure and 46% had at least one late seizure.[27]

## RISK FACTORS FOR THE DEVELOPMENT OF POSTCRANIOTOMY SEIZURES

Overwhelmingly, the most important determinant of the risk of postoperative seizure development is the operation type (Table 49.2), with a particularly pronounced risk after surgical treatment of abscesses. Increased manipulation of cerebral tissue during procedures increases the risk of postoperative seizures.[9] In the case of patients treated for glioma, the incidence of late postoperative seizures was reported at 48%, with low-grade histology and preoperative seizures being risk factors.[28] In those with surgically treated cerebral arteriovenous malformations with no history of preoperative seizures, 6% developed postoperative epilepsy in one study.[29] In one series of patients undergoing posterior fossa surgery, intraoperative positioning affected the risk of postoperative seizures, with seizure incidence being lower in the prone or lateral position than the sitting position.[24]

## INCIDENCE IN OTHER TYPES OF NEUROSURGICAL INTERVENTION

There is a low incidence of seizures in patients undergoing burr-hole drainage for management of chronic subdural hematoma.[30] According to Chen et al.[30] the incidence of seizures was 5.4% with the highest incidence occurring in those with mixed-density hematomas (16.2%), whereas it was 6.2% in patients with low-density hematomas and 2.4% in those with isodense hematomas. The highest risk—9.4%—occurred in the case of a left unilateral chronic subdural hematoma. There is a 15% incidence of postoperative seizures after cranioplasty performed to repair skull defects after decompressive craniectomy. In a series of 36 such patients, 7 had immediate seizures, 2 had early seizures, and 27 had late-onset seizures (after 7 days).[31]

## POSTTRAUMATIC SEIZURES

Posttraumatic epilepsy represents 20% of all symptomatic epilepsy.[32] Annegers et al.[33] performed a retrospective cohort study of patients with TBI and stratified the risk of new late posttraumatic seizures in the cohort of patients followed as follows: mild injury, 0.7%; moderate, 1.2%; and severe, 10.0% over 5 years—a correlation that had been described previously.[34] Over a 30-year period, 16.7% of those with severe injury, 4.2% with moderate injury, and 2.1% with mild injury developed new seizures. For those with mild head injury, the increased risk compared with the general population persisted for 5 years but not thereafter. Increased number of operative interventions in the management of trauma is correlated with increased risk of late posttraumatic seizures.[10] In penetrating brain injuries, the risk of posttraumatic epilepsy is 50%.[35]

**Table 49.2**  Incidence of New Onset of Seizures Postoperatively with Long-Term Follow-Up

| Type of patients | Incidence, percent | Comments |
|---|---|---|
| Craniotomies, supratentorial, overall | 8–17 | |
| Aneurysm, ruptured, overall | 3–26 | Lower rates in more recent studies; higher rates include some acute seizures |
| With ICH | 42 | at time of bleed |
| Without ICH | 19 | (ICH = intracerebral hemorrhage, parenchymal) |
| MCA aneurysm | 9–38 | (MCA = middle cerebral artery) |
| ACA aneurysm | 2–21 | (ACA = anterior cerebral artery) |
| ICA aneurysm | 8 | (ICA = internal carotid artery) |
| P. comm aneurysm | 7–9 | (P. comm = posterior communicating artery) |
| Basilar aneurysm | 6 | (Hunt and Hess grading scale) |
| Grade I | 2.5 | Unruptured data based on only 16 patients (17) |
| Grade II | 17 | |
| Grade III-IV | 33 | |
| Unruptured | 16 | |
| AVM | 8–57 | (AVM = arteriovenous malformation) |
| Tumors, supratentorial | 5–29 | Higher risk if parasagittal (33%) or parietal (42%) |
| Meningioma | 9 | At least some seizures due to tumor progression in patients with gliomas and |
| Glioma s/p biopsy | 20–36 | metastases |
| Glioma s/p surgery | 7–38 | Only with complications, e.g., hydrocephalus |
| Metastases | 0–21 | Probably due to temporal lobe retraction |
| Parasellar | 0–5 | |
| Posterior fossa | 22 | |
| Acoustic neuroma | 0–3 | |
| Subtemporal approach | | |
| Translabyrinthine | | |
| Infections | 69–92 | Risk remains high for >10 years |
| Abscess | 42–50 | May take years for first seizure to occur in both groups |
| Subdural empyema | | |
| Ventricular shunt insertion | 0–24 | |
| Single insertion | 6 | |
| ≥2 revisions | 24 | |
| Posterior fossa surgery | 0–5 | |
| Hemorrhage, intracerebral, spontaneous, nonaneurysmal | 20 | Based on only 15 patients |
| Carotid endarterectomy | 0–1 | Often part of hyperperfusion syndrome |
| Subdural hematoma, chronic | 2–22 | |
| Trauma, w/ or w/out surgery | 22–48 | (ICH = intracerebral hemorrhage of any type) |
| ICH | 22 | |
| Epidural | 42 | |
| Subdural | 48 | |
| Parenchymal | 3 | |
| No ICH | 15 | |
| Depressed skull fracture | 25–28 | |
| Early seizure | | |

Adapted from Batjer HH, Loftus CM, eds. *Textbook of Neurological Surgery: Principles and Practice.* Philadelphia: Lippincott Williams and Wilkins; 2003:741–53.

In those with severe TBI (defined as prolonged loss of consciousness, intracranial hematoma formation, or brain contusion on computed tomography [CT] or depressed skull fracture) the American Academy of Neurology (AAN) guidelines concluded that 7 days of prophylaxis with phenytoin decreases the risk of early posttraumatic seizures[36]—a conclusion that has been supported by metaanalysis.[37] Prophylaxis is not effective for longer than 7 days. Prophylaxis or treatment of early posttraumatic seizures is not known to influence the subsequent development of posttraumatic epilepsy or any other outcome measure. However, it is clear from many studies that longer prophylaxis (>1–2 weeks) does not prevent or delay late seizures or epilepsy, but does expose the patients to possible adverse effects and probably decreased rehabilitation potential.

# Prophylaxis

## Key Concepts

- The purpose of prophylactic treatment is to prevent immediate and early postoperative seizures—it does not reduce the risk of late seizures.
- There is no benefit described for any indication to continue postoperative seizure prophylaxis beyond 7 days postoperatively.
- Phenytoin is the most widely studied agent for seizure prophylaxis; however, levetiracetam is established as a viable alternative given its favorable side effect profile and the fact that it does not necessitate monitoring of serum levels.

## THE ARGUMENT FOR PROPHYLAXIS

There are well-defined guidelines for seizure prophylaxis in newly diagnosed brain tumors[38] and in severe TBI[36] but none for postoperative seizures after craniotomy. There is a paucity of randomized, controlled trials for seizure prophylaxis postcraniotomy.[39] Nevertheless, there are multiple reasons for pharmacological prophylaxis. The purpose of AED prophylaxis after craniotomy is threefold:

1) Prevent early seizures, which can lengthen postoperative recovery, cause neuronal injury, confound the neurological examination, and progress to status epilepticus.
2) Reduce the risk of postoperative epilepsy. There is no evidence to date that any AED prevents the development of epilepsy, despite multiple attempts to demonstrate this.[40]
3) Exploit the potential neuroprotectant effects of antiepileptic agents independent of their effect on seizure risk. Surgical insult causes free radical formation, which causes neuronal damage. AEDs tend to be neuroprotective—at least in animals—both by reducing the frequency of seizures and as a primary effect of the medication (suppressing anion movement across cell membranes). For instance, lamotrigine and felbamate have neuroprotective effects in experimental animals.[41] Unfortunately, to date there is no reliable evidence of this effect in humans.

## WHO SHOULD BE GIVEN PROPHYLACTIC TREATMENT?

Prior metaanalyses have not demonstrated a benefit in the use of AEDs for routine prophylaxis in patients undergoing supratentorial neurosurgery.[39,42] Therefore prophylaxis should be reserved for those who are at particularly high risk for seizures by the risk factors outlined earlier and should only be continued for 1 week postoperatively. Prior authors have suggested that if the seizure risk exceeds 10% to 15% or if a single seizure would have disastrous consequences, AED prophylaxis should be employed.[43] Short-term seizure prophylaxis is recommended in the following situations: patients with a previous history of epileptic seizures, long-term preoperative impairment of consciousness, those with evidence of localized neurological signs, cerebral contusion, or hemorrhage. The same group recommends prophylaxis against further seizure if there is an early postoperative seizure, although this does not apply in cases of TBI,[44] and we only support doing this during the acute critical illness; these people do not have epilepsy (only acute symptomatic seizures), and there is no evidence that prophylaxis will benefit them. In routine brain surgery for resection of tumors without prior seizures, the risk is low and prophylaxis is of questionable benefit.[45]

> ### Clinical Pearl
>
> Patients who develop seizures in the immediate or early postoperative period do not necessarily have a liability to further seizures and do not warrant long-term prophylaxis.

The AAN recommends not to treat people with resection of an intracranial neoplasm for more than 1 week if they have not had seizure postoperatively.[38] In the case of patients treated for glioma, the incidence of postoperative epilepsy was 48% with low-grade histology and preoperative seizures being risk factors.[28] Among patients with surgically treated cerebral aneurysms, the patients at highest risk for postoperative seizures were those with aneurysms of the middle cerebral artery, large intracerebral hematomas, postoperative vasospasm with late infarction, or shunt-dependent hydrocephalus.[46] Similarly, in patients who have suffered an intracranial hemorrhage (not necessarily intervened on surgically) and a single seizure, experts[47] do not recommend continuing antiepileptic therapy beyond 1 to 2 weeks. Brain Trauma Foundation guidelines recommend 1 week of phenytoin for seizure prophylaxis in cases of severe TBI.[44]

## OPTIONS FOR PHARMACOTHERAPY

Options for pharmacotherapy include the conventional AEDs, and because there is no strong evidence favoring one over the other, patient-specific factors should be used to determine the optimal drug (Table 49.3). For example, in patients with cerebral neoplasms, it is often better to avoid strong P450 enzyme inducers such as phenytoin, carbamazepine, phenobarbital, and primidone because they can lower the efficacy of steroids and chemotherapeutics.[48] This chapter will deal with the most extensively studied AEDs for use in postoperative prophylaxis. Some evidence is extrapolated from treatment of posttraumatic seizures.[49,50] In the context of emergence from anesthesia, the use of anesthetic drugs can be employed to control seizure until nonanesthetic AEDs can be initiated. Occasionally a patient may be transported to the ICU on an infusion of propofol, which is then slowly weaned off with addition of other AEDs.

**Table 49.3**   Pharmacotherapeutic Agents Used in the Prophylaxis of Postoperative Seizures

| Drug Name | Advantages | Disadvantages |
| --- | --- | --- |
| Phenytoin | 1. Wealth of data surrounding its use 2. Inexpensive 3. Does not cause impairment of consciousness | 1. Requires monitoring of serum levels 2. Causes hypotension if infused too rapidly |
| Levetiracetam | 1. Does not require monitoring of serum levels 2. Very few drug-drug interactions | 1. A newer agent so does not have as robust data as phenytoin |
| Phenobarbital | 1. Has strong anticonvulsant properties | 1. Causes hypotension 2. Causes sedation 3. Very long half-life |
| Propofol | 1. Has strong anticonvulsant properties 2. Very short half-life permits rapid titration | 1. Causes sedation 2. Requires ICU setting for use 3. Intravenous availability only |

## Clinical Pearl

In patients who will be undergoing chemotherapy, it is prudent to avoid antiseizure agents that induce the P450 system*because these can interfere with the efficacy of steroids and chemotherapeutics.

*The antiepileptic agents that induce the P450 enzymes are carbamazepine, phenobarbital, phenytoin, oxcarbazepine, topiramate and felbamate.[51]

## Phenytoin

Phenytoin has long been the standard for postoperative seizure prophylaxis. It is well studied, inexpensive, widely used, does not compromise level of consciousness, and is available intravenously. In addition, it is amenable to close monitoring of the serum levels. It is often the "gold-standard" comparison arm in trials of postoperative seizure prophylaxis.[20,50,52–53] Although effective for long-term seizure prophylaxis, it does not prevent epileptogenic focus formation.[54]

North et al.[55] conducted a trial of 12 months of treatment with phenytoin, beginning in the recovery room immediately postoperatively and continuing for a year afterward (a loading dose was given in the recovery room followed by 100 mg tid PO for 12 months), in which phenytoin reduced the incidence of seizures to 12.9% compared with the placebo group (of whom 18.4% had seizures) in 281 patients who underwent craniotomy (with the caveat that this study concerns patients exposed to surgical conditions from over 30 years ago). The rationale for its use postoperatively is partially extrapolated from its use in the prevention of late posttraumatic seizures.[49]

Its role in the prevention of seizures in the first postoperative week is less clear. De Santis et al.[56] conducted a prospective trial of phenytoin to examine its effect on seizures in the immediate postoperative period (7 days) in a cohort of patients, 90% of whom were already on AEDs. This trial exclusively concerned patients requiring elective craniotomy for supratentorial brain tumors and excluded patients with seizures in the 7 days prior to surgery, although 30% of both the treatment and control groups had a prior history of seizures at some point. On the day of surgery, a loading dose of 18 mg/kg of phenytoin was administered (this is in line with prior dosing regimens[57]), and administration continued for 7 days with a goal total serum concentration of 10 to 20 µg/mL. Thirteen percent of the treatment group experienced early seizures and 11% of the control group experienced them. This study was significant in that it exclusively concerned cases of brain tumor resection and did not include cases of head trauma (it is known independently that phenytoin can prevent early seizures in that population[49]). Although its side effect profile is acceptable with short-term use only,[58] there is likely no role for phenytoin in the prevention of early postoperative seizures in those undergoing craniotomy for supratentorial tumor resection. This was supported by Wu et al.[45] Its important adverse effects include allergic reactions, fever, enzyme induction, and possible impaired rehabilitation potential in the longer term. It is not recommended in patients after subarachnoid hemorrhage given its cognitive effects.[59]

Phenytoin causes hypotension and cardiac arrhythmias. In a hemodynamically unstable patient—such as after an operation with significant blood loss—it is important to be aware of this possibility and either be prepared to address blood pressure lability on an emergent basis or consider an alternative agent.

## Levetiracetam

Levetiracetam does not necessitate monitoring of serum levels, has very few drug interactions and a desirable side effect profile, and rarely causes allergic reactions. It may be given intravenously or orally. Its favorable pharmacokinetic profile makes it attractive for use in those undergoing concomitant chemotherapy for malignant neoplasms, and it may be substituted for phenytoin in the postoperative period.[60] Like phenytoin, however, it is unclear whether it should be given in patients at low risk for seizures because its effect was modest on seizure outcome in one cohort of postoperative patients with surgically treated high-grade gliomas.[61]

## Clinical Pearl

Levetiracetam use does not necessitate monitoring of serum levels, and it has very few drug interactions.

A trial by Kern et al.[53] demonstrated equivalent efficacy of levetiracetam and phenytoin in a group of 235 patients undergoing supratentorial neurosurgery who were deemed at risk for postoperative seizures and consequently planned for AED prophylaxis over a period of 5 days. Patients found to have contraindications to phenytoin (including depressed left ventricular ejection fraction, cardiac arrhythmias, or hypotension) were instead administered levetiracetam. The incidence of seizures in the 7 days postoperatively was 2.5% in the levetiracetam group versus 4.5% in the phenytoin group (p=0.66).

Milligan et al.[62] performed a retrospective study of nonepileptic patients undergoing supratentorial neurosurgery with at least a 7-day follow-up comparing monotherapy with levetiracetam to phenytoin. In this study, 9/210 patients taking phenytoin had a seizure within 7 days, whereas only 1/105 patients taking levetiracetam had a seizure within 7 days (however, the difference between these two agents did not attain statistical significance: p=0.17). Of note, however, adverse reactions were far less prevalent in those taking levetiracetam (p <0.001), resulting in greater compliance with levetiracetam after 12 months. It is not known whether levetiracetam's chief side effect (behavioral change) is relevant in the critically ill period. However, as patients recover, acute agitation could affect care in the ICU. The relationship between levetiracetam and possible emergence delirium is not known. It should be noted that this was a small, retrospective trial with an older population of patients in the phenytoin group.

## Phenobarbital

Phenobarbital is an IV barbiturate-derivative and is cumbersome to use because it leads to hypotension, sedation, and respiratory depression, and has a half-life of about 3 days.[63] It also has many drug interactions because it is a strong enzyme inducer (similar to phenytoin). One trial of 63 patients operated on for supratentorial neoplasms randomized patients to receive phenobarbital (4 mg/kg intravenously for 5 days followed by an oral switch) or phenytoin (10 mg/kg intravenously for 5 days followed by an oral switch) and suggested that they were equivalent in efficacy.[64]

## Carbamazepine

A small, single-center study[20] failed to demonstrate a benefit to giving carbamazepine (or phenytoin) for postoperative seizures in those who had a craniotomy for supratentorial surgery. They failed to show a benefit over a 6-month period in terms of seizure occurrence. Like phenytoin, carbamazepine is not known to exert an antiepileptogenic effect in experimental animals.[54] It is not currently available intravenously. It is a P450 enzyme inducer and causes frequent allergic reactions.

## Valproic Acid

Valproic acid has been studied extensively for treatment of the epilepsies and posttraumatic seizures and for seizure prophylaxis in patients with intracranial malignancies. With respect to postoperative seizure prophylaxis, its tendency to cause thrombocytopenia, platelet dysfunction, hypofibrinogenemia, and other bleeding tendencies is at least a theoretical concern.

Beenen et al.[52] demonstrated equivalent efficacy to phenytoin in a prospective, randomized, single-center trial with a year of treatment with each agent (there was no placebo arm in this study). However, fewer patients being treated with valproate stopped treatment due to adverse effects.

There is other pertinent evidence from related literature. Temkin et al.[50] reported a randomized, double-blind, single-center trial comparing valproate acid (given for 1 month or 6 months) with phenytoin (given for a week only) in the management of posttraumatic seizures (not necessarily postoperative). There was no difference in the rate of early or late postoperative seizures between those treated with phenytoin versus valproate. However, there was mortality of 13.4% in the valproate groups versus 7.2% in the phenytoin group—a difference that almost attained statistical significance (p=0.07). However, there was no difference in the rate of coagulopathies between the two drugs. It does not have a role in primary seizure prophylaxis in newly diagnosed intracranial tumors.[65] Valproate is well tolerated overall and has rare allergic reactions, but is highly protein bound, inhibits metabolism of some medications (in contrast to phenytoin), may exacerbate bleeding, and occasionally affects hepatic function.

## Oxcarbazepine

Oxcarbazepine has not been used widely in management of postoperative seizures. Mauro et al.[66] conducted a retrospective safety study of oxcarbazepine in the management of early postoperative seizures in patients undergoing resection of supratentorial gliomas. One hundred fifty patients were treated with 900 to 1200 mg oxcarbazepine daily in two divided doses starting 7 days prior to surgery. The seizure incidence within the first postoperative week was 2.7%. There was no comparison with placebo or standard of care in this preliminary study. One must be particularly vigilant to the possibility of hyponatremia, which is even more common with oxcarbazepine than with carbamazepine and can be an important issue in neurosurgical patients.

# Management

### Key Concepts

- Status epilepticus is defined as continuous seizures that last longer than 5 minutes or recurrent seizures without recovery of mental status between seizures. It can be either convulsive or nonconvulsive.
- Management of status epilepticus must proceed in parallel with an expedited workup given the emergent nature of the condition.
- Refractory status epilepticus (RSE) is present when a patient with status epilepticus does not respond to standard treatment regimens, typically the first two medications used.

In this section we will address the management of seizures that arise in the early postoperative period, including those that progress to status epilepticus, with emphasis on considerations specific to the postoperative patient. Although postoperative seizure liability can be expected to arise from cortical irritation at the site of operation, there are multiple other factors around surgery that can predispose to seizure activity, particularly in a vulnerable host. Consideration should be given not only to surgical complications (such as intracranial bleeding or hematoma formation), but also anesthetic and metabolic factors (such as hyponatremia that might occur in cerebral salt wasting syndrome) or the syndrome of inappropriate antidiuretic hormone secretion.

## DEFINITION

Status epilepticus is defined as a continuous clinical and/or electrographic seizure that lasts longer than 5 minutes or recurrent seizure activity with recovery of mental status between seizures.[67] Status epilepticus is divided into two principal types:

1) Generalized convulsive status epilepticus: Electrographic seizures correlated with rhythmic jerking of the extremities and altered mental status.
2) Nonconvulsive status epilepticus (NCSE): Electrographic seizures that are not associated with clinical evidence of seizure activity. In practice, there are two types of NCSE—one occurring in an ambulatory patient whose chief presentation is severe confusion versus the other, which occurs in a moribund ICU patient with altered mental status.[68]

## INVESTIGATIONS

Targeted towards addressing the etiology of post-operative seizures (Table 49.4). Initial testing:

- Laboratory studies:
  - Fingerstick glucose
  - Complete blood count
  - Basic metabolic panel
  - Calcium
  - Magnesium
  - Hepatic function panel
  - Albumin
  - Arterial blood gas analysis
  - Drug levels (if patient is on antiepileptic agents at baseline)
  - Troponin (to look for cardiac injury from status epilepticus)
- CT brain

Further testing (nonemergent and considered on a case-by-case basis):

- Magnetic resonance imaging brain
- Cerebrospinal fluid analysis by lumbar puncture
- Toxicology panel

**Table 49.4** Etiology of Postoperative Seizures

| Cause | Example |
|---|---|
| Local cortical irritation at the operative bed | |
| Vascular events | Intracerebral hemorrhage, extradural hematoma, or subdural hematoma |
| Metabolic disturbances | E.g., hypoglycemia, uremia, or hypocalcemia |
| Electrolyte disturbances | E.g., hyponatremia |
| Sepsis | |
| Pharmacological causes | |
| Seizure threshold-lowering anesthetics | E.g., meperidine, etomidate, ketamine,* and opioids |
| Withdrawal from alcohol or benzodiazepines | |
| AED mismanagement perioperatively | |
| Hypoxic brain injury | E.g., in the context of a cardiac arrest |
| Hypertensive encephalopathy | |
| Infectious processes | Encephalitis, intracerebral abscess, or meningitis |

*Like many anesthetic agents, ketamine is proconvulsant at low doses and anticonvulsant at higher doses.

## TREATMENT OF POSTOPERATIVE STATUS EPILEPTICUS

This section draws heavily from the Neurocritical Care Society Guidelines[67] for the management of status epilepticus. These are largely similar to guidelines from the European Federation of Neurological Societies,[70] except that they include recommendations for continuous EEG monitoring.

1. **Establish/maintain airway**
2. **Administer O₂**
3. **Continuous vital sign monitoring** (heart rate, blood pressure, respiratory rate, oxygen saturation, and temperature)
4. **Fingerstick (glucose)**
5. **Verify/maintain IV access**
6. **Correct hypoglycemia** (with attendant thiamine administration)
7. **Emergent initial AED therapy** – IV lorazepam is the optimal first-line agent.[71] The dose is 0.1 mg/kg per dose up to a maximum of 4 mg intravenously.
8. **Fluid resuscitation\***
9. **Further AED therapy** by the following algorithm:
   *Urgent Control Therapy*
   This is instituted even if seizure activity has been successfully controlled by emergent initial AED therapy. The goal for those who have responded to emergent initial therapy is to obtain therapeutic concentrations in the bloodstream in advance of continuing maintenance therapy. For those who have not responded to emergent initial therapy, its role is to terminate seizure activity. The choices include:
   A. IV phenytoin – 20 mg/kg IV
   B. IV fosphenytoin – 20 mg PE/kg IV
   C. Sodium valproate – 2 to 40 mg/kg IV (the high end of this range is typically used in patients in the ICU)
   D. Phenobarbital – 20 mg/kg IV
   E. Levetiracetam – 1000 to 3000 mg IV
   F. Midazolam or propofol – by continuous IV infusion
10. **Neurological examination**
11. **Correct underlying metabolic derangements**
12. **Continuous EEG:**
    The indications for continuous EEG (with interpretation by someone experienced at reading ICU EEGs) are outlined in Table 49.5.[67]

13. **Treatment of refractory status epilepticus** (which occurs in 40% of cases of status epilepticus):[72]
    A. Midazolam infusion
    B. Propofol infusion
    C. Pentobarbital infusion

**Table 49.5**   Indications for Continuous EEG Monitoring

| Indication | Rationale | Grade |
|---|---|---|
| Recent clinical seizure or SE without return to baseline >10 min | Ongoing nonconvulsive status despite cessation of motor activity 18%–50% | Class I, level B |
| Coma, including post-cardiac arrest | Frequent nonconvulsive seizures, 20%–60% | Class I, level B |
| Epileptiform activity or periodic discharged on initial 30 min EEG | Risk of nonconvulsive seizures, 40%–60% | Class I, level B |
| Intracranial hemorrhage including TBI, SAH, ICH | Frequent nonconvulsive seizures, 20%–35% | Class I, level B |
| Suspected nonconvulsive seizures in patients with altered mental status | Frequent nonconvulsive seizures, 10–30% | Class I, level B |

Reprinted from Brophy GM, et al. *Neurocrit Care.* 2012;17(1):3–23.

- The dosing of these drugs is determined by EEG findings. It is recommended that the level of anesthesia is titrated such that there is no evidence of electrographic seizures but not necessarily to a level that produces the so-called *suppression-burst pattern*.

Twenty-four to 48 hours of continuous EEG monitoring is recommended prior to withdrawal of continuous infusion AEDs for refractory status epilepticus (Fig. 49.1).

- There is no evidence to support a particular hematocrit goal in status epilepticus. However, in the critical care literature in general, a majority of studies favor a conservative transfusion strategy over a liberal one.[73] In acute coronary syndrome, a transfusion threshold of 8.0 g/dL is recommended[74] because transfusing at levels above that has been shown to increase mortality.

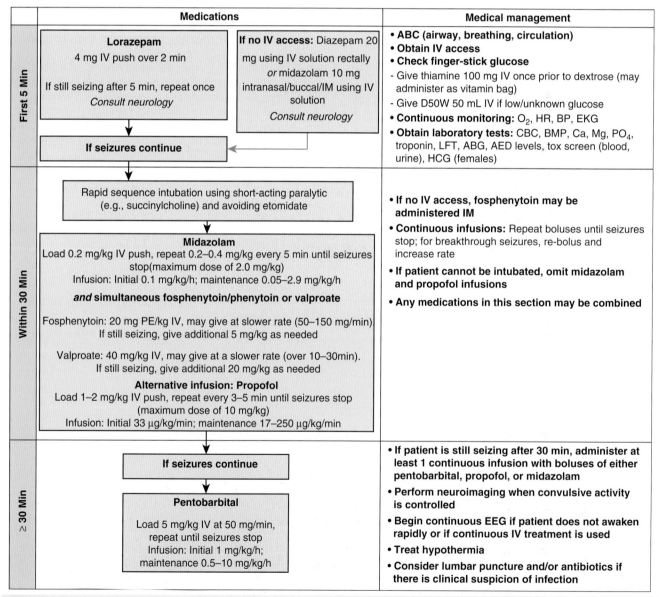

**Fig. 49.1** Status epilepticus treatment algorithm for adult patients in Yale-New Haven Hospital. (Courtesy of Yale-New Haven Hospital.)

## NONCONVULSIVE SEIZURES AND CONTINUOUS ELECTROENCEPHALOGRAPHY

### Key Concepts

- The majority of the literature on postoperative seizure management and prophylaxis concerns exclusively convulsive seizures. However, nonconvulsive seizures are a common, underrecognized phenomenon in hospitalized patients and are associated with worse outcomes.
- The clinical manifestations of nonconvulsive status epilepticus are variable, and continuous EEG monitoring is required for detection.
- Nonconvulsive status epilepticus should be treated in fundamentally the same way as convulsive status epilepticus. However, the nonconvulsive form does not have the same systemic physiological perturbances as the convulsive status epilepticus. Therefore it is safe to try more than one nonsedating AED prior to using anesthetics agents.[75]

The previous discussion—and indeed the majority of the literature on postoperative seizures—refers to convulsive seizures and convulsive status epilepticus. However, the majority of seizures in hospitalized patients, including the critically ill, are nonconvulsive.[76,77] The definition of nonconvulsive status epilepticus is continuous or near-continuous electrographic seizures for at least 30 minutes in duration, without overt clinical manifestations.

NCSE occurs in 10% of hospitalized patients with altered levels of consciousness.[78] After generalized convulsive status epilepticus, 48% of patients will have nonconvulsive seizures in the ensuing 24 hours.[79] Nonconvulsive seizure and status epilepticus are associated with poor outcomes, whereas early diagnosis improves outcomes.[80,81] Other seizure patterns, such as generalized periodic discharges, are not independently associated with worse outcome.[80]

### Clinical Pearl

After generalized convulsive status epilepticus, 48% of patients will have nonconvulsive seizures within the next 24 hours.

The clinical manifestations, if any, are variable and include subtle changes in behavior, face and limb myoclonus, eye deviation, autonomic instability, or delayed emergence from anesthesia. Continuous encephalography (cEEG) is required to detect NCSE. cEEG is used to guide treatment of nonconvulsive seizures, and nonconvulsive seizures are more common than convulsive ones.[77] A definitive diagnosis can be made by a trial of a low-dose, fast-acting antiepileptic agent, as in Box 49.1.[82]

Nonconvulsive seizures should always be considered if a patient remains persistently altered >10 to 30 minutes after convulsions cease or if emergence from anesthesia is delayed without explanation based on pharmacokinetics of the administered anesthetics or postoperative head imaging. Long-term monitoring is necessary because a short course will miss over half of cases.[83] Twenty-four hours

### Box 49.1 Benzodiazepine Trial for the Diagnosis of Nonconvulsive Status Epilepticus

*Patients*
  Rhythmic or periodic focal or generalized epileptiform discharged on EEG with neurological impairment
  *Monitoring*
  EEG, pulse oximetry, blood pressure, ECG, respiratory rate with dedicated nurse
  *Antiepileptic drug trial*

- Sequential small doses of rapidly acting short-duration benzodiazepine such as midazolam at 1 mg/dose
- Between doses, repeated clinical and EEG assessment
- Trial is stopped after any of the following
  - Persistent resolution of the EEG pattern (and examination repeated)
  - Definite clinical improvement
  - Respiratory depression, hypotension, or other adverse effect
  - A maximum dose is reached (such as 0.2 mg/kg midazolam, though higher may be needed if on chronic benzodiazepines)

  Test is considered positive if there is resolution of the potentially ictal EEG pattern AND either an improvement in the clinical state of the appearance of previously absent normal EEG patterns (e.g., posterior-dominant "alpha" rhythm). If EEG improves but patient does not, the result is equivocal.

Reprinted from Jirsch et al. *Clin Neurophysiol.* 2010;118(8):1660–70.

of cEEG monitoring is recommended in noncomatose patients and 48 hours is recommended in comatose patients. The treatment of nonconvulsive status epilepticus is the same as for convulsive status epilepticus with the exception that nonsedating AEDs should be used in preference to anesthetic agents to abort electrographic seizures.

### Clinical Pearl

Nonconvulsive seizures should always be considered if a patient remains persistently altered >10 to 30 minutes after convulsions cease.

## Summary

Seizures that arise in the postoperative period can be classified as immediate, early, and late, and there is a differing pathogenesis to these types. Immediate and early postoperative seizures occur due to tissue trauma with consequent free radical generation, neuronal hyperexcitability due to disturbance of the ionic milieu across the cell membrane, and alterations in the function of inhibitory interneuron function. The incidence of postoperative seizures varies between 17% and 37% across studies (and is up to 92% for certain subgroups of patients). The liability to seizure activity can be risk stratified based on the indication for surgery, operative approach, location, and type of surgery. Posttraumatic seizures represent 20% of all symptomatic epilepsy, and their incidence correlates with the severity of trauma. Observations in the genesis and incidence of epilepsy after TBI are likely relevant to nontraumatic intracranial surgery, and many of our guidelines are extrapolated from this literature.

Prophylaxis against postoperative seizures is not indicated routinely in patients postcraniotomy; however, given the low morbidity associated with at least a short course of an antiepileptic agent, it is common practice. Prophylaxis is reasonable for high-risk subgroups of patients during the acute setting only; high-risk generally refers to a patient deemed to have at least a 10% to 15% chance of early postoperative seizures. It is also reasonable to use AEDs acutely if one seizure could have disastrous consequences, as, for example, in patients with severe intracranial hypertension or an unsecured aneurysm. The most well-studied agent for prophylaxis is phenytoin, but levetiracetam seems to be as effective and better tolerated. Other agents exist, and choice of agent should depend on individual patient factors. All patients with persistently impaired mental status after a supratentorial procedure should undergo cEEG monitoring to assess for nonconvulsive seizures, particularly if they have had a clinical seizure. The management of postoperative status epilepticus has a number of considerations in postneurosurgical patients because the underlying etiology is likely to be different than in a nonsurgical host. However, the fundamental principles are the same: airway stabilization, optimization of hemodynamic parameters, promoting optimal gas exchange, and addressing the underlying cause while implementing a logical, stepwise approach to emergent pharmacotherapy.

## References

1. Hwang SL, Lieu AS, Kuo TH, et al. Preoperative and postoperative seizures in patients with astrocytic tumours: analysis of incidence and influencing factors. *J Clin Neurosci.* 2001;8(5):426–429.
2. Shaw MD, Foy PM. Epilepsy after craniotomy and the place of prophylactic anticonvulsant drugs: discussion paper. *J R Soc Med.* 1991;84(4):221–223.
3. Vespa P. Continuous EEG, monitoring for the detection of seizures in traumatic brain injury, infarction, and intracerebral hemorrhage: "to detect and protect" *J Clin Neurophysiol.* 2005;22(2):99–106.
4. Vespa PM, O'Phelan K, Shah M, et al. Acute seizures after intracerebral hemorrhage: a factor in progressive midline shift and outcome. *Neurology.* 2003;60(9):1441–1446.
5. Claassen J, Jetté N, Chum F, et al. Electrographic seizures and periodic discharges after intracerebral hemorrhage. *Neurology.* 2007;69(13):1356–1365.
6. Dube SK, Rath GP, Bharti SJ, et al. Causes of tracheal re-intubation after craniotomy: a prospective study. *Saudi J Anaesth.* 2013;7(4):410–414.
7. Jennett WB. Early traumatic epilepsy. Definition and identity. *Lancet.* 1969;1(7604):1023–1025.
8. Herman ST. Epilepsy after brain insult: targeting epileptogenesis. *Neurology.* 2002;59(9 suppl 5):S21–S26.
9. Honeybul S, Ho KM. Long-term complications of decompressive craniectomy for head injury. *J Neurotrauma.* 2011;28(6):929–935.
10. Englander J, Bushnik T, Duong TT, et al. Analyzing risk factors for late posttraumatic seizures: a prospective, multicenter investigation. *Arch Phys Med Rehabil.* 2003;84(3):365–373.
11. Mori A, Yokoi I, Noda Y, Willmore LJ. Natural antioxidants may prevent posttraumatic epilepsy: a proposal based on experimental animal studies. *Acta Med Okayama.* 2004;58(3):111–118.
12. Willmore LJ, Rubin JJ. Antiperoxidant pretreatment and iron-induced epileptiform discharges in the rat: EEG and histopathologic studies. *Neurology.* 1981;31(1):63–69.
13. Frantseva MV, Velazquez JL, Hwang PA, Carlen PL. Free radical production correlates with cell death in an in vitro model of epilepsy. *Eur J Neurosci.* 2000;12(4):1431–1439.
14. Nishizawa Y. Glutamate release and neuronal damage in ischemia. *Life Sci.* 2001;69(4):369–381.
15. Kofke WA, Dasheiff RM, Dong ML, Whitehurst S, Caldwell M. Anesthetic care during thiopental tests to evaluate epileptic patients for surgical therapy. *J Neurosurg Anesthesiol.* 1993;5(3):164–170.
16. Kofke WA, Attaallah AF, Kuwabara H, et al. The neuropathologic effects in rats and neurometabolic effects in humans of large-dose remifentanil. *Anesth Analg.* 2002;94(5):1229–1236. table of contents.
17. Sullivan PM, Sinz EH, Gunel E, Kofke WA. A retrospective comparison of remifentanil versus methohexital for anesthesia in electroconvulsive therapy. *J ECT.* 2004;20(4):219–224.
18. Kofke WA, Garman RH, Tom WC, Rose ME, Hawkins RA. Alfentanil-induced hypermetabolism, seizure, and histopathology in rat brain. *Anesth Analg.* 1992;75(6):953–964.
19. Foy PM, Copeland GP, Shaw MD. The incidence of postoperative seizures. *Acta Neurochir (Wien).* 1981;55(3–4):253–264.
20. Foy PM, Chadwick DW, Rajgopalan N, Johnson AL, Shaw MD. Do prophylactic anticonvulsant drugs alter the pattern of seizures after craniotomy? *J Neurol Neurosurg Psychiatry.* 1992;55(9):753–757.
21. Wang EC, Geyer JR, Berger MS. Incidence of postoperative epilepsy in children following subfrontal craniotomy for tumor. *Pediatr Neurosurg.* 1994;21(3):165–172. discussion 72–73.
22. Legg NJ, Gupta PC, Scott DF. Epilepsy following cerebral abscess. A clinical and EEG study of 70 patients. *Brain.* 1973;96(2):259–268.
23. Lee ST, Lui TN, Chang CN, Cheng WC. Early postoperative seizures after posterior fossa surgery. *J Neurosurg.* 1990;73(4):541–544.
24. Suri A, Mahapatra AK, Bithal P. Seizures following posterior fossa surgery. *Br J Neurosurg.* 1998;12(1):41–44.
25. Foy PM, Copeland GP, Shaw MD. The natural history of postoperative seizures. *Acta Neurochir (Wien).* 1981;57(1–2):15–22.
26. Kombogiorgas D, Jatavallabhula NS, Sgouros S, Josan V, Walsh AR, Hockley AD. Risk factors for developing epilepsy after craniotomy in children. *Childs Nerv Syst.* 2006;22(11):1441–1445.
27. Bartolini E, Lenzi B, Vannozzi R, Parenti GF, Iudice A. Incidence and management of late postsurgical seizures in clinical practice. *Turk Neurosurg.* 2012;22(5):651–655.
28. Pace A, Bove L, Innocenti P, et al. Epilepsy and gliomas: incidence and treatment in 119 patients. *J Exp Clin Cancer Res.* 1998;17(4):479–482.
29. Piepgras DG, Sundt TM, Ragoowansi AT, Stevens L. Seizure outcome in patients with surgically treated cerebral arteriovenous malformations. *J Neurosurg.* 1993;78(1):5–11.
30. Chen CW, Kuo JR, Lin HJ, et al. Early post-operative seizures after burr-hole drainage for chronic subdural hematoma: correlation with brain CT findings. *J Clin Neurosci.* 2004;11(7):706–709.
31. Lee L, Ker J, Quah BL, Chou N, Choy D, Yeo TT. A retrospective analysis and review of an institution's experience with the complications of cranioplasty. *Br J Neurosurg.* 2013;27(5):629–635.
32. Annegers JF, Coan SP. The risks of epilepsy after traumatic brain injury. *Seizure.* 2000;9(7):453–457.
33. Annegers JF, Hauser WA, Coan SP, Rocca WA. A population-based study of seizures after traumatic brain injuries. *N Engl J Med.* 1998;338(1):20–24.
34. Caveness WF, Meirowsky AM, Rish BL, et al. The nature of posttraumatic epilepsy. *J Neurosurg.* 1979;50(5):545–553.
35. Salazar AM, Jabbari B, Vance SC, Grafman J, Amin D, Dillon JD. Epilepsy after penetrating head injury. I. Clinical correlates: a report of the Vietnam Head Injury Study. *Neurology.* 1985;35(10):1406–1414.
36. Chang BS, Lowenstein DH. Neurology QSSotAAo. Practice parameter: antiepileptic drug prophylaxis in severe traumatic brain injury: report of the Quality Standards Subcommittee of the American Academy of Neurology. *Neurology.* 2003;60(1):10–16.
37. Schierhout G, Roberts I. Anti-epileptic drugs for preventing seizures following acute traumatic brain injury. *Cochrane Database Syst Rev.* 2001;4. CD000173.
38. Glantz MJ, Cole BF, Forsyth PA, et al. Practice parameter: anticonvulsant prophylaxis in patients with newly diagnosed brain tumors. Report of the Quality Standards Subcommittee of the American Academy of Neurology. *Neurology.* 2000;54(10):1886–1893.
39. Pulman J, Greenhalgh J, Marson AG. Antiepileptic drugs as prophylaxis for post-craniotomy seizures. *Cochrane Database Syst Rev.* 2013;2. CD007286.

40. Temkin NR. Antiepileptogenesis and seizure prevention trials with antiepileptic drugs: meta-analysis of controlled trials. *Epilepsia.* 2001;42(4):515–524.
41. Siniscalchi A, Zona C, Guatteo E, Mercuri NB, Bernardi G. An electrophysiological analysis of the protective effects of felbamate, lamotrigine, and lidocaine on the functional recovery from in vitro ischemia in rat neocortical slices. *Synapse.* 1998;30(4): 371–379.
42. Kuijlen JM, Teernstra OP, Kessels AG, Herpers MJ, Beuls EA. Effectiveness of antiepileptic prophylaxis used with supratentorial craniotomies: a meta-analysis. *Seizure.* 1996;5(4):291–298.
43. Deutschman CS, Haines SJ. Anticonvulsant prophylaxis in neurological surgery. *Neurosurgery.* 1985;17(3):510–517.
44. Bratton SL, Chestnut RM, Ghajar J, et al. Guidelines for the management of severe traumatic brain injury. XIII. Antiseizure prophylaxis. *J Neurotrauma.* 2007;(24 suppl 1):S83–S86.
45. Wu AS, Trinh VT, Suki D, et al. A prospective randomized trial of perioperative seizure prophylaxis in patients with intraparenchymal brain tumors. *J Neurosurg.* 2013;118(4):873–883.
46. Keränen T, Tapaninaho A, Hernesniemi J, Vapalahti M. Late epilepsy after aneurysm operations. *Neurosurgery.* 1985;17(6):897–900.
47. Gilmore E, Choi HA, Hirsch LJ, Claassen J. Seizures and CNS hemorrhage: spontaneous intracerebral and aneurysmal subarachnoid hemorrhage. *Neurologist.* 2010;16(3):165–175.
48. Oberndorfer S, Piribauer M, Marosi C, Lahrmann H, Hitzenberger P, Grisold W. P450 enzyme inducing and non-enzyme inducing antiepileptics in glioblastoma patients treated with standard chemotherapy. *J Neurooncol.* 2005;72(3):255–260.
49. Temkin NR, Dikmen SS, Wilensky AJ, Keihm J, Chabal S, Winn HR. A randomized, double-blind study of phenytoin for the prevention of post-traumatic seizures. *N Engl J Med.* 1990;323(8):497–502.
50. Temkin NR, Dikmen SS, Anderson GD, et al. Valproate therapy for prevention of posttraumatic seizures: a randomized trial. *J Neurosurg.* 1999;91(4):593–600.
51. Patsalos PN, Perucca E. Clinically important drug interactions in epilepsy: general features and interactions between antiepileptic drugs. *Lancet Neurol.* 2003;2(6):347–356.
52. Beenen LF, Lindeboom J, Kasteleijn-Nolst Trenité DG, et al. Comparative double blind clinical trial of phenytoin and sodium valproate as anticonvulsant prophylaxis after craniotomy: efficacy, tolerability, and cognitive effects. *J Neurol Neurosurg Psychiatry.* 1999;67(4):474–480.
53. Kern K, Schebesch KM, Schlaier J, et al. Levetiracetam compared to phenytoin for the prevention of postoperative seizures after craniotomy for intracranial tumours in patients without epilepsy. *J Clin Neurosci.* 2012;19(1):99–100.
54. Wada JA, Sato M, Wake A, Green JR, Troupin AS. Prophylactic effects of phenytoin, phenobarbital, and carbamazepine examined in kindling cat preparations. *Arch Neurol.* 1976;33(6):426–434.
55. North JB, Penhall RK, Hanieh A, Frewin DB, Taylor WB. Phenytoin and postoperative epilepsy. A double-blind study. *J Neurosurg.* 1983;58(5):672–677.
56. De Santis A, Villani R, Sinisi M, Stocchetti N, Perucca E. Add-on phenytoin fails to prevent early seizures after surgery for supratentorial brain tumors: a randomized controlled study. *Epilepsia.* 2002;43(2):175–182.
57. Levati A, Savoia G, Zoppi F, Boselli L, Tommasino C. Peri-operative prophylaxis with phenytoin: dosage and therapeutic plasma levels. *Acta Neurochir (Wien).* 1996;138(3):274–278. discussion 8–9.
58. Haltiner AM, Newell DW, Temkin NR, Dikmen SS, Winn HR. Side effects and mortality associated with use of phenytoin for early posttraumatic seizure prophylaxis. *J Neurosurg.* 1999;91(4):588–592.
59. Dewan MC, Mocco J. Current practice regarding seizure prophylaxis in aneurysmal subarachnoid hemorrhage across academic centers. *J Neurointerv Surg.* 2015;7(2):146–149.
60. Lim DA, Tarapore P, Chang E, et al. Safety and feasibility of switching from phenytoin to levetiracetam monotherapy for glioma-related seizure control following craniotomy: a randomized phase II pilot study. *J Neurooncol.* 2009;93(3):349–354.
61. Garbossa D, Panciani PP, Angeleri R, et al. A retrospective two-center study of antiepileptic prophylaxis in patients with surgically treated high-grade gliomas. *Neurol India.* 2013;61(2):131–137.
62. Milligan TA, Hurwitz S, Bromfield EB. Efficacy and tolerability of levetiracetam versus phenytoin after supratentorial neurosurgery. *Neurology.* 2008;71(9):665–669.
63. Tesoro EP, Brophy GM. Pharmacological management of seizures and status epilepticus in critically ill patients. *J Pharm Pract.* 2010;23(5):441–454.
64. Franceschetti S, Binelli S, Casazza M, et al. Influence of surgery and antiepileptic drugs on seizures symptomatic of cerebral tumours. *Acta Neurochir (Wien).* 1990;103(1–2):47–51.
65. Glantz MJ, Cole BF, Friedberg MH, et al. A randomized, blinded, placebo-controlled trial of divalproex sodium prophylaxis in adults with newly diagnosed brain tumors. *Neurology.* 1996;46(4): 985–991.
66. Mauro AM, Bomprezzi C, Morresi S, et al. Prevention of early postoperative seizures in patients with primary brain tumors: preliminary experience with oxcarbazepine. *J Neurooncol.* 2007;81(3):279–285.
67. Brophy GM, Bell R, Claassen J, et al. Guidelines for the evaluation and management of status epilepticus. *Neurocrit Care.* 2012;17(1):3–23.
68. Shorvon S. What is nonconvulsive status epilepticus, and what are its subtypes? *Epilepsia.* 2007;48(suppl 8):35–38.
69. Bleck TP. Refractory status epilepticus. *Curr Opin Crit Care.* 2005;11(2):117–120.
70. Meierkord H, Boon P, Engelsen B, et al. EFNS guideline on the management of status epilepticus in adults. *Eur J Neurol.* 2010;17(3):348–355.
71. Treiman DM, Meyers PD, Walton NY, et al. A comparison of four treatments for generalized convulsive status epilepticus. Veterans Affairs Status Epilepticus Cooperative Study Group. *N Engl J Med.* 1998;339(12):792–798.
72. Mayer SA, Claassen J, Lokin J, Mendelsohn F, Dennis LJ, Fitzsimmons BF. Refractory status epilepticus: frequency, risk factors, and impact on outcome. *Arch Neurol.* 2002;59(2):205–210.
73. Marik PE, Corwin HL. Efficacy of red blood cell transfusion in the critically ill: a systematic review of the literature. *Crit Care Med.* 2008;36(9):2667–2674.
74. Garfinkle M, Lawler PR, Filion KB, Eisenberg MJ. Red blood cell transfusion and mortality among patients hospitalized for acute coronary syndromes: a systematic review. *Int J Cardiol.* 2013;164(2):151–157.
75. Hirsch LJ, Gaspard N. Status epilepticus. *Continuum.* 2013;19(3 Epilepsy):767–794.
76. Claassen J, Mayer SA, Kowalski RG, Emerson RG, Hirsch LJ. Detection of electrographic seizures with continuous EEG monitoring in critically ill patients. *Neurology.* 2004;62(10):1743–1748.
77. Friedman D, Claassen J, Hirsch LJ. Continuous electroencephalogram monitoring in the intensive care unit. *Anesth Analg.* 2009;109(2):506–523.
78. Alroughani R, Javidan M, Qasem A, Alotaibi N. Non-convulsive status epilepticus; the rate of occurrence in a general hospital. *Seizure.* 2009;18(1):38–42.
79. Koubeissi M, Alshekhlee A. In-hospital mortality of generalized convulsive status epilepticus: a large US sample. *Neurology.* 2007;69(9):886–893.
80. Foreman B, Claassen J, Abou Khaled K, et al. Generalized periodic discharges in the critically ill: a case-control study of 200 patients. *Neurology.* 2012;79(19):1951–1960.
81. Chong DJ, Hirsch LJ. Which EEG patterns warrant treatment in the critically ill? Reviewing the evidence for treatment of periodic epileptiform discharges and related patterns. *J Clin Neurophysiol.* 2005;22(2):79–91.
82. Jirsch J, Hirsch LJ. Nonconvulsive seizures: developing a rational approach to the diagnosis and management in the critically ill population. *Clin Neurophysiol.* 2007;118(8):1660–1670.
83. Pandian JD, Cascino GD, So EL, Manno E, Fulgham JR. Digital video-electroencephalographic monitoring in the neurological-neurosurgical intensive care unit: clinical features and outcome. *Arch Neurol.* 2004;61(7):1090–1094.

# 50 Postoperative Neurosurgical Infections

ADARSH BHIMRAJ

## Key Concepts

- Postneurosurgical infections can range from simple incision site infections to complex infections like meningoventriculitis, cerebritis, central nervous system (CNS) abscesses, and neurological device infections.
- Gram-positive cocci like *Staphylococcus epidermidis* and *S. aureus* are the most common pathogens, followed by gram-negative rods (*Escherichia coli, Klebsiella, Pseudomonas,* and *Acinetobacter*) and anaerobes, especially *Proprionibacterium acnes*. The local incidence of different pathogens might differ considerably, so historical institutional data and susceptibility patterns should be considered when choosing empiric antimicrobials.
- The diagnosis of CNS infections may be elusive because noninfectious neurological conditions and neurosurgeries can cause similar clinical, cerebrospinal fluid (CSF), and imaging findings.
- Treatment of CNS infections, in addition to systemic antimicrobials, may require intraventricular or intrathecal administration of antimicrobials, because these infections can be refractory to IV antimicrobials alone.
- Often when neurosurgical devices like CSF shunts, CSF drains, deep brain stimulator leads, or cranioplasty meshes are infected, the devices need to be explanted. Focal collections like abscess and empyemas, especially when they are large or complex, need to be drained adequately.

## Introduction

Postoperative neurosurgical infections can range from skin and soft tissue infections at the incision site to deep infections like meningoventriculitis, cerebritis, or brain abscess. An anatomical classification of these infections would be clinically useful. Localization of inflammation should be based on history, examination, and imaging. The one caveat is that often discerning whether the cause of inflammation is an infection, the primary indication for the surgery (hemorrhage, tumor, or trauma), or neurosurgery itself (chemical meningitis) is not easy. The infections can be classified as shown in Figs. 50.1, 50.2, and 50.3:

- Incision site skin and soft tissue infections
- Subgaleal infections (postcraniotomy) or subfascial or subnuchal infections (postspinal surgery)
- Bone flap osteomyelitis (postcraniotomy) or vertebral osteomyelitis and discitis (postspinal surgery)
- Hardware- or device-related infections (cranioplasty mesh, spinal hardware, deep brain stimulator)
- Epidural abscess

- Subdural abscess
- Postneurosurgical, lumbar drain, or lumbar shunt meningitis (pia-arachnoidits)
- Cerebral ventricular shunt or drain related ventriculitis
- Cerebritis and brain abscess

This chapter will focus on diagnosis and management of health care–associated ventriculomeningitis (HCAM) or postneurosurgical and catheter-related meningitis. The management of osteomyelitis, device-related, and CNS focal suppurative infections will be briefly discussed. The risk factors, preventive measures including use of prophylactic antimicrobials, antimicrobial-impregnated catheters, surgical techniques, and infection prevention strategies will be discussed in Chapters 40 and 41.

## Epidemiology, Etiology, and Pathogenesis

Postcraniotomy infection rates range from 0% to 9%.[1-3] The incidence of CSF shunt infections is around 5% to 10%.[4,5] Ventricular drain infection rates are also around 10%.[6] Lumbar drain infection rates are 4.2%.[7] Postoperative spine infection rates are around 1% to 13%, with higher rates being associated with instrumentation.[8-11]

Organisms causing different postneurosurgical infections are fairly similar. During these surgeries, the skin, skull, and meninges, which act as natural barriers to pathogens, are breached. This makes it possible for microorganisms that colonize the skin, or those that live in the health care environment, to invade the skull, vertebrae, meninges, and CNS. In patients with ventriculoperitoneal (VP) shunts, organisms can rarely enter the ventricles by spreading up along the catheter after peritonitis. On the surface of catheters these organisms can form biofilms, which are thick polysaccharide layers that make them resistant to antimicrobial action.[12,13] The organisms that colonize skin, especially the scalp, are coagulase-negative Staphylococcus, *S. aureus* and *P. acnes*. The organisms that can be present in the health care environment are *S. aureus* (both methicillin-resistant and methicillin-susceptible strains) and gram-negative bacteria like *E. coli, Klebsiella, Pseudomonas,* and *Acinetobacter* species (some of the strains can be multidrug resistant).

Staphylococcal species are the most common organisms causing infections, with *S. epidermidis* (47%–64% of infections) being more common than *S. aureus* (12%–29% of infections).[4,6,14-16] Gram-negative bacteria account for

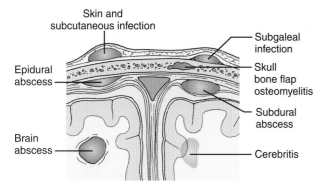

**Fig. 50.1** Postcraniotomy infections. (Modified from Lewin JJ, LaPointe M, Ziai WC. Central nervous system infections in the critically ill. *J Pharm Pract.* 2005;18(1):25–41.)

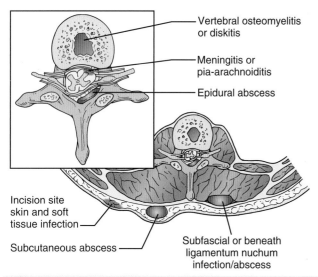

**Fig. 50.2** Postoperative spinal wound infections.

6% to 20% of the infections.[4,14,16,17] Diphtheroids (including *P. acnes*) have been reported to account for 1% to 14% of infections, but the reason for the low reported rates in some studies is probably due to inadequate culture techniques (i.e., anaerobic cultures with prolonged incubation are needed to detect *P. acnes*).[4–6,18–20] Fungal infections (e.g., due to *Candida*), although reported in the literature, are rare.[21] The local incidence of different pathogens might differ considerably, so historical institutional data and susceptibility patterns should be considered when choosing empiric antimicrobials.

## Clinical Pearl

*P. acnes* is a skin colonizer, especially in areas that are hairy, like the scalp and back. Because skin incisions for most neurosurgeries are in these areas, it is a common cause of post neurosurgical infections. It is often not detected on routine bacterial cultures or will have a Gram stain showing many gram-positive rods with no growth on cultures. Anaerobic cultures of the CSF and tissue should be done to detect *P. acnes*.

## Clinical Symptoms and Signs

Incision site infections often present with local features of inflammation like erythema, swelling, or purulent drainage from the incision or skin over subcutaneous components of devices and CSF catheters. A concomitant deeper focus of infection, such as a bone flap or an intracranial infection, may be present and is often difficult to rule out solely based on symptoms and signs.

The clinical presentation of HCAM can vary from acute and severe, if it is from virulent organisms like *S. aureus* or gram-negative bacteria, to more subtle and chronic if it is from less virulent organisms. Some organisms like

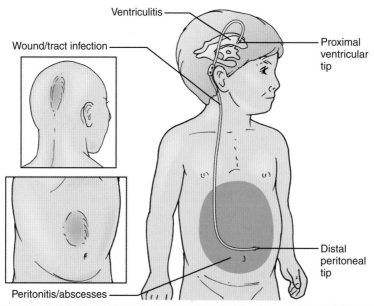

**Fig. 50.3** CSF (VP) shunt infections.

coagulase-negative staphylococci and *P. acnes* are indolent, evoke minimal inflammation, and are more pathogenic in the presence of prosthetic material.[12,13] Infected CSF shunts can cause ventriculitis without meningeal involvement, or only mechanical blockage as a result of biofilm formation in or on the catheter.[22] In CSF shunt infections, fever can be present only in about half the time (52%).[23] Headaches (31%) and changes in mental status (29%) can be present less than half the time.[23] Meningismus is rarely found (4%)[23] in these patients, and this is probably because this is mostly a ventriculitis rather than a meningitis. Clinical signs and symptoms are even less reliable in postcraniotomy and CSF drain–related ventriculomeningitis, because signs like changes in mental status, fever,[24] or meningismus could be a manifestation of other neurological diseases like intracranial hemorrhage or hydrocephalus from other causes.[25] Fever in the neurocritical care unit can be due to intracranial hemorrhage, brain dysfunction (central fever), thromboses, medications,[26] and non-CNS infection, like bloodstream infections, hospital-acquired pneumonias, and urinary tract infections.

CNS suppurative infections like epidural and brain abscesses often present with focal neurological symptoms or signs, but at times can present with no focal deficits. If the patient has preexisting deficits from an underlying neurological condition or from surgery, it is difficult to identify a superimposed focal suppurative CNS infection based on symptoms and signs alone.

## Diagnostic Studies

### ROUTINE LABORATORY AND CEREBROSPINAL FLUID DIAGNOSTIC TESTS

Studies have evaluated blood or serum markers, like procalcitonin, C-reactive protein (CRP), and peripheral white blood cell (WBC) counts, in patients with postneurosurgical infections.[24,27–30] In one open prospective study that recruited consecutive patients with ventricular drains, those with proven bacterial ventriculitis had significantly higher procalcitonin levels ($4.7 \pm 1.0$ vs. $0.2 \pm 0.01$ ng/mL, $p < .0001$), CRP levels ($134 \pm 29$ vs. $51 \pm 4$ mg/L, $p = .0005$), and peripheral WBC counts ($16.1 \pm 1.3$ vs. $10.7 \pm 0.3 \ 10^9$/L, $p = .0008$).[27] In one of these studies, a procalcitonin cut-off value of at least 1.0 ng/mL had a specificity of 77% and a sensitivity of only 68% for ventriculitis, although it had better diagnostic accuracy in community-acquired bacterial meningitis.[28] In another study, in children with suspected CSF shunt infections the values for serum CRP in infected individuals were higher than in noninfected ones ($91.8 \ +/- \ 70.2$ mg/L compared with $16.1 \ +/- \ 28.3$ mg/L, $p < 0.0001$).[31] Despite the statistically significant p values in some studies, the confidence intervals for calculated sensitivities were wide. Although these markers are easy to obtain and are often presumed to be sensitive indicators of infections, further well-designed prospective studies are required before they may be recommended for routine use to rule out postneurosurgical infections, especially from indolent organisms that cause minimal inflammation.

Studies have evaluated the diagnostic accuracy of CSF markers for HCAM. Like the blood marker studies, they have design and methodological limitations. One of the major limitations in interpreting these studies is the heterogeneous definition of the reference standard for the diagnosis of HCAM. To evaluate the diagnostic utility of CSF parameters or any other test, an independent comparison to an acceptable reference standard is required. Often CSF cultures are used as a reference standard in many studies, but diagnosing ventriculitis by a single positive CSF culture will run the risk of a false-positive diagnosis due to colonization or contamination. More specific diagnostic criteria like the presence of multiple CSF cultures with CSF pleocytosis or hypoglycorrhachia with attributable clinical signs and symptoms (fever, headache, photophobia, neck stiffness, decreased level of consciousness) would be clinically meaningful, but using that as a reference standard to calculate diagnostic accuracy, like sensitivity and specificity, would be erroneous because they are part of the definition of the reference standard and are not independent.

In CSF drain–related ventriculitis, the diagnostic utility of CSF leukocyte count, glucose, and protein is limited because noninfectious entities like intracranial hemorrhage and neurosurgical procedures can also cause abnormalities in these parameters. Schade et al.[32] performed a prospective study in a cohort of 230 consecutive patients with ventricular drains. Results from analyses of 1516 CSF samples showed no significant differences between the patients with external ventricular drain (EVD)–related ventriculitis and a control group without EVD-related ventriculitis with regard to CSF leukocyte count, protein concentration, glucose concentration, and CSF/blood glucose ratio. They evaluated the predictive and diagnostic value of the CSF parameters using Receiver Operations Characteristic (ROC) curves for different cut off values. For none of the CSF parameters could they establish a cutoff value with a sensitivity and specificity of at least 60%. Pfisterer et al.[33] conducted a prospective study over a 3-year period in patients with ventricular drains. Standard laboratory parameters, such as peripheral leukocyte count, CSF glucose, and CSF protein, were not reliable predictors for incipient ventricular catheter infection. The only parameter that significantly correlated with the occurrence of a positive CSF culture was an elevated CSF leukocyte count (unpaired t test, $p < 0.05$). In a prospective study, Pfausler et al.[34] looked at the utility of cell index (CI), which is the ratio of leukocytes to erythrocytes in CSF and leukocytes to erythrocytes in peripheral blood, in predicting ventriculitis. The study was done in patients with intraventricular hemorrhage who had EVDs. Diagnosis of bacterial ventriculitis by CI was possible up to 3 days prior to "conventional diagnosis," which was described as rise of CSF cell count, reduction of CSF/serum glucose, or a positive CSF culture.

Few studies have evaluated diagnostic accuracy of CSF parameters in CSF shunt infections. In a retrospective study that compared children with VP shunt infection (n = 10) to controls (n = 129), a CSF leukocyte count over 100/mm$^3$ had a 96% specificity and 60% sensitivity. CSF glucose of <40 mg/dL had a 93% specificity and 60% sensitivity.

The reference standard (shunt infection) in this study was defined as "clinical signs and symptoms with a positive CSF culture."[35] Often, less virulent organisms like *S. epidermidis* and *P. acnes* might not cause significant inflammation, so a lower cutoff for CSF leukocyte count would have probably increased the sensitivity, but that was not addressed in this study. However, CSF shunt infections can present with no CSF pleocytosis at times. In a retrospective analysis of CSF shunt infections in adults, the CSF WBC counts and lactate concentrations were normal in approximately 20% of episodes.[22] CSF parameter values might significantly differ depending on the site from which the CSF is obtained. In one study the leukocyte counts were significantly higher in CSF obtained by use of lumbar puncture (LP) (median leukocyte count, $573 \times 10(6)$ cells/L; $P = .001$) and valve puncture (median leukocyte count, $484 \times 10(6)$ cells/L; $P = .016$) than in ventricular CSF (median leukocyte count, $8.5 \times 10(6)$ cells/L).[22] The site of sampling should be considered when interpreting the values because the CSF pleocytosis from ventricular fluid might not be very high even in patients with CSF shunt–related ventriculitis.

There are limited studies on the diagnostic accuracy of CSF parameters in postcraniotomy meningitis and ventriculitis. Often the surgery itself causes "chemical meningitis" or postoperative meningitis, particularly posterior fossa surgeries. CSF leukocyte and glucose values can look very similar to infectious meningitis, making it hard to distinguish these entities based on these parameters. In one study, only extreme values of CSF leukocyte count >7500/microL ($7500 \times 10(6)$/L) and a glucose level of < 10 mg/dL were able to distinguish postneurosurgical chemical meningitis from bacterial meningitis.[36] Another caveat in postneurosurgical patients is that the CSF pleocytosis and low CSF glucose might be a result of a bone flap infection, subgaleal infection, or a deeper infection in the surgical bed like cerebritis or brain abscess.

## CEREBROSPINAL FLUID AND CENTRAL NERVOUS SYSTEM TISSUE MICROBIOLOGY STUDIES

CSF cultures are traditionally considered the reference standard for the diagnosis of meningitis and ventriculitis, and tissue cultures from the suspected site of infection (bone flap biopsy or abscess fluid) are the reference standard for deeper infections. In the context of community-acquired bacterial meningitis, positive CSF cultures for highly pathogenic organisms like pneumococcus or meningococcus are highly suggestive of meningitis. In the context of postneurosurgical infections, especially HCAM, the common pathogenic organisms like *S. epidermidis* and *P. acnes* are skin colonizers, and the possibility of contamination during specimen collection should be considered. Unlike organisms that cause acute community-acquired meningitis, those causing postneurosurgical infections are slow to grow on cultures and require anaerobic media. In a study on HCAM, a substantial number of positive CSF specimens grew bacteria after >3 days, with some requiring as long as 10 days.[37] CSF or other intraoperative specimens should be sent for both aerobic and anaerobic bacterial cultures. The cultures should also be held for 10 days to optimize the yield.

The site of specimen collection for microbiology studies is also important, particularly for CSF shunt infections. The site of CSF collection for ventricular catheter infection is ventricular fluid; for LP shunts, it is lumbar subarachnoid fluid; for postcraniotomy infection, it is either lumbar subarachnoid fluid or ventricular fluid obtained intraoperatively and tissue cultures. For VP shunt infection, the options are CSF by an LP, from a "shunt tap" (by accessing a subcutaneous reservoir underneath the scalp), or rarely, intraoperatively during shunt surgery. In VP shunt infection studies, direct aspiration of the shunt yielded a positive culture in 91% to 92%, whereas an LP CSF culture was positive in only around 45% to 67%.[22,38]

Polymerase chain reaction (PCR) might prove useful to detect organisms that are difficult or slow to grow in culture. In a study that used PCR to detect gram-positive bacteria in 86 specimens, 42 were culture negative but PCR positive.[39] There were no positive culture results in patients with a negative CSF PCR, suggesting that a negative PCR result is predictive of the absence of infection. More studies are needed, however, before routine use of PCR can be recommended in this setting.

## IMAGING

Imaging studies, like computed tomography (CT) and magnetic resonance imaging (MRI) of the brain or spine, are often considered when a deeper focus of infection is suspected. A head CT can show lytic areas or sclerosis in the skull, which is suggestive of a bone flap infection, but such changes can also be seen in old uninfected bone flaps. Thickening of the scalp with attenuation of fat in the superficial fascial layers or underlying subgaleal fluid collections in association with bony changes are suggestive of a bone flap infection. On MRI of the brain, if the diploic marrow shows decreased signal intensity on T1 and increased signal intensity on fat-suppressed T2-weighted images, that is suggestive of a bone flap infection.[40]

On head CT, epidural abscesses appear as lentiform fluid collections, often adjacent to the craniotomy flap, and subdural empyemas appear as crescentic fluid collections overlying the cerebral convexity or along the falx cerebri. On T1 MRI images, epidural and subdural abscesses are hypointense relative to the cortex and hyperintense relative to the CSF. On fluid attenuation inversion recovery images they are hyperintense relative to CSF. On both T1 and T2 images, abscesses are hypointense compared with chronic hematomas, and postcontrast T1 images show more peripheral enhancement in abscesses than hematomas.[40] Unlike in community-acquired focal suppurative CNS infections, diffusion-weighted imaging has proven to be less useful in postcraniotomy infection because the absence of restricted diffusion is not sufficient to exclude pyogenic postcraniotomy infection.[41,42] In the postcraniotomy patient, distinguishing postoperative changes from a subtle infection on CT and MRI is often difficult. Comparing serial imaging for progressively worsening radiological features, especially in conjunction with worsening clinical, laboratory, and CSF parameters, is diagnostically more useful.

For postspinal surgery infections, if the spine CT shows areas of bony destruction, soft tissue collections, or erosive changes at the endplates and disk space narrowing, it is suggestive of an infection. Interpretation is often limited due to instrumentation-related scatter/artifact. CT guidance can also be used to obtain a tissue biopsy of postoperative diskitis/osteomyelitis or needle aspiration of pus from abscess cavities for diagnostic studies.[16,43] Contrast-enhanced MRI imaging of the suspected area is the study of choice. Findings suggestive of discitis are a decreased signal on T1 and an increased signal on T2-weighted images in the disk space (Modic I changes) or increased T2 signal intensity of adjacent endplates. On MRI, an epidural abscess is seen as an area isointense with the cord or cauda equina on T1-weighted images and hyperintense on T2-weighted images, with peripheral enhancement on postcontrast imaging.[43,44] Subcutaneous and subfascial abscesses also appear as rim-enhancing lesions.

# Diagnostic Approach

The diagnosis of postneurosurgical infections, especially HCAM, is frequently difficult given the limitations of symptoms, signs, laboratory, CSF tests, and imaging studies. The approach suggested here is practical, using diagnostic criteria and cut-offs that are based on our clinical experience.

## CEREBROSPINAL FLUID DRAIN VENTRICULITIS

Lozier et al.[45] proposed a classification system for ventriculitis with a hierarchy of diagnoses based on suspected probability of infection. The diagnostic classification proposed here is a modification of that. In addition to being clinically helpful for deciding when to use antimicrobials, such classification would hopefully establish standard criteria for future research purposes.

- **Contamination:** An *isolated* positive CSF culture or Gram stain, with expected CSF cell count and glucose and *NO attributable symptoms or signs.*
- **Colonization:** *Multiple* positive CSF cultures or Gram stain, with expected CSF cell count ND glucose and *NO attributable symptoms or signs.*
- **Probable Ventriculitis:**
  - CSF WBC count or CSF/blood glucose ratio MORE abnormal than expected, but NOT an extreme value (CSF WBC count >1000/micro L) or CSF/blood glucose ratio <0.2 and STABLE (not progressively worsening), with attributable symptoms or signs and POSITIVE gram stain AND cultures.

  OR
  - Progressive rise in cell index or progressive decrease in CSF: blood glucose ratio or an extreme value for CSF WBC count (>1000/micro L) or CSF/ blood glucose ratio (<0.2), with attributable symptoms or signs, but NEGATIVE Gram stain AND cultures.
- **Definitive Ventriculitis:** Progressive rise in cell index or progressive decrease in CSF/ blood glucose ratio or an extreme value for CSF WBC count (>1000/micro L) or CSF/ blood glucose ratio (<0.2), with attributable symptoms or signs and a POSITIVE Gram stain AND cultures.

Contamination and colonization with skin colonizers generally does not mandate treatment. Antimicrobial treatment of contamination or colonization with virulent organisms is more controversial, but many clinicians might opt to treat positive CSF cultures for *S. aureus* or gram-negative rods. If the cultures and Gram stain are negative, antimicrobial treatment of a probable ventriculitis should be individualized depending on the circumstances, because at times chemical meningitis from subarachnoid hemorrhage or neurosurgery could cause extreme CSF poleocytosis or hypoglycorrhachia, which a clinician might prefer not to treat. Ventriculitis could be classified as probable ventriculitis when the CSF cultures are negative due to prior antimicrobial use or if the organism is slow to grow, which a clinician might chose to treat. Definitive ventriculitis would be treated with antimicrobials by most clinicians.

## POSTCRANIOTOMY INFECTIONS

Postcraniotomy meningitis can also be classified as possible, probable, and definitive using the previous criteria, because the confounding comorbidities and organism causing meningitis are similar to CSF drain infections.

Skin and soft tissue infections can be diagnosed if there is redness, swelling, or purulent drainage at the incision site.

Bone flap infections can be based on clinical and radiological findings (see imaging section) or based on intraoperative findings (bone appears necrotic with inflammatory features or pus in the adjacent area) or multiple positive bone flap cultures.

Epidural, subdural, or brain abscess is diagnosed based on radiological findings (see imaging section) or based on intraoperative findings (intracranial pus) with or without multiple positive cultures.

### Cerebrospinal fluid shunt ventriculitis

A diagnosis of CSF shunt–related ventriculitis should be considered when CSF WBC count (from a shunt tap) is greater than 10/microL OR CSF/serum glucose ratio is <0.4 with a positive CSF culture and attributable symptoms. The reason for using such a low cut-off for CSF WBC count is because most often indolent organisms cause minimal inflammation, but the decision to treat based on this should be individualized.

Another scenario suggestive of a shunt-related ventriculitis is when the CSF WBC count and glucose are normal, but there are multiple positive CSF cultures (from multiple shunt tap or explanted proximal shunt components) and attributable symptoms. CSF shunt infections can present as shunt blockage due to biofilms formed by an organism without significant inflammation.

### Postspinal surgical infections

The diagnostic approach for skin and subfascial infections will be similar to postcraniotomy infections. The diagnosis of vertebral osteomyelitis, discitis, and epidural abscess will be based on radiological findings (see imaging section) or on intraoperative findings (pus in the epidural space or necrotic bone) with or without multiple positive cultures.

# Principles of Management

Treatment of postneurosurgical infections, especially HCAM and CNS abscesses, is challenging for the following reasons:

1. It is difficult to achieve high CSF or brain antimicrobial levels with intravenous antimicrobials because of the blood–CSF and blood–brain barriers.
2. Organisms like Staphylococcus species and gram-negative rods tend to have higher minimum inhibitory concentrations (MICs) for antimicrobials than community-acquired organisms, making it harder to achieve therapeutically effective levels in the CSF and brain.
3. Organisms often form biofilms on prosthetic material and bone, which antimicrobials do not penetrate into well. This is especially an issue if the infected catheters, meshes, or devices are not removed.
4. It is difficult to achieve high antimicrobial levels in empyema and abscess fluid with intravenous antimicrobials, especially when they are large or complex.

## INTRAVENOUS ANTIMICROBIALS

The recommendations for intravenous antimicrobials in adults with a normal renal clearance (i.e., glomerular filtration rate) would be as follows.

### Empiric intravenous antimicrobial therapy

If HCAM is suspected, first obtain CSF cultures and then start empiric treatment with vancomycin (for gram-positive bacteria) as a continuous infusion or divided doses (two to three) of 60 mg per kg of body weight per day after a loading dose of 15 mg per kg of body weight, and ceftazidime 2 g IV q8h or cefepime 2 g IV q8h (for gram-negative bacteria).

In a penicillin-allergic patient, empiric coverage is with vancomycin (same dose as earlier) and aztreonam 2 g IV q6h.

In deep postcraniotomy or postspinal surgery infections, especially abscesses, empiric antimicrobial therapy should be delayed, if the patient is clinically stable, until a definitive culture is obtained either by open or minimally invasive procedures. This will increase the culture yield and the chance of detecting the pathogen. After microbiology specimens are obtained, or if the patient is severely ill, the same antimicrobials as for HCAM can be started.

### Organism-specific intravenous antimicrobial therapy

The medications in Box 50.1 can be started for specific organisms pending antimicrobial susceptibilities, but knowledge of the local antibiogram and susceptibilities at your institution should direct therapy.

---

### Box 50.1    Medications for Specific Organisms

- MRSA (methicillin-resistant *Staphylococcus aureus*) and MRSE (methicillin-resistant *S. epidermidis*) with a vancomycin MIC <= 1 µg/mL can be treated with vancomycin (same dose as earlier). If the catheter is retained, can add rifampin 300 mg IV q12h.
- MRSA and MRSE with a vancomycin MIC >1 µg/mL, or for patient with vancomycin allergy, can be treated with linezolid 600 mg IV or PO q12h.
- Specific treatment for MSSA (methicillin-susceptible *S. aureus*) and MSSE (methicillin-susceptible *S. epidermidis*) is nafcillin or oxacillin 2 g IV q4h.
- Specific treatment for *P. acnes* is penicillin G 2 to 4 MU IV q4h.
- Specific treatment for *Pseudomonas* spp. is ceftazidime 2 g IV q8h or cefepime 2 g IV q8h or meropenem 2 g IV q8h.
- Specific treatment for *E. coli* is ceftriaxone 2 g IV q12h or meropenem 2 g IV q8h (meropenem if there are epidemiological risk factors for prior colonization or infection with ESBL [extended-spectrum beta-lactamase] producers.
- Specific treatment for *Enterobacter* spp. or *Citrobacter* spp. is cefepime 2 g IV q8h or meropenem 2 g IV q8h.

---

### Clinical Pearl

A common mistake in treating CNS infections is not using the right intravenous antimicrobial or the right dose that adequately penetrates the CNS. For example, the right dose for ceftazidime to treat *Pseudomonal* meningitis is 2 g, which is twice the dose used for pneumonia. Certain antimicrobials, like Zosyn (piperacillin/tazobactam), can be reported to be susceptible in vitro, but should not be used because they do not adequately penetrate the CNS.

## INTRAVENTRICULAR AND INTRATHECAL ANTIMICROBIALS

Intraventricular or lumbar intrathecal (subarachnoid) administration of antimicrobials might be needed when patients do not respond to intravenous treatment or when organisms have high MICs to antimicrobials. This route of administration bypasses the blood–CSF barrier, with controlled delivery directly to the site of infection. CSF pharmacokinetic modeling studies[46–49] show that for most gram-negative bacteria, if the MIC for some cephalosporins is greater than 0.5 µg/mL, or for meropenem is greater than 0.25 µg/mL, and for gram-positive bacteria if the MIC for vancomycin is greater than 1 µg/mL, then the target pharmacokinetic-pharmacodynamic (PK-PD) parameters in the CSF may not be achieved with intravenous antimicrobials.

Although no antimicrobial agent has been approved by the U.S. Food and Drug Administration for intraventricular and intrathecal use, there have been several studies on their pharmacokinetics, safety, and efficacy, especially in adults.[50–56] CSF sterility and normalization of CSF parameters were achieved sooner with intraventricular and intravenous use compared with intravenous use alone.

However, use of intraventricular antimicrobial agents was not recommended in infants based on data in a recent Cochrane review.[57] A clinical trial found a three times higher relative risk of mortality when infants with gram-negative meningitis were treated with intraventricular gentamicin and intravenous antimicrobials, compared with intravenous therapy alone, although one half of the infants in the intraventricular gentamicin group had received only one dose, raising uncertainty about the cause of death.

Antimicrobial agents administered by the intraventricular or intrathecal route should be preservative free, and should be prepared and administered using strict sterile precautions. To avoid increasing the intracranial pressure (ICP), prior to instilling the drug, a volume of CSF equal to the volume of drug diluent and saline flush should be aspirated and discarded. After administering the drug via a CSF drain, a saline flush can be used to minimize the amount of drug remaining in the draining catheter. When administered through a CSF drain, the drain should be clamped for 15 to 60 minutes to allow the antimicrobial solution to equilibrate in the CSF before opening the drain.[58] During and after the procedure the patient's level of consciousness and ICP should be closely monitored. In treating CSF shunt ventriculitis, administration of the antimicrobials through the shunt reservoir may result in the agent draining distally into the peritoneal cavity; to avoid this issue, antimicrobials can be administered into the cerebral ventricles by placing a ventricular access device separate from the shunt reservoir.[59]

Determining the correct dosing regimen is challenging because the CSF concentrations obtained for the same intraventricular dose in pharmacokinetic studies have been highly variable, probably due to the differences among patients in either the volume of distribution, depending on ventricular size, or variable CSF clearance as a result of CSF drainage.[50–55,57] A consensus guideline by the British Society for Antimicrobial Chemotherapy Working Party on Infections in Neurosurgery has recommended that the initial dose of an intraventricular antimicrobial be based on ventricular volume.[60] In adults, the recommended dose of vancomycin is 5 mg in patients with slit ventricles, 10 mg in patients with normal-sized ventricles, and 15 to 20 mg in patients with enlarged ventricles. Using the same rationale, the initial dosing of an aminoglycoside can also be tailored to ventricular size. The same working party recommended that the frequency of dosing be based on the daily volume of CSF drainage: once-daily dosing if CSF drainage is >100 mL/day, every other day if the drainage is 50 to 100 mL/day, and every third day if drainage is <50 mL/day. The ranges of intraventricular or intrathecal dose/day for other antimicrobials are in Box 50.2.

Another approach, when drug levels can be monitored, is to base dosing on CSF drug concentrations after the initial intraventricular dose. However, there are very few studies that have evaluated CSF therapeutic drug monitoring, and given the variable CSF clearance of an antimicrobial agent, it is difficult to determine when to obtain CSF to measure peak and trough drug concentrations. A CSF drug concentration can be obtained 24 hours after administration of the first dose, which can be presumed to be the trough CSF concentration. The trough CSF concentration divided by the MIC of the agent for the isolated organism is termed the *inhibitory quotient*, which should exceed 10 to 20 for consistent CSF sterilization.[61,62]

> **Box 50.2 The Ranges of Intraventricular or Intrathecal Dose/Day for Other Antimicrobials**
>
> Gentamicin: 4–8 mg
> Tobramycin: 5–20 mg
> Amikacin: 5–30 mg
> Colistimethate sodium 10 mg by CMS units or 3.75 mg by CBA (colisitin base activity) units
> Daptomycin: 2–5 mg

> **Clinical Pearl**
>
> A common mistake is not using intraventricular antimicrobials early in severe ventriculomeningitis, especially in infections with virulent drug-resistant organisms. CSF cultures clear faster and CSF parameters normalize sooner with the addition of intraventricular antimicrobials.

## OPERATIVE MANAGEMENT

A general principle in infectious disease is that device or prostheses infections are difficult to cure without surgical removal of the infected device. Abscesses or necrotic tissue and bone infections are hard to treat without drainage and debridement. There are limited studies on postneurosurgical infections that evaluated different operative approaches or compared them to conservative treatment. Focal suppurative CNS infections, like cranial epidural, subdural and brain abscess, and post–spine surgery epidural abscess, should be adequately drained, especially when they are large with multiple loculations and thick walls. In the treatment of CSF drain infections, removal of the infected drain would be a prudent approach. Similarly, removing infected spinal hardware and other neurosurgical devices, if feasible, should be done, given the difficulty of treating them conservatively. In bone flap and cranioplasty mesh infections[25] treatment requires removal of the infected flap or mesh (craniectomy) and placement of a new mesh (cranioplasty) 3 to 6 months after disappearance of clinical signs and normalization of the CRP.

A range of surgical approaches on managing CSF shunt ventriculitis have been published.[63,64] A decision analysis[63] and a systematic review,[64] which synthesized results from many studies, showed cure rates were better with a two-stage surgical procedure, where the infected CSF shunt was removed with replacement of a new shunt in a second surgery after the ventriculitis cleared (88%–96%) compared with a one-stage procedure, where the infected CSF shunt was removed with new shunt placement in the same surgery (65%). Both operative approaches had better cure rates than treatment with antimicrobials alone, without removing the infected shunt (34%–36%).[63,64] In the two-stage approach there might be a need for a temporary CSF drain to treat raised ICP or hydrocephalus while waiting for CSF cultures to clear before reimplanting a new CSF shunt. The optimal timing of shunt reimplantation has not been studied. Early placement may increase the risk of relapse, but a delay in reimplantation may increase the risk of secondary infection of the EVD. The timing of reimplantation should be individualized based on the isolated organism, severity of ventriculitis, and improvement of CSF parameters and CSF sterilization in response to antimicrobial therapy. Most experts in the field would wait for at least 7 to 10 days after the CSF cultures become sterile to reimplant a new shunt.

## References

1. Savitz MH, Katz SS. Prevention of primary wound infection in neurosurgical patients: a 10-year study. *Neurosurgery*. 1986;18(6):685–688.
2. Blomstedt GC. Infections in neurosurgery: a retrospective study of 1143 patients and 1517 operations. *Acta Neurochir (Wien)*. 1985;78(3–4):81–90.
3. van Ek B, Bakker FP, van Dulken H, Dijkmans BA. Infections after craniotomy: a retrospective study. *J Infect*. 1986;12(2):105–109.
4. Tunkel A, Drake J. Cerebrospinal fluid shunt infections. In: Mandell G, Bennett J, Dolin R, eds. *Principles and Practice of Infectious Diseases*. 7th ed. Philadelphia: Churchill Livingstone; 2009:1231–1236.
5. Arnell K, Cesarini K, Lagerqvist-Widh A, Wester T, Sjolin J. Cerebrospinal fluid shunt infections in children over a 13-year period: anaerobic cultures and comparison of clinical signs of infection with Propionibacterium acnes and with other bacteria. *J Neurosurg Pediatr*. 2008;1(5):366–372.
6. Lozier AP, Sciacca RR, Romagnoli MF, Connolly Jr ES. Ventriculostomy-related infections: a critical review of the literature. *Neurosurgery*. 2008;62(suppl 2):688–700.
7. Coplin WM, Avellino AM, Kim DK, Winn HR, Grady MS. Bacterial meningitis associated with lumbar drains: a retrospective cohort study. *J Neurol Neurosurg Psychiatry*. 1999;67(4):468–473.
8. Weinstein MA, McCabe JP, Cammisa Jr FP. Postoperative spinal wound infection: a review of 2,391 consecutive index procedures. *J Spinal Disord*. 2000;13(5):422–426.
9. Fang A, Hu SS, Endres N, Bradford DS. Risk factors for infection after spinal surgery. *Spine*. 2005;30(12):1460–1465.
10. Kuo CH, Wang ST, Yu WK, Chang MC, Liu CL, Chen TH. Postoperative spinal deep wound infection: a six-year review of 3230 selective procedures. *J Chin Med Assoc*. 2004;67(8):398–402.
11. Mackenzie WG, Matsumoto H, Williams BA, et al. Surgical site infection following spinal instrumentation for scoliosis: a multicenter analysis of rates, risk factors, and pathogens. *J Bone Joint Surg Am*. 2013;95(9):800–806. S801–S802.
12. Snowden JN, Beaver M, Smeltzer MS, Kielian T. Biofilm-infected intracerebroventricular shunts elicit inflammation within the central nervous system. *Infect Immun*. 2012;80(9):3206–3214.
13. Braxton Jr EE, Ehrlich GD, Hall-Stoodley L, et al. Role of biofilms in neurosurgical device-related infections. *Neurosurg Rev*. 2005;28(4):249–255.
14. Wang KW, Chang WN, Shih TY, et al. Infection of cerebrospinal fluid shunts: causative pathogens, clinical features, and outcomes. *Jpn J Infect Dis*. 2004;57(2):44–48.
15. Dashti SR, Baharvahdat H, Spetzler RF, et al. Operative intracranial infection following craniotomy. *Neurosurg Focus*. 2008;24(6):E10.
16. Jimenez-Mejias ME, de Dios Colmenero J, Sanchez-Lora FJ, et al. Postoperative spondylodiskitis: etiology, clinical findings, prognosis, and comparison with nonoperative pyogenic spondylodiskitis. *Clin Infect Dis*. 1999;29(2):339–345.
17. Sells CJ, Shurtleff DB, Loeser JD. Gram-negative cerebrospinal fluid shunt-associated infections. *Pediatrics*. 1977;59(4):614–618.
18. Brook I. Meningitis and shunt infection caused by anaerobic bacteria in children. *Pediatr Neurol*. 2002;26(2):99–105.
19. Rekate HL, Ruch T, Nulsen FE. Diphtheroid infections of cerebrospinal fluid shunts. The changing pattern of shunt infection in Cleveland. *J Neurosurg*. 1980;52(4):553–556.
20. Nisbet M, Briggs S, Ellis-Pegler R, Thomas M, Holland D. Propionibacterium acnes: an under-appreciated cause of post-neurosurgical infection. *J Antimicrob Chemother*. 2007;60(5):1097–1103.
21. O'Brien D, Stevens NT, Lim CH, et al. Candida infection of the central nervous system following neurosurgery: a 12-year review. *Acta Neurochir (Wien)*. 2011;153(6):1347–1350.
22. Conen A, Walti LN, Merlo A, Fluckiger U, Battegay M, Trampuz A. Characteristics and treatment outcome of cerebrospinal fluid shunt-associated infections in adults: a retrospective analysis over an 11-year period. *Clin Infect Dis*. 2008;47(1):73–82.
23. Moores LE, Ellenbogen RG. Cerebrospinal fluid shunt infections. In: Hall WA, McCutcheon IE, AANS Publications Committee, eds. *Infections in Neurosurgery*. Park Ridge, IL: American Association of Neurological Surgeons; 2000:141–153.
24. Girgis F, Walcott BP, Kwon CS, et al. The absence of fever or leukocytosis does not exclude infection following cranioplasty. *Can J Neurol Sci*. 2015;42(4):255–259.
25. Bhaskar IP, Inglis TJ, Lee GY. Clinical, radiological, and microbiological profile of patients with autogenous cranioplasty infections. *World Neurosurg*. 2014;82(3-4):e531–e534.
26. Rabinstein AA, Sandhu K. Non-infectious fever in the neurological intensive care unit: incidence, causes and predictors. *J Neurol Neurosurg Psychiatry*. 2007;78(11):1278–1280.
27. Berger C, Schwarz S, Schaebitz WR, Aschoff A, Schwab S. Serum procalcitonin in cerebral ventriculitis. *Crit Care Med*. 2002;30(8):1778–1781.
28. Martinez R, Gaul C, Buchfelder M, Erbguth F, Tschaikowsky K. Serum procalcitonin monitoring for differential diagnosis of ventriculitis in adult intensive care patients. *Intensive Care Med*. 2002;28(2):208–210.
29. Vogelsang JP, Wehe A, Markakis E. Postoperative intracranial abscess—clinical aspects in the differential diagnosis to early recurrence of malignant glioma. *Clin Neurol Neurosurg*. 1998;100(1):11–14.
30. Khan MH, Smith PN, Rao N, Donaldson WF. Serum C-reactive protein levels correlate with clinical response in patients treated with antibiotics for wound infections after spinal surgery. *Spine J*. 2006;6(3):311–315.
31. Schuhmann MU, Ostrowski KR, Draper EJ, et al. The value of C-reactive protein in the management of shunt infections. *J Neurosurg*. 2005;103(3 suppl):223–230.
32. Schade RP, Schinkel J, Roelandse FW, et al. Lack of value of routine analysis of cerebrospinal fluid for prediction and diagnosis of external drainage-related bacterial meningitis. *J Neurosurg*. 2006;104(1):101–108.
33. Pfisterer W, Muhlbauer M, Czech T, Reinprecht A. Early diagnosis of external ventricular drainage infection: results of a prospective study. *J Neurol Neurosurg Psychiatry*. 2003;74(7):929–932.
34. Pfausler B, Beer R, Engelhardt K, Kemmler G, Mohsenipour I, Schmutzhard E. Cell index—a new parameter for the early diagnosis of ventriculostomy (external ventricular drainage)-related ventriculitis in patients with intraventricular hemorrhage? *Acta Neurochir (Wien)*. 2004;146(5):477–481.
35. Lan CC, Wong TT, Chen SJ, Liang ML, Tang RB. Early diagnosis of ventriculoperitoneal shunt infections and malfunctions in children with hydrocephalus. *J Microbiol Immunol Infect*. 2003;36(1):47–50.
36. Forgacs P, Geyer CA, Freidberg SR. Characterization of chemical meningitis after neurological surgery. *Clin Infect Dis*. 2001;32(2):179–185.
37. Desai A, Lollis SS, Missios S, et al. How long should cerebrospinal fluid cultures be held to detect shunt infections? Clinical article. *J Neurosurg Pediatr*. 2009;4(2):184–189.

38. Noetzel MJ, Baker RP. Shunt fluid examination: risks and benefits in the evaluation of shunt malfunction and infection. *J Neurosurg.* 1984;61(2):328–332.
39. Banks JT, Bharara S, Tubbs RS, et al. Polymerase chain reaction for the rapid detection of cerebrospinal fluid shunt or ventriculostomy infections. *Neurosurgery.* 2005;57(6):1237–1243. discussion 1237–1243.
40. Sinclair AG, Scoffings DJ. Imaging of the post-operative cranium. *Radiographics.* 2010;30(2):461–482.
41. Farrell CJ, Hoh BL, Pisculli ML, Henson JW, Barker 2nd FG, Curry Jr WT. Limitations of diffusion-weighted imaging in the diagnosis of postoperative infections. *Neurosurgery.* 2008;62(3):577–583 discussion 577–583.
42. Kim YJ, Moon KS, Kim SK, et al. The difference in diffusion-weighted imaging with apparent diffusion coefficient between spontaneous and postoperative intracranial infection. *Br J Neurosurg.* 2014;28(6):765–770.
43. Chaudhary SB, Vives MJ, Basra SK, Reiter MF. Postoperative spinal wound infections and postprocedural diskitis. *J Spinal Cord Med.* 2007;30(5):441–451.
44. Boden SD, Davis DO, Dina TS, Sunner JL, Wiesel SW. Postoperative diskitis: distinguishing early MR imaging findings from normal postoperative disk space changes. *Radiology.* 1992;184(3):765–771.
45. Lozier AP, Sciacca RR, Romagnoli MF, Connolly Jr ES. Ventriculostomy-related infections: a critical review of the literature. *Neurosurgery.* 2002;51(1):170–181. discussion 181–182.
46. Lodise TP, Nau R, Kinzig M, Drusano GL, Jones RN, Sorgel F. Pharmacodynamics of ceftazidime and meropenem in cerebrospinal fluid: results of population pharmacokinetic modelling and Monte Carlo simulation. *J Antimicrob Chemother.* 2007;60(5):1038–1044.
47. Lodise Jr TP, Rhoney DH, Tam VH, McKinnon PS, Drusano GL. Pharmacodynamic profiling of cefepime in plasma and cerebrospinal fluid of hospitalized patients with external ventriculostomies. *Diagn Microbiol Infect Dis.* 2006;54(3):223–230.
48. Nau R, Prange HW, Kinzig M, et al. Cerebrospinal fluid ceftazidime kinetics in patients with external ventriculostomies. *Antimicrob Agents Chemother.* 1996;40(3):763–766.
49. Ricard JD, Wolff M, Lacherade JC, et al. Levels of vancomycin in cerebrospinal fluid of adult patients receiving adjunctive corticosteroids to treat pneumococcal meningitis: a prospective multicenter observational study. *Clin Infect Dis.* 2007;44(2):250–255.
50. Wang JH, Lin PC, Chou CH, et al. Intraventricular antimicrobial therapy in postneurosurgical Gram-negative bacillary meningitis or ventriculitis: A hospital-based retrospective study. *J Microbiol Immunol Infect.* 2014;47(3):204–210.
51. Wilkie MD, Hanson MF, Statham PF, Brennan PM. Infections of cerebrospinal fluid diversion devices in adults: the role of intraventricular antimicrobial therapy. *J Infect.* 2013;66(3):239–246.
52. Ng K, Mabasa VH, Chow I, Ensom MHH. Systematic review of efficacy, pharmacokinetics, and administration of intraventricular vancomycin in adults. *Neurocrit Care.* 2014;20(1):158–171.
53. Tangden T, Enblad P, Ullberg M, Sjolin J. Neurosurgical gram-negative bacillary ventriculitis and meningitis: a retrospective study evaluating the efficacy of intraventricular gentamicin therapy in 31 consecutive cases. *Clin Infect Dis.* 2011;52(11):1310–1316.
54. Imberti R, Cusato M, Accetta G, et al. Pharmacokinetics of colistin in cerebrospinal fluid after intraventricular administration of colistin methanesulfonate. *Antimicrob Agents Chemother.* 2012;56(8):4416–4421.
55. Ziai WC, Lewin 3rd JJ. Improving the role of intraventricular antimicrobial agents in the management of meningitis. *Curr Opin Neurol.* 2009;22(3):277–282.
56. Remeš F, Tomáš R, Jindrák V, et al. Intraventricular and lumbar intrathecal administration of antibiotics in postneurosurgical patients with meningitis and/or ventriculitis in a serious clinical state. *J Neurosurg.* 2013;119:1596–1602.
57. Shah SS, Ohlsson A, Shah VS. Intraventricular antibiotics for bacterial meningitis in neonates. *Cochrane Database Syst Rev.* 2012;7 CD004496.
58. Cook AM, Mieure KD, Owen RD, Pesaturo AB, Hatton J. Intracerebroventricular administration of drugs. *Pharmacotherapy.* 2009;29(7):832–845.
59. Brown EM, Edwards RJ, Pople IK. Conservative management of patients with cerebrospinal fluid shunt infections. *Neurosurgery.* 2006;58(4):657–665. discussion 657–665.
60. The management of neurosurgical patients with postoperative bacterial or aseptic meningitis or external ventricular drain-associated ventriculitis. Infection in Neurosurgery Working Party of the British Society for Antimicrobial Chemotherapy. *Br J Neurosurg.* 2000;14(1):7–12.
61. Ellner PD, Neu HC. The inhibitory quotient. A method for interpreting minimum inhibitory concentration data. *JAMA.* 1981;246(14):1575–1578.
62. Tunkel AR, Hartman BJ, Kaplan SL, et al. Practice guidelines for the management of bacterial meningitis. *Clin Infect Dis.* 2004;39(9):1267–1284.
63. Schreffler RT, Schreffler AJ, Wittler RR. Treatment of cerebrospinal fluid shunt infections: a decision analysis. *Pediatr Infect Dis J.* 2002;21(7):632–636.
64. Yogev R. Cerebrospinal fluid shunt infections: a personal view. *Pediatr Infect Dis.* 1985;4(2):113–118.

# *Index*

Note: Page numbers followed by *b* indicate boxes, *f* indicate figures and *t* indicate tables.